Anatomy and Human Movement

Structure and Function

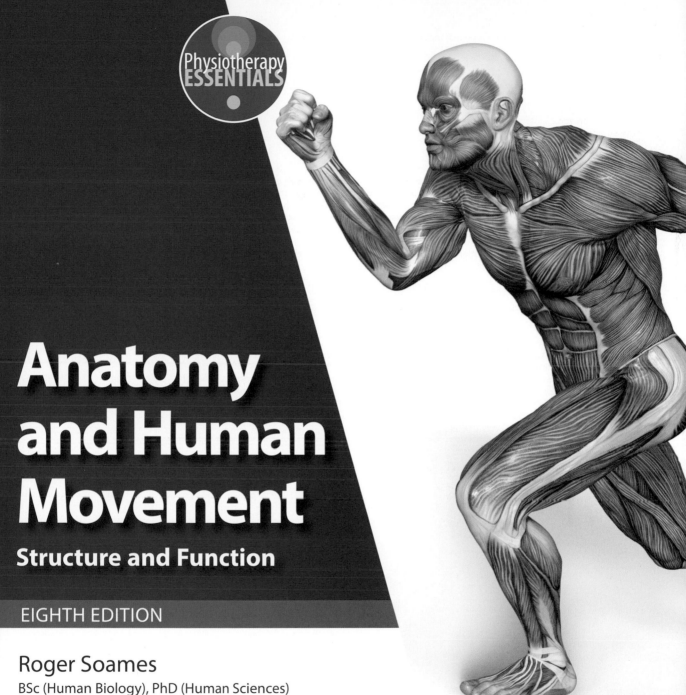

Physiotherapy
ESSENTIALS

Anatomy and Human Movement

Structure and Function

EIGHTH EDITION

Roger Soames

BSc (Human Biology), PhD (Human Sciences)
Professor Emeritus, University of Dundee, Dundee, United Kingdom

ELSEVIER

First edition 1989
First published as a paperback edition 1990
Second edition 1994
Third edition 1998
Fourth edition 2002
Fifth edition 2006
Sixth edition 2012
Seventh edition 2019

Notices

Practitioners and researchers must always rely on their own experience and knowledge in evaluating and using any information, methods, compounds or experiments described herein. Because of rapid advances in the medical sciences, in particular, independent verification of diagnoses and drug dosages should be made. To the fullest extent of the law, no responsibility is assumed by Elsevier, authors, editors or contributors for any injury and/or damage to persons or property as a matter of products liability, negligence or otherwise, or from any use or operation of any methods, products, instructions, or ideas contained in the material herein.

ISBN: 978-0-443-11327-7

Content Strategist: Chiara Giglio/Andrae Akeh
Content Project Manager: Shubham Dixit
Cover Designer: Amy Buxton
Illustration Manager: Muthukumaran Thangaraj
Marketing Manager: Deborah Watkins

Printed in India by Manipal Technologies Limited

Last digit is the print number: 9 8 7 6 5 4 3 2 1

Working together
to grow libraries in
developing countries

www.elsevier.com • www.bookaid.org

CONTENTS

We have designed and written this book for the student of anatomy who is concerned with the study of the living body and who wishes to use this knowledge functionally for a greater understanding of the mechanisms which allow movement to take place. Traditional anatomy texts are written as an adjunct to the study of the human body in the dissecting room, but only the surgeon has the advantage of directly viewing living musculoskeletal structures. The vast majority of students interested in musculoskeletal anatomy as well as those involved with human movement and its disorders are confronted by an intact skin and therefore must visualize the structures involved by palpation and analysis of movement. *Anatomy and Human Movement* presents the musculoskeletal structures as a living dynamic system – an approach lacking in many existing textbooks. The applied anatomy of the musculoskeletal system occupies the greater part of the book and is built up from a study of the bones and muscles (which are grouped according to their major functions, rather than as seen in the dissecting room) to a consideration of joints and their biomechanics. Anatomical descriptions of each joint are given with a detailed explanation of how it functions, the forces generated across it and how it might fail. We have placed great emphasis on the joints, as these are of major concern to those interested in active movement and passive manipulation, and we give examples of common traumatic or pathological problems affecting the structures described. Where possible, we describe palpation and analyse movement with respect to the joints and muscles involved, as well as any accessory movements.

The course and distribution of the major peripheral nerves and blood vessels, together with the lymphatic drainage of the region, are given at the end of each relevant section. There are separate chapters on embryology and the skin and its appendages, and we have included, in the introduction, a section on the terminology used in the book. There is also an account of the structure and function of the nervous system written by Nikolai Bogduk whose contribution has been extremely valuable. The format of the book matches a page of text to a page of illustrations, whenever possible, and we hope that this will allow the reader to confirm his or her understanding of the text with the visual information provided. The book is extensively illustrated with large, clear, fully labelled diagrams, all of which have been specially prepared. In the sections covering the joints and biomechanics, the illustrations have been drawn by Roger Soames, and these are particularly detailed as they pull together the anatomy from the previous parts of that chapter.

We hope that this new approach to the teaching of anatomy will serve to fill the gap which has always existed for those who have to learn their anatomy on a living subject and eventually have to determine their diagnoses and apply their treatments through an intact skin.

Nigel Palastanga
Derek Field
Roger Soames
1989

PREFACE TO EIGHTH EDITION

The eighth edition of *Anatomy and Human Movement* has undergone further re-organisation, which it is hoped will improve the usefulness of this already successful text. While the five major parts have been retained, only Part 1 (Introduction) remains essentially the same. In Parts 2 (Upper Limb) and 3 (Lower Limb) there has been minor re-organisation; however it is Parts 4 (Trunk and Neck) and 5 (Head and Brain) that have undergone substantial reorganisation. The neck content of Part 4 has been moved to Part 5, with the result that Part 4 is now concerned with the Trunk only and Part 5 the Neck and Head. In addition to the self-assessment questions following each section, a selection of self-assessment multiple choice questions is presented at the end of each part has been added.

The feedback of users (students, teachers, practitioners) of the book has been useful in making changes to the current edition. Enabling individuals to understand, remember and apply anatomy in practice has always been the prime purpose of this book.

In response to advances in the range of electronic aids to learning, the eighth edition is also available as an ebook via Elsevier's Evolve or other e-reader platforms. In addition, there is a separate supplementary e-learning course in functional human anatomy, which presents self-contained modules following the organisation of the book enabling students and others to study at their own pace and time. Information is delivered via outcome measures, animations, videos, quizzes, activity analyses and multiple choice question (MCQ) tests.

Whether the book is used by students, lecturers or practitioners the changes made to this edition are designed to make it more useful to your learning, teaching or practice. Changes to the way education is managed and delivered, especially since the pandemic, require students and educators to be flexible outside the classroom, therefore requiring the provision of high-quality material, both electronic and hard copy, to support learning wherever it is taking place. This edition of *Anatomy and Human Movement* and the accompanying electronic resources are designed to facilitate study in this new environment of varied learning spaces. The range of health professionals using *Anatomy and Human Movement* has grown extensively over the last 34 years, with its use spreading to other groups and disciplines interested in human movement.

Anatomy and Human Movement was initially conceived and written by authors experienced in teaching living anatomy and human movement. This remains the prime reason for producing the book, the appreciation of anatomy through the intact skin of the living is fundamental to the practice of a number of professions. I hope that this eighth will provide the reader with the stimulation and framework that will aid their understanding and learning of anatomy and their ability to apply the knowledge gained to human movement.

Roger Soames, 2023

ACKNOWLEDGEMENTS

I would like to acknowledge the tremendous contribution to the first four editions made by Derek Filed and to the first seven editions made by Nigel Palastanga. I am also extremely grateful to Dot Palastanga, formerly lecturer in Occupational Therapy at Cardiff University, who was involved in proofreading earlier editions.

The illustrations for the seventh edition, created by Paul Richardson, have been retained, as have the photographs showing the clinical examination and evaluation of various joints. The photographs were organised and provided by Stuart Porter of the University of Salford. Many thanks to Paul and Stuart, as well as to Ian Nixon, Sofia Gaspari, Tom Buckley and Claire Porter, who agreed to be models.

ABOUT THE AUTHOR

Roger Soames joined the Centre for Anatomy and Human Identification at the University of Dundee in 2007 as Principal Anatomist: he was formerly Associate Professor and Head of Anatomy at James Cook University in Queensland Australia. In 2009 he was appointed to a personal chair in Functional and Applied Anatomy and later the same year to the Cox Chair of Anatomy: he is currently Emeritus Professor of Functional and Applied Anatomy. His career has been entirely within the discipline of anatomy, teaching and examining on a wide range of undergraduate and postgraduate degree programmes and courses: he has also developed new programmes of study at both undergraduate and postgraduate levels. He retains research interests in the musculoskeletal system and continues to publish this area.

Introduction

OUTLINE

KEY CONCEPTS

- The anatomical position is an internationally accepted position to which directional terms refer, irrespective of the actual body position.
- Movement occurs in a plane perpendicular to the axis about which movement takes place.
- Somites, derived from paraxial mesoderm, divide into the sclerotome, which forms the axial skeleton; the myotome, which gives rise to all voluntary muscle of the trunk and limbs; and the dermatome, which forms the dermis over dorsal regions. The somatopleuric layer of the lateral plate mesenchyme forms the appendicular skeleton, connective tissues of the limbs and trunk, and dermis of the ventral body wall and limbs.
- Each somite is associated with a single spinal nerve: migration of cells of the dermatome or myotome carries this innervation with them, irrespective of their final destination.

- Skin is a tough, pliable, waterproof covering and sensory organ.
- Myelinated nerve fibres conduct impulses faster than non-myelinated nerve fibres.
- Bone ossifies either in membrane (intramembranous ossification) or from a precursor cartilage model (endochondral ossification).
- Bone growth and remodelling is a balanced process of removal by osteoclasts and deposition by osteoblasts.
- Skeletal (striated) muscle is under voluntary control and has a number of forms: fusiform for speed of movement and pennate for power.
- The more complex a joint (fibrous, cartilaginous, synovial), the greater the movement possible.
- Flexibility is joint specific.

OVERVIEW

This part is organised into six major sections: terminology; early embryology; nervous system; skin and its appendages; components of the musculoskeletal system; and flexibility and mobility.

In the terminology section, the standard anatomical position is introduced, and the terms used in descriptive anatomy and those describing movement are considered.

In the early embryology section, the stages in early development, mesodermal somites and development of the vertebrae and limbs are considered. In the nervous system section, cellular structure, interneural connections and myelination, together with the structure of peripheral nerves and the peripheral nervous system, are covered. In skin and its appendages, the basic organisation and structure of skin, including hair, nails and glands, are considered together with its blood supply and innervation; the clinical application of skin is addressed.

In the components of the musculoskeletal system section, the structure and types of muscular, connective and skeletal tissues are considered, as well as the classification and organisation of joints, the movements possible between articular surfaces and the principles of levers.

In the flexibility and mobility section, factors influencing joint flexibility, active and passive ranges of motion, the end feel to movement and the principles of measurement, including its validity and reliability, are covered.

At the end of each section is a summary of the main points followed by a selection of self-assessment questions. At the end of this part is a selection of self-assessment multiple choice questions.

TERMINOLOGY

LEARNING OUTCOMES

By the end of the section, you should be able to:
1. Describe the anatomical position and principal cardinal planes of the body
2. Describe the relationships between body structures and regions
3. Use appropriate terminology to describe the movement of one body segment with respect to another

ANATOMICAL TERMINOLOGY

It is essential for the study of anatomy and human movement to be familiar with an internationally accepted vocabulary allowing communication and understanding between members of the medical and paramedical professions throughout the world. Perhaps the single most important descriptive aspect of this vocabulary is the adoption of an unequivocal position of the human body (anatomical position). It is described as the body standing erect and facing forwards, the legs together with the feet parallel and toes pointing forwards, arms hanging loosely by the sides with the palms facing forwards and thumbs lateral (Fig. 1.1). All positional terminology uses this reference position irrespective of the actual position of the body (sitting down, lying prone, jumping).

A list of commonly used terms describing the position of anatomical structures is given below and shown in Fig. 1.2.

Anterior (ventral). Towards the front or in front: the patella lies anterior to the knee joint.

Posterior (dorsal). Towards the back or behind: gluteus maximus lies posterior to the hip joint. (Ventral and dorsal are used more commonly in quadrupeds.)

Superior (cephalic). Above: the head is superior to the trunk.

Inferior (caudal). Below: the knee is inferior to the hip.

Cephalic (head) and **Caudal** (tail). May be used in relation to the trunk and nervous system.

Lateral. Away from the median plane or midline: the thumb lies lateral to the index finger.

Medial. Towards the median plane or midline: the great toe lies medial to the little toe.

Distal. Further away from the trunk or root of the limb: the foot is distal to the knee.

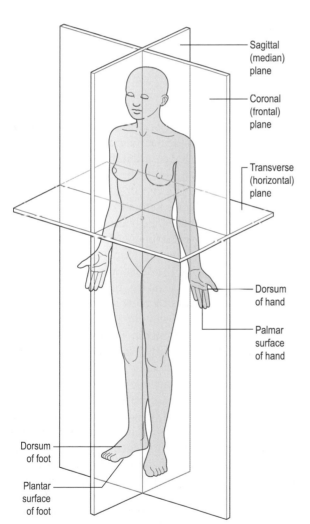

Fig. 1.1 Anatomical position of the body also showing the cardinal planes.

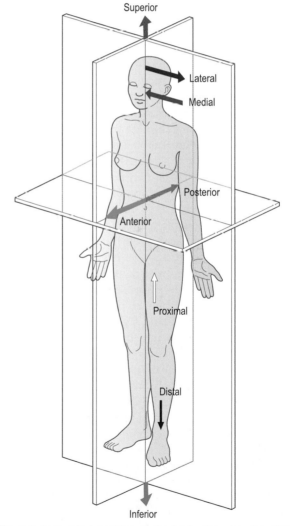

Fig. 1.2 Anatomical position of the body also showing directional terms.

Proximal. Closer to the trunk or root of the limb: the elbow is proximal to the hand.

Superficial. Closer to the surface of the body or skin: the ulnar nerve passes superficial to the flexor retinaculum at the wrist.

Deep. Further away from the body surface or skin: the tendon of tibialis posterior passes deep to the flexor retinaculum at the ankle.

To facilitate understanding the relationship of structures to each other, as well as the movement of one segment with respect to another, imaginary reference planes pass through the body in such a way that they are mutually perpendicular to each other (Fig. 1.1). Passing through the body from front to back, dividing it into symmetrical right and left halves, is the sagittal (median) plane: any plane parallel to this is a parasagittal (paramedian) plane.

A plane passing through the body from top to bottom, dividing it into anterior and posterior parts and perpendicular to the sagittal plane, is the coronal (frontal) plane; all planes dividing the body in this way are coronal planes. Finally, a plane passing through the body perpendicular to both the sagittal and coronal planes, dividing it into upper and lower parts, is a transverse (horizontal) plane. A whole family of parallel transverse planes exists. It is, therefore, usual when presenting a particular transverse section to specify the level at which it is taken. This may be done by specifying the vertebral level (C6) or position within the limb (mid-shaft of the humerus).

Within each plane, a single axis can be identified, usually in association with a particular joint, about which movement takes place. An anteroposterior axis in the sagittal or a paramedian plane allows movement in a coronal plane. Similarly, a vertical axis in a coronal plane allows movement in a transverse plane, while a transverse (right to left) axis in a coronal plane allows movement in a paramedian (parasagittal) plane.

By arranging these various axes to intersect at the centre of a joint, the movements possible at the joint can be broken down into simple components. It also becomes easier to understand how specific muscle groups produce particular movements and to determine the resultant movement of combined muscle actions.

TERMS USED TO DESCRIBE MOVEMENT

Rarely does movement of one body segment with respect to another take place in a single plane; it invariably occurs in two or three planes simultaneously, producing a complex pattern of movement. However, it is convenient to consider movements about each of the three defined axes separately. Movement about a transverse axis in a paramedian (parasagittal) plane is termed flexion and extension; that about an anteroposterior axis in a coronal (frontal) plane is termed abduction and adduction; and that about a vertical axis in a transverse plane is termed medial and lateral rotation.

All movements are described, unless otherwise stated, with respect to the anatomical position, this being the position of reference. In the anatomical position, joints are often referred to as being in a 'neutral position'.

Flexion. Bending of adjacent body segments in a paramedian (parasagittal) plane so that their two anterior/posterior surfaces are brought together; bending the elbow so that the anterior surfaces of the forearm and arm move towards each other (Fig. 1.3A). (In flexion at the knee joint, the posterior surfaces of the leg/calf and thigh move towards each other.)

Extension. The moving apart of two opposing surfaces in a paramedian (parasagittal) plane; the straightening of the flexed knee or elbow. Extension also refers to movement beyond the neutral position in a direction opposite to flexion; extension at the wrist occurs when the posterior surfaces of the hand and forearm move towards each other (Fig. 1.3B). (Flexion and extension of the foot at the ankle joint are usually referred to as plantarflexion and dorsiflexion, respectively.)

Plantarflexion. Moving the top (dorsum) of the foot away from the anterior surface of the leg (Fig. 1.3C).

Dorsiflexion. Bringing the dorsum of the foot towards the anterior surface of the leg (Fig. 1.3C).

Abduction. Movement of a body segment in a coronal (frontal) plane such that it moves away from the midline of the body; movement of the upper limb away from the side of the trunk (Fig. 1.3D).

Adduction. Movement of a body segment in a coronal (frontal) plane such that it moves towards the midline of the body; movement of the upper limb towards the side of the trunk (Fig. 1.3D).

Lateral flexion/bending. A term used to denote bending of the trunk (vertebral column) to one side; lateral flexion/bending of the trunk to the right (Fig. 1.3E); it occurs in the coronal (frontal) plane.

Medial rotation. Rotation of a limb segment about its longitudinal axis such that the anterior surface comes to face towards the midline of the body; turning the upper limb inwards so that the flexed forearm and hand point towards the midline (Fig. 1.3F).

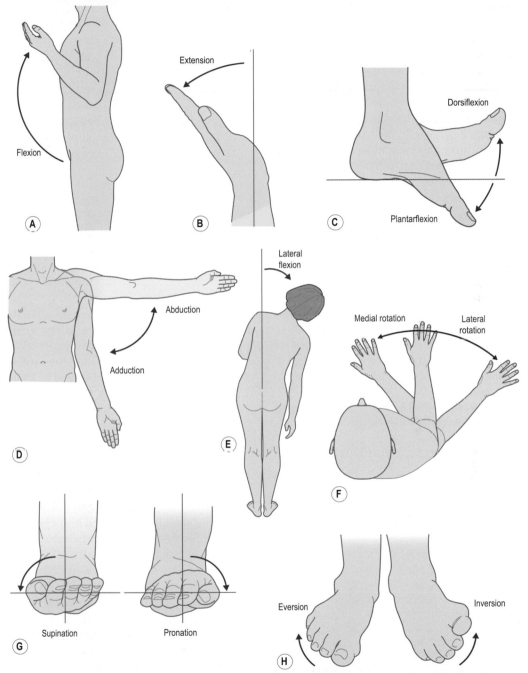

Fig. 1.3 (A) Flexion of the forearm at the elbow joint. (B) Extension of the hand at the wrist joint. (C) Plantarflexion and dorsiflexion of the foot at the ankle joint. (D) Abduction and adduction of the upper limb at the shoulder joint. (E) Lateral flexion of the trunk to the right. (F) Medial and lateral rotation of the upper limb at the shoulder joint. (G) Supination and pronation of the hand with the wrist flexed. (H) Inversion and eversion of the foot.

Lateral rotation. Rotation of a limb segment about its longitudinal axis so that its anterior surface faces away from the midline plane: turning the upper limb so that the flexed forearm and hand point away from the midline (Fig. 1.3F).

Supination and pronation are terms used in conjunction with the movements of the forearm and foot.

Supination. Movement of the forearm so that the palm of the hand faces forwards, with the wrist flexed the palm faces superiorly (Fig. 1.3G). In the foot, it is movement of the forefoot causing the sole to face medially: it is always accompanied by adduction of the forefoot.

Pronation. Movement of the forearm so that the palm of the hand faces backwards, with the wrist flexed the palm faces inferiorly (Fig. 1.3G). In the foot, it is movement of the forefoot causing the sole to face laterally: it is always accompanied by abduction of the forefoot.

Inversion and eversion are terms used to describe composite movements of the foot.

Inversion. Movement of the foot to make the sole face medially (Fig. 1.3H); it is the combined movements of supination and adduction of the forefoot.

Eversion. Movement of the foot to make the sole face laterally (Fig. 1.3H); it is the combined movements of pronation and abduction of the forefoot.

SECTION SUMMARY

Terminology
- Specific terms are used to describe the relationship of one body part/segment/region to another and are considered in relation to the anatomical position of the body.
- The anatomical position is standing erect facing forwards, legs together, toes pointing forwards, arms at the side and palms facing forwards.

Terms Describing Movement
- Specific terms refer to different types of movement between body parts/segments/regions.
- Flexion/extension occur about a transverse axis in a paramedian (parasagittal) plane; abduction/adduction occur about an anteroposterior axis in a coronal (frontal) plane; medial/lateral rotation occur about a vertical axis in a transverse plane.
- More specific terms are used for movements associated with some segments/regions: plantarflexion/dorsiflexion of the foot at the ankle joint; supination/pronation of the forearm; supination/pronation/inversion/eversion within the foot; and lateral flexion/bending of the vertebral column.

SELF-ASSESSMENT QUESTIONS

1. What is the standard anatomical position?
2. Which term describes one part of the upper limb being closer to the trunk than another?
3. Which term describes the movement of the lower limb away from the midline of the body?
4. Which plane divides the body into equal right and left halves?
5. If one part of the body lies below another, how is this described?
6. A transverse plane lies at right angles to which other plane(s)?
7. If part of the body is said to lie anterior to another part, what does this mean?
8. What movement is pronation of the forearm?
9. About which axis does medial and lateral rotation of a limb occur?
10. What movement is dorsiflexion of the foot at the ankle joint?

EARLY EMBRYOLOGY

LEARNING OUTCOMES

By the end of the section, you should be able to:
1. Describe the formation of the primary germ layers
2. Describe the fate of mesodermal somites
3. Describe the development of vertebrae
4. Describe the development and rotation of the limbs

STAGES IN DEVELOPMENT

The process of development begins with penetration of the zona pellucida of the ovum (egg) by the head of the sperm. This is fertilisation. It is this event which activates the ovum biochemically and leads approximately 40 weeks later to the birth of an infant. Between fertilisation and birth, a series of complicated changes gradually occur involving both differentiation and reorganisation, resulting in the appearance of different tissues, organs and organ systems to create a viable individual. This account is an introduction designed to help understand early human development. Unfortunately, many new and sometimes confusing terms are used, particularly when describing early development; where possible, these new terms are kept to a minimum.

Fertilisation and Cleavage

Fertilisation usually occurs within the fallopian (uterine) tubes (p. 612). It is not until 6 days later that the resulting

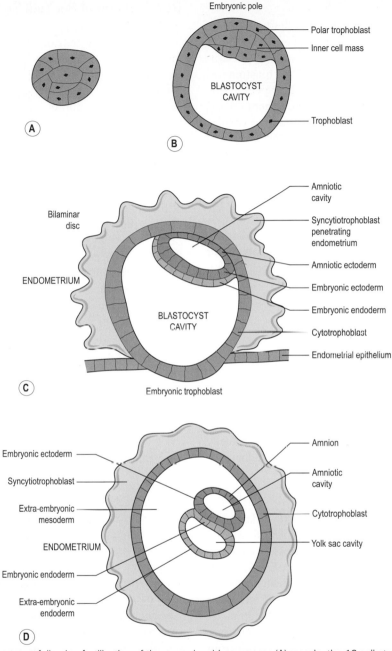

Fig. 1.4 Early stages following fertilisation of the ovum (egg) by a sperm: (A) morula, the 16-cell stage; (B) blasto-cyst; (C) implantation of the fertilised egg into the endometrium of the uterine wall; (D) appearance of the yolk sac.

cell mass becomes implanted in the uterine wall. During this time, considerable differentiation and organisation have already taken place. Within 12 hours of fertilisation, the male and female pronuclei have met and fused forming a zygote near the centre of the ovum. Within a further 12 hours cleavage occurs, consisting of repeated mitotic divisions of the zygote (still within the zona pellucida) resulting in the formation of increasing numbers of cells (blastomeres), but without an increase in total cytoplasmic mass, which is partitioned among the blastomeres. By the time there are 16 cells (after four divisions), the mass of cells is known as a morula (Fig. 1.4A).

Morula

Evidence suggests that the nuclei of individual cells lie in quantitatively and qualitatively different cytoplasmic environments; the initial circumstances of cellular differentiation have been created. The blastomeres of the future inner cell mass move with respect to one another, providing the basis for cell movement during gastrulation, and the possibility of inductive cellular interaction resulting from the acquisition of a new microenvironment by an individual cell is established.

At the 16-cell stage, the morula enters the uterus (p. 614) and the process of compaction occurs in which individual blastomeres become less distinct. Cells on the outside of the morula adhere to each other with a topographical difference established between the surface cells and those inside. Under the influence of the inner cell mass, the outer cells form the trophoectoderm, which eventually form the foetal membranes. The inner cell mass forms the embryonic cells and may contribute to the extra-embryonic membranes.

Blastocyst

Some 4–6 days after fertilisation, the morula takes in uterine fluid through the zona pellucida, forming a blastocyst cavity (Fig. 1.4B). This separates the inner cell mass from the trophoblast, except near the polar trophoblast overlying the inner cell mass (Fig. 1.4B). During blastocyst formation, the zona pellucida thins and is eventually shed, exposing the cells. The polar trophoblast adheres to the uterine wall and implantation begins.

Implantation

During the early stages of implantation (6–8 days), the inner cell mass differentiates and eventually forms the complete embryo. Initially, cells facing the blastocyst cavity form a single layer of primary embryonic endoderm. The remaining cells form another layer, which is the precursor of the embryonic ectoderm (Fig. 1.4C), also later giving rise to the embryonic mesoderm. The amniotic cavity appears between these cells and an overlying layer of cells forming the amniotic ectoderm, derived from the deep aspect of the polar trophoblast (Fig. 1.4C). The trophoblast forms the cytotrophoblast, surrounding the blastocyst cavity and syncytiotrophoblast, penetrating the endometrial lining of the uterus (Fig. 1.4C). The inner cell mass, from which cells of the future embryo arise, forms no more than a bilaminar disc, while the remaining blastocyst forms the foetal membranes.

Development of the Yolk Sac

As the amniotic cavity is formed, the blastocyst cavity becomes lined by cells of extra-embryonic endoderm. The blastocyst wall now consists of three layers: an outer trophoblast (extra-embryonic ectoderm) consisting of cytotrophoblast and syncytiotrophoblast, a loose reticular layer of extra-embryonic mesoderm and an inner cell layer of extra-embryonic endoderm: the space remaining is the yolk sac (Fig. 1.4D).

Prochordal Plate

The prochordal plate forms in a localised area in the roof of the yolk sac at the cranial end of the future embryo; it gives the bilaminar disc bilateral symmetry. At the same time, the extra-embryonic mesoderm develops fluid-filled spaces which join, forming a large cavity surrounding the whole of the yolk sac and amnion, except the mesodermal connecting stalk (Fig. 1.5A). This space (extra-embryonic coelom) splits the extra-embryonic mesoderm into visceral and parietal layers, separating the amniotic and yolk cavities from the outer wall of the conceptus (Fig. 1.5A).

Primary Germ Layers

The primary germ layers and supporting membranes have now been established. From the embryonic ectoderm, the outer covering of the embryo is formed, including the outer layers of the skin and its derivatives (hair, nails), the mucous membrane of the cranial and caudal ends of the alimentary canal (digestive/gastrointestinal tract), and the central and peripheral nervous systems, including the retina and part of the iris of the eye. In general terms, the embryonic endoderm forms epithelial tissues in the adult: the epithelial lining of the alimentary canal; parenchyma of its associated glands (liver, pancreas); lining of the respiratory system; and most of the epithelium of the bladder and urethra.

About 15 days after fertilisation, the trilaminar disc begins to form as a heaping up of cells in the upper layer of the bilaminar disc towards the posterior part of the midline, forming the primitive streak (Fig. 1.5B). The heaping up is mainly due to medial and backward migration of actively proliferating ectodermal cells spreading laterally and forward between the ectoderm and endoderm layers as the intra-embryonic mesoderm (Fig. 1.5C). At the lateral extremes of the migration, the mesodermal cells become continuous with the extra-embryonic

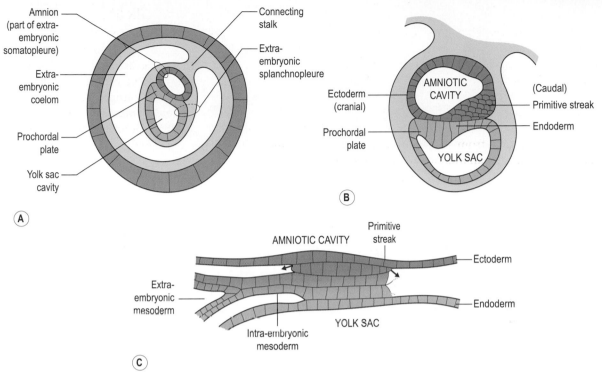

Fig. 1.5 (A) Site of development of the prochordal plate. (B) Further development of the prochordal plate and appearance of the primitive streak. (C) Trilaminar disc.

mesoderm (splanchnopleuric) covering the yolk sac and the amnion (somatopleuric). Anteriorly, the embryonic mesodermal cells become continuous across the midline in front of the prochordal plate.

Soon after the appearance of the primitive streak, which forms a line on the surface, further heaping up of cells occurs at the anterior end (primitive knot) from which the notochordal process extends forwards to the posterior edge of the prochordal plate. The ectoderm overlying the notochordal process, as well as that immediately anterior, becomes thickened (neural plate), from which the neural tube, and eventually the brain and spinal cord, develops.

On either side of the notochord, the mesoderm forms two longitudinal strips (paraxial mesoderm) (Fig. 1.6A), each becoming segmented forming approximately 44 blocks of mesoderm (somites), none of which are formed anterior to the notochord. Lateral to the paraxial mesoderm is a thinner layer (lateral plate mesoderm) continuous at its edges with the extra-embryonic mesoderm. Connecting the edge of the paraxial mesoderm to the lateral plate mesoderm is a longitudinal tract (intermediate mesoderm) from which arises the nephrogenic cord.

Within the lateral plate mesoderm, small fluid-filled spaces appear, which join together to form the intra-embryonic mesoderm, continuous across the midline (Fig. 1.6B). The intra-embryonic mesoderm forms the pericardial (heart), pleural (lung) and peritoneal (abdominal) cavities.

During the fourth week following fertilisation, the trilaminar disc bulges further into the amniotic cavity. Under its cranial and caudal parts, head and tail folds appear with marked folding along the lateral margins of the embryo (Fig. 1.7).

Development of the ear is outlined on page 703, eye on page 707, cardiovascular system on pages 582 to 584, respiratory system on page 590, digestive system on page 598, urinary system on page 606, genital system on page 611 and nervous system on pages 565 and 683.

MESODERMAL SOMITES

By the end of the third week following fertilisation, the paraxial mesoderm begins to divide (mesodermal somites), easily recognisable during the fourth and fifth

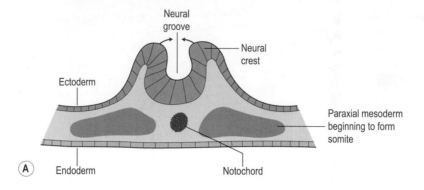

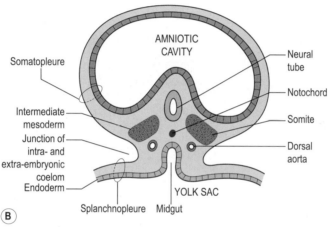

Fig. 1.6 (A) Formation of the neural groove. (B) Completion of neural tube formation showing the appearance of the paraxial (somite) and intermediate mesoderm.

weeks (Fig. 1.7). Eventually, approximately 44 pairs of somites develop, although not all are present at the same time; the cranial paraxial mesoderm of the embryo remains unsegmented. There are 4 occipital somites, 8 cervical, 12 thoracic, 5 lumbar, 5 sacral and 8–10 coccygeal somites. Growth and migration of the somitic cells are responsible for the thickening of the body wall, as well as the development of bone and muscle: the deeper layers of the skin are also of somitic origin. Somite-derived tissue spreads medially to form the vertebrae, dorsally to form the musculature of the back and ventrally into the body wall to form the ribs and the intercostal and abdominal muscles.

Soon after its formation, each somite differentiates into three parts. The ventromedial part forms the sclerotome, which migrates medially towards the notochord and neural tube to take part in the formation of

the vertebrae and ribs (Fig. 1.7). In the remaining part of the somite (dermomyotome) cells of the dorsal and ventral edges proliferate and move medially forming the myotome, whose cells migrate widely differentiating into myoblasts (primitive muscle cells), while the remaining thin layer of cells forms the dermatome, which spreads out to form the dermis of the skin.

The myotome of each somite receives a single spinal nerve which innervates all the muscles derived from that myotome irrespective of how far it eventually migrates. The dorsal aortae lie adjacent to the somites and give off a series of intersegmental arteries between them.

DEVELOPMENT OF VERTEBRAE

Soon after the formation of each somite, it differentiates into the three parts: the ventromedial sclerotome,

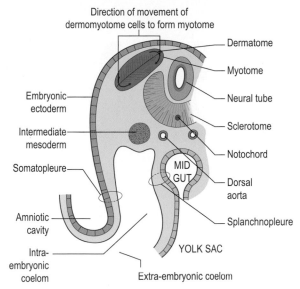

Fig. 1.7 Differentiation and migration of the somatic mesoderm.

the medial myotome and the thin lateral dermatome (Fig. 1.7). The sclerotomes surround the notochord followed by the myotomes. Each vertebra is formed from adjacent parts of two sclerotomes (Fig. 1.8) with the intervening part forming the outer part (annulus fibrosus) of the intervertebral disc; the nucleus pulposus of the intervertebral disc is derived from the notochord. As there are 8 cervical somites, there are also 8 cervical nerves, 12 in the thoracic region, 5 in the lumbar region and 5 in the sacral region. Because each vertebra is formed from adjacent somites, the cervical nerves come to lie above their correspondingly numbered vertebrae with the 8th cervical nerve lying below the 7th cervical vertebra. In the thoracic, lumbar and sacral regions, the spinal nerves all lie below their correspondingly numbered vertebrae.

The dermomyotome breaks up with cells moving both ventrally and dorsally. The original spinal nerve supplying the myotome divides into anterior and posterior primary rami, supplying the ventral (hypomere) and dorsal (epimere) parts of the myotome, respectively. The epimeres come to lie between the transverse and spinous processes, giving rise to the musculature of the trunk and neck. The hypomeres give rise to the prevertebral muscles (scalenes, quadratus lumborum, psoas, piriformis) and musculature of the thoracic and abdominal walls.

The occipital myotomes do not participate in the formation of the musculature of the trunk or neck: instead, they give rise to the muscle mass of the tongue. The unsegmented part of the paraxial mesoderm eventually becomes incorporated into the branchial (pharyngeal) arches, each of which is innervated by a cranial nerve. The musculature derived from these arches forms the muscles of the face, muscles associated with the mandible and muscles of the larynx and pharynx.

DEVELOPMENT OF THE LIMBS

The limbs initially appear as flipper-like projections (limb buds) with the forelimbs appearing first between 24 and 26 days. Each bud consists of a mass of mesenchyme covered by ectoderm with a thickened ectodermal ridge at the tip; the ectodermal ridge controls normal development of the limb, with damage to it resulting in trauma to the limb. At the beginning of the second month, the elbow and knee prominences project posterolaterally; at about the same time, the hand and foot plates appear as flattened expansions at the end of the limb bud. Between 36 and 38 days, five radiating thickenings forming the fingers/toes can be distinguished, and the webs between the thickenings disappear, freeing the digits. Appropriate spinal nerves grow into the limbs in association with migration of the myotomes: C5, C6, C7, C8 and T1 for the upper limb, and L4, L5, S1, S2 and S3 for the lower limb. The limb bones differentiate from the mesenchyme of the bud; the upper and lower limbs grow in such a way that they rotate in opposite directions, the upper limb laterally and lower limb medially (Fig. 1.9). Consequently, the thumb becomes the lateral digit of the hand, while the great toe is the medial digit of the foot.

During development, the limb bud appears as a swelling from the body wall (Fig. 1.10(i)). The upper limb bud at the level of the lower cervical and first thoracic segments, and lower limb bud at the level of the lower lumbar and upper sacral segments. At first, they project at right angles to the body surface, having ventral and dorsal surfaces and cephalic (preaxial) and caudal (postaxial) borders (Fig. 1.10(ii)). As the limbs increase in length, they become differentiated, during which time they are folded ventrally so that the ventral surface becomes medial (Fig. 1.10(iii)) with the convexities of the elbow and knee directed laterally (Fig. 1.10(iv)).

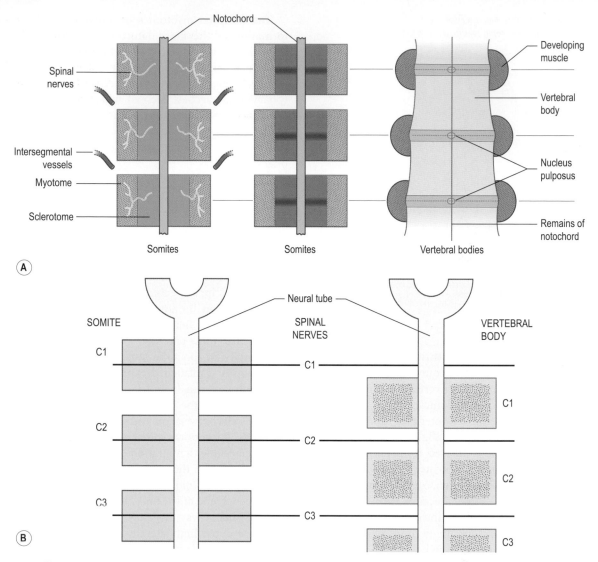

Fig. 1.8 (A) Development of vertebrae from the sclerotome component of the somite. (B) The relationship between spinal nerves and vertebrae.

At a later stage, the upper and lower limbs rotate in opposite directions so that the convexity of the elbow is directed towards the caudal end and that of the knee towards the cranial end of the body (Fig. 1.10(v)). Consequently, the thumb becomes the lateral digit of the hand, and the great toe, the medial digit of the foot.

As the limb bud develops, the primitive muscle mass becomes compartmentalised, foreshadowing the adult pattern with intermuscular septa extending outwards from the periosteum of the bones, dividing the limbs into anterior and posterior compartments. In the lower limb, some of the anterior compartment musculature becomes separated into an adductor group, while in the upper limb, this muscle mass has degenerated phylogenetically so all that remains is coracobrachialis. Adduction of the upper limb is a powerful action in humans served by great sheets of muscle (latissimus dorsi posteriorly, pectoralis major anteriorly) that have migrated into it. In the forearm and leg/calf, the preaxial (radius upper limb, tibia lower limb) and postaxial (ulna upper limb, fibula lower limb) bones

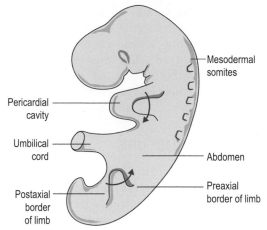

Fig. 1.9 Development of the upper and lower limb buds and the direction in which they rotate.

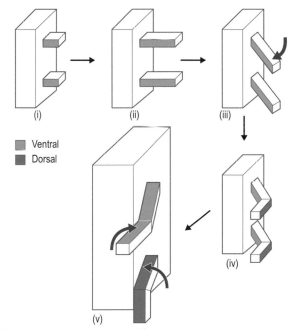

Ventral
Dorsal

Fig. 1.10 Rotation of the upper and lower limbs during development.

are connected by an interosseous membrane and to the investing fascia by intermuscular septa. The compartments formed enclose muscles of similar or related functions.

The ventral rami entering a limb bud pass anterior to the myotomes and eventually divide into dorsal and ventral divisions, which unite with the corresponding branches of adjacent ventral rami forming the nerves

of the dorsal and ventral aspects of the limb bud. These nerves respectively supply the sheets of muscle and overlying skin of the dorsal (extensor) and ventral (flexor) surfaces of the limbs prior to their rotation into the adult pattern. During folding and rotation of the limb and migration of muscle masses, these nerve-muscle connections are maintained.

SECTION SUMMARY

Stages in Development

Time From Ovulation		Event
Within	24 h	Fertilisation
	72 h	Passage of conceptus through isthmus of fallopian tubes
	80 h	Entry of conceptus into uterus
	4–6 days	Blastocyst formation
	7 days	Implantation
	9–13 days	Bilaminar embryonic disc
	14–15 days	Beginning of primitive streak; appearance of extra-embryonic coelom
	16 days	Beginning of notochord process
	17–18 days	Neural plate appears
	19–20 days	Intra-embryonic coelom begins to appear
	20–30 days	Formation of somites
	24 days	Head, tail and lateral body folds establish basic embryonic shape
	24–26 days	Limb buds appear
	5 weeks	Hands and feet begin to develop
	8 weeks	Primary ossification centres appear in long bones
	12 weeks	Formation of definitive body wall complete
	Birth	Vertebrae are in three parts (centrum and two neural arches); shafts of long bones are completely ossified; secondary ossification centres begin to appear (distal femur; proximal tibia)

❓ SELF-ASSESSMENT QUESTIONS

11. What are the three parts of a mesodermal somite?
12. What name is given to the fused male and female pronuclei?
13. What are the 44 blocks of tissue derived from the paraxial mesoderm known as?
14. From how many somites is each vertebral body derived?
15. How many pairs of cervical nerves are there and what is their relationship to the cervical vertebrae?
16. The dorsal part of the myotome (epimere) gives rise to which muscles?
17. The upper limb bud develops opposite which vertebral segments?
18. Following rotation of the limbs in which direction is the convexity of the knee directed?
19. When do the limb buds appear?
20. At birth, how many parts does each vertebra have and what are they?

NERVOUS SYSTEM

LEARNING OUTCOMES

By the end of the section, you should be able to:
1. Describe the structure of a nerve cell and the process of myelination
2. Describe the different types of synapses that occur and understand what happens at them
3. Describe the different types of nerve fibres within the peripheral nervous system
4. Describe the structure of a peripheral nerve and its constituent parts

INTRODUCTION

The nervous system consists of highly specialised cells designed to transmit information rapidly between various parts of the body. Topographically, it can be divided into two major components: the central nervous system (CNS) and peripheral nervous system (PNS). The brain and spinal cord constitute the CNS, which lies within the skull (p. 656) and vertebral canal (p. 564), while nerves in the PNS connect the CNS with all other parts of the body (p. 18).

The CNS is a massive collection of nerve cells connected in an intricate and complex way subserving higher order functions of the nervous system (thought, language, emotion, control of movement, analysis of sensation). It is isolated from the rest of the body, being located wholly within the skull and vertebral canal.

The PNS consists of cells connecting the CNS with other tissues of the body. These cells are aggregated into a large number of cable-like structures (nerves) threaded like wires throughout the tissues of the body.

CELLULAR STRUCTURE

The basic cellular unit of the nervous system is the nerve cell (neuron), which differs in size and shape according to its function and location within the nervous system. Different structural classes of neurons can be identified: multipolar neurons (motor neurons, central nervous system interneurons); bipolar neurons (sensory neurons in the retina, olfactory mucosa, inner ear); unipolar or pseudounipolar neurons (all other sensory neurons); and anaxonic neurons of the central nervous system which do not produce action potentials as they lack a true axon, but do regulate local electrical changes in adjacent neurons. Nevertheless, most neurons have three characteristic components: a cell body, an axon and dendrites (Fig. 1.11A).

The cell body is the expanded part of the cell containing the nucleus and apparatus necessary to sustain the cell's metabolic activities. The axon is a longitudinal tubular extension (process) of the cell membrane and cytoplasm, transmitting information away from the cell body; the cell membrane surrounding the axon is the axolemma. Dendrites are extensions of the cell membrane, radiating in various directions from the cell body; they are responsible for receiving information and transmitting it to the cell body.

Structurally, dendrites differ from axons as they typically undergo extensive branching close to the cell body, while axons remain singular for most of their course, only branching at their terminal ends. A neuron has only one axon but may have several dendrites; the length and calibre of axons and dendrites vary depending on the particular function of the neuron.

INTERNEURAL CONNECTIONS

Individual neurons convey information by conducting electrical action potentials along their cell membrane with communication between separate neurons occurring chemically at a specialised structure (synapse).

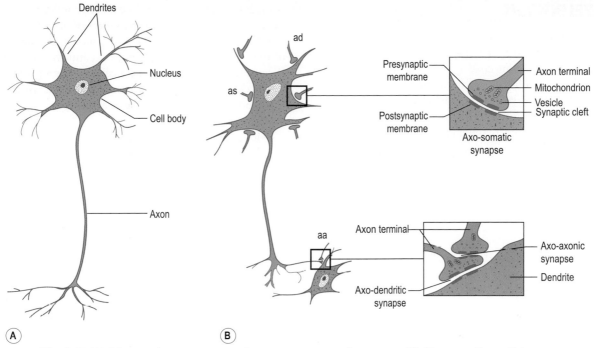

Fig. 1.11 (A) Microscopic appearance and component parts of a neuron. (B) Neuron with multiple axo-somatic (as), axo-dendritic (ad) and axo-axonic (aa) synapses with the insets showing the detailed structure of the synapse.

Synapses are formed by the close approximation of a small discrete area of the cell membrane of one neuron to a reciprocal area of the membrane of a second neuron (Fig. 1.11B); the apposed membranes are specially modified and separated by a gap (synaptic cleft) 0.02 μm in width. Across the synapse, one cell communicates with the next; communication is unidirectional. The membrane of the cell transmitting the information is the presynaptic membrane and that of the cell receiving the information the postsynaptic membrane.

Near the presynaptic membrane, the cytoplasm contains numerous small vesicles filled with chemicals (neurotransmitters), which vary according to the function of the neuron. In all cases, when an electrical signal arrives at the terminal end of an axon, the neurotransmitter is released through the presynaptic membrane into the synaptic cleft where it flows across to the postsynaptic membrane to exert its effect. The effect can be excitatory or inhibitory depending on the nature of the neurotransmitter and receptors on the postsynaptic membrane with which it interacts. Excitatory substances generate an action potential in the postsynaptic neuron, propagating the potential to its other end. Inhibitory

substances temporarily alter the electrical potential of the postsynaptic neuron, reducing its capacity to be stimulated by other neurons.

Synapses typically occur between the axon of one neuron and dendrite of another. However, they can also occur between axons and cell bodies, axons and axons, and even between dendrites and dendrites (Fig. 1.11B). Some neurons receive few synapses while others may receive thousands.

The purpose of synapses is not to relieve one neuron of information and simply pass it on to the next, but rather to allow the interaction of information from several sources onto a single neuron. The activity of any neuron may be influenced by many others and, conversely, by having several terminal branches to its axon, a single neuron may influence many other neurons.

By being connected to one another in diverse ways, groups of neurons are organised to serve different functions in the nervous system. The patterns of connections (circuits) vary in complexity; generally, the more sophisticated the function, the more complex the circuitry.

MYELINATION

Myelination is a process in which individual axons are wrapped in a lipid sheath (myelin), which serves as a protective and insulating coating for the axon, enhancing the speed of conduction of electrical impulses along it.

In the PNS, myelination is achieved by a Schwann cell curling an extension of its cell membrane around the shaft of the axon in a spiral manner (Fig. 1.12A). As the Schwann cell extension wraps around the axon, the cytoplasm in it

is squeezed out until only a double layer of Schwann cell membrane remains around the axon (Fig. 1.12A). In this way, the myelin sheath is formed by the lipid and protein of the Schwann cell membrane surrounding the axon. Peripheral to the myelin sheath, the axon is surrounded by the cytoplasm of the Schwann cell with the outermost Schwann cell membrane acting as a second membrane to the axon (neurolemma) (Fig. 1.12A).

Along its length, a given axon is surrounded in series by a large number of Schwann cells, but each Schwann

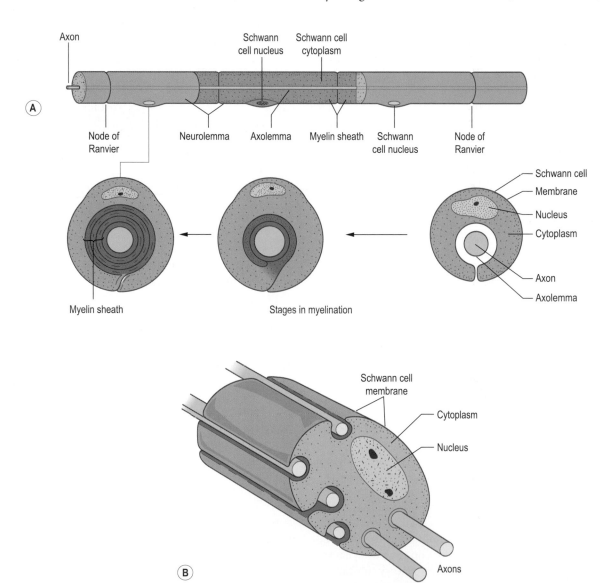

Fig. 1.12 (A) Myelinated axon in the peripheral nervous system and the stages in myelination. (B) Relationship between unmyelinated axons and Schwann cells.

cell is related only to a single axon (Fig. 1.12A). Junctions where the myelin sheath of one Schwann cell ends and the next sheath begins are nodes of Ranvier. An axon, its myelin sheath and the Schwann cells surrounding it make up a nerve fibre.

While many axons in the PNS are myelinated, a large number remain unmyelinated. Rather than being enveloped by a tightly spiralling sheath of myelin, they run embedded in invaginations of Schwann cell membranes; a single Schwann cell may envelop several axons (Fig. 1.12B). Unmyelinated axons have less physical protection than myelinated ones, but the major difference is that unmyelinated axons conduct impulses at much slower velocities.

In the CNS, myelination is performed by specialised cells (oligodendrocytes). The process is similar to that in the PNS, except that a given oligodendrocyte is usually involved in the simultaneous myelination of several separate axons (Fig. 1.13). Unmyelinated axons in the CNS run embedded in cytoplasmic extensions/processes of oligodendrocytes.

Several diseases can affect myelinating cells, including toxic and metabolic diseases, and most notably multiple sclerosis. In these diseases, neurons are not necessarily directly affected, but the loss of their myelin covering affects the conduction of action potentials, resulting in disordered neural function.

STRUCTURE OF PERIPHERAL NERVES

A peripheral nerve is formed by the parallel aggregation of myelinated and unmyelinated axons: the greater the number of axons, the larger the nerve. Microscopically within a peripheral nerve, myelinated axons are surrounded by their individual Schwann cell sheaths while unmyelinated axons run embedded in invaginations of the Schwann cell membrane. The axons are held together by sheaths of fibrous tissue, constituting additional coatings that protect them from external mechanical and chemical insults.

Individual myelinated axons are surrounded by a tubular sheath of fibrous tissue (endoneurium), while clusters of axons are held together by a larger fibrous sheath (perineurium) (Fig. 1.14). Unmyelinated axons are not enclosed by endoneurium but run in isolated bundles parallel to myelinated axons that are enclosed with them in the perineurial sheath.

A bundle of axons enclosed within a single perineurial sheath is a nerve fascicle (Fig. 1.14). Axons within a

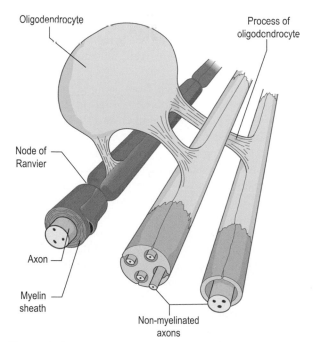

Fig. 1.13 Relationship between an oligodendrocyte and several myelinated and unmyelinated axons it ensheaths.

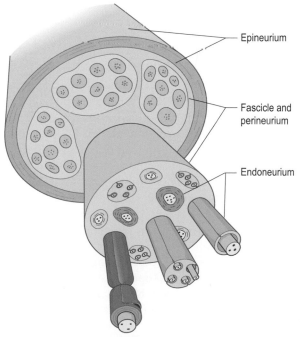

Fig. 1.14 Composition of a peripheral nerve.

fascicle largely remain within the same fascicle throughout the course of the nerve until their peripheral distribution. Nevertheless, along the course of a peripheral nerve, axons may leave one fascicle to enter and continue within an adjacent fascicle.

The fascicles within a peripheral nerve are bound together by an external sheath of fibrous tissue (epineurium) forming the external surface of the macroscopic nerve (Fig. 1.14). As a peripheral nerve passes through the body tissues, it gives branches composed of one or more fascicles of the parent nerve, which leave it to reach their particular destination. Along the course of a nerve, this process is repeated until all the fascicles and axons in the nerve have been distributed to their target tissues.

PERIPHERAL NERVOUS SYSTEM

Nerves that supply structural tissues such as bone, muscle and skin are somatic nerves. Groups of somatic nerves innervate specific areas or regions; they are considered in detail in the respective region.

Nerves supplying viscera such as the heart, lungs and digestive tract are visceral nerves. As the nervous functions concerning viscera are largely automatic and subconscious, that part of the nervous system innervating viscera is the autonomic nervous system (ANS). It has components in both the CNS and PNS and is described in detail on page 575.

Constituents of Peripheral Nerves

Peripheral nerves consist of different types of axons classified according to their size, function or physiological characteristics. The broadest classification of axons recognises afferent (sensory) and efferent (motor) fibres. The terms 'afferent' and 'efferent' refer to the direction in which axons conduct information: afferent fibres conduct towards and efferent fibres away from the CNS. The term 'sensory' refers to axons conveying information to the CNS about events occurring in the periphery: 'motor' fibres cause events in the periphery, usually as voluntary or smooth muscle contraction.

Axons are also classified according to their conduction velocities, which are proportional to their sizes (Fig. 1.15). By stimulating a peripheral nerve electrically and recording the evoked activity some distance along the nerve, a wave of electrical activity can be recorded. The wave is generated by summation of the electrical activity

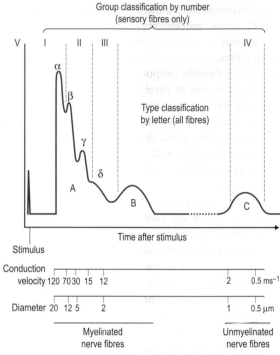

Fig. 1.15 Neurogram of an idealised peripheral nerve. Activity in different types of nerve fibres is reflected in depolarisations occurring at different times after the delivery of an electrical stimulus to the nerve.

in each axon in the nerve, its size being proportional to the number of axons present, while its shape reflects the type of axons present.

The waveform obtained from a nerve containing every known type of axon is shown in Fig. 1.15; it has three principal peaks (A, B and C waves). The A wave occurs soon after the triggering stimulus, produced by rapidly conducting axons with velocities in the range $12-120 \text{ ms}^{-1}$; these are the A fibres. The A wave is broken down into several secondary peaks (Aα, Aβ, Aγ and Aδ waves), each produced by a particular subgroup of rapidly conducting axons.

The B wave is produced by more slowly conducting, but nevertheless fast, fibres classified as B fibres. The C wave arrives at the recording electrode much later as it is produced by slowly conducting axons (C fibres) with conduction velocities of $0.5-2 \text{ ms}^{-1}$.

Not all peripheral nerves contain every type of fibre, therefore not all nerves show A, B and C waves: B fibres are not regularly present in all nerves, so they are not always recordable.

Myelinated axons conduct impulses faster than unmyelinated axons: among myelinated axons, those with larger diameters conduct impulses faster than those with smaller diameters. The conduction velocity of a myelinated axon is directly proportional to the overall diameter of the axon and its myelin sheath. A and B fibres are myelinated axons of various diameters and fast conduction velocities, while C fibres are unmyelinated axons with small diameters and slow conduction velocities.

Functionally, Aα and Aγ fibres represent motor fibres connected to voluntary muscles, but also include certain sensory fibres transmitting position sensation from skeletal muscles. Aβ fibres mediate the sensations of touch, vibration and pressure from skin; Aδ fibres are sensory fibres mediating pressure, pain and temperature sensations from the skin; pain and pressure from muscles; and pain, pressure and position sensation from ligaments and joints. B fibres are preganglionic sympathetic efferent fibres. C fibres are largely unmyelinated sensory fibres arising in virtually all body tissues and transmit pain, temperature and pressure sensations; however, some are postganglionic sympathetic neurons. Because Aβ fibres have large diameters, they are sometimes known as large-diameter afferent fibres, while Aδ and C fibres are known collectively as small-diameter afferent fibres.

Another system of axon classification relates specifically to sensory fibres in which they are classified according to their conduction velocities into groups I, II, III and IV; these groups have the same conduction velocities as type Aα, Aβ, Aδ and C fibres, respectively (Fig. 1.15), but do not include the Aα and Aβ motor fibres. The fibres of groups III and IV largely mediate pain and temperature sensations; group II constitutes fibres mediating pressure and touch, and fibres that form spray endings in muscle spindles (p. 32): group I is divided into Ia and Ib. Ia fibres are slightly larger and innervate muscle spindles, while Ib fibres innervate Golgi tendon organs (p. 32).

Nerve Endings

The terminals of axons in peripheral nerves have unique structures depending on their function. Motor axons have terminals designed to deliver a stimulus to muscle cells (p. 33), and sensory axons have terminals designed to detect particular types of stimuli. These terminals (receptors) and a diversity of morphological types can be found in the section on skin (p. 23).

SECTION SUMMARY

Nervous System
- Consists of specialised cells (neurons) concerned with the transmission of information throughout the body.
- Neurons have a cell body (expanded part of the cell), an axon (single long process arising from the cell body) and dendrites (multi-branching radiating processes arising from the cell body).
- Two parts: CNS comprises the brain, spinal cord and spinal nerves; PNS comprises nerves (peripheral and cranial) and sensory receptors.
- Connections (synapses) between neurons allow integration of information from several sources. The resultant effect may be excitatory or inhibitory depending on the type of neurotransmitter and type of receptors on the postsynaptic membrane.
- Axons may be myelinated or unmyelinated; myelinated axons have faster conduction velocities. In the PNS myelination is by Schwann cells and in the CNS by oligodendrocytes.

Peripheral Nerves
- Parallel aggregations of individual axons (fibres).
- Afferent (sensory) fibres transmit information towards and efferent (motor) away from the CNS.
- The larger the fibre diameter, the faster the nerve conduction velocity.

SELF-ASSESSMENT QUESTIONS

21. In the peripheral nervous system, which cell type is responsible for myelination of a nerve fibre?
22. What types of interneural connections are possible between individual nerves?
23. In the central nervous system, what cell type is responsible for the myelination of nerve fibres?
24. Which structure completely surrounds a nerve fibre?
25. What type of fibres are connected to voluntary muscle?
26. What are and what is the function of efferent fibres?
27. What is the function of synapses?
28. What are the components of the peripheral nervous system?
29. What is an axon?
30. What is a 'node of Ranvier'?

SKIN AND ITS APPENDAGES

LEARNING OUTCOMES

By the end of the section, you should be able to:
1. Describe the structure and function of skin
2. Describe the location and function of glands associated with the skin
3. Appreciate that incisions along cleavage lines leads to minimal scarring
4. Understand the process of wound healing
5. Appreciate that skin contains a variety of nerve endings with different functions

INTRODUCTION

Skin is a tough, pliable, waterproof covering of the body that blends with the more delicate lining membranes of the body at the mouth, nose, eyelids and urogenital and anal openings; it is the largest organ of the body. Not only does it provide a surface covering, it is also a sensory organ endowed with a host of nerve endings providing sensitivity to touch and pressure, and changes in temperature and painful stimuli; for general sensations, the skin is the principal source. The waterproofing function of skin is essentially concerned with preventing fluid loss from the body. Fatty secretions from sebaceous glands help maintain this waterproofing as well as being acted upon to produce vitamin D. However, the efficient waterproofing mechanism does not prevent the skin from having an absorptive function when certain drugs, vitamins and hormones are applied to it in suitable forms. Nor does it prevent the excretion of certain crystalloids through sweating; if sweating is copious, as much as 1 g of non-protein nitrogen can be eliminated in an hour. Because humans are warm-blooded, body temperature must be kept within relatively narrow limits despite large variations in environmental temperature. The reduction and control of body temperature is a special function of skin; because of the variability in its blood supply and the presence of sweat glands, heat is lost through radiation, convection and evaporation. Together with the lungs, skin accounts for more than 90% of total body heat loss. In addition to the ability of blood vessels to 'open up' to promote heat loss, they can also be 'closed down' in an attempt to conserve body heat in cool environments.

The metabolic functions of skin require a large surface area for effective functioning. In adults, the area is approximately 1.8 m^2, some seven times greater than at birth. Skin thickness also varies not only with age but also from region to region. It is thinnest over the eyelids (0.5 mm) and thickest over the back of the neck and upper trunk, palm of the hand and sole of the foot. It tends to be thicker over posterior and extensor surfaces than over anterior and flexor surfaces, usually being between 1 and 2 mm thick.

Total skin thickness depends on the thickness of both the epidermis and dermis. On the palms of the hands and soles of the feet, the epidermis is responsible for the skin thickness, the dermis being relatively thin. This arrangement provides protection for the underlying dermis, as the palms and soles are regions of great wear and tear. The character of flexor and extensor skin differs in more respects than just thickness; extensor skin of the limbs tends to be hairier, while flexor skin is usually far more sensitive as it has a rich nerve supply.

Skin is loosely applied to underlying tissues so that it is easily displaced. However, in some regions, it may be firmly attached to the underlying structures (cartilage of the ear and nose, subcutaneous periosteal surface of the tibia, deep fascia surrounding joints). In response to continued friction, skin reacts by increasing the thickness of its superficial layers; when wounded, it responds by increased growth and repair.

Skin in young individuals is extremely elastic, rapidly returning to its original shape and position: this elasticity is increasingly lost with increasing age so that unless it is firmly attached to the underlying tissues it stretches. Stretching tends to occur in one direction because of the orientation of the collagen fibres in the deeper layers, which run predominantly at right angles to the direction of stretch, parallel to the communicating grooves present on the skin surface. In some places, the skin is bound down to the underlying deep fascia, allowing freedom of movement without interference from subcutaneous fat and otherwise highly mobile skin; at flexion creases of joints, the skin is bound down to the underlying fibrous tissue. Where skin has to be pulled around a joint when it is flexed, it is bound down in loose folds which are taken up in flexion: the joints of the fingers clearly show this arrangement.

In adjusting to allow movement, skin follows the body contours. Although this is enabled by its intrinsic elasticity, it is nevertheless subjected to internal stresses, which vary from region to region: these stress lines are often referred to as cleavage (Langer) lines (Fig. 1.16).

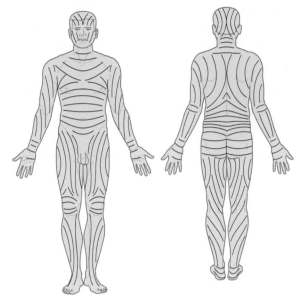

Fig. 1.16 Orientation of cleavage (Langer) lines along which incisions are made (if possible) to promote minimal scarring.

They are important because incisions along them heal with a minimum of scarring, while in wounds across them, the scar may become thicker with a risk of scar contraction because the wound edges are pulled apart by the internal stresses of the skin. Langer lines do not always correspond with the stress lines of life; they merely reflect the stresses within the skin at rest.

Skin colour depends on the presence of pigment (melanin) and the vascularity of the dermis. When hot, the skin appears reddened due to the reflection of large quantities of blood through the epidermis; similarly, when cold, it appears paler due to the reduction of blood flow to it. The degree of oxygenation of the blood also influences skin colour: anaemic individuals generally appear pale. Individual and racial variations in skin colour are dependent on the presence of melanin in the deepest layers of the epidermis; in darker-skinned races, melanin is distributed throughout the layers. In response to sunlight and heat, skin increases its pigmentation, making it appear darker. This physiological increase in pigment formation (tanning from exposure to sunlight) is widely sought after in some individuals. Some areas of the body show a constant deeper pigmentation (external genital and perianal regions, axilla, areola of the breast).

On the pads of the fingers and toes, and extending over the palm and sole, are a series of alternating ridges and depressions, the arrangement of which is highly individual so that even identical twins have different patterns; it is this patterning which forms the basis for identification through fingerprints. They are due to the specific arrangement of the large dermal papillae under the epidermis which act to improve grip and prevent slippage. Sweat glands open along the summits of these ridges; sebaceous glands and hair are absent on these surfaces.

The skin and subcutaneous tissues camouflage the deeper structures of the body. Nevertheless, it is often necessary to identify and manipulate these deeper structures through the skin as well as to test their function, effectiveness and efficiency. To do this, the examiner relies heavily on sensory information provided by their own skin, particularly that of the digits and hands. It is fortunate that the skin of this region is richly endowed with sensory nerve endings, allowing objects to be identified by touch alone, culminating in the ability of the blind to read with their fingers.

In addition to the functions of the skin discussed above, nails, hair, sebaceous and sweat glands are all derived from the epidermis. The delicate creases extending in all directions across the skin form irregular diamond-shaped regions; it is at the intersections of these creases that hairs typically emerge.

STRUCTURE

Skin consists of a superficial layer of ectodermal origin (epidermis) and a deeper mesodermal-derived layer (dermis) (Fig. 1.17).

Epidermis

Layer of stratified squamous epithelium of varying thickness (0.3–1.0 mm) composed of many layers of cells. The deeper cells are living and actively proliferating with the cells produced gradually passing towards the surface; as they do so, they become cornified (keratinised) and are ultimately shed as the skin rubs against clothing and other surfaces. The epidermis is avascular but is penetrated by sensory nerve endings. Its deep surface is firmly locked to the underlying dermis by projections into it (epidermal pegs) with reciprocal projections from the dermis (dermal papillae) (Fig. 1.17).

It is convenient to consider the epidermis as being divided into a number of layers, particularly in the so-called thick skin of the palm or sole. These layers are from within outwards the stratum basale, stratum

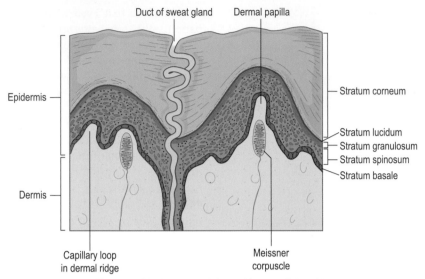

Duct of sweat gland   Dermal papilla

Epidermis —

— Stratum corneum

— Stratum lucidum
— Stratum granulosum
— Stratum spinosum
Stratum basale

Dermis —

Capillary loop
in dermal ridge

Meissner
corpuscle

Fig. 1.17 Epidermal and dermal layers of the skin.

spinosum, stratum granulosum, stratum lucidum and stratum corneum (Fig. 1.17).

The stratum basale is a single layer of cells adjacent to the dermis; it is in this layer, as well as the stratum spinosum, that new cells are produced, replacing those lost from the surface. The stratum spinosum consists of several layers of irregularly shaped cells, which become flattened as they approach the stratum granulosum. The stratum basale and stratum spinosum are together referred to as the germinal zone because of their role in new cell production.

Collectively, the remaining epidermal layers (granulosum, lucidum and corneum) are referred to as the horny layer. In the stratum granulosum, the cells become increasingly flattened and keratinisation begins: the cells are in the process of dying. A relatively thin transparent layer (stratum lucidum) lies between the granulosum and superficial stratum corneum. It is from the stratum corneum that the cells are shed; it is also mainly responsible for the thickness of the skin.

Epidermal melanocytes responsible for skin pigmentation lie within the deepest layers of the epidermis.

Dermis

The deeper interlacing feltwork of collagen and elastic fibres generally comprising the greater part of total skin thickness. It can be divided into a superficial finely textured papillary layer, which, although clearly separated from it, interdigitates with the epidermis, and a deeper coarser reticular layer, which gradually blends into the underlying subcutaneous connective tissue.

Projecting dermal papillae usually contain capillary networks, bringing blood into close association with the epidermis (Fig. 1.18). The ability to open up or close down these networks regulates heat loss through the skin, as well as causing individuals to blush in moments of embarrassment. Some papillae contain tactile receptors, which are more numerous in regions of high tactile sensitivity (fingers, lips) and less so in other regions (back).

The reticular layer of dermis is a dense mass of interweaving collagen and elastic connective tissue fibres; it gives the skin its toughness and strength. The fibres run in all directions but are generally tangential to the surface. There is, however, a predominant orientation of fibre bundles with respect to the skin surface, which varies in different regions of the body: it is this orientation which gives rise to the cleavage lines (Fig. 1.16).

The dermis contains numerous blood vessels and lymphatic channels, nerves and sensory nerve endings as well as a small amount of fat: it also contains hair follicles, sweat and sebaceous glands, and smooth muscle (arrector pili). The deep surface of the dermis is invaginated by projections of subcutaneous connective tissue serving partly for the entrance of nerves and blood vessels into the skin (Fig. 1.18).

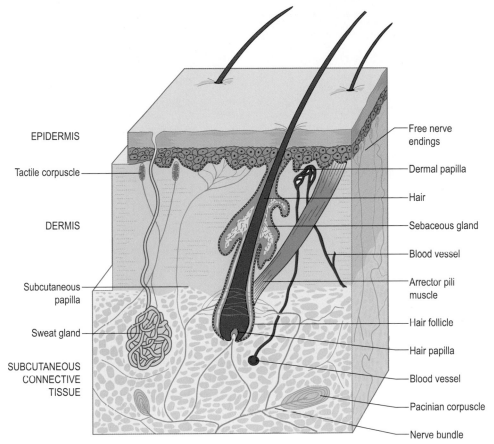

EPIDERMIS

Tactile corpuscle

DERMIS

Subcutaneous papilla

Sweat gland

SUBCUTANEOUS CONNECTIVE TISSUE

Free nerve endings

Dermal papilla

Hair

Sebaceous gland

Blood vessel

Arrector pili muscle

Hair follicle

Hair papilla

Blood vessel

Pacinian corpuscle

Nerve bundle

Fig. 1.18 Skin and the subcutaneous connective tissue layer showing the arrangement of hair and its component parts, glands and blood vessels.

Subcutaneous Connective Tissue

Layer of loosely arranged connective tissue containing fat and some elastic fibres. The amount of subcutaneous fat varies in different parts of the body, being completely absent in only a few regions (eyelid, scrotum, penis, nipple and areola). The distribution of subcutaneous fat differs between men and women, being a secondary sexual characteristic in women (breast, rounded contour of the hips). The subcutaneous connective tissue contains blood and lymph vessels, roots of hair follicles, secretory parts of sweat glands, cutaneous nerves and sensory endings (particularly Pacinian (pressure) corpuscles) (Figs 1.18 and 1.19).

In the subcutaneous tissue overlying joints, subcutaneous bursae exist, containing small amounts of fluid to facilitate skin movement in these regions.

Cutaneous Sensory Receptors

The nerve endings in skin vary from simple to complex. Simple nerve endings are those in which the axon terminates without branching or other elaboration. Complex endings are those in which the axons undergo a variety of changes, such as forming expansions, assuming a tangled appearance or becoming surrounded by additional specialised tissue. When an axon terminates by losing its myelin sheath to end as a naked axon, it is a free nerve ending.

The types of nerve endings found in skin are shown in Fig. 1.19. Simple free nerve endings occur within the epidermis and dermis. In the epidermis, they run as naked axons between the epidermal cells and may undergo branching; they are generally oriented perpendicular to the skin surface. In contrast, free nerve endings in the dermis run parallel to the skin surface. Free

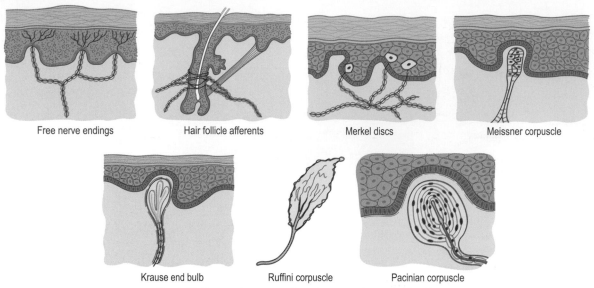

Free nerve endings   Hair follicle afferents   Merkel discs   Meissner corpuscle

Krause end bulb   Ruffini corpuscle   Pacinian corpuscle

Fig. 1.19 Types of nerve endings (receptors) present in skin.

nerve endings are thought to detect stimuli generating the sensations of pain and temperature, but many are also capable of responding to mechanical stimuli (touch, pressure) which deform the skin. Free nerve endings are also found surrounding the roots of hairs; these are stimulated by deformation of the hair and are involved in detecting coarse stimuli, causing the hairs on the skin to bend.

Merkel discs are complex endings formed when a free nerve ending terminates as a disc-like expansion under a specialised cell in the epidermis (Merkel (tactile) cell). They are found in hairless skin, particularly in the fingertips, and are thought to mediate the sensation of touch. Meissner corpuscles are complex encapsulated receptors formed by a spiralling axon surrounded by flattened Schwann cells, which in turn are surrounded by fibrous tissue continuous with the endoneurium of the axon. Meissner corpuscles are thought to be involved in the sensation of touch. Krause's end bulbs consist of an axon that forms a cluster of multiple short branches surrounded by a fibrous capsule; simpler varieties occur in which the axon does not undergo branching, forming only a bulbous ending surrounded by a poorly developed capsule. The function of these nerve endings is unclear, but they occur in the dermis and are thought to respond to the mechanical stimulation of skin.

Ruffini corpuscles consist of an axon that forms a flattened tangle of branches embedded in a bundle of collagen fibres; they occur in the dermis and respond to stretching of the collagen fibres when the skin is deformed by pressure. Pacinian corpuscles are the most complex of sensory nerve endings consisting of a single axon surrounded by several concentric laminae of modified Schwann cells all enclosed in a fibrous capsule; they are located in the dermis and are designed to respond to pressure stimuli.

Wound Repair

Lacerations of the skin are repaired by either primary or secondary union. Following surgical incisions, in which the wound is clean, uninfected and has its edges approximated by sutures, primary union occurs; however, in traumatic wounds with separated edges and more extensive cell and tissue loss, secondary union occurs. In both cases, repair involves the generation of large amounts of granulation tissue (specialised tissue formed during the repair process).

Repair of an incision or laceration to the skin involves stimulated growth of both the dermis and epidermis (Fig. 1.20). Dermal repair involves (i) formation of a blood clot; (ii) removal of damaged collagen fibres, mainly through macrophage activity associated with inflammation; (iii) the formation of granulation tissue; (iv) re-epithelialisation of the exposed surface; (v) proliferation and migration of fibroblasts and differentiation of myofibroblasts involved in wound contraction;

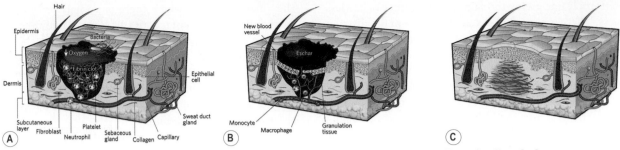

Fig. 1.20 Stages in wound repair: (a) inflammation; (b) proliferation; (c) remodeling. (From Geoffrey C. Gurtner et al., Wound repair and regeneration, Nature volume 453, pages 314–321 (2008).

and (vi) deposition and remodelling of the extracellular matrix of the underlying connective tissue. The use of sutures in primary union reduces the repair area through maximal closure of the wound, minimising scar formation. Epidermal repair involves proliferation of the basal cell layer in the surrounding undamaged site, with the wound site quickly being covered by a scab (dehydrated blood clot). The proliferating basal cells migrate (~0.5 mm/day) under the scab and across the wound surface; proliferation and differentiation occur behind the migration front restoring the multi-layered epidermis. As cells move towards the surface the overlying scab is freed, becoming detached from the periphery inwards. In full-thickness wounds of the epidermis, parts of hair follicles and the follicular bulge containing epidermal stem cells produce cells that migrate over the exposed surface to re-establish a complete epidermal layer.

If all epithelial structures of the skin have been destroyed, as in third-degree burns and extensive full-thickness abrasions, re-epithelialisation is prevented; in such cases, the wound can only be healed by skin (epidermal) grafting to cover the wounded area. Without a graft, the wound would re-epithelialise slowly and imperfectly due to ingrowth of cells from the margins of the wound.

APPENDAGES OF THE SKIN

These are nails, hairs, and sebaceous, sweat and mammary glands. All are derived from the epidermis.

Nails

An approximately rectangular plate of horny tissue on the dorsum of the terminal phalanx of the fingers, thumb and toes (Fig. 1.21). They are a special modification of

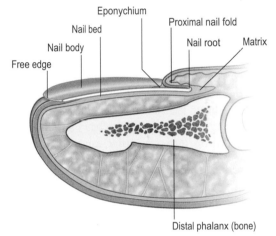

Fig. 1.21 Relationship of nails to the skin.

the two most superficial layers of the epidermis, particularly the stratum lucidum. Its transparency allows the pinkness of the underlying highly vascular nail bed to show through. The nail is partly surrounded by a fold of skin (nail wall) firmly adherent to the underlying nail bed with some fibres ending in the periosteum of the distal phalanx. It is this firm attachment which enables the nails to be used for scratching and as instruments for prying open various objects.

The proximal covered part (nail root) has an abundant supply of sensory nerve endings and blood vessels; the distal end of the nail is free. Nails grow at approximately 1 mm per week, being faster in summer than in winter.

Hairs

These are widely distributed over the body surface, notable exceptions being the palm of the hand and sole of the foot. Hairs vary in thickness and length; most are extremely fine giving the skin the appearance of hairless-ness. There is a marked sexual difference in the distribution of coarse hair, particularly on the face and trunk, and in its loss from the scalp. This coarse hair tends to become more prominent after puberty, particularly in the axilla, over the pubes and on the face in males.

Except for the eyelashes, all hairs emerge obliquely from the skin surface with the hairs in any one region doing so in the same direction. The part projecting from the skin surface is the shaft, which appears circular in cross-section; that part under the skin is the root, ensheathed in a sleeve of epidermis. The follicle extends into the subcutaneous tissue (Fig. 1.18). Throughout most of its length, hair consists of the keratinised remains of cells. Hair colour is due to melanin and a subtle red pigment in the hair cells, as well as air in the shaft. The hair of the head has a life span of between 2 and 4 years, while that of the eyelashes is only 3–5 months; all hairs are intermittently shed and replaced.

In growing hair, the deepest part of the follicle expands, forming a cap (bulb of the hair) almost completely surrounding loose vascular connective tissue (papilla). The follicle cells around the papilla proliferate forming the various layers of hair. In resting hair, follicles around the bulb and papilla shrink; the deepest part of the follicle is irregular in shape.

Associated with each hair are one or more sebaceous glands in the angle between the slanting hair follicle and skin surface, with their ducts opening into the neck of the follicle. Bundles of smooth muscle fibres (arrector pili) attach to the hair follicle sheath, deep to the sebaceous gland, passing to the papillary layers of dermis on the side towards which the hair slopes (Fig. 1.18). Contraction of the muscle fibres causes the hair to stand away from the skin, elevating it around the opening of the hair follicles, producing 'goose flesh'; this action also compresses the sebaceous glands causing them to empty their secretions onto the skin surface. The elevation of hairs traps a layer of air against the skin surface in an attempt to produce an insulating layer to reduce heat loss: the sebaceous secretions are important in 'water-proofing' the skin surface and aiding the absorption of fat-soluble substances through the skin.

Glands
Sebaceous Glands
These are associated with all hairs and hair follicles; between one and four are associated with each hair.

They may also exist where there is no hair (corner of the mouth and adjacent mucosa, lips, areola and nipple), opening directly onto the skin surface; they are absent from the skin of the palm, sole and dorsum of the distal segments of the digits. The glands vary in size between 0.2 and 2.0 mm in diameter. The gland cells are continuously destroyed (holocrine secretion) in the production of the oily secretions (sebum).

Inflammation and accumulation of secretion within the sebaceous glands give rise to acne. If plugging of the outlet is permanent, a sebaceous cyst may form in the duct and follicles, which may become so enlarged to require surgical removal. Sebaceous glands do not appear to be under nervous control.

Sweat Glands
These have a wide distribution throughout the body (Fig. 1.22), being more numerous on exposed parts, especially on the palms, soles and flexor surfaces of the digits; the ducts open onto the summits of the epidermal ridges. Each gland has a long tube extending into the

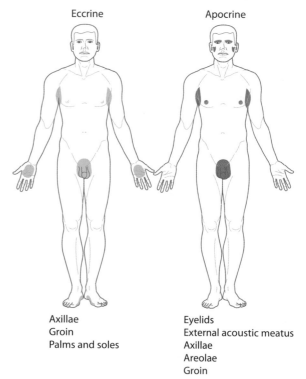

Eccrine	Apocrine
Axillae	Eyelids
Groin	External acoustic meatus
Palms and soles	Axillae
	Areolae
	Groin

Fig. 1.22 Distribution of eccrine and apocrine sweat glands in the body.

subcutaneous tissue where it coils, forming the secretory body of the gland (Fig. 1.18). The glands produce sweat, a clear fluid without any cellular elements, for secretion (eccrine secretion). The production of sweat is important in temperature regulation as its evaporation from the skin surface promotes heat loss. Eccrine sweat glands are innervated by sympathetic nerves; consequently, any disturbance in the sympathetic nervous system results in a dry warm skin (anhydrosis) either locally or extensively.

In the axilla, groin and around the anus are large, modified sweat glands between 3 and 5 mm in diameter lying deep in the subcutaneous layer. Their ducts may be associated with a hair follicle or they may open directly onto the skin surface; the secretions include some disintegration products of the gland cells (apocrine secretion). The odour associated with these glands is not from the secretion itself, but due to bacterial invasion and contamination from the skin. Pigment granules associated with axillary glands produce a slight colouration of the secretion. Apocrine glands vary with sexual development, enlarging at puberty; in females, they show cyclical changes associated with the menstrual cycle.

The glands opening at the margins of the eyelid (ciliary glands) are modified uncoiled sweat glands as are the glands of the external auditory meatus (ceruminous glands); ceruminous glands cells contain a yellowish pigment colouring the wax secretion (cerumen).

Mammary Gland (Breast)

Modified sweat glands, the mammary glands are an accessory to reproductive function in females, secreting milk (lactation) for the nourishment of the infant. In children prior to puberty and in adult males, the glands are rudimentary and functionless.

BLOOD SUPPLY AND LYMPHATIC DRAINAGE

The arterial supply to the skin is derived from vessels in the subcutaneous connective tissue, which form a network at the boundary between the dermis and subcutaneous tissue (Fig. 1.18). Branches from the network supply the fat, sweat glands and deep parts of hair follicles; branches within the dermis form a subpapillary plexus. Abundant arteriovenous anastomoses occur within the skin; the epidermis is avascular. Lymphatics of the skin begin in the dermal papillae as networks or blind outgrowths forming a dense mesh of lymphatic capillaries in the papillary layer. Larger lymphatic vessels pass deeply to the boundary between the dermis and subcutaneous tissue to accompany the arteries as they pass centrally.

INNERVATION

There are two types of nerves in skin: afferent somatic fibres mediating pain, touch, pressure, heat and cold (general sensations) and efferent autonomic (sympathetic) fibres supplying blood vessels, arrector pili and sweat glands. The sensory (afferent) endings have several forms. Free nerve endings extend between cells of the basal layer of the epidermis, terminating around and adjacent to hair follicles: they are receptive to general tactile sensation as well as painful stimuli. Enclosed tactile corpuscles sensitive to touch lie in the dermal papillae. Pacinian corpuscles (Figs 1.18 and 1.19) exist in the subcutaneous tissue, being particularly plentiful along the sides of the digits, acting as pressure receptors. Specific endings for heat and cold have been described, although general agreement on their identity has not been reached. Details of all of these receptors are given on page 23.

APPLICATION

The majority of physiotherapy techniques are applied either directly or indirectly via the individual's skin. Manual manipulations (massage, thermal treatments) have an effect on the skin. The skin provides an extremely important barrier restricting the penetration of damaging electromagnetic radiations in the ultraviolet spectrum. All but the very longest ultraviolet wavelengths are absorbed by the skin. If sufficiently high levels of ultraviolet light have been absorbed, the characteristic effects of erythema (thickening of the epidermis, increased pigmentation, peeling) will all occur.

The general dryness and natural greasiness of the skin surface give it a high electrical resistance: if electrical currents are to be applied directly to body tissues, this resistance must be reduced. This is usually successfully achieved by cleaning the skin and applying moist pads or conducting gels below the site of electrode attachment.

❓ SELF-ASSESSMENT QUESTIONS

31. Which layer of skin is the most superficial?
32. In which layers of the epidermis are new cells produced?
33. What are cleavage lines and what is their importance?
34. Where would you tend to find apocrine glands?
35. What type of glands are sweat glands?
36. In which layer of the skin are Pacinian corpuscles situated?
37. What determines the colour of hair?
38. On which part of the digit are nails found?
39. What sensation(s) do Ruffini corpuscles convey?
40. What needs to be done to the skin if electrical currents are to be applied to it?

COMPONENTS OF THE MUSCULOSKELETAL SYSTEM

An account of the major tissues of the musculoskeletal system (muscular, connective, skeletal) and of the types of joints enabling varying degrees of movement to occur is given as it will enhance understanding of the mobility and inherent stability of various segments. The initiation and coordination of movement is the responsibility of the nervous system.

LEARNING OUTCOMES

By the end of the section, you should be able to:
1. Describe the structure and arrangement of skeletal muscle
2. Demonstrate the action of skeletal muscle when it contracts
3. Describe the innervation of muscle, including muscle spindles and Golgi tendon organs
4. Describe the different types of fibrous tissue and where each is found
5. Describe the different types of skeletal tissue and their function
6. Describe the processes of bone growth and remodelling
7. Describe the structural organisation of bone tissue
8. Demonstrate and locate the diaphysis and epiphyses of a long bone
9. Understand different types of bone fracture and how they occur
10. Understand the process of fracture repair
11. Describe the different types of fibrous, cartilaginous and synovial joints and their function
12. Appreciate the type of movement that occurs between articulating surfaces
13. Understand the principle of levers

MUSCULAR TISSUE

There are three varieties of muscle within the human body: (i) smooth (involuntary, non-striated) muscle, (ii) cardiac muscle and (iii) skeletal (voluntary, striated) muscle. Smooth muscle forms the muscular layer in the walls of blood vessels and hollow organs such as the stomach. It is not under voluntary control, contracting more slowly and less powerfully than skeletal muscle; however, it is able to maintain its contraction longer. Cardiac muscle is also not under voluntary control; although it exhibits striations, it is considered to be different from skeletal muscle.

Smooth Muscle

Smooth muscle is specialised for slow, steady contraction controlled by involuntary mechanisms. Individual fibres are elongated and tapering (Fig. 1.23A), with the cells organised with the broadest part of one cell adjacent to the narrowest part of another. They are arranged

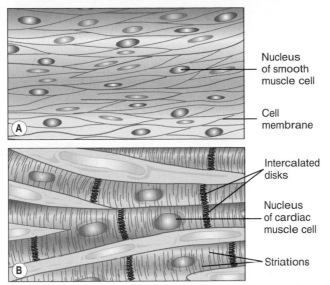

Fig. 1.23 Smooth (A) and cardiac (B) muscle. (From Medical Assistant: Introduction to Medical Assisting— MAIntro, Second Edition (2015). Elsevier.

in sheets or bundles containing many fibres, innervated by a single nerve.

It is regulated differently in the viscera, respiratory airways, and large and small blood vessels, involving the autonomic system (p. 575) and hormones, as well as local physiologic conditions (degree of stretch). Smooth muscle is most often spontaneously active without nervous stimulation; consequently, its innervation mainly modifies rather than initiates activity.

Cardiac Muscle

The cells are aligned in chainlike arrays forming complex junctions between interdigitating processes; cells within a fibre branch and bind to cells in adjacent fibres forming a syncytium (Fig. 1.23B). The heart, therefore, consists of interwoven bundles of cells showing a cross-striated banding pattern, enabling a characteristic wave of contraction to be propagated. Each cardiac muscle cell is surrounded by endomysium containing a rich capillary network. Cardiac muscle fibre contraction is intrinsic and spontaneous, with impulses for rhythmic contractions (heartbeat) being initiated, regulated and coordinated locally by nodes of unique myocardial fibres. The rate of contraction is modified by autonomic innervation of the conducting cells, with sympathetic activity increasing and parasympathetic activity decreasing the frequency of the impulses.

Skeletal Muscle

This comprises more than one-third of the total body mass; it consists of non-branching striated muscle fibres bound together by loose areolar tissue. Muscles have various forms: some are flat and sheet-like, some short and thick, and others long and slender. The length of a muscle, excluding its tendon(s), is closely related to the distance through which it needs to contract: muscle fibres have the ability to shorten to almost half their resting length. The arrangement of fibres within a muscle, therefore, determines how much it can shorten when it contracts. Irrespective of muscle fibre arrangement, all movement is brought about by muscle contraction (shortening) with the action across joints changing the relative positions of the bones involved.

Muscle Forms

The arrangement of the individual fibres within a muscle can be in one of two ways only: either parallel or oblique to the line of pull of the muscle as a whole. Fibres parallel to the line of pull are arranged as discrete bundles forming a fusiform muscle (biceps brachii) (Fig. 1.24A) or spread out as a broad thin sheet (external oblique of the abdomen) (Fig. 1.24B). When contraction occurs, it does so through the maximum distance allowed by the length of the muscle fibres; however, the muscle has limited power.

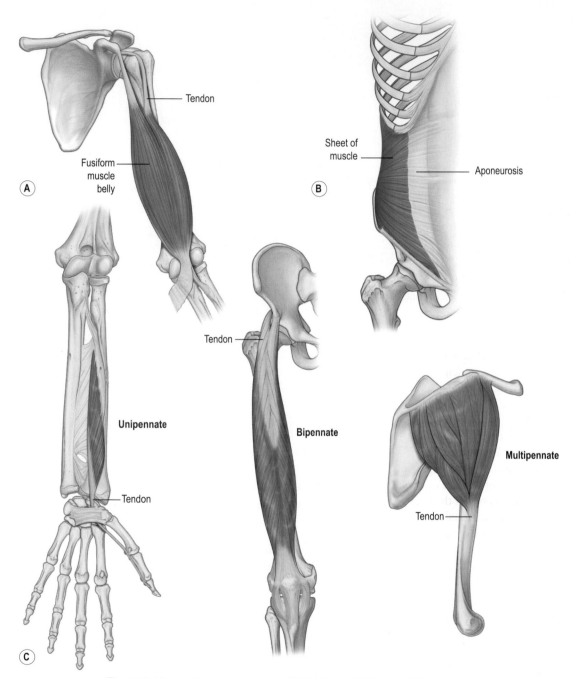

Fig. 1.24 Muscle fibre arrangements. (A) Fusiform. (B) Sheet. (C) Pennate.

Muscles with fibres oblique to the line of pull cannot shorten to the same extent, but because of the increased number of fibres in the same unit area, they are much more powerful. These pennate arrangements have three main patterns (Fig. 1.24C): in unipennate muscles, the fibres attach to one side of the tendon only (flexor pollicis longus); bipennate muscles have a central septum with muscle fibres attaching to both sides and to its continuous central tendon (rectus femoris); multipennate muscles possess several intermediate septa, each associated with a bipennate arrangement of fibres (deltoid).

Muscle Structure

Muscle consists of many individual fibres, each of which is a long, cylindrical, multinucleated cell of varying length and width. Each fibre has a delicate connective tissue covering (endomysium) separating it from its neighbour but connecting them together. Bundles of parallel fibres (fasciculi) are bound together by a denser connective tissue covering (perimysium). Groups of fasciculi are bound together forming whole muscles (Fig. 1.25) enclosed in a fibrous covering (epimysium), which may be thick and strong or thin and relatively weak.

Muscle Attachments

The attachment of muscle to bone or other tissue is always via its connective tissue elements; sometimes the perimysium and epimysium unite directly with the periosteum of bone or the joint capsule. Where the connective tissue element cannot readily be seen, the muscle has a fleshy attachment and leaves no mark on the bone, although the area is often flattened or depressed. In many cases, the connective tissue elements of the muscle fuse forming a tendon consisting of bundles of collagen fibres; there is no direct continuity between the muscle fibres and those of the tendon. Tendons can take various forms, all of which are generally strong: they can be round cords, flattened bands or thin sheets (aponeuroses). Attachments of tendon to bone nearly always leave a smooth mark; it is only when the attachment is by both fleshy and tendinous fibres, or when the attachment is via a long aponeurosis, that the bone surface is roughened.

Where a muscle or tendon passes over or around the edge of bone, it is usually separated from it by a bursa serving to reduce friction during movement. Bursae are saclike dilations which may communicate directly with an adjacent joint cavity or exist independently; they contain a fluid similar to synovial fluid.

When a tendon is subjected to friction, it may develop a sesamoid bone within it. Once formed, these have the effect of increasing the lever arm of the muscle, acting as a pulley, enabling a slight change in the direction of muscle pull (the patella and quadriceps tendon) (Fig. 1.26).

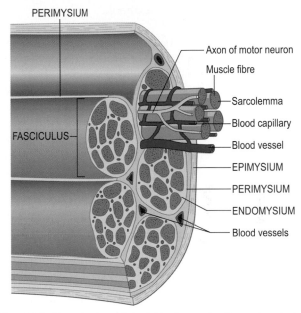

Fig. 1.25 Organisation of individual muscle fibres in whole muscles, together with their investing connective tissue layers.

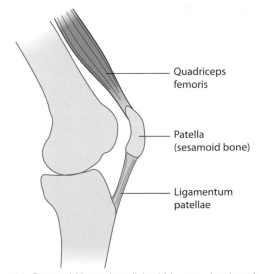

Fig. 1.26 Sesamoid bone (patella) within a tendon (quadriceps femoris).

Because each end of a muscle attaches to different bones, observing its principal action led to the designation of one end being the origin and the other the insertion; the insertion being to the bone showing the freest movement. Such a designation can be misleading as muscle contraction can cause either of the two attachments to move relatively freely. The term attachment is preferred and used in this textbook.

Muscle Action

When stimulated, muscle contracts bringing its two ends closer together. If this is allowed to happen, the length of the muscle changes, although the tension generated remains more or less constant (isotonic contraction). If the length of the muscle remains unaltered (isometric contraction) due to an externally applied force, the tension that develops usually increases in an attempt to overcome the resistance.

Isotonic contraction can be of two types: concentric, where the muscle shortens, or eccentric, where the muscle lengthens. Eccentric contraction occurs when the muscle is controlling the movement of a body segment against an applied force.

When a muscle or group of muscles contracts to produce a specific movement, it is a prime mover: muscles directly opposing this action are antagonists, while muscles preventing unwanted movements associated with the prime mover are synergists.

In all actions, part of the muscle activity (usually the larger part) is directed across the joint, stabilising it by pulling the two articular surfaces together (Fig. 1.27).

When testing muscle action to determine whether it is weakened or paralysed, the individual is usually asked to perform the principal action of the muscle against resistance; this may be insufficient to confirm muscle integrity. The only infallible guide is to palpate the muscle belly or its tendon(s) to determine whether it is contracting during the manoeuvre.

Sensory Receptors in Muscle

Muscles contain free nerve endings and two types of specialised receptors: Golgi tendon organs and muscle spindles. Free nerve endings are responsible for mediating pain; they are sparsely scattered throughout the muscle belly but more densely at the myotendinous junction.

Golgi tendon organs are formed by multiple terminal branches of an axon (nerve fibre) weaving between the

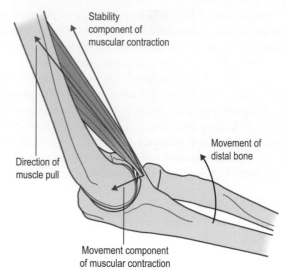

Fig. 1.27 Components of muscle contraction acting across a joint.

collagen fibres of the tendon with the region around the branches surrounded by a fibrous capsule (Fig. 1.28A). When a muscle contracts, the collagen fibres in the tendon stretch, bringing them closer together, compressing the nerve terminals and triggering the stimulus. In this way, Golgi tendon organs monitor the extent of muscle contraction, as well as the force exerted by the muscle.

Muscle spindles are highly elaborate structures essentially consisting of two types of modified muscle fibres (Fig. 1.28B); they are surrounded by a fibrous capsule and occur throughout the muscle belly.

The muscle fibres within a spindle monitor changes in muscle length. Because of this difference in function and because they are located within the fusiform capsule of the spindle, they are intrafusal muscle fibres. Muscle fibres producing movement on muscle contraction are the extrafusal fibres.

There are two types of intrafusal muscle fibres: nuclear bag fibres have their nuclei grouped into an expanded region in the middle of the fibre, and nuclear chain fibres have their nuclei spread along its length. At their middle, both nuclear bag and nuclear chain fibres are surrounded in a spiral fashion by branches of a group Ia sensory neuron. Group II neurons form similar spiral endings around nuclear chain fibres, but form spray-like endings on nuclear bag fibres (Fig. 1.28B).

As a muscle lengthens or shortens, the degree of stretching or relaxation of the intrafusal muscle fibres

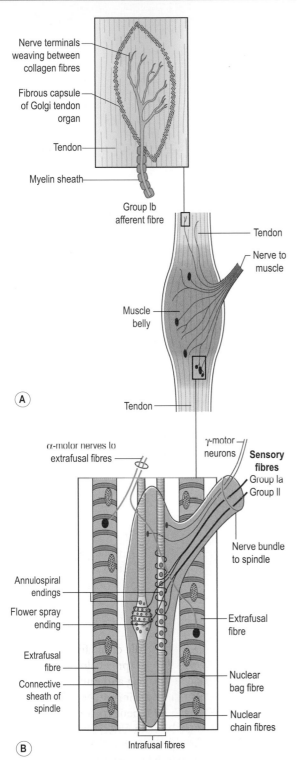

Nerve terminals weaving between collagen fibres

Fibrous capsule of Golgi tendon organ

Tendon

Myelin sheath

Group Ib afferent fibre

Tendon

Nerve to muscle

Muscle belly

Tendon

(A)

α-motor nerves to extrafusal fibres

γ-motor neurons

Sensory fibres
Group Ia
Group II

Nerve bundle to spindle

Annulospiral endings

Flower spray ending

Extrafusal fibre

Extrafusal fibre

Connective sheath of spindle

Nuclear bag fibre

Nuclear chain fibres

Intrafusal fibres

(B)

Fig. 1.28 Location and microscopic appearance of Golgi organs (A) and muscle spindles (B) within a muscle and its tendon.

alters activity in the Ia and II fibres innervating them. This activity is relayed to the CNS where the length of the muscle and its rate of lengthening or shortening are interpreted; indirectly, and in combination with other receptors, joint position is also determined. Various subgroups of nuclear bag and nuclear chain fibres have been identified with each responsible for detecting a different component of the change in muscle length or its rate of occurrence.

Muscle spindles also receive a motor innervation from γ-motor neurons. Terminals of γ-motor neurons end on intrafusal fibres either side of the central regions surrounded by the sensory neurons. Activity in the γ-motor neurons causes the peripheral ends of the intrafusal fibres to contract, stretching the central sensory region. This stretch alters the sensitivity or setting of the central region, allowing the sensory function of the spindle to remain in phase with the overall lengthening or shortening of the muscle as a whole as it relaxes or contracts.

Without γ activity, muscle spindles would respond to muscle stretch only when they were fully extended. Shortening the muscle would relieve the stretch with the muscle spindle with a cessation in signalling muscle length. By contracting, under the control of γ-motor neurons, intrafusal fibres keep the central sensory region of the spindle taut at all times, allowing it to monitor muscle length throughout the total range of movement.

Motor Nerve Endings

α-Motor neurons form endings designed to deliver stimuli to extrafusal muscle fibres; similar but smaller endings are formed by γ-motor neurons on intrafusal fibres. The junction (motor end plate, neuromuscular junction) between a motor neuron and muscle cell involves elaboration of the neuron, muscle cell and certain surrounding tissues (Fig. 1.29).

Structurally and functionally, neuromuscular junctions resemble synapses (Fig. 1.13B). As a motor axon approaches its target muscle cell, it loses its myelin sheath, forming a flattened expansion applied to the surface of the muscle membrane. The expansion is covered by a Schwann cell sheath insulating the neuromuscular junction from the external environment. The portion of the muscle cell to which the nerve is apposed is modified, creating a flattened bump on its surface, formed by the focal accumulation of cytoplasm (sarcoplasm) and organelles within the muscle cell, raising its membrane

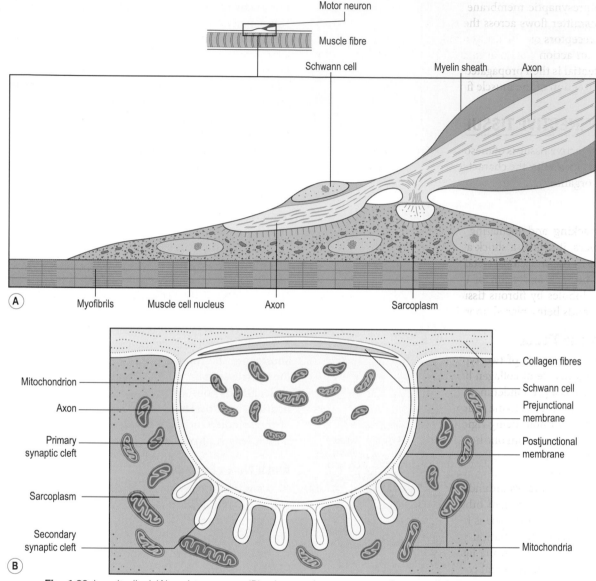

Fig. 1.29 Longitudinal (A) and transverse (B) microscopic appearance of motor end plates (neuromuscular junctions).

below the nerve terminal. That part of the muscle cell membrane applied to the nerve cell is the postjunctional membrane, with that part of the nerve cell membrane applied to the muscle cell being the prejunctional membrane (Fig. 1.29).

The postjunctional membrane forms troughs, in which are reciprocal folds of the prejunctional membrane. Within the troughs, the membranes of the nerve and muscle cells are separated by a synaptic cleft measuring 20–50 nm filled with an amorphous ground substance. In the floor of the trough, the postjunctional membrane is thrown into further folds (secondary synaptic clefts), increasing the surface area of the receptive muscle membrane (Fig. 1.29).

The terminal expansion of the motor neuron contains vesicles filled with the transmitter substance acetylcholine. When an action potential arrives at the nerve terminal, the vesicles release the acetylcholine through the presynaptic membrane into the synaptic cleft. The transmitter flows across the cleft to react with molecular receptors on the postjunctional membrane generating an action potential in the muscle membrane. This potential is then propagated into the muscle cell causing contraction of the muscle fibres.

CONNECTIVE TISSUE

Connective tissue is of mesodermal origin and has many forms in adults: the character of the tissue depending on the organisation of its constituent cells and fibres.

Fat

A packing and insulating material: in some circumstances, it acts as a shock absorber, an important function in the musculoskeletal system. Under the heel, in the buttock and palm of the hand, the fat is divided into lobules by fibrous tissue septa stiffening it for the demands being placed upon it.

Fibrous Tissue

Fibrous tissue is of two types: white fibrous tissue has an abundance of collagen bundles, while yellow fibrous tissue has a preponderance of elastic fibres.

White fibrous tissue is dense, providing considerable strength without being rigid or elastic. It forms (i) ligaments passing from one bone to another in the region of joints, uniting the bones and limiting joint movement; (ii) tendons for attaching muscles to bones; and (iii) protective membranes around muscle (perimysium), bone (periosteum) and many other structures.

Yellow fibrous tissue is highly specialised, capable of considerable deformation yet returning to its original shape. It is found in the ligamenta flava (p. 511) associated with the vertebral column, as well as in the walls of arteries.

SKELETAL TISSUE

Skeletal tissues are modified connective tissues in which the cells and fibres have a particular condensed organisation giving the tissue rigidity.

Cartilage

Supplementary to bone cartilage is formed wherever strength, rigidity and some elasticity are required. In foetal development, cartilage is often a temporary tissue later being replaced by bone; however, in many places cartilage persists throughout life. Although a rigid tissue, it is not as hard or strong as bone; it is also relatively avascular, being nourished by surrounding tissue fluids. A vascular invasion of cartilage results in death of the cells during the process of ossification of the cartilage and its eventual replacement by bone. Except for the articular cartilage of synovial joints, cartilage possesses a fibrous covering layer (perichondrium).

There are three main types of cartilage: hyaline cartilage, white fibrocartilage, yellow fibrocartilage.

Hyaline Cartilage

This forms the temporary skeleton of the foetus from which many bones develop; its remnants can be seen as the articular cartilages of synovial joints, epiphyseal growth plates between parts of an ossifying bone during growth, and the costal cartilages associated with the ribs. At joint surfaces, it provides a limited degree of elasticity offsetting and absorbing shocks, as well as providing a relatively smooth surface permitting free movement. With increasing age, hyaline cartilage tends to become calcified and occasionally ossified.

White Fibrocartilage

Containing bundles of white fibrous tissue, giving it great tensile strength combined with some elasticity, enables white fibrocartilage to resist considerable pressure. It is found at many sites within the musculoskeletal system: (i) within intervertebral discs between adjacent vertebrae; (ii) in the menisci of the knee joint; (iii) in the labrum surrounding and deepening the glenoid fossa of the shoulder joint and acetabulum of the hip joint; (iv) in articular discs of the radiocarpal (wrist), sternoclavicular, acromioclavicular and temporomandibular joints; and (v) as articular coverings of bones ossifying in membrane (clavicle, mandible). White fibrocartilage may calcify and ossify.

Yellow Fibrocartilage

Containing bundles of elastic fibres with little or no white fibrous tissue, yellow fibrocartilage neither calcifies or ossifies and is not found within the musculoskeletal system.

Bone

Extremely hard with a certain amount of resilience, it is essentially an organic matrix of fibrous connective tissue impregnated with mineral salts. The connective tissue gives bone its toughness and elasticity, while the mineral salts provide hardness and rigidity; the two are skilfully blended together. The mineral component provides a ready store of calcium, which is continuously exchanged with that in body fluids: the rate of exchange and overall balance of these mineral ions is influenced by several factors, including hormones.

Each bone is enclosed in a dense layer of fibrous tissue (periosteum) with its form and structure adapted to the functions of support and the resistance of mechanical stresses. As a living tissue, bone continually remodels to meet these demands; this is particularly evident during growth. The structure of a bone cannot be satisfactorily considered in isolation; it is dependent upon its relationship to adjacent bones and the type of articulation between them, as well as the attachment of muscles, tendons and ligaments.

Its internal architecture reveals a system of struts and plates (trabeculae) running in many directions (Fig. 1.30) and organised to resist compressive, tensile and shearing stresses. Surrounding the trabecular systems, which tend to be found at the extremities of long bones, is a thin layer of condensed or compact bone (Fig. 1.30). Because of its appearance, the network of the trabeculae is known as cancellous or spongy bone. The shaft of a long bone has an outer relatively thick ring of compact bone surrounding a cavity containing bone marrow.

Red and white blood cells are formed in red bone marrow, which after birth is the only source of red blood cells and the main source of white blood cells. In infants, the cavities of all bones contain red marrow; this gradually becomes replaced by yellow fat marrow so that, at puberty, red marrow is only found in cavities associated with cancellous bone. With increasing age, many of these red marrow-containing regions are replaced by yellow marrow; nevertheless, red marrow tends to persist throughout life in the vertebrae, ribs, sternum and proximal ends of the femur and humerus.

For descriptive purposes, bones are classified according to their shape:

1. Long bones are found within the limbs; each consists of a shaft (diaphysis) and two expanded ends (epiphyses).
2. Short bones are those of the wrist (carpus) and part of the foot (tarsus).
3. Flat bones are thin and tend to be curved in spite of their classification; they include the bones of the skull

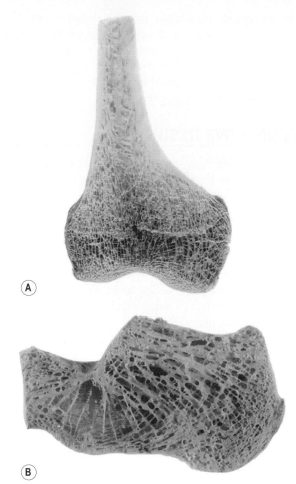

(A)

(B)

Fig. 1.30 Trabecular organisation within bone. (A) Coronal section through the distal end of the femur. (B) Sagittal section through the calcaneus.

vault and ribs. Structurally, they consist of two layers of compact bone enclosing cancellous bone (diploe).
4. Irregular bones are those fitting none of the previous categories; they include the vertebrae and many bones of the skull and face.

Both irregular and short bones consist of a thin layer of compact bone surrounding cancellous bone.

Development

Bone develops either directly in the mesoderm by the deposition of mineral salts (intramembranous ossification) or in a previously formed cartilage model (endochondral ossification). Intramembranous ossification is the process of calcification and then ossification without an intervening cartilage model, the resulting bone is

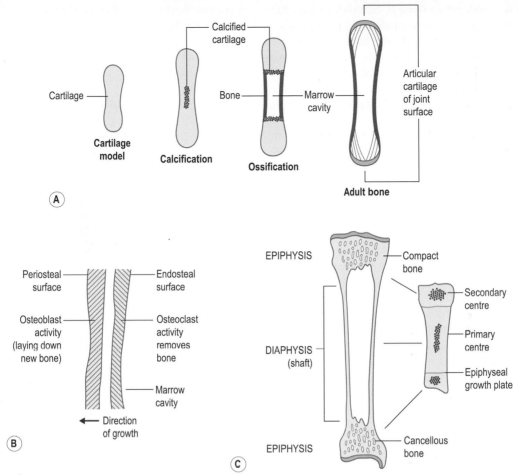

Fig. 1.31 (A) Stages in the calcification and ossification of bone from a cartilage model. (B) Osteoblast and osteoclast activity. (C) Sites of ossification centres in long bones and the parts which develop from each.

referred to as membrane bone. Where there is an intervening cartilage model, the resulting bone is referred to as cartilage bone. The latter process is the most common.

Intramembranous ossification. The site of bone formation is initially indicated by a condensation of cells and collagen fibres accompanied by the laying down of organic bone matrix, which becomes impregnated with mineral salts. The formation of new bone continues in a manner similar to bone developed in cartilage. Intramembranous ossification occurs in certain bones of the skull, the mandible and clavicle.

Endochondral ossification. The first step in the process is the accumulation of mesodermal cells in the region where the bone is to develop. A cartilage model of the future bone develops from these mesodermal cells (Fig. 1.31A). In long bones, the cartilage model grows principally at its ends so that the oldest part is near the middle. As time progresses, the cartilage matrix in the older region is impregnated with mineral salts so that it becomes calcified; the cartilage cells are cut off from their nutrient supply and die. The greater part of the calcified cartilage is subsequently removed, and bone is formed around its few remaining spicules (Fig. 1.31A). The continual process of excavation of calcified cartilage and deposition of bone leads to complete removal of the calcified cartilage (Fig. 1.31A).

The cartilage at the extremities of the bone continues to grow due to multiplication of its cells; however, the deeper layers gradually become calcified and replaced by bone. The increase in length of a long bone is due to active cartilage at its ends, while an increase in width is by deposition of new bone on already existing bone.

When first laid down, bone is cancellous in appearance, having no particular organisation (woven bone). In the repair of fractures (p. 39), the newly formed bone also has this woven appearance. However, in response to stresses applied to the bone by muscles, tendons and ligaments, as well as the forces transmitted across joints, the woven bone gradually assumes a specific pattern in response to these stresses.

Ossification Centres

Regions where bone begins to be laid down are known as ossification centres; it is from these centres that ossification spreads. The earliest and usually principal ossification centre is the primary ossification centre. These appear at different times in different bones, but are relatively constant between individuals, they also appear in an orderly sequence. The majority of primary centres appear between the 7th and 12th week of intrauterine life; virtually all are present before birth. In long bones, the primary ossification centre appears in the shaft of the bone (Fig. 1.31C).

Secondary ossification centres appear much later than primary centres, usually after birth, appearing in parts of the cartilage model into which ossification from the primary centre has not spread (Fig. 1.31C). All long bones in the body, and many others, have secondary centres of ossification: the bone formed is almost entirely cancellous.

The part of a long bone ossifying from the primary centre is the diaphysis, while that from a secondary centre is an epiphysis. The plate of cartilage between these two regions (epiphyseal growth plate) is where the diaphysis continues to grow in length (Fig. 1.31C). When the growth plate disappears, the diaphysis and epiphysis fuse and growth in bone length ceases.

Growth and Remodelling

During growth, there is an obvious change in the shape of a bone. It should be remembered that, even in adults, bone is continuously remodelled, principally under the direct control of hormones to stabilise blood calcium levels, but also in response to long-term changes in the pattern of stresses applied to the bone.

Both growth and remodelling depend on the balanced activity of two cell types, one removing bone tissue (osteoclasts) and one laying down new bone (osteoblasts). In a growing bone, new bone is laid down around the circumference of the shaft increasing its diameter; at the same time, the deepest layers of bone are removed, maintaining a reasonable thickness of cortical bone but enlarging the marrow cavity (Fig. 1.31B). Should the process of deposition and removal fail to match, then either a very thick or a very thin shaft results.

Fractures

A fracture is a break in a bone: it can range from a thin crack to a complete break, with most fractures occurring when a bone is impacted by more force than it can support. A closed fracture is where the skin is not broken; it is often referred to as a simple fracture. In contrast, an open fracture is when the bone breaks through the skin or there is a deep wound exposing the bone: it is often referred to as a compound fracture. A partial fracture is an incomplete break in the bone, while in complete fractures the bone is separated into two or more parts. In stable fractures the two ends of the bone are aligned and not moved out of place, while in displaced fractures there is a gap between the broken ends; displaced fractures often require surgery.

Types of fracture.

Transverse fracture: straight line break across the bone (Fig. 1.32), often caused by falls and traffic accidents.

Spiral fracture. These spiral around the bone (Fig. 1.32), being caused by twisting injuries, often sustained during sports; they occur in long bones of the lower (femur, tibia, fibula) and upper (humerus, radius, ulna) limbs.

Greenstick fracture. A partial fracture in which the bone bends and breaks but does not separate into two separate pieces (Fig. 1.32); it occurs mostly in children as their bones tend to be softer and more flexible.

Stress (hairline) fracture. Appears as a crack which can be difficult to diagnose (Fig. 1.32); they are often caused by repetitive motions (running).

Compression fracture. Occurs when bones are crushed, with the broken bone being wider and flatter than before the injury, occurring most often in the spine causing vertebrae to collapse; osteoporosis is the most common cause.

Oblique fracture. A diagonal break across the bone occurring most frequently in long bones (Fig. 1.32); they are often due to a sharp blow at an angle due to a fall or other trauma. A longitudinal fracture occurs along the length of a long bone (Fig. 1.32).

Impacted fracture. A break in which the broken ends of the bone are forced together by the force of the injury causing the fracture (Fig. 1.32).

Segmental fracture. Two breaks in the same bone leaving a 'floating' segment between the breaks (Fig. 1.32);

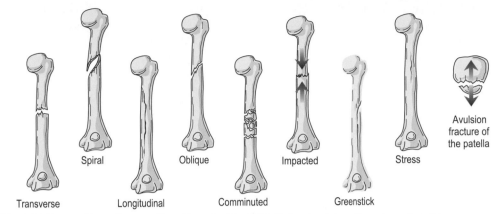

Fig. 1.32 Types of bone fracture. From Banasik, J.L., 2021. Pathophysiology. Saunders, Elsevier.

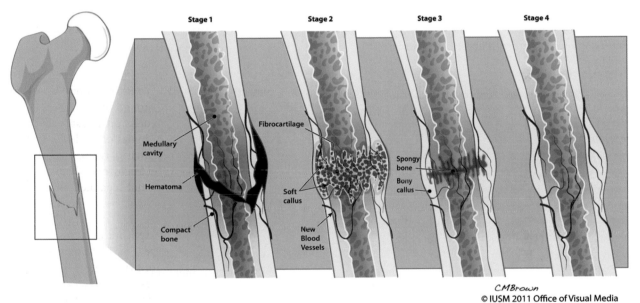

CMBrown
© IUSM 2011 Office of Visual Media

Fig. 1.33 Stages in fracture repair. From Burr, D.B. and Allen, M.R. eds., 2019. Basic and applied bone biology. Academic Press.

they often occur in long bones and can take longer to heal and can cause complications.

Comminuted fracture. Three or more breaks in the same bone with bone fragments at the fracture site (Fig. 1.32); they are due to high-impact trauma as in a road traffic accident.

Avulsion fracture. Occurs when a fragment is pulled off the bone by a tendon/ligament (Fig. 1.32), being more common in children than adults; in children the fracture can be through the growth plate.

Fracture repair. Repair of fractured bone occurs through four main stages (Fig. 1.33) using mechanisms in place for bone remodelling. At the fracture site the torn blood vessels release blood that clots producing a large fracture haematoma (stage 1), which is gradually removed by macrophages and replaced by a soft fibrocartilage-like mass of procallus tissue rich in collagen and fibroblasts (stage 2); if disrupted the periosteum re-establishes continuity over this tissue. The soft procallus is invaded by ingrowing blood vessels and osteoblasts; over the next few weeks the fibrocartilage is gradually replaced by woven bone forming a hard callus throughout the original fracture site (stage 3). Finally, the woven bone is remodelled as compact and cancellous bone in continuity with the adjacent non-injured areas, with a fully functional vasculature being established (stage 4).

JOINTS

The bones of the body come together to form joints. It is through these articulations that movement occurs, with the type and extent of movement possible depending on the structure and function of the joint, which can and do vary considerably. Nevertheless, variation in the form and function of the joints of the body allows them to be grouped into well-defined classes (fibrous, cartilaginous, synovial), with the extent of movement possible gradually increasing from fibrous to synovial.

Fibrous Joints

These are of three types: suture, gomphosis, syndesmosis.

Suture

A form of fibrous joint between the bones of the skull permitting no movement as the edges of the articulating bones are often highly serrated, as well as being united by an intermediate layer of fibrous tissue (Fig. 1.34A). Either side of the fibrous tissue, the inner and outer periosteal layers of the bones are continuous constituting the main bond between them.

Sutures are not permanent joints as they usually become partially obliterated after age 30.

Gomphosis

In this type of fibrous joint, a peg fits into a socket being held in place by a fibrous ligament or band. The roots of the teeth held within their sockets in the maxilla and mandible are examples (Fig. 1.34B), with the fibrous band connecting tooth and bone being the periodontal ligament (periodontal membrane).

Syndesmosis

In a syndesmosis, the uniting fibrous tissue is greater in amount than in a suture, constituting a ligament or interosseous membrane (Fig. 1.34C). In adults, examples are (i) the inferior tibiofibular joint, where the two

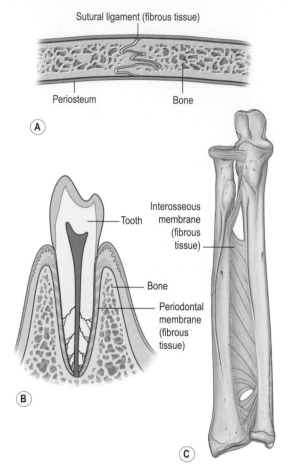

Fig. 1.34 Types of fibrous joints. (A) Suture. (B) Gomphosis. (C) Syndesmosis.

bones are held together by an interosseous ligament, and (ii) the interosseous membrane between the radius and ulna and that between the tibia and fibula. Flexibility of the membrane or twisting and stretching of the ligament permit movement at the joint; however, the movement allowed is controlled and restricted.

Cartilaginous Joints

In these joints, the two bones are united by a continuous pad of cartilage. There are two types of cartilaginous joint: primary (synchondrosis) and secondary (symphysis).

Primary Cartilaginous

Between the ends of the bones involved is a continuous layer of hyaline cartilage (Fig. 1.35A). They occur at the epiphyseal growth plates of growing and developing

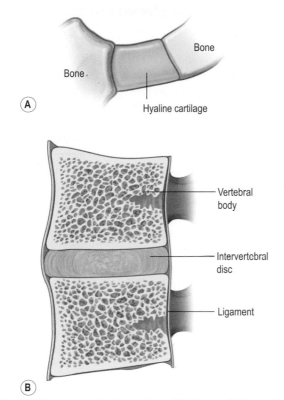

Fig. 1.35 Types of cartilaginous joints. (A) Primary. (B) Secondary.

bone, becoming obliterated with fusion of the diaphysis and epiphysis. Because the plate of hyaline cartilage is relatively rigid, such joints exhibit no movement. There is one such joint in adults (1st sternocostal joint) which is slightly modified because, by virtue of its structure, it enables slight movement to occur.

Secondary Cartilaginous

These occur in the midline of the body and are slightly more specialised enabling a small amount of controlled movement to take place. Hyaline cartilage covers the articular surfaces of the bones involved, between which is a pad of fibrocartilage. Examples are (i) the joints between the bodies of adjacent vertebrae (Fig. 1.35B), where the fibrocartilaginous pad is the intervertebral disc, and (ii) the joint between the bodies of the pubic bones (symphysis pubis).

Synovial Joints

These are a class of freely mobile joints with movement limited by the associated joint capsule, ligaments and muscles crossing the joint; the majority of joints in the limbs are synovial. In synovial joints, the articular surfaces are covered with articular (hyaline) cartilage, which because of its hardness and smoothness enable the bones to move against each other with minimum friction. Surrounding the joint, attaching either at or away from the articular margins, is a fibrous articular capsule, often strengthened by ligaments or the deeper parts of muscles crossing the joint. Lining the deep surface of the capsule is the synovial membrane covering all non-articular surfaces within the capsule (Fig. 1.36A). The synovial membrane secretes synovial fluid into the joint space (joint cavity) enclosed by the capsule, serving to lubricate and nourish the articular cartilage, as well as the opposing joint surfaces. Bursae are often associated with synovial joints, sometimes communicating directly with the joint space. During movement, the joint surfaces either glide or roll past each other.

If the bones involved originally ossified in membrane (p. 37), the articular cartilage has a large fibrous element. In addition, a complete or incomplete intra-articular disc separates the two articular surfaces enclosed by the capsule (Fig. 1.36B).

Because of the large number of synovial joints within the body and their differing forms, they can be classified according to the shape of their articular surfaces and the movement(s) permitted.

Plane Joint

The joint surfaces are flat or relatively flat and of approximately equal extents. The movement possible is either a single gliding or twisting of one bone against the other, usually within narrow limits (acromioclavicular joint).

Saddle Joint

The two surfaces are reciprocally concavoconvex, such as a rider sitting on a saddle. The principal movements occur about two mutually perpendicular axes; because of the nature of the joint surfaces, there is usually a small amount of movement about a third axis (carpometacarpal joint of the thumb).

Hinge Joint

The surfaces are arranged to allow movement about one axis only, with the 'fit' of the articular surfaces usually being good (elbow joint); the joint is also supported by strong collateral ligaments. The knee joint is

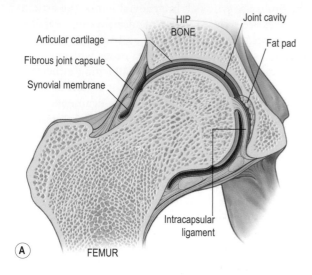

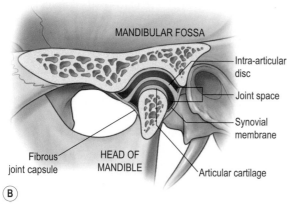

Fig. 1.36 Structure of synovial joints without (A) and with (B) an intra-articular disc.

considered to be a modified hinge joint as it permits some movement about a second axis; in this case, the movement is possible because of the poor fit of the articular surfaces.

Pivot Joint

Movement occurs about a single axis with the articular surfaces arranged so that one bone rotates within a fibro-osseous ring (atlantoaxial joint).

Ball and Socket Joint

As the name suggests, the 'ball' of one bone fits into the 'socket' of the other; it allows movement about

three principal mutually perpendicular axes (hip joint).

Condyloid Joint

A condyloid joint is a modified form of ball and socket joint, allowing active movement to occur about two perpendicular axes (metacarpophalangeal joints); passive movement may occur about the third axis.

Ellipsoid Joint

Another form of ball and socket joint, although the surfaces are ellipsoid; movement is only possible about two perpendicular axes (radiocarpal joint).

Receptors in Joints and Ligaments

Joints and ligaments typically have three types of receptors: free nerve endings believed to be responsible for mediating pain; nerve endings resembling the Ruffini corpuscles; and Pacinian corpuscles found in skin. The latter are not as well developed as the Pacinian corpuscles in skin, being referred to as paciniform endings. Ruffini-type and paciniform endings are responsible for detecting stretch of and pressure in joint capsules and/or ligaments and so are involved in position sense.

SPIN, ROLL AND SLIDE

The movements occurring between articular surfaces can be complex, with the terms spin, roll and slide being used to help explain them. Spin, in which one surface spins relative to the other, occurs about a fixed central axis (Fig. 1.37A). Roll is where one surface rolls across the other so that new parts of both surfaces continually come into contact with each other, as in a wheel rolling along the ground (Fig. 1.37A). Slide occurs when one surface slides over the other so that new points on one surface make contact with the same point on the other surface, as in a wheel sliding across an icy surface (Fig. 1.37A).

Spin, roll and slide do not normally occur separately as they complement one another to facilitate the complex movements occurring at joints. Combinations of spin, roll and slide are the basic components underlying movement at all joints. This can best be illustrated at the knee joint, a modified hinge joint, because of the type of movement available: a true

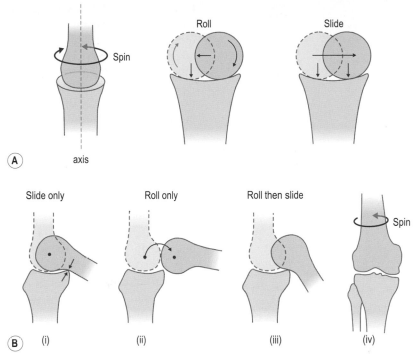

Fig. 1.37 (A) Spin, roll and slide between articular surfaces. (B) The effect of (i) pure sliding or (ii) rolling and (iii) a combination of rolling then sliding at the knee joint, together with (iv) the spin that accompanies full extension.

hinge joint would permit slide only as one surface moves past the other about a fixed axis. For example, if only sliding movements were possible at the knee, the movement would soon become restricted because of contact of the popliteal surface of the femur with the posterior part of the tibial condyle (Fig. 1.37B(i)). Similarly, if the femoral condyles only rolled over the tibial plateaux, a situation would soon be reached where the femur would hypothetically roll off the tibia because the profile of the femoral articular condyle is much longer than that of the tibial plateaux (Fig. 1.37B(ii)). The actual movement at the knee joint is a combination of both rolling and sliding between the two articular surfaces under the control of the associated ligaments, allowing a greater range of movement to be achieved (Fig. 1.37B(iii)). Spin also occurs as full extension is approached as the femur spins about its longitudinal axis on the tibia so that the medial femoral condyle moves backwards (Fig. 1.37B(iv)); the resultant effect is to put the knee into its close-packed position of maximum congruity between the

joint surfaces. As with the combination of rolling and sliding, the joint ligaments are primarily responsible for bringing about spin at the knee. See also page 345 where movements of the knee are described in more detail.

LEVERS

An understanding of the action and principle of levers is important when considering movement at joints through muscle action, as well as the forces applied to bones. The following is a simplified description of the mechanics of levers and how they are applied in the body.

A lever may be considered as a simple rigid bar with no account taken of its shape or structure. Most long bones appear as rigid bars, although many bones, such as those of the skull, are far from the usual concept of a lever, yet they can still act in this way.

The fulcrum is the point about which the lever rotates. The part of the lever between the fulcrum and between the load and force arms; a second-class lever has the fulcrum at one end and the applied force at the other, with the load situated between them; a third-class lever again has the fulcrum at one end but the load at the other with the applied force between (Fig. 1.38B).

All three classes of lever are found within the body: the fulcrum is usually situated at the joint; the load may be body weight or some external resistance; the force is usually produced by muscular effort. It is the complex arrangement of all three classes of lever that produces movement.

A first-class lever is used in balancing weight and/or changing the direction of pull. There is usually no gain in mechanical advantage. When standing on the right lower limb, the fulcrum is the right hip joint, the load is body weight applied to the left of the hip and the force is provided by contraction of the right gluteus medius and minimus.

A second-class lever (the principle on which weight is lifted in a wheelbarrow) gains mechanical advantage, allowing large loads to be moved but with a loss of speed. Rising up onto the toes is an example of such a system; the metatarsal heads act as the fulcrum, the weight of the body acting down through the tibia is the load and the leg/calf muscles contracting produces the required force. The load arm is the distance from the tibia to the metatarsal heads, while the force arm is the distance between the attachment of the leg/calf muscles to the calcaneus and the metatarsal heads.

A third-class lever is most commonly found within the body; it works at a mechanical disadvantage moving less weight but often at great speed. Biceps brachii acting across the elbow joint is an example of a third-class lever. The elbow joint is the fulcrum, the weight is the forearm and hand being supported with the force provided by the contraction of biceps. The load arm is the distance between the elbow and centre of mass of the forearm and hand, and the force arm is the distance between the elbow joint and the attachment of biceps.

All movements are dependent on the interaction of these three classes of lever. When studying the structure of the human body, it is important to remember the relationship between the joint, the attachment of relevant muscles and the load to be moved as this will lead to an understanding of functional anatomy and, with it, human movement.

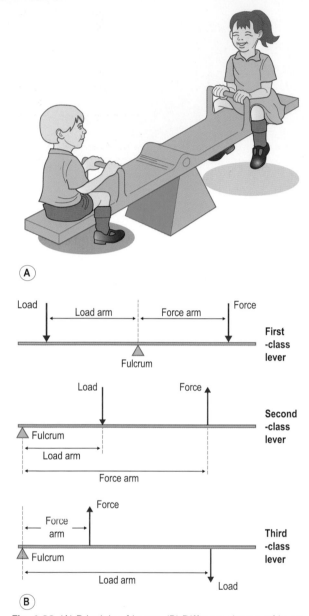

Fig. 1.38 (A) Principle of levers. (B) Different classes of lever.

point of application of the force is the force arm, while that between the fulcrum and point of application of the load is the load arm; this concept is easy to understand when applied to a child's see-saw (Fig. 1.38A). Different arrangements of the fulcrum, load and force arms produce different classes of lever. There are three possible arrangements: a first-class lever has the fulcrum

SECTION SUMMARY

Muscular Tissue

- There are three varieties of muscle: smooth, associated with viscera and blood vessels; cardiac, associated with the heart; and skeletal.
- Muscle fibres are either aligned with (fusiform) or oblique to (pennate) the direction of pull.
- Fusiform muscles can shorten quickly over a large distance but have limited power; pennate muscles are more powerful but cannot shorten to the same extent.
- Muscles attach either directly to bones or via a tendon.
- Isotonic muscle contraction involves a change in muscle length often under constant force generation; in concentric contraction, the muscle shortens, while in eccentric contraction it lengthens.
- Isometric contraction involves no change in muscle length but is usually associated with a change in the tension generated.
- Prime movers are responsible for producing a specific movement, antagonists oppose the movement and synergists help prevent unwanted movements.
- Muscles contain free nerve endings (which mediate pain), Golgi tendon organs (which monitor the extent and force of contraction) and muscle spindles (which monitor changes in muscle length).
- Muscle spindles (intrafusal fibres) are of two types (nuclear bag and nuclear chain fibres).
- Innervation of muscle spindles by γ-motor neurons maintains their length in relation to the overall muscle length, keeping them taut throughout the full range of movement.
- Motor end plates (neuromuscular junctions) are specialised endings between nerve and muscle.
- Transmission of the neural impulse to muscle occurs at the motor end plate (neuromuscular junction).

Skeletal Tissues

Cartilage

- Supplementary to bone providing strength, rigidity and some elasticity.
- Hyaline cartilage forms the temporary skeleton of bone and the articular surfaces of synovial joints.
- White fibrocartilage has great tensile strength and is able to resist compressive stresses.
- Yellow fibrocartilage contains elastic fibres.

Bone

- An organic matrix of cells and fibres impregnated with mineral salts surrounded by periosteum.
- Compact bone is found in the shaft (diaphysis) of long bones and as a thin shell covering cancellous bone.
- Cancellous bone is found in the ends (epiphyses) of long bones, short and flat bones.
- Bone develops by either intramembranous or endochondral ossification initiated from a series of primary and secondary ossification centres.

Joints

- The articulation between two or more bones, classed as fibrous, cartilaginous and synovial joints.

Fibrous joints

- Three types (sutures, gomphoses, syndesmoses) generally permitting little or no movement.

Cartilaginous Joints

- Two types (primary, secondary) permitting some limited and controlled movement.
- In primary cartilaginous joints, a layer of hyaline cartilage separates the bones.
- In secondary cartilaginous joints, a fibrocartilage pad separates the hyaline cartilage layers.

Synovial Joints

- Freely mobile joints as there is no direct connection between the articular surfaces; movement is limited by the joint capsule, ligaments and muscles crossing the joint.
- Surrounded by fibrous capsule lined with synovial membrane, which secretes synovial fluid to lubricate and nourish the articulating surfaces.
- Different surface shapes permit different types of movement.
- Subdivisions are plane, saddle, hinge, pivot, ball and socket, condyloid and ellipsoid.

Levers

- Three classes of lever are found within the body, with the third class being the most common.
- First-class levers have the load and muscle action on opposite sides of the joint (fulcrum); second-class levers have the load between the joint and the muscle attachment; third-class levers have the muscle attachment between the load and the joint.

❓ SELF-ASSESSMENT QUESTIONS

41. Where in adults would you find a syndesmosis?
42. What type of joint is found between adjacent vertebral bodies?
43. Which part(s) of a long bone develops from a secondary ossification centre?
44. What is the function of hyaline cartilage in (a) the foetus, (b) the growing child and (c) the fully grown adult?
45. What type of fibrous tissue is tendon composed of?
46. The internal architecture of the ends of a long bone consists of plates and struts known as what?
47. In what type of ossification is there no cartilage model?
48. What are the bones of the skull referred to as?
49. What is the name given to the outer covering of a muscle?
50. What name is given to a bone which develops in a tendon?
51. What is the function of muscle spindles?
52. What is a motor end plate (neuromuscular junction)?
53. What happens to a muscle when it contracts eccentrically?
54. What is the role of prime movers?
55. What type of synovial joint is the carpometacarpal joint of the thumb?
56. Which type of lever is most commonly found in the body?
57. What is the characteristic of a second-class lever?
58. What type of movement occurs at a pivot joint?
59. What are the functions of synovial fluid within a joint?
60. What and where are gomphoses?

FLEXIBILITY AND MOBILITY

LEARNING OUTCOMES

At the end of the section, you should be able to:

1. Describe the factors producing soft, firm and hard end feels to movement
2. Describe the influence that both age and gender may have on the range of movement at a joint
3. Understand that flexibility is joint specific
4. Demonstrate and appreciate the difference in range of movement at a joint when produced actively and passively

5. Understand the importance of reliability in joint measurement

INTRODUCTION

Determination of the range of movement at a joint (its flexibility) is influenced by a number of factors including age, gender and whether the movement is performed actively or passively. In addition, factors such as activity in opposing muscles, temperature of the surroundings and whether there has been a sufficient 'warm-up' period also influence the measured range of movement.

Flexibility tends to be joint specific. It is not necessarily the case that because an individual has great flexibility at one joint that all joints will be equally flexible. Although studies have shown that in healthy individuals the range of movement is more or less equivalent on the right and left sides (Roass and Andersson, 1982; Murray et al., 1985; Ahlberg et al., 1988; Svenningsen et al., 1989), it appears that the active range responds to the habitual activity of that joint, particularly if there has been trauma to the corresponding joint of the opposite limb (Poulis et al., 2000). This should be borne in mind when assessing the range of movement and using the opposite joint as a reference, especially during rehabilitation.

AGE

This can have a major influence on the range of joint movement, with younger individuals being more flexible than older individuals. Several studies have reported on the ranges of movement in infants and young children (Watanabe et al., 1979; Waugh et al., 1983; Drews et al., 1984), with the observations being joint specific and not influenced by gender. With increasing age, the range of movement decreases at most, if not all, joints. Mean ranges of movement have been published for specific age groups (Walker et al., 1984; Downey et al., 1991) and should, where possible, be used as a standard against which measurement is evaluated. These mean values for each joint are given in the relevant sections of Parts 2, 3, 4 and 5; however, the tabulated required ranges for specific activities given are not age specific. They are provided as a guide to the range of movement required to undertake a particular task or activity.

Factors influencing these age-related ranges of movement include changes in activity level, muscle strength and neuromuscular coordination, degenerative disease and trauma, each of which will vary from individual to individual. In general, more physically active individuals tend to have greater ranges of movement than those who are less active.

GENDER

This does appear to be joint specific with the differences between men and women being relatively small. No attempt has been made to quantify these differences; nevertheless differences have been reported (Moll and Wright, 1971; Beighton et al., 1973; O'Driscoll and Thomenson, 1982).

ACTIVE RANGE OF MOTION

The range of movement achieved during voluntary motion and provides information about coordination, muscle strength and the willingness to move; the movement may be limited due to pain or the expectation of pain. The active range of movement tends to be less than that achieved passively.

PASSIVE RANGE OF MOTION

The range achieved by the examiner without any contribution from the individual is the passive range of motion. It is normally greater than the active range as each joint permits an additional amount of movement not under voluntary control. Testing the passive range of motion provides information about the integrity of the articular surfaces, as well as the extensibility of the soft tissues associated with the joint.

END FEEL TO MOVEMENT

The end feel to movement during passive testing may give an indication of the factors restricting further motion. Normally the end feel will be soft, due to soft tissue contact; firm, due to tension developed in the joint capsule, associated ligaments and muscles; or hard, due to bony contact. If the range of movement is prematurely arrested, the end feel can still be soft, firm or hard. If soft, this may indicate soft tissue oedema or synovitis; if firm, this may indicate either soft tissue contracture or increased muscle tone; if hard, this may indicate osteoarthritis, loose bodies within the joint space or a

fracture. Occasionally, there may be no end feel because pain limits joint movement: such situations may indicate joint inflammation, bursitis, an abscess, a fracture or be psychosomatic.

PRINCIPLES OF MEASUREMENT

Joint motion can be estimated visually; however, this provides no permanent objective record making comparisons between different assessment sessions difficult. Using an objective method of measurement is important for evaluating the effectiveness of a specific treatment regime or rehabilitation programme. In a clinical setting, a simple two-arm goniometer may be the most appropriate; however, specific devices may be readily available for some joints or regions. Irrespective of the equipment used, specific procedures must be followed ensuring correct alignment and positioning so that the movement of interest is being measured.

Before taking any measurements, the relevant bony landmarks must be accurately identified and palpated, and the examiner must be aware of the most appropriate position in which to place the individual as well as stabilising other body segments. The measurement of joint motion should be undertaken and recorded as accurately as possible, with the movement recorded as the maximum number of degrees the joint moves in a particular plane.

VALIDITY AND RELIABILITY

To provide meaningful data, the measurement must be valid and reliable. Validity is the extent to which the device measures what it is supposed to measure, and reliability is the consistency between successive measurements of the same individual under the same conditions.

Validity is often taken for granted without being specifically assessed. The assumption is that aligning the goniometer with specific landmarks and measuring the change in angle during movement represents the angular change at the joint. This takes no account of changing axes of motion or changes in the overlying soft tissues with respect to the underlying bony landmarks. The issue of validity has led to the establishment of criterion-based validity for various types of goniometers used in clinical applications, often based on comparisons with an accepted 'gold standard'. Nevertheless, in practice, and providing specific relevant landmarks have been identified, the measurement can be deemed to be valid.

A measurement is reliable if successive measurements under the same conditions give the same result. A highly reliable measurement has little measurement error; conversely, a measurement with poor reliability contains a large amount of measurement error. Measurements with poor reliability cannot be relied upon and should be avoided.

The measurement of range of motion is subject to several sources of error: changes in position of the axis of movement; variations in the individual's effort when assessing active range of motion; and variation in the force applied when assessing passive range of motion. Measuring a fixed joint position is more reliable than measuring a range of movement. Reliability also varies from joint to joint (Boone et al., 1978), being higher for the limbs (Low, 1976; Hellebrandt et al., 1985) than for the vertebral column (Fitzgerald et al., 1983; Tucci et al., 1986; Youdas et al., 1991). In general, the more complex the joint the less reliable the measurement.

Reliability has also been observed to be higher when successive measurements are made by the same examiner (intratester reliability) rather than by different examiners (intertester reliability). Intertester reliability can be improved if all examiners use consistent, well-defined positions and measurement techniques. An additional factor influencing reliability is the time interval between successive measurements, with longer time intervals (days and weeks rather than hours) being less reliable.

Reliability can be improved by (i) using consistent well-defined test positions and landmarks; (ii) applying the same amount of force to the body segment when assessing passive range of motion; (iii) encouraging the individual to exert the same effort to perform a movement when assessing active range of motion; (iv) taking repeat measurements with the same measuring device to reduce the variability of the measurement; and (v) having the same examiner take successive measurements.

When assessing the effects of a treatment or rehabilitation regime it has been suggested that there should be at least a 5-degree difference in joint motion before a true increase or decrease in the range of movement is accepted (Boone et al., 1978).

SECTION SUMMARY

- Joint flexibility is influenced by factors such as age, gender, whether movement is performed actively or passively, the tone in opposing muscles and the temperature of the surroundings.
- Flexibility is joint specific.
- Active movement provides information about coordination, muscle strength and willingness to move.
- Passive movement provides information about the articular surfaces and extensibility of the surrounding soft tissues.
- The end feel to movement can be soft due to soft tissue contact, firm due to tension developed in the joint capsule and associated ligaments and muscles, or hard due to bony contact.
- Validity of measurement is the extent to which the device measures what it is supposed to.
- Measurement is reliable if successive measurements under the same conditions give similar results.

❓ SELF-ASSESSMENT QUESTIONS

61. Define the terms (a) validity and (b) reliability related to joint measurement.
62. What influence can age have on joint flexibility?
63. What is the difference between active and passive range of movement?
64. Which tend to be more reliable intratester or intertester measurements?
65. Give five ways in which reliability of joint measurement can be improved.

▌SELF-ASSESSMENT MULTIPLE CHOICE QUESTIONS

1. A muscle which acts as an antagonist during movement:
   a. is the principal muscle producing the movement.
   b. aids the movement being undertaken.
   c. is working concentrically.
   d. opposes the movement being undertaken.
   e. is working isometrically.

2. The passive range of movement at a joint:
   a. is less than the active range of movement.
   b. provides information about muscle strength.
   c. is not joint specific.
   d. is not influenced by the temperature of the surroundings.

e. provides information about the extensibility of surrounding tissues.
3. Concerning skin, which of the following statements is correct?
   a. The epidermis lies deep to the dermis.
   b. Sweat glands are derived from the epidermis.
   c. The epidermis can be considered as a number of distinct layers.
   d. Projecting dermal papillae contain hair follicles.
   e. Has a surface area in excess of 4 m².
4. Which of the flowing statements concerning skeletal muscle is NOT correct?
   a. Can have a pennate arrangement of fibres.
   b. Is innervated by peripheral nerves.
   c. Contains intercalated discs between individual fibres.
   d. Develops from the sclerotome of the somite.
   e. Is often attached to bone by an intervening tendon.
5. Concerning bone, which of the following statements is NOT correct?
   a. Osteoblasts remove bone tissue.
   b. Long bones grow in length at the epiphyses.
   c. Not all bones in adults contain red bone marrow.
   d. The epiphyses contain cancellous bone.
   e. All bones develop from a primary ossification centre.
6. Which of the following is a type of synovial joint?
   a. Gomphosis
   b. Synchondrosis
   c. Suture
   d. Condyloid
   e. Symphysis
7. Which of the following is NOT associated with synovial joints?
   a. Joint capsule
   b. Synovial membrane
   c. Direct connection between the articular surfaces
   d. Synovial fluid
   e. Joint space
8. Concerning joints, which of the following statements is NOT correct?
   a. Ellipsoid joints permit active movement in two mutually perpendicular directions.
   b. In adults, sutures allow no movement between adjacent bones.
   c. A synchondrosis contains a fibrocartilaginous pad of tissue connecting the hyaline cartilage covering the bone surfaces.

d. Symphyses are found in the midline of the body.
e. The joint between the distal ends of the radius and ulna is a syndesmosis.
9. Which of the following bones ossifies in membrane?
   a. Scapula
   b. Femur
   c. Hyoid
   d. Ulna
   e. Clavicle
10. Concerning the peripheral nervous system, which of the following statements is NOT correct?
    a. All peripheral nerves arise from the spinal cord.
    b. The autonomic nervous system has sympathetic and parasympathetic components.
    c. Each peripheral nerve is surrounded by an epineurium.
    d. Peripheral nerves contain both motor and sensory fibres.
    e. Bundles of axons enclosed within a single perineurial sheath is a nerve fascicle.
11. Which of the following types of nerve ending is NOT found in skin?
    a. Free nerve endings
    b. Merkel disc
    c. Pacinian corpuscle
    d. Golgi organ
    e. Krause end bulb
12. Which of the following is NOT a type of connective tissue?
    a. Blood
    b. Muscle
    c. White fibrous tissue
    d. Cartilage
    e. Bone
13. In terms of movement what is the role of a muscle that acts as a synergist?
    a. Acts to oppose the movement
    b. Contracts eccentrically
    c. Initiates the movement
    d. Contracts isometrically
    e. Helps produce the movement
14. Concerning movement, which of the following statements is NOT correct?
    a. Active movement at a joint provides information about coordination.
    b. A measurement of movement is only valid if successive measurements under the same conditions give the same result.

    c. Active movement at a joint provides information about the extensibility of the surrounding tissues.

    d. Movement at a joint is influenced by gender.

    e. When the end feel to a movement is firm it is due to tension developed in the associated joint capsule, ligaments and muscles.

15. Which of the following statements is correct?

    a. Pennate muscles are not as powerful as fusiform muscles.

    b. When a muscle contracts isotonically the force generated changes.

    c. During eccentric contraction muscle length decreases.

    d. Isometric contraction involves no change in muscle length.

    e. Fusiform muscles cannot shorten as much as pennate muscles during contraction.

REFERENCES

Ahlberg, A., Moussa, M., Al-Nahidi, M., 1988. On geographical variations in the range of joint motion. Clin. Orthop. 234, 229–231.

Beighton, P., Solomon, L., Soskolne, C.L., 1973. Articular mobility in an African population. Ann. Rheum. Dis. 32, 413–418.

Boone, D.C., Azen, S.P., Lin, C.M., et al., 1978. Reliability of goniometric measurements. Phys. Ther. 58, 1355–1390.

Downey, P.A., Fiebert, J., Stackpole-Brown, J.B., 1991. Shoulder range of motion in persons aged sixty and older. Phys. Ther. 71, S75.

Drews, J.E., Vraciu, J.K., Pellino, G., 1984. Range of motion of the lower extremities of newborns. Phys. Occup. Ther. Pediatr. 4, 49–62.

Fitzgerald, G.K., Wynveen, K.J., Rheault, W., et al., 1983. Objective assessment with establishment of normal values for lumbar spine range of motion. Phys. Ther. 63, 1776–1781.

Hellebrandt, F.A., Duvall, E.N., Moore, M.L., 1985. The measurement of joint motion. Part III. Reliability of goniometry. Phys. Ther. Rev. 65, 1339.

Low, J.L., 1976. The reliability of the joint measurement. Physiotherapy 62, 227–229.

Moll, J.M., Wright, V., 1971. Normal range of spinal mobility: an objective clinical study. Ann. Rheum. Dis. 30, 381–386.

Murray, M.P., Gore, D.R., Gardner, G.M., et al., 1985. Shoulder motion and muscle strength of normal men and women in two age groups. Clin. Orthop. 192, 268–273.

O'Driscoll, S.L., Thomenson, J., 1982. The cervical spine. Clin. Rheum. Dis 8, 617–630.

Poulis, S., Poulis, A., Soames, R.W., 2000. Torque characteristics of the ankle plantarflexors and dorsiflexors during eccentric and concentric contraction in healthy young males. Isokinet. Exerc. Sci. 8, 195–202.

Roass, A., Andersson, G.B., 1982. Normal range of motion of the hip, knee and ankle joint in male subjects 30-40 years of age. Acta Orthop. Scand. 3, 205–208.

Svenningsen, S., Terjesen, T., Auflem, M., et al., 1989. Hip motion related to age and sex. Acta Orthop. Scand. 60, 97–100.

Tucci, S.M., Hicks, J.E., Gross, E.G., et al., 1986. Cervical motion assessment: a new simple and accurate method. Arch. Phys. Med. Rehabil. 67, 225–230.

Walker, J.M., Sue, D., Miles-Elkousy, N., et al., 1984. Active mobility of the extremities in older subjects. Phys. Ther. 64, 919–923.

Watanabe, H., Ogata, K., Amano, T., et al., 1979. The range of joint motions of the extremities in healthy Japanese people: the difference according to age. Nippon. Seikeigeka Gakkai Zasshi 53, 275–281.

Waugh, K.G., Minkel, J.L., Parker, R., et al., 1983. Measurement of selected hip, knee, and ankle joint motions in newborns. Phys. Ther. 63, 1616–1621.

Youdas, J.W., Carey, J.R., Garrett, T.R., 1991. Reliability of measurements of cervical spine range of motion: comparison of three methods. Phys. Ther. 71, 98–104.

Upper Limb

KEY CONCEPTS

- From proximal to distal, the bones of the upper limb are organised to permit increasing function of the hand.
- From proximal to distal, the joints of the upper limb are organised to provide increasing flexibility while maintaining stability.

- Joint stability is maintained by the shape of the articular surfaces and associated ligaments, reinforced by muscle activity.
- Innervation of the muscles of the anterior arm is by the musculocutaneous nerve; the anterior forearm by the median nerve (with exceptions); the posterior

arm and forearm by the radial nerve; and the hand by the ulnar nerve (with exceptions).
- Flexor muscles are supplied by the anterior divisions of the trunks of the brachial plexus by the musculocutaneous, median and ulnar nerves; extensor muscles are supplied by posterior divisions of the trunks of the brachial plexus by the radial nerve.
- Innervation of the skin of the upper limb reflects its outpouching from the trunk (axial skeleton): preaxial arm (C5, C6); preaxial forearm (C7); hand (C8); postaxial forearm (T1); postaxial arm (T2).

- Muscles crossing more than one joint promote coordinated movement and function.
- Combinations of activity in different muscles crossing a joint produce a wide range of movement in many directions.
- The role of most muscles is to stabilise the joints they cross; producing movement is a secondary function.
- The hand has a very rich blood and nerve supply subserving its function as a tactile and manipulative structure.
- The upper limb is adapted to enable the hand to be placed anywhere in space yet remain functional.

OVERVIEW

This part considers the anatomy and function of the upper limb, including its examination though palpation and clinical evaluation. It is organised into seven major sections: pectoral girdle; shoulder; elbow; forearm; wrist; hand and digits; and brachial plexus and nerves of the upper limb. In addition, there is a section on blood supply and lymphatic drainage, as well as a consideration of simple activities of the upper limb.

In each section, the individual bones are considered, including their palpation, followed by the joints between the bones, their palpation, the movements possible and the muscles producing each movement. For each muscle mentioned, its attachments, innervation, action and palpation are given. The clinical examination and evaluation of movement of each joint are given, including its measurement and the end feel of the movement. At the end of each section, there is a summary of the bones, joints and muscles (including root value of the innervation) involved, as well as the clinical examination. Also at the end of each section is a selection of self-assessment questions, while at the end of the chapter, there are a series of self-assessment multiple-choice questions.

INTRODUCTION

The upper limb has almost no locomotor function, except in cases of pathology and/or trauma to the lower limb. With the evolutionary adaptation of bipedalism, it has acquired a great degree of freedom of movement, developing into a highly mobile organ used for grasping and manipulation. Nevertheless, the upper limb still retains its ability to act as a locomotor prop, as when grasping an immobile object and pulling the body towards the hand. Alternatively, it may be used in conjunction with a walking aid to support the body during gait. However, the bones of the upper limb are not as robust as their counterparts in the lower limb.

The pectoral girdle attaches the upper limb to the trunk; it consists of the scapula and the clavicle, with the only point of articulation with the axial skeleton being at the sternoclavicular joint. The scapula sits in a sea of muscles attaching it to the head, neck and thorax, while the clavicle acts as a strut holding the upper limb away from the trunk. Between the trunk and hand are a series of highly mobile joints and a system of levers, which enable the hand to be brought to any point in space and held there steadily and securely while performing tasks. The development of the hand as a sensitive instrument of precision and power is the acme of human evolution. The importance of the opposability of the thumb in providing effective grasping and manipulating skills makes the hand the most efficient tool in the animal kingdom. In grasping, the thumb is equal in value to the other four digits; loss of the thumb is as disabling as the loss of all four fingers. To support these skills, the hand has a rich motor and sensory nerve supply. It is no coincidence that the hand has large representations in both the motor and sensory regions of the cerebral cortex. The adoption of a bipedal gait during human evolution freed the upper limbs for functions other than locomotion; this is one reason why the brain developed and enlarged to its present form. Not to be overlooked in the functional effectiveness of the hand is the important contribution made by the extensive vascular network in supporting its metabolic requirements.

As the upper limb is also used for carrying loads and supporting the body, the question arises as to how these forces are transmitted to the axial skeleton. The usual means is by tension developed in the muscles and ligaments crossing the various joints. However, because the upper limb itself is heavy, every movement that it makes has to be accompanied by postural contractions and adjustments of the muscles of the trunk and lower limb to compensate for shifts in the body's centre of gravity.

With the upper limb in the anatomical position, the anterior preaxial compartments are in a continuous plane with the muscles supplied by branches from the lateral and medial cords of the brachial plexus (p. 225), which are derived from the anterior divisions of the nerve trunks. Similarly, the posterior postaxial compartment muscles are all supplied by branches of the posterior cord, derived from the posterior divisions of the nerve trunks.

The median, musculocutaneous and ulnar nerves are responsible for preaxial innervation, while the radial nerve supplies all postaxial musculature of the upper limb below the shoulder. Within the pectoral girdle, the clavicle is the anterior preaxial bone, and the scapula, with the exception of the coracoid process (which is also an anterior bone), is the posterior postaxial bone. The distinction with respect to the coracoid process is that, phylogenetically, it is a separate bone: its fusion with the scapula is secondary. Consequently, muscles arising from the clavicle or coracoid process belong to the preaxial group and are, therefore, supplied by preaxial branches of the brachial plexus. Similarly, muscles arising from the remainder of the scapula are part of the postaxial group and are innervated by postaxial branches of the plexus.

There is a serial arrangement of the nerves in the brachial plexus with respect to both their motor and sensory innervation; the order is retained from the primitive serial morphology of the embryo. Remembering that the skin has essentially been stretched over the developing limb, the fifth cervical nerve (C5) in adults is sensory to the cranial part of the limb and the first thoracic nerve (T1) to its caudal part, with the seventh cervical nerve (C7) lying in the middle of the limb. The pattern of motor innervation, in simple terms, progresses from C5 for shoulder movements to T1 for intrinsic hand movements, with the elbow served by C5 and C6, the forearm by C6, the wrist by C6 and C7, and the fingers and thumb by C7 and C8.

As in the lower limb, many muscles cross two or more joints and are, therefore, able to act on all of them. Consequently, a complex system of synergists and fixators is required to prevent or restrict unwanted movements. Procedures for testing for the loss of muscle action, as in paralysis, can thus be quite complicated.

The upper limit of the upper limb is not so easily defined as in the lower limb. Despite muscle attachments to the head, neck and thorax, the upper limit can be conveniently considered as the superior surface of the clavicle anteriorly and the superior border of the scapula posteriorly. The free upper limb is divided into the arm between the shoulder and elbow, forearm between the elbow and wrist, and the hand beyond the wrist; the hand has an anterior (palmar) and posterior (dorsal) surface (Fig. 2.1).

The bones of the upper limb are the clavicle and scapula of the pectoral girdle, the humerus in the arm, the lateral radius and medial ulna in the forearm, the eight carpal bones of the wrist, the five metacarpals of the hand and the phalanges of the digits, two in the thumb and three in each finger (Fig. 2.1).

The upper limb develops as a swelling of the body wall opposite the lower cervical and first thoracic segments, projecting at right angles to the body surface with ventral and dorsal surfaces, and cephalic (preaxial) and caudal (postaxial) borders. With increases in length, the limb becomes folded ventrally, so the ventral surface becomes medial with the convexity of the elbow directed laterally. Further details of limb development can be found on page 11: see also Fig. 1.10.

Fasciae of the Upper Limb

Superficial fascia surrounds the upper limb like a sleeve but shows regional differences between the shoulder and hand. In the pectoral (shoulder) region and arm, it contains a variable amount of fat: in females, there is deposition of fat in this region (secondary sexual characteristic) with the amount tending to increase after middle age. At the elbow, a subcutaneous bursa is present between the skin and olecranon process, which can become enlarged in individuals who tend to lean on their elbows, giving rise to a condition known as 'student's elbow'. There is nothing particularly noteworthy about the superficial fascia in the forearm. However, in the hand, there are several specialisations, most of which enhance the hand's tactile or prehensile capabilities: these are considered on page 177.

REGIONS

BONES

JOINTS

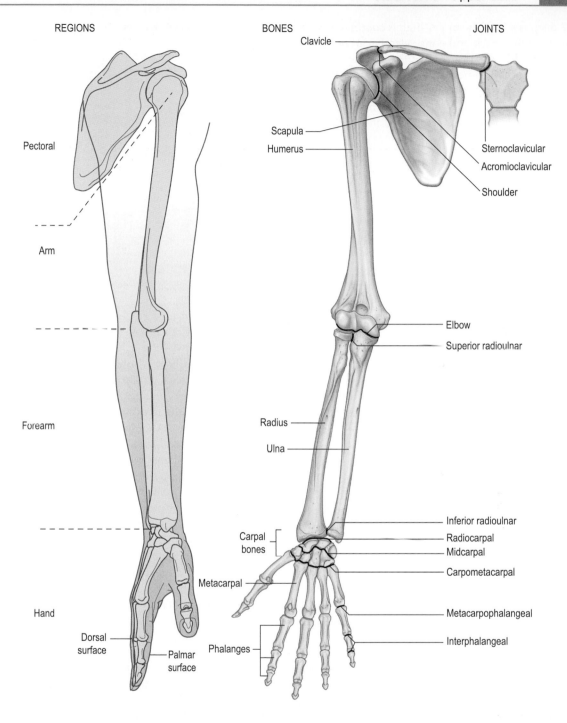

Pectoral

Arm

Forearm

Hand

Dorsal
surface

Palmar
surface

Clavicle

Scapula

Humerus

Radius

Ulna

Carpal
bones

Metacarpal

Phalanges

Sternoclavicular

Acromioclavicular

Shoulder

Elbow

Superior radioulnar

Inferior radioulnar

Radiocarpal

Midcarpal

Carpometacarpal

Metacarpophalangeal

Interphalangeal

Fig. 2.1 Regions, bones and joints of the upper limb.

The deep fascia of the upper limb is continuous with that of the upper back and consequently can be traced superiorly to the superior nuchal line on the occipital bone (p. 656), the ligamentum nuchae in the posterior midline of the cervical region (p. 633) and the supraspinous and interspinous ligaments in the thoracic region (p. 511). The deep fascia is considered in detail in the appropriate section.

PECTORAL GIRDLE

LEARNING OUTCOMES

By the end of the section, you should be able to:
1. Identify, palpate and examine the scapula and clavicle
2. Describe the bones, joints and muscles of the pectoral girdle
3. Describe and explain the movements possible, as well as their restraints, at the sternoclavicular and acromioclavicular joints
4. Locate, palpate and examine the muscles associated with the pectoral girdle, and give their attachments, action and innervation
5. Examine and assess movements of the pectoral girdle
6. Appreciate the role of the pectoral girdle and its joints in movement of the shoulder joint
7. Appreciate the influence of pathology and/or trauma on the function of the pectoral girdle

INTRODUCTION

The upper limb has become highly specialised in its functions of prehension and manipulation. Evolution has produced a limb which is extremely mobile without losing the stability required to give this acquired mobility force and precision. The result of this evolutionary development is an upper limb which has no locomotor function except in infants and in individuals who, of necessity, use walking aids.

All vertebrates possess four limbs of one form or another, these being connected to the axial skeleton by the pectoral and pelvic girdles. In humans, the pelvic girdle is firmly anchored to the vertebral column, providing the stability necessary for bipedal locomotion. In contrast, the pectoral girdle does not articulate with the vertebral column: it articulates only with the thoracic cage (Fig. 2.2), which, although providing a mechanism whereby forces generated in the upper limb

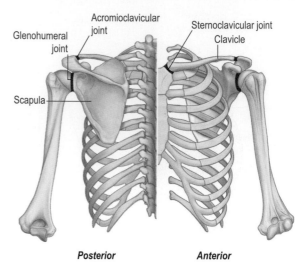

Fig. 2.2 Relationship of the pectoral girdle to the thorax.

can be partially transferred to the axial skeleton, does not unduly restrict movement of the pectoral girdle as a whole.

The shoulder blade (scapula) and clavicle are the bones of the pectoral girdle. The shoulder blade is usually referred to as the scapula in descriptive anatomy: morphologically, the term has a slightly more restricted meaning (see later). Although movements of the shoulder joint accompany nearly all movements of the joints of the pectoral girdle, it is not part of the pectoral girdle. The shoulder blade is slung in muscle from the thoracic cage, while the clavicle is interposed between the shoulder blade and thorax providing a strut which steadies and braces the pectoral girdle during movements, particularly adduction. The clavicle articulates with the thorax by the sternoclavicular joint (Fig. 2.2) and with the shoulder blade by the acromioclavicular joint (Fig. 2.2). The humerus articulates with the shoulder blade at the glenohumeral (shoulder) joint. It is the summation of the mobility of these three individual, yet mutually interdependent, joints which gives the upper limb its freedom of movement; consequently, the ultimate range of movement of the shoulder complex is much greater than that of the equivalent joint (hip) in the lower limb. The clavicle moves with respect to the sternum, the shoulder blade with respect to the clavicle, the humerus with respect to the shoulder blade and the shoulder blade with respect to the thoracic wall. This arrangement favours mobility of the shoulder–arm complex; however, it makes stabilisation of the upper limb against the axial skeleton more

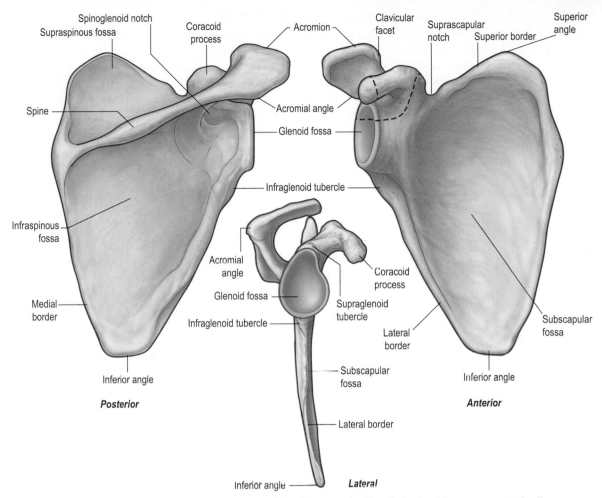

Fig. 2.3 Posterior, anterior and lateral aspects of the right scapula. The dashed red lines represent the lines of fusion between the embryological parts of the scapula.

difficult. Stability is achieved by the powerful musculature attaching the pectoral girdle to the thorax, vertebral column, and head and neck. Furthermore, this musculature acts as a shock absorber when body weight is received by the upper limbs.

Just as the innominate of the pelvis consists of three parts which meet and fuse at the acetabulum, so there are three parts of the shoulder blade (Fig. 2.3). The broad, flat, dorsal part of the shoulder blade is the scapula, and the ventral part is the coracoid process, the two joining together in the upper part of the glenoid fossa. (These are the counterparts of the ilium and ischium, respectively.) A small piece of bone (precoracoid) ossifying separately at the tip of the coracoid process is the counterpart of the pubis.

The clavicle has no counterpart in the pelvic girdle. Forces from the upper limb are transmitted via trapezius to the cervical spine and by the clavicle to the axial skeleton by the coracoclavicular and costoclavicular ligaments so that normally neither end of the clavicle transmits much force.

SCAPULA

Large, flat, triangular plate of bone on the posterolateral aspect of the thorax, overlying the 2nd to 7th ribs. Suspended in muscles, the scapula is held in position by the strut-like clavicle yet retains great mobility relative to the thorax. Being a triangular bone, it has three angles, three borders and two surfaces which support three bony processes (Fig. 2.3).

The costal surface (subscapular fossa), which faces the ribs, is slightly hollowed and ridged with a smooth, narrow strip along its entire medial border.

The dorsal surface faces posterolaterally and is divided by the spine of the scapula into a smaller supraspinous fossa above and a larger infraspinous fossa below. The supraspinous and infraspinous fossae communicate via the spinoglenoid notch between the lateral end of the spine and neck of the scapula. The spine of the scapula has superior and inferior free borders which diverge laterally enclosing the acromion.

The thin medial border lies between the inferior and superior angles, being slightly angled at the medial end of the spine. The lateral border is thicker, being deeply invested in muscles, and runs inferiorly from the infraglenoid tubercle inferior to the glenoid fossa to meet the medial border at the inferior angle. The thin and sharp superior border is the shortest and has the suprascapular notch at the junction with the root of the coracoid process.

Inferiorly, the thick inferior angle lies over the seventh rib and is easily palpated. The superior angle lies at the junction of the medial and superior borders, while the lateral angle is truncated and broadened to support the head and glenoid fossa of the scapula.

The head of the scapula is an expanded part of the bone joined to a flat blade by a short inconspicuous neck. The glenoid fossa (cavity) is on the head and presents as a shallow, pear-shaped concavity facing anterolaterally; it is broader inferiorly and articulates with the head of the humerus forming the shoulder (glenohumeral) joint. Immediately superior to the glenoid fossa is the supraglenoid tubercle.

The acromion (expanded lateral end of the spine) is large and quadrilateral and projects anteriorly at right angles to the spine. The inferior border of the crest of the spine continues as the lateral border of the acromion, with the junction of these two borders forming the palpable acromial angle. The superior border of the crest is continuous with the medial border of the acromion and carries an oval facet for articulation with the clavicle at the acromioclavicular joint. The superior surface of the acromion is flattened and subcutaneous.

The coracoid process is a hooklike projection with a broad base directed superiorly and anteriorly from the superior part of the head, and a narrow more horizontal part which passes anterolaterally from the upper edge of the base. The tip lies below the junction of the middle and lateral thirds of the clavicle.

Ossification

The scapula ossifies from a number of centres. The primary ossification centre appears in the region of the neck by the 8th week *in utero*, so that, at birth, the coracoid process, acromion, glenoid fossa, medial border and inferior angle are still cartilaginous. Secondary ossification centres appear in each of these regions, except the coracoid, between the ages of 12 and 14 years, fusing with the body between 20 and 25 years. In contrast, the secondary centre for the coracoid process appears during the first year and fuses with the body between 12 and 14 years.

Palpation

Starting at the lowest point, the inferior angle can be readily gripped between the thumb and index finger and, if the individual is sufficiently relaxed, can be lifted away from the thorax. The medial border can be followed along its whole length between the inferior and superior angles. The spine of the scapula can be palpated as a small triangular area medially, increasing in size as the fingers move laterally along it; the flat crest with its upper and lower borders can be identified. Continuing along the lower border of the crest to its most lateral point, the sharp 90 degrees acromial angle can be felt continuing as the palpable lateral border of the acromion. Running onto this lateral border, the flat upper surface of the acromion can be felt above the shoulder joint. The coracoid process can be palpated as an anterior projection below the junction of the middle and lateral thirds of the clavicle: it is a useful reference point for surface-marking the shoulder joint as it lies just medial to the joint line.

CLAVICLE

A subcutaneous bone, the clavicle runs horizontally from the sternum to the acromion (Fig. 2.4). It acts as a strut holding the scapula laterally, enabling the arm to be clear of the trunk – an essential feature in primates. The scapula and clavicle together form the pectoral (shoulder) girdle, transmitting the weight of the upper limb to the axial skeleton and facilitating a wide range of movement of the upper limb.

The medial two-thirds of the clavicle is convex anteriorly and roughly triangular in cross-section. The lateral one-third is concave anteriorly and flattened from superior to inferior. The medial convexity conforms to the

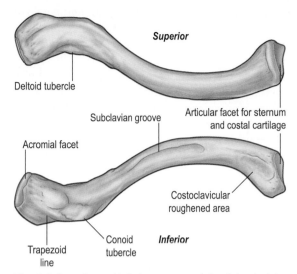

Deltoid tubercle

Superior

Subclavian groove

Articular facet for sternum and costal cartilage

Acromial facet

Costoclavicular roughened area

Conoid tubercle

Inferior

Trapezoid line

Fig. 2.4 Superior and inferior aspects of the right clavicle.

curvature of the superior thoracic aperture (thoracic inlet) and the lateral concavity to the shape of the shoulder.

The lateral (acromial) end of the clavicle is the most flattened part with a small deltoid tubercle on its anterior border. Inferiorly, the rounded conoid tubercle lies on the posteroinferior edge with the rough trapezoid line running anteriorly and laterally away from it (Fig. 2.4). The conoid tubercle and trapezoid line give attachment to the conoid and trapezoid parts of the coracoclavicular ligament, which bind the clavicle and scapula together. Laterally is a small oval facet, facing obliquely inferolaterally, for the acromion.

The medial (sternal) end of the clavicle is enlarged and faces inferomedially. The lower three-quarters is bevelled and articulates with the clavicular notch of the manubrium and 1st costal cartilage, forming the sternoclavicular joint. The cylindrical clavicle projects above the shallow notch on the sternum; this can be confirmed by palpation. The upper quarter of the sternal end is roughened for attachment of the intra-articular disc and ligaments of the sternoclavicular joint. Between the lateral and medial ends, the superior surface is smooth, whereas the inferior surface is marked by a rough subclavian groove centrally and a large, oval, roughened area for the costoclavicular ligament medially. The anterior and posterior borders are roughened by muscle attachments.

The clavicle is often fractured by the direct violence of a blow or by indirect forces transmitted up the limb after a fall on an outstretched arm. The fracture usually occurs at the junction of the two curvatures with the medial fragment overriding the lateral at the fracture site due to the weight of the arm pulling the shoulder inferomedially.

Ossification

The clavicle ossifies in membrane, being the first bone in the body to begin ossification and the last to completely fuse. Two primary centres appear during the 5th week *in utero* which unite, with ossification spreading towards each end of the bone. A secondary centre appears in the medial end between 14 and 18 years, fusing with the main part of the bone as early as 18–20 years in females and 23–25 years in males. An additional centre may appear in the lateral end at puberty; however, it soon fuses with the main bone.

Palpation

In slender individuals, the whole length of the clavicle can often be seen directly beneath the skin. Initially, the enlarged medial end of the clavicle can be palpated with the fingers with the line of the sternoclavicular joint also being identified. Moving laterally, almost the whole length of the clavicle can be gripped between the finger and thumb. At the lateral end, the line of the acromioclavicular joint should be palpable, particularly from above, although the bulk of deltoid may require deeper pressure to be applied.

STERNOCLAVICULAR JOINT

The synovial sternoclavicular joint provides the only point of bony connection between the pectoral girdle, upper limb and trunk. Although functionally a ball-and-socket joint, it does not have the form of such a joint.

Palpation

The line of the sternoclavicular joint can be easily identified through the skin and subcutaneous tissues at the medial end of the clavicle. The projection of the medial end of the clavicle above the sternum can also be palpated.

Articular Surfaces

The medial end of the clavicle articulates with the clavicular notch at the superolateral angle of the sternum (p. 551) and adjacent superior medial surface of the 1st costal cartilage. The clavicular articular surface tends to be larger than that on the sternum; consequently, the medial end of the clavicle projects above the upper margin of the manubrium sterni.

The articular surfaces are reciprocally concavoconvex, although they do not usually have similar radii of curvature. The joint is not particularly congruent, congruence being partly improved by the presence of an intra-articular fibrocartilaginous disc. The articular surface on the manubrium sterni is set approximately 45 degrees to the vertical; it is markedly concave from superior to inferior and convex from posterior to anterior, it is covered with hyaline cartilage. The clavicular articular surface is convex vertically and flattened or slightly concave horizontally with the concavity being continued over the inferior surface of the shaft for articulation with the 1st costal cartilage. The greater horizontal articular surface of the clavicle overlaps the sternocostal surface anteriorly and especially posteriorly; the whole joint surface is covered with fibrocartilage rather than hyaline cartilage.

Joint Capsule and Synovial Membrane

A fibrous capsule surrounds the joint like a sleeve, attaching to the articular margins of both the clavicle and sternum with its inferior part passing between the clavicle and superior surface of the 1st costal cartilage (Fig. 2.5). Except for this inferior part, which is weak,

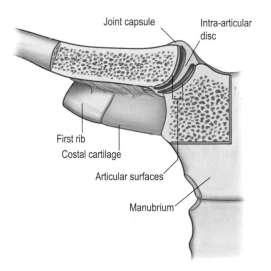

Fig. 2.5 Coronal section (viewed anteriorly) through the right sternoclavicular joint showing the articular surfaces, intra-articular disc and attachments of the joint capsule.

the joint capsule is relatively strong, strengthened anteriorly, posteriorly and superiorly by capsular thickenings (anterior and posterior sternoclavicular and interclavicular ligaments, respectively).

Because there are two separate cavities associated with the joint, there are two synovial membranes. A relatively loose lateral membrane lines the capsule, reflected from the articular margin of the medial end of the clavicle to the margins of the intra-articular disc. Similarly, the medial membrane attaches to the articular margins on the sternum and the margins of the intra-articular disc.

Intra-Articular Structures

A complete, intra-articular, fibrocartilaginous disc divides the joint into two separate synovial cavities (Fig. 2.5). The disc is flat, round and thinner centrally than peripherally: it may occasionally be perforated permitting communication between the two cavities. It is attached at its circumference to the joint capsule, particularly anteriorly and posteriorly. More importantly, however, the disc is firmly attached superiorly and posteriorly to the superior border of the medial end of the clavicle and inferiorly to the 1st costal cartilage near its sternal end (Fig. 2.5). Consequently, as well as providing some cushioning between the articular surfaces from forces transmitted from the upper limb and compensating for the incongruity of the joint surfaces, the disc also has an important ligamentous action. Although mainly fibrocartilaginous, the disc is fibrous or ligamentous at its circumference holding the medial end of the clavicle against the sternum. It prevents the clavicle from moving superomedially along the sloping sternochondral surface under the influence of strong, thrusting forces transmitted from the limb or when the lateral clavicle is depressed, as by a heavy weight carried in the hand.

Ligaments

The joint capsule is strengthened anteriorly, posteriorly and superiorly by the anterior and posterior sternoclavicular and interclavicular ligaments, respectively. In addition, an accessory ligament (costoclavicular ligament) binds the clavicle to the 1st costal cartilage just lateral to the joint.

Anterior Sternoclavicular Ligament

Strong, broad band of fibres attaching to the superior and anterior parts of the medial end of the clavicle, passing obliquely inferomedially to the anterior aspect of the superior aspect of the manubrium sterni (Fig. 2.6); it is reinforced by the tendinous attachment of sternomastoid.

Posterior Sternoclavicular Ligament

Although not as strong as the anterior ligament, it is also a broad band running obliquely inferomedially (Fig. 2.6B). Laterally, the ligament attaches to the superior and posterior parts of the medial end of the clavicle, while medially it is attached to the posterior aspect of the superior aspect of the manubrium sterni. The sternal

attachment of sternohyoid extends across the ligament reinforcing it.

Interclavicular Ligament

This strengthens the capsule superiorly (Fig. 2.6), being formed by fibres attaching to the superior aspect of the sternal end of one clavicle passing across the jugular notch to join similar fibres from the opposite side; some fibres attach to the floor of the jugular notch.

Costoclavicular Ligament

An extremely strong, extracapsular, short, dense band of fibres (Fig. 2.6) attached to the superior surface of the 1st costal cartilage near its lateral end and to a roughened area on the posterior aspect of the inferior surface of the medial end of the clavicle. The ligament has two laminae, usually separated by a bursa, which attach to the anterior and posterior lips of the clavicular rhomboid impression. The anterior fibres run superolaterally, while those of the posterior lamina run superomedially giving the fibres a cruciate arrangement. The direction of fibres in the two laminae is the same as those in the external and internal intercostal muscles of the thorax, respectively.

The costoclavicular ligament essentially limits elevation of the clavicle; however, it is also active in preventing excessive anterior or posterior movement of the medial end of the clavicle. Its position and strength compensate for the weakness of the adjacent inferior part of the joint capsule.

Blood Supply, Lymphatic Drainage and Innervation

The arterial supply to the sternoclavicular joint is from branches of the internal thoracic artery, superior thoracic branch of the axillary artery, clavicular branch of the thoracoacromial trunk and suprascapular artery. Venous drainage is to the axillary and external jugular veins. Lymphatics from the joint pass to the lower deep cervical group of nodes (supraclavicular nodes) and then to the jugular trunk. A few lymphatics may pass to the apical group of axillary nodes (p. 241).

The nerve supply to the joint is by twigs from the medial supraclavicular nerve (C3, C4) and the nerve to subclavius (C5, C6).

Relations

The tendinous attachment of the sternal head of the sternomastoid overlies the joint anteriorly (Fig. 2.7), while

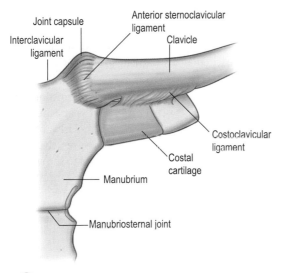

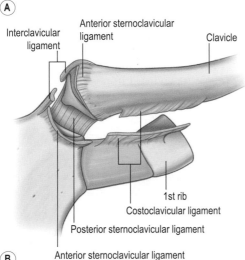

Fig. 2.6 (A) Anterior aspect of the left sternoclavicular joint and associated ligaments. (B) The joint opened out and capsule removed.

posteriorly it is separated from the brachiocephalic vein and common carotid artery on the left and the brachiocephalic trunk on the right by sternohyoid and sternothyroid (Fig. 2.7). The superior vena cava, formed by the union of the two brachiocephalic veins, lies just inferior to the right joint at the inferior border of the 1st costal cartilage (Fig. 2.7).

On the right, the phrenic and vagus nerves lie lateral to the joint as they enter the thorax from the neck; however, on the left, the vagus may pass posterior to the joint as it descends between the common carotid and subclavian arteries.

Stability

Only a limited amount of security for the joint is provided by the shape of the articular surfaces and the surrounding musculature. Joint stability is primarily dependent on the strength and integrity of its ligaments, particularly the costoclavicular ligament. Unfortunately, when dislocation of the joint occurs it is liable to recur.

Movements

Although the articular surfaces do not conform to those of a ball-and-socket joint, the sternoclavicular joint, nevertheless, has three degrees of freedom of movement: elevation and depression; protraction and retraction; axial rotation. The fulcrum of these movements, except axial rotation, is not at the joint centre but through the costoclavicular ligament. Consequently, elevation and depression and protraction and retraction involve gliding between (i) the clavicle and intra-articular disc and (ii) the intra-articular disc and sternum.

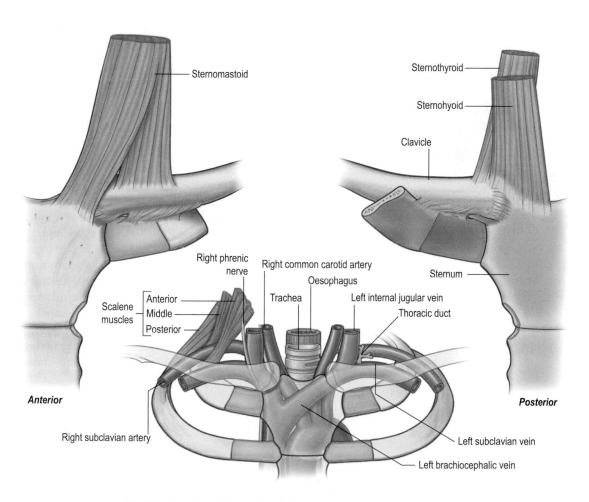

Fig. 2.7 Anterior and posterior relationships of the sternoclavicular joint.

Elevation and Depression

The axis of rotation for elevation and depression runs horizontally and slightly obliquely anterolaterally through the costoclavicular ligament (Fig. 2.8A). It has been suggested that two axes of rotation can be identified for elevation and depression, one for gliding of the clavicle with respect to the disc and the other for gliding of the disc against the sternum; functionally the combined axis of movement runs through the costoclavicular ligament.

Because the axis of movement is not at the centre of the joint, as the lateral end of the clavicle moves in one direction, its medial end moves in the opposite direction (Fig. 2.8A). Consequently, elevation of the lateral end of the clavicle causes the medial end to move inferolaterally. The range of movement of the lateral end of the clavicle is approximately 10 cm for elevation and 3 cm for depression, giving a total angular range of movement of some 60 degrees. Elevation is limited by tension in the costoclavicular ligament and tone in subclavius. Depression of the clavicle, in which the medial end moves superomedially, is limited by tension in the interclavicular ligament and by the intra-articular disc. If these two mechanisms fail, then movement is eventually limited by contact between the clavicle and superior surface of the 1st rib.

Protraction and Retraction

The axis of movement for protraction and retraction lies in a vertical plane running obliquely inferolaterally through the middle part of the costoclavicular ligament (Fig. 2.8B). Again, the ends of the clavicle move in opposite directions because of the position of the fulcrum about which movement takes place (Fig. 2.8B); in protraction of the lateral end, the medial end moves posteriorly and vice versa. In these movements, the medial end of the clavicle and intra-articular disc tend to move as a single unit against the sternum. The range of movement of the lateral end of the clavicle is approximately 5 cm for protraction (anterior movement) and 2 cm for retraction (posterior movement), giving a total angular range of movement of about 35 degrees. Anterior movement is limited by tension in the anterior sternoclavicular and costoclavicular ligaments, while posterior movement is limited by the posterior sternoclavicular and costoclavicular ligaments.

Axial Rotation

While elevation, depression, protraction and retraction of the clavicle are active movements brought about by direct muscle action, axial rotation (Fig. 2.8C) is entirely passive, produced by rotation of the scapula transmitted to the clavicle by the coracoclavicular ligament. Pure axial rotation of the clavicle is not possible in the living; it always accompanies movements in other planes. The axis about which rotation occurs passes through the

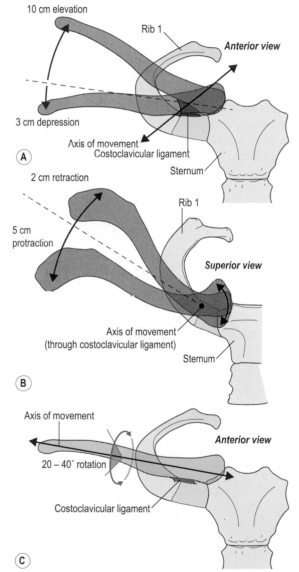

Fig. 2.8 Movements of the clavicle at the sternoclavicular joint during (A) elevation and depression, (B) protraction and retraction (viewed from above) and (C) axial rotation.

centre of the articular surfaces of the sternoclavicular and acromioclavicular joints.

The range of movement is small when the clavicle is in the coronal plane, but increases considerably when the lateral end of the clavicle is carried posteriorly. The degree of axial rotation possible is between 20 and 40 degrees depending on the position of the clavicle.

That there should be any axial rotation possible at the sternoclavicular joint is due to (i) the relative incongruity of the articular surfaces, (ii) the presence of an intra-articular disc and (iii) the relative laxness of the capsular thickenings.

Accessory Movements

With the individual lying supine, downward pressure by the thumb on the medial end of the clavicle produces a posterior gliding of the clavicle against the sternum.

ACROMIOCLAVICULAR JOINT

Plane synovial joint between the clavicle and shoulder blade. The role it plays in movements of the pectoral girdle is considered by some to be greater than that of the sternoclavicular joint, particularly for movements in or close to the sagittal plane.

Palpation

The line of the acromioclavicular joint can be palpated from above by applying a downward pressure to the lateral end of the clavicle.

Articular Surfaces

The articulation is between an oval flat or slightly convex facet on the lateral end of the clavicle and a similarly shaped flat or slightly concave facet on the anteromedial border of the acromion; both surfaces are covered with fibrocartilage. The major axis of both facets runs from anterolateral to posteromedial so that the clavicular facet faces posterolaterally, with that on the acromion facing anteromedially. Consequently, the lateral end of the clavicle tends to override the acromion which, together with the slope of their articulating surfaces, favours displacement of the acromion inferiorly under the clavicle in dislocations.

Joint Capsule and Synovial Membrane

A relatively loose strong fibrous capsule surrounds the joint attaching to the articular margins; its coarse fibres run in parallel fasciculi from one bone to the other. The capsule is thickest and strongest superiorly where it is reinforced by the fibres of trapezius. Some contend that the joint capsule is reinforced by two strong ligaments (superior and inferior acromioclavicular ligaments) passing between the adjacent surfaces of the two bones (Fig. 2.9). In reality, these are no more than capsular thickenings, which show varying degrees of thickening between individuals.

Synovial membrane lines the deep surface of the capsule attaching to the margins of the articular surfaces.

Intra-Articular Structures

A wedge-shaped, fibrocartilaginous intra-articular disc partially divides the cavity in most joints (see Fig. 2.9). When present, it is attached to the superior deep aspect of the capsule extending inferiorly between the two articulating surfaces; only rarely does the disc form a complete partition within the joint. The presence of the articular disc partially compensates for the small degree of incongruity between the joint surfaces.

Ligaments

Apart from the capsular thickenings, the strength and stability of the acromioclavicular joint are provided by the extracapsular coracoclavicular ligament.

Coracoclavicular Ligament

An extremely powerful ligament situated medial to the acromioclavicular joint; it anchors the lateral end of the clavicle to the coracoid process, thus stabilising the

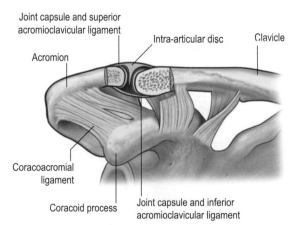

Joint capsule and superior acromioclavicular ligament

Intra-articular disc

Clavicle

Acromion

Coracoacromial ligament

Coracoid process

Joint capsule and inferior acromioclavicular ligament

Fig. 2.9 Coronal section through the right acromioclavicular joint showing the intra-articular disc and capsular attachments.

clavicle with respect to the acromion. It is in two parts, the posteromedial conoid and anterolateral trapezoid ligaments (Fig. 2.10), named according to their shapes. The two parts tend to be continuous with each other posteriorly but are separated anteriorly by a small gap in which is found a synovial bursa.

The apex of the fan-shaped conoid ligament attaches posteromedially to the 'elbow' of the coracoid process (Fig. 2.10). From here, it widens as it passes superiorly, more or less in the coronal plane, to attach to the conoid tubercle on the inferior surface of the clavicle.

The stronger, more powerful trapezoid ligament is a flat quadrilateral band attached inferiorly to a roughened ridge on the superior surface of the coracoid process (Fig. 2.10). Its wider superior surface is attached to the trapezoid line on the inferior surface of the clavicle, which runs anterolaterally from the conoid tubercle. Although the two surfaces of the trapezoid ligament are set obliquely, it lies in a more or less sagittal plane, being more nearly horizontal than vertical.

Because the conoid and trapezoid ligaments lie in different planes, being almost at right angles to each other, and because the posterior edge of the trapezoid ligament is usually in contact with the lateral edge of the conoid ligament, a solid angle facing anteromedially is formed between them.

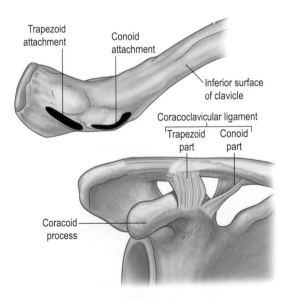

Fig. 2.10 Attachments of the parts of the right coracoclavicular ligament to the coracoid process of the scapula and clavicle.

The two parts of the coracoclavicular ligament are set to restrain opposite movements of the scapula with respect to the clavicle: the conoid ligament limits anterior movement, the trapezoid ligament posterior movement. The importance of these limiting movements is discussed more fully in the section on movements of the pectoral girdle (p. 69). Both ligaments, especially the trapezoid ligament, prevent the acromion from being carried medially under the lateral end of the clavicle when laterally directed forces are applied to the shoulder.

Blood Supply, Lymphatic Drainage and Innervation

The arterial supply to the joint is by branches from the suprascapular branch of the subclavian artery and acromial branch of the thoracoacromial trunk. Venous drainage is to the external jugular and axillary veins. Lymphatic drainage is to the apical group of axillary nodes (p. 241).

The nerve supply to the joint is by twigs from the lateral supraclavicular, lateral pectoral, suprascapular and axillary nerves, from roots C4, C5 and C6.

Relations

The attachments of trapezius and deltoid cover the posterosuperior and anterosuperior aspects of the joint, respectively. Medial to the coracoclavicular ligament, the transverse superior scapular ligament converts the suprascapular notch into a foramen through which passes the suprascapular nerve; the suprascapular vessels usually pass above the transverse ligament. The lateral supraclavicular nerve crosses the clavicle medial to the acromioclavicular joint.

Although not directly associated with the joint, the coracoacromial ligament (p. 87), as its name suggests, is attached to both the coracoid and acromion processes.

Stability

The stability of the joint is essentially provided by the coracoclavicular ligament. Because trapezius and deltoid cross the joint, they also provide some stability during movements at the joint.

Movements

These are entirely passive as there are no muscles connecting the clavicle and shoulder blade which could cause one to move with respect to the other. Muscles which move the shoulder blade cause it to move on the clavicle; indeed, all movements of the shoulder blade involve movement at both the acromioclavicular and sternoclavicular joints. All movements at the acromioclavicular joint, except axial rotation, are gliding movements with the coracoclavicular ligament limiting movement.

The acromioclavicular joint has three degrees of freedom of motion about three axes. Because the joint constantly changes its relation to the trunk, movement is best described in terms of its relation to the shoulder blade rather than with respect to the cardinal axes of the body. The most important function of the joint is to provide an additional range of movement for the pectoral girdle after the range of movement at the sternoclavicular joint has been exhausted.

About a Vertical Axis

This is associated with protraction and retraction of the shoulder blade; the axis of movement passes vertically through the lateral end of the clavicle midway between the joint and coracoclavicular ligament (Fig. 2.11A). As the acromion glides posteriorly with respect to the clavicle, the angle between the clavicle and shoulder blade increases; similarly, as the acromion glides anteriorly the angle decreases (Fig. 2.11A). Posterior movement of the acromion is checked by the anterior joint capsule and actively limited by the trapezoid ligament as it becomes stretched. Anterior movement is checked by the posterior joint capsule and limited by the conoid ligament. Towards the end of the anterior movement of the acromion, the trapezoid ligament may also be put under tension and, therefore, help to limit the movement. Compensatory movements of the clavicle at the sternoclavicular joint accompany those at the acromioclavicular joint.

About a Sagittal Axis

Movement about a sagittal axis (Fig. 2.11B) occurs when the shoulder blade is elevated or depressed with the total range of movement being no more than 15 degrees. Elevation is limited by tension in both parts of the coracoclavicular ligament, with the conoid ligament coming into play first; depression is checked by the coracoid process coming into contact with the inferior surface of the clavicle.

Axial Rotation

This is associated with medial and lateral rotation of the shoulder blade (when the glenoid fossa faces inferiorly

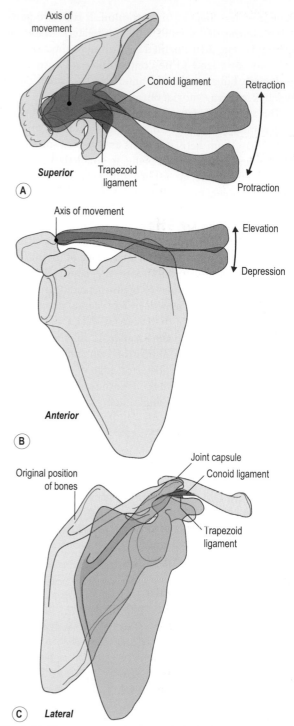

Fig. 2.11 Movements at the acromioclavicular joint during (A) protraction/retraction of the scapula about a vertical axis, (B) elevation/depression of the scapula about a sagittal axis and (C) axial rotation of the scapula.

or superiorly, respectively). The range of rotation of the shoulder blade with respect to the clavicle is approximately 30 degrees and occurs about an axis passing through the conoid ligament and acromioclavicular joint (Fig. 2.11C). It allows the flexed arm to be fully elevated. Restraints to rotation are provided by both parts of the coracoclavicular ligament.

Accessory Movements

With the individual lying supine, downward pressure applied with the thumb on the lateral end of the clavicle causes it to glide posteriorly against the acromion.

MOVEMENTS OF THE PECTORAL (SHOULDER) GIRDLE

The pectoral girdle provides the link between the upper limb and axial skeleton via the shoulder (glenohumeral) and sternoclavicular joints, respectively, serving to increase the range of movement of the shoulder joint by changing the relative position of the glenoid fossa with respect to the chest wall. During movement, the glenoid fossa travels in an arc of a circle whose radius is the clavicle; however, the medial border of the scapula, held against the chest wall, travels in a curve of shorter radius. Consequently, the relative positions of the clavicle and shoulder blade must be capable of changing, this occurs at the acromioclavicular joint; a rigid union between the clavicle and shoulder blade would severely limit mobility of the upper limb.

In all movements, the clavicle acts as a strut holding the shoulder away from the trunk securing greater freedom of movement of the upper limb. It should be remembered that movements of the pectoral girdle accompany virtually all movements of the shoulder joint (p. 93).

The flattened triangular scapula provides attachment for many muscles, some of which anchor the pectoral girdle to the thorax while others control the position of the upper limb. Because of the connections (both muscular and ligamentous) between the scapula and clavicle, movements of the pectoral girdle, either independently or in association with the upper limb, means that both are always involved. The position and movement of the scapula are determined by activity of the muscles attached to it. An individual muscle, when acting in concert with combinations of other muscles, will be involved in producing different movements of the pectoral girdle. Movements between the scapula and thorax are allowed because the fascia covering adjacent layers of muscles facilitates gliding and sliding movements.

Movements of the shoulder girdle are described as taking place from the anatomical position, where the scapula lies obliquely over the 2nd to 7th ribs on the posterior thoracic wall with the coracoid process pointing anteriorly. The movements are:

Retraction and Protraction

Retraction is medial movement of the scapula, whilst maintaining its vertical position, such that its medial border approaches the vertebral column, as in bracing the shoulder; the glenoid fossa comes to face more laterally (Fig. 2.12A and B). Protraction is lateral movement of the scapula anteriorly around the chest wall, as in rounding the shoulders; there may be some associated lateral rotation; the glenoid fossa comes to face more directly anteriorly (Fig. 2.12A and B).

These extreme positions of the scapula form a solid angle of 40–45 degrees with the coronal plane (Fig. 2.12A). Furthermore, the angle between the clavicle and shoulder blade decreases to approximately 60 degrees on full lateral movement of the shoulder blade, increasing to approximately 70 degrees on full medial movement (Fig. 2.12A). The total range of linear translation of the shoulder blade around the chest wall is about 15 cm.

Elevation and Depression

In elevation the pectoral girdle is lifted superiorly as in shrugging the shoulders; in depression, it is pulled inferiorly (Fig. 2.12C).

Elevation and depression of the shoulder blade has a linear range of some 10–12 cm; it is usually accompanied by some rotation so that, in elevation, the glenoid fossa comes to face increasingly superiorly and in depression the fossa points increasingly inferiorly.

Lateral (Forward) and Medial (Backward) Rotation of the Scapula

These are complex movement of the pectoral girdle. In lateral rotation, the inferior angle of the scapula moves laterally around the chest wall, while the strut-like clavicle results in a concomitant superior movement of the scapula causing the glenoid fossa to be turned increasingly superiorly (Fig. 2.12D). Medial rotation returns

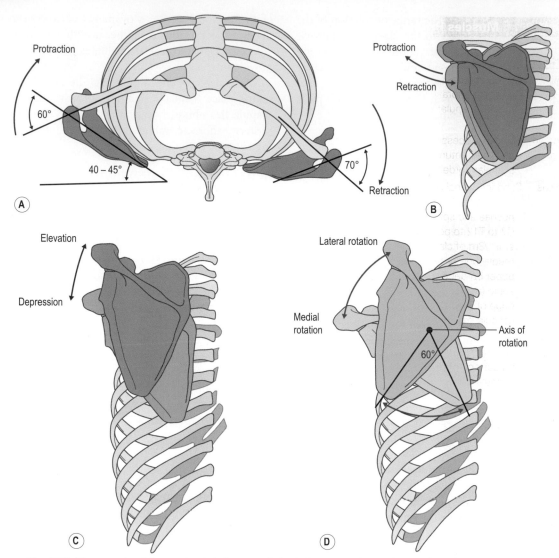

Fig. 2.12 Movements of the pectoral girdle as a whole during protraction and retraction, viewed from above (A) and behind (B); (C) elevation and depression; and (D) axial rotation.

the scapula to its resting position from lateral rotation (Fig. 2.12D).

Rotation of the shoulder blade against the chest wall does so about an axis perpendicular to the plane of the scapula, situated a little below the spine close to the superomedial angle. The total range of angular rotation of the scapula amounts to 60 degrees, involving displacement of the inferior angle of the scapula some 10–12 cm and of the superolateral angle some 5–6 cm.

Abduction and/or flexion of the arm causes the clavicle to rotate about its long axis so that its superior surface becomes increasingly directed posteriorly. Towards the end of rotation of the scapula against the clavicle, the coracoclavicular ligament becomes taut transmitting the rotating force to the clavicle, accounting for scapular rotation on the chest wall. Any impairment to clavicular rotation at either the sternoclavicular or acromioclavicular joints interferes with the free movement of the shoulder blade and upper limb as a whole.

TABLE 2.1 Muscles Producing Movement of and Stabilising the Pectoral Girdle

Muscle	Attachments	Action	Innervation (root value)
Rhomboid major	Spinous processes of T2 to T5 and adjacent supraspinous ligament to medial scapular border below root of spine	Retraction and medial rotation of scapula: important stabiliser when other muscle groups are active	Dorsal scapular nerve (C5)
Rhomboid minor	Spinous processes of C7 and T1, and ligamentum nuchae to medial scapular border near root of spine	Retraction and medial rotation of scapula: important stabiliser when other muscle groups are active	Dorsal scapular nerve (C5)
Trapezius	Superior nuchal line and external occipital protuberance, ligamentum nuchae and spinous processes of C7 to T12 to posterior border of lateral 1/3rd of clavicle (upper fibres), medial border of acromion and upper border of crest of scapular spine (middle fibres), and inferior edge of medial end of spine of scapula (lower fibres)	Stabilises scapula during movements of upper limb: upper fibres elevate pectoral girdle to maintain the level of the shoulders against the effects of gravity or when carrying a weight, they can also laterally flex neck and with the lower fibres produce lateral rotation of scapula; middle fibres retract pectoral girdle (may be aided by upper and lower fibres); lower fibres pull down medial part of scapula, especially against resistance	Motor, spinal part of the accessory nerve (XI): sensory, C3 and C4
Serratus anterior	Lateral surfaces of upper 8/9 ribs and intervening fascia to costal surface of medial border of scapula	Stabilises scapula during movements of upper limb by holding medial border against chest wall; protraction of pectoral girdle (involved in all thrusting, pushing and punching movements); with upper fibres of trapezius the lower digitations rotate scapula laterally	Long thoracic nerve (C5, C6, C7)
Pectoralis minor	Lateral surfaces of 3rd, 4th and 5th ribs to coracoid process	Pulls coracoid process (and scapula) anteriorly and inferiorly; helps transfer weight of trunk to upper limbs when leaning on hands; with scapula fixed it can act as an accessory muscle of respiration	Medial pectoral nerve (C6, C7, C8)
Levator scapulae	Transverse processes of C1 to C3/C4 to medial border of scapula above root of spine	Elevation and retraction of pectoral girdle; also resists inferior movement when carrying a load; with trapezius both sides extend the neck	Dorsal scapular nerve (C5) and directly from C3 and C4
Subclavius	1st rib near its junction with costal cartilage to inferior surface of clavicle	Steadies clavicle against sternum during movements of pectoral girdle	Nerve to subclavius (C5, C6)

It is important to remember that movements of the pectoral girdle are not pure movements; all are composite movements involving some degree of each.

The major muscles producing movements of the pectoral girdle are given in Table 2.1. Further details of each muscle can be found in following sections.

BIOMECHANICS

Stresses on the Clavicle

The clavicle is subjected to both compression and tension stresses, which under normal conditions are absorbed within it; these stresses only become apparent when the integrity of the pectoral girdle is compromised (fracture, dislocation, muscular imbalance). Unlike the pelvic girdle, it is not a complete bony ring, the intrinsic stresses require the cooperation of muscles attached to it in order to maintain equilibrium.

A compressive stress along the length of the clavicle directed medially towards the sternoclavicular joint is produced by the action of trapezius and pectoralis minor as they pull the clavicle towards the sternum. Forces transmitted medially from the upper limb to the glenoid fossa are transmitted from the scapula to the clavicle by the trapezoid ligament and from the clavicle to the 1st rib by the costoclavicular ligament. Consequently, falling on an outstretched hand or elbow puts little or no strain on the joints at either end of the clavicle. If the clavicle fractures as a result, it does so between these two ligaments with the fragments tending to override one another. Compressive stresses are increased when lying on the side.

Tension stresses within the clavicle are produced, under the action of deltoid, when the upper limb is abducted; hanging and swinging forwards by the arms increases these tensile stresses. If sufficiently large, they may lead to some discontinuity of the pectoral girdle; however, joint dislocation is much more likely to occur than a fracture.

A rotational force transmitted through the scapula to the clavicle tends to damage the acromioclavicular and/ or sternoclavicular joints and their associated ligaments rather than causing the clavicle to fracture. Downward forces applied to the lateral end of the clavicle create bending stresses within it, which, if sufficiently large or if the clavicle comes into contact with the coracoid process, may lead to it fracturing.

MUSCLES RETRACTING THE PECTORAL (SHOULDER) GIRDLE

Rhomboid minor
Rhomboid major
Trapezius

Rhomboid Minor

Small quadrilateral muscle (Fig. 2.13) whose fibres run obliquely inferolaterally from the spinous processes

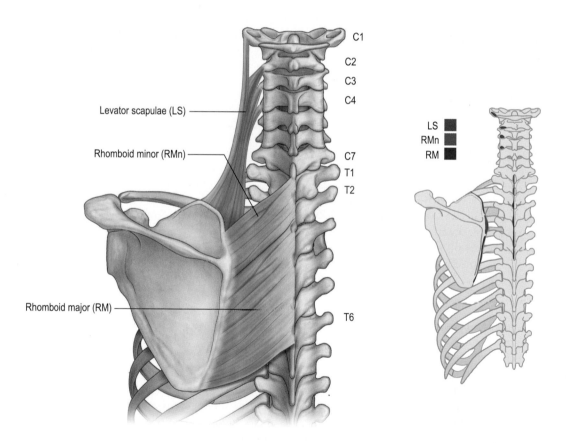

Fig. 2.13 Posterior aspect of the cervical and upper thoracic vertebrae and left scapula showing the attachments of levator scapulae, rhomboid minor and rhomboid major. *LS*, Levator scapulae; *RMn*, rhomboid minor; *RM*, rhomboid major.

of C7 and T1, intervening supraspinous ligament and inferior part of the ligamentum nuchae to attach to the medial border of the smooth triangular area at the base of the spine of the scapula.

Rhomboid Major

Larger than rhomboid minor, rhomboid major may be continuous with it (Fig. 2.13); it arises by tendinous slips from the spinous processes of T2 to T5 and intervening supraspinous ligament. The muscle fibres run obliquely inferolaterally to attach to the medial border of the scapula between the base of the spine and inferior angle.

Both rhomboids lie superficial to the long back muscles, being themselves covered by trapezius, except for the lower border of rhomboid major which forms the floor of the 'triangle of auscultation'.

Innervation

Both rhomboids are supplied by the dorsal scapular nerve (root value C5).

Action

Acting principally to retract the scapula, both muscles are also active in medial rotation of the pectoral girdle. In addition, they act as important stabilisers of the scapula when other muscle groups are active.

Palpation

With the individual's hand placed in the small of the back (to relax trapezius), the rhomboids can be palpated through trapezius when the hand is moved posteriorly. Contraction of the rhomboids can be felt (and occasionally seen) between the medial border of the scapula and vertebral column.

Trapezius

Large, flat triangular sheet of muscle extending from the skull and vertebral column medially to the pectoral girdle laterally (Fig. 2.14). It is the most superficial muscle in the upper trunk and, with its fellow of the opposite side, it forms a trapezium, hence its name.

The medial attachment runs from the medial one-third of the superior nuchal line and external occipital protuberance of the occipital bone, ligamentum nuchae and spinous processes of C7 to T12 and intervening supraspinous ligaments. The majority of this attachment is by direct muscular slips; however, a triangular

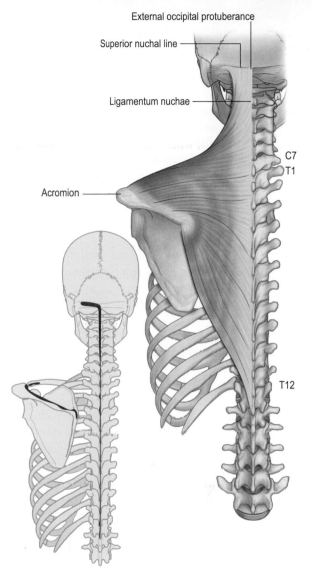

Fig. 2.14 Posterior aspect of the skull, vertebral column and left scapula showing the position and attachments of trapezius.

aponeurosis exists between C6 and T3 corresponding to a hollow seen in the living.

From this extensive medial attachment, there is a continuous line of attachment to the clavicle and scapula: the upper fibres run inferolaterally, the middle fibres almost horizontally and the lower fibres superolaterally. The upper fibres descend to the posterior border of the lateral one-third of the clavicle, the middle fibres to the medial border of the acromion and superior border of the crest of the spine of the scapula, separated from the smooth area on the medial part of the spine by a small bursa, while the lower fibres converge to a tendon attaching to the tubercle on the inferior edge at the medial end of the spine of the scapula.

The superior free margin of trapezius forms the posterior border of the posterior triangle of the neck, while the inferior free border forms the medial boundary of the triangle of auscultation. (The triangle of auscultation is an area on the chest wall free of bony obstruction by the scapula and thinly covered by muscle; its other boundaries are the superior border of latissimus dorsi inferiorly and the medial border of the scapula laterally.)

Innervation

The motor supply is via the spinal part of the accessory nerve (XI) which enters it from the posterior triangle. It also receives sensory fibres from the ventral rami of C3 and C4 via the cervical plexus; skin over trapezius is supplied by the dorsal rami of C3 to T12.

Action

Trapezius has an important function in stabilising the scapula during movements of the upper limb. The middle horizontal fibres retract the scapula towards the midline, which may be aided by the upper and lower fibres contracting together to produce a 'resolved' force towards the midline. The upper fibres elevate the pectoral girdle and maintain the level of the shoulders against the effect of gravity or when a weight is carried in the hand. When both left and right muscles contract, they can extend the neck, but when acting individually, the upper fibres produce lateral flexion/bending of the neck. The lower fibres pull down the medial part of the scapula lowering the shoulder, especially against resistance (using the arms to get out of a chair). Together, the upper and lower fibres produce lateral rotation of the scapula about a point towards the base of the spine. Trapezius is, therefore, important in the overall function of the upper limb as its action increases the range of movement possible.

Paralysis of trapezius, particularly its upper part, results in the scapula moving anteriorly around the chest wall with the inferior angle moving medially. The usually smooth curve of its superior border between the occiput and acromion may become markedly angulated.

Palpation

To demonstrate and palpate all three parts of trapezius, the individual should abduct both arms to 90 degrees, flex the elbows to 90 degrees and then rotate them laterally so that the fingers are pointing superiorly. In this position, the three sets of fibres can be readily palpated; in lean individuals, contraction of the various parts of the muscle can be seen. Contraction of the lower fibres can be further enhanced by asking the individual to clasp their hands together above the head and pull hard.

Soft tissue techniques are often applied to the upper muscular fibres of trapezius in the presence of muscle spasm secondary to neck pain with the aim of inducing relaxation. Deep transverse frictions can also be applied to the tendinous attachment of trapezius on the superior nuchal line when this is the site of a lesion causing pain in the neck or occipital region.

MUSCLES PROTRACTING THE PECTORAL (SHOULDER) GIRDLE

Serratus anterior
Pectoralis minor

Serratus Anterior

Large, flat, sheet of muscle covering the lateral aspect of the thorax situated between the ribs and scapula (Fig. 2.15). To facilitate free movement of the scapula loose fascia exists between its deep surface and the ribs or intercostal fascia, as well as between its superficial surface and subscapularis. Serratus anterior forms the medial wall of the axilla and is partly covered by the breast inferolaterally. The upper digitations lie behind the clavicle, while latissimus dorsi crosses its inferior border.

Serratus anterior attaches by fleshy digitations to the lateral surfaces of the upper eight or nine ribs and intervening intercostal fascia just anterior to the midaxillary line. The upper digitation arises from the 1st and 2nd ribs while the remaining digitations arise from a single rib. The lower four digitations interdigitate with the costal attachment of external oblique of the abdomen.

From this extensive attachment, the muscle fibres run posteriorly to attach to the costal surface of the medial border of the scapula between the superior and inferior angles. However, the digitations are not evenly distributed in their attachment; the 1st passes almost horizontally to the superior angle, while the lower four condense attaching to the inferior angle with the intervening digitations spread along the medial border.

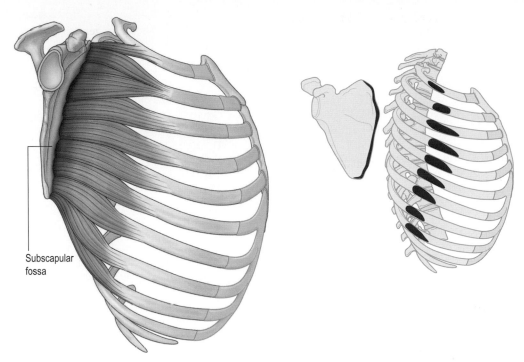

Fig. 2.15 Lateral thoracic wall with the right scapula lifted posteriorly showing the position and attachments of serratus anterior.

Innervation

By the long thoracic nerve (root value C5, C6 and C7), with the first two digitations supplied by C5, the next two by C6 and the remaining four by C7; the nerve enters the muscle on its superficial aspect. Skin over the accessible parts of the muscle is supplied by nerves with root values T3 to T7.

Action

Serratus anterior is a major protractor of the pectoral girdle and, as such, is involved in all thrusting, pushing and punching movements where the scapula is driven forwards carrying the upper limb with it. (Note the massive development of this muscle in boxers.)

It plays a vital role in stabilising the scapula during movements of the upper limb and contracts strongly to hold the medial border of the scapula against the chest wall when the arm is flexed or when a weight is carried in front of the body. Failure to perform this action, as when paralysed, results in 'winging' of the scapula in which the medial border stands away from the chest wall, severely affecting the function and mobility of the upper limb.

The lower digitations of the muscle work with trapezius to rotate the scapula laterally, so that the glenoid fossa faces superomedially. When paralysed, loss of the rotating action of serratus anterior means that the upper limb cannot be abducted by more than approximately 90 degrees, seriously limiting the functional capacity of the upper limb. There is some controversy as to whether serratus anterior acts as an accessory muscle of inspiration during respiratory distress. The line of action of the muscle fibres, except perhaps for the first two digitations and maybe the last, are not directed to cause elevation of the ribs; indeed, they are more likely to cause depression of the ribs.

Palpation

In a muscular individual, the digitations of serratus anterior can be felt and often seen running anteriorly in the region of the midaxillary line, especially when performing 'press-ups'.

Pectoralis Minor

Thin, flat, triangular muscle is situated on the anterior chest wall deep to pectoralis major (Fig. 2.16). Inferiorly,

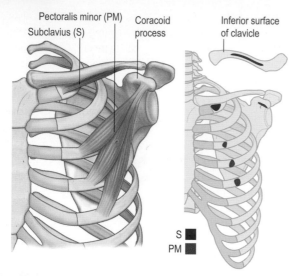

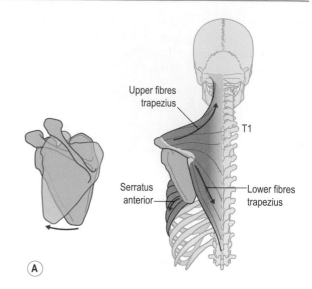

Fig. 2.16 Anterior aspect of the thorax, left clavicle and scapula showing the position and attachments of subclavius and pectoralis minor.

it attaches to the lateral surfaces of the 3rd, 4th and 5th ribs, close to their costal cartilages, and the intervening intercostal fascia; there may be additional attachments to the 2nd or 6th rib, or more rarely to both. The fibres converge to a short, flat tendon as they pass superolaterally to attach to the superior surface and medial border of the coracoid process of the scapula.

Innervation

By the medial pectoral nerve, which pierces it; however, within the axilla, the medial and lateral pectoral nerves communicate, so that pectoralis minor is supplied by both nerves; the segmental supply is by nerve roots C6, C7 and C8.

Action

When pectoralis minor exerts a strong pull on the coracoid process, the scapula can be pulled anteriorly and inferiorly during pushing and punching movements. When leaning on the hands, it helps to transfer the weight of the trunk to the upper limb. Its attachment to the coracoid process allows it to help produce medial rotation of the scapula against resistance (Fig. 2.17B). With the scapula and upper limb fixed, pectoralis minor may be used as an accessory muscle of inspiration during respiratory distress.

Palpation

Lying deep to the bulk of pectoralis major, contraction of pectoralis minor is difficult to palpate.

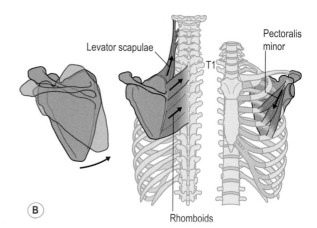

Fig. 2.17 Movement of the scapula shown diagrammatically indicating the direction of pull of the principle muscles in (A) lateral (forward) rotation and (B) medial (backward) rotation.

MUSCLES ELEVATING THE PECTORAL (SHOULDER) GIRDLE

Trapezius (upper fibres) (p. 73)
Levator scapulae

Levator Scapulae

Situated in the posterior part of the neck, the superior part of levator scapulae lies deep to sternomastoid and the inferior part deep to trapezius (Fig. 2.13); its middle portion forms part of the floor of the posterior triangle. It lies superficial to the extensor muscles of the neck and attaches by tendinous slips to the transverse processes of the upper three or four cervical vertebrae (attaching to the posterior tubercles of the lower two) posterior to the attachment of scalenus medius. From here, the fibres run inferolaterally to attach to the medial margin of the scapula between the superior angle and base of the spine.

Innervation

Partly from the dorsal scapular nerve (C5) and directly from the ventral rami of C3 and C4.

Action

Working with trapezius, levator scapulae can produce elevation and retraction of the pectoral girdle or resist its inferior movement, as when carrying a load in the hand. In addition, when working with trapezius, contraction of both sides produces extension of the neck, while one side produces lateral flexion/bending of the neck. Levator scapulae also helps stabilise the scapula and is active in producing medial scapular rotation.

Palpation

The muscle can be palpated when trapezius is not contracting (similar to the rhomboids) with the individual erect and the hands in the small of the back. Levator scapulae can be felt anterior to trapezius in the posterolateral part of the neck when the individual's hand is moved posteriorly with the elbow flexed.

MUSCLES DEPRESSING THE PECTORAL (SHOULDER) GIRDLE

Trapezius (lower fibres) (p. 73)
Pectoralis minor (p. 75)

From the position of elevation in the anatomical position, depression is usually produced by gravity controlled by eccentric contraction of the elevators. However, in situations requiring inferior movement of the pectoral girdle against resistance (using crutches, pushing up from a chair) trapezius and pectoralis minor can produce active depression.

MUSCLES LATERALLY ROTATING THE SCAPULA

Trapezius (p. 73)
Serratus anterior (p. 74)

As can be seen in Figs 2.14 and 2.15, both muscles are well positioned to pull the inferior angle of the scapula laterally around the thoracic wall. The clavicle, acting as a strut, restricts movement at the acromion, so that the overall effect of their action is to elevate the acromion and move the inferior angle laterally, enabling the glenoid fossa to face more directly superiorly. This movement of the pectoral girdle is extremely important for increasing the range of movement possible, particularly in terms of abduction and flexion of the upper limb at the shoulder joint (p. 93).

Trapezius contributes to the rotation by contraction of its upper fibres, which lift the lateral end of the clavicle and acromion superiorly, while at the same time its lower fibres pull inferiorly on the medial end of the spine of the scapula.

Serratus anterior, the more important of the muscles in this movement, pulls the inferior angle of the scapula, where the majority of its muscle fibres attach, laterally around the chest wall. The notional axis about which this rotation takes place is just below the spine of the scapula towards the base. The resultant movements are shown in Fig. 2.17.

MUSCLES MEDIALLY ROTATING THE SCAPULA

Rhomboid major (p. 73)
Rhomboid minor (p. 72)
Pectoralis minor (p. 75)
Levator scapulae (p. 76)

Movement of the inferior angle of the scapula towards the vertebral column is frequently produced by the action of gravity, controlled by the eccentric contraction of trapezius and serratus anterior. However, the muscles contract strongly if the pectoral girdle is medially rotated against resistance, as when moving the weight of the body from a position of hanging from a beam to a full chin-up. The notional axis of rotation is just below the spine of the scapula, towards the base. Pectoralis minor exerts an inferior pull on the lateral side of this axis via its attachment to the coracoid process, while the rhomboids and levator scapulae pull superiorly on the medial side; the resultant movements are shown in Fig. 2.17. Details of the movements of the individual joints of the pectoral girdle can be found on pages 64 and 67.

MUSCLES STABILISING THE CLAVICLE

Subclavius

Subclavius

Small muscle lying entirely inferior to the clavicle deep to pectoralis major (see Fig. 2.16); the fleshy belly attaches to the floor of the subclavian groove on the inferior surface of the clavicle. The fibres converge and pass medially, becoming tendinous, attaching to the 1st rib near its junction with the costal cartilage.

Innervation

By the nerve to subclavius (root value C5, C6) from the upper trunk of the brachial plexus.

Action

The principal action of subclavius is to steady the clavicle by pulling it towards the disc of the sternoclavicular joint and sternum during movements of the pectoral girdle. This action tends to depress the lateral end of the clavicle. Paralysis of subclavius has no demonstrable effect.

Section Summary

Scapula
- Triangular bone located on the posterolateral aspect of the thorax.
- Has superior, lateral and inferior angles; medial, lateral and superior borders; posterior spine; laterally projecting acromion; and anteriorly projecting coracoid process.
- Articulates with clavicle at acromion forming acromioclavicular joint; head of the humerus at glenoid fossa forming the shoulder (glenohumeral) joint.

Clavicle
- Curved bone: medially convex anteriorly, laterally concave anteriorly.
- Has smooth superior surface; roughened inferior surface; and expanded medial and flattened lateral ends.
- Articulates with acromion of scapula laterally forming acromioclavicular joint; sternum medially forming sternoclavicular joint.

Sternoclavicular Joint

Type	Saddle-shaped synovial, but functionally a ball-and-socket joint
Articular surfaces	Medial end of clavicle, clavicular notch of sternum and 1st costal cartilage; a complete intra-articular disc divides the joint into two separate compartments
Capsule	Complete fibrous capsule
Ligaments	Anterior and posterior sternoclavicular; interclavicular; costoclavicular
Stability	Mainly provided by costoclavicular ligament
Movements	Active elevation/depression and protraction/retraction; passive axial rotation

Acromioclavicular Joint

Type	Synovial plane joint
Articular surfaces	Lateral end of clavicle and acromion of scapula; an incomplete intra-articular disc is often present between the two bones
Capsule	Fibrous capsule attached to articular margins
Ligaments	Coracoclavicular (conoid and trapezoid parts)
Stability	Mainly provided by coracoclavicular ligament
Movements	Passive gliding during movements of pectoral girdle

Movements at Pectoral (Shoulder) Girdle

The pectoral (shoulder) girdle is capable of a range of independent movements produced by the following muscles:

Movement	Muscles (root value of nerve supply)
Retraction	Rhomboid major (C5)
	Rhomboid minor (C5)
	Trapezius (CN XI)
Protraction	Serratus anterior (C5, C6, C7)
	Pectoralis minor (C6, C7, C8)
Elevation	Trapezius (upper fibres) (CN XI)
	Levator scapulae (C3, C4, C5)
Depression	Pectoralis minor (C6, C7, C8)
	Trapezius (lower fibres) (CN XI)
Lateral rotation	Trapezius (CN XI)
	Serratus anterior (C5, C6, C7)
Medial rotation	Rhomboid major (C5)
	Rhomboid minor (C5)
	Levator scapulae (C3, C4, C5)
	Pectoralis minor (C6, C7, C8)

- It is important to consider the effect of gravity or resistance on these movements and muscle work; the elevators may work concentrically against gravity or resistance to raise the pectoral girdle, but eccentrically to lower it back down.
- The muscles, especially serratus anterior, act to hold the scapula against the thorax.
- Movements of the pectoral girdle increase the range of movement of the upper limb by combining with that available at the shoulder joint during functional activities.

❓ SELF-ASSESSMENT QUESTIONS

1. Which muscle attaches to the costal surface of the medial border of the scapula?
2. Which of the following muscles does NOT attach to the coracoid process? A, coracobrachialis; B, pectoralis major; C, pectoralis minor; D, biceps brachii
3. Which nerve, including its root value, supplies serratus anterior?
4. Which structures primarily stabilises the acromioclavicular joint?
5. Which muscles lies anterior to the sternoclavicular joint?
6. Which structure(s) act(s) as the fulcrum of movement at the sternoclavicular joint during elevation/depression and protraction/retraction?
7. Which structure unites the medial ends of the right and left clavicles?
8. What are the attachments of the intra-articular disc within the sternoclavicular joint?
9. What is the function/role of the clavicle?
10. Which muscles are responsible for producing medial rotation of the scapula?
11. What type of joint is the acromioclavicular joint?
12. Approximately how much rotation is there of the inferior angle of the scapula between full medial and full lateral rotation?
13. In medial and lateral rotation of the scapula, where is the axis of rotation located?
14. By approximately how much does the scapula move around the chest wall during protraction?
15. Which muscle stabilises the clavicle?
16. What is the nerve supply, including root value, of levator scapulae?
17. Which muscle acts principally to keep the scapula against the chest wall?
18. What are the principal functions of the pectoral girdle?

▌SHOULDER

LEARNING OUTCOMES

By the end of the section, you should be able to:
1. Identify, palpate and examine the scapula and proximal humerus
2. Describe the bones, joints and muscles of the shoulder region
3. Describe and explain the movements possible, and their restraints, at the shoulder joint
4. Locate, palpate and examine the muscles associated with the shoulder and describe their attachments, action and innervation
5. Examine and assess movements of the shoulder joint
6. Appreciate the influence of pathology and/or trauma on the function of the shoulder
7. Describe the boundaries and contents of the axilla

INTRODUCTION

The shoulder (glenohumeral) joint is the articulation between the head of the humerus and glenoid fossa of the scapula (Fig. 2.18). The intracapsular presence of the epiphyseal line between the ventral coracoid and dorsal scapula in the upper part of the glenoid fossa facilitates adjustments of the joint surface during the growth of the bone. Similar arrangements are also to be found in the elbow and hip joints.

It is a ball-and-socket synovial joint with the head of the humerus forming the ball and glenoid fossa the socket; freedom of movement at the joint has been developed at the expense of stability. Mobility of the upper limb is partly due to changes in the shoulder joint which have occurred with freeing the upper limbs from locomotor activity, and partly due to the mobility of the pectoral girdle linking the upper limb to the trunk. Comparison of the shoulder and hip joints, equivalent joints in the upper and lower limbs, together with their mode of attachment to the axial skeleton, reveals significant and important differences between them, even though their basic features are similar.

In the coronal plane, the axis of the head and neck of the humerus forms an angle of 135–140 degrees (angle of inclination) with the long axis of the shaft (Fig. 2.19A). Because of this angulation, the centre of the humeral head lies about 1 cm medial to the long axis of the humerus. Although the anatomical and mechanical axes of the humerus do not exactly coincide, unlike in the femur (p. 287), they both lie inside the bone (Fig. 2.19A). Consequently, the action of muscle groups producing movement at the shoulder joint, especially medial and lateral rotation, is more easily understood.

As well as being set at an angle to the shaft of the humerus, the axis of the head and neck is rotated posteriorly with respect to the shaft 30–40 degrees (angle of retroversion) (Fig. 2.19B); the extent of retroversion is said to vary both with age and race. It is suggested that this angle has increased with the attainment of bipedalism, in which there has also been flattening of the thoracic cage anteroposteriorly and a posterior displacement of the scapula, the result being that, as the glenoid fossa came to be directed more laterally, the head and

Anteroposterior radiograph of right shoulder

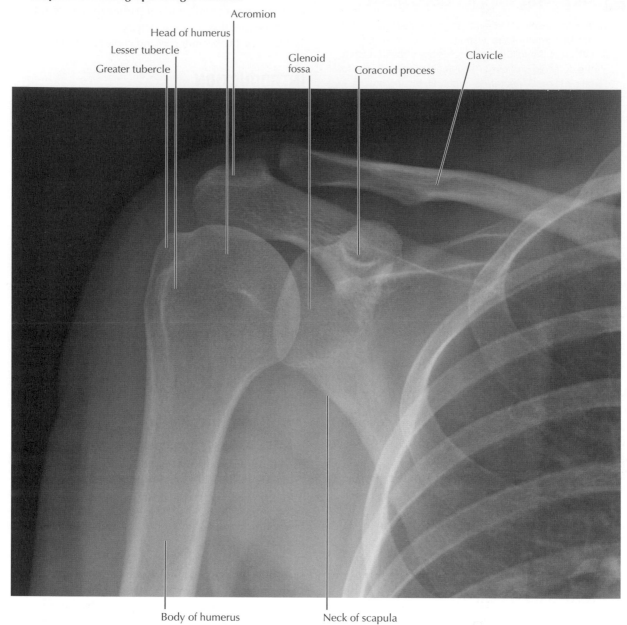

Fig. 2.18 Anteroposterior radiograph of the right shoulder. (From Frank, H.N., 2022. Netter Atlas of Human Anatomy: Classic Regional Approach. Elsevier.)

neck of the humerus became more twisted in an attempt to maintain maximum joint contact between the articulating surfaces. Structurally, this adaptation was not entirely successful, which to some extent was fortuitous because, in humans, the use of the upper limb gradually changed from one of support to one of manipulation.

Fascia Around the Shoulder

In the shoulder region, the deep fascia is extremely strong over infraspinatus and teres minor, firmly attaching to the medial and lateral borders of the scapula. Superiorly, a sheath is formed for deltoid, which attaches to the clavicle, acromion and spine of the scapula.

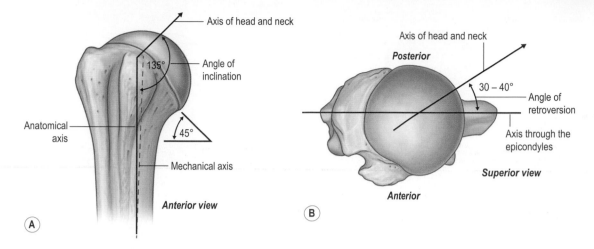

Fig. 2.19 Proximal end of the humerus viewed anteriorly (A) and from above (B) showing the angles of inclination and retroversion.

The deep fascia covering pectoralis major attaches superiorly to the clavicle and may be traced, via the clavicle, into the neck; inferiorly it is continuous with the fascia of the anterior abdominal wall. Medially, the deep fascia is firmly attached to the sternum, while laterally it becomes thickened as the axillary fascia forming the floor of the axilla; further laterally it becomes continuous with the deep fascia of the arm.

Deep to pectoralis major is the clavipectoral fascia, which attaches medially to the 1st costal cartilage and passes to the coracoid process and coracoclavicular ligament laterally. The clavipectoral fascia splits to surround subclavius superiorly to attach to the inferior surface of the clavicle; it also splits to enclose pectoralis minor inferiorly. An extension of the fascia from the lateral border of pectoralis minor passes into the axilla attaching to the axillary floor (suspensory ligament of the axilla). The deep surface of the clavipectoral fascia is connected to the axillary sheath surrounding the axillary vessels and brachial plexus.

In the arm, the deep fascia forms an investing layer around the muscles. At the elbow, it attaches to the medial and lateral epicondyles of the humerus and the olecranon process, becoming continuous with the deep fascia of the forearm. Two intermuscular septa arise from the deep surface of this investing layer attaching to the supracondylar ridges of the humerus: the medial and lateral intermuscular septa are found only in the distal half of the arm. Besides separating the arm into flexor and extensor compartments, the septa also give attachment to muscles in each compartment; of the two, the medial intermuscular septum is the stronger.

SCAPULA

Details of the scapula can be found on page 59.

HUMERUS

Largest bone in the upper limb (Fig. 2.20), the humerus is a typical long bone with a shaft (body) and proximal and distal extremities (epiphyses); proximally, it articulates with the glenoid fossa of the scapula forming the shoulder (glenohumeral) joint and distally with the radius and ulna forming the elbow joint.

Proximally, the major feature is the almost hemispherical head with its smooth, rounded, articular surface facing posterosuperomedially; it is considerably larger than the socket formed by the glenoid fossa. The head is joined to the proximal end of the shaft by the anatomical neck, a slightly constricted region encircling the bone at the articular margin, separating it from the greater and lesser tubercles.

Adjacent to the head is a prominence (greater tubercle) on the proximal lateral part of the bone, marked by three distinct impressions for muscular attachment; it merges with the shaft inferiorly. The greater tubercle projects laterally past the margin of the acromion, being the most lateral bony point at the shoulder.

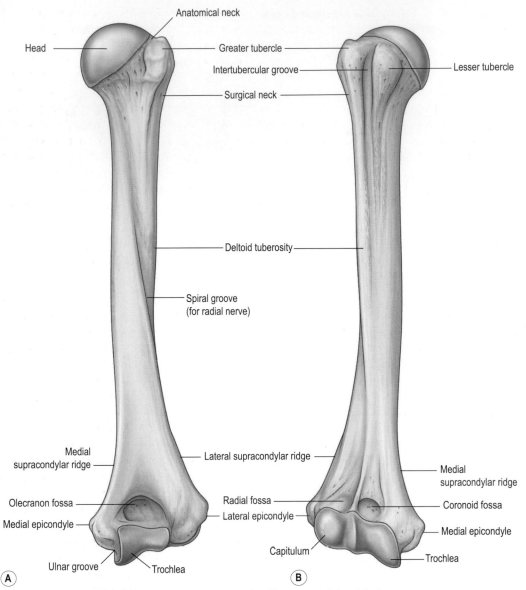

Fig. 2.20 Posterior (A) and anterior (B) aspects of the right humerus.

The smaller lesser tubercle is a distinct prominence on the anterior aspect below the anatomical neck; it has a well-marked impression on its medial side for muscular attachment. Between the greater and lesser tubercles and passing onto the shaft is the deep intertubercular groove (sulcus). The crests of the greater and lesser tubercles continue inferiorly from the anterior borders of the tubercles to form the lateral and medial lips of the intertubercular groove, between which is the floor.

There is a definite constriction (surgical neck) below where the head and tubercles join the shaft; fractures often occur here, particularly in the elderly.

The shaft of the humerus is almost cylindrical proximally, becoming triangular in its distal part with distinct medial and lateral borders. It presents three borders (anterior, medial and lateral), although they are frequently rounded and indistinct, between which are the three surfaces (anteromedial, anterolateral and posterior) of the shaft. The intertubercular groove is continuous with the anteromedial surface; the medial border begins as the crest of the lesser tubercle and ends by curving towards the medial epicondyle. The smooth anterolateral surface is marked near its middle by the deltoid tuberosity. The posterior surface is crossed obliquely from superomedial to inferolateral by the spiral (radial) groove, which reaches the lateral border below the deltoid tuberosity; it is often poorly marked.

The distal end of the humerus is expanded laterally, flattened anteroposteriorly and curves slightly anteriorly; it presents two articular surfaces separated by a ridge. The lateral rounded convex articular surface (capitulum) is situated anteroinferiorly, being less than a hemisphere in size; it articulates with the radius, making its greatest contact when the elbow is fully flexed. Medial to the capitulum is a grooved surface like a pulley (trochlea) for articulation with the ulna. The medial edge of the trochlea projects further distally and anteriorly than the lateral causing the ulna also to project laterally, resulting in the creation of an angle (carrying angle) between the humerus and ulna (see Fig. 2.48B).

On the medial side of the trochlea is the large medial epicondyle; its posterior surface is smooth with a shallow groove for the ulnar nerve. The sharp medial supracondylar ridge, comprising the distal one third of the medial border, runs superiorly onto the shaft. On the lateral side of the capitulum is the lateral epicondyle with the lateral supracondylar ridge, comprising the distal one-third of the lateral border, which also runs superiorly onto the shaft.

Just above the articular surfaces, the distal end of the humerus presents three fossae for the bony processes of the radius and ulna. Posteriorly is the deep olecranon fossa, which on full elbow extension receives the olecranon process of the ulna. Anteriorly are two fossae, the lateral radial and medial coronoid fossae, which on full elbow flexion receive the head of the radius and coronoid process of the ulna, respectively. Many of the bony features described above can be seen in Fig. 2.47.

Ossification

A primary ossification centre appears in the shaft in the 8th week *in utero* and spreads until, at birth, only the ends are cartilaginous. Secondary centres appear in the head early in the 1st year and in the greater and lesser tubercles at about 3 and 5 years, respectively. These fuse to form a single cap of bone between the ages of 6 and 8 years, finally fusing with the shaft between 18 and 20 years in females and 20 and 22 years in males.

At the distal end of the humerus, secondary centres appear for the capitulum during the 2nd year, for the trochlea between 9 and 10 years and for the lateral epicondyle between 12 and 14 years. These join together at about 14 years, fusing with the shaft at 15 years in females and 18 years in males. A separate centre for the medial epicondyle appears between 6 and 8 years and fuses between 15 and 18 years with a spicule of bone projecting inferiorly from the shaft medial to the trochlea; this latter ossification centre lies entirely outside the joint capsule. Most of the growth in length of the humerus occurs at its proximal end.

Palpation

At the proximal end of the humerus, the most lateral bony point at the shoulder is the greater tubercle, whose quadrilateral superior, anterior and posterior surfaces can be felt. Further differentiation can be made by palpating the lateral margin of the acromion (p. 60) and then running the fingers onto the greater tubercle. The rounded lesser tubercle can be felt through deltoid, being just lateral to the tip of the coracoid process. Lateral to the lesser tubercle, the impression of the intertubercular sulcus can usually be felt. The shaft of the humerus is covered with thick muscle but can be palpated on its medial and lateral aspects. At the distal end, the prominent medial epicondyle is the most obvious bony landmark; the ulnar nerve can be rolled in the groove behind it ('funny bone'). Running superiorly from the medial epicondyle, the sharp medial supracondylar ridge can be palpated. The lateral epicondyle can be palpated at the base of a dimple on the lateral aspect of the elbow, as can the lateral supracondylar ridge running superiorly from it. Posteriorly, if the relaxed elbow is flexed, the olecranon fossa can be felt through the triceps tendon.

Articular Surfaces

The articular surfaces of the shoulder joint are the shallow glenoid fossa and rounded head of the humerus. The adaptation of these surfaces contributes very little, if at all, to the stability and security of the joint. As in the majority of synovial joints, the articular surfaces are covered by hyaline cartilage.

Glenoid Fossa

Situated at the superolateral angle of the scapula, the glenoid fossa faces anterolaterally and slightly superiorly.

It is pear-shaped with the narrower region superiorly, being concave both vertically and transversely. However, the concavity of the joint is irregular and less deep than the convexity of the head of the humerus. In the plane of the axis of the head and neck of the humerus, the curvature of the glenoid fossa, with its larger radius, subtends an angle of approximately 75 degrees. The articular surface of the fossa is little more than one-third that of the humeral head, being deepened to some extent by the presence of the glenoid labrum (p. 87).

Head of the Humerus

The head of the humerus represents two-fifths of a sphere and faces superomedially and posteriorly (Fig. 2.20). With its smaller radius of curvature, the articular surface subtends an angle of approximately 150 degrees in the plane of the axis of the head and neck. Regardless of the position of the joint, only one-third of the humeral head makes contact with the glenoid fossa at any time. It is essentially the mismatch in coaptation of the articular surfaces which gives the joint its mobility.

Palpation

The line of the shoulder joint cannot be directly palpated due to the surrounding mass of muscles. However, the surface projection of the joint line can be estimated first by identifying the surface projection of the midpoint of the joint, which is approximately 1 cm lateral to the apex of the coracoid process. A vertical line, slightly concave laterally, through this point gives an indication of the joint line.

Joint Capsule and Synovial Membrane

The fibrous joint capsule forms a loose cylindrical sleeve between the two bones (Fig. 2.21). The majority of the capsular fibres pass horizontally between the scapula and humerus, but some oblique and transverse fibres are also present. Although it is thick and strong in parts, particularly anteriorly, the capsule provides little stability to the joint because of its laxness. On the scapula, the capsule attaches just outside the glenoid labrum anteriorly and inferiorly, and to the labrum superiorly and posteriorly. Recesses formed between the anterior capsular attachment and the glenoid labrum may have pathological significance in shoulder joint trauma.

On the humerus, the capsule attaches to the anatomical neck, around the articular margins of the head, medial to the greater and lesser tubercles, except inferiorly where it joins the medial surface of the shaft about 1 cm below the articular margin. The inferomedial extension of the capsular attachment means that the medial end of the proximal epiphyseal line of the humerus is intracapsular.

The anterior part of the capsule is thickened and strengthened by the presence of three glenohumeral ligaments, which can only be seen on its inner aspect. The superoposterior part is strengthened near its humeral attachment by the coracohumeral ligament. The tendons of the 'rotator cuff' muscles spread out over the capsule, blending with it near their humeral attachments; these short scapular muscles act as extensible ligaments and are extremely important in maintaining joint integrity.

With the arm in the anatomical position, the inferior part of the joint capsule is lax forming a redundant fold; when the arm is abducted, this part of the capsule becomes increasingly taut.

There are two openings in the fibrous capsule (Fig. 2.22A); there may also be a third opening. One opening is at the proximal end of the intertubercular groove to allow the long head of biceps brachii to pass into the arm. This part of the capsule is thickened, forming the transverse humeral ligament, arching over the tendon as it emerges from the capsule. The second opening is in the anterior part of the capsule, between the superior and middle glenohumeral ligaments, and communicates with the subscapular bursa deep to the tendon of subscapularis. The third opening is posterior, allowing a communication between the joint cavity and infraspinatus bursa.

Capsular Ligaments

The anterior part of the joint capsule is reinforced by three longitudinal bands of fibres (glenohumeral ligaments) (Fig. 2.21). They are seldom prominent and, when present, radiate from the anterior glenoid margin, extending inferiorly from the supraglenoid tubercle.

Superior glenohumeral ligament. Slender ligament arising from the superior part of the glenoid margin and adjacent labrum immediately anterior to the attachment of the tendon of the long head of biceps brachii; it runs laterally parallel to the biceps tendon to the superior surface of the lesser tubercle.

Middle glenohumeral ligament. Arising below the superior ligament it attaches to the humerus on the anterior aspect of the lesser tubercle below the attachment of subscapularis.

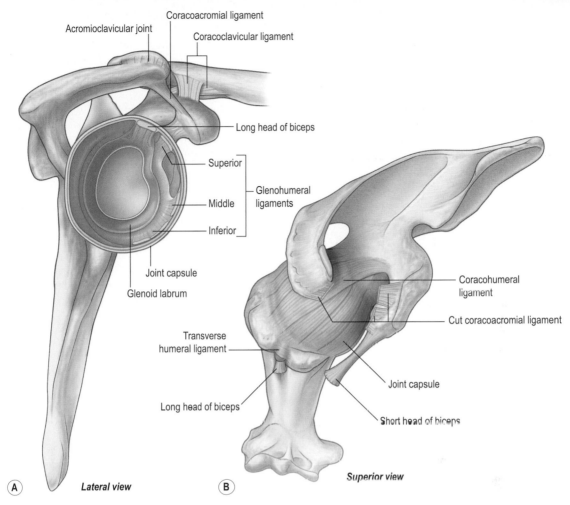

Fig. 2.21 (A) Lateral aspect of the glenoid fossa with the humeral head removed showing the joint capsule and coracoacromial, coracoclavicular and glenohumeral ligaments. (B) Superior aspect of the shoulder joint showing the transverse humeral, coracohumeral and coracoacromial ligaments.

Inferior glenohumeral ligament. From the glenoid margin below the notch on its anterior border and the adjacent anterior border of the glenoid labrum, it descends slightly obliquely to the humerus to attach to the antero-inferior part of the anatomical neck; it is usually the most well developed of the ligaments, although it is occasionally absent. As it passes from the scapula to the humerus, the upper part of the inferior ligament may merge with the lower part of the middle glenohumeral ligament.

Although they have no real stabilising function, certain movements of the shoulder joint will tend to increase the tension in some or all of the glenohumeral ligaments. Lateral rotation of the humerus puts all three ligaments under tension, while medial rotation relaxes them. In abduction, only the middle and inferior ligaments become taut, while the superior ligament becomes relaxed.

Transverse humeral ligament. At the proximal end of the intertubercular groove, the transverse humeral ligament bridges the gap between the greater and lesser tubercles (Fig. 2.21B); it is formed by transverse capsular fibres and serves to hold the biceps brachii tendon in the intertubercular groove as it leaves the shoulder joint.

Synovial Membrane

Synovial membrane lines the capsule and also extends inferiorly as a pouch when the arm is hanging by the

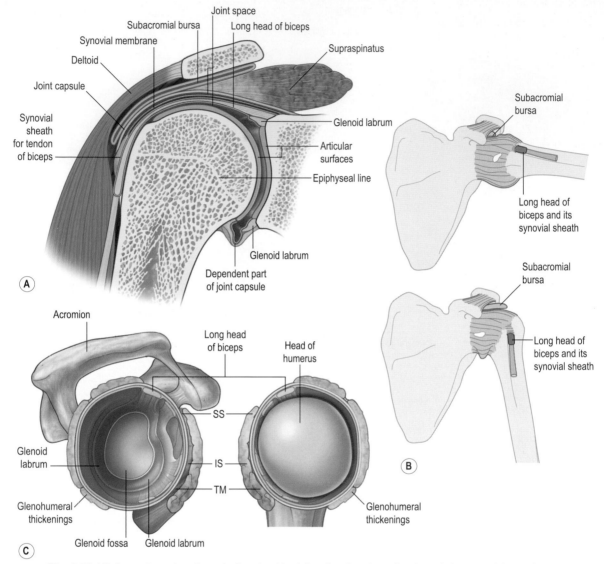

Fig. 2.22 (A) Coronal section through the shoulder joint showing the reflection of the synovial membrane around the long head of biceps brachii. (B) Withdrawal of the subacromial bursa and protrusion of the synovial sheath surrounding biceps brachii from the joint capsule when the arm is abducted. (C) The shoulder joint opened showing the rotator cuff muscles blending with the capsule. *IS*, Infraspinatus; *SS*, supraspinatus; *TM*, teres minor.

side (Fig. 2.22A). It attaches to the articular margins of both bones and is, therefore, reflected superiorly on the medial side of the humeral shaft to its attachment. Although the medial part of the epiphyseal line is intracapsular, it is extrasynovial (Fig. 2.22A). The synovial membrane extends through the anterior opening of the capsule forming the subscapularis bursa. It may be limited in extent to the posterior surface of the subscapularis

tendon; however, it may be sufficiently large to extend above the upper border of the tendon and come to lie inferior to the coracoid process; the superior extension may be replaced by a separate subcoracoid bursa. The posterior extension of the membrane through the joint capsule forms the infraspinatus bursa.

The intracapsular part of the long head of biceps brachii is enclosed within a double-layered tubular sheath of synovial membrane continuous with that of the joint at its glenoid attachment (Fig. 2.21A). The sheath surrounds the biceps brachii tendon as it passes deep to the transverse humeral ligament into the intertubercular groove, extending some 2 cm into the arm (Fig. 2.22B).

The subacromial bursa is an important, but non-communicating, bursa associated with the shoulder joint (Fig. 2.22A and B) lying between and separating, the coracoacromial arch and deltoid from the superolateral aspect of the shoulder joint. That part of the bursa extending laterally deep to deltoid is usually referred to as the subdeltoid bursa.

Some of these bursae are of clinical significance as adhesions may form preventing free gliding movements. This is particularly true for the bicipital sheath and subdeltoid bursa; the subdeltoid bursa may become inflamed (bursitis) and affect the underlying tendon of supraspinatus, leading to its rupture in some cases.

Intra-Articular Structures
Glenoid Labrum
The glenoid fossa is deepened by the presence of a triangular fibrocartilaginous rim (glenoid labrum) (Fig. 2.22C); it has a thin free edge and is about 4 mm deep. The base of the labrum attaches to the margin of the glenoid fossa; the outer surface gives attachment to the joint capsule posteriorly and superiorly, while the inner (joint) surface is in contact with the head of the humerus and is lined by cartilage continuous with that of the glenoid fossa. The superior part of the labrum may not be completely fixed to the bone so that its inner edge may project into the joint like a meniscus.

The outer margin of the labrum gives attachment to the tendon of the long head of biceps brachii superiorly, while inferiorly the tendon of the long head of triceps brachii partly arises from it.

Long Head of Biceps Brachii
The tendon of the long head of biceps brachii runs intracapsularly from its attachment to the supraglenoid tubercle and adjacent superior margin of the glenoid labrum until it emerges from the shoulder joint deep to the transverse humeral ligament (Fig. 2.21). During its intracapsular course, and for some 2 cm beyond, the tendon is enclosed within a synovial sleeve.

Accessory Ligaments
In addition to the capsular ligaments, two further ligaments are associated with the shoulder joint. Both are considered to be accessory ligaments, although the coracohumeral ligament blends with the joint capsule; the coracoacromial ligament completes the fibro-osseous arch above the joint.

Coracohumeral Ligament
Fairly strong, broad band arising from the lateral border of the coracoid process near its root. As it passes laterally, it becomes flattened with the margins diverging above the intertubercular groove to attach to the proximal part of the anatomical neck in the region of the greater and lesser tubercles and intervening transverse humeral ligament (Fig. 2.21B).

The anterior border of the medial part is free, but as it passes laterally it fuses with the tendon of subscapularis as it blends with the joint capsule before attaching to the lesser tubercle. The posterior part of the ligament blends with the tendon of supraspinatus as it attaches to the superior facet on the greater tubercle of the humerus.

Coracoacromial Ligament
Not directly associated with the joint, but together with the coracoid process and acromion, the coracoacromial ligament forms a fibro-osseous arch superior to the head of the humerus. It is a strong, triangular ligament, with the anterior and posterior borders tending to be thicker than the intermediate part. Occasionally, the tendon of pectoralis minor is prolonged and pierces the base of the ligament to become continuous with the coracohumeral ligament. The coracoacromial ligament is attached by a broad base to the lateral border of the horizontal part of the coracoid process with the blunt apex attaching to the apex of the acromion anterior to the acromioclavicular joint (Fig. 2.21B). Superiorly are the clavicle and deltoid, while inferiorly it is separated from the tendon of supraspinatus and the shoulder joint by the subacromial bursa.

The arch formed by the ligament and bony processes increase the surface area upon which the head of the humerus is supported when force is transmitted superiorly along the humerus.

Blood Supply, Lymphatic Drainage and Innervation
The arterial supply is from numerous sources as there is an important anastomosis around the scapula involving vessels from the subclavian and axillary arteries and the descending aorta (Fig. 2.23). The supply to the shoulder joint is by branches from the suprascapular branch of

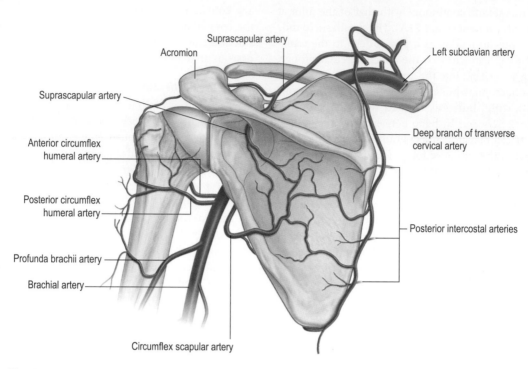

Fig. 2.23 Posterior aspect of the left scapula and humerus showing vessels involved in supplying the shoulder region, together with those contributing to the scapular collateral anastomosis.

the subclavian artery, the acromial branch of the thoracoacromial artery and branches from the anterior and posterior circumflex humeral arteries; the latter three are branches of the axillary artery. Venous drainage is by similarly named veins which drain into the external jugular and axillary veins.

Lymphatic drainage of the joint is to lymph nodes within the axilla, eventually passing via the apical group of nodes into the subclavian lymph trunk.

The nerve supply to the shoulder joint is by twigs from the suprascapular, axillary, subscapular, lateral pectoral and musculocutaneous nerves, with a root value of C5, C6 and C7.

Relations

The shoulder joint is almost completely surrounded by muscles passing between the pectoral girdle and humerus (Fig. 2.24); these serve to protect the joint by helping to suspend the upper limb from the pectoral girdle providing a degree of stability to the joint, with some muscles being more important in this respect than others. The anterior, superior and posterior parts of the joint are directly related to the tendons of subscapularis,

supraspinatus, infraspinatus and teres minor, respectively, all of which blend with the humeral part of the joint capsule; because of their action on the shoulder joint (pp. 99, 105–107), they are known as the rotator cuff. Covering the superolateral part of the joint is deltoid, giving the shoulder its rounded appearance (Fig. 2.24). The tendon of the long head of biceps brachii passes directly superior to the joint within the capsule. Superiorly and separated from the joint by the tendon of supraspinatus is the coracoacromial arch. Inferiorly, arising from the infraglenoid tubercle is the long head of triceps brachii as it passes into the arm almost parallel to the humerus.

Immediately inferior to the shoulder joint is the quadrangular space, bounded superiorly by teres minor, inferiorly by teres major, medially by the long head of triceps brachii and laterally by the shaft of the humerus (Fig. 2.25). Passing through this space from anterior to posterior are the axillary nerve and posterior circumflex humeral artery. Inferior dislocation of the head of the humerus or prolonged upwardly applied pressure (falling asleep with the arm hanging over the back of a chair) may cause temporary or permanent damage to the nerve

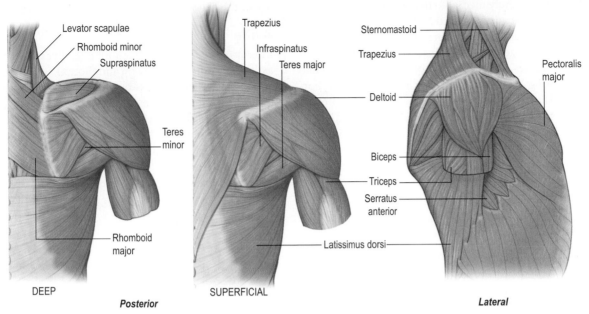

Fig. 2.24 Muscles of the shoulder region.

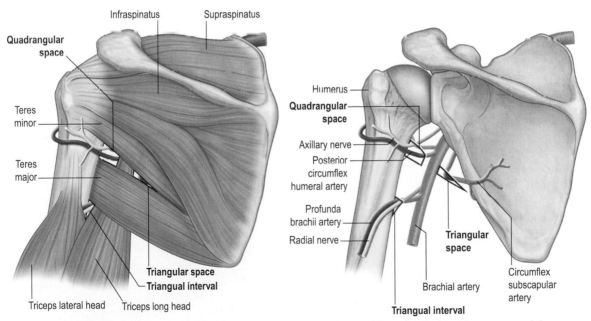

Fig. 2.25 Posterior aspect of the left shoulder region showing the quadrilateral and triangular spaces and the triangular interval together with their contents.

and consequent loss of function of deltoid and teres minor. Immediately medial to the quadrangular space is the triangular space, bounded by teres minor and major, and the long head of triceps brachii, through which pass the circumflex scapular vessels (Fig. 2.25). The triangular interval lies inferior to the quadrilateral space and has the long head of triceps brachii as its medial border, the shaft of the humerus laterally and lower border of teres major as its base (Fig. 2.25); it is an important region as the radial nerve and profunda brachii vessels pass through it to gain access to the posterior compartment of the arm. Fractures of the shaft of the humerus, or pressure from the axillary pad of an incorrectly used crutch, may involve the radial nerve, resulting in radial

nerve palsy (wrist drop), which will affect the functional use of the hand.

Axilla

Inferomedial to the shoulder joint is the pyramid-shaped axilla (space between the arm and thorax), which enables vessels and nerves to pass between the neck and upper limb (Fig. 2.26). The apex of the axilla is formed by the clavicle anteriorly, scapula posteriorly and lateral border of the 1st rib medially. Its concave base (floor) is formed by deep fascia extending from over serratus anterior to the deep fascia of the arm, attached to the margins of the axillary folds anteriorly and posteriorly, and supported by the suspensory ligament of the axilla, itself

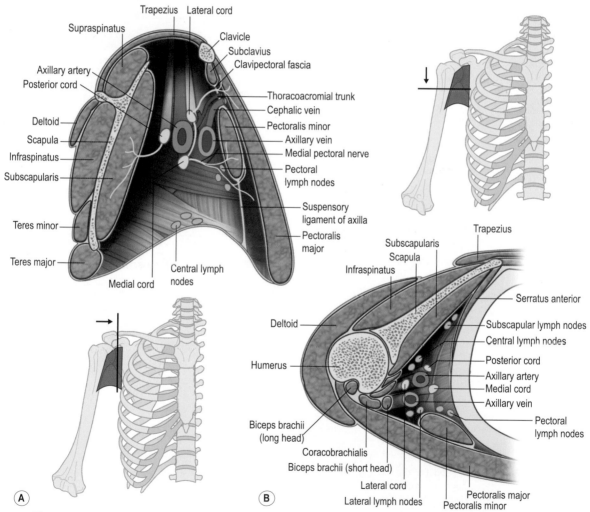

Fig. 2.26 Sagittal (A) and transverse (B) sections through the right axilla showing its boundaries and contents.

an inferior extension of the clavipectoral fascia below pectoralis minor (Fig. 2.26A). The anterior axillary wall is formed by pectoralis major, the lower rounded fold formed by twisting of the muscle fibres as they pass from the chest wall to the humerus (p. 102). The posterior wall extends more inferiorly than the anterior, being formed by subscapularis and teres major, with the tendon of latissimus dorsi twisting around teres major (Fig. 2.26A). The medial wall is formed by serratus anterior and the lateral wall by the floor of the intertubercular groove (Fig. 2.26B). The anterior and posterior axillary folds can both be easily palpated. A vertical line midway between the folds passing down the thoracic wall is the mid-axillary line.

When the arm is fully abducted, the axillary folds virtually disappear as the muscles forming them run almost parallel to the humerus; the axillary hollow may be replaced by a bulge.

The principal contents of the axilla are the blood vessels and nerves passing between the neck and upper limb (Fig. 2.26). These are the axillary artery and its branches, the axillary vein and its tributaries, and the brachial plexus and its terminal branches; together with various groups of lymph nodes, these structures are surrounded by fat and loose areolar tissue. The tendon of the long head of biceps brachii runs in the intertubercular groove and so lies just within the axilla. Also within the axilla are the short head of biceps brachii and coracobrachialis. The major vessels and nerve trunks are enclosed within the axillary sheath, a fascial extension of the prevertebral layer of the cervical fascia. The axillary sheath is adherent to the clavipectoral fascia posterior to pectoralis minor, while just beyond the second part of the axillary artery, it blends with the tunica adventitia of the vessels.

The axillary artery runs through the axilla superior and posterior to the vein; its position is indicated on the surface of the abducted arm by a straight line passing between the middle of the clavicle and the medial prominence of coracobrachialis. With the arm hanging by the side, the artery describes a gentle curve with the concavity facing inferomedially.

The axillary artery is crossed anteriorly by the tendon of pectoralis minor, dividing it into three parts. Superior to the first part of the artery are the lateral and posterior cords of the brachial plexus and posterior is the medial cord; it is crossed by a communicating loop between the medial and lateral pectoral nerves. The second part of the axillary artery, posterior to pectoralis minor, has the

various cords of the brachial plexus in their named positions. The third part of the artery, lying laterally against coracobrachialis, has the musculocutaneous nerve laterally, the median nerve anteriorly, the ulnar and medial cutaneous nerves of the arm and forearm medially, and the axillary and radial nerves posteriorly.

Axillary lymph nodes are widely distributed within the axillary fat but may be conveniently divided into five groups (Fig. 2.26; see also Figs 2.145 and 2.146). The lateral nodes lie along and superior to the axillary vein and receive the majority of the lymphatic drainage of the upper limb. The posterior (subscapular) nodes lie along the subscapular artery and receive lymph from the scapular region and back above the level of the umbilicus. The anterior (pectoral) nodes, alongside the lateral thoracic artery, receive lymph from the anterior chest wall including the breast. These groups of nodes drain to a central group, which lie above the axillary floor. From here, efferents pass to the apical group (the only group lying superior to the tendon of pectoralis minor) and then to the subclavian lymph trunk.

Because of the involvement of the axillary nodes in the lymphatic drainage of the breast, they may be subjected to radiotherapy treatment in an attempt to limit the secondary spread of cancer from the breast. It is important to remember that the lateral group of nodes lie above the axillary vein so that they can be excluded from treatment programmes, otherwise severe problems with lymphatic drainage of the upper limb may result.

Stability

Incongruity of the articular surfaces, together with laxness of the joint capsule, suggests that the shoulder joint is not very stable. Although dislocation is common, it is by no means an everyday occurrence. What factors are responsible for conferring stability to the joint? The glenoid labrum, as well as deepening the fossa, also improves joint congruency and thus becomes a significant stabilising factor. Fracture of the glenoid or tearing of the labrum often results in dislocation.

The most important factor; however, is the tone in the short scapular (rotator cuff) muscles (supraspinatus, infraspinatus, teres minor and subscapularis). Not only do they attach close to the joint, but they also fuse with the lateral part of the joint capsule (Fig. 2.27). In this way, they act as ligaments of variable length and tension and prevent the lax capsule and its synovial lining from becoming trapped between the articulating surfaces.

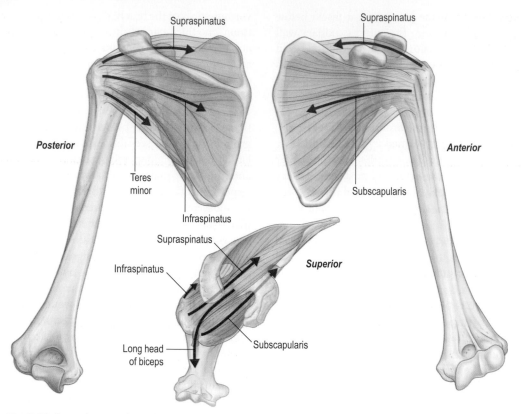

Fig. 2.27 Posterior, anterior and superior aspects of the scapula and humerus showing the action of the rotator cuff muscles in stabilising the shoulder joint.

The inferior part of the capsule is the weakest as it is not supported by muscles; however, as the arm is gradually abducted, the long head of triceps brachii and teres major become increasingly applied to this aspect of the joint.

In addition to the rotator cuff muscles, all muscles passing between the pectoral girdle and humerus assist in maintaining joint stability; particularly important are the long heads of biceps brachii and triceps brachii. The tendon of the long head of biceps brachii, which is partly intracapsular, acts as a strong support for the joint superiorly, while the long head of triceps brachii gives support inferiorly when the arm is abducted.

Superior displacement of the head of the humerus is resisted by the coracoacromial arch. Although not part of the joint, the arch, separated from the joint by the subacromial bursa, functions mechanically as an articular surface. It is so strong that an upward thrust on the humerus will fracture either the clavicle or the humerus before compromising the arch.

Dislocation of the shoulder is more common than for many joints as a consequence of the need to have the joint as mobile as possible; furthermore, the long humerus has great leverage in dislocating forces. In anterior dislocation, which is the more common, the head of the humerus comes to lie inferior to the coracoid process, producing a bulge in the region of the clavipectoral groove; at the same time, the roundness of the shoulder is lost. In such dislocations, the humeral head usually comes through the joint capsule between the long head of triceps brachii and the inferior glenohumeral ligament.

As the glenoid fossa faces anterolaterally, it is better situated to resist posteriorly directed forces; infraspinatus and teres minor reinforce the capsule posteriorly. Posterior dislocation may result when a large force is applied to the long axis of the humerus when the arm is medially rotated and abducted. The joint capsule tears in the region of teres minor, with the head of the humerus coming to lie inferior to the spinous process of the scapula.

MOVEMENTS OF THE ARM AT THE SHOULDER JOINT

The anatomy of the shoulder joint gives it a greater range of movement than any other joint in the body; its ball-and-socket shape means that movement can take place around an infinite number of axes intersecting at the centre of the head of the humerus. For descriptive purposes, the shoulder joint is capable of flexion and extension, abduction and adduction, and medial and lateral rotation. However, the axes about which these movements occur have to be carefully defined as the plane of the glenoid fossa does not coincide with any of the cardinal planes of the body; it is inclined approximately 45 degrees to both the coronal and sagittal planes. It is, therefore, possible to define two sets of axes about which movements occur, one with respect to the cardinal planes of the body (Fig. 2.28A) and another with respect to the plane of the glenoid fossa (Fig. 2.28B). If the cardinal planes are used, flexion and extension occur about a transverse axis, abduction and adduction about an anteroposterior axis, and medial and lateral rotation about the longitudinal axis of the humerus, passing between the centre of the head and centre of the capitulum (Fig. 2.28A). However, if movement is considered with respect to the plane of the scapula, then flexion and extension take place about an axis perpendicular to the plane of the glenoid fossa, abduction and adduction about an axis parallel to the plane of the glenoid fossa, and medial and lateral rotation about the longitudinal axis of the humerus (Fig. 2.28B). Although the presentation of these two sets of axes may initially appear to be confusing, the importance of those with respect to the plane of the glenoid fossa is that, in the treatment of some shoulder injuries, the position of the joint which will not create asymmetric tension on the joint capsule is when it is abducted to 90 degrees with respect to the plane of the glenoid fossa.

Irrespective of the orientation of these axes, the incongruity of the joint surfaces means that all movements,

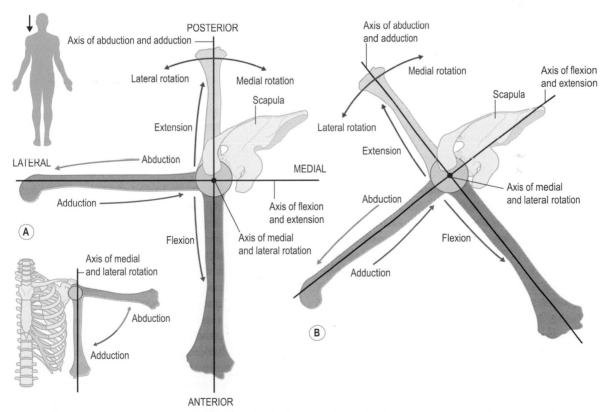

Fig. 2.28 Movements at the shoulder joint with the axes about which movement occurs aligned with the cardinal axes of the body (A) and with the plane of the glenoid fossa (B).

except axial rotation, are a combination of gliding and rolling of the articular surfaces against each other. However, unlike the knee, it is not possible to define the extent of each type of motion in each movement. Although the range of movement at the shoulder joint is relatively large, the mobility of the upper limb against the trunk is increased by movements of the pectoral girdle. Indeed, flexion and extension, as well as abduction and adduction, may be considered to be always accompanied by scapular and clavicular movements, except perhaps for the initial stages. Movement at the shoulder joint is more concerned with bringing the arm to the horizontal position, while pectoral girdle movements, principally that of the scapula, are more concerned with bringing the arm into a vertical position.

The association of shoulder and pectoral girdle movements also increases the power of the movement. The rotator cuff muscles, which are attached close to the axes of movement, have a poor mechanical advantage compared with muscles acting on the scapula, which have considerable leverage and are generally more powerful. In individuals with fused or fixed shoulder joints, a large degree of upper limb mobility with respect to the trunk is still possible due to movement of the pectoral girdle.

Movements of the Arm at the Shoulder Joint in the Plane of the Glenoid Fossa

The ranges of shoulder joint motion associated with some common activities are given in Table 2.2.

Abduction and Adduction

These occur about an oblique horizontal axis in the same plane as the glenoid fossa; in abduction, the arm moves anterolaterally away from the trunk (Fig. 2.29A). The total

range of movement at the shoulder joint is 120 degrees; however, only the first 25 degrees occurs without accompanying rotation of the scapula, consequently between 30 and 180 degrees scapula rotation augments shoulder abduction in the ratio of 1:2. The terminal part of shoulder joint abduction is accompanied by lateral rotation of the humerus, not to prevent bony contact between the greater tubercle and acromion, but rather to provide

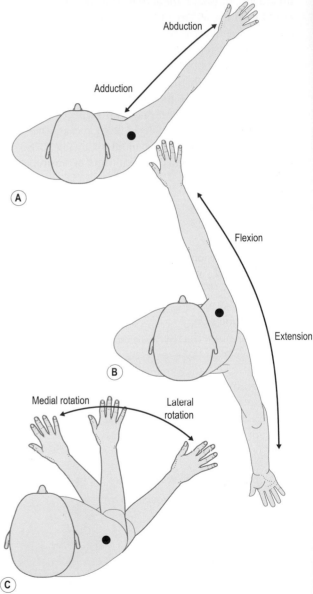

Fig. 2.29 Movements of the arm at the shoulder joint with respect to the plane of the glenoid fossa. (A) Abduction and adduction. (B) Flexion and extension. (C) Medial and lateral rotation.

TABLE 2.2 Required Range of Shoulder Joint Movement During Some Common Activities

	Flexion (°)	Abduction (°)	Medial rotation (°)
Eating	35	25	20
Drinking	45	35	25
Combing hair	110	100	45

Adapted from Safaee-Rad, R., Shwedyk, E., Quanbury, A.O., Cooper, J.E., 1990. Normal functional range of motion of the upper limb during performance of three feeding activities. Arch. Phys. Med. Rehabil. 71, 505–509.

further articular surface for the head of the humerus with the glenoid fossa. Abduction of the medially rotated humerus is limited by tension in the posterior joint capsule and lateral rotators. Adduction beyond the neutral joint position is not possible because of the presence of the trunk. At all ages, females tend to have a greater range of movement than males (Clarke et al., 1975).

Abduction is initiated by supraspinatus which, although nowhere near as strong as deltoid, is better placed to act on the humerus. With the arm hanging at the side, the fibres of deltoid, particularly the middle fibres, run almost parallel to the shaft of the humerus so that on contraction they pull it superiorly. Once the arm has been pulled away from the trunk, deltoid can take over and continue the movement. Supraspinatus is required for the initial 20 degrees of abduction; if deltoid is paralysed, supraspinatus is not strong enough to abduct the upper limb fully; however, if supraspinatus is paralysed, deltoid cannot initiate abduction. Passive abduction of approximately 20 degrees, or leaning to the affected side so that the limb hangs away from the body, enables deltoid to continue the movement. In some circumstances, biceps brachii can be re-educated to take over the initiating role of a paralysed supraspinatus. As abduction proceeds, both teres minor and major prevent superior movement of the head of the humerus by the pull of deltoid, while together with subscapularis and infraspinatus, they stabilise the humeral head against the glenoid fossa.

Lateral rotation of the scapula accompanying abduction of the humerus is produced by the force couple of the lower part of serratus anterior, acting on the inferior angle of scapula, and the upper fibres of trapezius pulling on the acromion.

Adduction from an abducted position of the upper limb is produced by the eccentric contraction of serratus anterior, trapezius, deltoid and supraspinatus, under the action of gravity. If adduction is resisted, then a forceful movement is produced by pectoralis major, teres major, latissimus dorsi and coracobrachialis.

Flexion and Extension

These occur about an axis perpendicular to the plane of the glenoid fossa, so that, in flexion, the arm moves anteromedially at an angle of approximately 45 degrees to the sagittal plane (Fig. 2.29B). In extension, it is carried posterolaterally (Fig. 2.29B); extension is limited by the greater tubercle of the humerus making contact with the coracoacromial arch. The range of flexion is approximately 110 degrees and of extension 70 degrees, both of which may be extended by movements of the pectoral girdle so that flexion of the upper limb with respect to the trunk can reach 180 degrees and extension just exceeds 90 degrees. The range of flexion and extension changes with age. In neonates, the passive range of flexion is between 172 and 180 degrees and of extension between 79 and 89 degrees, decreasing to 169 and 69 degrees, respectively, by age 5 (Watanabe et al., 1979). The passive range of movement continues to decrease so that, by age 60, flexion is 160 degrees and extension is 38 degrees (Walker et al., 1984).

Flexion is produced by the anterior fibres of deltoid, the clavicular head of pectoralis major, coracobrachialis and biceps brachii. Passive extension from the flexed position is essentially due to the eccentric contraction of these same muscles. Beyond the neutral position; however, extension is produced by the posterior fibres of deltoid, teres major and latissimus dorsi; there may be additional extension due to the long head of triceps brachii and the sternal fibres of pectoralis major when active extension is performed from a flexed position.

Medial and Lateral Rotation

Rotation takes place about the longitudinal axis of the humerus described earlier (p. 93). In lateral rotation, the anterior surface of the humerus is turned laterally (Fig. 2.29C), produced by infraspinatus, teres minor and the posterior fibres of deltoid; it has a maximum range of 80 degrees. In medial rotation, the anterior surface of the humerus is turned medially (Fig. 2.29C), produced by subscapularis, pectoralis major, latissimus dorsi, teres major and the anterior fibres of deltoid; it has a maximum range in excess of 90 degrees. However, to reach this value with the elbow flexed, the forearm has to be pulled behind the trunk to prevent contact between the trunk and forearm limiting movements. The combined range of rotation varies with the position of the arm, being greatest when the arm is by the side, decreasing to 90 degrees with the arm horizontal and negligible as the arm approaches the vertical. With increasing age, the range of rotation decreases; in neonates, lateral rotation is between 118 and 134 degrees and medial rotation between 72 and 90 degrees (Watanabe et al., 1979). At age 5, the mean range has reduced to 110 and 71 degrees, respectively, decreasing to 80 and 65 degrees at age 60 and above (Downey et al., 1991). At all ages, females tend to have a greater range of movement than males (Walker et al., 1984).

Rotation is limited by the extent of the articular surfaces and tension in the appropriate part of the joint capsule and opposing musculature; it is the movement most commonly affected by pathology of or injury to the shoulder joint. When assessing the range of rotation possible at the joint, the elbow must be flexed to exclude the possibility of pronatory or supinatory action of the forearm.

How the above movements are related to movements of the upper limb in the cardinal planes is discussed below. Reference is made to functional movements which combine some of these movements.

Movements of the Arm at the Shoulder Joint with Respect to the Cardinal Planes of the Body

Although movements of the arm at the shoulder joint have been considered with respect to the plane of the glenoid fossa, it is often more convenient to test the range of movement possible with respect to the cardinal planes of the body.

Movements of the arm about a transverse axis through the humeral head produce what are termed 'flexion' and 'extension'; strictly speaking, these movements are a combination of flexion and abduction, and extension and adduction, with the extent of each depending on the position of the scapula on the chest wall. Forward 'flexion' has a range of 180 degrees, while backward 'extension' is limited to 50 degrees.

In relation to an anteroposterior axis, the movements produced are termed 'abduction' and 'adduction'. 'Abduction' is a combination of abduction and extension, having a range of 180 degrees with scapula rotation. 'Adduction' is the combined movement of adduction and flexion; the movement is limited by the trunk so that adduction beyond the neutral joint position is not possible. However, with protraction of the pectoral girdle, 30 degrees of 'adduction' is possible as the arm is brought across the front of the chest. Similarly, retraction of the pectoral girdle allows a minimal amount of 'adduction' to occur behind the back.

Although the terminology used to describe these movements of the arm at the shoulder joint is of little practical significance, it is important to understand the context in which it is being used. It is also important to be fully aware which movements are being tested when

asking individuals to perform certain actions. Two simple activities that demonstrate the mobility of the shoulder joint and pectoral girdle are (i) combing the hair and (ii) putting on a coat or jacket.

With respect to the cardinal planes, when the arm is flexed at 45 degrees, abducted 60 degrees and neither medially nor laterally rotated, it is said to be in the position of function of the shoulder. This corresponds to the position of equilibrium of the short scapular muscles, hence its use when immobilising fractures of the humeral shaft.

Accessory Movements

When the individual is lying supine, the muscles around the shoulder are relatively relaxed. In this position, the relative laxity of the ligaments and joint capsule allows an appreciable range of accessory movements. By placing the hand high up in the axilla and applying a lateral force to the proximal medial aspect of the arm, the head of the humerus can be lifted away from the glenoid fossa by as much as 1 cm.

Proximal and distal gliding movements of the head of the humerus against the glenoid fossa can be produced by forces applied along the shaft of the humerus. Similarly, anterior and posterior gliding movements can be produced by applying pressure in an appropriate direction to the region of the surgical neck of the humerus.

The major muscles producing movements of the arm at the shoulder joint are shown in Table 2.3; further details of each muscle can be found in following sections.

BIOMECHANICS

The rotator cuff muscles are active during abduction and lateral rotation, providing stability at the shoulder joint; however, they are also involved in the pathogenesis of dislocation of the shoulder. In any equilibrium analysis of the joint, certain assumptions have to be made. The following is based on an account given by Morrey and Chao (1981). The assumptions made were:

1. Each muscle contributing to the equilibrium acts with a force proportional to its cross-sectional area (6.2 kg/cm^2).
2. Each muscle is equally active.
3. Each active muscle contracts along a straight line connecting the centres of its two areas of attachment.

TABLE 2.3 Muscles Producing Movement of the Arm at the Shoulder Joint

Muscle	Attachments	Action	Innervation (root value)
Pectoralis major[a]	Medial ½ of anterior surface of clavicle, anterior surface of sternum and upper 6 costal cartilages to lateral lip of the intertubercular groove of humerus	Powerful adductor and medial rotator of arm at shoulder joint	Medial (C8, T1) and lateral (C5, C6, C7) pectoral nerves
Deltoid[a]	Anterior border of lateral 1/3rd of clavicle (anterior fibres), lateral margin of acromion (middle fibres) and lower border of crest of scapular spine (posterior fibres) to deltoid tuberosity of the humerus	Involved in all movements of arm at shoulder joint except adduction	Axillary nerve (C5, C6)
Biceps brachii	Supraglenoid tubercle above glenoid fossa of scapula (long head) and coracoid process of scapula (short head) to radial tuberosity	Weak flexor of arm at shoulder joint; its main action is flexion of forearm at elbow joint and supination of forearm at superior and inferior radioulnar joints	Musculocutaneous nerve (C5, C6)
Coracobrachialis	Coracoid process of scapula to medial aspect of humeral shaft	Adductor and weak flexor of arm at shoulder joint	Musculocutaneous nerve (C6, C7)
Latissimus dorsi[a]	Thoracolumbar fascia and spinous processes of T7 to S5, lateral lip of iliac crest, outer surfaces of lower 3 or 4 ribs and inferior angle of scapula (via fascia) to floor of intertubercular groove of humerus	Strong adductor and medial rotator of arm at shoulder joint; strong extensor of flexed arm; with scapula fixed it retracts pectoral girdle	Thoracodorsal nerve (C6, C7, C8)
Teres major[a]	Dorsal surface of scapula near inferior angle to medial lip of intertubercular groove on humerus	Adducts and medially rotates arm at shoulder joint; also helps extend flexed arm	Lower subscapular nerve (C6, C7)
Triceps brachii	Infraglenoid tubercle below glenoid fossa of scapula (long head), proximal and lateral to spiral groove of humerus (lateral head) and posterior surface of humerus distal and medial to spiral groove (medial head) to posterior aspect of proximal surface of olecranon of ulna and deep fascia of forearm; all heads unite	Long head extends and adducts flexed arm at shoulder joint; its main action is extension of forearm at elbow joint	Radial nerve (C6, C7, C8)
Subscapularis[b]	Medial 2/3rd of subscapular fossa of scapula to lesser tubercle of humerus	Strong medial rotator of arm at shoulder joint; also assists adduction	Upper and lower subscapular nerves (C5, C6, C7)
Teres minor[a,b]	Proximal 2/3rd of lateral border of scapula to lower facet on greater tubercle of humerus	Laterally rotates arm at shoulder joint; also adducts abducted arm	Axillary nerve (C5, C6)
Infraspinatus[a,b]	Medial 2/3rd of infraspinous fossa of scapula to middle facet on greater tubercle of humerus	Laterally rotates arm at shoulder joint	Suprascapular nerve (C5, C6)

[a]Shown in Figure 2.24.
[b]'Rotator cuff' muscles.

While none of these assumptions is necessarily true, they provide a framework within which to work. When the unloaded arm is laterally rotated and abducted to 90 degrees, there is a compressive force of approximately 70 kg between the articular surfaces, with anterior and inferior shear forces of 12 and 14 kg, respectively; these forces are produced by muscles actively resisting the weight of the arm. The resultant force is directed 12 degrees anteriorly with a magnitude of 72 kg.

In addition to being abducted and laterally rotated, if the arm is also extended 30 degrees and loaded so that the muscles are contracting maximally, then the magnitude of the forces across the joint increases dramatically. The compressive force between the articular surfaces rises to 210 kg, and the anterior and inferior shear forces to 42 and 58 kg, respectively; the resultant force is directed 36 degrees anteriorly with a magnitude of 222 kg. Because the glenoid fossa is too shallow to provide much constraint to prevent anterior dislocation, the shearing forces must be balanced by the joint capsule and its associated ligaments. As the tensile strength of the capsule and ligaments is approximately 50 kg, an imbalance of forces may occur leading to joint dislocation. Once the anterior part of the capsule has been torn, less force is then required for subsequent dislocations.

The above force analysis is similar to the situation when an individual slips when walking on ice and puts out an arm to break a backward fall.

Velocity of Movement

Because the shoulder joint is extremely mobile, some movements are performed at fairly high velocities. In many instances (when studying natural or artificial joints and their lubrication) knowledge of the sliding velocities at the articulating surfaces is important.

Using filming techniques and suitable trigonometric relationships, the maximum sliding velocities at the shoulder joint in some common activities have been determined (Table 2.4). In activities requiring fast and forceful movement at the shoulder, (tennis serve) the sliding velocities will be much greater. The demands made upon the lubricating fluid and articular surfaces in such situations are high; consequently, it is not surprising that sometimes the system breaks down resulting in joint trauma.

Shoulder Joint Replacement

Pathologies of the shoulder joint do not all require surgical intervention; arthroplasty is only considered as a

TABLE 2.4 **Velocity of Shoulder Joint Movement During Common Activities**

Activity	Velocity of movement (mm/s)
Hanging out clothes	100
Sweeping	34
Bedmaking	40
Arm swing during walking	30
Eating	13
Dressing	25

last resort after conservative treatments give little or no improvement in pain relief. Replacement of a damaged or arthritic humeral head may offer the immediate relief of pain; however, an intact rotator cuff and normal glenoid fossa are often prerequisites for hemiarthroplasty. Replacement after a severe fracture of the humeral head should be done as soon as possible, and certainly not later than 4 weeks following injury because of the extensive development of scar tissue and subsequent limitation of movement.

Total shoulder arthroplasty replaces both articular surfaces with prosthetic components which mimic normal shoulder anatomy, except for reverse shoulder arthroplasty in which the glenoid fossa is replaced with a glenosphere and the humeral head is changed into a concave humerosocket. Constrained prostheses do not rely on the surrounding tissues to provide support as the two components are physically linked; however, there is limited joint movement and tend to be used as a last resort. Semiconstrained prostheses, which have a hooded glenoid component to restrict superior migration of the humeral head, are also rarely used. Unconstrained total arthroplasty is extensively used in the treatment of primary avascular necrosis, fractures of the humeral head and especially glenohumeral osteoarthritis; however, the primary cause of failure in such prostheses is glenoid component loosening. Interpositional arthroplasty, although not new, has been and continues to be developed. This involves resurfacing the glenoid fossa with a meniscus, tendon or fascia lata allograft and can be performed with hemiarthroplasty of the humeral head or independently via arthroscopy to improve joint congruence.

All forms of total shoulder arthroplasty are inefficient at restoring function in individuals with rotator cuff tears or arthropathy. Interpositional arthroplasty appears to be more promising with some reports stating that it exceeds the functional results of conventional hemiarthroplasty. Nevertheless, superior migration and subluxation of the humeral head remain a problem.

MUSCLES ABDUCTING THE ARM AT THE SHOULDER JOINT

Supraspinatus
Deltoid

Supraspinatus

Arising from the medial two-thirds of the supraspinous fossa and deep surface of the dense fascia covering the muscle and tendon, which forms within it, supraspinatus passes laterally deep to trapezius, the acromion and coracoacromial ligament to pass over the superior aspect of the shoulder joint (Fig. 2.30). The deep surface of the tendon blends with the joint capsule before attaching to the upper facet on the greater tubercle of the humerus.

Innervation

By the suprascapular nerve (root value C5, C6), a branch from the upper trunk of the brachial plexus. Skin over the muscle is supplied from roots C4 and T2.

Action

Supraspinatus initiates abduction at the shoulder joint, being more important during the early part of the movement than later when deltoid takes over. Its role is probably twofold: (i) bracing the head of the humerus firmly against the glenoid fossa to prevent superior shearing (this has been likened to a 'foot on the ladder' where a small force applied at one end will produce a rotatory rather than a shearing movement), and (ii) producing abduction. After the initial 20 degrees of abduction, when the stronger deltoid takes over, supraspinatus acts to hold the humeral head against the glenoid fossa.

Functional Activity

Supraspinatus is one of the four muscles forming a musculotendinous (rotator) cuff around the head of the humerus; they function to keep the head of the humerus in the glenoid fossa during movements of the shoulder joint.

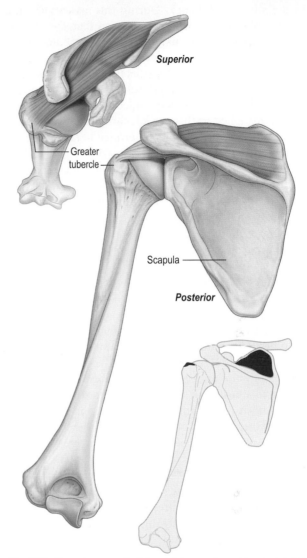

Fig. 2.30 Superior aspect of the right scapula and humerus and posterior aspect of the left scapula and humerus showing the position and attachments of supraspinatus.

Palpation

Contraction of supraspinatus can be felt through trapezius if the examiner's fingers are pressed into the medial part of the supraspinous fossa when the individual initiates abduction. In the anatomical position, the tendon of supraspinatus is covered by the acromion but can be palpated if the individual medially rotates the shoulder with the hand resting passively in the small of the back. During this manoeuvre, the greater tubercle moves anteriorly so that the tendon can now be rolled against the bone by a medial to lateral pressure of the examiner's finger against the tubercle. The tendon of supraspinatus is the most frequently damaged soft tissue in the shoulder region; techniques such as transverse frictions, injection and ultrasound are often applied to this exact location. In severe cases, the tendon may be sufficiently eroded to cause its rupture, which then affects the ease with which abduction can occur. In such cases, or when supraspinatus is paralysed, the individual can still initiate abduction by leaning to the side, using gravity. Alternatively, the individual may use the opposite arm to push the affected limb away from the side or jerk the hips to 'kick' the elbow out. Each of these actions produces a small yet sufficient degree of abduction to enable the powerful deltoid to take over.

Deltoid

Coarse, thick, triangular muscle (Fig. 2.31) giving the shoulder its rounded contour. Functionally, it is divided into three parts (anterior, middle and posterior) of which only the middle part is multipennate. It has an extensive attachment to the pectoral girdle; anteriorly, fibres attach to the anterior border of the lateral one-third of the clavicle and posteriorly to the lower lip of the crest of the spine of the scapula. The most anterior and posterior fibres both run obliquely in an uninterrupted manner to the deltoid tuberosity on the lateral surface of the shaft of the humerus.

The middle muscle fibres are more complex because of their multipennate arrangement (Fig. 2.31); these shorter oblique fibres run from four tendinous slips attached to the lateral margin of the acromion to join three intersecting tendinous slips which ultimately run to the deltoid tuberosity of the humerus. The shorter more numerous middle fibres, working under considerable mechanical disadvantage when active, give this part of the muscle great strength.

Deltoid is separated from the coracoacromial arch and superior and lateral aspects of the shoulder joint, as well as the tendons lying on it, by the subacromial bursa.

Innervation

By the axillary nerve (root value C5 and C6) from the posterior cord of the brachial plexus. Skin over deltoid is supplied by roots C4 and C5.

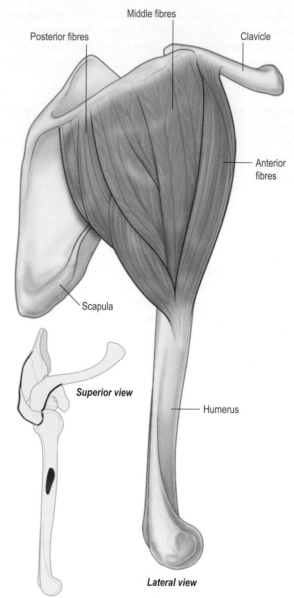

Fig. 2.31 Lateral aspect of the right clavicle, scapula and humerus showing the position and attachments of deltoid.

Action

Deltoid is the principal abductor of the arm at the shoulder joint, the movement being produced by its middle multipennate fibres; however, it can only produce this movement efficiently after it has been initiated by supraspinatus.

The true plane of abduction is in line with the blade of the scapula and, for this, the anterior and posterior fibres are active to maintain the plane of abduction by acting as 'guy ropes'. The tendency for deltoid to produce a superior shearing of the humeral head is resisted by the rotator cuff muscles (subscapularis anteriorly; teres minor and infraspinatus posteriorly; supraspinatus superiorly).

The anterior part of deltoid is a strong flexor and medial rotator of the arm and can help in transferring the strain of heavy weights carried in the hand to the pectoral girdle. The posterior part is a strong extensor and lateral rotator, being active during adduction of the arm to counteract the medial rotation produced by pectoralis major and latissimus dorsi.

Functional Activity

Deltoid is active in abduction when the middle fibres contract concentrically, but the massive development and multipennate nature of the muscle is most likely due to the fact that many activities involving the upper limb require it to be maintained or 'held' in this position for long periods of time. Consequently, the middle fibres contract isometrically when performing activities with the arm in front of the trunk; they then lower the arm back to the side by working eccentrically.

Palpation

With the individual seated and the arm raised to 60 degrees abduction in the plane of the scapula, the triangular bulk of deltoid can be seen and felt. Palpating the superior surface of the acromion and moving the fingers laterally from its edge, the depressions in the muscle caused by the tendinous intersections can be felt if anteroposterior pressure is applied by the fingers.

The anterior and posterior fibres can be made to stand out more clearly if, in the same position, the individual is asked to maintain the position against resistance, first anteriorly and then posteriorly.

Paralysis of deltoid severely affects the functioning of the shoulder joint and, therefore, the upper limb.

MUSCLES ADDUCTING THE ARM AT THE SHOULDER JOINT

Coracobrachialis

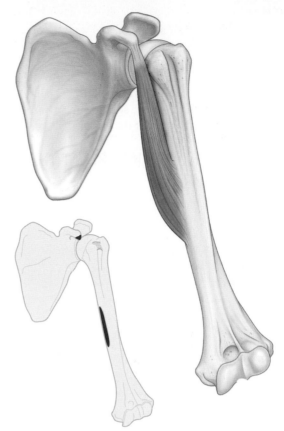

Fig. 2.32 Anterior aspect of the left scapula and humerus showing the position and attachments of coracobrachialis.

Coracobrachialis

The only true representative of the adductor group of muscles in the arm, coracobrachialis (Fig. 2.32) arises via a rounded tendon, in conjunction with the short head of biceps brachii, from the apex of the coracoid process of the scapula and attaches by a flat tendon to the medial side of the shaft of the humerus at its midpoint, between triceps brachii and brachialis. Some fibres may continue onto the medial intermuscular septum of the arm.

Innervation

By the musculocutaneous nerve (root value C6, C7) from the lateral cord of the brachial plexus. However, as it pierces the muscle, the nerve to coracobrachialis may arise directly from the lateral cord of the brachial plexus. Skin over the muscle is supplied by roots T1 and T2.

Action

Coracobrachialis is an adductor and weak flexor of the arm at the shoulder joint.

Palpation

When the fully abducted arm is adducted against resistance, coracobrachialis can be seen and felt as a rounded ridge on the medial aspect of the arm.

MUSCLES FLEXING THE ARM AT THE SHOULDER JOINT

Pectoralis major
Deltoid (anterior fibres) (p. 100)
Biceps brachii – long head (p. 129)
Coracobrachialis (p. 101)

Pectoralis Major

Thick, triangular muscle located on the upper half of the anterior surface of the thorax (Fig. 2.33) having clavicular and sternocostal parts, which, although usually continuous with each other, may be separated by a groove. As the fibres pass towards the humerus, they twist forming the rounded anterior axillary fold.

The smaller clavicular part attaches to the medial half of the anterior surface of the clavicle, while the larger sternocostal attachment is from the anterior surface of the manubrium and body of the sternum, anterior aspects of the upper six costal cartilages, anterior part of the 6th rib and the aponeurosis of the external oblique muscle of the abdomen.

From this large medial attachment, the muscle narrows and attaches via a laminated tendon into the lateral

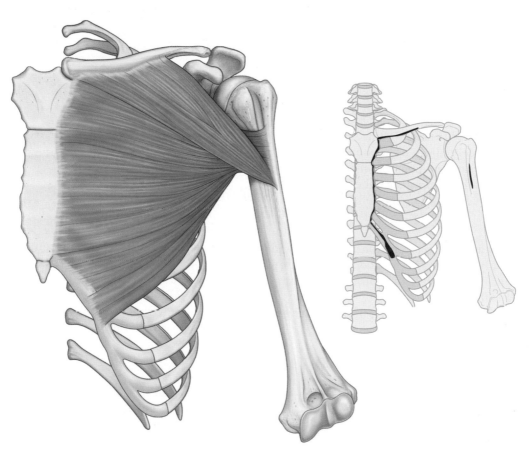

Fig. 2.33 Anterior aspect of the thorax and left humerus showing the position and attachments of pectoralis major.

lip of the intertubercular groove of the humerus. The anterior lamina (clavicular part) runs to the distal part of the humeral attachment, while the posterior lamina (sternocostal part) passes superiorly posterior to the anterior lamina to the proximal part of the humeral attachment; the tendon resembles a U in cross-section. The posterior fibres blend with the shoulder joint capsule, while the anterior clavicular fibres blend with the attachment of deltoid.

As the most superficial muscle of the anterior thoracic wall, pectoralis major lies superficial to pectoralis minor, the upper ribs and serratus anterior. In females, the muscle is covered by the breast with the fibrous septa of the breast attaching to the deep fascia overlying the muscle. Pectoralis major is separated from deltoid by the deltopectoral groove (infraclavicular fossa) in which lie the cephalic vein and branches from the thoracoacromial artery.

Innervation

By the medial (C8, T1) and lateral (C5, C6, C7) pectoral nerves, the clavicular part by roots C5 and C6, and sternocostal part by C7, C8 and T1. Skin over pectoralis major is supplied by roots T2 to T6.

Action

As a whole pectoralis major is a powerful adductor and medial rotator of the arm at the shoulder joint. In addition, the clavicular part can flex the arm to the horizontal, while the sternocostal fibres, because of their direction, can extend the flexed arm, particularly against resistance in the anatomical position. With the arm fixed (gripping a bed, table, or chair back) pectoralis major pulls on the upper ribs to assist inspiration during respiratory distress.

Functional Activity

Pectoralis major is a major climbing muscle. With the arms fixed above the head, its power can be used to pull the trunk superiorly, assisted by latissimus dorsi. In pushing, punching and throwing movements, pectoralis major acts to move the arm forcefully forward, while serratus anterior and pectoralis minor simultaneously protract the pectoral girdle.

In exercises, such as the 'press-up', pectoralis major contracts concentrically on the upward phase to raise the body, and eccentrically on the downward phase when lowering the body.

Palpation

With the arm flexed to 60 degrees and held against downward pressure the clavicular part can be readily palpated, while the sternocostal part is best palpated if this same position is maintained against upward pressure. The integrity of the muscle can be tested by adduction of the arm against resistance.

MUSCLES EXTENDING THE ARM AT THE SHOULDER JOINT

Latissimus dorsi
Teres major
Pectoralis major (p. 102)
Deltoid (posterior fibres) (p. 100)
Triceps brachii (long head) (p. 132)

Latissimus Dorsi

Large, flat, triangular sheet of muscle, latissimus dorsi extends between the trunk and arm (Fig. 2.34); consequently, it acts on the shoulder joint. The superior border forms the inferior border of the triangle of auscultation, while its lateral border forms the medial border of the lumbar triangle.

Latissimus dorsi arises from the posterior layer of the thoracolumbar fascia, which attaches to the spinous processes of the lower six thoracic and all lumbar and sacral vertebrae, as well as the intervening supraspinous and interspinous ligaments; that part arising from the lower six thoracic vertebrae is covered by trapezius. In addition to its vertebral attachment, latissimus dorsi also arises from the posterior part of the lateral lip of the iliac crest, most laterally by direct muscular slips. As these fibres pass superolaterally across the lower part of the thorax they attach to the lateral surfaces of the lower three or four ribs and via fascia to the inferior angle of the scapula. From this widespread attachment, the fibres converge as they pass towards the humerus forming a thin, flattened tendon, which winds around the lower border of teres major, to attach to the floor of the intertubercular groove of the humerus anterior to the tendon of teres major, separated from it by a bursa. The effect of the muscle twisting through 180 degrees means that the anterior surface of the tendon becomes continuous with the posterior surface of the rest of the muscle; consequently, fibres with the lowest attachment on the trunk gain the highest attachment on the humerus.

Latissimus dorsi has an important function in rowing and during the downstroke in swimming. Its attachment to the ribs means that it is active in violent expiration; it can be felt pressing forcibly inwards during a cough or sneeze as it acts to compress the thorax and abdomen.

The attachment to the inferior angle of the scapula allows latissimus dorsi to assist in holding it against the thorax during movements of the upper limb.

If the arm becomes the fixed point when standing (using crutches) latissimus dorsi is able to pull the trunk forwards relative to the arms; this is associated with lifting of the pelvis. In individuals with paralysis of the lower half of the body, the fact that latissimus dorsi attaches to the pelvis means it can be used to produce movement of the pelvis and trunk, provided it is still innervated. Consequently, individuals wearing callipers and using crutches can produce a modified gait by fixing the arms and hitching the hips by alternate contractions of each latissimus dorsi.

Palpation

In a lean individual, with the arm raised to 90 degrees flexion and held steady against an upwardly directed pressure, latissimus dorsi can be made to stand out relative to the thorax. It can be felt contracting if the posterior axillary fold is held between the finger and thumb while the individual coughs. Adduction of the abducted arm against resistance also enables latissimus dorsi to be seen and felt.

Teres Major

Thick, chunky muscle forming the posterior fold of the axilla with latissimus dorsi; in the posterior part of the axilla, teres major (Fig. 2.35) forms the inferior boundary of both the triangular and quadrangular spaces (Fig. 2.25). It arises from an oval area on the dorsal surface of the scapula near the inferior angle and fascia between it and adjacent muscles. The fibres adjacent to latissimus dorsi run superolaterally forming a broad, flat tendon attaching along the medial lip of the intertubercular groove of the humerus. The tendon is separated from that of latissimus dorsi by a bursa; latissimus dorsi virtually covers the whole of the muscle.

Innervation

By the lower subscapular nerve (root value C6, C7) from the posterior cord of the brachial plexus.

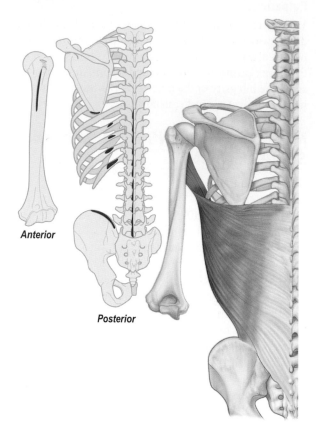

Anterior

Posterior

Fig. 2.34 Posterior aspect of the trunk and left humerus showing the position and attachments of latissimus dorsi.

Innervation

By the thoracodorsal nerve (root value C6, C7, C8) from the posterior cord of the brachial plexus; the nerve enters the muscle on its deep surface. Skin covering the muscle is supplied by the ventral and dorsal rami of roots T4 to T12 and the dorsal rami of L1 to L3.

Action

Latissimus dorsi is a strong extensor of the flexed arm; however, if the humerus is fixed relative to the scapula, it retracts the pectoral girdle. It is also a strong adductor and medial rotator of the arm at the shoulder joint.

Functional Activity

Functionally, latissimus dorsi is a climbing muscle so that, in conjunction with pectoralis major, with the arms fixed above the head, it can pull the trunk upwards.

Action

Teres major adducts and medially rotates the arm at the shoulder joint; in addition, it can help to extend the flexed arm.

Functional Activity

Teres major is a climbing muscle working with latissimus dorsi and pectoralis major to pull the trunk superiorly when the arms are fixed. In conjunction with latissimus dorsi and pectoralis major, teres major is important in stabilising the shoulder joint.

Palpation

Teres major is covered by latissimus dorsi, as these two muscles have similar actions caution must be exercised when it is tested. First, find the inferior angle of the scapula, then move the fingers superolaterally into the posterior wall of the axilla. Ask the individual to abduct the arm to 90 degrees and then adduct against an upwardly directed resistance; the rounded contour of teres major should now be palpable. During this same manoeuvre, the flattened tendon of latissimus dorsi, as it twists around teres major, may also be felt.

MUSCLES MEDIALLY ROTATING THE ARM AT THE SHOULDER JOINT

Subscapularis
Teres major (p. 104)
Latissimus dorsi (p. 103)
Pectoralis major (p. 102)
Deltoid (anterior fibres) (p. 100)

Subscapularis

Forming the greater part of the posterior wall of the axilla, subscapularis (Fig. 2.36) lies close to teres major

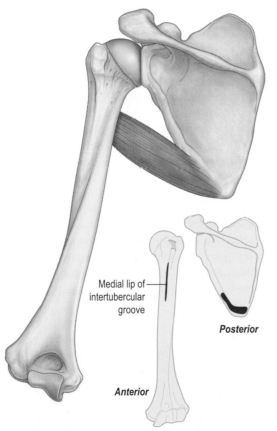

Medial lip of intertubercular groove

Posterior

Anterior

Fig. 2.35 Posterior aspect of the left scapula and humerus showing the position and attachment of teres major.

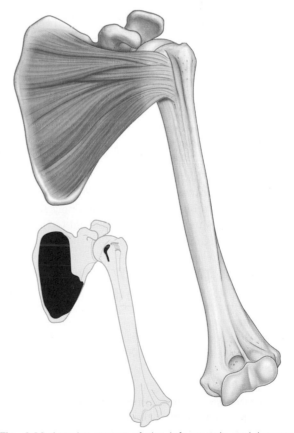

Fig. 2.36 Anterior aspect of the left scapula and humerus showing the position and attachments of subscapularis.

and latissimus dorsi; its anterior surface lies on serratus anterior. Viewed anteriorly, it forms the superior boundary of the triangular and quadrangular spaces (Fig. 2.25).

Subscapularis is a multipennate muscle arising from the medial two-thirds of the subscapular fossa and tendinous septa, which reinforce the muscle, which are attached to bony ridges in the fossa; there is also an attachment to the fascia covering the muscle. The fibres narrow forming a broad, thick tendon which attaches to the lesser tubercle of the humerus, shoulder joint capsule and anterior aspect of the humerus inferior to the tuberosity. A bursa, which communicates directly with the shoulder joint, separates the tendon from the neck of the scapula.

Innervation

By the upper and lower subscapular nerves (root value C5, C6, C7) from the posterior cord of the brachial plexus.

Action

Subscapularis is a strong medial rotator of the arm at the shoulder joint; it may also assist in adduction of the arm.

Functional Activity

As part of the 'rotator cuff', subscapularis plays an important role in maintaining the integrity of the shoulder joint during movement by keeping the head of the humerus within the glenoid fossa. It also resists superior displacement of the humeral head when deltoid, biceps brachii and the long head of triceps brachii are active.

Palpation

The muscle belly cannot be palpated as it lies deep to the scapula. However, careful deep palpation may allow the tendon to be felt just before its attachment to the lesser tuberosity of the humerus.

MUSCLES LATERALLY ROTATING THE ARM AT THE SHOULDER JOINT

Teres minor
Infraspinatus
Deltoid (posterior fibres) (p. 100)

Teres Minor

Viewed posteriorly, teres minor (Fig. 2.37) forms the superior boundary of both the triangular and quadrangular spaces (Fig. 2.25). It is a thin muscle arising by two heads, separated by a groove for the circumflex scapular artery, from the superior two-thirds of the lateral border

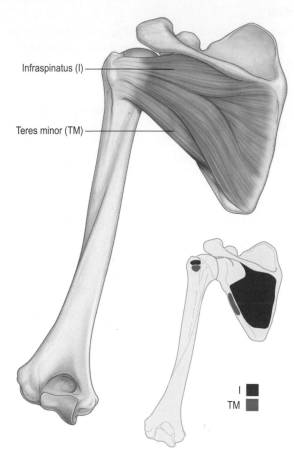

Fig. 2.37 Posterior aspect of the left scapula and humerus showing the position and attachments of infraspinatus *(IM)* and teres minor *(TM)*.

of the scapula and the fascia between it and teres major (inferior) and infraspinatus (superior). The fibres run superolaterally forming a narrow tendon attaching to the inferior facet on the greater tubercle of the humerus and bone immediately inferior. The tendon reinforces and blends with the inferior posterior part of the shoulder joint capsule.

Innervation

By the axillary nerve (root value C5, C6) from the posterior cord of the brachial plexus. Skin over the muscle is supplied by roots T1, T2 and T3.

Action

In the anatomical position, teres minor laterally rotates the arm at the shoulder joint, but when the arm is abducted, it laterally rotates and adducts.

Palpation

By placing the fingers halfway up the lateral border of the scapula and the arm, then actively laterally rotating the arm teres minor can be felt contracting; the tendon lies just inferior to that of infraspinatus.

Infraspinatus

Thick triangular muscle, infraspinatus (Fig. 2.37) arises from the medial two-thirds of the infraspinous fossa of the scapula, tendinous intersections attached to ridges in this fossa and the thick fascia covering the muscle. The fibres converge to a narrow tendon attaching to the middle facet on the greater tubercle of the humerus and posterior aspect of the shoulder joint capsule. A bursa, which occasionally communicates with the shoulder joint, separates the muscle from the neck of the scapula. The upper part of the muscle lies deep to trapezius, deltoid and the acromion process; the lower part is superficial.

Innervation

By the suprascapular nerve (root value C5, C6) from the upper trunk of the brachial plexus. Skin over the muscle is supplied by the dorsal rami of T1 to T6.

Action

Infraspinatus is a lateral rotator of the arm at the shoulder joint.

Functional Activity

Infraspinatus and teres minor are important when the arm is fully abducted. During the latter part of the movement, the humerus is laterally rotated so that the greater tubercle moves clear of the coracoacromial arch, thereby enabling the remaining part of the humeral head to come into contact with the glenoid fossa and full abduction to occur.

Palpation

When the arm is laterally rotated, contraction of infraspinatus can be felt in the medial part of the infraspinous fossa. Its tendon can be palpated if the greater tubercle is moved from below the acromion. To accomplish this, the individual lies prone supporting themselves on the elbows and forearms; the arm is then laterally rotated 25 degrees and slightly adducted. The tendon can then be palpated just below the acromial angle; it is at this point that soft tissue techniques (transverse frictions, electrical treatments) are applied if the tendon becomes inflamed.

Teres minor, infraspinatus, supraspinatus and subscapularis, the musculotendinous 'rotator cuff' of extensible ligaments around the shoulder joint, are all concerned with its stability; the proximity of their tendons to the joint enhances their effect. During movement of the head of the humerus against the glenoid fossa, the interplay between these muscles reduces the sliding and shearing movements which tend to occur. When carrying a weight in the hand, these same muscles brace the head of the humerus against the glenoid fossa.

CLINICAL EXAMINATION AND EVALUATION

Evaluating the full range of motion of the arm at the shoulder requires free movement at the shoulder joint itself, as well as at the acromioclavicular and sternoclavicular joints; there also needs to be free movement of the scapula against the chest wall. Depending on the extent of stabilisation, either shoulder joint movement separately or with associated pectoral girdle movement can be determined.

Abduction

With the individual lying supine:

- Place the shoulder in neutral flexion/extension and full lateral rotation with the palm facing anteriorly and elbow extended.
- Stabilise the scapula to prevent lateral rotation and elevation during abduction (Fig. 2.38A).
- Stabilise the thorax to prevent lateral flexion of the trunk if shoulder abduction and associated pectoral girdle movement are being determined.

The end feel to abduction is firm due to tension in the middle and inferior glenohumeral ligaments, inferior joint capsule, latissimus dorsi and pectoralis major. When assessing abduction and pectoral girdle movement, the end feel is also firm due to tension in rhomboid minor, rhomboid major, and the middle and inferior parts of trapezius.

To measure abduction, the centre of the goniometer is placed over the anterior aspect of the acromion process with the proximal arm parallel to the midline of the sternum and the distal arm aligned with the medial midline of the humerus. Measurement can also be taken with the individual standing (Fig. 2.38B) or lying prone. When sitting or standing, the centre of the goniometer is placed over the

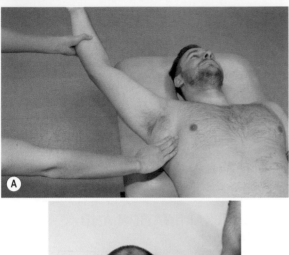

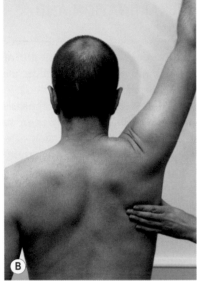

Fig. 2.38 Evaluation of the range of abduction of the arm at the shoulder joint with the individual lying supine (A) and standing (B).

posterior aspect of the acromion process with the proximal arm parallel to the vertebral spinous processes and the distal arm in line with the lateral epicondyle of the humerus.

Adduction

With the individual lying supine:
- Flex the shoulder sufficiently to allow the arm to pass in front of the chest and medially rotate to 90 degrees.
- Stabilise the scapula to prevent lateral rotation and elevation when the arm is adducted across the front of the chest (Fig. 2.39A).
- Stabilise the thorax to prevent lateral flexion of the trunk if shoulder adduction and associated pectoral girdle movement is to be assessed.

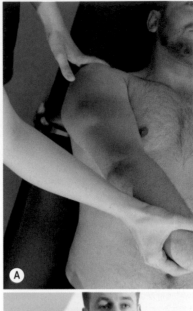

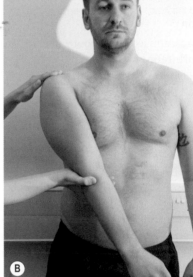

Fig. 2.39 Evaluation of the range of adduction of the arm at the shoulder joint with the individual lying supine (A) and standing (B).

The end feel to adduction is firm due to tension in the superior glenohumeral ligament, superior joint capsule, and middle and posterior fibres of deltoid. When assessing adduction and pectoral girdle movement, the end feel is also firm due to tension in the superior and middle parts of the trapezius.

To measure adduction, place the centre of the goniometer over the anterior aspect of the acromion process

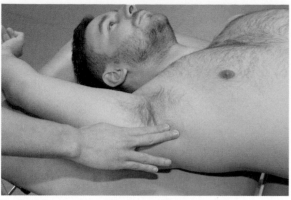

Fig. 2.40 Evaluation of the range of flexion of the arm at the shoulder joint with the individual lying supine.

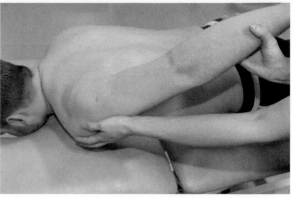

Fig. 2.41 Evaluation of the range of extension of the arm at the shoulder joint with the individual lying prone.

with the proximal arm parallel to the midline of the sternum and the distal arm in line with the lateral epicondyle of the humerus. Adduction can also be measured with the individual sitting or standing (Fig. 2.39B) with the same stabilisation and goniometer placements.

Flexion

With the individual lying supine:
- Flex the knees to flatten the lumbar spine.
- Place the shoulder in neutral abduction/adduction and rotation.
- Place the forearm in mid pronation/supination with the palm against the body.
- Stabilise the scapula to prevent elevation, posterior tilting and lateral rotation when the arm is flexed (Fig. 2.40).

When measuring flexion and associated pectoral girdle movement, the thorax should also be stabilised to prevent extension of the vertebral column. The end feel to flexion is firm due to tension in the posterior band of the coracohumeral ligament, posterior joint capsule, teres minor, teres major and infraspinatus. When assessing flexion and associated pectoral girdle movement, the end feel is also firm due to tension in latissimus dorsi and pectoralis major.

To measure flexion, the centre of the goniometer is placed over the lateral aspect of the acromion process with the proximal arm aligned along the mid-axillary line and the distal arm in line with the lateral epicondyle of the humerus.

Extension

With the individual lying prone:
- Turn the head away from the shoulder being tested.

- Place the shoulder in neutral abduction/adduction and rotation, and the elbow in slight flexion.
- Place the forearm in mid pronation/supination with the palm facing the body.
- Stabilise the scapula to prevent its posterior elevation and anterior tilting when the arm is extended (Fig. 2.41).

When measuring extension and associated pectoral girdle movement, the thorax should also be stabilised to prevent flexion of the vertebral column. The end feel to extension is firm due to tension in the anterior band of the coracohumeral ligament and anterior joint capsule. When assessing extension and associated pectoral girdle movement, the end feel is also firm due to tension in pectoralis major and serratus anterior.

To measure extension, the centre of the goniometer is placed over the lateral aspect of the acromion process with the proximal arm aligned with the mid-axillary line and the distal arm in line with the lateral epicondyle of the humerus.

Lateral Rotation

With the individual lying supine:
- Abduct the shoulder to 90 degrees, flex the elbow to 90 degrees and pronate the forearm.
- Stabilise the distal end of the humerus, as well as the scapula, towards the end of the movement to prevent posterior tilting, then laterally rotate the arm (Fig. 2.42A).

When measuring lateral rotation and associated pectoral girdle movement, the thorax should also be stabilised to prevent extension of the vertebral column towards the end of the movement. The end feel to lateral

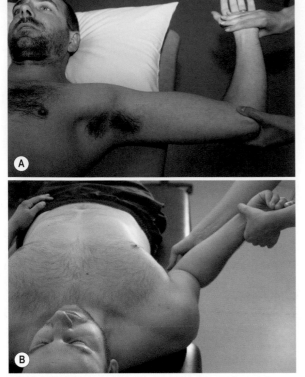

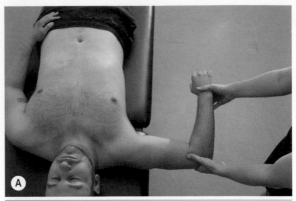

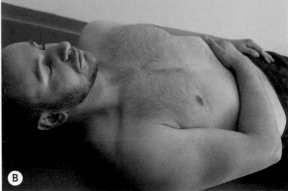

Fig. 2.42 Evaluation of the range of lateral rotation of the arm at the shoulder joint with the individual lying supine and shoulder abducted 90 degrees (A) and in neutral (B).

Fig. 2.43 Evaluation of the range of medial rotation of the arm at the shoulder with the individual lying supine and shoulder abducted 90 degrees (A) and in neutral (B).

rotation is firm due to tension in the glenohumeral and coracohumeral ligaments, anterior joint capsule, subscapularis, pectoralis major, latissimus dorsi and teres major. When assessing lateral rotation and associated pectoral girdle movement, the end feel is also firm due to tension in serratus anterior and pectoralis minor.

To measure lateral rotation, the centre of the goniometer is placed over the olecranon process, with the proximal arm either parallel or perpendicular to the supporting surface and the distal arm in line with the ulnar styloid process.

Alternatively, the range of lateral rotation can be determined with the individual sitting or standing with the shoulder in neutral flexion/extension and abduction/adduction, elbow flexed 90 degrees and forearm in mid pronation/supination, the distal end of the humerus is stabilised as the forearm is moved away from the midline (Fig. 2.42B). To measure lateral rotation, the centre of the goniometer is placed over the olecranon process with the proximal arm aligned in the sagittal plane and the distal arm in line with the ulnar styloid process.

Medial Rotation

With the individual lying supine:

- Adduct the shoulder to 90 degrees, flex the elbow to 90 degrees and pronate the forearm.
- Stabilise the distal end of the humerus, as well as the scapula, towards the end of the movement to prevent elevation and anterior tilting, then medially rotate the arm (Fig. 2.43A).

When measuring medial rotation and associated pectoral girdle movement, the thorax should also be stabilised to prevent flexion of the vertebral column towards the end of the movement. The end feel to medial rotation is firm due to tension in the posterior joint capsule, infraspinatus and teres minor. When assessing medial rotation and associated pectoral girdle movement, the end feel to movement is also firm due to tension in the rhomboids and the middle and inferior parts of trapezius.

To measure medial rotation of the arm at the shoulder joint and associated pectoral girdle movement, the centre of the goniometer is placed over the olecranon process with the proximal arm either parallel or perpendicular to the supporting surface and the distal arm in line with the ulnar styloid process.

Alternatively, medial rotation can be determined with the individual sitting or standing, the shoulder in neutral flexion/extension and abduction/adduction, elbow flexed 90 degrees and forearm in mid pronation/supination and the distal end of the humerus stabilised as the forearm is moved towards the midline (Fig. 2.43B). To measure medial rotation, the centre of the goniometer is placed on the olecranon process with the proximal arm aligned in the sagittal plane and the distal arm in line with the ulnar styloid process.

A third method of assessing medial rotation is to determine the extent of posterior reach; in addition to shoulder movement, this also requires movement at the elbow, wrist and thumb (Fig. 2.44). Posterior reach is defined as the highest segment of the trunk that can be reached by the thumb, which can reach as high as T4 in females and T5 in males; the adult range is usually between T6 and T10.

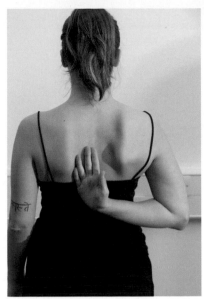

Fig. 2.44 Medial rotation of the arm at the shoulder joint assessed by determining the extent of posterior reach: this method also requires movement at the elbow, wrist and thumb.

Section Summary

Scapula
- Articulates with head of humerus at glenoid fossa forming the shoulder (glenohumeral) joint; clavicle at acromion forming acromioclavicular joint.

Humerus
- Head articulates with glenoid fossa of scapula forming shoulder (glenohumeral) joint.

Shoulder Joint

Type	Synovial ball-and-socket joint
Articular surfaces	Head of humerus, glenoid fossa (deepened by glenoid labrum) of scapula
Capsule	Loose attaching to articular margins of both bones but, on humerus, attaches a short way inferiorly onto shaft medially
Ligaments	Superior, middle and inferior glenohumeral (reinforce capsule); transverse humeral (spans intertubercular groove); coracohumeral; coracoacromial (with acromion and coracoid process forms an arch above joint)
Stability	Effectively provided by rotator cuff muscles (supraspinatus, infraspinatus, subscapularis, teres minor)
Movements	Can be described with respect to the plane of the scapula or cardinal planes of the body: flexion/extension; abduction/adduction; medial/lateral rotation

Movements of Arm at Shoulder Joint

The shoulder joint consists of the head of humerus and glenoid fossa of the scapula. It is capable of a wide range of independent movements produced by the following muscles:

Movement	Muscles (root value of nerve supply)
Abduction	Supraspinatus (C5, C6)
	Deltoid (C5, C6)
Adduction	Coracobrachialis (C6, C7)
	Pectoralis major (C5, C6, C7, C8, T1)
	Latissimus dorsi (C6, C7, C8)
	Teres major (C6, C7)

Continued

Section Summary—Cont'd

Movement	Muscles (root value of nerve supply)
Flexion	Pectoralis major (C5, C6, C7, C8, T1)
	Deltoid (anterior fibres) (C5, C6)
	Coracobrachialis (C6, C7)
	Biceps (long head) (C5, C6)
Extension	Latissimus dorsi (C6, C7, C8)
	Teres major (C6, C7)
	Pectoralis major (to midline) (C5, C6, C7, C8, T1)
	Deltoid (posterior fibres) (C5, C6)
	Triceps (long head) (C6, C7, C8)
Medial rotation	Subscapularis (C5, C6, C7)
	Teres major (C6, C7)
	Latissimus dorsi (C6, C7, C8)
	Pectoralis major (C5, C6, C7, C8, T1)
	Deltoid (anterior fibres) (C5, C6)
Lateral rotation	Teres minor (C5, C6)
	Infraspinatus (C5, C6)
	Deltoid (posterior fibres) (C5, C6)

- All the muscles listed above contribute to the stability of the shoulder joint.
- It is important to consider the effects of gravity or resistance on these movements and muscle work: adduction against resistance is produced by the adductors listed above; however, when lowering the arm (adduction) with gravity producing the movement, the abductors work eccentrically to control the rate of descent.

Clinical Examination and Evaluation

Movement and Maximum Range	End Feel to Movement
Abduction 120° (with pectoral girdle 180°)	Firm
Adduction 35°	Firm
Flexion 110° (with pectoral girdle 180°)	Firm
Extension 70° (with pectoral girdle 90°)	Firm
Lateral rotation 80°	Firm
Medial rotation 90°	Firm

? SELF-ASSESSMENT QUESTIONS

19. Which structures form the shoulder joint?
20. Which muscles attach to the facets on the greater tubercle of the humerus?
21. What is the angle of inclination of the humerus? Give a normal value in degrees.
22. What type of joint is the shoulder joint?
23. Which structure deepens the glenoid fossa of the scapula?
24. Name the rotator cuff muscles.
25. The tendon of which muscle passes through the shoulder joint capsule?
26. Which structures strengthen the anterior aspect of the shoulder joint capsule?
27. Which structures pass through the quadrangular space?
28. What are the boundaries of the triangular space?
29. What is the sequence of muscle activity when abducting the arm at the shoulder joint?
30. What is the nerve supply, including root value, of teres major?
31. Which muscles laterally rotate the arm at the shoulder joint?
32. Which muscles flex the arm at the shoulder joint?
33. Which muscle forms the anterior axillary fold?
34. What are the attachments of teres major?
35. What are the actions of latissimus dorsi?
36. What are the attachments of subscapularis?
37. What forms the medial wall of the axilla?
38. In which part of the shoulder joint capsule are the glenohumeral ligaments?
39. What is the axillary sheath?
40. In which direction does the head of the humerus most commonly dislocate?
41. What is meant by the term 'cardinal plane' when referring to movements of the shoulder joint?
42. Which structure passes deep to the transverse humeral ligament?
43. What is the angle of retroversion?
44. Which of the glenohumeral ligaments is usually most well developed?
45. What is the root value of nerves supplying the shoulder joint?
46. Which muscle passes anterior to the axillary artery in the axilla?
47. What is the function/role of the rotator cuff muscles?
48. What is the surface marking of the shoulder joint line?

ELBOW

LEARNING OUTCOMES

By the end of the section, you should be able to:

1. Identify, palpate and examine the distal humerus, proximal radius and ulna
2. Describe the bones, joints and muscles of the elbow region
3. Describe and explain the movements possible, and their restraints, at the elbow joint
4. Locate, palpate and examine the muscles associated with the elbow and know their attachments, action and innervation
5. Examine and assess movements of the elbow joint
6. Appreciate the influence of pathology and/or trauma on the function of the elbow

INTRODUCTION

The elbow joint is the intermediate joint of the upper limb, between the arm and forearm; it can be considered to be subservient to the hand in that it enables the hand and fingers to be properly placed in space. The elbow joint is responsible for shortening and lengthening the upper limb; the ability to carry food to the mouth is due to flexion at the elbow. If situations arise in which the hand and forearm are unable to move, then the arm and trunk can move towards the hand.

The elbow joint shows the fundamental characteristics of all hinge joints. The articular surfaces are reciprocally shaped; it has strong collateral ligaments, and the muscles are grouped at the sides of the joint where they do not interfere with movement.

The deep fascia of the elbow is very strong because many of the muscles arising from either the common flexor or extensor origins are also attached to the overlying fascia. The bicipital aponeurosis helps to strengthen the fascia anteriorly, while the triceps brachii attachment does so posteriorly.

HUMERUS

Details of the humerus can be found on page 81.

RADIUS

Lying lateral to the ulna in the forearm the radius is the shorter of the two bones (Fig. 2.45A and B). It articulates proximally with the capitulum of the humerus, distally with the scaphoid and lunate of the proximal row of the carpus, and at each end with the ulna. It has a shaft and two ends, the inferior being the larger.

The head is a thick disc with a concave superior surface for articulation with the capitulum: the outer, articular surface of the head is flattened, articulating with a fibro-osseous ring formed by the radial notch of the ulna and the annular ligament. Inferior to the head is the constricted neck, which slopes medially as it approaches the shaft; where the shaft joins the neck, it is round, becoming triangular distally. Together with the neck, the shaft has a slight medial convexity in its proximal quarter with a lateral convexity in the remaining distal part. The radial tuberosity lies antero-medially on the proximal part of the shaft at the maximum convexity of the medial curve. The majority of the shaft presents three borders (anterior, posterior and interosseous) and three surfaces (lateral, anterior and posterior).

The sharp interosseous border, to which the interosseous membrane attaches, faces medially and extends from just inferior to the radial tuberosity to the medial side of the distal end of the radius, splitting into two ridges which become continuous with the anterior and posterior margins of the ulnar notch. The anterior and posterior borders pass obliquely inferolaterally from either side of the radial tuberosity to the roughened area for pronator teres inferiorly. The anterior border becomes distinct distally, while the posterior border becomes more rounded; these borders enclose the lateral, anterior and flatter posterior surfaces.

The distal end of the radius is expanded with five distinct surfaces. The lateral surface, extending to the styloid process, has a shallow groove anteriorly for the tendons of abductor pollicis longus and extensor pollicis brevis. The medial surface forms the concave ulnar notch for articulation with the head of the ulna; it has a roughened triangular area superiorly. The posterior surface is convex and grooved by tendons with the prominent ridge (dorsal (Lister's) tubercle) in the middle; the lateral half of the surface continues onto the styloid process. The anterior surface is smooth and curves anteriorly to a distinct anterior margin. The distal articular surface is concave extending onto the styloid process, divided by a ridge into two areas: a triangular lateral area for articulation with the scaphoid and a quadrilateral medial area for articulation with the lunate (Fig. 2.45C).

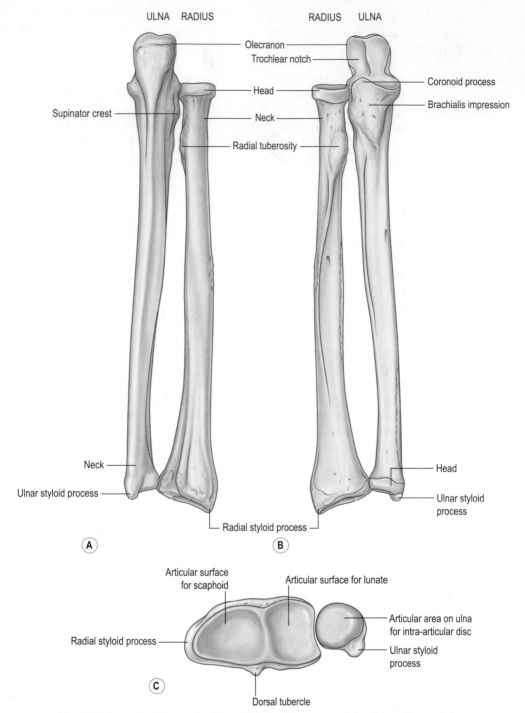

Fig. 2.45 Posterior (A), anterior (B) and inferior (C) aspects of the right radius and ulna.

Ossification

A primary ossification centre appears in the shaft during the 8th week *in utero*, so that, at birth, only the head, distal end and radial tuberosity are cartilaginous. The first secondary centre appears in the distal end during the 1st year of life, fusing with the shaft between 20 and 22 years. The secondary centre for the head appears at about 6 years, fusing with the shaft between 15 and 17 years. A secondary centre usually appears in the radial tuberosity between 14 and 15 years, soon fusing with the shaft.

Palpation

The head of the radius can be palpated in a 'dimple' on the posterolateral aspect of the elbow, particularly when the elbow joint is extended as it overhangs the capitulum; it can be felt rotating during pronation and supination. The shaft of the radius can be palpated on its lateral side in the distal half of the forearm. Distally, on the posterior aspect, the dorsal tubercle can be identified proximal to the wrist, as can the styloid process laterally between the extensor tendons of the thumb within the 'anatomical snuffbox'.

ULNA

Lying medial to the radius the ulna is the longer of the two bones in the forearm; it has a shaft and two ends, of which the proximal is the larger, presenting as a hook-like projection for articulation with the trochlea of the humerus. The smaller rounded distal end is the head of the ulna (Fig. 2.45A and B); it does not articulate directly with the carpus. The ulna articulates laterally at each end with the radius.

The large proximal end of the ulna has two projecting processes, enclosing a concavity. The olecranon process is the larger, forming the proximal part of the bone (Figs 2.45A and B and 2.46A) and has thickened and roughened borders; it is beak-shaped and directed anteriorly, being continuous inferiorly with the shaft. Posteriorly, it is smooth and subcutaneous, while anteriorly it is concave forming the superior part of the articular surface of the trochlear notch.

The coronoid process projects from the anterior aspect of the shaft and has a superior articular surface completing the trochlear notch (Figs 2.45 and 2.46B). These surfaces are often separated by a roughened non-articular area running horizontally across the notch.

The trochlear notch is divided into larger medial and smaller lateral parts by a vertical ridge; the lateral part is continuous over its outer edge with the articular surface of the radial notch on the lateral side of the coronoid process. A small tubercle, where the medial and anterior edges of the articular surface of the coronoid process meet, gives attachment to the anterior part of the ulnar collateral ligament. The irregular, anterior surface of the coronoid ends below at the rough tuberosity of the ulna; both this surface and the tuberosity give attachment to brachialis. At the superior medial part of the coronoid is the small sublime tubercle from which the pronator ridge runs inferolaterally.

The concave radial notch on the lateral side of the coronoid process receives the head of the radius. Inferior to this and extending onto the shaft is the triangular supinator fossa bound posteriorly by the distinct supinator crest; the medial border of this area forms a prominent ridge with a small tubercle at its proximal end.

The prominent interosseous border gives attachment to the interosseous membrane; it runs inferiorly from the apex of the supinator fossa. The anterior border runs inferiorly from the medial margin of the coronoid process but is indistinct. The sinuous, subcutaneous posterior border, prominent in its proximal part, is continuous with the subcutaneous region of the olecranon and the proximal part of the shaft. Between these borders are three surfaces (anterior, medial and posterior), the anterior and medial being continuous at the rounded anterior border; the distal quarter of the anterior surface is marked by an oblique ridge running inferomedially. On the posterior surface, an oblique ridge runs postero-inferiorly from the radial notch to the posterior border; the remaining posterior surface has faint ridges laterally but is smooth medially.

The distal end of the ulna has a narrowed neck which expands into a small, rounded head which has a smooth articular surface for the radius on its anterior and lateral aspects: the distal surface is smooth and almost flat, articulating with an articular disc between it and the triquetral (carpal bone). From the posteromedial part of the head, the conical styloid process projects inferiorly.

Ossification

A primary ossification centre appears in the shaft during the 8th week *in utero*; the body, coronoid process and major part of the olecranon ossify from this primary centre. A secondary centre appears in the head during

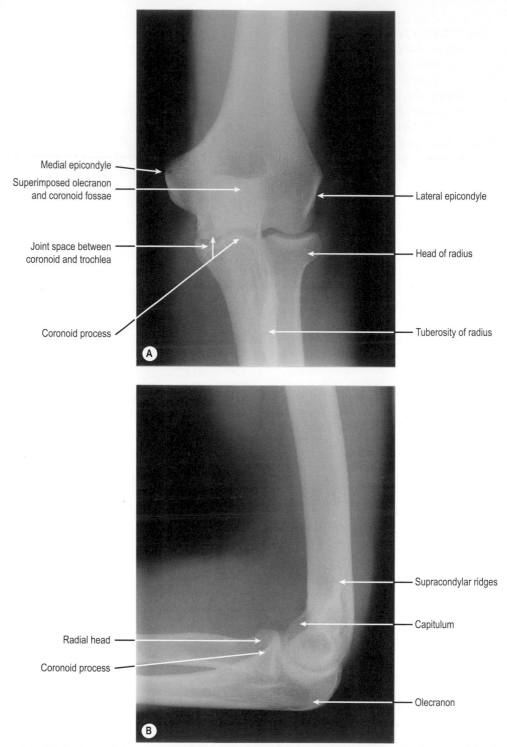

Fig. 2.46 (A) Posteroanterior radiograph of the right elbow in full extension. (B) Lateral radiograph of the right elbow in flexion.

the 5th year fusing with the shaft between 20 and 22 years. The secondary centre for the remainder of the olecranon appears at about 11 years, with fusion occurring between 16 and 19 years; there may be several secondary centres for the olecranon.

Palpation

At the superior and posterior aspect of the elbow, the outline of the olecranon can be identified; in flexion, it forms the 'point' of the elbow. Running inferiorly from this point, the posterior border can be palpated throughout its length. At the distal end, the neck, head and styloid process can all be palpated with the styloid process being the most posterior. When the forearm is fully pronated, the rounded head of the ulna is prominent on the posterior aspect of the wrist.

ELBOW JOINT

Articular Surfaces

The articulation at the elbow joint involves three bones: the distal end of the humerus and the proximal ends of the radius and ulna. The distal end of the humerus shows two joined articular regions, the grooved trochlea medially and rounded capitulum laterally, separated by a groove of variable depth (Fig. 2.47A and B). The whole of this complex surface is covered by a continuous layer of hyaline cartilage. The trochlea articulates with the trochlear notch of the ulna and the capitulum with the cupped head of the radius; both surfaces are covered with hyaline cartilage.

Viewed laterally, the distal end of the humerus projects anteroinferiorly at an angle of 45 degrees so that the trochlea lies anterior to the axis of the shaft (Fig. 2.48A).

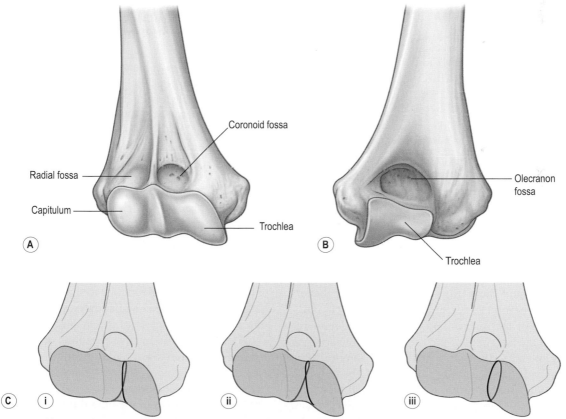

Fig. 2.47 Anterior (A) and posterior (B) aspects of the right humerus showing the articular surfaces participating in the elbow joint. (C) Anterior aspect of the right distal humerus showing variations in the trochlear groove.

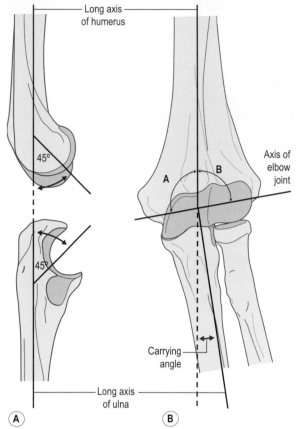

Fig. 2.48 Lateral aspect of the right elbow (A) and anterior aspect of the left elbow (B) showing the relationship of the axes of the elbow joint and formation of the carrying angle.

Similarly, the trochlear notch of the ulna projects anterosuperiorly at an angle of 45 degrees, also lying anterior to the axis of the shaft of the ulna (Fig. 2.48A). These projections of the articular surfaces facilitate a large range of flexion at the elbow joint by delaying contact between the humerus and ulna. In addition, it provides a space between them to accommodate the musculature until the bones are almost parallel. Without these two features, particularly the former, flexion beyond 90 degrees would be severely limited.

In spite of the anterior projections of the humerus and ulna, the long axes of the two bones coincide when viewed laterally. However, when viewed anteriorly, the ulnar axis deviates laterally from that of the humerus (Fig. 2.48B); this deviation is referred to as the carrying angle, being approximately 10 to 15 degrees in males and 20 to 25 degrees in females. Normally, the transverse axis of the elbow joint bisects this angle so that, when it is fully flexed, the forearm overlies the arm and the hand

covers the shoulder joint. If, however, the bisected parts of the carrying angle (A and B, Fig. 2.48B) are not equal, then the hand will be lateral (A < B) or medial (A > B) to the shoulder on full flexion of the joint.

The transverse axis of the elbow joint runs from inferoposteromedial to superoanterolateral, passing approximately through the middle of the trochlea. Because of this slight obliquity, there is some debate as to whether the joint exhibits a pure hinge movement, especially as this axis oscillates slightly during flexion and extension. Nevertheless, for practical purposes, it can be considered as a pure hinge joint.

Trochlea of the Humerus

The pulley-shaped trochlea with its groove presents a concave surface in the coronal plane; it is convex in a parasagittal plane. It forms an almost complete circle separated by a thin wall of bone, which itself may be perforated so that 320 to 330 degrees of the surface is cartilage-covered (Fig. 2.47A and B). The medial free border is not circular but describes part of a helix with a radially directed slant. The trochlea groove is limited by a sharp prominent ridge medially and a lower blunter ridge laterally, which blends with the articular surface of the capitulum (Fig. 2.47A); the tilt on the trochlea is partly responsible for the carrying angle of the elbow.

Although the trochlear groove appears to lie in the sagittal plane, it runs obliquely and shows individual variation; however, the most common form is with the anterior part of the groove running vertically and the posterior part obliquely inferolaterally. As a whole, the groove runs in a spiral around the transverse axis of the trochlea (Fig. 2.47C(i)); occasionally, it runs obliquely superolaterally anteriorly and inferolaterally posteriorly forming a true spiral (Fig. 2.47C(ii)); rarely, the groove runs obliquely proximally anteromedially and distally posterolaterally forming a circle (Fig. 2.47C(iii)). The functional significance of these variations in trochlea angulation is minimal; the only observable difference is in the magnitude of the carrying angle and the relative positions of the arm and forearm in full flexion at the elbow joint.

Immediately superior to the trochlea anteriorly is the concave coronoid fossa (Fig. 2.47A), which receives the coronoid process of the ulna during flexion. Posteriorly, in a similar position, is the olecranon fossa which receives the olecranon during extension (Fig. 2.47B). If these two fossae are particularly deep the intervening

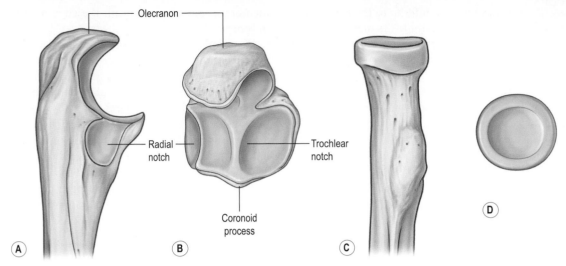

Fig. 2.49 Lateral (A) and superior (B) aspects of the right ulna showing the articular surfaces participating in the elbow joint; anterior (C) and superior (D) aspects of the right radius showing the articular surfaces participating in the elbow joint.

thin plate of bone may be perforated, allowing the fossae to communicate with each other.

Capitulum

The capitulum is not a complete sphere but a hemisphere on the anteroinferior aspect of the humerus (Fig. 2.47A); it does not extend posteriorly like the trochlea. Although considered hemispherical, its radius of curvature is not constant, increasing slightly from proximal to distal. The cartilage covering the capitulum is thickest centrally, where it may be 5 mm thick. The medial border of the capitulum is truncated, forming the capitulotrochlear groove. Superior to the capitulum anteriorly is the radial fossa, which receives the rim of the head of the radius during flexion (Fig. 2.47A).

Trochlear Notch of the Ulna

The proximal end of the ulna has the deep trochlear notch (Fig. 2.49A and B) for articulation with the trochlea of the humerus. It has a rounded, curved, longitudinal ridge extending from the tip of the olecranon superiorly to the tip of the coronoid process inferiorly. This ridge fits snugly into the groove of the trochlea, on either side of which is a concave surface for the trochlea. The cartilage of the trochlear notch is interrupted by a transverse line across its deepest part, providing two separate surfaces, one on the olecranon and the other on the coronoid process.

Head of the Radius

The concave superior surface of the head of the radius articulates with the capitulum and the raised margin with the capitulotrochlear groove (Fig. 2.49C and D). The cartilage of this surface is continuous with that around the sides of the head, being thickest in the middle of the concavity.

Because of the articulations between the radius and ulna, their proximal surfaces may be considered as constituting a single articular surface. However, because of movement between the bones, they do not maintain the same relative positions with respect to the humerus, nor does the radius always maintain contact with the humerus (p. 126).

While the articular surface of the trochlea has an angular value of 330 degrees and the capitulum 180 degrees, the angular values of the articular surfaces of the trochlear notch of the ulna and the head of the radius are much smaller (190 and 40 degrees, respectively). The difference in angular values between corresponding parts of the elbow joint is approximately 140 degrees, a value close to the range of flexion/extension possible at the joint.

Palpation

Palpation of the joint line anteriorly is not possible because of its deepness within the cubital fossa and the overlying muscles. Nevertheless, it can be approximated by a line joining a point 1 cm inferior to the lateral epicondyle with a point 2 cm inferior to the medial epicondyle. Posteriorly, the gap between the head of the radius and capitulum can be palpated in the large dimple present on the posterior aspect of the extended elbow.

Posteriorly, the olecranon is subcutaneous and can be readily palpated, either side of which the medial and lateral epicondyles form easily recognisable bony landmarks.

Joint Capsule and Synovial Membrane

A single fibrous capsule completely encloses the elbow and superior radioulnar (p. 138) joints. The capsule has no openings in it, but slight pouching of the synovial membrane may occur beneath the edge of the capsule in some areas.

Anteriorly, it arises from the medial epicondyle away from the articular surface of the trochlea, arching superolaterally to attach to the margins of the coronoid and radial fossae and the articular margin of the capitulum as it reaches the lateral epicondyle. Posteriorly, the capsule follows the lateral margins of the capitulum arching superiorly around the olecranon fossa, returning to the medial epicondyle some distance from the edge of the trochlear surface (Fig. 2.50).

Distally, the capsule attaches to the margins of the trochlear notch, around the olecranon and coronoid processes. As it reaches the radial notch, it passes onto

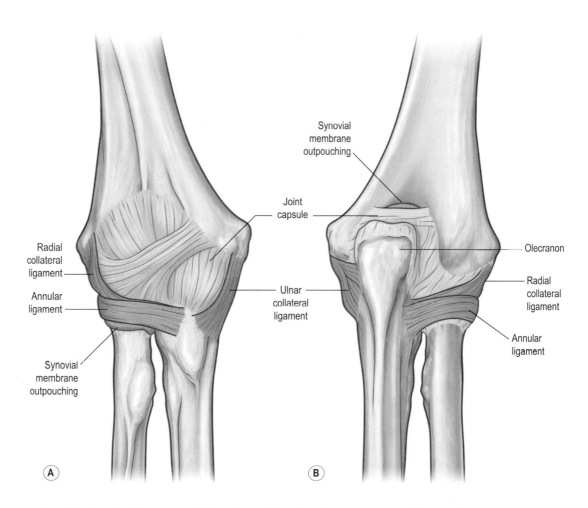

Fig. 2.50 Anterior (A) and posterior (B) aspects of the right elbow showing the joint capsule and outpouchings of the synovial membrane; also shown are the radial and ulna collateral ligaments.

and attaches to the annular ligament (p. 138); medially and laterally it blends with the collateral ligaments of the joint (Fig. 2.50). The joint capsule has no direct attachment to the radius; if this was the case movement between the radius and ulna would be severely limited.

Because the capsule blends with the collateral ligaments, it is strengthened in these regions; however, it is relatively weak anteriorly and posteriorly. Anteriorly, the capsule consists mainly of longitudinal fibres running from above the coronoid and radial fossae to the anterior border of the coronoid process and the anterior aspect of the annular ligament (Fig. 2.50A). Some bundles among these longitudinal fibres run obliquely mediolaterally (Fig. 2.50A). Consequently, this part of the capsule is thicker centrally than at the sides and is often referred to as a capsular ligament. Some deep fibres of brachialis attach to the anterior aspect of the capsule as the muscle crosses the joint; this serves to pull the capsule and underlying synovial membrane away from the articulating bones preventing them from becoming trapped during flexion.

The posterior part of the capsule is thin and membranous, being mainly composed of transverse fibres extending loosely between the margins of the olecranon and edges of the olecranon fossa. Some fibres stretch across the fossa as a transverse band with a free superior border without attaching to the olecranon (Fig. 2.50B); it does not extend as far as the superior margin of the fossa. Posteriorly, the capsule passes laterally from the lateral epicondyle to the posterior border of the radial notch and posterior aspect of the annular ligament. The weakest part of the capsule posteriorly is centrally; however, here it blends with the deep part of the tendon of triceps brachii, which supports it during extension of the joint, having a similar function to the deep part of brachialis.

Synovial Membrane

The synovial membrane lining the joint capsule is extensive, attaching to the articular margins of the humerus and ulna, reflected onto the humerus to cover the coronoid and radial fossae anteriorly and olecranon fossa posteriorly. Distally, it is prolonged onto the superior part of the deep surface of the annular ligament. The membrane continues into the superior radioulnar articulation covering the inferior part of the annular ligament and then reflected onto the neck of the radius. Below the inferior border of the annular ligament, the membrane emerges as a redundant fold (Fig. 2.50A) giving freedom of movement to the head of the radius. This inferior reflection is supported by a few loose fibres passing from the inferior border of the annular ligament to the neck of the radius. The synovial membrane is supported by the quadrate ligament (p. 140) as it passes from the medial side of the neck of the radius to the inferior border of the radial notch, preventing herniation of the membrane between the anterior and posterior free edges of the annular ligament.

Various synovial folds project into the recesses of the joint between the edges of the articular surfaces. An especially constant fold forms an almost complete ring overlying the periphery of the radial head, projecting into the gap between it and the capitulum. Slight outpouching of the membrane may occur below the inferior borders of the annular ligament and the transverse band of the ulnar collateral ligament, as well as superior to the transverse capsular fibres crossing the superior part of the olecranon fossa (Fig. 2.50B).

Well-marked extrasynovial fat pads lie adjacent to the articular fossae. In extension, they fill the radial and coronoid fossae and, in flexion, the olecranon fossa; they are displaced when parts of the ulna or radius occupy the fossae.

Ligaments

The collateral ligaments associated with the elbow joint are strong triangular bands blending with the sides of the joint capsule. They span the axis of movement in all positions of the joint, therefore, they are relatively tense in all positions of flexion and extension; they impose strict limitations on abduction, adduction and axial rotation.

Ulnar Collateral Ligament

Fanning out from the medial epicondyle, the ulnar collateral ligament has thick anterior and posterior bands united by a thinner intermediate central portion (Fig. 2.51A). The anterior band passes from the anterior aspect of the medial epicondyle to the medial edge of the coronoid process; it is intimately associated with the common tendon of the superficial forearm flexors, giving attachment to some fibres of flexor digitorum superficialis. The posterior band runs from the posterior aspect of the medial epicondyle to the medial edge of the olecranon. The apex of the thinner intermediate part is attached to the inferior surface of the medial epicondyle

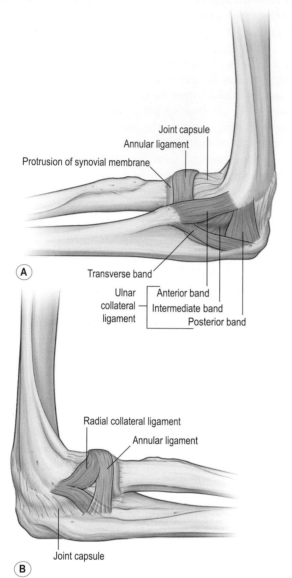

Joint capsule
Annular ligament
Protrusion of synovial membrane

Ⓐ

Transverse band

Ulnar
collateral
ligament

Anterior band
Intermediate band
Posterior band

Radial collateral ligament
Annular ligament

Joint capsule
Ⓑ

Fig. 2.51 Medial (A) and lateral (B) aspects of the right elbow showing the joint capsule and radial and ulnar collateral ligaments.

and its base to the transverse band passing between the attachments of the anterior and posterior bands (Fig. 2.51A). Synovial membrane protrudes inferior to the free edge of the transverse ligament during movement at the joint. The intermediate grooved part of the ligament is crossed by the ulnar nerve as it passes posterior to the medial epicondyle to enter the forearm.

Radial Collateral Ligament

Strong triangular band attaching superiorly to a depression on the anteroinferior aspect of the lateral epicondyle deep to the overlying common extensor tendon (Fig. 2.51B); inferiorly it blends with the annular ligament of the radius. The slightly thicker anterior and posterior margins pass anteriorly and posteriorly to attach to the margins of the radial notch of the ulna (Fig. 2.51B); it is less distinct than the ulnar collateral ligament.

Blood Supply, Lymphatic Drainage and Innervation

The arterial supply to the joint is from an extensive anastomosis around the elbow involving the brachial artery and its terminal branches. Descending inferiorly are the superior and inferior ulnar collateral branches of the brachial artery, and the radial and middle collateral branches of the profunda brachii. These anastomose on the surface of the joint capsule, as well as with the anterior and posterior recurrent branches of the ulnar artery, the radial recurrent branch of the radial artery and the interosseous recurrent branch of the common interosseous artery (Fig. 2.52).

Venous drainage, by vessels accompanying the arteries, is into the radial, ulnar and brachial veins. Lymphatic drainage is predominantly to the deep cubital nodes at the bifurcation of the brachial artery, the efferents of which pass to the lateral group of nodes in the axilla. Some lymphatics from the joint may pass to small nodes situated along the interosseous, ulnar, radial or brachial arteries and then to the lateral axillary group of nodes.

The joint is innervated by twigs derived from the musculocutaneous, median and radial nerves anteriorly, and the ulnar nerve and radial nerve, by its branch to anconeus, posteriorly; the root value of these nerves is C5, C6, C7 and C8.

Relations

Anteriorly is the cubital fossa, a triangular space bounded superiorly by an imaginary line between the medial and lateral epicondyles, and at the sides by the converging medial borders of brachioradialis laterally and pronator teres medially (Fig. 2.53A). The floor of the fossa is formed mainly by brachialis with supinator inferolaterally (Fig. 2.53A); the roof is the deep fascia of the forearm, reinforced medially by the bicipital aponeurosis passing from the tendon of biceps

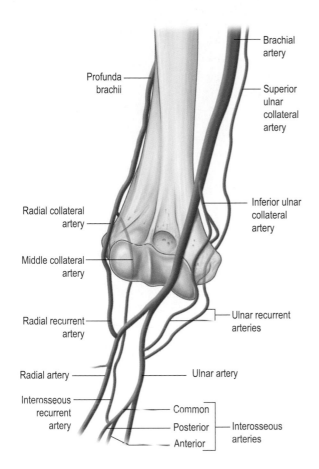

Fig. 2.52 Anterior aspect of the right distal humerus showing the arterial anastomosis around the elbow.

nerve of the forearm (terminal branch of the musculocutaneous nerve). Crossing the median cubital vein and running with the basilic vein and its tributaries are branches of the medial cutaneous nerve of the forearm (Fig. 2.53B).

Lying within the cubital fossa deep to the deep fascia are several structures passing into the forearm. The most medial is the median nerve as it passes distally through the fossa to emerge between the two heads of pronator teres to enter the forearm (Fig 2.53A; see also Fig. 2.140). While in the fossa, the median nerve gives a branch to pronator teres and the anterior interosseous nerve as it passes through pronator teres. Lateral to the median nerve is the brachial artery, which bifurcates at the neck of the radius in the inferior part of the fossa into the ulnar and radial arteries (Figs 2.52 and 2.53A). The ulnar artery passes inferomedially deep to pronator teres, giving the common interosseous artery and recurrent branches to the elbow joint. The radial artery passes inferolaterally over the tendon of biceps brachii deep to brachioradialis, giving a recurrent branch to the elbow joint. Through the central region of the fossa, lateral to both the brachial artery and median nerve, the tendon of biceps brachii passes towards its attachment to the radial tuberosity (see Fig. 2.53A). As it passes through the fossa, the tendon twists on itself so that its anterior surface comes to face laterally. The radial nerve is the most lateral structure passing through the fossa lying between brachialis and brachioradialis: in the superior part of the fossa it supplies both muscles, then divides into its terminal branches, superficial radial and posterior interosseous (deep radial) nerves. The superficial branch continues distally into the forearm deep to brachioradialis, while the posterior interosseous nerve passes posteriorly around the lateral aspect of the radius to enter the forearm between the two heads of supinator.

The ulnar nerve passes posterior to the medial epicondyle of the humerus on the intermediate part of the ulnar collateral ligament posteromedial to the elbow joint; it does not pass through the cubital fossa.

Stability

The shape of the articular surfaces of the humerus (trochlea and capitulum), ulna (trochlear notch) and radial head confer some stability to the elbow joint. Nevertheless, without strong collateral ligaments and the muscular cuff of triceps brachii, biceps brachii,

brachii inferomedially to the deep fascia of the forearm (Fig. 2.53B). The deep fascia separates the superficial veins and nerves from the deeper more important structures (Fig. 2.53B).

This region is of considerable importance because the large superficial veins are frequently used for venepuncture, while the deeper brachial artery is used for determining blood pressure. The main superficial veins are the cephalic laterally, basilic medially and median cubital passing obliquely superomedially between them (see Fig. 2.53B). It is not unusual for the median cubital vein to lie towards the lateral side of the fossa or be joined by the median vein of the forearm. Occasionally, the median cubital vein is absent, with the median vein of the forearm dividing into lateral and medial branches to join with the cephalic and basilic veins, respectively. Lateral to the cephalic vein runs the lateral cutaneous

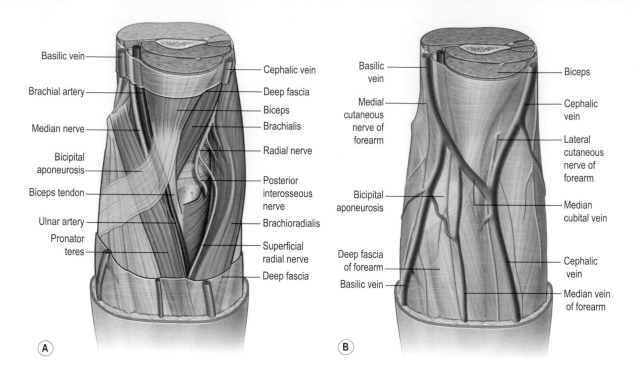

Fig. 2.53 Anterior aspect of the left cubital fossa showing the deep (A) and superficial (B) structures.

brachialis and brachioradialis, together with the common tendons of the superficial flexors and extensors arising from the medial and lateral epicondyles of the humerus, respectively, the elbow joint cannot be considered an inherently stable joint. The bony surfaces are in closest contact with the forearm flexed to 90 degrees in a position of mid pronation/supination. This is the position of greatest joint stability; it is the position naturally assumed when fine manipulation of the hand and fingers is required (writing).

In spite of ligaments and muscles crossing the joint, dislocation of the elbow can and does occur. In young children, because the head of the radius is small relative to the annular ligament, it is commonly dislocated by traction forces applied to the forearm and hand. In older individuals, a fall on the hand with the forearm extended may tear the annular ligament, with a consequent anterior displacement of the head of the radius (Fig. 2.54A). The radial head may also be dislocated by tearing the annular ligament in extreme pronation. In both cases, the head of the radius can be palpated in the cubital fossa.

The majority of elbow dislocations involve posterior movement of the ulna through the relatively weak posterior capsule, often associated with fracture of the coronoid process (Fig. 2.54B). The radius and ulna may be displaced together due to their connections at the superior radioulnar joint; this posterior displacement can lead to pressure on the brachial artery, which may go into spasm reducing the blood supply to the forearm and hand. Pressure on the brachial artery can also occur in supracondylar fractures as the distal fragment moves anteriorly. Either of these events can also lead to injury to the median nerve, with a consequent loss of pronation and reduced function of the hand. Both dislocations and supracondylar fractures result in considerable swelling in the region of the elbow. The alignment of the humeral epicondyles and olecranon can be used to determine the nature of the trauma in an individual with a swollen elbow; the alignment remains unchanged in supracondylar fractures (Fig. 2.54C), but changes in dislocations (Fig. 2.54D). When an apparently dislocated joint cannot be reduced, fracture of the olecranon should be considered, particularly if the joint is extremely unstable.

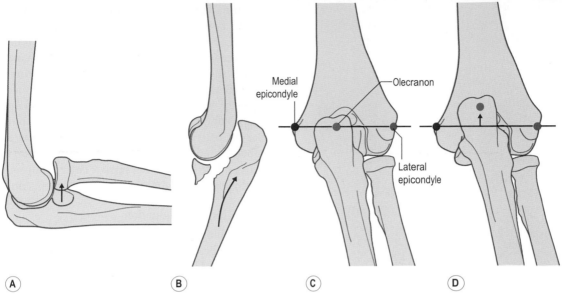

Fig. 2.54 (A) Dislocation of the head of the radius into the cubital fossa. (B) Posterior dislocation of the ulna accompanying fracture of the coronoid process. (C) Normal alignment. (D) Malalignment of the olecranon and humeral epicondyles.

A forceful abduction applied to the forearm may be sufficient to rupture the ulnar collateral ligament, or more commonly result in avulsion of the medial epicondyle; the ulnar nerve is especially liable to damage at the time of injury. If the fracture does not unite or the ligament does not heal, the forearm tends to become more and more abducted, with a consequent stretching of the ulnar nerve leading to sensory disturbances and muscle weakness/paralysis.

MOVEMENTS OF THE FOREARM AT THE ELBOW JOINT

Flexion and extension are possible at the elbow joint, which take place about a transverse axis through the humeral epicondyles (Fig. 2.48B). The axis is not at right angles to the long axis of the humerus or forearm as it bisects the carrying angle at the elbow (Fig. 2.48B); its medial end is, therefore, slightly lower than the lateral. Except at the extremes of flexion and extension, movement between the humerus and the radius and ulna is one of sliding. It is only at the extremes of movement, when the axis changes slightly, that the sliding motion changes to rolling between the articular surfaces. The collateral ligaments remain tense in all positions of the joint.

TABLE 2.5 Required Range of Flexion at the Elbow Joint During Some Common Activities

Activity	Flexion (°)
Eating/drinking	130
Opening door	60
Reading	105
Using phone	135
Rising from a chair	95
Pouring from a jug/bottle	60

Adapted from Safaee-Rad, R., Shwedyk, E., Quanbury, A.O., Cooper, J.E., 1990. Normal functional range of motion of the upper limb during performance of three feeding activities. Arch. Phys. Med. Rehabil. 71, 505–509.

The range of elbow joint motion associated with some common activities is given in Table 2.5.

Flexion and Extension

Movement of the forearm anteriorly is flexion (Fig. 2.55A) continuing until contact between the forearm and arm prevents further movement. The active range of flexion is 145 degrees; however, 160 degrees of flexion can be attained passively. In neonates, the range of active flexion may be as large as 155 degrees but decreases to

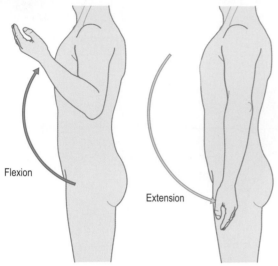

Fig. 2.55 Flexion and extension of the elbow joint.

145 degrees by age 5 (Watanabe et al., 1979); it is not until after age 60 that the range decreases slightly to 140 degrees. There is no difference in the range of flexion between males and females.

Because of the obliquity of the axis about which flexion occurs, the hand moves medially coming to lie over the shoulder during flexion. Flexion is produced by brachialis, biceps brachii and brachioradialis. In slow gentle movements, brachialis is the main muscle used, while in rapid and forceful movements, all three muscles, as well as the superficial forearm flexors, are used. Flexion is primarily limited by apposition of the anterior aspects of the arm and forearm, together with tension in the posterior part of the joint capsule and triceps brachii; impact of the bony surfaces is insignificant.

Extension is movement of the forearm posteriorly, best defined as returning the forearm to the anatomical position (Fig. 2.55B); there may be a small amount (5 degrees) of hyperextension. Strictly speaking, the range of extension possible at the joint is zero as full extension corresponds to the anatomical position; relative extension is always possible from any position of the joint. Active extension is brought about by triceps brachii and anconeus, while passive extension is due to gravity controlled by the eccentric contraction of the elbow flexors, particularly when a weight is held in the hand. Extension is usually limited by tension in the anterior joint capsule and flexor muscles, and to some extent by the anterior parts of the collateral ligaments.

Limitation of either flexion or extension is rarely due to bony contact, although the presence of small cartilage-covered facets at the inferior part of the coronoid fossa and sides of the olecranon fossa in some individuals suggests that bony contact occurs during life.

Small changes in the position of the axis of movement at the extremes of the range results in a small degree of axial rotation due to the configuration of the humeroulnar articulation and ligamentous constraints. During initial flexion, the forearm may medially rotate up to 5 degrees, laterally rotating up to 5 degrees during terminal flexion; although small, these movements do occur.

Abduction and Adduction

Being a hinge joint, the only movements expected at the elbow are described above; however, during pronation and supination of the forearm, there is a small degree of abduction and adduction, respectively, between the trochlear notch of the ulna and trochlea of the humerus. Full details of these movements can be found on page 143.

Accessory Movements

With the elbow almost fully extended, a small degree of abduction and adduction at the joint is possible. Holding the distal part of the arm steady and applying alternate medial and lateral pressure to the distal end of the forearm will produce these accessory movements; this is best demonstrated with the individual lying supine.

The major muscles producing movements of the forearm at the elbow joint are shown in Table 2.6; further details of each muscle can be found in following sections.

BIOMECHANICS
Contact Areas

Because of the rounded ridge extending from the tip of the olecranon to the tip of the coronoid process, as well as the transverse ridge observable on the articular cartilage, the trochlear notch can be conveniently divided into four quadrants (Fig. 2.56A). Direct observation reveals that the contact area on the humerus changes during flexion and extension. In general, the humeroulnar contact area increases from full extension to full flexion; at the same time, the head of the radius establishes greater contact with the capitulum as it moves proximally during flexion. The increasing area of contact supports the view that stability at the joint increases with flexion.

TABLE 2.6	Muscles Producing Movement of the Forearm at the Elbow Joint		
Muscle	Attachments	Action	Innervation
Biceps brachii	Supraglenoid tubercle above glenoid fossa of scapula (long head) and coracoid process of scapula (short head) to radial tuberosity	Flexor of forearm at elbow joint and supinator of forearm at superior and inferior radioulnar joints; also a weak flexor of arm at shoulder joint	Musculocutaneous nerve (C5, C6)
Brachialis	Distal 2/3rd of anterior surface of shaft of humerus and medial and lateral intermuscular septa to inferior part of coronoid process of ulna	Flexor of forearm at elbow joint	Musculocutaneous nerve (C5, C6)
Brachioradialis	Proximal 2/3rd of lateral supracondylar ridge of humerus to lateral aspect of radius above styloid process	Flexor of forearm at elbow joint, especially when forearm is mid pronated/supinated; helps return forearm to the mid position from extremes of either pronation or supination	Radial nerve (C5, C6)
Pronator teres	Distal part of medial supracondylar ridge (upper head) and medial epicondyle of humerus (lower head) to pronator ridge on ulna	Pronator of forearm at radioulnar joints; also weak flexor of forearm at elbow joint	Median nerve (C6, C7)
Triceps brachii	Infraglenoid tubercle below glenoid fossa of scapula (long head), proximal and lateral to spiral groove of humerus (lateral head) and posterior surface of humerus distal and medial to spiral groove (medial head) to posterior aspect of proximal surface of olecranon and deep fascia of forearm; all heads unite	Extensor of forearm at elbow joint; also adductor and extensor of flexed arm at shoulder joint	Radial nerve (C6, C7, C8)
Anconeus	Lateral epicondyle of humerus to olecranon and proximal quarter of posterior surface of ulna	Assists extension of forearm at elbow joint	Radial nerve (C7, C8)

In full extension, the contact areas are in the inferior part of the trochlear notch with concentrations on the medial aspects (Fig. 2.56A); there is no contact between the radius and capitulum. At 90 degrees flexion, the contact area becomes a diagonal strip running from the inferior medial to superior lateral quadrants. Small parts of the superior surface of the coronoid process and inferior surface of the olecranon also show contact; there is some contact between the capitulum and the head of the radius (Fig. 2.56B). It is only when the elbow is fully flexed that a definite area of contact between the radius and capitulum can be identified (Fig. 2.56B). Trochlear notch contact areas, although of a similar diagonal orientation, are larger and extends into the superior medial quadrant (Fig. 2.56A).

The general increase in contact area across the joint reduces the pressure applied to the cartilage helping to protect it, particularly when loading is supported with the elbow flexed or when fine manipulative movements are performed, when many muscles crossing the joint may be active.

Efficiency of Muscular Action

As a group, the flexor muscles are more powerful than the extensors; therefore, with the arm hanging loosely by the side, the elbow tends to be slightly flexed. Not only does the power of the muscle groups vary with the position of the shoulder, because of the attachment of biceps brachii and triceps brachii to the supra- and infraglenoid tubercles, respectively, the degree of rotation of the forearm is also an important factor. The flexors are more powerful when the forearm is pronated because biceps brachii is stretched, thus increasing the efficiency of its action. The flexor efficiency ratio of biceps brachii for pronation and supination is approximately 5:3.

Biceps brachii works most efficiently between 80 and 90 degrees, brachialis between 90 and 100 degrees, and brachioradialis between 100 and 110 degrees; as a whole, the flexor muscles work at their best when the

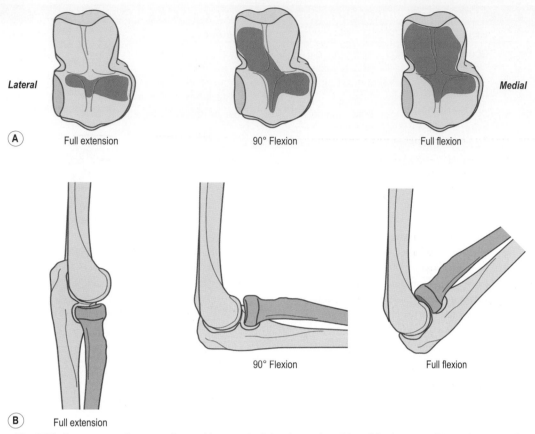

Fig. 2.56 Contact areas between the trochlear notch of the ulna and trochlea of the humerus (A), and between the head of the radius and capitulum of the humerus (B) in extension, 90-degree flexion and full flexion of the elbow.

elbow is flexed at 90 degrees. In this position, the muscles are at their optimal lengths and their direction of pull (line of action), particularly for biceps brachii and brachialis, is almost at 90 degrees to the forearm. Most of the force of contraction, therefore, moves the forearm and is involved in maintaining the integrity of the elbow joint. The reverse is true when the elbow is extended, because, in this position, the direction of pull is nearly parallel to the forearm rather than perpendicular to it. Because the attachment of the flexor muscles, between the fulcrum (elbow joint) and the resistance (weight of the forearm and hand together with any applied load), conforms to that of a third-class lever, it follows that the flexors favour range and speed of movement at the expense of power.

Triceps brachii is most efficient when the elbow is flexed to between 20 and 30 degrees. As flexion increases, its tendon becomes wound around the

superior surface of the olecranon, which acts as a pulley. At the same time, the muscle fibres become passively stretched; both help to compensate for the loss of efficiency in flexion. Triceps brachii is more powerful when the shoulder is flexed and also when both the elbow and shoulder are simultaneously extended from a flexed position (when executing a karate chop). On the other hand, triceps brachii is weakest when the elbow is extended at the same time as the shoulder is being flexed.

There are, therefore, preferential positions of the upper limb in which the muscle groups achieve maximum efficiency. For extension, this is with the arm and forearm hanging by the side with an angle of 20–30 degrees between them. For flexion, it is with the arm and forearm above the shoulder. The muscles of the upper limb have retained their adaptation for climbing, developed in the dawn of human evolution.

Elbow Joint Replacement

Total elbow arthroplasty is a well-established procedure for any condition leading to elbow dysfunction, with pain, stiffness and instability after traumatic or arthritic conditions being the main indicators. A common pathology leading to replacement is rheumatoid arthritis; however, osteoarthritis and fracture of the distal humerus may also require total joint replacement. Initial designs were one of two types (linked and unlinked); however, a new generation of modular implants have been introduced. The advantage of linked prostheses is their inherent stability; consequently, they are generally used where there is also traumatic soft tissue pathology. Linked prostheses are also used in revision procedures because osseous and ligamentous integrity is often compromised. In unlinked prostheses, there is no physical connection between the components; however, they require precise insertion to ensure correct alignment and tracking of the components. Semiconstrained implants consist of two components which are almost congruent but not physically linked, often replicating the normal anatomy. Modular implant systems offer the advantage of interchangeability between linked and unlinked designs, allowing more precise restoration of the anatomical flexion-extension axis and soft tissue balance, promoting the reproduction of normal elbow kinematics likely to decrease mechanical failure.

MUSCLES FLEXING THE FOREARM AT THE ELBOW JOINT

Biceps brachii
Brachialis
Brachioradialis
Pronator teres (p. 146)

Biceps Brachii

Prominent fusiform muscle on the anterior aspect of the arm (Fig. 2.57), biceps brachii arises by two tendinous heads (long and short) at its proximal end and has tendinous and aponeurotic attachments at its distal end. The proximal end is covered by deltoid and pectoralis major, but the main part of the muscle is only covered by skin and subcutaneous fat.

The long head arises from the supraglenoid tubercle of the scapula and adjacent glenoid labrum of the shoulder joint and the short head by a flat tendon, shared with coracobrachialis, from the apex of the coracoid process

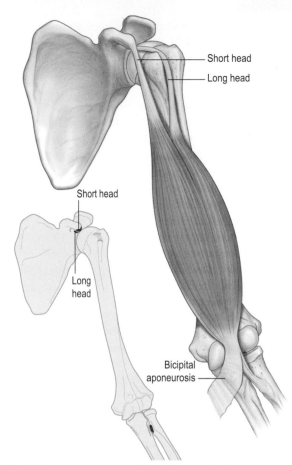

Fig. 2.57 Anterior aspect of the left scapula, humerus, proximal radius and ulna showing the position and attachments of biceps brachii.

of the scapula. The tendon of the long head runs through the shoulder joint enclosed within a synovial sleeve and enters the intertubercular groove by passing deep to the transverse humeral ligament (Fig. 2.21). The two fleshy bellies fuse as they continue towards the elbow forming a single muscle just below the middle of the arm. At the elbow, a single flattened tendon is formed which twists through 90 degrees before attaching to the posterior part of the radial tuberosity; a bursa separates the tendon from the remainder of the radial tuberosity. The prominent bicipital aponeurosis, a strong membranous band arising from the lateral side of the main tendon, runs inferomedially across the cubital fossa, superficial to the brachial artery and median nerve and deep to the superficial veins (Fig. 2.53), to attach to the deep fascia on the ulnar side of the forearm (Fig. 2.57).

Innervation

By the musculocutaneous nerve (root value C5, C6) from the lateral cord of the brachial plexus. Skin over biceps brachii is supplied by roots C5, C6, T2 and T3.

Action

Biceps brachii is not only an important flexor of the forearm at the elbow joint but also a powerful supinator of the forearm; however, the supinating action of the biceps is lost when the elbow is fully extended. Often these two actions are performed together with any unwanted actions cancelled by antagonists. Maximum power is achieved for both flexion and supination with the elbow flexed to 90 degrees. Biceps brachii also flexes the shoulder joint; the fact that the long head crosses the superior aspect of the shoulder joint means it has an important stabilising role.

Functional Activity

Biceps brachii may use its supinatory and flexing actions sequentially in an activity (inserting a corkscrew and pulling out the cork). During this activity, the head of the ulna may move medially due to the force of the biceps contraction transmitted to its posterior border via the bicipital aponeurosis.

When deltoid is paralysed, the long head of biceps can be re-educated to abduct the shoulder; this is achieved by laterally rotating the arm at the shoulder joint putting the long head into a more appropriate position.

Palpation

With the elbow flexed to 90 degrees and the forearm pronated, the muscle can be felt contracting in the middle of the arm when supination against resistance is attempted.

The distal part of the muscle is easily palpated through the skin. Proximally, each tendon may be palpated but with some difficulty. The tendon of the long head lies between the greater and lesser tubercles of the humerus; having located these, firm deep pressure between them is needed to locate the tendon. This is the point at which deep transverse frictions or electrical treatments are applied when the tendon becomes inflamed.

The short head can be found by first palpating the apex of the coracoid process and then placing the fingers just below it; as the elbow is flexed, the tendon can be felt to stand out.

At the elbow, the distal tendon is best palpated with the elbow flexed to 20 degrees when it can be easily gripped between the index finger and thumb. If, in this same position, the individual is asked to resist a strong downward pressure on the forearm, the upper border of the bicipital aponeurosis can be seen and felt as a crescentic border running inferomedially from the main tendon.

The distal tendon of biceps is the point at which the biceps reflex is tested, often by the examiner placing their thumb over the tendon and then tapping with a patella hammer. The resultant reflex contraction can be felt below the thumb; biceps brachii may be seen contracting if the reflex is brisk enough.

Brachialis

Lying deep to biceps brachii in the distal half of the anterior compartment of the arm (Fig. 2.58), brachialis arises from the distal two-thirds of the anterior surface of the shaft of the humerus extending onto the medial and lateral intermuscular septa. The fibres are separated from the distal part of the lateral intermuscular septum by brachioradialis, with which it may be partly fused, and extensor carpi radialis longus. The fibres converge to a thick tendon which forms the floor of the cubital fossa and attaches to the rough triangular brachialis impression on the inferior part of the coronoid process and tuberosity of the ulna. Some deeper fibres attach to the elbow joint capsule pulling it away from the moving bones during flexion to prevent it from becoming trapped.

Innervation

Mainly by the musculocutaneous nerve (root value C5, C6) from the lateral cord of the brachial plexus, but also by a branch from the radial nerve from the posterior cord of the brachial plexus (root value C5, C6) as it runs along the lateral border of the muscle. However, this latter branch is thought to be almost entirely sensory.

Action

Brachialis is the main flexor of the elbow joint.

Functional Activity

Although brachialis flexes the elbow, it is important in controlling extension under the influence of gravity. In

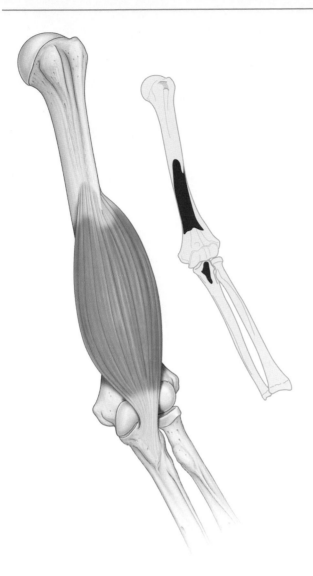

Fig. 2.58 Anterior aspect of the left humerus and proximal radius and ulna showing the position and attachments of brachialis.

this situation, the flexors of the elbow control the movement by eccentric contraction.

Palpation

With the elbow flexed when biceps brachii has been identified (p. 130), brachialis can be felt extending either side of its belly. The tendon can be palpated by applying deep pressure just above the coronoid process of the ulna.

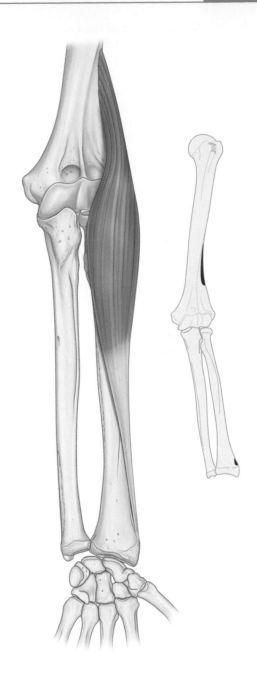

Fig. 2.59 Anterior aspect of the left distal humerus, radius, ulna and wrist showing the position and attachments of brachioradialis.

Brachioradialis

Superficial muscle on the lateral aspect of the forearm extending almost as far as the wrist (Fig. 2.59). It forms the lateral border of the cubital fossa, covered in its proximal part by brachialis with which it may be partly fused. Its proximal attachment is to the proximal two-thirds of the anterior aspect of the lateral supracondylar ridge of the humerus and adjacent part of the lateral intermuscular septum. From here, the fibres run inferiorly forming a long, narrow, flat tendon in the middle of the lateral aspect of the forearm. The tendon is crossed by those of abductor pollicis longus and extensor pollicis brevis before it attaches to the lateral aspect of the radius just superior to the styloid process.

Innervation

By a branch from the radial nerve (root value C5, C6) from the posterior cord of the brachial plexus, which enters its medial side proximal to the elbow. Skin over the muscle is also supplied by roots C5 and C6.

Action

Brachioradialis flexes the elbow joint, particularly when the forearm is in mid pronation/supination. It also helps to return the forearm to this midposition from the extremes of either pronation or supination; this can be confirmed by palpation.

Functional Activity

Brachioradialis acts primarily to maintain the integrity of the elbow joint as its fibres run more or less parallel to the radius. It also works eccentrically as an extensor of the forearm at the elbow joint in activities such as hammering.

Palpation

With the elbow flexed to 90 degrees and the forearm in mid-pronation, brachioradialis can be felt along the superior aspect of the forearm when this position is maintained against resistance. Using firm pressure, the tendon can be palpated proximal to the radial styloid process. The brachioradialis reflex can be elicited by firmly tapping its tendon just above the wrist.

MUSCLES EXTENDING THE FOREARM AT THE ELBOW JOINT

Triceps brachii
Anconeus

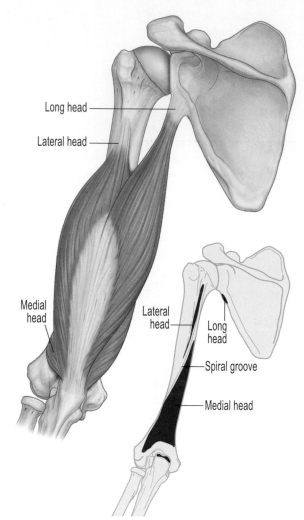

Fig. 2.60 Posterior aspect of the left scapula, humerus, proximal radius and ulna showing the position and attachments of triceps brachii.

Triceps Brachii

Situated on the posterior aspect of the arm triceps brachii, as its name suggests, arises by three heads (long, lateral and medial) (Fig. 2.60). One head arises from the scapula and two from the humerus, separated by the spiral groove; it attaches via a tendon to the olecranon of the ulna.

The tendinous long head arises from the infraglenoid tubercle of the scapula and adjacent glenoid labrum, blending with the inferior part of the shoulder joint capsule. The most medial of the three heads, the fibres run distally superficial to the medial head before joining the tendon. As it descends, the long head passes anterior to teres minor and posterior to teres major. In its course, it forms the medial border of the quadrangular space and triangular interval, and lateral border of the triangular space (Fig. 2.25).

The fleshy lateral head arises proximal and lateral to the spiral groove on the posterior surface of the humerus between the attachments of teres minor and deltoid. As the fibres pass to join with those of the medial head, they cover the spiral groove.

The large, fleshy medial head is the deepest arising from the posterior surface of the humerus, distal and medial to the spiral groove as far distally as the olecranon fossa; it has an additional attachment to the posterior aspect of the medial and lateral intermuscular septa.

The three heads together form a broad laminated tendon, the superficial part of which covers the posterior aspect of the distal one-third of the muscle, while the deeper part arises from within the substance of the muscle. This arrangement provides a larger surface area for the attachment of the muscle fibres. Both laminae blend to form a single tendon which attaches to the posterior aspect of the proximal surface of the olecranon of the ulna and deep fascia of the forearm on either side. Some fibres from the medial head attach to the posterior aspect of the elbow joint capsule pulling it clear of the moving bones during extension, preventing it from becoming trapped.

Innervation

All three parts of the muscle are supplied separately by branches from the radial nerve from the posterior cord of the brachial plexus. The branch to the lateral head is derived from C6, C7 and C8, those to the long and medial heads from C7 and C8. Of these, the medial head receives two branches, one of which accompanies the ulnar nerve for some distance before entering the distal part of the muscle. The other branch enters more proximally, continuing through the muscle to end in and supply anconeus. Skin over the muscle is supplied by roots C5, C7, T1 and T2.

Action

Triceps brachii extends the forearm at the elbow joint; the long head can also adduct the arm and extend it from a flexed position.

Functional Activity

Once the elbow has been flexed, gravity often provides the necessary force for extension with the elbow flexors working eccentrically to control the movement. Triceps brachii only becomes active in this form of extension when the speed of movement becomes important as in executing a karate chop. Triceps brachii works strongly in pushing and punching activities and when performing 'press-ups'. In the latter, it is working concentrically in the upward phase and eccentrically in the downward phase. It works in a similar manner when using the arms when getting out of or lowering oneself into a chair with arms or when using crutches or parallel bars to relieve body weight from the legs during walking. When using a wheelchair, triceps brachii works strongly to push the wheel around to propel the chair forwards.

Triceps brachii is also an important extensile 'ligament' on the inferior aspect of the shoulder joint capsule during abduction of the arm.

Palpation

The bulk of triceps brachii is easy to see and feel on the posterior aspect of the arm (Fig. 2.24). All three heads can be felt contracting if the individual flexes the elbow to 90 degrees with the hand resting on a table and then alternately pressing downwards and then relaxing. The long head can be felt high up on the posterior aspect of the arm almost at the axilla; with careful palpation, it can be traced almost to its attachment on the scapula. The lateral head can be felt on the proximal lateral part of the arm, extending as far around as biceps brachii, while the medial head, covered by the other two heads, can be felt contracting just proximal to the olecranon.

The thick tendon of triceps brachii can be easily gripped between the thumb and index finger just proximal to the olecranon of the ulna. The triceps brachii reflex is elicited by tapping the tendon just above its attachment with the elbow slightly flexed.

Anconeus

Small triangular muscle situated immediately posterior to the elbow joint, anconeus almost appears to be part of triceps brachii (Fig. 2.61). It arises from the posterior aspect of the lateral epicondyle of the humerus and the adjacent part of the elbow joint capsule. The fibres pass medially and distally to attach to

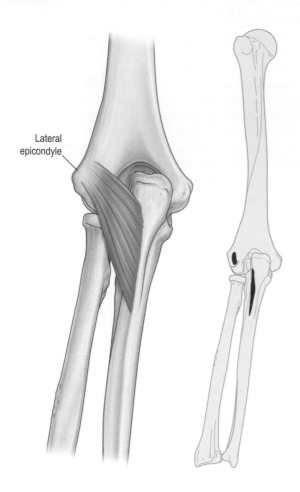

Lateral
epicondyle

Fig. 2.61 Posterior aspect of left distal humerus and proximal radius and ulna showing the position and attachments of anconeus.

the lateral surface of the olecranon and the proximal quarter of the posterior surface of the ulna and covering fascia.

Innervation

By a branch of the radial nerve (root value C7, C8) to the medial head of the triceps brachii. Skin over anconeus is supplied by root T1.

Action

Anconeus assists in extension of the forearm at the elbow joint.

Functional Activity

By virtue of its long attachment on the ulna, it is thought that anconeus produces lateral movement (abduction) and extension at its distal end. These movements occur during pronation and are essential if a tool (screwdriver) is being used. Movement of the ulna with respect to the radius allows the axis of pronation and supination to change, enabling the forearm to rotate about a single axis, which does not describe an arc; this can be appreciated on an articulated skeleton. This action allows the rotatory movement of the forearm to be transmitted along the screwdriver into the head of the screw.

Palpation

Anconeus can be palpated between the lateral epicondyle of the humerus and proximal part of the ulna during pronation and supination, particularly if the axis of rotation is maintained through the extended index finger. As a practical exercise, it can be demonstrated that anconeus alters the axis of pronation and supination by making each of the fingers, in turn, the axis of rotation.

CLINICAL EXAMINATION AND EVALUATION

Except at the extremes of flexion and extension, where it changes to rolling, movement between the humerus, radius and ulna is one of gliding. When fully extended, some accessory abduction/adduction at the joint is possible when pressure is applied to the distal end of the forearm.

Flexion

With the individual lying supine:
- Place the shoulder in neutral flexion/extension and abduction/adduction and fully supinate the forearm.
- Stabilise the distal end of the humerus, then flex the elbow (Fig. 2.62A).

The end feel is usually soft due to compression of the flexors of the arm and forearm; in muscle atrophy, the end feel may be hard due to contact between the coronoid process and coronoid fossa and the radial head and radial fossa. Tension in the posterior capsule and triceps brachii arrests movement before contact of the flexors, in which case the end feel is firm.

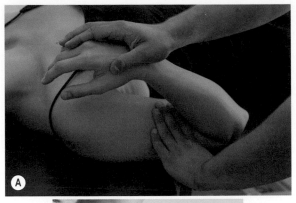

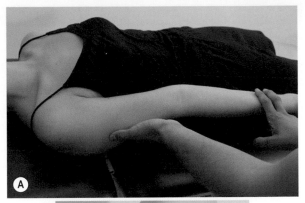

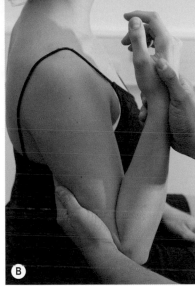

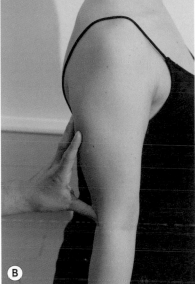

Fig. 2.62 Evaluation of the range of flexion at the elbow joint with the individual lying supine (A) and standing (B).

Fig. 2.63 Evaluation of the range of extension at the elbow joint with the individual lying supine (A) and standing (B).

Alternatively, flexion can be determined with the individual sitting or standing (Fig. 2.62B).

To measure flexion, the centre of the goniometer is placed over the lateral epicondyle of the humerus with the proximal arm aligned with the centre of the lateral aspect of the acromion process and the distal arm in line with the radial styloid process.

Extension

With the individual lying supine and a pad under the distal end of the humerus:
• Place the shoulder in neutral flexion/extension and abduction/adduction and fully supinate the forearm.

• Stabilise the distal end of the humerus, then extend the elbow (Fig. 2.63A).

The end feel is usually hard due to contact between the olecranon and olecranon fossa. Tension in the anterior joint capsule, collateral ligaments, biceps brachii and brachialis results in the end feel being firm.

Alternatively, extension can be determined with the individual sitting or standing (Fig. 2.63B).

To measure extension, the centre of the goniometer is placed over the lateral epicondyle of the humerus with the proximal arm aligned with the centre of the lateral aspect of the acromion process and the distal arm in line with the radial styloid process.

Section Summary

Humerus
• Capitulum and trochlea of distal end.

Radius
• Head (proximal end) articulates with capitulum forming lateral part of elbow joint: with radial notch of ulna forms superior radioulnar joint.

Ulna
• Trochlear notch (proximal end) articulates with trochlea forming medial part of elbow joint.

Type	Synovial hinge joint
Articular surfaces	Capitulum and trochlea of humerus, head of radius and trochlear notch of ulna
Capsule	Complete fibrous capsule surrounds the joint including the superior radioulnar joint, radial, olecranon and coronoid fossae
Ligaments	Ulnar collateral; radial collateral
Stability	Provided by shape of articular surfaces, collateral ligaments and muscles crossing joint
Movements	Flexion and extension

Movements at Elbow Joint
The elbow joint consists of the distal end of the humerus and proximal ends of the radius and ulna. It is capable of only two major movements produced by the following muscles:

Movement	Muscles (root value of nerve supply)
Flexion	Biceps brachii (C5, C6)
	Brachialis (C5, C6)
	Brachioradialis (C5, C6)
	Pronator teres (C6, C7)
	Superficial forearm flexors:
	Flexor digitorum superficialis (C7, C8, T1)
	Flexors carpi radialis (C6, C7)
	Flexor carpi ulnaris (C7, C8)
	Palmaris longus (C8)

Movement	Muscles (root value of nerve supply)
Extension	Triceps (C6, C7, C8)
	Anconeus (C7, C8)
	Superficial forearm extensors:
	Extensor carpi radialis longus (C6, C7)
	Extensor carpi radialis brevis (C6, C7)
	Extensor carpi ulnaris (C7, C8)
	Extensor digitorum (C7, C8)
	Extensor digiti minimi (C7, C8)

• The muscles shown in italics have their primary action at the wrist or in the digits; once this has been achieved, they can also aid movement at the elbow joint due to their attachment to the humerus.
• During many functional activities, extension of the elbow is produced by gravity and is controlled by eccentric work of the flexors.
• Anconeus can move the ulna into slight abduction to alter the axis for pronation/supination during some fine movements.

Clinical Examination and Evaluation

Movement and Maximum Range	End Feel to Movement
Flexion 145° (passive range 160°)	Soft (hard with muscle atrophy); firm with tension in posterior capsule and triceps
Extension 0°	Hard; firm with tension in anterior capsule, collateral ligaments, biceps and brachialis

❓ SELF-ASSESSMENT QUESTIONS

49. What are the action(s) of biceps brachii?
50. With what does the head of the radius articulate?
51. What are the attachments of the radial collateral ligament?
52. What are the boundaries of the cubital fossa?
53. From medial to lateral what is the arrangement of major structures passing through the cubital fossa?
54. What is the distal attachment of pronator teres?
55. How does the ulnar nerve enter the forearm?
56. What is the distal attachment of triceps brachii?
57. Which muscle is the main flexor of the elbow joint?
58. What is the nerve supply of brachioradialis?
59. Which structure separates the deep and superficial structures in the cubital fossa?

SELF-ASSESSMENT QUESTIONS—CONT'D

60. Which muscle has an attachment to the infraglenoid tubercle?
61. What is the distal attachment of brachioradialis?
62. Which muscle attaches to the radial tuberosity?
63. Which ligament of the elbow joint consists of three parts?
64. What accessory movements are possible at the elbow joint?
65. How does the contact area between the humerus and ulna change with increasing elbow joint flexion?
66. What is the nerve supply to triceps brachii?
67. What are the attachments of triceps brachii?
68. What are the attachments of anconeus?

FOREARM

LEARNING OUTCOMES

By the end of the section, you should be able to:
1. Describe, identify and palpate the bones and joints of the forearm
2. Describe and explain the movements possible, and their restraints, at the superior and inferior radioulnar joints
3. Locate, palpate and examine the muscles associated with the forearm and know their attachments, action and innervation
4. Examine and assess movements of the forearm
5. Appreciate the influence of pathology and/or trauma on the function of the forearm

INTRODUCTION

The bones of the forearm are the radius laterally and the ulna medially. Both are long bones, the ulna being expanded proximally and the radius distally (Fig. 2.45A and B). The shaft of the radius is convex laterally, allowing it to move around the ulna, carrying the hand with it in pronation of the forearm. As well as articulating independently with the humerus at the elbow joint, the radius and ulna also articulate with each other at their proximal and distal ends by synovial pivot joints (Fig. 2.45) and by an interosseous membrane along their shafts in the manner of a syndesmosis. The predominant movement between them is rotation of the radius around the ulna so that they cross in space producing pronation; the reverse movement brings the bones into parallel alignment producing supination. In pronation and supination, the hand is carried with the forearm, giving a further axis of movement of the hand at the wrist. In functional terms, the combination of pronation and supination of the forearm and

movements at the wrist means that the hand is effectively connected to the forearm by a universal joint. The fact that several joints are involved and that the axes about which movement occurs do not all pass through a common point gives stability to the hand when performing delicate tasks.

Without freely movable joints between the radius and ulna, perhaps the evolutionary development of the hand as a manipulative tool would not have been so successful, nor perhaps would so much development and enlargement of the brain have occurred particularly the cerebral cortex.

The deep fascia of the forearm is strong and thick where it attaches to the posterior border of the ulna, giving attachment to the flexor digitorum profundus and flexor and extensor carpi ulnaris.

RADIUS AND ULNA

Details of the radius and ulna can be found on pages 113 and 115, respectively.

Interosseous Membrane

Strong, fibrous sheet stretching between the interosseous borders of the radius and ulna; the fibres pass predominantly obliquely inferomedially (Fig. 2.64). Deficient superiorly, the free oblique border attaches 2–3 cm inferior to the radial tuberosity passing to a slightly more distal level on the ulna. Inferiorly, the membrane is continuous with the fascia on the posterior aspect of pronator quadratus, attaching to the posterior of the two lines into which the radial interosseous border divides. An opening in the distal part of the membrane permits the anterior interosseous vessels to gain access to the posterior compartment of the forearm. On the posterior aspect of the membrane are a number of fibrous bands which pass obliquely inferolaterally (Fig. 2.64). During pronation and supination,

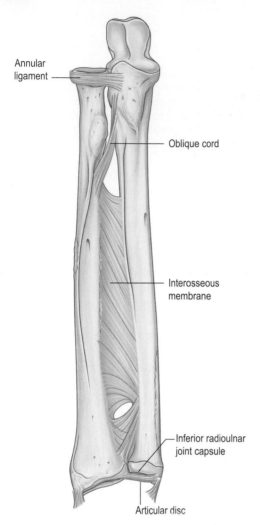

Annular ligament

Oblique cord

Interosseous membrane

Inferior radioulnar joint capsule

Articular disc

Fig. 2.64 Anterior aspect of the right radius and ulna showing the position of the interosseous membrane and direction of its fibres.

tension in the membrane varies, being greatest in the mid-prone position.

The oblique direction of its fibres transmits forces from the radius to the ulna. Through its articulation at the radiocarpal joint, the radius receives impacts and forces from the scaphoid and lunate. At the elbow, however, the radius has a rather ineffective articulation with the humerus, whereas the ulna has a large firm articulation; the membrane serves to transmit forces received by the hand through the radius to the ulna and then to the elbow joint and humerus.

As well as providing a firm connection between the radius and ulna, the interosseous membrane separates the anterior and posterior compartments of the forearm, as well as increasing the area of attachment for the deep muscles in each compartment.

Above the proximal free border of the interosseous membrane, an oblique cord passes superomedially from the radius to the ulna (Fig. 2.64); it is a slender, flattened, fibrous band thought to represent a degenerated part of flexor pollicis longus or supinator, attaching just inferior to the radial tuberosity and lateral border of the ulnar tuberosity. In the gap between the oblique cord and interosseous membrane, the posterior interosseous vessels pass to and from the posterior compartment of the forearm.

SUPERIOR RADIOULNAR JOINT

Articular Surfaces

The articulation is between the head of the radius rotating within the fibro-osseous ring formed by the radial notch of the ulna and annular ligament.

Head of the Radius

The bevelled circumference of the radial head forms a smooth surface for articulation with the ulna and annular ligament; it is covered by hyaline cartilage continuous with that on its proximal concave surface (Fig. 2.65). The anterior, medial and posterior parts of the circumference tend to be wider than the lateral part for direct articulation with the ulna. The head of the radius is slightly oval with the major axis lying obliquely anteroposteriorly; the major and minor axes have a length ratio of approximately 7:6.

Radial Notch of the Ulna

The hyaline-covered radial notch is continuous with the trochlear of the ulna on its lateral aspect, separated from it by a blunt ridge (Fig. 2.49A and B); it forms approximately one-fifth of the articular fibro-osseous ring, being concave anteroposteriorly but almost flat vertically.

Annular Ligament

Strong, flexible, well-defined fibrous band attaching to the anterior and posterior margins of the radial notch of the ulna completing the remaining four-fifths of the

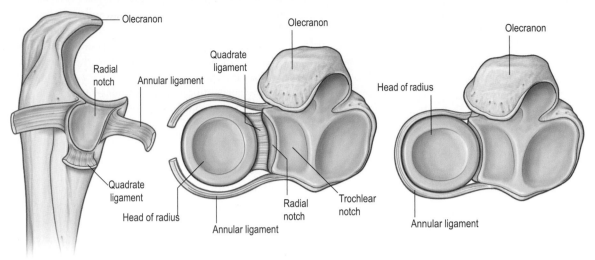

Fig. 2.65 Articular surfaces of the right superior radioulnar joint also showing the quadrate ligament.

articular surface encircling the head and neck of the radius (Fig. 2.65); its flexibility enables the oval radial head to rotate freely during pronation and supination. Posteriorly, the ligament widens where it attaches to adjacent areas of the ulna superior and inferior to the posterior margin of the radial notch. The distal diameter is narrower than that proximally, cupping under the head of the radius and acting as a restraining ligament preventing its inferior displacement through the fibro-osseous ring.

Superiorly, the annular ligament is supported by the radial collateral ligament and blending of the lateral part of the fibrous capsule of the elbow joint anteriorly and posteriorly (Fig. 2.51B). Inferiorly, it is attached to the neck of the radius beyond the epiphyseal line by a few loose fibres; these fibres are too loose to interfere with movements at the joint but give some support to a dependent fold of synovial membrane. The proximal part of the ligament is lined with fibrocartilage continuous with the hyaline cartilage of the radial notch; the distal part is lined by synovial membrane.

Palpation

The line of the superior radioulnar joint can be palpated posteriorly. Having identified the head of the radius in the depression on the posterolateral aspect of the elbow, a vertical groove between the radius and ulna can be felt medially; this is the joint line. During pronation and

supination, the head of the radius can be felt rotating against the ulna.

Joint Capsule and Synovial Membrane

As the superior radioulnar joint is continuous with the elbow joint, it shares the same joint capsule (Fig. 2.66); the capsular attachments can be found on page 120. The synovial membrane associated with the elbow part of the joint space attaches to the superior margin of the fibrocartilage lining of the annular ligament. From the inferior border of the fibrocartilage, and lining the lower part of the annular ligament, the synovial membrane extends below the distal border of the ligament as a redundant fold which has a loose attachment to the neck of the radius (Fig. 2.66). The membrane lies on the superior surface of the quadrate ligament, which limits and supports it, passing medially from the radius to attach to the distal border of the radial notch of the ulna. The redundancy of the synovial membrane inferior to the annular ligament permits twisting of the membrane accompanying rotation of the radius.

Ligaments

Although the annular ligament provides an important support for the head of the radius, it is not sufficient by itself to provide the only support to the superior radioulnar joint because of its need to change shape during pronation and supination. The constant need to

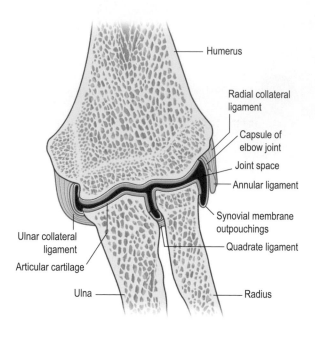

Fig. 2.66 Coronal section through the left elbow and superior radioulnar joints.

accommodate to the changing orientation of the head of the radius may lead to stretching of the ligament. Consequently, additional structures provide support to the joint, namely the quadrate ligament and interosseous membrane (p. 137).

Quadrate Ligament

Passing between the distal border of the radial notch of the ulna and adjacent medial aspect of the neck of the radius proximal to the radial tuberosity (Fig. 2.65), the fibres run in a criss-cross manner; irrespective of their relationship, some fibres are always under tension. Its two borders are strengthened by fibres from the distal border of the annular ligament. The overall tension within the ligament remains relatively constant in all positions of pronation and supination.

Blood Supply, Lymphatic Drainage and Innervation

The arterial supply is by branches from vessels supplying the lateral part of the elbow joint, being the middle and radial collateral branches from the profunda brachii, and the radial and interosseous recurrent branches from

the radial and common interosseous arteries. Venous drainage is by similarly named vessels eventually draining to the brachial vein. Lymphatic drainage is by vessels accompanying the arteries to small nodes associated with the main arteries and then to the lateral group of axillary nodes.

The nerve supply to the joint is by twigs from the posterior interosseous branch of the radial nerve, the musculocutaneous and median nerves, with a root value of C5, C6 and C7.

Relations

Anteriorly, the joint is crossed by the tendon of biceps brachii passing to its attachment to the radial tuberosity, and posteriorly is the fleshy belly of anconeus. Medial to the tendon of biceps brachii is the brachial artery proximally and radial artery distally.

Stability

The joint has reasonable inherent stability; however, in children, the head of the radius may be pulled from the confines of the annular ligament in traction dislocation. Tears of the annular ligament will also result in dislocation at the joint. Further details can be found on page 123.

Movements

The main movement that occurs at the superior radioulnar joint is rotation of the head of the radius within the fibro-osseous ring of the annular ligament and radial notch of the ulna (Fig. 2.67A); movement is limited by tension developed in the quadrate ligament.

In addition to this principal movement there are four other related movements:

1. rotation of the superior concave surface of the radial head in relation to the capitulum
2. gliding of the bevelled ridge of the radial head against the capitulotrochlear groove
3. lateral displacement of the head of the radius as its major axis comes to lie transversely (Fig. 2.67A)
4. inferolateral tilting of the plane of the radial head during pronation due to the radius moving obliquely around the ulna (Fig. 2.67B).

Accessory Movements

With the head of the radius gripped between the thumb and index finger, it can be moved anteroposteriorly with respect to both the ulna and capitulum.

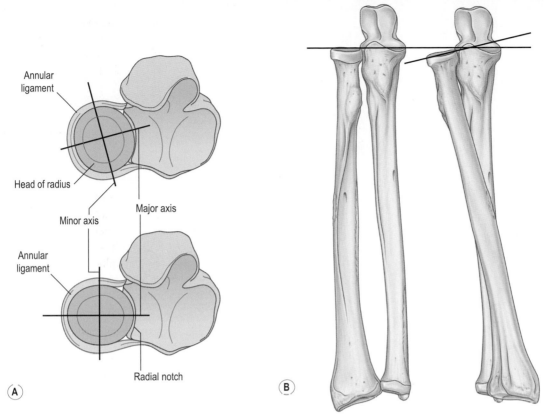

Annular
ligament

Head of radius

Minor axis

Major axis

Annular
ligament

Radial notch

(A)

(B)

Fig. 2.67 Superior (A) and anterior (B) aspects of the right superior radioulnar joint showing movement of the head of the radius during pronation and supination.

INFERIOR RADIOULNAR JOINT

Articular Surfaces

Between the head of the ulna and ulnar notch on the distal end of the radius, the inferior radioulnar joint is closed inferiorly by an articular disc between the radius and ulna, separating the inferior radioulnar joint from the radiocarpal joint of the wrist.

Head of the Ulna

Slightly expanded distal end of the ulna (Fig. 2.68), the crescent-shaped articular surface is situated on its anterior and lateral aspects and covered with hyaline cartilage continuous with that on the distal end of the ulna over a rounded border. The distal end of the head of the ulna articulates with an articular disc.

Ulnar Notch of the Radius

Situated between the two edges of its interosseous border, the ulnar notch of the radius faces medially (Fig. 2.68). Concave anteroposteriorly and plane or slightly concave vertically, the ulnar notch is lined by hyaline cartilage.

Articular Disc

A triangular, fibrocartilaginous articular disc is the principal structure uniting the radius and ulna. It attaches by its apex to the lateral aspect of the root of the ulna styloid process and by its base to the sharp inferior edge of the ulnar notch between the ulnar and carpal surfaces of the radius (Fig. 2.68B). The disc is thicker peripherally than centrally; it is rarely perforated.

The disc is an essential part of the total bearing surface of the joint by its articulation with the distal surface

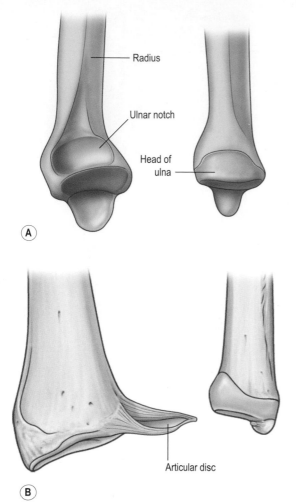

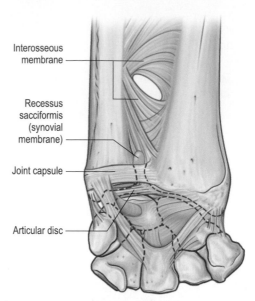

Fig. 2.69 Anterior aspect of the left distal radius and ulna and carpus showing the inferior radioulnar joint capsule, recessus sacciformis and interosseous membrane. (The dashed lines show the positions of the distal radius and ulna, and some of the carpus.)

Fig. 2.68 (A) Articular surfaces of the inferior radioulnar joint; (B) also showing the articular disc.

of the head of the ulna; inferiorly, it participates in the radiocarpal joint. Perforation of its central part leads to communication between the inferior radioulnar and radiocarpal joints.

Palpation

The line of the inferior radioulnar joint can be palpated on the posterior aspect of the wrist, running vertically between the two bones.

Joint Capsule and Synovial Membrane

A relatively weak, loose, fibrous capsule is formed by transverse bands of fibres attaching to the anterior and posterior margins of the ulnar notch of the radius and corresponding regions on the head of the ulna (Fig. 2.69). The inferior margins of the bands blend with the anterior and posterior edges of the articular disc; however, superiorly, they remain separated.

The synovial membrane is large in relation to the size of the joint, extending superiorly above the margins of the joint capsule between the radius and ulna anterior to the interosseous membrane (recessus sacciformis).

Blood Supply, Lymphatic Drainage and Innervation

The arterial supply to the joint is by branches from the anterior and posterior interosseous arteries and the dorsal and palmar carpal networks, which themselves receive branches from the radial and ulnar arteries. Venous drainage is by similarly named vessels into the deep system of veins. Lymphatic drainage of the joint is by vessels accompanying the deeper blood vessels, some of which pass to nodes in the cubital fossa, but most go directly to the lateral group of axillary nodes.

The nerve supply to the joint is by twigs from the anterior and posterior interosseous nerves with a root value of C7 and C8.

Relations

The tendon of extensor digiti minimi, enclosed within its synovial sheath, passes directly posterior to the joint on its way to the little (5th digit) finger (see Fig. 2.86). Anteriorly lies the lateral part of flexor digitorum profundus enclosed within the common flexor sheath. Proximal to the joint anteriorly, pronator quadratus passes between the radius and ulna, holding them together, and protecting the joint.

Stability

Although the loose joint capsule permits movement between the radius and ulna, the inferior radioulnar joint is extremely stable and rarely dislocated. Joint stability is mainly due to the articular disc, but also to the interosscous membrane and pronator quadratus attaching to the radius and ulna.

A fall on the outstretched hand with the wrist extended frequently results in a transverse fracture in the distal 2 or 3 cm of the radius (Colles' fracture), the fragment being displaced posteriorly. The ulna is usually not involved except that its styloid process may be avulsed. In a Colles' fracture, the hand is displaced laterally and dorsally. Alternatively, the fall may result in dislocation at the radiocarpal but not the inferior radioulnar joint.

Movements

The main movement at the joint is rotation of the distal end of the radius around the head of the ulna during pronation and supination. During everyday activities, the axis of pronation and supination coincides with the axis of the hand along the middle finger; radial rotation is also accompanied by movement of the head of the ulna. As the radius rotates about the ulna, the ulna is also displaced with respect to the radius (Fig. 2.70); the displacement is the result of two elementary movements, slight extension and medial displacement of the ulna at the elbow joint. The slight side-to-side movement possible between the trochlea of the humerus and trochlear notch of the ulna is mechanically amplified at the distal end of the ulna to become a movement of appreciable magnitude. Extension and lateral displacement of the ulna are both brought about by the action of anconeus and occur simultaneously during pronation. The arc of the movement described by the head of the ulna does not involve rotation; it remains parallel to

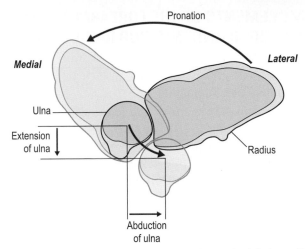

Fig. 2.70 Movement of the radius and ulna at the inferior radioulnar joint during pronation.

TABLE 2.7 Required Range of Pronation and Supination of the Forearm During Some Common Activities

Activity	Pronation (°)	Supination (°)
Eating/drinking	45	
Opening door	35	25
Reading	50	
Using phone	40	25
Rising from a chair	35	
Pouring from a jug/ bottle	45	25

Adapted from Morrey, B.F., Askew, L.J., Chao, E.Y., 1981. A biomechanical study of normal functional elbow motion. J. Bone Joint Surg. Am. 53A, 872–877.

itself throughout with the ulnar styloid process remaining posteromedial (Fig. 2.70).

The total range of pronation and supination in neonates can be as much as 190 degrees, approximately 95 degrees each way. With increasing age, the range decreases to 65 degrees pronation and 80 degrees supination at age 60. The range of pronation and supination associated with some common activities is given in Table 2.7.

Accessory Movements

With the distal ends of the radius and ulna gripped firmly, the head of the ulna can be moved anteroposteriorly with respect to the radius.

MOVEMENTS OF THE FOREARM AT THE SUPERIOR AND INFERIOR RADIOULMNAR JOINTS

Pronation and Supination

In supination the bones of the forearm lie parallel to one another (Fig. 2.71A); in the anatomical position, the palm of the hand, therefore, faces anteriorly. In the prone position, the radius and ulna cross one another (Fig. 2.71A) with the radius lying anterior to the ulna; with reference to the anatomical position, the palm faces posteriorly. Pronation is the movement causing the radius to cross the ulna, while supination is the movement bringing them to lie parallel to each other. Movements between the radius and ulna occur at the superior and inferior radioulnar joints; these movements are considered on pages 140 and 143, respectively.

Muscles producing pronation are pronators teres and quadratus, with pronator teres being the more powerful; flexor carpi radialis, because of its oblique course, can and does assist in pronation. Supination is produced by supinator and biceps brachii, of which biceps brachii is by far the stronger. However, with the elbow fully extended, biceps brachii is unable to act as a supinator as its tendon lies almost parallel to the shaft of the radius and cannot produce radial rotation. Of the two movements, supination is the more powerful; because the majority of the population is right-handed, screws have a right-hand thread. If you are trying to remove a particularly stubborn screw from a cabinet or door frame, ask a left-handed friend to do it for you! Both

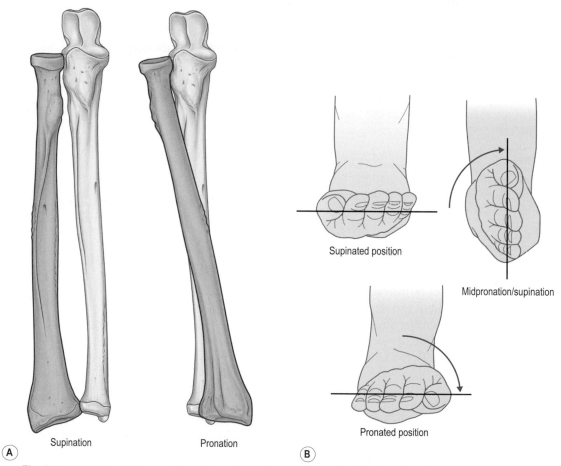

Supination   Pronation

(A)

Supinated position

Midpronation/supination

Pronated position

(B)

Fig. 2.71 (A) Relation between the radius and ulna in pronation and supination of the forearm. (B) Movement of the right hand in pronation and supination with the elbow joint flexed to 90 degrees.

pronation and supination are most powerful when the elbow is flexed to 90 degrees.

The axis of pronation and supination varies depending about which finger the movement is occurring. It always passes through the centre of the head of the radius, but at the wrist, it can pass through any point between the ulnar and radial styloid processes. Nevertheless, it tends to lie in the medial half of this region in most cases; to state that the axis runs between the centre of the radial head and base of the ulnar styloid process is not strictly correct. When rotation occurs at a more laterally placed centre at the wrist, ulnar movement at the trochlea is insufficient. Consequently, with the elbow flexed, the movement is supplemented by rotation of the humerus.

The forearm can be pronated through almost 180 degrees without medial rotation of the humerus (Fig. 2.71). The constraint to further movement comes predominantly from the passive resistance of the opposing muscles and not from ligamentous ties. However, if the humerus is allowed to rotate, then it becomes possible to turn the hand through almost 360 degrees.

Pronation and supination are frequently used movements in many activities; loss of the ability to pronate and supinate can be a marked disability. When these movements are lost, it is less disabling if the forearm is fixed in mid pronation/supination with the palm facing medially.

The major muscles involved in pronating and supinating the forearm are given in Table 2.8; further details of each muscle can be found in following sections.

MUSCLES SUPINATING THE FOREARM

Supinator
Biceps brachii (p. 129)
Brachioradialis (p. 131)

TABLE 2.8 Major Muscles Involved in Pronation and Supination of the Forearm

Muscle	Attachments	Action	Innervation (root value)
Pronator teres	Distal part of medial supracondylar ridge (upper head) and medial epicondyle of humerus (lower head) to pronator ridge on ulna	Pronator of forearm at radioulnar joints; also weak flexor of forearm at elbow joint	Median nerve (C6, C7)
Pronator quadratus	Fibres pass transversely between distal quarter of anterior surfaces of ulna and radius	Initiates pronation of forearm at superior and inferior radioulnar joints	Anterior interosseous branch of median nerve (C8, T1)
Biceps brachii	Supraglenoid tubercle above glenoid fossa of scapula (long head) and coracoid process of scapula (short head) to radial tuberosity	Flexor of forearm at elbow joint and supinator of forearm at superior and inferior radioulnar joints; also a weak flexor of arm at shoulder joint	Musculocutaneous nerve (C5, C6)
Supinator	Inferior aspect of lateral epicondyle of humerus, lateral collateral and annular ligaments (upper head) and supinator crest and fossa of ulna (lower head) to posterior, lateral and anterior aspects of radius between neck and attachment of pronator teres	Supinates forearm at radioulnar joints; most powerful with elbow flexed to 120°	Posterior interosseous branch of the radial nerve (C5, C6)
Brachioradialis	From proximal 2/3rd of lateral supracondylar ridge of humerus to lateral surface of radius above styloid process	Flexor of forearm at elbow joint, especially when forearm is in mid pronation/ supination; helps return forearm to this mid position from the extremes of either pronation or supination	Radial nerve (C5, C6)

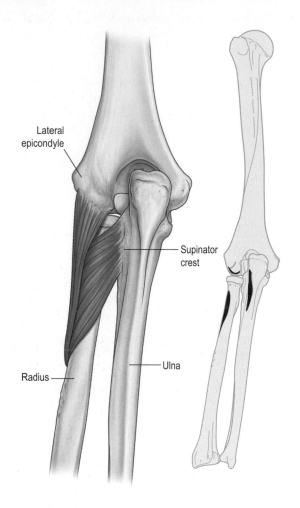

Fig. 2.72 Posterior aspect of the left distal humerus, and proximal radius and ulna showing the position and attachments of supinator.

Supinator

Deep in the proximal part of the forearm, supinator (Fig. 2.72) lies deep to the superficial muscles as it passes around the proximal radius. Its two heads arise in a continuous manner from the inferior aspect of the lateral epicondyle of the humerus, the radial collateral and annular ligaments, supinator crest and fossa of the ulna. It is convenient; however, to think of supinator as arising by two heads (humeral and ulnar) between which passes the posterior interosseous (deep radial)

nerve to gain access to the extensor compartment of the forearm. From this extensive origin, the fibres pass inferolaterally to wrap around the proximal one-third of the radius, attaching to the posterior, lateral and anterior aspects of the radius as far anteriorly as the anterior margin between the neck and attachment of pronator teres.

Innervation

By the posterior interosseous branch of the radial nerve (root value C5, C6). Skin overlying supinator is supplied by roots C5, C6 and T1.

Action

Supinator supinates the forearm causing an anterolateral movement of the distal end of the radius around the ulna so that the two bones come to lie parallel to each other. Unless a particularly powerful supinatory action is required, supinator is probably the prime mover; however, in powerful movements, biceps brachii is also recruited. It must be remembered that biceps brachii cannot function as a supinator with the elbow fully extended; consequently, powerful supinatory movements are performed with the elbow flexed to approximately 120 degrees.

Palpation

With the arm fully extended at the elbow and the forearm in mid-pronation, supinator can be felt contracting over the posterior aspect of the proximal one-third of the radius when the arm is supinated against resistance.

MUSCLES PRONATING THE FOREARM

Pronator teres
Pronator quadratus
Brachioradialis (p. 131)

Pronator Teres

Forming the medial border of the cubital fossa at the elbow, pronator teres (Fig. 2.73) is the most lateral of the superficial muscles in the flexor compartment of the forearm. It arises by humeral and ulnar heads; the humeral head from the distal part of the medial supracondylar ridge and adjacent intermuscular septum, as well as from the common flexor origin on the medial

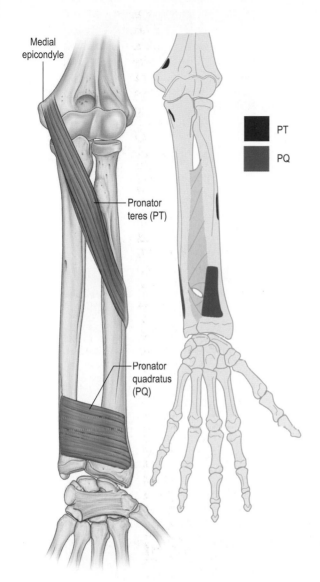

Fig. 2.73 Anterior aspect of the left distal humerus, radius, ulna and carpus showing the position and attachments of pronator teres *(PT)* and pronator quadratus *(PQ)*.

a roughened oval area on the middle of the lateral surface of the radius.

Innervation

By the median nerve (root value C6, C7) from the medial and lateral cords of the brachial plexus. Skin over the muscle is supplied by roots C6 and T1.

Action

Pronator teres pronates the forearm by producing an anteromedial movement of the distal end of the radius across the ulna, carrying the hand with it. Pronator teres is also a weak flexor of the elbow.

Palpation

The muscle can be palpated running along the medial border of the cubital fossa between the medial epicondyle of the humerus and middle of the radius. Pronator teres can then be most easily felt, and occasionally seen when resisting pronation of the forearm.

Pronator Quadratus

Fleshy, quadrangular muscle in the flexor compartment of the forearm (Fig. 2.73), pronator quadratus passes transversely from the distal quarter of the anterior surface of the ulna to the distal quarter of the anterior surface of the radius. Some deeper fibres attach to the triangular area superior to the ulnar notch of the radius.

Innervation

By the anterior interosseous branch of the median nerve (root value C8, T1). Skin overlying the muscle is supplied by roots C6, C7 and C8.

Action

Pronator quadratus initiates pronation of the forearm. The transverse fibres allow the distal ends of the radius and ulna to be held together when upward pressure is applied (when the hand is weight-bearing) protecting the inferior radioulnar joint.

Palpation

Pronator quadratus is difficult to palpate because of its deep position, but if firm pressure is applied between the long flexor tendons in the distal part of the forearm, contraction of the muscle may be felt when it acts against resistance.

epicondyle of the humerus and covering fascia; the ulnar head from the pronator ridge on the ulna, which runs distally from the medial part of the coronoid process, joins the humeral head on its deep surface. The median nerve passes between the two heads. The muscle fibres pass inferolaterally attaching via a flattened tendon into

CLINICAL EXAMINATION AND EVALUATION

Movement at the radioulnar joints involves rotation of the radius about the ulna at both joints producing pronation and supination. Accessory movements are possible at both joints; proximally, the radial head can be moved anteroposteriorly with respect to both the ulna and capitulum, and distally the head of the ulna can be moved anteroposteriorly with respect to the radius.

Pronation and Supination

With the individual seated or standing:
- Place the shoulder in neutral flexion/extension, abduction/adduction and rotation.
- Flex the elbow to 90 degrees.
- Support the forearm in mid pronation/supination with the thumb pointing superiorly.
- Stabilise the distal end of the humerus, then pronate (Fig. 2.74A) or supinate (Fig. 2.74B) the forearm.

The end feel to pronation is firm due to tension in the posterior radioulnar ligaments, interosseous membrane, supinator and biceps brachii; if there is contact between the radius and ulna, the end feel is hard. The end feel to supination is also firm due to tension in the anterior radioulnar ligaments, interosseous membrane, oblique cord, and pronators teres and quadratus.

To measure pronation, the centre of the goniometer is placed lateral to the ulnar styloid process with the proximal arm parallel to the anterior midline of the humerus and the distal arm across the posterior aspect of the forearm just proximal to the radial and ulnar styloid processes. To measure supination, the centre of the goniometer is placed medial to the ulnar styloid process with the proximal arm parallel to the anterior midline of the humerus and the distal arm across the anterior aspect of the forearm just proximal to the radial and ulnar styloid processes.

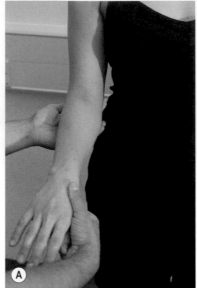

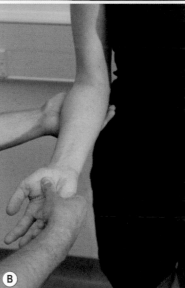

Fig. 2.74 Evaluation of the range of pronation (A) and supination (B) of the forearm.

Section Summary

Radius
- Head articulates with capitulum forming lateral part of elbow joint and with radial notch of ulna forming superior radioulnar joint.

Ulna
- Radial notch articulates with head of radius forming superior radioulnar joint.

- Head articulates with ulnar notch of radius forming inferior radioulnar joint and with intra-articular disc proximal to radiocarpal joint.

Superior Radioulnar Joint

Type	Synovial pivot joint
Articular surfaces	Rounded head of radius, fibro-osseous ring formed by radial notch of ulna and annular ligament

Section Summary—cont'd

Capsule	Continuous with that of elbow joint
Ligaments	Annular; quadrate
Stability	Mainly due to ligaments

Inferior Radioulnar Joint

Type	Synovial pivot joint
Articular surfaces	Head of ulna and ulnar notch of radius and intra-articular disc
Capsule	Weak and loose
Stability	Very stable due to articular disc, interosseous membrane and pronator quadratus
Movements	Pronation and supination, which occur at the superior and inferior radioulnar joints

Movements at Radioulnar Joints

The radius and ulna articulate at their proximal and distal ends at the superior and inferior radioulnar joints. The distal end of the radius is moved around the ulna by the following muscles.

Movement	Muscles (root value of nerve supply)
Supination	Supinator (C5, C6)
	Biceps brachii (C5, C6)
	Brachioradialis (C5, C6)

Movement	Muscles (root value of nerve supply)
Pronation	Pronators teres (C6, C7)
	Pronator quadratus (C8, T1)
	Brachioradialis (C5, C6)

- Movement of the radius around the ulna carries the hand with it and is, therefore, an important component of hand function.
- The proximal end of the radius remains lateral to the ulna, while the distal end crosses to the medial side during pronation and returns during supination.

Clinical Examination and Evaluation

Movement and Maximum Range	End Feel to Movement
Pronation 85°	Firm (hard if contact between the radius and ulna occurs)
Supination 85°	Firm

SELF-ASSESSMENT QUESTIONS

69. Which is the stronger movement, supination or pronation?
70. Which muscle initiates pronation?
71. Which nerve innervates pronator quadratus?
72. What type of joint is the inferior radioulnar joint?
73. Which structure holds the head of the radius in the radial notch of the ulna?
74. What is the innervation of supinator?
75. Which structure unites adjacent borders of the radius and ulna?
76. Which tendon passes directly posterior to the inferior radioulnar joint?
77. In which direction do the fibres of the interosseous membrane run?
78. What is the approximate range of pronation of the forearm?
79. With rotation of the humerus, what is the approximate range of pronation?
80. What is the most important structure stabilising the inferior radioulnar joint?
81. In which position of the forearm do the radius and ulna lie parallel to each other?
82. What are the attachments of brachioradialis?
83. What is the action of brachioradialis?
84. What is the function of the interosseous membrane?
85. Which muscle(s) can act to alter the axis of pronation/supination?
86. Where is the quadrate ligament in relation to the superior radioulnar joint?
87. What name is given to the proximal synovial outpouching at the inferior radioulnar joint?
88. What is the name given to a fracture where the distal fragment of the wrist is displaced posteriorly?

WRIST

LEARNING OUTCOMES

By the end of the section, you should be able to:

1. Identify, palpate and examine the distal ends of the radius and ulna, the scaphoid, lunate, triquetral, pisiform, hamate, capitate, trapezoid and trapezium
2. Describe the bones forming the radiocarpal, midcarpal and intercarpal joints
3. Describe and explain the movements possible, and their restraints, at the radiocarpal and midcarpal joints
4. Locate, palpate and examine the muscles acting at the wrist and know their attachments, action and innervation
5. Examine and assess movements of the wrist
6. Appreciate the influence of pathology and/or trauma on the function of the wrist

INTRODUCTION

The wrist joint is not a single joint but comprises the articulations between the carpal bones (midcarpal and intercarpal joints) and the articulation with the forearm (radiocarpal joint) (Fig. 2.75). Functionally, the eight carpal bones are arranged and move as two independent rows which articulate with each other at the midcarpal joint, a sinuous articular area convex laterally and concave medially (Fig. 2.75). The distal surface of the distal row of carpal bones articulates with the bases of the metacarpals.

Because of the functional interdependence of the wrist and hand, all movements of the hand are accompanied by movement at the radiocarpal, midcarpal and intercarpal joints. The wrist complex is capable of movement in two directions: when combined with pronation and supination of the forearm the hand appears to be connected to the forearm by a ball-and-socket joint with great intrinsic stability because of the separation of the three axes about which movements occur.

Fascia at the Wrist

At the wrist, the deep fascia becomes thinner, although thickenings of the transverse fibres form the flexor and extensor retinacula, which serve to hold the tendons entering the hand in place preventing 'bowstringing'.

Flexor Retinaculum and Synovial Sheaths

Anterior to the carpus, the flexor retinaculum converts the carpal sulcus into a tunnel (Figs 2.76A and 2.85A), acting to retain the long flexor tendons. The flexor retinaculum attaches to the tubercle of the scaphoid and both lips of the groove on the trapezium laterally, and to the pisiform and hook of the hamate medially. Flexor carpi radialis passes deep to the flexor retinaculum in a separate compartment laterally surrounded by its synovial sheath. Medially, the single tendon of flexor pollicis longus lies within its synovial sheath, while in a common synovial sheath, all eight tendons of flexors digitorum superficialis and profundus pass deep to the retinaculum. The median nerve also enters the hand by passing deep to the flexor retinaculum, lying anterior to the superficialis tendons; it is here that it may become compressed if the synovial sheaths become inflamed, giving rise to 'carpal tunnel syndrome' ('median nerve palsy').

Extensor Retinaculum and Synovial Sheaths

On the posterior aspect of the forearm and wrist, the extensor retinaculum is a thickening of the deep fascia attaching laterally to the distal part of the anterior surface of the radius and medially to the distal end of the ulna, pisiform, triquetral and ulnar collateral ligament of the wrist. Septa run from its deep surface to the distal ends of the radius and ulna, converting the grooves on the dorsum of the wrist into six separate tunnels, each of which is lined by a synovial sheath (see Fig. 2.85A). From lateral to medial, the compartments transmit: abductor pollicis longus and extensor pollicis brevis; extensors carpi radialis longus and brevis; extensor pollicis longus; extensors digitorum and indicis; extensor digiti minimi; and extensor carpi ulnaris. The synovial sheaths extend just proximal to the extensor retinaculum (see Fig. 2.86B). All except that surrounding extensor pollicis longus, which extends almost as far as the metacarpophalangeal joint of the thumb, end at the middle of the dorsum of the hand. The extensor retinaculum functions to retain the extensor tendons in their positions preventing bowstringing.

RADIUS AND ULNA

Details of the radius and ulna can be found on pages 113 and 115, respectively.

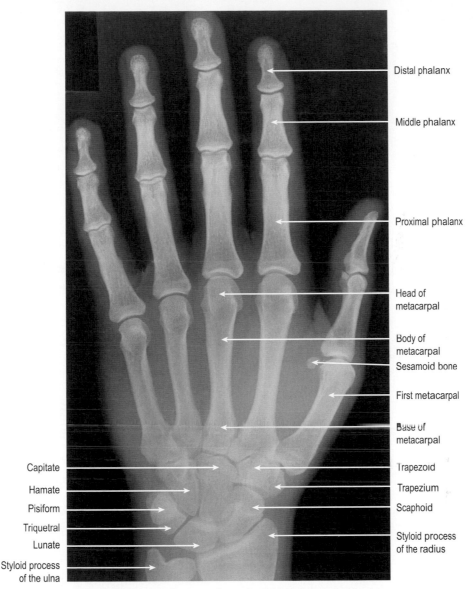

Fig. 2.75 Anteroposterior radiograph of the right hand and wrist.

CARPUS

The carpus consists of eight separate bones arranged around the capitate, but commonly described as being in two rows each of four bones. Three of the bones in the proximal row articulate proximally with the radius or articular disc at the radiocarpal joint, while distally they articulate with the distal row of bones forming the midcarpal joint. The four carpal bones of the distal row articulate with the bases of the five metacarpals via the carpometacarpal joints. Intercarpal joints are present between adjacent carpal bones in each row.

The bones are bound together by ligaments forming a compact mass, which has a posterior convexity and pronounced anterior concavity (carpal sulcus); the sulcus is converted into a canal (carpal tunnel) by the flexor retinaculum.

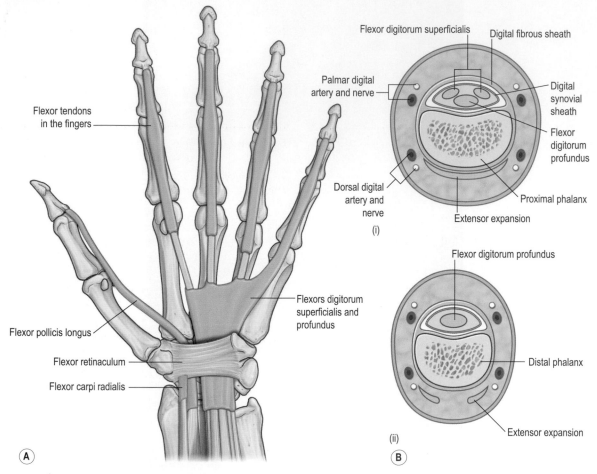

Fig. 2.76 (A) Flexor tendons of the left wrist and hand and their associated synovial sheaths (in *green*) passing deep to the flexor retinaculum. (B) Cross-sections at the level of the (i) proximal and (ii) distal phalanx within a digit showing the arrangement of the tendons and synovial sheaths.

Individual carpal bones are clinically important because they are often injured, especially the scaphoid and lunate, and because they provide recognisable bony landmarks in the wrist region.

From lateral to medial, the proximal and distal rows are arranged as follows (Figs 2.75 and 2.77):

Proximal: scaphoid, lunate, triquetral, pisiform

Distal: trapezium, trapezoid, capitate, hamate

The three lateral bones of the proximal row form a convex articular surface facing proximally, fitting into the concavity formed by the radius and articular disc. Individually, each bone has a characteristic shape and articular surfaces.

Scaphoid

Marked anteriorly by a prominent palpable tubercle the scaphoid has a narrowed waist around its centre. Articular surfaces are present proximally for the radius, medially for the lunate and more distally for the head of the capitate, and, lateral to the tubercle, for the trapezium and trapezoid. The small non-articular surface of the tubercle is the only region available for the entry of blood vessels; it is a common site of fracture.

Lunate

Has a smooth convex palmar surface larger than its dorsal surface. On its medial side is a square articular

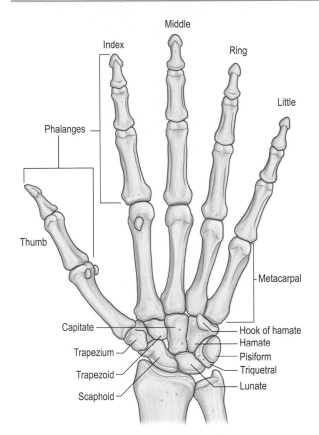

Index

Middle

Ring

Little

Phalanges

Thumb

Metacarpal

Capitate

Trapezium

Trapezoid

Scaphoid

Hook of hamate

Hamate

Pisiform

Triquetral

Lunate

Fig. 2.77 Anterior aspect of the left distal radius and ulna, wrist and hand.

surface for the triquetral and laterally a crescent-shaped area for the scaphoid. Distally is a deep concavity for the head of the capitate, while proximally the bone is convex where it articulates with the radius and articular disc.

Triquetral

Lying in the angle between the lunate and hamate, with which it articulates via a sinuous surface, is the triquetral; the square lateral articular surface is for the lunate. The triquetral is distinguished by a circular articular surface for the pisiform. The proximal part enters the radiocarpal joint during adduction of the hand.

Pisiform

Small, round, sesamoid bone in the tendon of flexor carpi ulnaris; it articulates with the palmar surface of the triquetral. The anterior surface projects distally and laterally forming the medial part of the carpal tunnel.

The distal row of carpal bones presents a more complex proximal articular surface, as it is flat laterally and convex medially; individually, the bones have characteristic shapes.

Trapezium

The most irregular of the carpal bones with a palpable tubercle and groove medially on its anterior aspect, the trapezium has articular surfaces proximally for the scaphoid and trapezoid set at an angle to each other. Its main feature is the saddle-shaped articular surface for the base of the 1st metacarpal, which faces distally anterolaterally; it makes a major contribution to the mobility of the carpometacarpal joint of the thumb.

Trapezoid

Small irregular bone articulating with the 2nd metacarpal; it lies in the space bounded by the metacarpal, scaphoid, capitate and trapezium, articulating with each.

Capitate

Largest of the carpal bones, and it is centrally placed with a rounded head articulating with the concavities of the lunate and scaphoid. Medially and laterally are flatter articular surfaces for the hamate and trapezoid, respectively. The dorsal surface is flat, but the palmar aspect is roughened by ligamentous attachments. The distal surface articulates mainly with the base of the 3rd metacarpal, but also by narrow surfaces with the bases of the 2nd and 4th metacarpals.

Hamate

Wedge-shaped with a large curved palpable hook projecting from its palmar surface near the base of the 5th metacarpal; the hook is concave medially forming part of the carpal tunnel. The distal base of the wedge articulates with the bases of the 4th and 5th metacarpals with the wedge passing between the capitate and triquetral to reach the lunate. The articular surface for the capitate is flat while that for the triquetral is sinuous.

Overall, the carpus presents a deep transverse concavity on the palmar aspect of the wrist. The flexor retinaculum bridges this concavity, attaching to the tubercles of the scaphoid and trapezium laterally and to the pisiform and hook of hamate medially; it forms the roof of the carpal tunnel.

Ossification

Each carpal bone ossifies from a single centre, all of which appear after birth. During the first year the centres for the capitate and hamate appear followed by centres for the triquetral between 2 and 4 years; the lunate between 3 and 5 years; the scaphoid, trapezium and trapezoid between 4 and 6 years; and finally the pisiform between 9 and 14 years. Ossification is not complete until between 20 and 25 years; the hook of the hamate may remain separate. Small additional nodules may also be present. The shape of the individual carpal bones, and not their size, can be used to determine the age of an individual.

Palpation

Starting on the medial side of the palmar aspect of the wrist at the proximal part of the hypothenar eminence, the pisiform can be distinguished with the tendon of flexor carpi ulnaris running proximally from it. Immediately distal and slightly lateral to the pisiform, the hook of the hamate can be palpated if sufficient pressure is applied through the hypothenar muscles.

On the lateral side of the carpus proximal to the distal wrist crease, the prominent tubercle of the scaphoid can be palpated, immediately distal to which is the tubercle of the trapezium. The scaphoid can be 'pinched' between the palpating thumb and index finger if these are placed on the tubercle and in the 'anatomical snuffbox' at the base of the thumb on its dorsal surface.

RADIOCARPAL JOINT

Synovial ellipsoid joint permitting movement in two planes, the radiocarpal joint is formed proximally between the distal surfaces of the radius and articular disc and distally between the scaphoid, lunate and triquetral of the proximal row of carpal bones.

Articular Surfaces

Distal Surface of the Radius and Articular Disc

The radius and articular disc form a continuous, concave, ellipsoid surface shallower about its longer transverse axis than about its shorter anteroposterior axis (Fig. 2.78A). The articular cartilage on the radius is divided by a low ridge into a triangular lateral and quadrangular medial area.

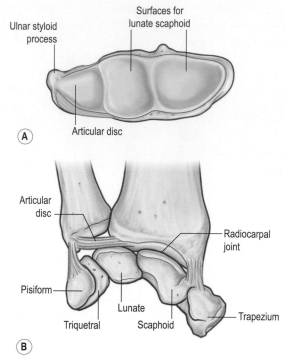

Fig. 2.78 Articular surfaces of radiocarpal joint. (A) Radius and articular disc. (B) Anterior aspect showing the proximal row of carpal bones.

Proximal Carpal Row

The proximal row of carpal bones presents an almost continuous, convex, articular surface (Fig. 2.78B). The three carpal bones are closely united by interosseous ligaments continuous with the cartilage on the proximal surfaces of the bones. In the anatomical position, the scaphoid lies opposite the lateral area on the radius, the lunate opposite the medial radial area and the articular disc, while the triquetral is in contact with the medial part of the joint capsule (Fig. 2.78B).

Surface-Marking. The position of the joint is indicated by a line slightly convex proximally between the radial styloid process and head of the ulna, so that the concavity of the radius and articular disc face distally, anteromedially.

Joint Capsule and Synovial Membrane

A fibrous capsule completely encloses the joint (Fig. 2.69) attaching to the distal edges of the radius and ulna anteriorly and posteriorly, and the radial and ulnar styloid processes laterally and medially, respectively.

Distally, the capsule is firmly attached anteriorly and posteriorly to the margins of the articular surfaces of the proximal row of carpal bones. Medially, it passes to the medial side of the triquetral and laterally to the lateral side of the scaphoid. The anterior and posterior aspects of the capsule are both thickened and strengthened; at the sides the capsule blends with the collateral carpal ligaments.

Capsular Ligaments

Distinct bands of fibres passing between specific bones. In addition to strengthening the capsule, their arrangement determines that the hand follows the radius in its movements and displacements.

Synovial Membrane

A relatively lax synovial membrane lines the joint capsule attaching to the margins of all articular surfaces; it has numerous folds, especially posteriorly. Because of the articular disc of the inferior radioulnar joint and the completeness of the interosseous ligaments uniting the proximal surfaces of the proximal carpal row, the synovial cavity is limited to the radiocarpal space. Only occasionally does it communicate with the inferior radioulnar joint via a perforation in the articular disc or with the midcarpal joint via an incomplete interosseous ligament.

Ligaments

At both sides of the radiocarpal joint, collateral ligaments reinforce and strengthen the joint capsule. They are active in limiting abduction and adduction at the joint; in adduction, the radial collateral ligament becomes taut while the ulnar collateral ligament relaxes, the reverse occurring in abduction.

Dorsal Radiocarpal Ligament

From the posterior edge of the distal end of the radius to the posterior surface of the scaphoid, lunate and triquetral (Fig. 2.79A); the fibres run inferomedially,

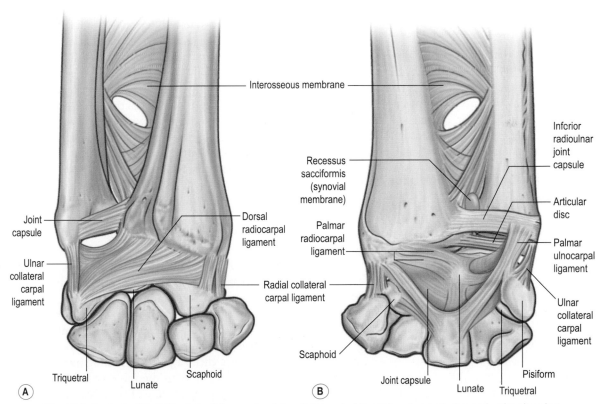

Fig. 2.79 Posterior (A) and anterior (B) aspects of the distal end of the left radius and ulna and wrist showing the capsular and collateral ligaments of the radiocarpal joint.

principally to the triquetral, being continuous with the dorsal intercarpal ligaments.

Palmar Radiocarpal Ligament

Broad band of fibres passing distally and slightly medially from the anterior edge of the distal end of the radius and its styloid process to the anterior surfaces of the proximal row of carpal bones (Fig. 2.79B); some fibres are prolonged to attach to the capitate.

Palmar Ulnocarpal Ligament

Formed by fibres extending distally and laterally from the anterior edge of the articular disc and base of the ulnar styloid process to the anterior surfaces of the proximal carpal bones, mainly the capitate (Fig. 2.79B).

The anterior and posterior capsular ligaments become taut in extension and flexion of the radiocarpal joint, respectively.

Radial Collateral Carpal Ligament

Running from the tip of the radial styloid process to the lateral aspect of the scaphoid the radial collateral carpal ligament lies immediately adjacent to its proximal articular surface and lateral side of the trapezium (Fig. 2.79).

Ulnar Collateral Carpal Ligament

Rounded cord attached to the ulnar styloid process proximally and to the base of the pisiform and medial and posterior non-articular surfaces of the triquetral distally (Fig. 2.79). By its attachment to the pisiform, it blends with the medial part of the flexor retinaculum.

Blood Supply, Lymphatic Drainage and Innervation

The arterial supply to the joint is by branches from the dorsal and palmar carpal arches with venous drainage to the deep veins of the forearm. Lymphatic drainage of the joint follows the deep vessels.

The nerve supply to the joint is by twigs from the anterior interosseous branch of the median nerve, the posterior interosseous branch of the radial nerve, and dorsal and deep branches of the ulnar nerve with root values C7 and C8.

Movements

Flexion and extension, and adduction and abduction are possible at the radiocarpal joint with each being contributed to by movements between the proximal and distal row of carpal bones at the midcarpal joint.

Flexion and Extension

These occur about a transverse axis more or less in the coronal plane so that the hand moves towards the anterior and posterior aspects of the forearm, respectively. Flexion is freer than extension with a maximum range of 50 degrees; extension has a maximum range of 35 degrees (Fig. 2.80). The movements are checked by the margins of the radius; as the posterior margin extends further distally than the anterior, extension is checked earlier than flexion.

During flexion, the scaphoid and lunate move within the concave distal surface of the radius so that the proximal surfaces come to face posterosuperiorly. In addition, the scaphoid twists about its long axis with the tubercle becoming less prominent in full flexion; during extension the tubercle becomes more prominent.

Abduction and Adduction

Lateral and medial movements, respectively, of the proximal row of bones in relation to the distal end of the radius, also referred to as radial and ulnar deviation (Fig. 2.80). The radial styloid process extends further distally than the ulnar styloid process; consequently, abduction is more limited at the radiocarpal joint having a range of only 7 degrees; in contrast, adduction has a range of 30 degrees. In adduction, the scaphoid rotates with its tubercle moving away from the radial styloid process, enabling the lunate to move laterally coming to lie entirely distal to the radius; the triquetral lies distal to the articular disc. In abduction, the triquetral moves medially and distally to be clear of the radius, the lunate follows so that its centre lies distal to the inferior radioulnar joint; movement is limited by impact of the scaphoid tubercle against the radial styloid process.

Accessory Movements

An anteroposterior gliding of the proximal row of carpal bones against the radius and articular disc can be produced by firmly gripping the distal end of the radius and ulna with one hand and the proximal row of carpal bones with the other. Alternate anterior and posterior pressure elicits a palpable gliding movement at the radiocarpal joint. With the same grip, a longitudinally applied force along the line of the forearm pulls the carpal bones away from the radius and articular disc.

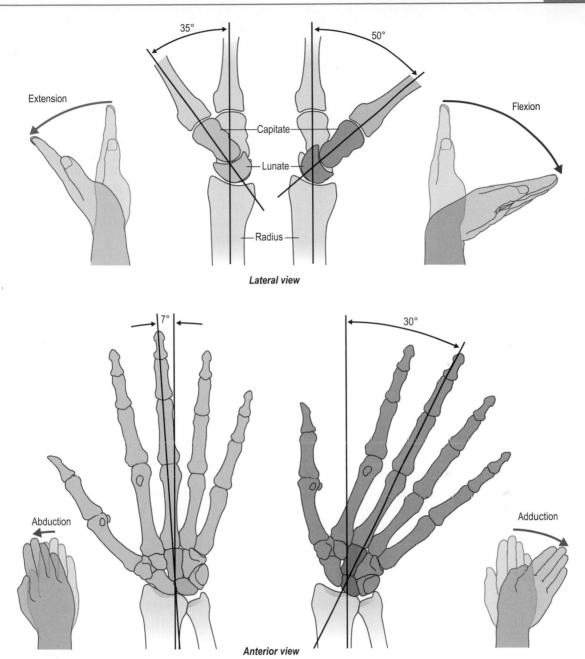

Fig. 2.80 Movement of the proximal row of carpal bones at the radiocarpal joint.

MIDCARPAL JOINT

The midcarpal joint is the articulation between the proximal and distal rows of carpal bones, each of which is considered to act as a single functional unit (Fig. 2.81). The lateral part of the joint consists of two plane surfaces arranged to form a slight convexity directed distally; the larger medial part of the joint is concave distally in all directions.

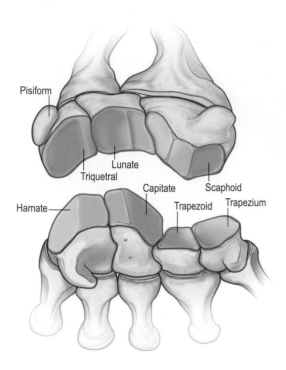

Fig. 2.81 Articular surfaces of the proximal and distal rows of carpal bones at the midcarpal joint.

Articular Surfaces

Laterally, plane surfaces on the trapezium and trapezoid articulate with the slightly rounded distal surface of the scaphoid. The head of the capitate articulates with the scaphoid and lunate in the central part of the joint. The apex of the hamate also articulates with the lunate, while its ulnar surface articulates with the triquetral (Figs 2.81 and 2.82).

Joint Capsule and Synovial Membrane

A fibrous capsule surrounds the midcarpal joint, composed primarily of irregular bands of fibres running between the two rows of bones. Anteriorly and posteriorly, the bands constitute the palmar and dorsal intercarpal ligaments; at the sides, the capsule is strengthened by collateral ligaments.

Synovial Cavity

The joint cavity is large and complex (Fig. 2.82) extending between the two rows of bones; however, it may be partially or completely interrupted by an interosseous ligament between the scaphoid and capitate. Extensions of the cavity pass proximally between the scaphoid, lunate and triquetral as far as the intervening interosseous ligaments (Fig. 2.82); rarely is there communication with the radiocarpal joint cavity. Further extensions extend distally between the trapezium, trapezoid, capitate and hamate. If the intervening interosseous ligaments do not extend the full depth of the articulation or one is missing (usually that between trapezium and trapezoid), the intercarpal joint cavity communicates with the carpometacarpal joint and is prolonged between the bases of the medial four metacarpals (Fig. 2.82). The intercarpal synovial cavity does not communicate with the first carpometacarpal or the pisiform–triquetral joint spaces.

Synovial membrane lines the capsule and all nonarticular surfaces attaching to the margins of all joint surfaces.

Ligaments
Palmar Intercarpal Ligament

Passing from the bones of the proximal row predominantly to the head of the capitate (Fig. 2.83); it is sometimes referred to as the radiate capitate ligament.

Dorsal Intercarpal Ligament

Passes from the bones of one row to those of the other.

Radial Collateral Ligament

Strong distinct band passing from the scaphoid to the trapezium (Fig. 2.83); it is a continuation of the radial collateral carpal ligament of the radiocarpal joint.

Ulnar Collateral Ligament

Connects the triquetral and hamate, being a continuation of the ulnar collateral carpal ligament of the radiocarpal joint (Fig. 2.83).

Interosseous Ligament

Occasional slender interosseous ligament that runs from the lateral side of the capitate to the scaphoid near its trapezoid articular surface (Fig. 2.83).

Movements

Movements possible at the midcarpal joint are flexion and extension, and abduction and adduction, which

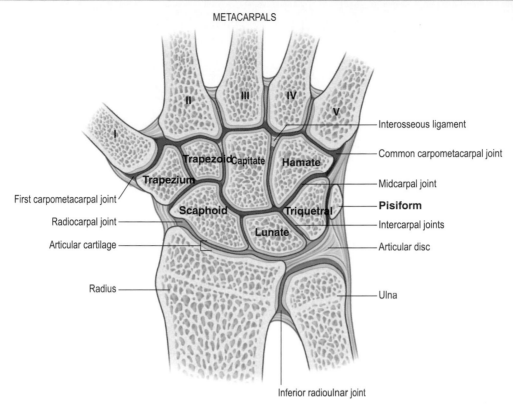

Fig. 2.82 Coronal section through the left wrist showing the relationship between the radiocarpal, midcarpal, intercarpal and first and common carpometacarpal joints.

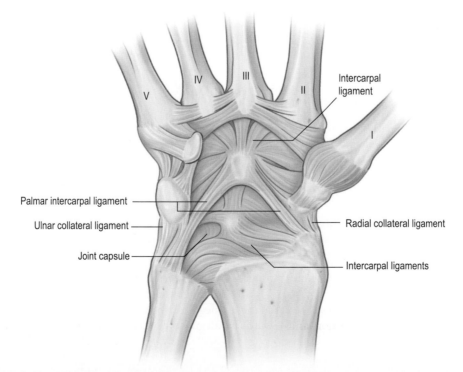

Fig. 2.83 Palmar aspect of the right wrist region showing the ligaments associated with the midcarpal joint.

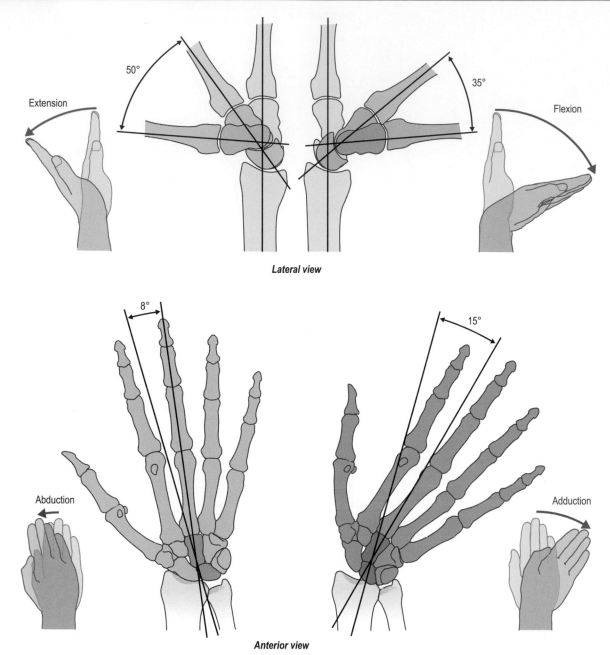

Fig. 2.84 Movement of the distal row of carpal bones at the midcarpal joint.

occur about transverse and anteroposterior axes through the head of the capitate.

At the midcarpal joint, the hand moves towards the anterior aspect of the forearm in flexion and towards the posterior aspect in extension (Fig. 2.84); extension is freer than flexion having a maximum range of 50 degrees, with flexion having a maximum range of 35 degrees. In these movements, the head of the capitate rotates within the concavity formed by the scaphoid and lunate, while the hamate rotates against the triquetral. Accompanying these movements is a compensatory swing of the scaphoid on the lunate to receive the head of the capitate.

The ranges of abduction and adduction are 8 and 15 degrees, respectively, with the principal limit to abduction being closing of the lateral part of the joint space between the scaphoid and trapezium. During adduction, the capitate rotates so that its distal part moves medially; the hamate approaches the lunate and separates from the triquetral (Fig. 2.84). In abduction, the capitate comes close to the triquetral, separating the hamate from the lunate. Accompanying abduction and adduction is a complex movement of torsion between the two rows of bones. During abduction, the distal row undergoes a 'rotation' in the direction of supination and extension, while the proximal row 'rotates' in the direction of pronation and flexion. Twisting of the scaphoid delays its impact on the radial styloid process by bringing its tubercle forwards; it also makes the tubercle more easily palpable. In adduction, a reverse twisting motion occurs so that the proximal row 'rotates' in the direction of supination and extension, while the distal row moves in the direction of pronation and flexion. It must be emphasised that these movements are extremely small; it is debatable whether they contribute much in the normal functioning of the wrist.

Accessory Movements

Anteroposterior movement at the midcarpal joint can be elicited using a similar technique to that described for the radiocarpal joint (p. 156). A firm circular grip is applied around each carpal row; with the proximal row stabilised the distal row can be moved anteroposteriorly. Applying the same grip, a longitudinally applied force separates the joint surfaces.

INTERCARPAL JOINTS

Between the adjacent individual carpal bones, the majority of joints are plane synovial permitting only slight movement between the bones involved; the capitate is the only bone with appreciable movement.

Joints of the Proximal Row

Plane synovial joints exist between the distal parts of the adjacent surfaces of the scaphoid, lunate and triquetral (Fig. 2.82); because the bones are bound together by interosseous, dorsal and palmar intercarpal ligaments, there is minimal movement between them.

The interosseous intercarpal ligaments are short bands attaching to the margins of the joint surfaces involved in the radiocarpal articulation (Fig. 2.82), uniting the bones along their whole anteroposterior lengths. The palmar and dorsal intercarpal ligaments are transverse bands from the scaphoid to lunate and from the lunate to triquetral on the anterior and posterior aspects of the individual bones.

The pisiform rests on the palmar surface of the triquetral, having a separate synovial joint with it completely enclosed by a thin but strong fibrous capsule. The pisiform is also anchored to the hook of the hamate by the pisohamate ligament and to the base of the 5th metacarpal by the pisometacarpal ligament. These two ligaments resist the pull of flexor carpi ulnaris transferring its action to the hamate and base of the 5th metacarpal; in this way, the ligaments form extensions of the muscle.

Joints of the Distal Row

As in the proximal row, the bones of the distal row are united by interosseous, palmar and dorsal intercarpal ligaments with the joints between the individual bones being plane synovial. Because of the ligaments, movement between adjacent bones is minimal.

The interosseous ligaments are not as extensive as in the proximal row, leaving clefts between the bones which communicate with the midcarpal joint proximally and with the common carpometacarpal joint distally (Fig. 2.82). Occasionally, the midcarpal and common carpometacarpal joints communicate between the bones of the distal row, occurring when an interosseous ligament is incomplete; communication is around the borders of the ligament or when one ligament is absent (most commonly that between the trapezium and trapezoid). Dorsal and palmar ligaments generally run transversely across the appropriate surfaces of the bones, uniting trapezium to trapezoid, trapezoid to capitate and capitate to hamate.

Blood Supply, Lymphatic Drainage and Innervation

The arterial supply to all intercarpal joints is by branches from the palmar and dorsal carpal arches, with venous drainage to the deep veins of the forearm. Lymphatic drainage follows the deep vessels.

The nerve supply to the joints is by twigs from the anterior and posterior interosseous nerves and the deep and dorsal branches of the ulnar nerve; the root value is C7 and C8.

Movements

Movements at the intercarpal joints are small accompanying and facilitating movements at the radiocarpal and midcarpal joints.

Accessory Movements

Anteroposterior gliding movements of any two adjacent carpal bones can be produced if one is stabilised and the other moved; this can be achieved by gripping each bone between thumb and index finger.

Relations

All structures entering or leaving the hand have to cross the wrist; some lie directly against the carpal bones, and others are separated by intervening soft tissues. The nature of the arrangement of the carpal bones, which form part of a fibro-osseous canal, makes the anterior aspect of the wrist an extremely important region.

The carpal bones of each row form a transverse arch with a palmar concavity (Fig. 2.85A). The principal structure maintaining the bones in this position is the flexor retinaculum; it is considered by some to be an

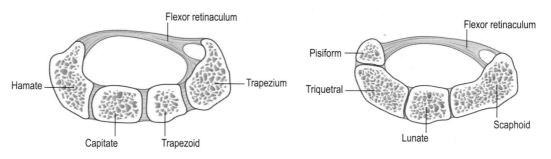

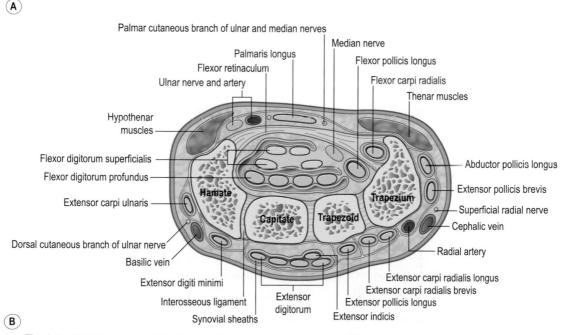

Fig. 2.85 (A) Attachment of the flexor retinaculum to the proximal and distal rows of carpal bones. (B) Transverse section through the left wrist showing the relationships of the structures passing into the hand.

accessory ligament to the intercarpal joints. The flexor retinaculum attaches medially to the pisiform and hook of the hamate, and laterally to the scaphoid tubercle and both lips of the groove on the trapezium, which forms a small lateral compartment separate from the rest of the canal. Passing through this lateral compartment is the tendon of flexor carpi radialis enclosed within its own synovial sheath (Fig. 2.85B). Through the larger main part of the canal pass:

- the tendon of flexor pollicis longus most laterally, medial to the trapezium
- the four tendons of flexor digitorum profundus lying side by side directly over the capitate
- the four tendons of flexor digitorum superficialis overlying those of profundus with those to the 3rd and 4th digits anterior to those of the 2nd and 5th: the tendons of flexors digitorum superficialis and profundus are enclosed within the same synovial sheath
- the median nerve lying lateral to the superficialis tendons (Fig. 2.85B)

Inflammation of the synovial sheaths within the carpal tunnel may lead to compression of the median nerve, giving rise to carpal tunnel (median nerve) syndrome, leading to paraesthesia and loss of sensory acuity in the region of the nerve's sensory distribution, loss of power and limitation of some thumb movements, together with some wasting of the thenar eminence. Passing anterior to and blending with the flexor retinaculum is the tendon of palmaris longus. Passing superficial to the flexor retinaculum medially is the ulnar nerve with the ulnar artery medial to it. In addition, the palmar cutaneous branches of the median and ulnar nerves and the superficial palmar branch of the radial artery enter the hand by crossing anterior to the retinaculum.

On the posterior aspect of the carpal bones, the extensor tendons pass into the hand separated by fibrous septa passing from the deep surface of the extensor retinaculum to ridges on the radius, ulna and capsular tissues of the wrist joint (Fig. 2.85B). The six longitudinal compartments formed transmit the tendons of the nine muscles of the extensor compartment.

Most laterally, over the lateral aspect of the radial styloid process and continuing over the scaphoid and trapezium, pass the tendons of abductor pollicis longus and extensor pollicis brevis within the same synovial sheath (Fig. 2.86A). In the adjacent compartment, posterior to the radius lateral to the dorsal tubercle, and then posterior to the scaphoid and the most medial part of the trapezium and trapezoid, pass the tendons of extensors carpi radialis longus and brevis (Fig. 2.86A). In the third compartment in a groove on the medial side of the dorsal tubercle is the tendon of extensor pollicis longus (Fig. 2.86A); however, because the tendon uses the dorsal tubercle as a pulley, it deviates laterally towards the thumb to cross the scaphoid and trapezium between the tendons of the two previous compartments. Passing over the most medial part of the dorsum of the radius, and then over the adjacent parts of the scaphoid, lunate and capitate, are the four tendons of extensor digitorum with the tendon of extensor indicis deep to them (Fig. 2.86B); all five tendons are enclosed within a common synovial sheath. Crossing the posterior surface of the inferior radioulnar joint, lunate and adjacent surfaces of the capitate and hamate is the tendon of extensor digiti minimi (Fig. 2.86B). Finally, the tendon of extensor carpi ulnaris passes in a groove on the posterior aspect of the ulna and onto the triquetral before attaching to the base of the 5th metacarpal (Fig. 2.86B).

Crossing superficial to the extensor retinaculum to enter the dorsum of the hand on its medial and lateral sides are the dorsal branch of the ulnar nerve and terminal branches of the superficial radial nerve, respectively. The other major structure to enter the hand is the radial artery; it does so by a convoluted route (Figs 2.85 and 2.86). In the forearm proximal to the flexor retinaculum, the radial artery can be palpated lateral to the tendon of flexor carpi radialis. It then turns laterally to pass superficial to the radial collateral carpal ligament, scaphoid and trapezium, being deep to the tendons of abductor pollicis longus and extensors pollicis brevis and longus before passing into the palm of the hand between the two heads of the first dorsal interosseous. With the thumb extended the hollowed region between the tendons of abductor pollicis longus and extensor pollicis brevis laterally and extensor pollicis longus medially is known as the 'anatomical snuffbox' (Fig. 2.86A). The radial artery crosses the floor of this hollow, formed proximal to distal by the radial styloid process, scaphoid, trapezium and base of the 1st metacarpal; its pulsations can be felt by applying firm pressure between the tendons.

Stability

Because of the attachment of the flexor retinaculum and the many tendons crossing the joint anteriorly and

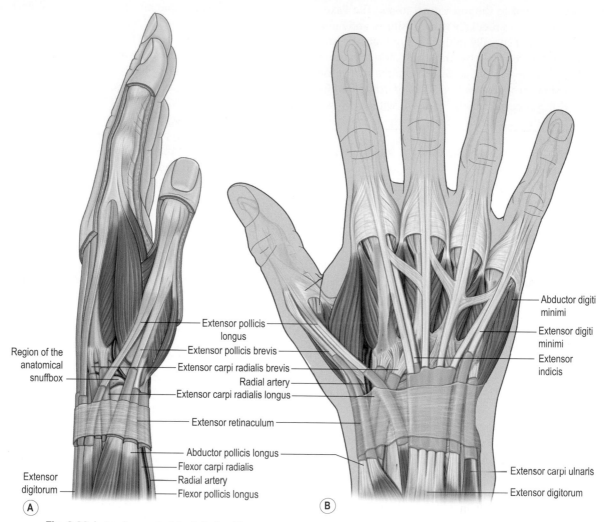

Fig. 2.86 Lateral aspect of the left distal forearm and hand (A) and posterior aspect of the right distal forearm and hand (B) showing the principal relations of the wrist region.

posteriorly (Figs 2.85 and 2.86), the wrist is a relatively stable region. Nevertheless, abnormal stresses applied to the region may result in dislocation or fracture.

A fall on an outstretched hand may result in dislocation at the radiocarpal and/or midcarpal joints, involving anterior dislocation of the lunate; this can usually be reduced by manipulation. Care must be taken; however, in not confusing a dislocation with a Colles' fracture. A fall on the hand is more likely to result in the force being transmitted through the trapezium and trapezoid to the scaphoid, which tends to fracture at its waist. Persistent pain on applying pressure in the anatomical snuffbox is characteristic of scaphoid fracture. When setting the

fracture care must be taken to ensure that the two fragments are aligned and in contact, otherwise non-union and/or avascular necrosis may result if viable blood vessels reach only one fragment; in the majority of individuals the blood supply to the scaphoid is from distal to proximal.

MOVEMENTS OF THE HAND AT THE WRIST

Flexion and Extension

Movement at the radiocarpal and midcarpal joints takes place simultaneously, with the maximum ranges of flexion

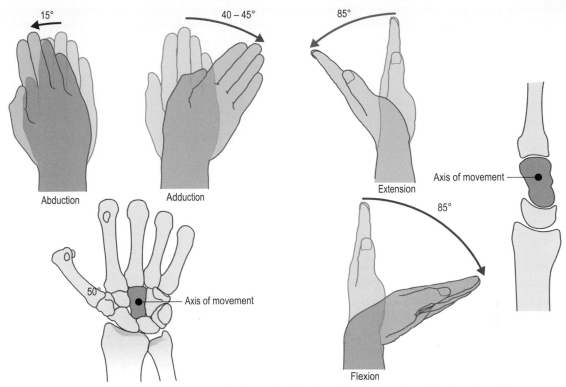

Fig. 2.87 Ranges of flexion, extension, abduction and adduction of the hand at the wrist; also shown the axes about which movement occurs.

and extension each being 85 degrees (Fig. 2.87). In neonates, the total range may exceed 180 degrees, up to 96 degrees flexion and 89 degrees extension (Watanabe et al., 1979); however, by late teens, this decreases to 75 and 73 degrees, respectively. With increasing age, both flexion and extension continue to decrease, so that by age 70, the range of flexion is 62 degrees and extension 61 degrees (Walker et al., 1984). At all ages, females tend to have a greater range of motion than males. Flexion is limited by tension in the extensor tendons and is greatly reduced if the fingers are fully flexed. The main muscles producing flexion are flexors carpi radialis and ulnaris, while those producing extension are extensors carpi ulnaris and radialis longus and brevis. Cineradiography shows that flexion and extension at the wrist occur about a single transverse axis through the head of the capitate (Fig. 2.87).

Abduction and Adduction

Abduction and adduction at the radiocarpal and midcarpal joints also occur simultaneously, with the range possible being 15 degrees abduction and 45 degrees adduction (Fig. 2.87). In young children, the ranges are 25 degrees abduction and 40 degrees adduction, decreasing to 15 and 35 degrees respectively by age 20. Further decreases with increasing age result in a range of 15 degrees abduction and 25 degrees adduction at age 60 (Walker et al., 1984). The movements occur about a single anteroposterior axis passing through the head of the capitate, slightly more distal to the axis for flexion and extension (Fig. 2.87). Abduction is more limited than adduction primarily because the radial styloid process projects further distally than the ulnar styloid process. Abduction is produced by flexor carpi radialis and extensors carpi radialis longus and brevis, while adduction is produced by flexor and extensor carpi ulnaris.

The ranges of flexion/extension and abduction/adduction associated with some common activities are given in Table 2.9.

Accessory Movements

The functional interdependence of the wrist and hand means that movements at both the radiocarpal and

TABLE 2.9 Required Range of Movement at the Wrist During Some Common Activities

Activity	Flexion (°)	Extension (°)	Abduction (°)	Adduction (°)
Eating/drinking	5	40		
Writing		15		10
Using phone		45	15	
Rising from chair		65	15	
Pouring from jug/bottle	10	30	10	
Placing hand on:				
Neck	5		10	
Waist	15			
Chest	20			
Back of head		15		
Shoe		15		

Adapted from Brumfield, R.H., Champoux, J.A., 1984. A biomechanical study of normal functional wrist motion. Clin. Orthop. Relat. Res. 187, 23–25.

midcarpal joints accompany all movements of the hand. Both radiocarpal and midcarpal joints permit flexion/extension and abduction/adduction with movement occurring simultaneously at both joints about single axes passing through the head of the capitate (Fig. 2.87). Accessory anteroposterior movements are possible at both joints if either the radius and ulna or proximal row of carpal bones are stabilised. Applying a longitudinal force separates the proximal row from the radius and articular disc, and the joint surfaces of the proximal and distal rows.

The major muscles producing movement of the hand at the wrist are given in Table 2.10; further details of each muscle can be found in following sections.

BIOMECHANICS

The lines of action of the muscles of the wrist are always oblique with respect to the axes about which of movement occurs (Fig. 2.88). The movement produced by a single muscle is not pure (contraction of flexor carpi radialis produces flexion and abduction at the wrist); to produce pure flexion, the unwanted abduction has to be cancelled by also contracting flexor carpi ulnaris. By combining various forces acting in different directions, any desired movement of the wrist can be produced within the complete range of motion of the joint.

The carpal flexors and extensors fix the wrist during extension or flexion of the fingers to prevent the digital muscles from losing power and efficiency, which would occur if they also acted on the radiocarpal and midcarpal joints. When powerful movements of the fingers are required, the flexors and extensors of the wrist contract simultaneously. The importance of such actions is obvious when attempting to grip strongly with the finger flexors when the wrist is already flexed; extending the wrist stretches these muscles so that they now exert considerable power. Slight extension of the wrist is the position naturally adopted when the hand is used for gripping; look at your own wrist when writing or picking up a mug. If the wrist is to be fixed through disease, it should be secured in slight extension so that a powerful and precise grip can still be achieved.

The extrinsic finger flexors are the major force-producing muscles during exertions of the hand. Deviation of the wrist causes the tendons to move against the adjacent walls of the carpal tunnel; in flexion, the tendons are supported by the flexor retinaculum and, in extension, by the carpal bones. The force between the tendons and retinaculum may compress the median nerve and be an important factor in carpal tunnel syndrome; such compression has been confirmed by direct pressure measurement. In addition to the median nerve, the synovial sheaths surrounding the flexor tendons are also compressed in both flexion and extension; this may lead to their inflammation and subsequent swelling, leading to further compression of the median nerve. Taking into account wrist size, loading of the flexor retinaculum in flexion is 14% greater in females than males. This may be one reason why carpal tunnel

TABLE 2.10   Major Muscles Producing Movement of the Hand at the Wrist

Muscle	Attachments	Action	Innervation (root value)
Flexor carpi radialis	Medial epicondyle of humerus via common flexor origin to palmar surfaces of bases of 2nd and 3rd metacarpals	Flexor and abductor of hand at wrist	Median nerve (C6, C7)
Flexor carpi ulnaris	Medial epicondyle of humerus via common flexor origin (humeral head) and proximal 2/3rd of posterior border of ulna (ulnar head) to hook of hamate and base of 5th metacarpal; it also attaches to and invests the pisiform	Flexor and adductor of hand at wrist	Ulnar nerve (C7, C8)
Palmaris longus	Medial epicondyle of humerus via common flexor origin to superficial aspect of flexor retinaculum and apex of palmar aponeurosis	Flexor of hand at wrist; by tightening palmar fascia it may also cause slight flexion at metacarpo-phalangeal joints	Median nerve (C8)
Extensor carpi radialis longus	Distal 1/3rd of lateral supracondylar ridge to posterior surface of base of 2nd metacarpal	Extensor and abductor of hand at wrist	Radial nerve (C6, C7)
Extensor carpi radialis brevis	Lateral epicondyle of humerus via common extensor tendon and lateral collateral ligament to posterior surface of base of 3rd metacarpal	Extensor and abductor of hand at wrist	Posterior interosseous branch of the radial nerve (C6, C7)
Extensor carpi ulnaris	Lateral epicondyle of humerus via common extensor tendon and posterior border of ulna to tubercle on medial side of base of 5th metacarpal	Extensor and adductor of hand at wrist	Posterior interosseous branch of the radial nerve (C7, C8)

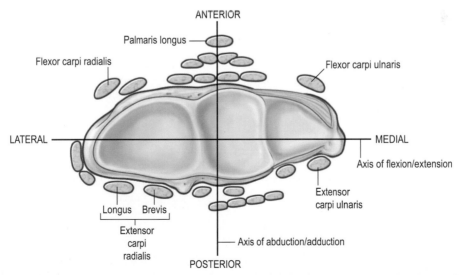

Fig. 2.88 Inferior surface of the right radius and articular disc of the radiocarpal joint showing the relationship of the tendons of muscles producing movement at the wrist to the axes of flexion/extension and abduction/adduction.

syndrome is between 2 and 10 times more prevalent in women than men.

In some cases of limitation or absence of movement at the wrist, often associated with persistent pain, total wrist arthroplasty can relieve the pain and improve mobility.

MUSCLES FLEXING THE HAND AT THE WRIST

Flexor carpi ulnaris
Flexor carpi radialis
Palmaris longus
Flexor digitorum superficialis (p. 193)
Flexor digitorum profundus (p. 194)
Flexor pollicis longus (p. 211)

Flexor Carpi Ulnaris

Lying along the medial border of the forearm, flexor carpi ulnaris (Fig. 2.89) is the most medial of the superficial flexor group of muscles. It arises from the humerus and ulna; the humeral head from the common flexor origin on the medial epicondyle of the humerus and adjacent fascia, and ulnar head from the medial border of the olecranon and, by an aponeurotic attachment, the proximal two-thirds of the posterior border of the ulna. Between these two heads, the ulnar nerve passes gaining access to the medial side of the flexor compartment of the forearm.

The muscle forms a long tendon halfway down the forearm which attaches to and invests the pisiform; the tendon is prolonged to the hook of the hamate and base of the 5th metacarpal by the pisohamate and pisometa-carpal ligaments, respectively. Occasionally, some fibres may be prolonged into abductor digiti minimi. Lateral to the tendon are the ulnar nerve and blood vessels.

Innervation

By several branches from the ulnar nerve (root value C7 and C8) from the medial cord of the brachial plexus. Skin overlying the muscle is supplied by roots C8 and T1.

Action

In conjunction with flexor carpi radialis, and to some extent palmaris longus, flexor carpi ulnaris flexes the hand at the wrist; however, when working with extensor carpi ulnaris, it produces adduction (ulnar deviation) of the hand at the wrist. It also plays an important role in stabilising the pisiform during abduction of the little

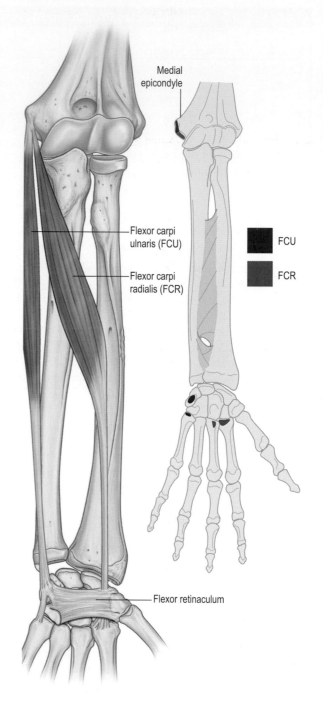

Fig. 2.89 Anterior aspect of the left distal humerus, radius, ulna, wrist and proximal metacarpals showing the position and attachments of flexor carpi ulnaris *(FCU)* and flexor carpi radialis *(FCR)*.

finger, providing abductor digiti minimi with a firm base from which to work. As with flexor carpi radialis, flexor carpi ulnaris is an important synergist in extension of the fingers, preventing unwanted extension of the wrist.

Palpation

The tendon can be identified running proximally from the pisiform where it can be pinched between the thumb and index finger. In the proximal medial part of the forearm, the muscle belly can be palpated when the wrist is flexed against resistance.

Flexor Carpi Radialis

A fusiform muscle, flexor carpi radialis (Fig. 2.89) is the most lateral of the superficial flexors in the distal half of the forearm. It arises from the medial epicondyle of the humerus via the common flexor origin and adjacent fascia. Halfway down the forearm, the muscle fibres condense to form a long tendon which passes deep to the flexor retinaculum, where it lies in its own lateral compartment within the carpal tunnel surrounded by its own synovial sheath as it grooves the trapezium. Distally, the tendon attaches to the palmar surface of the bases of the 2nd and 3rd metacarpals. Its course in the forearm is oblique, running from medial to lateral, and from proximal to distal; at the wrist, the tendon lies between the radial vessels laterally and median nerve medially.

Innervation

By the median nerve (root value C6 and C7) from the medial and lateral cords of the brachial plexus. Skin over the muscle is supplied by roots C6 and T1.

Action

Working with palmaris longus and flexor carpi ulnaris, flexor carpi radialis flexes the wrist. Abduction (radial deviation) of the wrist is produced by the combined action of flexor carpi radialis and extensors carpi radialis longus and brevis. Because of its oblique course in the forearm, flexor carpi radialis may aid pronation; it can also help flex the elbow. It works in a similar way to flexor carpi ulnaris in preventing unwanted extension of the wrist when extending the fingers.

Palpation

With the wrist flexed and abducted, the tendon of flexor carpi radialis can be palpated as the most lateral of the tendons on the anterior aspect of the wrist at the level of the radial styloid process.

Palmaris Longus

Small vestigial muscle, palmaris longus (Fig. 2.90) is absent in approximately 10% of the population. Lying centrally among the superficial flexors of the forearm, it arises from the anterior aspect of the medial epicondyle of the humerus via the common flexor origin. The short muscle fibres soon form a long slender tendon passing distally to attach to the superficial surface of the flexor retinaculum attaching to the apex of the palmar aponeurosis. At the wrist, the tendon lies superficial to the median nerve.

Innervation

By the median nerve (root value C8) from the medial and lateral cords of the brachial plexus. Skin over the muscle is supplied by roots C7 and T1.

Action

Palmaris longus is a weak flexor of the wrist; however, because of its attachment to the palmar aponeurosis, it may produce slight flexion of the metacarpophalangeal joints as it tightens the palmar fascia.

Palpation

The tendon of palmaris longus can be identified just proximal to the wrist, where it is the most central structure when flexion of the wrist is resisted; the tendon lies on the medial side of flexor carpi radialis.

MUSCLES EXTENDING THE HAND AT THE WRIST

Extensor carpi radialis longus
Extensor carpi radialis brevis
Extensor carpi ulnaris
Extensor digitorum (p. 197)
Extensor indicis (p. 199)
Extensor digiti minimi (p. 198)
Extensor pollicis longus (p. 212)
Extensor pollicis brevis (p. 213)

Extensor Carpi Radialis Longus

Lying on the lateral side of the posterior compartment of the forearm, extensor carpi radialis longus (Fig. 2.91)

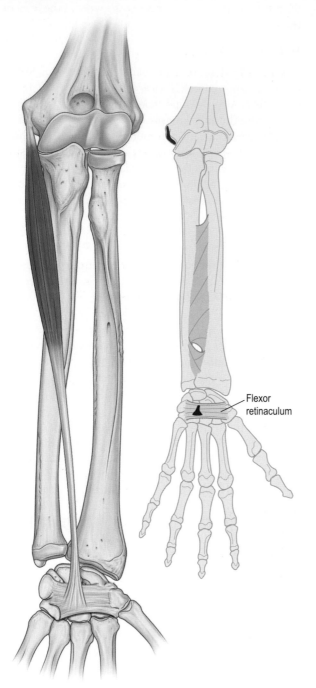

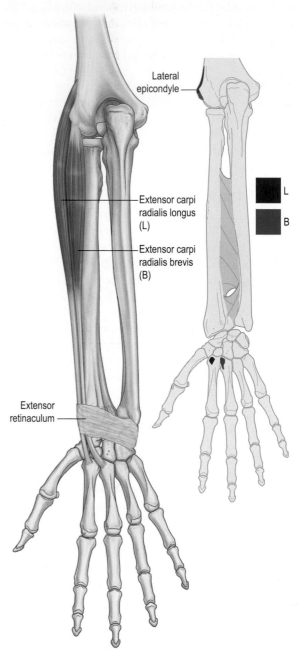

Fig. 2.90 Anterior aspect of the left distal humerus, radius, ulna, wrist and proximal metacarpals showing the position and attachments of palmaris longus.

Fig. 2.91 Posterior aspect of the left distal humerus, radius, ulna, wrist and hand showing the position and attachments of extensor carpi radialis longus (L) and extensor carpi radialis brevis (B).

is partly covered by brachioradialis. It arises from the anterior aspect of the distal one-third of the lateral supracondylar ridge of the humerus and adjacent intermuscular septum; occasionally there may be an attachment to the lateral epicondyle by the common extensor tendon. Approximately in the middle of the forearm, the muscle forms a flattened tendon which runs distally over the lateral surface of the radius. In the distal one-third of the forearm, the tendon, together with that of extensor carpi radialis brevis, is crossed by the tendons of abductor pollicis longus and extensor pollicis brevis. The tendons of extensor carpi radialis longus and brevis pass deep to the extensor retinaculum in a common synovial sheath (Fig. 2.86B); together they groove the posterior surface of the radial styloid process. The tendon of extensor carpi radialis longus attaches to the posterior surface of the base of the 2nd metacarpal.

Innervation

By the radial nerve (root value C6, C7) from the posterior cord of the brachial plexus, which enters the muscle above the elbow. Skin over the muscle is supplied by roots C5 and C6.

Action and Palpation

These are considered with extensor carpi radialis brevis.

Extensor Carpi Radialis Brevis

Lying adjacent to and partly covered by extensor carpi radialis longus, to which it may be partly fused, is extensor carpi radialis brevis (Fig. 2.91). It arises from the lateral epicondyle of the humerus via the common extensor tendon, lateral ligament of the elbow joint and adjacent fascia. The tendon forms halfway down the forearm running with that of extensor carpi radialis longus deep to abductor pollicis longus and extensor pollicis brevis. It passes deep to the extensor retinaculum, in a common synovial sheath, to attach to the posterior surface of the base of the 3rd metacarpal.

Innervation

By the posterior interosseous branch of the radial nerve (root value C6 and C7). Skin over the muscle is supplied by roots C5, C6 and C7.

Action

Working with extensor carpi ulnaris, extensors carpi radialis longus and brevis produce extension of the wrist; however, working with flexor carpi radialis they produce abduction (radial deviation) of the wrist. In addition, extensor carpi radialis longus may help flex the forearm at the elbow joint.

Functional Activity

Functionally, the wrist extensors work strongly in gripping where they have a synergistic role; this is a vital factor in gripping. By maintaining the wrist in an extended position, flexion of the wrist by flexors digitorum superficialis and profundus is prevented so that they act on the fingers. If the wrist is allowed to flex, the flexor tendons cannot shorten sufficiently to produce effective movement at the interphalangeal joints, creating a state of active insufficiency.

If the radial nerve is damaged, the individual is unable to produce an effective grip because the wrist extensors are paralysed. However, with the wrist splinted in extension, the tendons of flexors digitorum superficialis and profundus act on the fingers and a functional grip can be obtained (p. 231).

Palpation

With the wrist extended and abducted against resistance, both extensors carpi radialis longus and brevis can be palpated in the superior lateral aspect of the posterior aspect of the forearm. The tendons, particularly longus, can be palpated in the floor of the 'anatomical snuffbox' if the same movement is carried out.

Extensor Carpi Ulnaris

Extensor carpi ulnaris (Fig. 2.92) arises from the lateral epicondyle of the humerus via the common extensor tendon and adjacent fascia; there is also a strong attachment via a common aponeurosis shared with flexor digitorum profundus and flexor carpi ulnaris from the posterior border of the ulna. The tendon forms near the wrist and passes deep to the extensor retinaculum in its own synovial sheath and compartment (Fig. 2.85B) in a groove next to the ulnar styloid process. The tendon attaches to a tubercle on the medial side of the base of the 5th metacarpal.

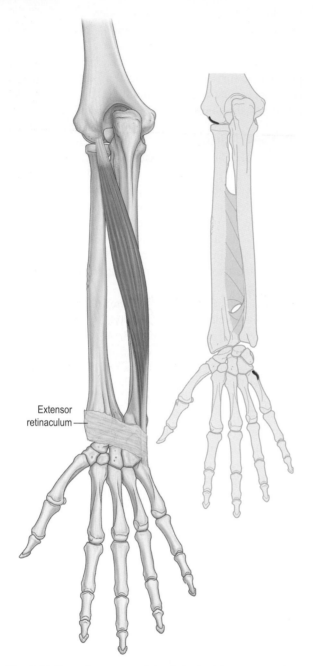

Extensor
retinaculum

Fig. 2.92 Posterior aspect of the left distal humerus, radius, ulna, wrist and hand showing the position and attachments of extensor carpi ulnaris.

Innervation

By the posterior interosseous branch of the radial nerve (root value C7, C8). Skin over the muscle is supplied by roots C6, C7 and C8.

Action

Working with extensors carpi radialis longus and brevis, extensor carpi ulnaris extends the wrist; the functional significance of this has been described in the actions of extensor carpi radialis muscles. Working with flexor carpi ulnaris, it produces adduction (ulnar deviation) at the wrist.

Palpation

The tendon of extensor carpi ulnaris can be identified on the dorsum of the wrist when it is extended and adducted against resistance, lying on the lateral side of the ulnar styloid process.

MUSCLES ABDUCTING THE HAND AT THE WRIST

Flexor carpi radialis (p. 169)
Extensor carpi radialis longus (p. 169)
Extensor carpi radialis brevis (p. 171)

MUSCLES ADDUCTING THE HAND AT THE WRIST

Flexor carpi ulnaris (p. 168)
Extensor carpi ulnaris (p. 171)

CLINICAL EXAMINATION AND EVALUATION

Flexion and Extension

With the individual seated:
- Abduct the shoulder to 90 degrees and flex the elbow to 90 degrees.
- Support the forearm in mid pronation/supination with the hand free to move.
- Stabilise the radius and ulna, then flex (Fig. 2.93A) or extend the wrist (Fig. 2.94A) while preventing abduction/adduction.

The end feel to flexion is firm due to tension in the dorsal intercarpal ligament and posterior joint capsule; if the fingers are flexed, the range of movement is reduced due to tension in extensors digitorum, indicis and digiti minimi. The end feel to extension is also firm due to tension in the palmar intercarpal ligament and anterior joint capsule; if the fingers are flexed, the range of extension is reduced due to

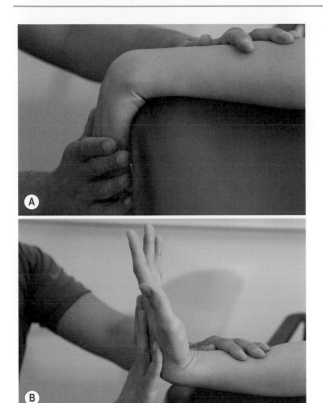

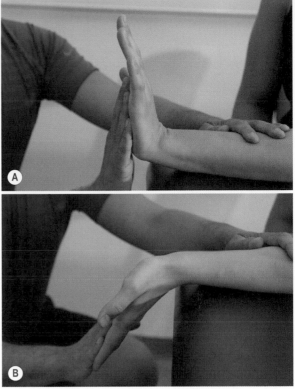

Fig. 2.93 Evaluation of the range of flexion of the wrist with the individual seated and the forearm in (A) mid pronation/supination and (B) supinated.

Fig. 2.94 Evaluation of the range of extension at the wrist with the individual seated and the forearm in (A) mid pronation/supination and (B) supinated.

tension in flexors digitorum superficialis and profundus. However, the end feel to extension may be hard due to contact between the radius and the scaphoid and lunate.

To measure flexion, the centre of the goniometer is placed over the medial aspect of the wrist distal to the ulnar styloid process, with the proximal arm along a line joining the ulnar styloid and olecranon processes and the distal arm along the 5th metacarpal. Alternatively, with the forearm supinated (Fig. 2.93B), the centre of the goniometer is placed over the middle of the posterior aspect of the wrist, with the proximal arm along the posterior midline of the forearm and the distal arm along the 3rd metacarpal. To measure extension, the centre of the goniometer is placed over the middle of the posterior aspect of the wrist, with the proximal arm along a line joining the ulnar styloid and olecranon processes and the distal arm along

the 5th metacarpal. Alternatively, with the forearm supinated (Fig. 2.94B), the centre of the goniometer is placed over the middle of the posterior aspect of the wrist, with the proximal arm along the posterior midline of the forearm and the distal arm along the 3rd metacarpal.

Abduction and Adduction

With the individual seated:
- Abduct the shoulder to 90 degrees and flex the elbow to 90 degrees.
- Support the forearm in mid pronation/supination with the hand free to move.
- Stabilise the radius, ulna and elbow joint, then either abduct (Fig. 2.95A) or adduct (Fig. 2.95B) the wrist.

The end feel to abduction is usually hard due to contact between the scaphoid and radial styloid process; however, it may be firm due to tension in the ulnar

Section Summary

Radius
- Distally articulates with the scaphoid and lunate as part of the radiocarpal joint of the wrist, and by the ulnar notch with the head of the ulna forming the inferior radioulnar joint.

Ulna
- Head articulates with the ulnar notch of the radius forming the inferior radioulnar joint and with the articular disc proximal to the radiocarpal joint.

Carpus
- Eight small bones arranged as two rows situated between the forearm and hand. Proximal row (lateral to medial): scaphoid, lunate, triquetral, pisiform (sesamoid bone). Distal row (lateral to medial): trapezium, trapezoid, capitate, hamate.
- Proximal row articulates with the distal end of the radius and articular disc forming the radiocarpal joint.
- Distal row articulates with the proximal row (except pisiform) forming the midcarpal joint and with bases of the metacarpals forming carpometacarpal joints.
- Adjacent carpal bones articulate via intercarpal joints.

Radiocarpal Joint

Type	Synovial ellipsoid joint
Articular surfaces	Distal surface of radius and articular disc, proximal surfaces of scaphoid, lunate and triquetral of the proximal row of carpal bones
Capsule	Complete fibrous capsule reinforced by ligaments
Ligaments	Dorsal radiocarpal; palmar radiocarpal; radial collateral carpal; ulnar collateral carpal
Movements	Flexion and extension; abduction (radial deviation) and adduction (ulnar deviation)

Midcarpal Joint

Type	Complex synovial joint
Articular surfaces	Distal surfaces of scaphoid, lunate, triquetral with proximal surfaces of trapezium, trapezoid, capitate and hamate
Capsule	Complete fibrous capsule reinforced by ligaments
Ligaments	Palmar intercarpal; dorsal intercarpal; radial collateral; ulnar collateral
Movements	Flexion and extension; abduction (radial deviation) and adduction (ulnar deviation)

- Movements at the radiocarpal and midcarpal joints combine to give a greater range of movement at the wrist.

- Stability at the wrist is mainly due to ligaments and tendons crossing the joints.

Movements at Wrist Joint

The wrist joint consists of the distal ends of the radius and ulna (via an articular disc) and the proximal row of carpal bones. In addition to the prime movers working on the joint, other muscles crossing the wrist (destined for the fingers and thumb) also contribute to movement.

Movement	Muscles (root value of nerve supply)
Flexion	Flexor carpi ulnaris (C7, C8)
	Flexor carpi radialis (C6, C7)
	Palmaris longus (C8)
	Flexor digitorum superficialis (C7, C8, T1)
	Flexor digitorum profundus (C7, C8, T1)
	Flexor pollicis longus (C8, T1)
Extension	Extensor carpi ulnaris (C7, C8)
	Extensor carpi radialis longus (C6, C7)
	Extensor carpi radialis brevis (C6, C7)
	Extensor digitorum (C7, C8)
	Extensor indicis (C7, C8)
	Extensor digiti minimi (C7, C8)
	Extensor pollicis longus (C7, C8)
	Extensor pollicis brevis (C7, C8)
Abduction (radial deviation)	Flexor carpi radialis (C6, C7)
	Extensor carpi radialis longus (C6, C7)
	Extensor carpi radialis brevis (C6, C7)
Adduction (ulnar deviation)	Flexor carpi ulnaris (C7, C8)
	Extensor carpi ulnaris (C7, C8)

- The muscles shown in italics have the primary function of flexing or extending the digits; once this has been achieved, they can act to move the wrist in a continued action.
- The wrist extensors have an important functional action during gripping. Acting as synergists, they prevent unwanted continued action of the finger flexors at the wrist. Holding the wrist in extension during gripping prevents active insufficiency of the finger flexors.

Clinical Examination

Movement and Maximum Range	End Feel to Movement
Flexion 85°	Firm
Extension 85°	Firm; may be hard if contact is between bones
Abduction 15°	Hard; may be firm if contact is not between bones
Adduction 45°	Firm

collateral and ulnar collateral carpal ligaments and medial part of the joint capsule. The end feel to adduction is firm due to tension in the radial collateral and radial collateral carpal ligaments and lateral part of the joint capsule.

To measure both abduction and adduction, the centre of the goniometer is placed over the middle of the posterior aspect of the wrist (over the capitate), with the proximal arm along the posterior midline of the forearm and the distal arm along the 3rd metacarpal.

? SELF-ASSESSMENT QUESTIONS

89. From medial to lateral, which bones form the distal row of carpal bones?
90. Which bones articulate with the radius?
91. Through which bone do the axes of flexion/extension and abduction/adduction of the wrist occur?
92. Which muscles produce abduction at the wrist?
93. Which structure converts the anterior concavity of the carpal bones into the carpal tunnel?
94. The midcarpal joint is between which structures?
95. What type of joints are the intercarpal joints?
96. What is the range of flexion and extension at the radiocarpal joint?
97. How many tendons cross the dorsal surface of the wrist?
98. Which tendons pass over the posterior surface of the radial styloid process?
99. Which carpal bone does not participate in the midcarpal joint?
100. Which tendon passes through the flexor retinaculum?
101. Which nerve passes through the carpal tunnel?
102. What is the innervation of flexor carpi ulnaris?
103. What is the innervation of extensor carpi ulnaris?
104. Which tendon(s) pass over the dorsal aspect of the ulna?
105. At the wrist, does the ulnar nerve lie medial or lateral to the ulnar artery?
106. Which tendon(s) lie directly anterior to the capitate?
107. In which activity do the wrist extensors work strongly as synergists?
108. Which bones can be palpated in the floor of the 'anatomical snuffbox'?

▌HAND AND DIGITS

LEARNING OUTCOMES

By the end of the section, you should be able to:
1. Identify, palpate and examine the distal row of carpal bones, metacarpals and phalanges
2. Describe the bones, joints, muscles and fascia of the hand
3. Describe and explain the movements possible, and their restraints, at the common and first carpometacarpal joints, and at the metacarpophalangeal and interphalangeal joints of the fingers and thumb
4. Locate, palpate and examine the muscles associated with the fingers and thumb, and know their attachments, action, function and innervation
5. Examine and assess movements at the first carpometacarpal, metacarpophalangeal and interphalangeal joints of the fingers and thumb

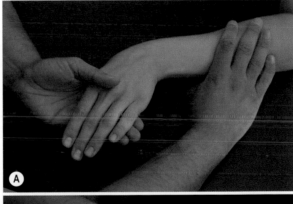

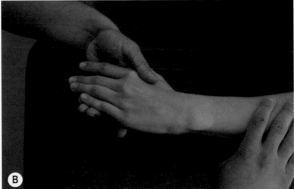

Fig. 2.95 Evaluation of the range of (A) abduction and (B) adduction at the wrist with the individual seated and the forearm in mid pronation/supination.

6. Appreciate the influence of pathology and/or trauma on the function of the hand, fingers and thumb

INTRODUCTION

Just as the foot has evolved as an organ of support and locomotion, so the hand has developed into an instrument of manipulation endowed with fine sensory discrimination. It is often hard to accept that the hand and wrist and the foot and ankle have similar building blocks in terms of bony and muscular constituents, patterns of innervation and blood supply. Refinements in the hand have followed its release from the burden of supporting the body during locomotion. The extent to which the hand is used indicates its importance in everyday life; it is used to grip and manipulate objects facilitating dressing, eating, playing instruments and games. The hand has to be capable of applying large gripping forces between the fingers and thumb, while at other times undertake precision movements. Its sensory functions must not be overlooked as it relays information regarding texture and surface contour, warns against extremes of hot and cold, and prevents collisions, especially when sight is compromised. These motor and sensory functions require considerable representation in the motor and sensory cortices of the brain (see Figs 5.52 and 5.53). As the hand developed, so did the cerebral cortex enlarge to obtain maximum benefit for the new, freely mobile, sensitive structure.

Much of the motor functioning of the hand is due to its ability to grip objects; however, prehension can be observed in many animals, from the pincers of crabs to the hand of the great apes. It is the concomitant development of the hand and brain forming an interacting functional pair that has led to human dominance in the animal kingdom. Because of the uses to which the hand is put, it is particularly disabling when part or all of it is injured; it is particularly vulnerable because it is not protected. Lesions of the peripheral and central nervous systems, infections, accidental amputations, burns, lacerations and penetrating wounds, as well as diseases of the joints all disable the hand.

In many respects, the arrangement of bones and the intervening joints are simpler in the hand than the foot, principally because the carpus is limited to the wrist (Figs 2.75 and 2.77). The metacarpals articulate with the wrist at the carpometacarpal joints, of which the first is separate and different from the remainder, and with each other via the intermetacarpal joints. The head of each metacarpal articulates with the base of the proximal phalanx at the metacarpophalangeal joint (Figs 2.75 and 2.77), while adjacent phalanges articulate via interphalangeal joints (Figs 2.75 and 2.77). Because the thumb has only two phalanges, it has only one interphalangeal joint; the fingers have three phalanges and two interphalangeal joints.

Care has to be taken when using the terms fingers and digits as confusion can arise. There are four fingers and a thumb or five digits. If 'finger' and 'thumb' are the preferred terminology, then to avoid confusion, the use of an appropriate prefix is advised, that being 'index', 'middle', 'ring' and 'little' from lateral to medial.

The axis of the hand runs along the middle finger (3rd digit) and is in line with the long axis of the forearm (Fig. 2.96); certain movements of the digits are made with reference to this axis. In describing movements of the thumb, remember that it is rotated 90 degrees with respect to the remaining digits.

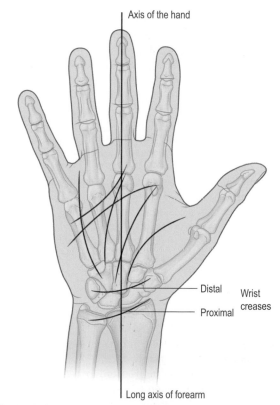

Fig. 2.96 Anterior aspect of the right hand showing the relationship of the underlying bones to the surface creases of the wrist and palm.

The fine movements produced in the hand must be controlled from a stable base; the attachment of the intrinsic hand muscles remains fixed by the muscles of the forearm which are brought into play. The attachments of the forearm muscles in turn require fixation at the elbow by muscles of the arm, and these in turn require stabilisation at the shoulder and pectoral girdle. Even writing involves the use of the shoulder muscles, as well as those of the fingers and thumb.

Fascia in the Hand

The superficial fascia on the dorsum of the hand is loose and thin and can be easily lifted away from the underlying tissue. It is in the palm, as well as the palmar surfaces of the digits, where specialisations of the fascia can be seen. In the centre of the palm, strong bands of connective tissue connect the skin to the palmar aponeurosis (thickening of the deep fascia) (see Fig. 2.126). Overlying the thenar and hypothenar regions, fixation of the skin to the deep fascia is less marked, but here the superficial fascia is thicker and less fibrous to facilitate the gripping actions of the hand. This is because it can adapt to the contours of the object being held. Palmaris brevis lies in the superficial fascia overlying the hypothenar eminence; by wrinkling the skin it improves the grip. Similar less fibrous pads of tissue are also found opposite the metacarpophalangeal joints, where the superficial transverse metacarpal ligament (band of transverse fibres) connects to the palmar surfaces of the fibrous flexor sheaths of the fingers.

The pads on the palmar surfaces of the distal phalanges are highly specialised regions housing numerous tactile nerve endings; here the skin is firmly attached to the distal two-thirds of the distal phalanx. The blood supply to the distal phalanx passes through this highly specialised pad; if it becomes infected, there may be compression of the artery with death of this part of the bone. On the dorsum of the distal phalanx is the nail (p. 25): it has no superficial fascia deep to it.

There are two layers of deep fascia in the palm of the hand: the more superficial layer is strong and forms the palmar aponeurosis centrally, the deeper layer covers the interossei and also encloses adductor pollicis. On each side of the aponeurosis, the fascia thins out to cover the thenar and hypothenar muscles. The palmar aponeurosis strengthens the hand for gripping, yet also protects the underlying vessels and nerves. It is a dense, thick, triangular structure bound to the overlying superficial

fascia; its apex is at the wrist and base at the webs of the fingers. From the base, four slips pass into the fingers becoming continuous with the digital sheaths of the flexor tendons. Each slip further divides having attachments to the deep transverse metacarpal ligament, capsule of the metacarpophalangeal joint and sides of the proximal phalanx; the slips pass anterior to the lumbricals and digital vessels and nerves.

In some individuals, often the elderly, the medial part of the palmar aponeurosis and the fibrous flexor sheaths of the little and ring fingers become contracted (shortened), leading to progressive flexion of the fingers at the metacarpophalangeal and proximal interphalangeal joints, pulling the fingers towards the palm. The distal phalanx is not flexed because the tip of the finger is pressed against the palm. In severe cases, the distal interphalangeal joint may become hyperextended; there is an inability to extend the fingers, even passively. Treatment usually involves removal of the offending fibrous tissue. However, there is a tendency for it to reform and contract again; the condition is Dupuytren's contracture (Fig. 2.97).

Palmar Regions, Compartments and Spaces

From the medial and lateral borders of the palmar aponeurosis, septa pass towards and fuse with the fascia covering the interossei, dividing the palm into three compartments. Of these, the medial and lateral compartments contain the hypothenar and thenar muscles, respectively; the intermediate compartment contains the long flexor tendons and lumbricals surrounded by loose connective tissue. A further septum, although often incomplete, runs from the deep aspect of this connective tissue to the shaft of the 3rd metacarpal dividing the compartment into two potential spaces (lateral and medial midpalmar spaces).

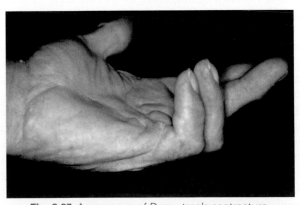

Fig. 2.97 Appearance of Dupuytren's contracture.

Proximally, they communicate deep to the flexor tendons with a similar potential space anterior to pronator quadratus; distally, they are prolonged around each lumbrical as the lumbrical canal which passes into the web of the fingers. The web space, in turn, is in free communication with the subaponeurotic space on the dorsum of the hand deep to the extensor tendons, as well as with the dorsal subcutaneous space. Accumulations of fluid in the midpalmar spaces, following injury or infection of the hand, can track back in the deep part of the flexor compartment, or via the web spaces of the fingers, to the posterior forearm in the loose superficial fascia.

The common synovial sheath for the flexor digitorum superficialis and profundus tendons extends from 2 cm proximal to the flexor retinaculum distally through the carpal tunnel to end in the midpalmar region. Only the synovial sheath of the little finger is continuous with the common synovial sheath in the palm; the synovial sheaths lining the fibro-osseous canals of the other three fingers are separated from it (Fig. 2.76A). The single synovial sheath of flexor pollicis longus has the same proximal limit but continues distally through the carpal tunnel and along the fibro-osseous canal of the thumb (Fig. 2.76A).

Fibro-Osseous Canals, Retinacula and Synovial Sheaths of the Flexors of the Wrist and Digits

The tendons of the digital flexors are held close to the phalanges by fibrous sheaths (Fig. 2.76B) to prevent them bowstringing, ensuring that their pull produces movement at the interphalangeal joints. The canals are formed by a shallow groove on the anterior surface of the phalanges, and a fibrous sheath attached to the raised lateral and medial margins of the palmar surfaces of the proximal and middle phalanges, and palmar surface of the distal phalanx. The canal is closed distally by attaching to the distal phalanx but is open proximally deep to the palmar aponeurosis. Most fibres of the sheath are arranged transversely, but at the interphalangeal joints, they have a criss-cross arrangement to permit flexion at the joint (Fig. 2.98). All five fibro-osseous canals are lined with a synovial sheath surrounding the enclosed tendons. In the fingers, the synovial sheath surrounds the tendons of flexors digitorum superficialis and profundus, and it is connected to them by vinculae. The sheath of the thumb contains only the tendon of flexor pollicis longus within a synovial covering.

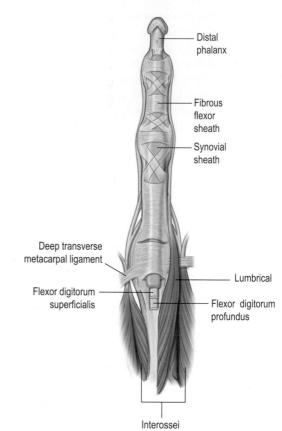

Fig. 2.98 Anterior aspect of a finger showing the fibrous flexor and synovial sheaths.

In 'trigger finger', a swelling of the flexor tendons proximal to the fibro-osseous canal means that, when the digit is flexed, the swelling moves into the canal causing difficulty during extension. In Dupuytren's contracture, the medial portion of the palmar aponeurosis and fibrous sheaths of the ring and little fingers may become shortened, in which case the fingers are pulled towards the palm (Fig. 2.97). In severe cases, the tips of the fingers may become pressed into the palm; the lateral two fibrous sheaths are less commonly affected.

FUNCTIONAL ACTIVITY

The arrangement of bones, tendons and ligaments within the hand is such that, in the so-called position of rest, the palm is hollowed, the fingers flexed and thumb slightly opposed; flexion of the fingers increases progressively from index to little finger. Underlying the

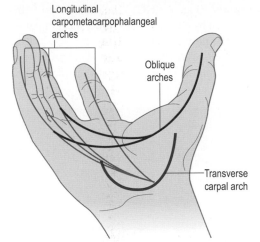

Longitudinal carpometacarpophalangeal arches

Oblique arches

Transverse carpal arch

Fig. 2.99 Arch arrangements of the bony elements of the wrist and hand.

hollowing of the palm and facilitating gripping movements, the bony skeleton forms a series of arches running in three different directions (Fig. 2.99).

The transverse carpal arch is maintained by the flexor retinaculum; it continues distally as far as the metacarpal heads (metacarpal arch); the long axis of this 'gutter' crosses the lunate, capitate and 3rd metacarpal. The concavity of this arch at the level of the metacarpal heads is much shallower and more widespread than at the level of the carpal bones; the shallowness at the metacarpal heads can be seen and appreciated in the relaxed hand. Running longitudinally are the carpometacarpophalangeal arches extending from the wrist, formed for each digit by the corresponding metacarpal and phalanges; these arches are concave on their palmar surface with the keystone of each being at the level of the metacarpophalangeal joint. Consequently, muscular imbalance at this point interferes with the concavity of the arch. Of these longitudinal arches, the two most important are those of the middle and index fingers. During opposition of the thumb to the fingers, oblique arches are formed running from the thumb into the finger being opposed; the most important oblique arch is that linking thumb and index finger because of its use in holding objects (pen).

When the palm is hollowed, an oblique gutter (palmar gutter) runs across the oblique arches formed with the thumb from the base of the hypothenar eminence, where the pisiform can be palpated, to the head of the 2nd metacarpal; it is the direction taken by the handle of a tool when fully grasped by the hand.

In use, the hand does not always utilise the various arches. When carrying large and heavy flat objects, the hand spreads out and becomes flattened so that contact with the object is made at the thenar and hypothenar eminences, metacarpal heads and anterior surfaces of the phalanges. This provides a large area of contact and support, with movement of the object limited by friction between it and the skin.

The digits may be used individually as circumstances dictate; being functionally separate from the remaining digits, the thumb can be moved and used independently. Although not completely separate, the index finger has a considerable freedom (it can be used independently in pointing and gesturing); this relative freedom is important in grasping. The remaining fingers cannot be used independently throughout their full range of movement, principally because of the linkage between the tendons of the extensor digitorum on their dorsal surfaces.

Prehension (Grip)

The way in which the hand is used to grip an object depends upon several factors, not least being the size, shape and weight of the object, as well as the use to which it is being put. In general terms, the grip can be classified as being either a 'precision grip' or a 'power grip'. The thumb and the fingers combine in various ways to produce the former, while the hand becomes involved in the latter.

Hand movements are extremely precise, and the ability to manipulate small objects and carry out very intricate tasks is one of the characteristics of human development.

Precision Grip

In precision grips, the object is usually small and sometimes fragile; it is seized between the pads of the digits, which spread around the object conforming to its shape. The action involves rotation at the carpometacarpal joint of the thumb and the metacarpophalangeal joints of the thumb and finger(s) involved. Several types of precision grip can be identified (Fig. 2.100).

Terminal opposition (pincer) grip. The tips of the pads, or sometimes the edges of the nails, are used to pick up fine objects (pin) (Fig. 2.100A); it is the finest and most precise of all precision grips and, therefore, the most easily upset in trauma of the hand.

Subterminal opposition. A grip in which the palmar surfaces of the thumb, index and possibly other fingers come into contact. The most common example is the tripod grip (Fig. 2.100B) in which the thumb, index and middle finger come into contact (holding a pen).

Pinch grip. This involves the pads of the thumb and index finger when they oppose (gripping a clothes peg or tweezers) (Fig. 2.100C). The efficiency of this grip can be tested by attempting to pull a sheet of paper from between the thumb and index finger.

Subtermino-lateral opposition (key) grip. Where the pad of the thumb presses against the side of the index

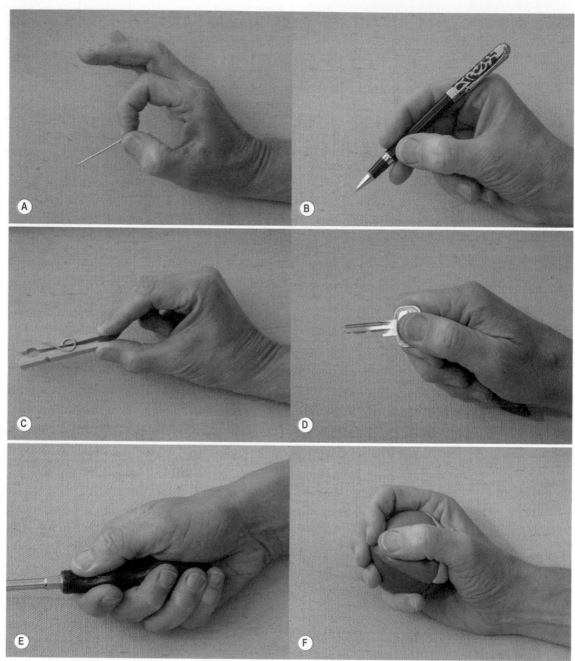

Fig. 2.100 Types of grip. (A) Pincer. (B) Tripod. (C) Pinch. (D) Key. (E) Oblique palmar. (F) Ball.

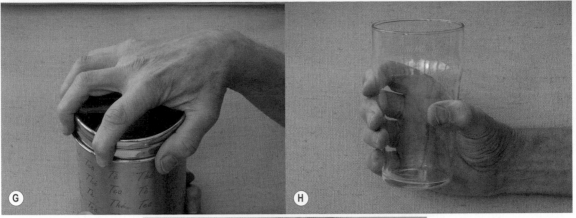

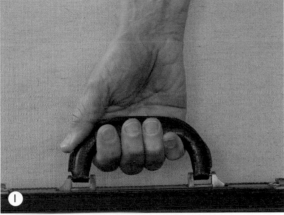

Fig. 2.100, cont'd (G) Span. (H) Cylinder. (I) Hook.

finger to hold an object (key, plate) between them (Fig. 2.100D). It is less fine but strong and can replace other precision grips when the distal phalanx of the index finger has been lost.

The position of the wrist and the muscle work involved are the same as for the power grip, with the muscles involved being the small muscles of the hand, as well as flexors digitorum profundus and superficialis and pollicis longus. Depending upon the activity, there are varying degrees of flexion and extension in the joints of the fingers and thumb. In writing the pen is held between the thumb, index and middle finger. The muscle work involved is similar to that for the power grip, but the strength of contraction is much less. In addition to the long flexors of the fingers and thumb holding the pen, the lumbricals and interossei produce and control the very fine movements of the fingers, which, together with movements of the thumb, allow the pen to be moved to write.

Power Grip

In power grips, where considerable force may be required, the hand is used in addition to the digits. The flexors and extensors of the wrist work strongly to fix its position, and the long finger flexors and intrinsic muscles of the hand work to grip the object.

Oblique palmar grip. The most powerful power grip in which the whole hand and fingers wrap around the object (Fig. 2.100E), whose long axis lies obliquely across the palm. The thumb acts as a buttress, with the fingers closing around the object, the size of which determines the strength of the grip. The shapes of tool handles are sculpted to facilitate this grip, which is maximal when the thumb can still touch the index finger, such as when using a screwdriver.

Ball grip. Used to accommodate a ball-shaped object, which is enclosed by the palm, fingers and thumb (Fig. 2.100F); the fingers and thumb are increasingly abducted as the diameter of the object increases.

Span grip. If the object is circular but flat (lid of a canister or jar) the palm may not make contact with the object (Fig. 2.100G); this increases the power needed in the fingers and thumb to maintain the grip whilst opening.

Cylinder grip. A grip where an object is held transversely across the palm, fingers and thumb, the hand and digits (Fig. 2.100H), with the cylindrical shape of the hand allowing variations in the size of the object and the power applied to it.

There is little movement involved in the above power grips. The distal and proximal interphalangeal joints of the fingers are flexed by flexors digitorum profundus and superficialis, respectively; the metacarpophalangeal joints are flexed by the lumbricals and long flexors; the thumb is strongly held against the flexed fingers by flexor pollicis longus and the intrinsic thumb muscles; the wrist is held in extension by the synergistic action of extensors carpi radialis longus, brevis and carpi ulnaris. This wrist position prevents the continued contraction of the long flexors pulling the wrist into flexion, preventing loss of power in the gripping fingers by 'active insufficiency' of the flexor muscles. Once in the gripping position, all of the above muscles are working isometrically with the joint positions determined by the size of the object being held.

Hook grip. In this type of grip, the object (suitcase handle) is held across the palmar surfaces of the flexed fingers (Fig. 2.100I). The thumb plays no part in a true hook grip, but should the weight of the object increase, the grip will change to a palmar grip. A hook grip is relatively secure but only in one direction (towards the fingers). In this grip, the wrist is maintained in a similar position of extension. The fingers are hooked through or around the handle to allow carrying, as when holding a suitcase. The distal and proximal interphalangeal joints are flexed by flexors digitorum profundus and superficialis, respectively, working isometrically to maintain the grip. The metacarpophalangeal joints are held in a neutral position.

One activity in which both types of grip can be seen, albeit in different hands, is when hammering in a nail; the nail is held precisely between the thumb and index finger of one hand, while the hammer is firmly held using a palmar grip in the other.

HAND

METACARPUS

The metacarpus consists of five bones (metacarpals), one corresponding to each digit and numbered in sequence from lateral (1st) to medial (5th). Each is a long bone with a proximal quadrilateral base, shaft (body) and distal rounded head (Fig. 2.101); variations in the shape of

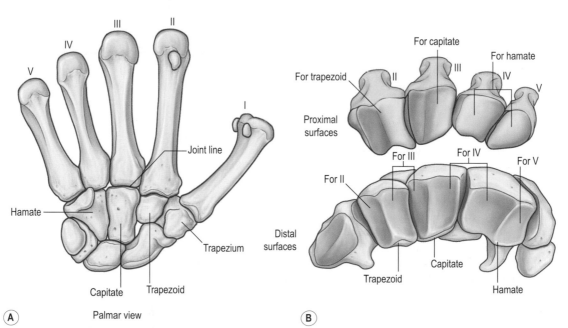

Fig. 2.101 (A) Anterior aspect of the right carpus and metacarpals. (B) Articular surfaces of the common carpometacarpal joint.

the bases provides a means by which each can be distinguished. The base of the 1st metacarpal has a saddle-shaped articular surface which fits a corresponding surface on the trapezium; that of the 2nd articulates with the trapezium, trapezoid and capitate; that of the 3rd has a single articulation with the capitate; and those of the 4th and 5th articulate with the hamate. The bases of the 2nd to 5th also articulate with the adjacent metacarpals, having articular facets in appropriate positions.

The metacarpal heads are smooth and rounded, extending further onto the palmar surface; the palmar articular margin is notched in the midline. The head of the 1st metacarpal is wider than the others having two sesamoid bones, usually in the short tendons crossing the joint anteriorly, which articulate with the palmar part of the joint surface, occasionally grooving it. The head fits into a concavity on the base of the proximal phalanx at the metacarpophalangeal joint. The metacarpal shaft is slightly curved with a longitudinal palmar concavity; that of the 1st is nearly as wide as the base and has a rounded dorsal surface. The palmar surface is divided by a blunt ridge into larger lateral and smaller medial parts.

Ossification

Primary ossification centres appear in the shaft in the 9th week *in utero*, so that the bones are well ossified at birth. Secondary centres appear in the heads of the 2nd to 5th metacarpals between 2 and 3 years; a secondary centre for the base of the 1st metacarpal appears slightly later. Fusion of the epiphysis with the shaft occurs between 17 and 19 years for all metacarpals. Occasionally, a secondary centre may appear in the head of the 1st metacarpal.

Palpation

If the fingers are flexed to form a fist, the metacarpal heads can be palpated as the knuckles. Running proximally on the dorsal surface of the hand, the shafts can be distinguished, at the proximal end of which the gap between the base of the metacarpal and carpus can be palpated as the line of the carpometacarpal joint.

COMMON CARPOMETACARPAL JOINT

The carpometacarpal joints are the sites of articulation between the carpus and metacarpals. The bases of the medial four metacarpals and the medial three carpal bones of the distal row form the common carpometacarpal joint; it has an irregular joint line (Fig. 2.101A).

The joints are plane synovial with the exception of the slightly bevelled joint surfaces between the hamate and base of the 5th metacarpal.

Articular Surfaces

The base of the 2nd metacarpal fits into a recess formed by the medial side of the trapezium, distal surface of the trapezoid and anterolateral corner of the capitate; that of the 3rd only with the distal surface of the capitate; that of the 4th mainly with the anterolateral distal surface of the hamate, but also with the anteromedial corner of the capitate; and that of the 5th with the anteromedial part of the distal surface of the hamate (Fig. 2.101).

Joint Capsule and Synovial Membrane

A fibrous capsule surrounds the common carpometacarpal joint; various capsular thickenings can be identified. Synovial membrane, attaching to the articular margins, lines the capsule and all non-articular surfaces. The joint cavity extends proximally between the carpal bones and usually communicates with the midcarpal joint (p. 157). Distally, the joint space extends between the bases of the medial four metacarpals.

Ligaments

The dorsal and palmar carpometacarpal ligaments are little more than thickenings of the joint capsule.

Dorsal Carpometacarpal Ligaments

These are a series of fibrous bands passing from the distal row of carpal bones to the bases of the metacarpals, with each metacarpal generally receiving two bands. Those to the 2nd metacarpal come from the trapezium and trapezoid; those to the 3rd from the trapezoid and capitate; and those to the 4th from the capitate and hamate. The base of the 5th metacarpal receives a single band from the hamate.

Palmar Carpometacarpal Ligaments

The arrangement of the fibrous bands of the palmar carpometacarpal ligaments is similar to that for the dorsal ligaments, except that the base of the 3rd metacarpal receives three bands arising from the trapezoid, capitate and hamate (Fig. 2.83).

Interosseous Ligament

A short interosseous ligament is usually present, passing from the adjacent inferior angles of the capitate and hamate to the base of the 3rd or 4th metacarpal or both; occasionally, it divides the joint space into medial and lateral compartments.

Blood Supply and Innervation

The arterial supply to the joint is from the palmar and dorsal carpal networks, and the nerve supply is by twigs from the anterior and posterior interosseous nerves and the deep and dorsal branches of the ulnar nerve (root value C7 and C8).

Relations

The common carpometacarpal joint lies deep to the tendons of flexors digitorum superficialis and profundus. Most laterally on the palmar surface, the tendon of flexor carpi radialis crosses the joint to attach to the base of the 2nd metacarpal, while the tendon of flexor carpi ulnaris passes most medially. Also overlying the joint medially are the muscles of the hypothenar eminence.

On the posterior aspect of the joint are the extensor tendons as they pass into the hand. From lateral to medial these are extensors carpi radialis longus and brevis, extensor pollicis longus, extensor indicis, extensors digitorum and digiti minimi and extensor carpi ulnaris.

Stability

The joint is extremely stable, providing a firm base between the joints of the wrist and those of the hand.

Movements

Little movement at the carpometacarpal joints of the fingers is possible. The 2nd and 3rd metacarpals are essentially immobile, while a slight gliding may occur between the 4th metacarpal and hamate. Only the 5th metacarpal has any appreciable movement as it glides on the hamate because of the bevelled joint surfaces. The movement that does occur is flexion, seen during a tight grasp, as well as in opposition of the thumb to the little finger; there is also slight rotation during opposition due to the action of opponens digiti minimi.

Accessory Movements

A slight degree of anteroposterior gliding can be produced between the base of the metacarpal and adjacent carpal bone if the appropriate pressure is applied.

INTERMETACARPAL JOINTS

The intermetacarpal joints are plane synovial joints between adjacent sides of the bases of the 2nd and 3rd, 3rd and 4th, and 4th and 5th metacarpals. The joints are closed anteriorly, posteriorly and distally by palmar and dorsal metacarpal and interosseous ligaments, respectively, that pass transversely between adjacent bones (Fig. 2.82). The joint spaces are continuous with the common carpometacarpal joint proximally. The blood and nerve supply to the joints is similar to that for the common carpometacarpal joint. Movements at the intercarpal joints accompany movements of the metacarpals against the distal row of carpal bones. In accessory movements, a small amount of anteroposterior gliding can be produced between any two metacarpal bases by appropriately applied pressure.

FINGERS

In general, the fingers act in one plane to close around an object forming a pincer action with the opposed thumb. The size of the object grasped determines whether and to what extent two-dimensional movement at the metacarpophalangeal joints occurs.

The articulation of the 2nd to 5th metacarpals with the distal row of carpal bones has already been considered (p. 183); this section considers the metacarpophalangeal joints and the two interphalangeal joints of each finger.

PHALANGES

There are 14 phalanges in each hand, 3 in each finger (2nd to 5th digits) and 2 for the thumb (1st digit) (Figs 2.75 and 2.77). As long bones, each phalanx has a shaft, larger proximal end (base) and smaller distal end (head) (Fig. 2.102A); the phalanges of the thumb are shorter and broader than those of the fingers.

The proximal phalanx has a concave oval facet on its base for articulation with the head of the metacarpal. The rounded head, which extends further onto the palmar surface, has a wide pulley-shaped articular surface for the base of the next phalanx. The shaft is curved along its length, being convex dorsally; it is convex from side to side on its dorsal surface and flat on the palmar surface. The middle and distal phalanges are similar to the proximal phalanx; however, the base of the distal

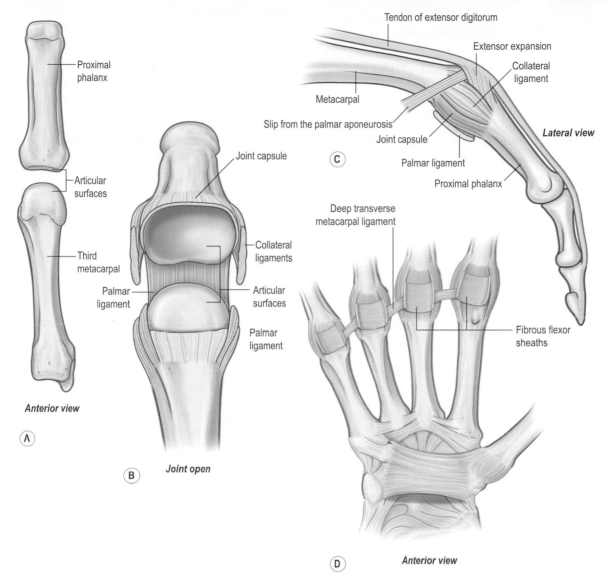

Fig. 2.102 (A) Articular surfaces of the metacarpophalangeal joints of the fingers. (B and C) Ligaments associated with the metacarpophalangeal joint. (D) Anterior aspect of the wrist, metacarpals and 2nd to 4th phalanges showing the deep transverse metacarpal ligament.

phalanx is large and the head expanded to support the pulp pad of the digits.

By convention, the digits are described by name rather than by number and are, from lateral to medial: thumb; index, middle, ring and little fingers.

Ossification

Primary ossification centres appear in the shafts of the phalanges between the 8th and 12th week *in utero* with the distal phalanges ossifying first. Secondary centres appear in the bases of the phalanges during the 2nd and 3rd year, fusing with the shaft between 17 and 19 years. Occasionally, a secondary centre may appear in the head as well as in the base.

Palpation

By flexing the fingers into a fist, the heads of the proximal and middle phalanges can be palpated. The shafts of the phalanges are also easily followed throughout their length, especially on their dorsal surface.

METACARPOPHALANGEAL JOINTS

Articular Surfaces

The articular surface of the metacarpal head is biconvex, with the curvatures being unequal transversely and anteroposteriorly; it is broader anteriorly than posteriorly with the hyaline cartilage extending further proximally on its anterior aspect (Fig. 2.102A).

The base of the proximal phalanx is biconcave having a smaller articular surface than the metacarpal head (Fig. 2.102A); the surface area is increased by the presence of the palmar ligament attached to the anterior margin of the articular surface (Fig. 2.102B and C).

Joint Capsule and Synovial Membrane

The fibrous capsule surrounding the joint is loose and attached closer to the articular margins on the posterior aspects of the bone than anteriorly. On each side, it is strengthened by collateral ligaments and replaced anteriorly by the palmar ligament (Fig. 2.102B and C); posteriorly, the extensor expansion of the long extensor tendon replaces the capsule, blending at the sides with the collateral ligaments. The posterior part of the capsule also receives fibres from the distal slips of the palmar aponeurosis (Fig. 2.102C).

The capsule is lined by synovial membrane, covering all non-articular surfaces. Synovial-lined anterior and posterior recesses of the capsule permit freedom of movement, particularly during flexion.

Ligaments

In addition to the collateral and palmar ligaments associated with each metacarpophalangeal joint, the heads of the 2nd to 5th metacarpals are united by the deep transverse metacarpal ligaments.

Collateral Ligaments

These pass from the tubercle and adjacent depression on the side of the metacarpal head to the palmar aspect of the side of the base of the proximal phalanx (Fig. 2.102B and C); they are strong and fan out as they pass from metacarpal to phalanx. Anteriorly, they blend with the palmar ligament, while posteriorly the extensor expansion joins them.

Palmar Ligament

A dense fibrocartilaginous plate firmly attached to the anterior margin of the base of the proximal phalanx (Fig. 2.102B and C. Proximally, it is loosely attached to the neck of the metacarpal by the joint capsule; on each side, it receives fibres from the collateral ligaments. The palmar ligament acts as a mobile articular surface facilitating flexion at the joint.

Deep Transverse Metacarpal Ligaments

Series of short ligaments connecting the palmar ligaments of the four metacarpophalangeal joints of the fingers (Fig. 2.102D), being continuous with the palmar interosseous fascia and blending with the fibrous flexor sheaths. They act to bind the heads of the four medial metacarpals together, limiting their movement apart. (There is no ligament between the 1st and 2nd metacarpal, thus the independence and freedom of movement of the thumb.) The deep transverse metacarpal ligaments also receive fibres from the distal slips of the palmar aponeurosis, as well as part of the extensor expansion as it passes forwards on each side of the metacarpal head.

Passing posterior to the deep transverse metacarpal ligaments are the tendons of the dorsal and palmar interossei; the lumbrical tendons pass anteriorly.

Blood Supply and Innervation

The arterial supply to the joints is by branches from adjacent digital arteries, while the nerve supply is by twigs from the median, possibly the radial nerve for the index and middle finger, and the ulnar nerve for the ring and little fingers. Root value of the nerve supply is C7.

Relations

On the posterior aspect of the joint is the expansion of the long extensor tendon (Fig. 2.103A and C), part of which passes around the sides of the metacarpal head blending with the deep transverse metacarpal ligament. The tendon of the lumbrical passes lateral to the joint (see Fig. 2.103A and C), anterior to the deep transverse metacarpal ligament, before attaching to the base of the proximal phalanx and extensor expansion. Exactly which interosseous tendons pass medial and lateral to each metacarpophalangeal joint depends on which finger is being considered:

1. For the index finger, the 1st dorsal interosseous is lateral and 1st palmar interosseous medial.

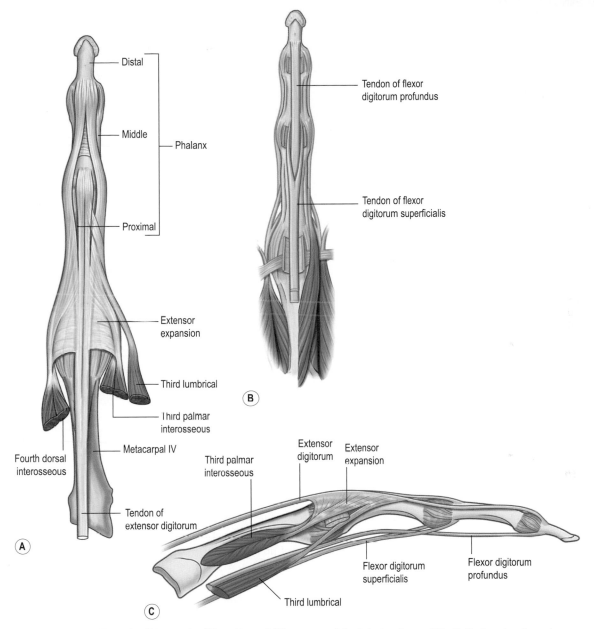

Fig. 2.103 Posterior (A), anterior (B) and lateral (C) aspects of the left ring finger (4th digit) showing the relations of the metacarpophalangeal joint.

2. For the middle finger, the 2nd and 3rd dorsal interossei are lateral and medial, respectively.
3. For the ring finger, the 2nd palmar interosseous is lateral and 4th dorsal interosseous medial (Fig. 2.103A).
4. For the little finger, the 3rd palmar interosseous is lateral and the tendon of abductor digiti minimi medial.

Immediately anterior to the joint is the tendon of flexor digitorum profundus, anterior to which is the tendon of flexor digitorum superficialis, the latter splitting into two at the level of the joint (Fig. 2.103B and C). Flexor digiti minimi brevis is situated on the anterolateral aspect of the joint of the little finger. Digital branches from the dorsal and palmar metacarpal arteries, together with digital branches from the median, ulnar and radial nerves (depending on the finger) pass either side of the metacarpophalangeal joint (Fig. 2.76B).

Stability

The metacarpophalangeal joint is stabilised primarily by the long flexor and extensor tendons crossing the joint, as well as by the lumbricals and interossei. Dislocation of the joint does occur; however, it can often be reduced by manipulation.

MOVEMENTS OF THE FINGERS AT THE METACARPOPHALANGEAL JOINTS

Active movement at the metacarpophalangeal joint occurs about two axes, each located in the metacarpal head approximately 9/10th of the midline length of the metacarpal from its base. The movements are flexion and extension, and abduction and adduction; passive axial rotation also occurs.

Flexion and Extension

These occur about a transverse axis through the metacarpal head. The geometry of the articular surfaces dictates that the intersection of the longitudinal axes of the proximal phalanx and metacarpal moves distally during flexion. In extension, the anterior surface of the metacarpal head articulates with the palmar ligament (Fig. 2.104), which moves past the metacarpal head turning upon itself to glide along the palmar surface of the shaft (Fig. 2.104). As this is occurring, the capsule and its synovial lining unfold so as not to limit movement prematurely. The range of flexion is slightly less than 90 degrees for the index finger but progressively increases towards the little finger. Flexion of one joint in isolation is limited by tension developed in the deep transverse metacarpal ligaments; flexion is ultimately resisted by tension in the collateral ligaments. The range of active extension is variable between individuals but may reach 50 degrees; passive extension may reach as much as 90 degrees in individuals with lax ligaments. The total ranges of flexion/extension for each finger are given in Table 2.11.

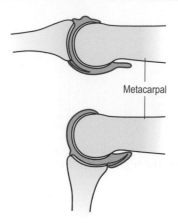

Fig. 2.104 Movements of the fingers at the metacarpophalangeal joints.

	Flexion/	Abduction/
Finger	**Extension (°)**	**Adduction (°)**
Index	148/155	50/62
Middle	145/151	40/53
Ring	149/159	38/55
Little	152/172	57/68

TABLE 2.11 Ranges of Active/Passive Flexion/Extension and Abduction/Adduction at the Metacarpophalangeal Joint of Each Finger

Taken from Youm, Y., Gillespie, T.E., Flatt, A.E., Sprague, B.L., 1978. Kinematic investigation of normal MCP joint. J. Biomech. 11, 109–118.

Flexion at the metacarpophalangeal joints is brought about primarily by the lumbricals, aided by the tendons of flexors digitorum profundus and superficialis, as well as the interossei. In the little finger, flexor and abductor digiti minimi also contribute to the movement. Extension is achieved at all metacarpophalangeal joints by extensor digitorum with the addition of extensor indicis in the index finger and extensor digiti minimi in the little finger.

Abduction and Adduction

These occur about an anteroposterior axis through the metacarpal head with the movement away from (abduction) or towards (adduction) the middle finger (3rd digit). The movement is easier and has a greater range when the fingers are extended, being as much as 30 degrees in each direction. Tension in the collateral ligaments in flexion of the joint severely limits the side-to-side movement, so much so that, at 90 degrees flexion, the total range of abduction/adduction may be no more than 10 degrees. The total ranges of active/passive abduction/adduction with the fingers in neutral are given in Table 2.11.

Abduction at the joint is brought about by the dorsal interossei for the index, middle and ring fingers, and by abductor digiti minimi for the little finger. At the index and middle fingers, the movement may be assisted by the 1st and 2nd lumbricals, respectively, via their attachment to the extensor expansion. If the joint is hyperextended, then extensor digitorum also aids abduction. Adduction towards the middle finger (3rd digit) is achieved by the palmar interossei and can be assisted by the 3rd and 4th lumbricals for the ring and little fingers. If the joint is simultaneously flexed, then adduction is assisted by flexors digitorum superficialis and profundus.

Rotation

Active rotation is not possible except in the little finger; however, because of the shape of the joint surfaces and relative laxity of the associated ligaments, some passive rotation is possible with a maximum range of 60 degrees. In the index finger, the range of medial rotation is approximately 45 degrees, while lateral rotation is negligible; the range of medial and lateral rotation in the remaining fingers is approximately equal.

INTERPHALANGEAL JOINTS

Because each finger has three phalanges, it has two interphalangeal joints: proximal between the head of the proximal and base of the middle phalanx, and distal between the head of the middle and base of the distal phalanx. Both proximal and distal joints are hinge joints permitting flexion and extension only, with the articular surfaces covered by hyaline cartilage.

Articular Surfaces

Between the pulley-shaped head of the phalanx and two shallow facets separated by a ridge on the base of the immediately distal phalanx (Fig. 2.105). The groove and ridge on the head and base respectively do not lie exactly in a parasagittal plane, except for the joints of the index finger. In all other joints, they run slightly obliquely

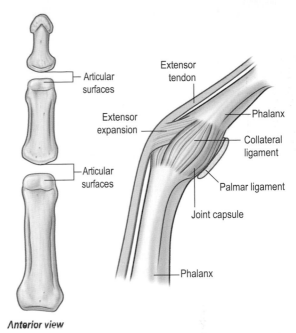

Anterior view

Fig. 2.105 Articular surfaces and ligaments of the interphalangeal joints of the fingers.

from posterolateral to anteromedial with the obliquity increasing from the middle to little finger.

The articular surface of the phalangeal head is greater than that on the adjacent base, extending further distally on its anterior aspect; the head is also wider anteriorly than posteriorly. A fibrocartilaginous plate (palmar ligament) similar to that associated with the metacarpophalangeal joint acts as a mobile articular surface.

Joint Capsule and Synovial Membrane

A loose fibrous capsule surrounds the joint, strengthened at the sides by collateral ligaments and partly replaced anteriorly and posteriorly by the palmar ligament and extensor expansion, respectively (Fig. 2.105). Synovial membrane lines all non-articular surfaces, including the anterior and posterior recesses of the capsule.

Ligaments
Collateral Ligaments

These attach to the sides of the head of the most proximal phalanx and sides of the base of the adjacent more distal phalanx, blending with the margins of the palmar ligament (Fig. 2.105). They tend not to be as obliquely orientated as the collateral ligaments of the metacarpophalangeal joints; they become increasingly tense with flexion at the joint.

Palmar Ligament

A mobile fibrocartilaginous plate attached to the anterior margin of the base of the adjacent phalanx; it is loosely attached by the joint capsule to the anterior aspect of the neck of the immediately preceding phalanx (Fig. 2.105). Also attaching to the palmar ligament is the fibrous flexor sheath of the digit.

Blood Supply, Lymphatic Drainage and Innervation

The arterial supply to the joints is by branches from the digital arteries running along the sides of each finger. Anteriorly, the digital arteries arise from the palmar metacarpal arteries, and posteriorly from the dorsal metacarpal arteries. Venous drainage is by similarly named vessels, eventually draining into the venae comitantes associated with the radial and ulnar arteries. Posteriorly, some venous drainage passes to the dorsal venous plexus on the dorsum of the hand and then into the basilic and cephalic veins. Lymphatic drainage from the joints is by vessels which follow the arteries, with the majority of lymph draining to the lateral group of axillary nodes, although some may pass to cubital or brachial nodes.

The nerve supply to each joint is by twigs from adjacent digital nerves (root value C7). For the index, middle and lateral side of the ring fingers, the digital nerves are branches of the median nerve anteriorly and radial nerve posteriorly; for the medial side of the ring and the little fingers, the digital nerves arise from the ulnar nerve.

Relations

On the anterior aspect of the proximal interphalangeal joint are the tendons of flexors digitorum superficialis and profundus enclosed within the fibrous flexor sheath (Fig. 2.76B(i)); only the tendon of profundus lies anterior to the distal interphalangeal joint (Fig. 2.76B(ii)). The fibrous flexor sheaths are relatively thin and loose over the interphalangeal joints with a cruciate arrangement of fibres as they pass from the side of one phalanx to the opposite side of the preceding phalanx (Fig. 2.98). Immediately beyond the distal interphalangeal joint, the flexor sheath attaches to the palmar surface of the distal phalanx.

Posterior to the proximal interphalangeal joint is the central slip of the extensor expansion (Fig. 2.103A). On the posterior aspect of the middle phalanx, the two collateral slips of the extensor expansion come together forming a single tendon that crosses the posterior aspect of the distal interphalangeal joint (Fig. 2.103A).

Stability

The interphalangeal joints are fairly stable because of the presence of the long flexor and extensor tendons crossing them; nevertheless, dislocation can and does occur, but can often be reduced by manipulation.

MOVEMENTS OF THE FINGERS AT THE INTERPHALANGEAL JOINTS

Because of the nature of the joint surfaces, the only active movement possible at the interphalangeal joints are flexion and extension; however, a small degree of passive side-to-side movement is possible, particularly at the distal interphalangeal joint.

Flexion and Extension

These occur about a transverse axis, which for the middle, ring and little fingers runs with increasing obliquity from proximomedially to distolaterally. Each axis is approximately perpendicular to the groove on the phalangeal head so that when the medial fingers are flexed at the interphalangeal joints, the movement does not occur in a sagittal plane but enables these fingers to oppose the thumb more easily: flexion of the index finger, however, occurs in a sagittal plane.

The range of flexion at the proximal interphalangeal joint is greater than 90 degrees for all fingers, gradually increasing towards the little finger which is capable of 135 degrees flexion. At the distal interphalangeal joint, the range of flexion for the little finger is 90 degrees, gradually decreasing towards the index finger. Active extension at the interphalangeal joints is minimal, no more than 5 degrees at the distal and only 1 or 2 degrees at the proximal interphalangeal joints; passive extension may be considerably greater.

Flexion at the proximal interphalangeal joint is primarily due to the action of flexor digitorum superficialis, assisted by flexor digitorum profundus; only profundus flexes the distal interphalangeal joint. Extension of the interphalangeal joints is produced by the lumbricals and interossei via their attachments to the extensor expansion. They are assisted in each finger by extensor digitorum and in the index and little fingers by extensors indicis and digiti minimi, respectively.

Simultaneous flexion at one interphalangeal joint and extension at the other are produced by a controlled balance between the activity of the flexor and extensor muscles; flexion of the wrist facilitates extension of the fingers and opening the fist. The functional position of the wrist (extension) puts the finger flexors beyond their natural length enabling greater tension to be developed in them, facilitating a powerful grip. Similarly, flexing the interphalangeal joints places the extensors of the wrist under increased tension. In stabilising the wrist, a certain amount of flexor strength and extensor power is sacrificed. Only 70% of the strength of the finger flexors is available from flexion of the interphalangeal joints. Weakness of the wrist extensors, by failing to maintain the position of

function, greatly interferes with the strength of the finger flexors and the ability to carry out forceful closure of the fist.

Accessory Movements of the Joints of the Fingers

Similar accessory movements of anteroposterior gliding and rotation are possible at each of the metacarpophalangeal and interphalangeal joints of all four fingers. With the proximal component stabilised between the thumb and index finger, the more distal segment can be made to execute the accessory movements.

Muscles involved in producing movement at the metacarpophalangeal, and interphalangeal joints of the fingers are given in Table 2.12; further details of each muscle can be found in following sections.

TABLE 2.12 Muscles Producing Movements at the Metacarpophalangeal and Interphalangeal Joints of the Fingers

Muscle	Attachments	Action	Innervation (root value)
Flexor digitorum superficialis	Medial epicondyle via common flexor origin, ulnar collateral ligament and coronoid process of the ulna (humeroulnar head) and proximal 2/3rd of anterior surface of radius (radial head) to palmar surface of middle phalanx of finger after splitting to allow tendon of flexor digitorum profundus to pass through	Flexor of metacarpophalangeal and proximal interphalangeal joints; assists flexion at wrist joint	Median nerve (C7, C8, T1)
Flexor digitorum profundus	Coronoid process, proximal ¾ of anterior and medial surfaces of ulna and adjacent anterior surface of interosseous membrane to base of palmar surface of distal phalanx after passing through tendon of flexor digitorum superficialis	Flexor of distal interphalangeal joint; assists in flexing proximal interphalangeal, metacarpophalangeal and wrist joints	Anterior interosseous branch of the median nerve (C7, C8, T1)
Flexor digiti minimi brevis[a]	Hook of hamate and adjacent flexor retinaculum to base of proximal phalanx of little finger	Flexor of metacarpophalangeal joint of little finger	Deep branch of the ulnar nerve (T1)
Extensor digitorum	Lateral epicondyle of humerus via common extensor tendon dividing into four tendons near wrist, each expanding over posterior aspect of metacarpophalangeal joint with central tendon attaching to dorsal surface of base of middle phalanx and lateral tendons to dorsal aspect of base of distal phalanx	Extensor of metacarpophalangeal joint; assists extension of both interphalangeal joints of fingers	Posterior interosseous branch of the radial nerve (C7, C8)
Extensor indicis	Posterior surface of ulna and adjacent interosseous membrane to extensor expansion of index finger	Assists extensor digitorum in index finger, enabling it to extend independently; also aids extension at wrist	Posterior interosseous branch of the radial nerve (C7, C8)

Continued

TABLE 2.12   Muscles Producing Movements at the Metacarpophalangeal and Interphalangeal Joints of the Fingers—cont'd

Muscle	Attachments	Action	Innervation (root value)
Extensor digiti minimi	Lateral epicondyle of humerus via common extensor tendon to extensor expansion of little finger	Assists extensor digitorum in little finger, enabling it to extend independently; also aids extension at wrist	Posterior interosseous branch of the radial nerve (C7, C8)
Abductor digiti minimi[a]	Pisiform, pisohamate ligament and tendon of flexor carpi ulnaris to extensor expansion and ulnar side of proximal phalanx of little finger	Abducts little finger away from ring finger; aids extension of interphalangeal joints	Deep branch of the ulnar nerve (T1)
Opponens digiti minimi[a]	Hook of hamate and adjacent flexor retinaculum to medial ½ of palmar surface of 5th metacarpal	Pulls little finger towards palm at same time rotating it laterally at carpometacarpal joint	Deep branch of the ulnar nerve (T1)
Dorsal interossei	Sides of adjacent metacarpals to extensor expansion and proximal phalanx; two attach to middle finger and one each to index and ring fingers	Abducts index, middle and ring fingers away from long axis of hand; also assist lumbricals	Deep branch of the ulnar nerve (T1)
Palmar interossei	Shaft of metacarpal to extensor expansion and base of proximal phalanx of same digit	Adducts thumb, index, ring and little finger towards middle finger; also assist lumbricals	Deep branch of the ulnar nerve (T1)
Lumbricals	Lateral side of tendon of flexor digitorum profundus to lateral margin of extensor expansion	Flexor of metacarpophalangeal and extensor of interphalangeal joints	Lateral 2 by median nerve (T1), medial 2 by ulnar nerve (T1)

[a]Muscles of the hypothenar eminence

BIOMECHANICS

Joint Forces

Because of the size and weight of many objects carried or manipulated, the forces transmitted across various joints within the hand and fingers can reach considerable magnitudes. An estimation of the magnitudes of these forces is necessary to refine finger prostheses. Joint reactions at the carpometacarpal, metacarpophalangeal, proximal and distal interphalangeal joints are on average twice, 3 times, 10 times and 6 times the applied load, respectively. The magnitude and direction of action of these forces at various joints have led to predictions of clinical deformities and joint damage.

Pathology

Due to the delicate balance between the soft tissues of the hand, it is highly susceptible to trauma and disability; more than half of all injuries leading to disability involve the hand and fingers. Various bones may be fractured and/or joints dislocated with the most common injuries being accidental amputation of all or part of the hand and/or finger(s), burns, tendon lacerations, penetrating wounds and nerve injuries.

The most common deformity in rheumatoid arthritis is induced by synovitis of the metacarpophalangeal joint leading to narrowing of the articular cartilage and attenuation of the collateral ligaments. Under the influence of these two effects, palmar subluxation of the proximal phalanx on the metacarpal head occurs creating laxity of the flexor complex. Under the pull of the flexor tendons, there may be further subluxation of the proximal phalanx associated with an ulnar deviation, particularly in the index and middle fingers.

Joint Replacement

As with all joint replacements, the primary object is the relief of pain and restoration of as full a range of movement as possible. However, when considering finger joint replacements, the main problem appears to be maintenance of the cortical bone. Stresses on the endosteal surface of the bone have a tendency to produce gradual deformity and sometimes erosion so that the prosthesis protrudes through the shaft of the bone; the inserted foreign material may be a contributory factor in this erosion through disruption of the endosteal arterial supply.

In normal bone, the tensile stresses applied to the outer surface of the bone by ligamentous and periosteal attachments make a significant contribution to maintaining the integrity of the cortical bone. When these stresses are replaced by prostheses that depend on transmission of stress by the endosteal surface, the bone is clearly reacting and remodelling to an entirely different pattern of stresses.

MUSCLES FLEXING THE FINGERS

Flexor digitorum superficialis
Flexor digitorum profundus
Lumbricals
Flexor digiti minimi brevis

Flexor Digitorum Superficialis

Large muscle (Fig. 2.106A) lying in the anterior compartment of the forearm deep to pronator teres, palmaris longus and flexors carpi radialis and ulnaris, and superficial to flexor digitorum profundus and flexor pollicis longus. It arises by a long linear attachment but may be considered to arise by two heads. The humeroulnar (medial) head arises from the medial epicondyle of the humerus via the common flexor tendon, the anterior aspect of the ulnar collateral ligament and the sublime tubercle at the superior medial aspect of the coronoid process of the ulna. The radial (lateral) head arises from the proximal two-thirds of the anterior border of the radius, which runs inferolaterally from the radial tuberosity.

Approximately halfway down the forearm, the muscle narrows forming four separate tendons which pass deep to the flexor retinaculum where they are arranged in two pairs to enter the hand (Fig. 2.85B); the superficial pair pass to the middle and ring fingers, and deep pair to the index and little fingers. Within the carpal tunnel, the tendons of flexor digitorum superficialis lie superficial to those of flexor digitorum profundus with which they share a common synovial sheath (Fig. 2.85B). In the palm, the tendons separate and pass towards their

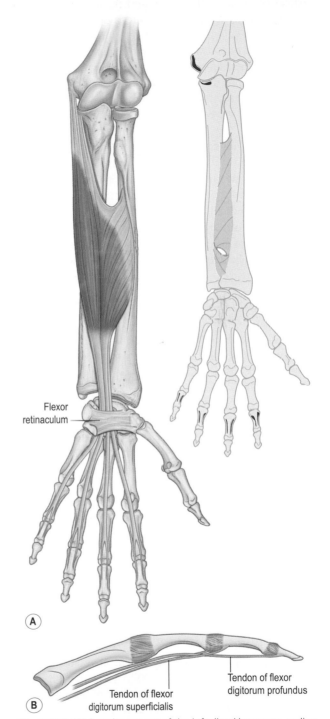

Flexor retinaculum

Tendon of flexor digitorum superficialis

Tendon of flexor digitorum profundus

(A)

(B)

Fig. 2.106 (A) Anterior aspect of the left distal humerus, radius, ulna, wrist and hand showing the position and attachments of flexor digitorum superficialis. (B) Lateral aspect of the hand showing the relationship of the long flexor tendons in the hand and fingers.

respective fingers, still lying superficial to the profundus tendons. At the level of the metacarpophalangeal joint, each superficialis tendon splits longitudinally into two parts, which pass around the profundus tendon, twisting so that their lateral surfaces unite forming a groove along which the tendon of flexor digitorum profundus passes. Prior to attaching to either side of the palmar surface of the base of the middle phalanx, the tendon splits again.

This arrangement provides a tunnel allowing the profundus tendon to become superficial (Fig. 2.106B); the arrangement also increases the lever arm of flexor digitorum profundus at the proximal interphalangeal joint, enabling a powerful grip of the fingers to be developed. As well as their main attachment to the middle phalanx, the tendons of flexor digitorum superficialis also provide attachments for the vincula tendinum which convey blood vessels to the tendon.

Innervation

By the median nerve (root value C7, C8 and T1) from the medial and lateral cords of the brachial plexus. Skin overlying the muscle and its tendons are supplied by roots C6, C7, C8 and T1.

Action

The muscle is primarily a flexor of the finger at the metacarpophalangeal and proximal interphalangeal joints. Because it crosses the wrist joint, it also aids flexion of the hand at the wrist if its action is continued.

Palpation

Contraction of the muscle can be felt by applying deep pressure through the superficial flexor muscles in the proximal part of the forearm with the fingers flexed; the tendons can be palpated in a similar manner proximal to the flexor retinaculum. It can be tested specifically by asking the individual to flex the proximal interphalangeal joint without flexing the distal interphalangeal joint.

Flexor Digitorum Profundus

Lying deep to flexor digitorum superficialis on the medial aspect of the forearm (Fig. 2.107A), flexor digitorum profundus attaches to the medial side of the coronoid process of the ulna, the proximal three-quarters of the anterior and medial surfaces of the ulna, and the medial middle one-third of the anterior surface of the adjacent interosseous membrane; it also has an attachment to the

aponeurosis attaching flexor carpi ulnaris to the posterior border of the ulna.

That part of the muscle from the interosseous membrane forms a separate tendon about halfway down the forearm which passes to the index finger; the remaining tendons are not usually formed until just proximal to the flexor retinaculum. The separate tendons pass deep to the flexor retinaculum where they lie side by side, deep to those of flexor digitorum superficialis but within the same synovial sheath (Fig. 2.85B). In the palm, the four tendons pass to their respective fingers. At first, they travel deep to superficialis but then pass through the tunnel formed by its tendon at the level of the metacarpophalangeal joint (Fig. 2.106B).

The tendon of flexor digitorum profundus attaches to the base of the palmar surface of the distal phalanx having passed through a fibro-osseous tunnel (Fig. 2.76B). Like the tendons of flexor digitorum superficialis, the profundus tendons are provided with vincula tendinum.

Innervation

Flexor digitorum profundus has a dual nerve supply. The lateral part of the muscle giving tendons to the index and middle fingers is supplied by the anterior interosseous branch of the median nerve (root value C7, C8 and T1); the medial part giving tendons to the ring and little fingers is supplied by the ulnar nerve (root value C8, T1) from the medial cord of the brachial plexus. Skin over the muscle is supplied by roots C7, C8 and T1.

Action

The primary action of flexor digitorum profundus is flexion of the distal interphalangeal joint. However, because it crosses several other joints during its course, it also aids in flexion of the proximal interphalangeal, metacarpophalangeal and wrist joints.

Palpation

The muscular part of flexor digitorum profundus can be palpated immediately medial to the posterior border of the ulna, where its contraction can be felt as the fingers are fully flexed from a position of extension.

Lumbricals

Four small round muscles located in the palm in association with the tendons of flexor digitorum profundus. The lateral two lumbricals are frequently unipennate arising from the lateral side of the flexor digitorum profundus

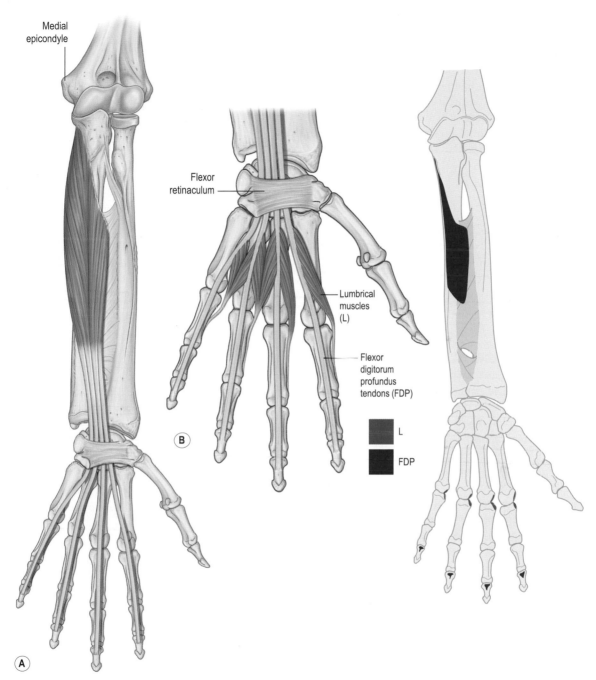

Medial epicondyle

Flexor retinaculum

Lumbrical muscles (L)

Flexor digitorum profundus tendons (FDP)

L

FDP

A

B

Fig. 2.107 (A) Anterior aspect of the left distal humerus, radius, ulna, wrist and hand showing the position and attachments of flexor digitorum profundus *(FDP)*. (B) Position and attachments of the lumbricals *(L)*.

tendons, while the medial two are bipennate arising from the adjacent sides of the tendons of the middle and ring, and ring and little fingers (Fig. 2.107B).

From this proximal attachment, the muscles pass distally to their respective fingers, anterior to the deep transverse metacarpal ligament, and then obliquely on the lateral side of the metacarpophalangeal joint to attach to the lateral margin of the extensor expansion at the side of the proximal phalanx. A few fibres make their way to the middle phalanx, but the majority can be traced to the base of the distal phalanx via the extensor expansion (Fig. 2.103C).

Innervation

The nerve supply varies, but the most common arrangement is for the lateral two lumbricals to be supplied by the median nerve (root value T1) from the medial and lateral cords of the brachial plexus and the medial two by the ulnar nerve (root value T1) from the medial cord of the brachial plexus.

Action

The lumbricals in the hands, as well as those in the feet, are unique muscles as they pass between the flexor and extensor tendons. Their anatomical position means that, in the hand, they flex the metacarpophalangeal joint and extend both interphalangeal joints of the corresponding finger ('lumbrical action'). In theory, the lumbricals should be able to rotate their respective fingers at the metacarpophalangeal joint; however, this only appears evident in the index finger so that the pad faces medially; the 1st dorsal interosseous is also involved in producing this movement. Functionally, the lumbricals are involved in the coordination of complex activities of the fingers involving both flexion and extension (writing). As a group, they have major functional significance in the dexterity of the hand, which is further enhanced by their rich sensory innervation.

Palpation

They are too deep to palpate, but their actions can be demonstrated by accurate electrical stimulation.

Flexor Digiti Minimi Brevis

Not always present, but when it is, it lies lateral to abductor digiti minimi arising from the hook of the hamate and adjacent flexor retinaculum. It attaches, together with abductor digiti minimi, to the base of the proximal phalanx of the little finger on its ulnar side (Fig. 2.108).

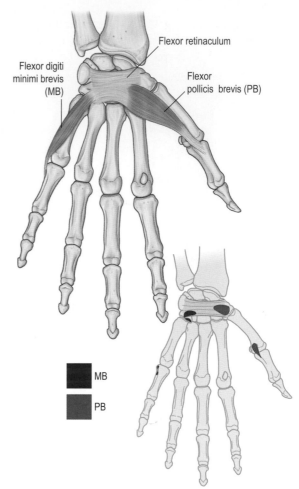

Fig. 2.108 Anterior aspect of the left wrist and hand showing the position and attachments of flexor pollicis brevis *(PB)* and flexor digiti minimi brevis *(MB)*.

Innervation

By the deep branch of the ulnar nerve (root value T1) from the medial cord of the brachial plexus.

Action

Flexion of the metacarpophalangeal joint of the little finger.

MUSCLES EXTENDING THE FINGERS

Extensor digitorum
Extensor digiti minimi
Extensor indicis
Palmar interossei (p. 200)
Dorsal interossei (p. 201)
Lumbricals (p. 194)

Extensor Digitorum

Extensor digitorum (Fig. 2.109A) is centrally placed within the posterior compartment of the forearm. It arises from the lateral epicondyle of the humerus via the common extensor tendon, the covering fascia and intermuscular septa at its sides. In the distal part of the forearm, it forms four tendons which pass deep to the extensor retinaculum in a synovial sheath shared with

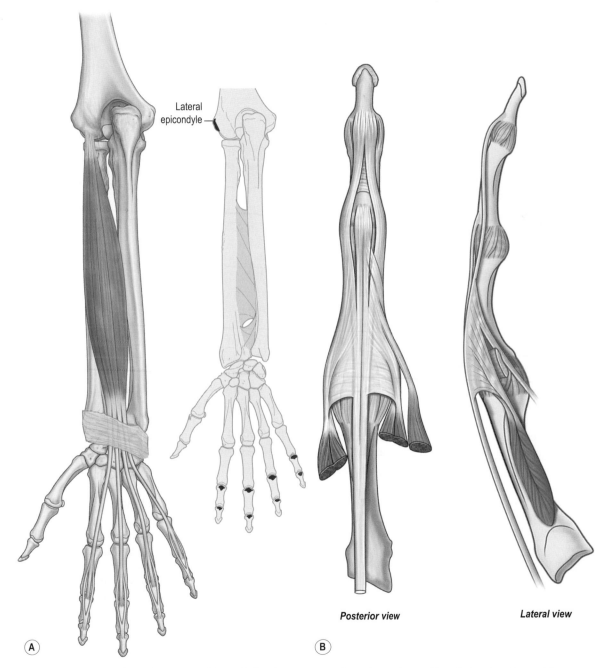

Lateral epicondyle

Posterior view

Lateral view

(A)

(B)

Fig. 2.109 (A) Posterior aspect of the left distal humerus, radius, ulna, wrist and hand showing the position and attachments of extensor digitorum. (B) The extensor expansion.

the tendon of extensor indicis (Fig. 2.85B). On the dorsum of the hand, the tendons diverge towards the medial four digits, interconnected by obliquely running fibrous bands; the arrangement of these bands is variable. The tendons for the ring and little fingers usually remain attached until just proximal to the metacarpophalangeal joints; the tendon to the index finger may not be attached to that of the middle finger.

The distal attachment of extensor digitorum is complex in that each tendon helps to form an aponeurosis over the dorsum of the finger (extensor expansion). In its simplest form, it is best considered as a movable triangular expansion, the base of which lies proximally over the metacarpophalangeal joint; from here, the sides of the expansion wrap around the proximal phalanx with the apex directed distally. The extensor expansion forms the dorsal part of the capsule of the metacarpophalangeal joint, extending either side of the metacarpal head to fuse with the deep transverse metacarpal ligament. As the extensor expansion approaches the proximal interphalangeal joint, it narrows and is reinforced on either side by the interossei and lumbrical associated with that finger; at the distal end of the proximal phalanx, the extensor expansion divides into three parts (Fig. 2.109B). The central part is directly continuous with the extensor tendon and attaches to the base of the middle phalanx on its dorsal aspect; the two collateral parts, continuous with the tendons of the interossei and lumbrical, reunite to attach to the base of the distal phalanx on its dorsal aspect. There may be an attachment to the base of the proximal phalanx, but this is unusual.

The way in which the extensor expansion wraps around the phalanges towards the palm facilitates the attachment of the lumbricals and interossei, enabling the complex coordinated movements of the fingers involving flexion of some joints and extension of others (writing). The overall arrangement of this complex structure is shown in Fig. 2.109B. Detachment or rupture of the extensor expansion from the distal phalanx gives rise to 'mallet finger'.

Innervation

By the posterior interosseous branch of the radial nerve (root value C7, C8). Skin over the muscle is supplied by roots C6, C7 and C8.

Action

The principal action of extensor digitorum is extension of the metacarpophalangeal joint, and it also helps to extend both interphalangeal joints; however, the main extensors of these joints are the interossei and lumbricals, which also help to prevent hyperextension of the metacarpophalangeal joint. When these small muscles are paralysed, extensor digitorum hyperextends the metacarpophalangeal joint and is then unable to extend the interphalangeal joints. Extensor digitorum also extends the wrist.

Palpation

The tendons of extensor digitorum can be palpated on the dorsum of the hand when the fingers are extended; it may also be possible to identify the fibrous interconnections between some of the tendons. Contraction of the muscle belly can be palpated in the posterior central part of the proximal part of the forearm during the same movement.

Extensor Digiti Minimi

Small muscle on the medial side of extensor digitorum (Fig. 2.110A) arising from the lateral epicondyle of the humerus via the common extensor tendon and surrounding fascia. In the distal forearm, it forms a single tendon which passes deep to the extensor retinaculum in a separate compartment in its own synovial sheath (Fig. 2.85B). Deep to the extensor retinaculum, it lies immediately posterior to the inferior radioulnar joint. On the dorsum of the hand, the tendon splits into two with both parts attaching to the extensor expansion of the little finger. The double tendon of extensor digiti minimi lies medial to that of extensor digitorum.

Innervation

By the posterior interosseous branch of the radial nerve (root value C7, C8). Skin over the muscle is supplied by roots C8 and T1.

Action

Extensor digiti minimi assists extensor digitorum extend the metacarpophalangeal joint of the little finger and, via the extensor expansion, the interphalangeal joints; it can also cause ulnar deviation of the little finger. It also aids extension of the wrist.

Palpation

The tendon of extensor digiti minimi can be palpated just distal to the inferior radioulnar joint when the little finger is extended. The muscle belly can be palpated

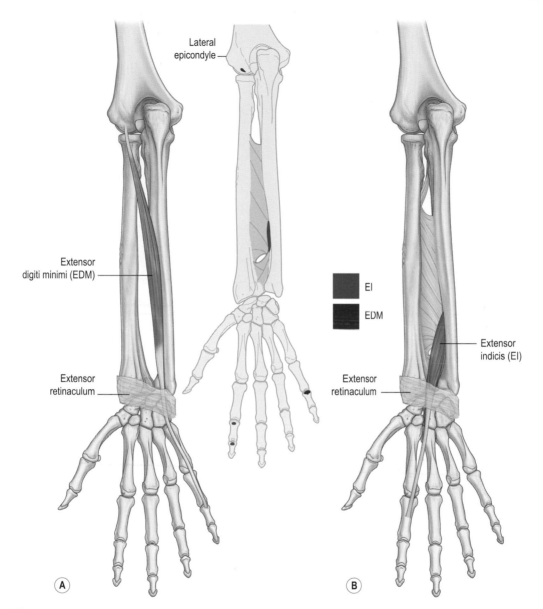

Fig. 2.110 Posterior aspect of the left distal humerus, radius, ulna, wrist and hand showing the position and attachments of extensor digiti minimi *(EDM)* (A) and extensor indicis *(EI)* (B).

medial to that of extensor digitorum when the same movement is performed.

Extensor Indicis

Lying deep to extensor digitorum, extensor indicis (Fig. 2.110B) arises from the distal part of the posterior surface of the ulna and adjacent interosseous membrane. It forms a single tendon which passes deep to the extensor retinaculum in the same synovial sheath as extensor digitorum. On the dorsum of the hand, the tendon lies on the medial side of extensor digitorum, attaching to the extensor expansion on the

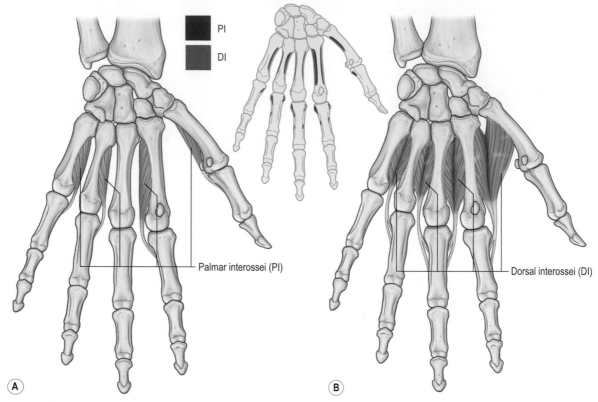

PI

DI

Palmar interossei (PI)

Dorsal interossei (DI)

Ⓐ

Ⓑ

Fig. 2.111 Anterior aspect of the left distal radius and ulna, wrist and hand showing the position and attachments of the palmar interossei (PI) (A) and dorsal interossei *(DI)* (B).

posterior aspect of the proximal phalanx of the index finger.

Innervation

By the posterior interosseous branch of the radial nerve (root value C7, C8). Skin over the muscle is supplied by roots C6 and C7.

Action

Extensor indicis assists extensor digitorum in its actions with respect to the joints of the index finger, enabling it to be used independently; it also aids wrist extension.

Palpation

Lying medial to that of extensor digitorum, the tendon of extensor indicis can be palpated on the dorsum of the hand when the index finger is extended. The muscle

belly can be palpated by deep pressure over the distal part of the ulna during the same movement.

MUSCLES ABDUCTING/ADDUCTING/OPPOSING THE FINGERS

Palmar interossei
Dorsal interossei
Abductor digiti minimi
Opponens digiti minimi

Palmar Interossei

Situated between the metacarpals are the four palmar interossei (Fig. 2.111A) with one running each to the thumb, index, ring and little finger. Each muscle arises from the shaft of the metacarpal of the digit on which it acts, attaching to the extensor expansion and base of the proximal phalanx of the same digit.

The 1st palmar interosseous lies on the medial side of the thumb and passes between the 1st dorsal interosseous and oblique head of adductor pollicis to attach to the medial side of the base of its proximal phalanx with adductor pollicis. Of the remaining palmar interossei, the 2nd lies on the medial side of the index finger, while the 3rd and 4th lie on the lateral side of the ring finger and little finger, respectively. The tendons of all but the 1st palmar interosseous pass posterior to the deep transverse metacarpal ligament on their way to the extensor expansion.

Innervation

All are supplied by the deep branch of the ulnar nerve (root value T1).

Action

The palmar interossei adduct the thumb, index, ring and little finger towards the middle finger (3rd digit). The 1st palmar interosseous also assists flexor pollicis brevis in flexing the thumb at the metacarpophalangeal joint. The three remaining interossei, via their attachment to the extensor expansion, assist the lumbricals in flexing the metacarpophalangeal joint and extending both interphalangeal joints.

Palpation

The palmar interossei are too deep to palpate, but their actions can be demonstrated by accurate electrical stimulation.

Dorsal Interossei

Lying superficially in the spaces between the metacarpals on the dorsum of the hand are the four dorsal interossei (Fig. 2.111B). Two attach to the middle finger and one each to the index and ring fingers; each is a bipennate muscle arising from the sides of adjacent metacarpals. The 1st and 2nd dorsal interossei lie on the lateral side of the index and middle finger, respectively, and the 3rd and 4th on the medial side of the middle and ring fingers, respectively. After passing posterior to the deep transverse metacarpal ligament all dorsal interossei attach to the proximal phalanx and extensor expansion of the appropriate finger.

Innervation

All are supplied by the deep branch of the ulnar nerve (root value T1). Skin overlying the muscles is supplied by roots C6, C7 and C8.

Action

The dorsal interossei are abductors of the index, middle and ring fingers. In addition, the 1st dorsal interosseous can rotate the index finger at the metacarpophalangeal joint and may assist adductor pollicis in adducting the thumb. Their attachment to the extensor expansion means that, like the palmar interossei, they assist the lumbricals in producing flexion of the metacarpophalangeal joint and extension at the interphalangeal joint.

Palpation

During resisted abduction of the index, middle or ring fingers, the dorsal interossei can be palpated on the dorsum of the hand between the metacarpals; the 1st dorsal interosseous may be seen contracting against resistance in the thumb web.

Abductor Digiti Minimi

Most superficial of the hypothenar muscles, lying in series with the dorsal interossei. It arises from the pisiform, pisohamate and pisometacarpal ligaments, and tendon of flexor carpi ulnaris, to attach by a tendon into the ulnar side of the proximal phalanx of the little finger and its extensor expansion (Fig. 2.112).

Innervation

By the deep branch of the ulnar nerve (root value T1).

Action

Abductor digiti minimi moves the little finger away from the ring finger into a position of abduction; it also helps flex the metacarpophalangeal joint. By its attachment to the extensor expansion, it may help extend the interphalangeal joints. It is a powerful muscle playing an important role in grasping large objects with outspread fingers.

Opponens Digiti Minimi

Lying deep to abductor digiti minimi, opponens digiti minimi (Fig. 2.113A) arises from the hook of the hamate and adjacent flexor retinaculum attaching to the medial half of the palmar surface of the 5th metacarpal.

Innervation

By the deep branch of the ulnar nerve (root value T1).

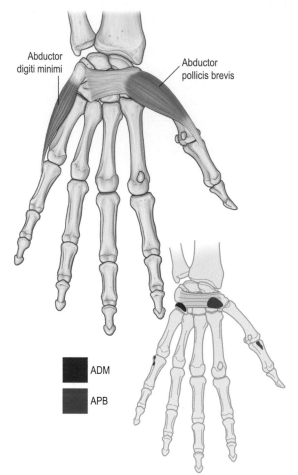

Abductor digiti minimi

Abductor pollicis brevis

ADM

APB

Fig. 2.112 Anterior aspect of the left distal radius and ulna, wrist and hand showing the position and attachments of abductor pollicis brevis *(APB)* and abductor digiti minimi *(ADM)*.

Action

Opponens digiti minimi moves the little finger anteriorly towards the palm, rotating it laterally at the carpometacarpal joint. The movement deepens the hollow of the hand and is a necessary part of opposition of the little finger.

Palpation

The hypothenar muscles are closely related to one another making individual palpation difficult. Resistance to abduction of the little finger enables abductor digiti minimi to be palpated on the ulnar border of the hand. For flexion and opposition of the little finger, it is difficult to localise the action of the

remaining hypothenar muscles, so accurate palpation is hard to achieve.

CLINICAL EXAMINATION AND EVALUATION

There is little movement at the common carpometacarpal joint, being flexion only: the 2nd and 3rd metacarpals are essentially immobile, the 4th glides slightly against the hamate, with only the 5th having any appreciable gliding movement against the hamate during a tight grasp and in opposition of the thumb to the little finger.

Metacarpophalangeal Joints

The shape of the joint surfaces permits active flexion/extension in the sagittal plane and abduction/adduction in the coronal plane, as well as passive axial rotation; active rotation is possible in the little finger.

Flexion and Extension

With the individual seated:
- Support the forearm in mid pronation/supination.
- Place the wrist in neutral flexion/extension and abduction/adduction.
- Place the metacarpophalangeal joint in neutral abduction/adduction.
- Stabilise the metacarpal with the hand resting on a supporting surface, then flex (Fig. 2.114A) or extend (Fig. 2.114B) the metacarpophalangeal joint; the other metacarpophalangeal joints should be free to move to not restrict movement.

The end feel to flexion is usually firm due to tension in the posterior joint capsule and collateral ligaments but may be hard due to contact between the palmar aspects of the proximal phalanx and metacarpal. The end feel to extension is firm due to tension in the anterior joint capsule and palmar ligament.

To measure flexion or extension, the centre of the goniometer is placed over the posterior aspect of the metacarpophalangeal joint with the proximal arm in line with the metacarpal and the distal arm in line with the proximal phalanx.

Abduction and Adduction

With the individual seated:
- Support the forearm in mid pronation/supination.
- Place the wrist in neutral flexion/extension and abduction/adduction.

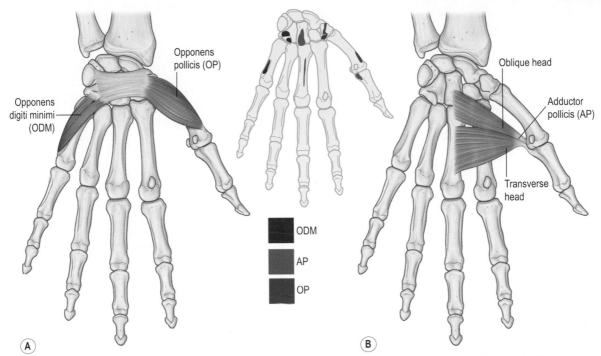

Fig. 2.113 Anterior aspect of the left distal radius and ulna, wrist and hand showing the position and attachments of (A) opponens pollicis *(OP)* and opponens digiti minimi *(ODM)*, and (B) adductor pollicis *(AP)*.

- Place the metacarpophalangeal joint in neutral flexion/extension.
- Stabilise the metacarpal with the hand resting on a supporting surface, then either abduct (Fig. 2.115A) or adduct (Fig. 2.115B) the metacarpophalangeal joint.

The end feel to both abduction and adduction is firm due to tension in the collateral ligaments, the fascia of the web space between the fingers and appropriate palmar interosseous (abduction) or dorsal interosseous (adduction) muscles.

To measure abduction or adduction, the centre of the goniometer is placed flat over the posterior aspect of the metacarpophalangeal joint with the proximal arm in line with the metacarpal and the distal arm in line with the proximal phalanx.

Proximal Interphalangeal Joints

The joint permits only flexion/extension.

With the individual seated:

- Support the forearm in mid pronation/supination.
- Place the wrist and metacarpophalangeal joints in neutral flexion/extension and abduction/adduction.

- Stabilise the proximal phalanx with the hand resting on a supporting surface, then either flex (Fig. 2.116A) or extend (Fig. 2.116B) the proximal interphalangeal joint.

The end feel to flexion is usually hard due to contact between the palmar aspects of the middle and proximal phalanges; however, it may be firm due to tension in the posterior joint capsule and collateral ligaments, or soft due to compression of the soft tissue between the middle and proximal phalanges. The end feel to movement in extension is firm due to tension in the anterior joint capsule and palmar ligament.

To measure both flexion and extension, the centre of the goniometer is placed over the posterior aspect of the proximal interphalangeal joint with the proximal and distal arms in line with the proximal and middle phalanges, respectively.

Distal Interphalangeal Joint

The joint permits only flexion/extension.

With the individual seated:

- Support the forearm in mid pronation/supination.
- Place the wrist and metacarpophalangeal joints in neutral flexion/extension and abduction/adduction.

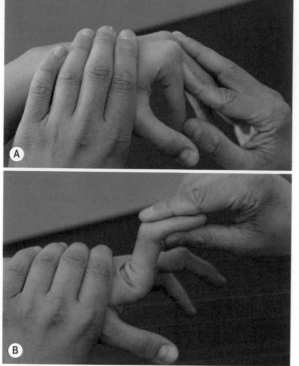

Fig. 2.114 Evaluation of the range of flexion (A) and extension (B) at the metacarpophalangeal joint of the index finger.

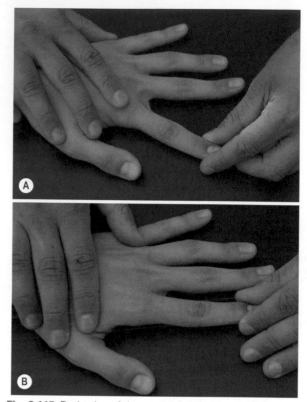

Fig. 2.115 Evaluation of the range of abduction (A) and adduction (B) at the metacarpophalangeal joint of the index finger.

- Flex the proximal interphalangeal joint to 90 degrees.
- Stabilise the middle phalanx with the hand resting on a supporting surface, then either flex (Fig. 2.117A) or extend (Fig. 2.117B) the distal interphalangeal joint.

The end feel to flexion is firm due to tension in the posterior joint capsule and collateral ligaments, and to extension is also firm due to tension in the anterior joint capsule and palmar ligament, respectively.

To measure both flexion and extension, the centre of the goniometer is placed over the posterior aspect of the proximal interphalangeal joint with the proximal and distal arms in line with the middle and distal phalanges, respectively.

THUMB

The thumb is an extremely mobile and specialised digit, both of which are important prerequisites for the movement of opposition and for the normal prehensile functioning of the hand.

SCAPHOID, 1st METACARPAL AND PHALANGES

Details of the scaphoid, 1st metacarpal and phalanges can be found on pages 152, 182 and 184, respectively.

FIRST CARPOMETACARPAL JOINT

Although extremely mobile, the carpometacarpal joint of the thumb nevertheless provides a stable base from which it can work effectively and efficiently; it plays a vital role allowing movement of the thumb in three dimensions.

Articular Surfaces

Between the trapezium and base of the 1st metacarpal (Fig. 2.118A and B) it provides the best example in the body of a saddle type of synovial joint with the two surfaces being reciprocally concavoconvex and covered with hyaline cartilage.

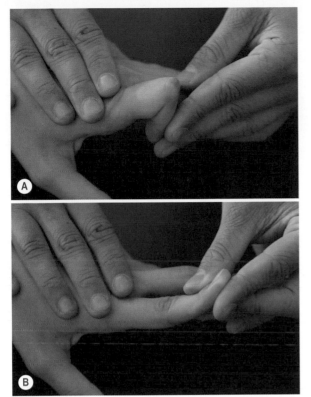

Fig. 2.116 Evaluation of the ranges of flexion (A) and extension (B) at the proximal interphalangeal joint of the index finger.

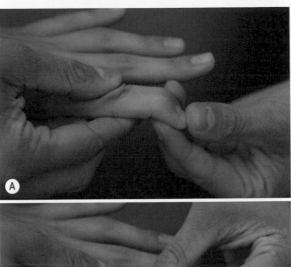

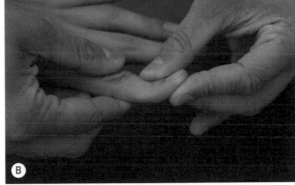

Fig. 2.117 Evaluation of the ranges of flexion (A) and extension (B) at the distal interphalangeal joint of the index finger.

The articular surface of the trapezium is concave in a more or less anteroposterior direction and convex perpendicularly; the base of the 1st metacarpal has reciprocal curvatures. The concavities and convexities of the surfaces do not lie strictly within the transverse and anteroposterior planes as will become evident when the axes about which movement occurs are considered.

Joint Capsule and Synovial Membrane

A loose but strong fibrous capsule lined with synovial membrane completely encloses the joint attaching to the articular margins of both bones (Fig. 2.118C). The capsule is thickened laterally by the radial carpometacarpal ligament, and anteriorly and posteriorly by anterior and posterior oblique ligaments.

Ligaments
Radial Carpometacarpal Ligament
Between the adjacent lateral surfaces of the trapezium and 1st metacarpal (Fig. 2.118C).

Anterior and Posterior Oblique Ligaments
These pass from their respective surfaces of the trapezium to the medial aspect of the 1st metacarpal converging as they do so (Fig. 2.118C); the posterior oblique ligament becomes taut in flexion and the anterior during extension.

Blood Supply and Innervation

The arterial supply to the joint is by branches from the palmar and dorsal carpal networks, with venous drainage into vessels accompanying the arteries. The nerve supply is by twigs from the anterior and posterior interosseous nerves (root value C7 and C8).

Relations

The joint lies deep to the thenar muscles which cover its anterior aspect. The tendon of flexor pollicis longus lies medial, while those of extensors pollicis longus and brevis lie laterally.

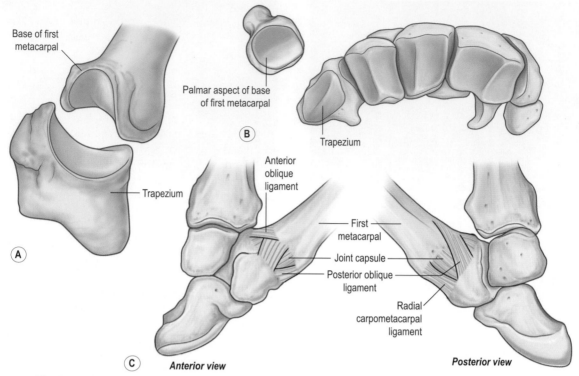

Base of first
metacarpal

Palmar aspect of base
of first metacarpal

B

Trapezium

Trapezium

A

Anterior
oblique
ligament

First
metacarpal

Joint capsule

Posterior oblique
ligament

Radial
carpometacarpal
ligament

C   *Anterior view*

Posterior view

Fig. 2.118 Articular surfaces (A and B) of the first carpometacarpal joint of the left thumb, together with the associated ligaments (C).

Stability

The joint is principally stabilised and the surfaces kept in apposition by the tone of the muscles whose tendons cross it. The shape of the articular surfaces and looseness of the fibrous capsule give the joint its large degree of mobility, playing only a minor role in stability.

MOVEMENTS OF THE THUMB AT THE CARPOMETARCARPAL JOINT

Because the thumb is rotated approximately 90 degrees with respect to the plane of the hand, the terminology used to describe its movements can at first appear to be confusing. The terms flexion, extension, abduction and adduction are used as if the thumb were in line with the fingers; however, this is not the case, as can clearly be seen when observing your own hand. The thumbnail faces almost laterally while the fingernails face posteriorly. Thus flexion and extension of the thumb occur in a coronal plane as with abduction and adduction of the fingers; abduction and adduction occur in a sagittal

plane as with flexion and extension of the fingers. Due to the nature of the joint surfaces and looseness of the joint capsule, some rotation is also possible at the joint. Because movements at the joint are brought about mainly by muscles whose tendons lie parallel to the metacarpal, movement is always accompanied by compression across the opposing surfaces. The joint surfaces, therefore, tend to grind against each other rather than there being a rolling or gliding between them.

Flexion and Extension

This occurs in the plane of the palm of the hand so that, in flexion, the thumb moves medially, and in extension, laterally (Fig. 2.119). The axis about which the movement occurs passes through the base of the 1st metacarpal at the centres of curvature of the concave trapezium and the convex metacarpal. It does not lie exactly in an anteroposterior plane but is set slightly obliquely from posterior, lateral and proximal to anterior, medial and distal.

The total range of flexion and extension is between 40 and 50 degrees. Towards the end of full flexion, tension

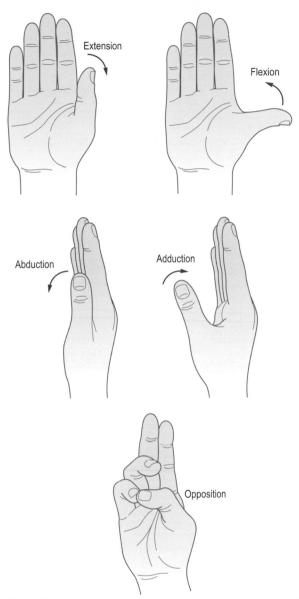

Extension

Flexion

Abduction

Adduction

Opposition

Fig. 2.119 Movement of the thumb at the carpometacarpal joint.

developed in the posterior oblique ligament causes medial rotation of the metacarpal so that the palmar surface of the thumb faces posteriorly. Conversely, towards the end of full extension, lateral rotation of the metacarpal occurs because of tension developed in the anterior oblique ligament. Flexion occurs as a secondary action of flexors pollicis longus and brevis on the interphalangeal and metacarpophalangeal joints, respectively.

Similarly, extension is a secondary action of extensors pollicis longus and brevis on the interphalangeal and metacarpophalangeal joints, respectively.

Abduction and Adduction

These occur at right angles to the palm so that in abduction the thumb moves away from the palm and in adduction, it moves towards the palm (Fig. 2.119). The axis about which movement occurs is perpendicular to that for flexion and extension, passing through the trapezium at the centres of curvature of the concave metacarpal and convex trapezium, running slightly obliquely distally from posteromedial to anterolateral proximally.

The range of abduction and adduction is approximately 80 degrees, adduction being the return of the thumb so that it lies in the plane of the palm. Abduction is by the direct action of abductor pollicis longus on the joint and by the secondary action of abductor pollicis brevis on the metacarpophalangeal joint; adduction is brought about by adductor pollicis pulling on the proximal phalanx.

Opposition

Opposition is movement in which the distal pad of the thumb is brought against the distal pad of any of the remaining digits (Fig. 2.119); it is an essential movement of the hand. The loss of opposition markedly reduces the hand's functional capacity. The movement is complex involving flexion, abduction and rotation of the thumb, followed by adduction at the carpometacarpal joint, as well as movements at other joints of the thumb.

Essentially, opposition consists of three elementary movements. Initially, flexion and abduction occur simultaneously at the carpometacarpal joint by flexors pollicis longus and brevis and abductor pollicis longus; this produces passive medial axial rotation of the metacarpal due to the posterior oblique ligament becoming taut and looseness of the joint capsule. At some point during this movement, opponens pollicis contracts producing active rotation of the metacarpal; this is the second elementary movement. Finally, adduction occurs, produced by adductor pollicis, bringing the metacarpal towards the plane of the palm. During opposition, the metacarpal rotates approximately 40 degrees.

Movements at the metacarpophalangeal joint contribute significantly to the overall movement of opposition of the thumb. At the same time as the carpometacarpal joint is being flexed and abducted, so is the metacarpophalangeal joint; simultaneous movement of the proximal phalanx also result in some axial rotation. The pad of the thumb, therefore, comes to face postero-medially.

Returning the thumb to the anatomical position has no specific name; perhaps it should be referred to as exposition. It is brought about mainly by contraction of the extensor muscles of the thumb.

METACARPOPHALANGEAL JOINT

Articular Surfaces

Between the rounded head of the metacarpal and the shallow oval concavity of the base of the proximal phalanx (Fig. 2.120); both surfaces are covered with hyaline cartilage. The biconvex metacarpal head is wider anteriorly than posteriorly, with the articular surface not extending very far on the posterior surface; in addition, the curvature of the metacarpal head is greater transversely than anteroposteriorly. The base of the proximal phalanx has a much smaller articular area than the metacarpal head but is increased anteriorly by the palmar ligament, a fibrocartilaginous plate (Fig. 2.120) attached to the anterior surface of the base of the phalanx by a small fibrous band which functions like a hinge.

Joint Capsule and Synovial Membrane

A loose fibrous capsule surrounds the joint, attached closer to the articular margins posteriorly than anteriorly (Fig. 2.120); it is strengthened at its sides by collateral ligaments. Anteriorly, the capsule is mainly replaced by the palmar ligament, which has a weak attachment to the neck of the metacarpal. Posteriorly, the capsule is strengthened or entirely replaced by the expansion of extensor pollicis longus.

Synovial membrane lines all non-articular surfaces of the joint, presenting anterior and posterior recesses when the joint is extended.

Ligaments
Collateral Ligaments

Strong ligaments on either side of the joint attach proximally to the tubercle and adjacent depression on the side of the metacarpal head passing to the palmar aspect of the side of the base of the proximal phalanx (Fig. 2.120). Although cordlike in appearance, they fan out slightly from proximal to distal, gaining attachment to

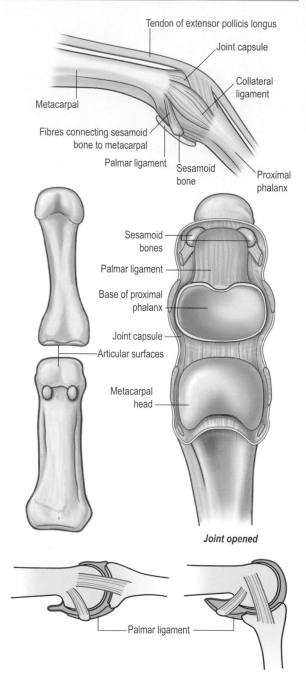

Fig. 2.120 Articular surfaces and ligaments associated with the metacarpophalangeal joint of the thumb.

the margins of the palmar ligament. The collateral ligaments are relatively lax during extension, becoming increasingly taut as the joint flexes.

Palmar Ligament

Dense fibrocartilaginous pad increasing the phalangeal articular surface anteriorly; it is firmly attached to the anterior surface of the base of the proximal phalanx and loosely attached to the anterior aspect of the neck of the metacarpal (Fig. 2.120). The palmar ligament contains two small sesamoid bones attached to the phalanx and metacarpal by straight and cruciate fibres; it is grooved on its anterior aspect by the tendon of flexor pollicis longus. The collateral ligaments of the joint blend with the margins of the palmar ligament.

Blood Supply and Innervation

The arterial supply to the joint is by branches from the princeps pollicis artery, with the venous drainage by accompanying veins. The nerve supply is by twigs from the median nerve (root value C7).

Stability

The joint is stabilised by the collateral ligaments and the tendons of flexor and extensor pollicis longus as they pass anterior and posterior to the joint to their attachments on the distal phalanx. Flexor and extensor pollicis brevis and abductor pollicis brevis also cross the joint attaching to the base of the proximal phalanx.

MOVEMENTS OF THE THUMB AT THE METACARPOPHALANGEAL JOINT

Being a condyloid joint, the metacarpophalangeal joint has two degrees of freedom of movement: flexion/extension and abduction/adduction. However, as in the carpometacarpal joint, passive axial rotation occurs due to the small degree of elasticity of the associated ligaments.

Flexion and Extension

Occurs about a single fixed axis passing transversely through the metacarpal at approximately 9/10th of its midline length from its base. In going from flexion to extension, the area of contact shifts from the palmar aspect of the phalangeal base to its distal end.

Flexion has a range of 60 degrees (American Association of Orthopaedic Surgeons, 1994); extension is zero under normal circumstances, both actively and passively (Fig. 2.121). Only in full extension does the anterior part of the metacarpal head articulate with the palmar ligament. As flexion increases, the palmar ligament

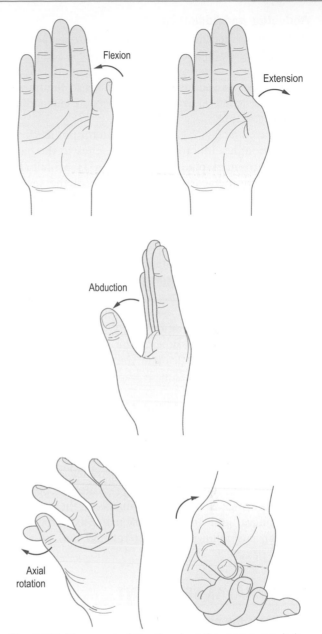

Fig. 2.121 Movement of the thumb at the metacarpophalangeal joint.

gradually loses contact with the metacarpal head; at the same time, the synovial recesses become progressively unfolded (Fig. 2.120).

Flexion is primarily by flexor pollicis brevis, aided by flexor pollicis longus. Similarly, extension from the flexed position is primarily due to extensor pollicis brevis with some help from extensor pollicis longus.

Abduction and Adduction

These are limited due to the width of the metacarpal head; 15 degrees of abduction and negligible adduction occur about an anteroposterior axis through the metacarpal head. As well as bony limitations to the movements, the collateral ligaments also become taut adding to the restriction.

Abduction (Fig. 2.121) is by abductor pollicis brevis. Although adductor pollicis attaches to the base of the proximal phalanx, its action is principally at the carpometacarpal joint because of the severe limitation of adduction at the metacarpophalangeal joint.

Axial Rotation

Some degree of axial rotation is possible, which is important during opposition (Fig. 2.121). Active rotation is produced by flexor and abductor pollicis brevis, or passively as when pressing the thumb against the index finger. Active rotation is always directed medially, while passive rotation can be in either direction depending on which side of the thumb comes into contact with the finger.

Movements at the Joint During Opposition

These include a secondary flexion at the metacarpophalangeal joint following that at the carpometacarpal joint. At the same time, there is abduction at the joint, which continues after the metacarpal becomes adducted; abduction is greatest when contact is made with the pad of the little finger. Flexion and abduction at the metacarpophalangeal joint initially cause active axial rotation; however, any following contact rotation may be augmented passively.

INTERPHALANGEAL JOINT

Because the thumb only contains two phalanges, there is only one interphalangeal joint. Like those of the fingers, it is a synovial hinge joint permitting movement in one direction only.

Articular Surfaces

Between the pulley-shaped head of the proximal phalanx and base of the distal phalanx, which has a median ridge separating two shallow facets (Fig. 2.122). As in

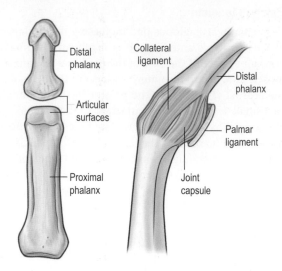

Fig. 2.122 Articular surfaces and associated ligaments of the interphalangeal joint of the thumb.

the metacarpophalangeal joint, a fibrocartilaginous plate (palmar ligament) is attached to the anterior margin of the base of the distal phalanx.

Joint Capsule

A fibrous capsule completely surrounds the joint, replaced by the palmar ligament anteriorly and strengthened at the sides by the collateral ligaments (Fig. 2.122).

Ligaments
Collateral Ligaments

Attached to the sides of the head of the proximal phalanx the collateral ligaments pass to the palmar aspect of the base of the distal phalanx, blending with the lateral margins of the palmar ligament.

Palmar Ligament

Fibrocartilaginous plate, as in the metacarpophalangeal joint, the palmar ligament is attached to the anterior margin of the base of the distal phalanx, and loosely attached to the anterior aspect of the neck of the proximal phalanx by the joint capsule.

Blood Supply and Innervation

The same as for the metacarpophalangeal joint (p. 209).

MOVEMENTS OF THE THUMB AT THE INTERPHALANGEAL JOINT

Being a hinge joint supported by strong collateral ligaments, movement is allowed in one plane only.

Flexion and Extension

These occur about a transverse axis passing approximately through the neck of the proximal phalanx; flexion is in excess of 90 degrees, while extension is limited to no more than 10 degrees. Passive hyperextension may be marked in some individuals who apply large forces using the thumb (butchers, physiotherapy manipulators).

Accessory Movements at the Joints of the Thumb

Carpometacarpal joint. Gripping the trapezium between the thumb and index finger of one hand and the base of the 1st metacarpal with the other, the metacarpal base can be moved anteroposteriorly and mediolaterally. With the same grip, longitudinal gapping and rotation can be achieved.

Metacarpophalangeal and interphalangeal joints. If the principle of stabilising the proximal bone and moving the distal one is employed, then anteroposterior gliding movements can be demonstrated at both the metacarpophalangeal and interphalangeal joints. Best results are obtained when each bone is held firmly between thumb and index finger. A good range of rotation, as well as longitudinal gapping, is also possible at the metacarpophalangeal joint.

Muscles producing movement of the thumb are given in Table 2.13; further details of each muscle can be found in following sections.

MUSCLES FLEXING THE THUMB

Flexor pollicis longus
Flexor pollicis brevis

Flexor Pollicis Longus

Lying on the lateral side of flexor digitorum profundus, flexor pollicis longus (Fig. 2.123) arises from the anterior surface of the radius between the radial tuberosity proximally and pronator quadratus distally, and the adjacent anterior surface of the interosseous membrane; occasionally, it also arises by a small slip from the medial border of the coronoid process of the ulna. The fibres pass almost to the wrist before a single tendon is formed, which continues deep to the flexor retinaculum in its own synovial sheath (Fig. 2.85B), attaching to the palmar surface of the base of the distal phalanx of the thumb.

Innervation

By the anterior interosseous branch of the median nerve (root value C8 and T1).

Action

Flexor pollicis longus is the only flexor of the interphalangeal joint of the thumb and is thus vital for all gripping activities of the hand; it also flexes the metacarpophalangeal and wrist joints.

Palpation

When only the thumb is flexed, contraction of flexor pollicis longus can be felt in the distal one-third of the forearm immediately lateral to the superficial flexor tendons.

Flexor Pollicis Brevis

The most medial of the three thenar muscles, flexor pollicis brevis (Fig. 2.108) is usually partly fused with opponens pollicis. It arises from the distal border of the flexor retinaculum and tubercle of the trapezium (superficial part) with a deeper attachment to the capitate and trapezoid. Both parts form a single tendon, containing a sesamoid bone, which attaches to the radial side of the base of the proximal phalanx of the thumb.

Innervation

By the median nerve (root value T1) from the medial and lateral cords of the brachial plexus; frequently, the deep part is supplied by the ulnar nerve (root value T1) from the medial cord of the brachial plexus. Skin over the muscle is supplied by root C6.

Action

Flexes the thumb at the metacarpophalangeal and carpometacarpal joints; its continued action produces medial rotation of the thumb, as flexion of the carpometacarpal joint automatically involves this movement.

Palpation

The muscle can be palpated in the medial part of the thenar eminence if flexion of the thumb is resisted.

TABLE 2.13   Muscles Producing Movements at the Metacarpophalangeal and Interphalangeal Joints of the Thumb

Muscle	Attachments	Action	Innervation (root value)
Flexor pollicis longus	Anterior surface of radius and adjacent interosseous membrane to palmar surface of base of distal phalanx of thumb	Flexor of interphalangeal joint of thumb; assists in flexion of metacarpophalangeal and wrist joints	Anterior interosseous branch of the median nerve (C8, T1)
Flexor pollicis brevis[a]	Distal border of flexor retinaculum, trapezium, capitate and trapezoid to base of proximal phalanx of thumb	Flexor of thumb at metacarpophalangeal and carpometacarpal joints; its continued action medially rotates thumb	Median nerve (T1)
Extensor pollicis longus	Lateral aspect of middle 1/3rd of posterior surface of ulna and adjacent interosseous membrane to dorsal surface of base of distal phalanx of thumb	Extensor of all joints of thumb; assists in extension and abduction at wrist	Posterior interosseous branch of the radial nerve (C7, C8)
Extensor pollicis brevis	Middle part of posterior surface of radius and adjacent interosseous membrane to dorsal surface of base of proximal phalanx of thumb	Extensor of carpometacarpal and metacarpophalangeal joints of thumb	Posterior interosseous branch of the radial nerve (C7, C8)
Abductor pollicis longus	Proximal part of ulna and radius and adjacent interosseous membrane to base of 1st metacarpal	Abductor and extensor of carpometacarpal joint of thumb	Posterior interosseous branch of the radial nerve (C7, C8)
Abductor pollicis brevis[a]	Flexor retinaculum, scaphoid and trapezium to base of proximal phalanx of thumb	Abductor of thumb at metacarpophalangeal and carpometacarpal joints	Median nerve (T1)
Opponens pollicis[a]	Flexor retinaculum and trapezium to lateral ½ of anterior surface of 1st metacarpal	Opposition of thumb	Median nerve (T1)
Adductor pollicis	Sheath of tendon of flexor carpi radialis, bases of 2nd, 3rd and 4th metacarpals, trapezoid and capitate (transverse head) and longitudinal ridge on anterior surface of shaft of 3rd metacarpal (oblique head) to base of proximal phalanx of thumb	Adductor of thumb	Deep branch of the ulnar nerve (T1)

[a]Muscles of the thenar eminence.

MUSCLES EXTENDING THE THUMB

Extensor pollicis longus
Extensor pollicis brevis

Extensor Pollicis Longus

Lying deep to extensor digitorum in the posterior compartment of the forearm, extensor pollicis longus (Fig. 2.124) arises from the lateral aspect of the middle one-third of the posterior surface of the ulna and adjacent interosseous membrane proximal to extensor indicis. Proximal to the wrist, it forms a single tendon which

passes in its own synovial sheath deep to the extensor retinaculum (Fig. 2.85B), lying in the groove on the posterior aspect of the radius medial to the dorsal tubercle. Winding around the tubercle, the tendon changes direction and crosses superficial to the tendons of extensor carpi radialis longus and brevis (Fig. 2.86) and the radial artery. As the tendon crosses the metacarpophalangeal joint, it forms the dorsal part of the joint capsule, where it is joined by slips from abductor pollicis brevis laterally and adductor pollicis medially. This arrangement forms a triangular expansion, not unlike that of extensor digitorum; the expansion may be joined by extensor pollicis

Innervation

By the posterior interosseous branch of the radial nerve (root value C7 and C8). Skin over the muscle is supplied by roots C6 and C7.

Action

It extends all joints of the thumb, as well as assisting extension and abduction at the wrist. Once this has been achieved, the obliquity of its tendon pulls the 1st metacarpal into a laterally rotated and abducted position. In full abduction or extension of the thumb, extensor pollicis longus can act as an adductor. It may also contribute slightly to supination due to its oblique course across the distal part of the forearm.

Palpation

The tendon of extensor pollicis longus is easily identified as the medial border of the 'anatomical snuffbox' with the thumb extended. The tendon frequently ruptures in conditions such as rheumatoid arthritis or post-Colles' fracture, with the individual being incapable of extending the interphalangeal joint of the thumb.

Extensor Pollicis Brevis

It lies on the lateral side of and adjacent to extensor pollicis longus, and distal to abductor pollicis longus to which it closely adheres (Fig. 2.124); it arises from the middle part of the posterior surface of the radius and adjacent interosseous membrane. The tendon is formed proximal to the wrist and runs with that of abductor pollicis longus deep to the extensor retinaculum in a common synovial sheath (Fig. 2.85B) in the groove on the lateral aspect of the radial styloid process. Distal to this point, the two tendons form the lateral boundary of the 'anatomical snuffbox'. The tendon partly replaces the dorsal part of the metacarpophalangeal joint capsule and attaches to the dorsal surface of the base of the proximal phalanx; occasionally, it may be prolonged to run with and attach to the tendon of extensor pollicis longus.

Innervation

By the posterior interosseous branch of the radial nerve (root value C7 and C8). Skin over the muscle is supplied by roots C6 and C7.

Action

Extensor pollicis brevis extends both the carpometacarpal and metacarpophalangeal joints of the thumb; it may also help extend and abduct the wrist, particularly against resistance.

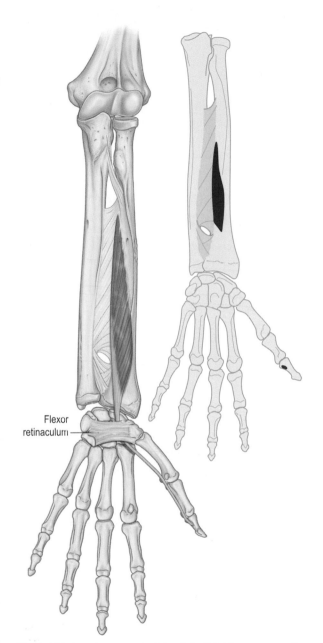

Fig. 2.123 Anterior aspect of the left distal humerus, radius, ulna, wrist and hand showing the position and attachments of flexor pollicis longus.

brevis. The tendon then attaches to the dorsal surface of the base of the distal phalanx of the thumb. As it passes across the posterior aspect of the hand, the tendon forms the medial boundary of a region known as the 'anatomical snuffbox'.

Flexor retinaculum

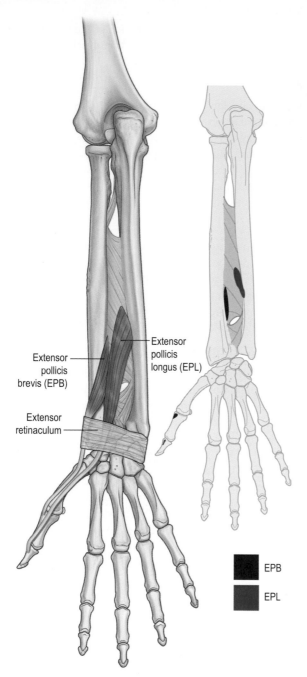

Extensor
pollicis
brevis (EPB)

Extensor
pollicis
longus (EPL)

Extensor
retinaculum

EPB

EPL

Fig. 2.124 Posterior aspect of the left distal humerus, radius, ulna, wrist and hand showing the position and attachments of extensors pollicis longus and brevis (*EPL* and *EPB*).

Palpation

The tendons of extensor pollicis brevis and abductor pollicis longus run together from the distal lateral aspect of the radius where they form the lateral boundary of the 'anatomical snuffbox'. Both tendons can be palpated when the thumb is extended, that of abductor pollicis longus being the most anterior.

Application

The synovial sheath of extensor pollicis brevis and abductor pollicis longus frequently becomes inflamed in the region of the radial styloid process (de Quervain's syndrome). Techniques (transverse frictions, ultrasound, injections) can be usefully applied to this region.

MUSCLES ABDUCTING/ADDUCTING/OPPOSING THE THUMB

Abductor pollicis longus
Abductor pollicis brevis
Opponens pollicis
Adductor pollicis
Palmaris brevis

Abductor Pollicis Longus

Lying deep to extensor digitorum in the posterior compartment of the forearm, abductor pollicis longus (Fig. 2.125) arises from the proximal part of the posterior surface of the ulna distal to anconeus, the middle one-third of the posterior surface of the radius distal to supinator and intervening interosseous membrane.

Passing distally, abductor pollicis longus emerges from its deep position to lie superficially in the distal part of the forearm. The tendon forms proximal to the wrist and passes, with that of extensor pollicis brevis, in the same synovial sheath deep to the extensor retinaculum (Fig. 2.85B), where it lies in the groove on the lateral aspect of the radial styloid process. The tendon attaches primarily to the radial side of the base of the 1st metacarpal, with a slip passing to the trapezium and another to abductor pollicis brevis and the fascia over the thenar eminence.

Innervation

By the posterior interosseous branch of the radial nerve (root value C7 and C8). Skin over the muscle is supplied by roots C6 and C7.

Action

By itself, the muscle puts the thumb into a mid extended and abducted position. Working with the extensors, abductor pollicis longus helps to extend the thumb at the carpometacarpal joint, while, with abductor pollicis brevis, it abducts the thumb.

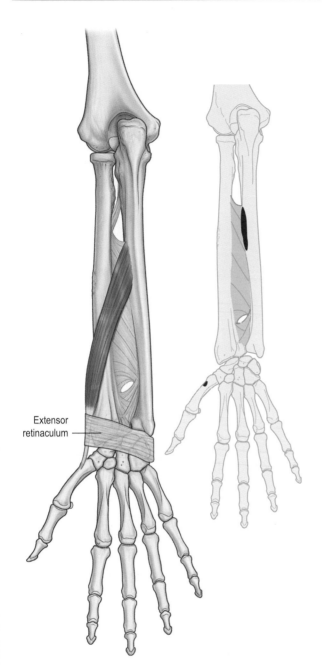

Extensor
retinaculum

Fig. 2.125 Posterior aspect of the left distal humerus, radius, ulna, wrist and hand showing the position and attachments of abductor pollicis longus.

Palpation

Palpation of the muscle is described with that of extensor pollicis brevis (p. 213).

Abductor Pollicis Brevis

The most lateral and superficial of the three muscles forming the thenar eminence (Fig. 2.112). It arises mainly from the anterior aspect of the flexor retinaculum, extending onto the tubercles of the scaphoid and trapezium with an occasional contribution from the tendon of abductor pollicis longus. It forms a short tendon which attaches to the radial side of the base of the proximal phalanx of the thumb, with some fibres reaching the expansion of the extensor pollicis longus tendon.

Innervation

By the median nerve (root value T1) from the medial and lateral cords of the brachial plexus. Skin over the muscle is supplied by root C6.

Action

It abducts the thumb at both the carpometacarpal and metacarpophalangeal joints, causing it to move anteriorly at right angles to the palm. To achieve this, there must be some medial rotation at the carpometacarpal joint, the remainder occurring at the metacarpophalangeal joint. This movement is of great significance in terms of the function of the hand as the thumb can be moved towards the fingertips (opposition), where it can carry out precision tasks that require a pincer grip. Because of its partial attachment to the extensor pollicis longus tendon, abductor pollicis brevis can aid flexion of the metacarpophalangeal joint and extension of the interphalangeal joint.

Palpation

The three muscles forming the thenar eminence lie closely together and are covered with tough fascia which makes the identification of individual muscles difficult. However, if the thenar eminence is carefully palpated during resisted movements, all but opponens pollicis can be identified. If abduction (movement away from the palm in a plane at 90 degrees to the palm) of the thumb is resisted, abductor pollicis brevis can be identified in the lateral part of the thenar eminence.

Opponens Pollicis

Covered by abductor pollicis brevis, opponens pollicis (Fig. 2.113A) arises from the flexor retinaculum and tubercle of the trapezium; it attaches to the whole length of the lateral half of the anterior surface of the 1st metacarpal.

Innervation

By the median nerve (root value T1) from the medial and lateral cords of the brachial plexus; occasionally, it may be supplied by the ulnar nerve. Skin over the muscle is supplied by root C6.

Action

It produces the complex movement of the thumb called opposition where the 1st metacarpal is drawn antero-medially in an arc towards the fingers. The movement involves, in order of action, abduction, medial rotation and finally flexion and adduction at the carpometacarpal joint of the thumb. The importance of this action is that the tip of the thumb can be brought into contact with the tip of any finger, thus allowing for very precise action of the hand.

Adductor Pollicis

Located in the web space of the thumb on its palmar aspect, adductor pollicis (Fig. 2.113B) has oblique and transverse heads. The oblique head arises from the sheath of the tendon of flexor carpi radialis, bases of the 2nd, 3rd and 4th metacarpals, trapezoid and capitate; the transverse head arises from the longitudinal ridge on the anterior surface of the shaft of the 3rd metacarpal. The radial artery passes between the two heads to gain access to the palmar aspect of the hand. Both heads attach to the medial side of the base of the proximal phalanx of the thumb by a tendon containing a sesamoid bone.

Innervation

By the deep branch of the ulnar nerve (root value C8, T1). Skin over the muscle is supplied by roots C6 and C7.

Action

A strong muscle returning the thumb to the palm from a position of abduction; it is also active in the later stages of opposition. Functionally, its strength can be demonstrated when the tip of the index finger and thumb are held together in a pincer grip and an attempt is made to pull them apart. Adductor pollicis is, therefore, an important muscle in maintaining the precision grip of the hand.

Palpation

Located in the web between the thumb and index finger adductor pollicis can be felt on the palmar aspect when adduction is resisted.

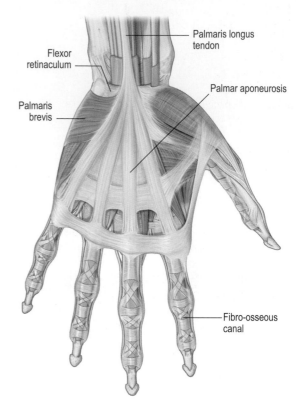

Fig. 2.126 Anterior aspect of the left distal radius and ulna, wrist and hand showing the position of the palmar aponeurosis and palmaris brevis.

Palmaris Brevis

Superficial muscle covering the hypothenar eminence (Fig. 2.126) arising from the medial border of the palmar aponeurosis and anterior aspect of the flexor retinaculum attaching to the skin of the medial border of the hand.

Innervation

By the superficial branch of the ulnar nerve (root value T1). Skin over the muscle is supplied by root C8.

Action

Contraction of palmaris brevis wrinkles the skin on the ulnar side of the hand. It is included in this section as its main function is to assist the thumb in producing a good grip.

CLINICAL EXAMINATION AND EVALUATION

The thumb is rotated approximately 90 degrees with respect to the remaining digits; therefore, its movements are in different planes to those of the other digits. It is an extremely mobile and specialised digit, both of which are important prerequisites for the prehensile functioning of the hand.

First Carpometacarpal Joint

Due to the shape of the articular surfaces and looseness of the joint capsule, the joint is highly mobile allowing flexion/extension, abduction/adduction and axial rotation (opposition). Flexion/extension and abduction/adduction are in the plane of the palm and perpendicular to the palm, respectively.

Flexion and Extension

With the individual seated:

- Support the forearm in supination.
- Place the wrist in neutral flexion/extension and abduction/adduction.
- Place the carpometacarpal joint in neutral abduction/adduction, and the metacarpophalangeal and interphalangeal joints in neutral flexion/extension.
- Stabilise the carpus with the hand resting on a supporting surface, then either flex (Fig. 2.127A) or extend (Fig. 2.127B) the carpometacarpal joint.

The end feel to flexion is usually soft due to compression of the thenar eminence against the palm of the hand; however, it may be firm due to tension in the posterior joint capsule, extensor and abductor pollicis brevis. The end feel to extension is firm due to tension in the anterior joint capsule, flexor pollicis brevis, adductor pollicis, opponens pollicis and the 1st dorsal interosseous.

To measure flexion and extension, the centre of the goniometer is placed over the palmar aspect of the carpometacarpal joint with the proximal arm along a line joining the radial styloid process and radial head and the distal arm along the anterior midline of the 1st metacarpal. The initial goniometer reading may not read 0 degrees, if so, the difference between the initial and final readings gives the range.

Abduction

With the individual seated:

- Support the forearm in mid pronation/supination.
- Place the wrist in neutral flexion/extension and abduction/adduction.

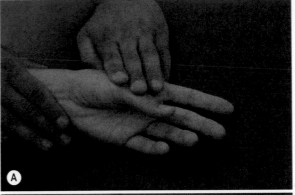
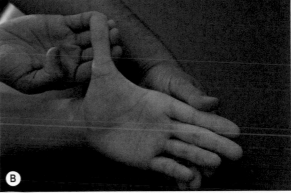

Fig. 2.127 Evaluation of the range of flexion (A) and extension (B) at the carpometacarpal joint of the thumb.

- Place the carpometacarpal, metacarpophalangeal and interphalangeal joints in neutral flexion/extension.
- Stabilise the carpus and 2nd metacarpal with the hand resting on a supporting surface, then abduct the carpometacarpal joint (Fig. 2.128).

The end feel is firm due to tension primarily in the fascia and skin of the web space between the thumb and index finger; there may also be tension in adductor pollicis and the 1st dorsal interosseous.

To measure abduction, the centre of the goniometer is placed over the lateral aspect of the radial styloid process with the proximal and distal arms in line with the midlines of the 2nd and 1st metacarpals, respectively.

Metacarpophalangeal Joint

Because of the shape of the articular surfaces, active movement is permitted in two planes, flexion/extension in the coronal plane and abduction/adduction in the sagittal plane, as well as passive axial rotation accompanying simultaneous flexion and abduction or when pressing the thumb against the index finger. Active

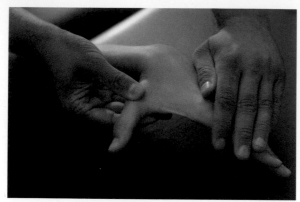

Fig. 2.128 Evaluation of the range of abduction at the carpo-metacarpal joint of the thumb.

rotation is always medially directed, while passive rotation can be in either direction.

Flexion and Extension

With the individual seated:
- Support the forearm in supination.
- Place the wrist and carpometacarpal joints in neutral flexion/extension and abduction/adduction, and the interphalangeal joint in neutral flexion/extension.
- Stabilise the 1st metacarpal with the hand resting on a supporting surface, then either flex (Fig. 2.129A) or extend (Fig. 2.129B) the metacarpophalangeal joint.

The end feel to flexion is usually firm due to tension in the posterior joint capsule, collateral ligaments and extensor pollicis brevis; however, it may be hard due to contact between the palmar aspect of the proximal phalanx and 1st metacarpal. The end feel to extension is firm due to tension in the anterior joint capsule, palmar ligament and flexor pollicis brevis.

To measure flexion and extension (hyperextension), the centre of the goniometer is placed over the posterior aspect of the metacarpophalangeal joint with the proximal and distal arms in line with the metacarpal and proximal phalanx, respectively.

Abduction

With the individual seated:
- Place the forearm in mid pronation/supination with the medial border resting on a supporting surface.
- Place the wrist and carpometacarpal joints in neutral flexion/extension and abduction/adduction, and the interphalangeal joint in neutral flexion/extension.

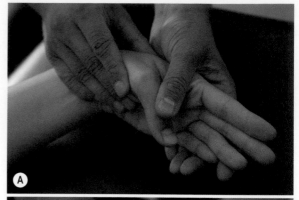

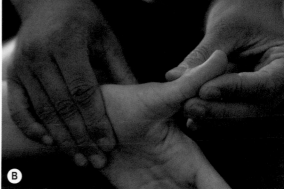

Fig. 2.129 Evaluation of the range of flexion (A) and extension (B) at the metacarpophalangeal joint of the thumb.

- Stabilise the 1st metacarpal with the medial border of the hand resting on a supporting surface, then abduct the metacarpophalangeal joint (Fig. 2.130A).

The end feel is firm due to tension in the medial joint capsule and collateral ligaments.

To measure abduction, the centre of the goniometer is placed over the posterior aspect of the metacarpophalangeal joint with the proximal and distal arms in line with the metacarpal and proximal phalanx, respectively.

Opposition

With the individual seated:
- Support the forearm in supination.
- Place the wrist in neutral flexion/extension and abduction/adduction, and the interphalangeal joint in neutral.
- Stabilise the 5th metacarpal with the hand resting on a supporting surface, then oppose the thumb (Fig. 2.130B).

The end feel may be soft due to compression of the thenar eminence against the palm of the hand or firm

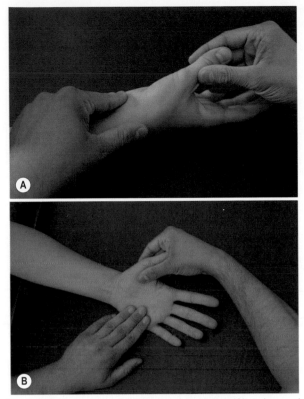

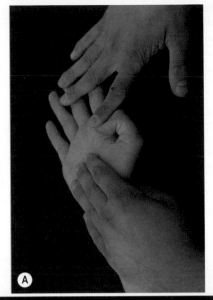

Fig. 2.130 Evaluation of the range of abduction (A) and opposition (B) of the metacarpophalangeal joint of the thumb.

due to tension in the joint capsule and extensor pollicis brevis.

The distance between the tips of the thumb and little finger or between the tip of the thumb and base of the 5th metacarpal is measured with a ruler. If movement is allowed at the metacarpophalangeal and interphalangeal joints of the little finger, the tips of the thumb and little finger usually meet. The thumb can also be opposed to the index, middle and ring fingers.

Interphalangeal Joint

The interphalangeal joint is a synovial hinge joint permitting flexion and extension only.

Flexion and Extension

With the individual seated:
- Support the forearm in supination.
- Place the wrist and carpometacarpal joints in neutral flexion/extension and abduction/adduction, and the metacarpophalangeal joint in neutral flexion/extension.

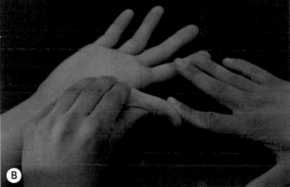

Fig. 2.131 Evaluation of the range of flexion (A) and extension (B) at the interphalangeal joint of the thumb.

- Stabilise the proximal phalanx with the hand resting on a supporting surface, then either flex (Fig. 2.131A) or extend (Fig. 2.131B) the interphalangeal joint.

The end feel to flexion is usually firm due to tension in the collateral ligaments and posterior joint capsule but may be hard due to contact between the palmar aspect of the distal phalanx, palmar ligament and proximal phalanx. The end feel to extension is usually firm due to tension in the anterior joint capsule and palmar ligament.

To measure flexion and extension, the centre of the goniometer is placed over the posterior aspect of the interphalangeal joint with the proximal and distal arms in line with the proximal and distal phalanges respectively.

Section Summary

Metacarpus

- Five long bones (metacarpals) in hand, each with a proximal quadrilateral base; shaft, distal rounded head.
- Bases articulate with the distal row of carpal bones forming the carpometacarpal joints and with adjacent metacarpals forming intercarpal joints.
- Heads articulate with the base of corresponding proximal phalanx forming the metacarpophalangeal joints.

Phalanges

- Fourteen individual bones with three in each finger (proximal, middle and distal) and two in the thumb (proximal and distal) each having proximal base; shaft; distal head (flattened pad in distal phalanges).
- Bases of the proximal phalanges articulate with heads of the metacarpals forming the metacarpophalangeal joints.
- Interphalangeal joints formed between the heads and bases of adjacent phalanges.

Joints of the Hand

Common Carpometacarpal Joint

Type	Synovial plane
Articular surfaces	Distal surfaces of trapezium, trapezoid, capitate and hamate with bases of 2nd, 3rd, 4th and 5th metacarpals
Capsule	Complete and surrounds joint
Ligaments	Dorsal carpometacarpal; palmar metacarpal; interosseous
Movements	Some flexion and rotation of the 5th metacarpal only

Metacarpophalangeal Joints of Fingers

Type	Synovial condyloid
Articular surfaces	Head of metacarpal with base of proximal phalanx
Capsule	Loose but reinforced by ligaments
Ligaments	Palmar; collateral; deep transverse metacarpal (index to little finger)
Stability	Mainly by tendons crossing joint
Movements	Flexion and extension; abduction and adduction

Interphalangeal Joints of Fingers

Type	Synovial hinge
Articular surfaces	Head of proximal phalanx with base of middle phalanx and head of middle phalanx with base of distal phalanx
Capsule	Encloses joint, replaced by palmar ligament anteriorly
Movements	Flexion and extension

First Carpometacarpal Joint (Thumb)

Type	Synovial saddle
Articular surfaces	Distal surface of trapezium with base of 1st metacarpal
Capsule	Loose but strong
Ligaments	Radial carpometacarpal; anterior and posterior oblique
Stability	Good due to tendons crossing joint
Movements	Flexion and extension; abduction and adduction; axial rotation/opposition

Metacarpophalangeal Joint of Thumb

Type	Synovial condyloid
Articular surfaces	Head of metacarpal with base of proximal phalanx
Capsule	Loose but reinforced by ligaments
Ligaments	Palmar; collateral
Stability	Mainly by tendons crossing joint
Movements	Flexion and extension; abduction and adduction; axial rotation/opposition

Interphalangeal Joint of Thumb

Type	Synovial hinge
Articular surfaces	Head of proximal phalanx with base of middle phalanx and head of middle phalanx with base of distal phalanx
Capsule	Encloses joint, replaced by palmar ligament anteriorly
Movements	Flexion and extension

Movements at Joints of Fingers and Thumb

Each finger comprises three joints, the distal (DIP) and proximal (PIP) interphalangeal joints, and metacarpophalangeal (MCP) joint. The thumb has one interphalangeal (IP) joint, a metacarpophalangeal (MCP) joint and a carpometacarpal (CMJ) joint. The joints that the muscles produce movement at are given.

Movement (fingers)	Muscles (root value of nerve supply)
Flexion	Flexor digitorum profundus at DIP, PIP and MCP (C7, C8, T1)
	Flexor digitorum superficialis at PIP and MCP (C7, C8, T1)
	Lumbricals at MCP (T1)
	Interossei at MCP (T1)
Extension	Extensor digitorum at DIP, PIP and MCP (C7, C8)
	Extensors indicis at DIP, PIP and MCP of index finger (C7, C8)
	Extensor digit minimi at DIP, PIP and MCP of little finger (C7, C8)

Section Summary—Cont'd

Movement (fingers)	Muscles (root value of nerve supply)
Abduction	Dorsal interossei at MCP (T1)
	Abductor digiti minimi at MCP (T1)
Adduction	Palmar interossei at MCP (T1)
Opposition	Opponens digiti minimi at CMJ of little finger (T1)

Movement (thumb)	Muscles (root value of nerve supply)
Flexion	Flexor pollicis longus at IP and MCP (C8, T1)
	Flexor pollicis brevis at MCP (T1)
Extension	Extensor pollicis longus at IP and MCP (C7, C8)
	Extensor pollicis brevis at MCP (C7, C8)
Abduction	Abductor pollicis longus at CMJ (C7, C8)
	Abductor pollicis brevis at CMJ (T1)
Adduction	Adductor pollicis at CMJ (C8, T1)
Opposition	Opponens pollicis at CMJ (T1)

Many of the muscles above cross several joints and are involved in complex combined movements; considering individual muscles is somewhat artificial.

Interaction of the extrinsic and intrinsic muscles of the fingers and thumb allows the wide range of complex grips and functions possible in the human hand.

Clinical Examination

Movement and Maximum Range	End Feel to Movement
MCP Fingers	
Flexion 90°–110° depending on finger	Firm; may be hard if bone contact
Extension 10°	Firm
Abduction 30°	Firm
Adduction 30°	Firm
PIP Fingers	
Flexion 90°–135° depending on finger	Usually hard; may be soft due to soft tissue contact
Extension <2°	Firm
DIP Fingers	
Flexion 90°	Firm
Extension <5°	Firm
1st Carpometacarpal	
Flexion 30°	Usually soft; may be firm
Extension 15°	Firm
Abduction 80°	Firm
MCP Thumb	
Flexion 60°	Usually firm; may be hard due to bone contact
Extension 0°	Firm
Abduction 15°	Firm
Adduction 0°	Soft
IP Thumb	
Flexion >90°	Firm; may be hard due to bone contact
Extension 10°	Firm

SELF-ASSESSMENT QUESTIONS

109. Which muscle(s) in the hand are supplied by the median nerve?
110. What is the root value of the nerve supplying adductor pollicis?
111. What is the action of the dorsal interossei?
112. With which bone does the trapezium articulate distally?
113. What movements are possible at the carpometacarpal joint of the thumb?
114. What type of joint is the proximal interphalangeal joint?
115. What is opposition of the thumb?
116. With which joint are the anterior and posterior oblique ligaments associated?
117. Which bones are involved in the common carpometacarpal joint?

118. How many phalanges are there in each finger?
119. What is the action of the lumbricals?
120. Which muscles attach to the extensor expansion of extensor digitorum of the middle finger?
121. Which muscles constitute the hypothenar muscles?
122. Which artery pass between the two heads of adductor pollicis?
123. The common synovial sheath in the hand contains the tendons of which muscle(s)?
124. What is the function of the palmar ligaments?
125. Which tendons pass anterior and posterior to the deep transverse metacarpal ligaments?
126. What is the relationship of the long flexor tendons in the fingers?
127. What movements are possible at the proximal interphalangeal joint?

Continued

SELF-ASSESSMENT QUESTIONS—CONT'D

128. Which is the most powerful grip possible?
129. Which grip would be used to hold a key to insert it into a lock?
130. Which type of grip is used to carry a bag by its handle?
131. What is the distal attachment of flexor pollicis longus?
132. How do the tendons of extensor digitorum enter the hand?
133. Which major nerve enters the hand superficial to the flexor retinaculum?

134. What causes Dupuytren's contracture?
135. In radial nerve palsy, what action of the hand is lost and which function is severely affected?
136. What movements are possible at the common carpometacarpal joint?
137. What is the proximal attachment of extensor carpi radialis brevis?
138. What is the distal attachment of flexor digitorum superficialis?

SIMPLE ACTIVITIES OF THE UPPER LIMB

INTRODUCTION

This section provides a simple analysis of some common activities to show how different muscle groups cooperate in producing a desired movement. The analysis describes the starting position (omitting muscle work) and then describes the sequence of movements involved, giving the joints and muscles responsible, ending with a description of how the muscles work with respect to joint movement. These general principles can be applied to any movement.

Abduction of the Arm Through to Full Elevation
Starting Position
The movement begins with the individual standing in the anatomical position.

Sequence of Movements
Abduction of the humerus is initiated by supraspinatus, raising the upper limb by approximately 10 degrees putting it into a position to enable deltoid to produce a rotatory force (torque) to continue abduction. Upward shearing of the humeral head against the glenoid fossa is prevented by the rotator cuff muscles, acting isometrically as stabilisers with the exception of supraspinatus, which shortens concentrically. Deltoid also works concentrically, with the principal force being exerted by its middle multipennate fibres, with the anterior and posterior fibres acting as guides controlling the plane of abduction.

At 30 degrees of abduction, lateral rotation of the scapula begins, turning the glenoid fossa to face superiorly and increasing the total range of movement. For every 15 degrees of abduction from this point onwards, approximately 10 degrees occurs at the shoulder joint and 5 degrees from lateral rotation of the scapula. Lateral rotation of the scapula is produced by concentric contraction of the upper and lower fibres of trapezius and the lower half of serratus anterior; other muscles assist by holding the scapula against the chest wall.

As shoulder joint movement approaches 90 degrees (120 degrees abduction), lateral rotation of the humerus occurs to prevent it: (i) coming into contact with the coracoacromial arch, and (ii) stopping further movement. Lateral rotation brings the inferior part of the articular surface of the humeral head into contact with the glenoid fossa, brought about by concentric contraction of teres minor and infraspinatus.

As the clavicle is firmly anchored to the acromion, lateral scapular rotation elevates the lateral end of the clavicle producing an inferior movement of the medial end of the clavicle at the sternoclavicular joint. There is also some rotation of the clavicle about its long axis, which takes place at both the acromioclavicular and sternoclavicular joints.

Throwing a Ball Overarm
Techniques for throwing a ball overarm vary enormously depending on the distance, height and direction of the throw. The type, weight and size of the ball will influence the grip used, while the surface of the ball may affect its trajectory and resultant movement as it hits the ground.

In the following analysis, a cricket ball is thrown with some force from the boundary of a cricket field towards the wicket keeper.

Starting Position

Drawing the arm posteriorly prior to the throw is an important factor in determining the velocity of the ball. The starting position is with the ball in the right hand and arm at the side of the body. As this position has little to do with the actual throw, the muscle work and joint position are not described; however, it is from this position that the activity begins.

Sequence of Movements

Stretch phase. To achieve maximum power in the throw, the muscles involved must be stretched as much as possible. The pectoral girdle is retracted and depressed by the middle and lower fibres of trapezius, thus stretching the protractors and elevators. The shoulder joint is extended by the posterior fibres of deltoid, latissimus dorsi, teres major and possibly the long head of triceps brachii stretching the flexors. The shoulder joint is also abducted by the middle fibres of deltoid, and laterally rotated by the posterior fibres of deltoid and infraspinatus. The elbow is extended by triceps brachii and anconeus. The wrist is extended by extensors carpi radialis longus and brevis, extensor carpi ulnaris and the long digital extensors, and adducted by extensor and flexor carpi ulnaris. All muscles producing these movements are working concentrically.

The ball is usually held in the ulnar side of the hand in a type of power grip with the fingers flexed around it by the long digital flexors. The distal and proximal interphalangeal and metacarpophalangeal joints are flexed by flexors digitorum profundus and superficialis and lumbricals, respectively. To obtain a better grip, the little finger is often opposed to the ball by opponens digiti minimi. The thumb is flexed at the interphalangeal, metacarpophalangeal and carpometacarpal joints by flexors pollicis longus and brevis. The thumb is also abducted and opposed; abduction is due to the shape of the ball with the adductors working to grip the ball, while opposition is by opponens pollicis. The muscles of the hand are working isometrically.

Movements of the upper right limb are accompanied by rotation of the trunk to the right with right lateral flexion and extension by the concentric contraction of the right internal oblique, left external oblique,

right quadratus lumborum and postvertebral muscles, respectively; movements of the lower limbs are not covered in this analysis but are considerable.

Trajectory phase. Muscles producing movement in this phase are working concentrically unless otherwise stated. The pectoral girdle is rapidly protracted by serratus anterior and pectoralis minor, and elevated by the upper fibres of trapezius and levator scapulae. The shoulder joint is flexed by the anterior fibres of deltoid and pectoralis major (clavicular head), and medially rotated by the anterior fibres of deltoid and pectoralis major, aided by latissimus dorsi and teres major acting as a 'drag' on the medial side of the arm. During this movement, the shoulder passes through abduction, produced by deltoid, initially by the posterior and middle fibres, then the middle fibres and finally the middle and anterior fibres.

The elbow moves from full extension into a variable degree of flexion according to technique, brought about by biceps brachii and brachialis. When the upper limb moves in front of the trunk, the elbow is fully extended by triceps brachii and anconeus.

The precise trajectory of the movement of the upper limb is determined by the required elevation of the ball. At the top of the trajectory, the ball is released by extension of the fingers by extensor digitorum aided by the lumbricals and interossei, and extension and abduction of the thumb by extensors pollicis longus and brevis and abductors longus and brevis.

At the same time as the trajectory phase of the upper limb, the trunk powerfully flexes with lateral flexion and rotation to the left. Flexion is by the oblique abdominal muscles and rectus abdominis of the left side, left rotation by the left internal oblique and right external oblique, and lateral flexion by the left quadratus lumborum. All movements are accompanied by powerful actions of the lower limbs with body weight transferred from the back of the right foot to the front of the left foot. There is also considerable movement of the neck to maintain the face and eyes looking in the direction the ball is being thrown.

Pushing or Punching
Starting Position
The shoulder joint is abducted 90 degrees and fully extended and the elbow joint fully flexed. The hand is either open for pushing or closed for punching. For this activity, the muscle work and joint positions of the hand are not considered.

Sequence of Movements

Abduction and flexion of the shoulder are by isometric contraction of the middle fibres of deltoid, then rapidly flexed by the anterior fibres of deltoid and pectoralis major assisted by coracobrachialis and the long head of biceps brachii, all working concentrically.

Protraction of the scapula and extension of the forearm increases the force and range of the movement brought about by strong concentric contraction of serratus anterior and pectoralis minor. At the same time, forceful contraction of triceps brachii produces rapid extension of the forearm at the elbow joint.

The major difference between pushing and punching is the velocity of the movement, with the latter being more rapid and explosive.

Press-Ups
Starting Position

The individual lies prone with the palmar surfaces of the hands on the ground below the shoulders, which are abducted 90 degrees and in slight extension; the elbows are fully flexed. It is assumed that static muscle work in the legs and trunk maintains their neutral position throughout.

Sequence of Movements

Upward movement. Initially, this is simultaneous elbow extension by triceps brachii and anconeus, and shoulder flexion by pectoralis major and anterior fibres of deltoid, assisted by coracobrachialis and long head of biceps brachii. The pectoral girdle is strongly protracted by serratus anterior and pectoralis minor, the arms are straight and shoulders are protracted. All muscles work concentrically.

From this position, the downward movement can now be considered.

Downward movement. There is simultaneous movement at both the elbow and shoulder joints under the influence of gravity. The elbows are flexed under the eccentric contraction of triceps brachii and anconeus working to control the rate of descent. At the shoulder joint, extension is controlled by eccentric contraction of pectoralis major and anterior fibres of deltoid with the assistance of the long head of biceps brachii and coracobrachialis. The pectoral girdle retracts under the eccentric action of serratus anterior and pectoralis minor.

It is worth remembering that the same muscles are involved in producing both movements, upwards by shortening and downwards by lengthening.

Pulling
Starting Position

The individual stands with the shoulder flexed to 90 degrees, the elbow in full extension and hand firmly gripping the object to be pulled.

Sequence of Movements

The elbow is flexed by concentric contraction of biceps brachii and brachialis, while the shoulder is extended by the strong concentric action of teres major, latissimus dorsi and posterior fibres of deltoid. The pectoral girdle is retracted by concentric contraction of trapezius and rhomboids major and minor.

Rowing

Rowing can be a pleasurable activity whether it takes place on a lake, river or sea; the type of rowing, however, varies considerably according to its purpose. Rowing machines are also frequently used for exercising.

This brief outline of the joint movement and muscle work involved in rowing is based on an amateur oarsman in an ordinary rowing boat with a sliding seat and rowlocks to extend the fulcrum of the oars. As styles vary considerably, no attempt is made to recommend any particular technique.

The description begins in the fully forward position with the arms straight, the grip tightening on the oar, the trunk fully flexed, the neck slightly flexed and the head slightly extended on the neck. The moveable seat is fully forward with the ankles dorsiflexed and knees and hips fully flexed. Description of activities in the lower limb is considered in the section on the lower limb (p. 465).

Starting Position

The blades of the oars are in the water at right angles to the surface. The hands are placed on the ends of the oars with the fingers and palms over the top and thumbs below the oars. The interphalangeal and metacarpophalangeal joints of all fingers are in a semiflexed position around the oars, held by the static muscle work of flexor digitorum profundus, and all other joints by flexors digitorum superficialis and profundus.

The thumb grips the underside of the oars due to the isometric action of adductors pollicis longus and brevis. Semiflexion of the interphalangeal joints is due to the isometric action of flexor pollicis longus and semiflexion of the metacarpophalangeal joint by flexors pollicis longus and brevis. There is also abduction at the carpometacarpal joint due to the thickness of the oar.

The wrists are in a neutral position with both the flexors and extensors working isometrically. The elbows are in full extension with triceps brachii working isometrically; the shoulders are flexed and in almost full elevation due to the isometric action of the anterior and middle fibres of deltoid and clavicular head of pectoralis major. The trunk is held in full flexion by the abdominal muscles, particularly rectus abdominis aided by the abdominal obliques.

Sequence of Movements

Stroke phase. At the beginning of this phase, the grip is tightened on the oars as they are pulled backwards by flexion of the elbows, brought about by powerful concentric action of biceps brachii, brachialis and brachioradialis. The shoulders are extended through abduction by the concentric action of latissimus dorsi and teres major aided by the middle and posterior fibres of deltoid. The pectoral girdle is retracted by the concentric activity of rhomboid major and minor and middle fibres of trapezius, and depressed by the lower fibres of trapezius.

The trunk is almost fully extended by erectores spinae (iliocostalis, longissimus and spinalis) aided by quadratus lumborum and latissimus dorsi all working concentrically. The neck is extended to the neutral position by concentric contraction of the upper fibres of trapezius, splenius cervicis and semispinalis; the head is stabilised in neutral.

The powerful stroke is arrested by the oar coming into contact with the upper abdomen. The oars are then released from the water by strong extension of the wrists by the concentric action of extensors carpi radialis longus and brevis and extensor carpi ulnaris. During the stroke phase, the lower limbs are powerfully extended (p. 465).

Recovery phase. The grip on the oars is maintained but relaxed a little. Extension of the wrists is maintained until the end of the recovery phase and brought about by static muscle work of the wrist extensors.

The elbows are extended fully by the concentric contraction of triceps brachii. The shoulders are flexed into almost full elevation by the anterior fibres of deltoid, clavicular head of pectoralis major, coracobrachialis and long head of biceps brachii. Both pectoral girdles are protracted by the concentric action of pectoralis minor and serratus anterior and partially elevated by the upper fibres of trapezius and levator scapulae.

The trunk is flexed by the powerful concentric action of the abdominal muscles, particularly rectus abdominis. The neck is partially flexed by concentric contraction of sternomastoid and the prevertebral muscles. The head is slightly extended by the posterior suboccipital muscles (rectus capitis posterior major and minor) and upper fibres of trapezius.

During this recovery phase, the lower limbs are flexing and drawing the seat forward on the slide ready for the next stroke (p. 465).

Finally, when the individual has come as far forward as possible without leaving the seat, the wrists are flexed to the neutral position and the blade of the oar put cleanly into the water ready for the next stroke phase.

BRACHIAL PLEXUS AND NERVES OF THE UPPER LIMB

LEARNING OUTCOMES

By the end of the section, you should be able to:
1. Describe the formation of the brachial plexus from its roots to its terminal branches
2. Give the root value of each terminal branch
3. State the muscles supplied by each branch
4. Describe the course and distribution of each branch
5. Describe the sensory innervation of the upper limb
6. Appreciate the influence of pathology and/or trauma to the brachial plexus and its terminal branches

INTRODUCTION

Knowledge of the distribution of the major peripheral nerves of the upper limb is necessary in clinical practice for the diagnosis and assessment of peripheral nerve injuries and other neurological disorders. The course and distribution of the peripheral nerves are described in detail later in this section; their cutaneous

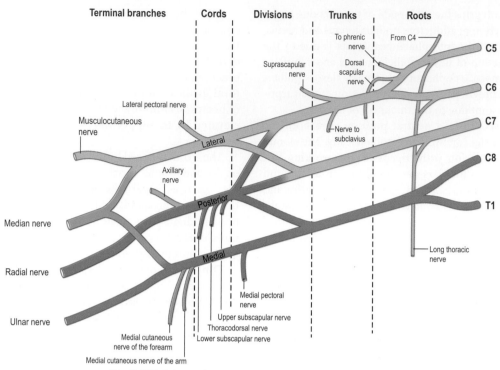

Fig. 2.132 Schematic representation of the brachial plexus.

distribution follows and complements the segmental dermatome arrangement.

A prerequisite for learning the muscular distribution of the major peripheral nerves is to appreciate the groupings of muscles into compartments; the upper limb is divided into four compartments. In the arm, there is an anterior compartment containing coracobrachialis, biceps brachii and brachialis supplied by the musculocutaneous nerve, and a posterior compartment containing triceps brachii and anconeus supplied by the radial nerve. In the forearm, there are also two compartments; an anterior compartment containing the flexors of the wrist, long flexors of the digits, pronators teres and quadratus supplied by the median and ulnar nerves, and a posterior compartment containing the extensors of the wrist and digits, abductor pollicis longus, supinator and brachioradialis supplied by the radial nerve. The intrinsic muscles of the hand are supplied by the median and ulnar nerves.

Nerves supplying the structures in the upper limb are all derived from the brachial plexus, a complex of intermingling nerves originating in the neck from the ventral rami of the lower four cervical nerves and first thoracic

nerve, giving it a root value of C5, C6, C7, C8 and T1. Occasionally, there may be a contribution from C4, T2 or both (Fig. 2.132).

The ventral (anterior) rami are the anterior divisions of the spinal nerves, formed just outside the intervertebral foramen, and situated between scalenus anterior and medius; they are collectively termed the roots of the plexus. Each spinal nerve receives an autonomic contribution; C5 and C6 receive grey rami communicantes from the middle cervical ganglion and C7, C8 and T1 receive them from the inferior or cervicothoracic ganglion.

Generally, the upper two roots (C5 and C6) unite forming the upper trunk, C7 continues as the middle trunk and the lower two roots (C8 and T1) form the lower trunk. The three trunks are found between the scalene muscles and superior border of the clavicle in the posterior triangle of the neck. The lower trunk may groove the superior surface of the 1st rib posterior to the subclavian artery; the T1 root is always in contact with the rib.

Immediately superior to the clavicle, each trunk divides into anterior and posterior divisions which supply the flexor and extensor compartments of the arm, respectively. The three posterior divisions unite forming the posterior cord, the anterior divisions of the upper and middle trunks unite forming the lateral cord, and the anterior division of the lower trunk continues as the medial cord. The cords pass into the axilla, initially posterolateral to the axillary artery and then in their named positions with respect to the second part of the axillary artery posterior to pectoralis minor. The cords and axillary artery are bound together in an extension of the prevertebral fascia layer of the cervical fascia (axillary sheath) which extends into the axilla.

Applied Anatomy

The brachial plexus is subject to direct injury; an understanding of its formation is, therefore, helpful in determining which parts and at what levels the damage has occurred. Traction injuries occur when the roots are torn from the spinal cord or when the constituent parts are partially or completely torn. If the upper roots are completely torn, Erb's paralysis (palsy) affecting the musculature of the arm is produced, while if the lower roots are completely torn, Klumpke's paralysis (palsy) affecting the hand and forearm results. In extreme cases, the whole plexus may be disrupted producing a completely denervated upper limb.

Nerves Arising From the Brachial Plexus and their Distribution

The simplest way to describe the nerves of the brachial plexus is to consider them in relation to the part of the plexus from which they originate (and to indicate their root value).

Branches From the Roots

Nerves to the scalene and longus colli muscles. These arise by twigs from the upper surface of the anterior rami of C5, C6, C7 and C8 as they emerge from the intervertebral foramina; they supply the scalene and longus colli muscles directly entering them.

Branch to the phrenic nerve. The C5 contribution to the phrenic nerve arises at the lateral border of scalenus anterior.

Dorsal scapular nerve. The dorsal scapular nerve (C5) (Fig. 2.132) passes through scalenus medius to the deep surface of levator scapulae, from where it runs onto the anterior surface of the rhomboids. It supplies rhomboid major, rhomboid minor and levator scapulae.

Long thoracic nerve. The C5 and C6 roots of the long thoracic nerve (Fig. 2.132) unite after piercing scalenus medius and are joined by the C7 root on its anterior surface. The nerve passes posterior to the trunks of the plexus between the 1st rib and axillary artery to the lateral (axillary) surface of serratus anterior, which it supplies; the upper two digitations are supplied by C5, the next two by C6 and remaining four by C7.

The long thoracic nerve may be damaged by direct pressure on it from above the shoulder. The resulting paralysis of serratus anterior causes the characteristic 'winged' scapula with the inability to perform activities (abduction of the upper limb) where the scapula is stabilised or laterally rotated.

Branches From the Trunks

Nerve to subclavius. Small branch ((C4), C5 and C6) from the upper trunk, it descends anterior to the subclavian artery to supply subclavius. It may communicate with the phrenic nerve.

Suprascapular nerve. Large branch from the upper trunk, the suprascapular nerve ((C4), C5 and C6) (Fig. 2.132) passes inferolaterally superior and parallel to the trunks through the suprascapular notch deep to trapezius to enter the supraspinous fossa of the scapula. It then runs deep to supraspinatus entering the infraspinous fossa via the spinoglenoid notch. The suprascapular nerve supplies both supraspinatus and infraspinatus and gives articular filaments to the shoulder and acromioclavicular joints.

All of the above branches arise superior to the clavicle, while those following all arise in the axilla inferior to the level of the clavicle.

Branches From the Divisions

No nerves arise from the divisions.

Branches From the Cords

Lateral Cord

Lateral pectoral nerve. Arising from the lateral cord with a root value C5, C6 and C7 (Fig. 2.132), the lateral pectoral nerve crosses medially anterior to the axillary artery, giving a branch to the medial pectoral nerve, before piercing the clavipectoral fascia to gain the deep surface of pectoralis major which it supplies.

Musculocutaneous nerve. Details of its origin, course and distribution can be found on page 229.

Lateral head of the median nerve. Details of its origin, course and distribution can be found on page 234.

Posterior Cord

Upper and lower subscapular nerves. Both (Fig. 2.132) arise from the posterior cord with root values (C4), C5, C6, (C7) and C5, C6, respectively. From posterior to the axillary artery, they descend towards the subscapular fossa where they both supply subscapularis. In addition, the lower subscapular nerve enters and supplies teres major.

Thoracodorsal nerve. Arising from the posterior cord (root value (C6), C7 and C8) between the two subscapular nerves (Fig. 2.132) the thoracodorsal nerve passes inferomedially along the posterior wall of the axilla and anterolateral surface of latissimus dorsi before entering its deep surface to supply it.

Axillary nerve. Details of its origin, course and distribution can be found on page 229.

Radial nerve. Details of its origin, course and distribution can be found on page 230.

Medial Cord

Medial pectoral nerve. From the medial cord, with a root value C8 and T1, the medial pectoral nerve (Fig. 2.132) receives a contribution from the lateral pectoral nerve. It passes between the axillary artery and vein to the deep surface of pectoralis minor, which it supplies; it then the pierces pectoralis minor to end in and supply pectoralis major.

Medial cutaneous nerve of the arm. Small nerve (Fig. 2.132) arising from the medial cord (root value T1) descending through the axilla on the medial side of the axillary vein, then along the medial side of the brachial artery. It pierces the deep fascia to supply skin and fascia on the medial side of the proximal half of the arm, extending onto both the anterior and posterior surfaces (Fig. 2.133); it may be partly or entirely replaced by the intercostobrachial nerve (root value T2 and 3).

Medial cutaneous nerve of the forearm. Arising directly from the medial cord with a root value of C8 and T1, the medial cutaneous nerve of the forearm descends on the medial side of the axillary and bra-

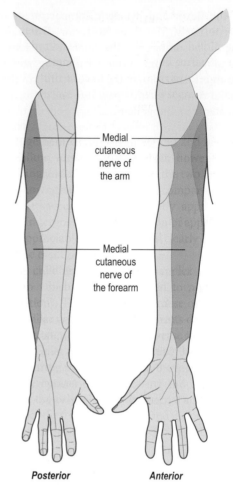

Medial cutaneous nerve of the arm

Medial cutaneous nerve of the forearm

Posterior   Anterior

Fig. 2.133 Distribution of the medial cutaneous nerves of the arm and of the forearm.

chial arteries. It pierces the deep fascia, together with the basilic vein, in the middle of the arm, descending with it to the elbow, where it divides into anterior and ulnar branches. The medial cutaneous nerve of the forearm supplies skin over the distal part of biceps brachii, medial side of the forearm as far as the wrist and part of the medial side of the posterior surface of the forearm (Fig. 2.133).

Ulnar nerve. Details of its origin, course and distribution can be found on page 232.

Medial head of the median nerve. Details of its origin, course and distribution can be found on page 234.

MUSCULOCUTANEOUS NERVE

Arising from the lateral cord of the brachial plexus with a root value C5, C6, C7, the musculocutaneous nerve (Fig. 2.134) initially lies lateral to the axillary artery descending between the artery and coracobrachialis, which it supplies and pierces, before running distally between biceps brachii and brachialis to reach the lateral aspect of the arm. At the elbow, it pierces the deep fascia between biceps brachii and brachioradialis as the lateral cutaneous nerve of the forearm.

In the arm, it supplies both heads of biceps brachii and two-third of brachialis, as well as coracobrachialis.

The lateral cutaneous nerve of the forearm divides into anterior and posterior branches. The anterior branch supplies skin on the lateral half of the forearm as far as the ball of the thumb; the posterior branch supplies a variable area over the extensor muscles of the forearm, wrist and occasionally the 1st metacarpal (Fig. 2.134B).

AXILLARY NERVE

From the posterior cord with a root value of C5 and C6, in the axilla the axillary nerve descends posterior to the axillary artery anterior to subscapularis, at the distal border of which it passes posteriorly close to the inferior part of the shoulder joint in company with the posterior circumflex humeral vessels. It then passes through the quadrilateral space (Fig. 2.25) where it supplies the shoulder joint and divides into anterior and posterior branches. The anterior branch winds around the surgical neck of the humerus, deep to and as far as the anterior part of deltoid, which it supplies (Fig. 2.135); the posterior branch supplies teres minor and the posterior part of deltoid.

It then passes around deltoid as the upper lateral cutaneous nerve of the arm, piercing the deep fascia to supply skin over the distal part of deltoid and lateral head of triceps brachii as far as the middle part of the arm (Fig. 2.135B).

Applied Anatomy

The axillary nerve is frequently injured when the shoulder is dislocated because of its close proximity

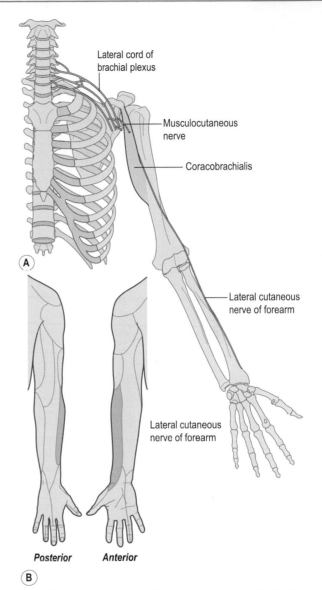

Fig. 2.134 Anterior aspect of the thorax and upper limb showing the course (A) and cutaneous distribution (B) of the musculocutaneous nerve.

to the joint. Paralysis of deltoid and teres minor is the result, with an inability to abduct the arm beyond that possible by the action of supraspinatus. This, together with an area of anaesthesia over the posterior part of deltoid and lateral head of triceps brachii, allows a differential clinical diagnosis of nerve injury to be made.

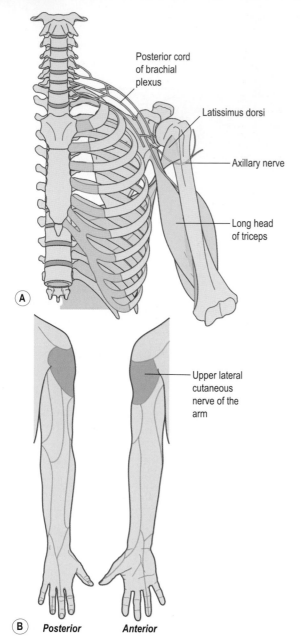

Posterior cord of brachial plexus

Latissimus dorsi

Axillary nerve

Long head of triceps

Upper lateral cutaneous nerve of the arm

(A)

(B)   *Posterior*   *Anterior*

Fig. 2.135 Anterior aspect of the thorax and upper limb showing the course (A) and cutaneous distribution (B) of the axillary nerve.

RADIAL NERVE

The major nerve arising from the posterior cord, with a root value of C5, C6, C7, C8 and (T1); it is one of the terminal branches. In the axilla, it lies posterior to the axillary and proximal part of the brachial

arteries, passing anterior to the tendons of subscapularis, latissimus dorsi and teres major (Fig. 2.136). Together with the profunda brachii artery, it enters the posterior compartment of the arm through the triangular interval formed by the humerus laterally, long head of triceps brachii medially and teres major superiorly (Figs 2.25 and 2.136). In passing through this space, the nerve enters the spiral (radial) groove of the humerus, descending obliquely between the lateral and medial heads of triceps brachii, reaching the lateral border of the humerus in the distal one-third of the arm. It pierces the lateral intermuscular septum to enter the anterior compartment, where it lies in a muscular groove between brachialis and brachioradialis. Anterior to the lateral epicondyle of the humerus, the radial nerve divides into its terminal superficial and deep branches (Fig. 2.136).

In the arm, the radial nerve supplies the three heads of triceps brachii, anconeus, lateral part of brachialis, brachioradialis and extensor carpi radialis longus. The branches to triceps brachii all arise before the nerve enters the spiral groove; anconeus is supplied by a branch to the medial head of triceps brachii.

The radial nerve also gives articular branches to the elbow joint and has three cutaneous branches supplying the skin on the posterior aspects of the arm and forearm (Fig. 2.136B).

The posterior cutaneous nerve of the arm arises in the axilla, piercing the deep fascia near the posterior axillary fold supplying skin on the posterior surface of the proximal one-third of the arm.

The lower lateral cutaneous nerve of the arm arises before the radial nerve enters the spiral groove, pierces the lateral intermuscular septum, becoming cutaneous just inferior to deltoid. It supplies skin over the distal lateral part of the arm and a small area on the forearm.

The posterior cutaneous nerve of the forearm arises just inferior to the lower lateral cutaneous nerve of the arm and supplies a variable area of skin on the dorsum of the forearm as far as the wrist, or occasionally beyond.

The superficial branch is the direct continuation of the radial nerve, passing anterior to the lateral epicondyle before passing along the anterolateral side of the forearm; it is entirely sensory. It lies on supinator, pronator teres, flexor digitorum superficialis and flexor of brachioradialis piercing the deep fascia to become superficial. It supplies skin on the dorsum of the wrist, lateral dorsal surface of the hand and dorsum of the thumb (Fig. 2.136B), then divides into four or five digital nerves. The digital nerves supply skin on the dorsum of the thumb, index, middle and adjacent half of the ring finger as far as the distal interphalangeal joint. The digital branches also give articular branches to the metacarpophalangeal and proximal interphalangeal joints of all five digits.

The deep branch (posterior interosseous nerve) is entirely muscular and articular. It begins anterior to the lateral epicondyle of the humerus, entering the posterior compartment of the forearm by passing between the two heads of supinator, curving around the lateral and posterior surfaces of the radius; during its course, it supplies both extensor carpi radialis brevis and supinator. It then descends between the deep and superficial groups of extensor muscles, accompanied by the posterior interosseous artery, supplying all muscles in the extensor compartment of the forearm (extensor digitorum, extensor digiti minimi, extensor carpi ulnaris, extensor pollicis longus, extensor indicis, abductor pollicis longus, extensor pollicis brevis).

In the distal part of the forearm, the posterior interosseous nerve lies on the interosseous membrane ending in a flattened expansion, giving articular branches to the intercarpal joints.

Applied Anatomy

The radial nerve is often injured in its course close to the humerus, either as the result of a fracture or by pressure from a direct blow or the incorrect use of a crutch. Triceps brachii usually escapes paralysis as it derives its innervation from branches given off proximally in the arm, but total paralysis of the extensors of the wrist and digits leads to the deformity of 'dropped wrist' (Fig. 2.137A). Attempts to grip or make a fist leads to increased wrist flexion and an inability to carry out effective movement due to the loss of the synergic action of the wrist extensors, which usually prevent the unwanted wrist flexion produced by the continued action of the finger flexors.

The interphalangeal joints of the fingers can be extended by the lumbricals and interossei because of their attachment to the extensor expansion; however, proper use of the hand requires an effective form of dynamic splint (Fig. 2.137B) which compensates for the paralysed muscles. The dynamic splint holds the wrist

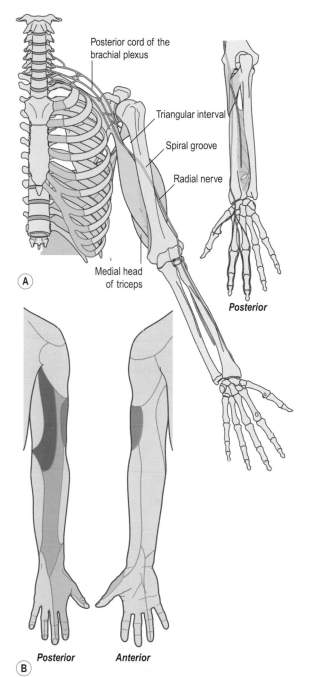

Fig. 2.136 Anterior aspect of the thorax and upper limb showing the course (A) and cutaneous distribution (B) of the radial nerve.

pollicis longus covered by brachioradialis with the radial artery medial to it. In the distal one-third of the forearm, it emerges posteriorly from deep to the tendon

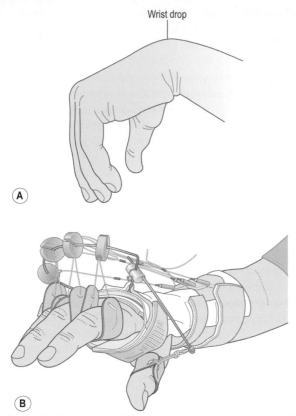

Fig. 2.137 (A) Typical radial nerve deformity of the hand. (B) Example of a dynamic radial nerve splint.

in extension and recoils to pull the fingers and thumb from flexion into extension, allowing the grip to release. Even though the sensory distribution of the radial nerve on the dorsum of the hand appears extensive, overlap by adjacent cutaneous nerves means that the area of exclusive radial nerve supply is a small patch on the dorsum of the thumb web.

ULNAR NERVE

Terminal branch of the medial cord of the brachial plexus, the ulnar nerve has root value C8 and T1; it frequently contains C7 fibres. Descending on the medial side of the axillary artery posterior to the medial cutaneous nerve of the forearm, it continues inferiorly medial to the brachial artery, anterior to triceps brachii (Fig. 2.138). In the distal half of the arm, the ulnar nerve passes posteriorly piercing the medial intermuscular septum to enter the posterior compartment of the arm, where it lies on the anterior aspect of the medial head of triceps brachii. Continuing

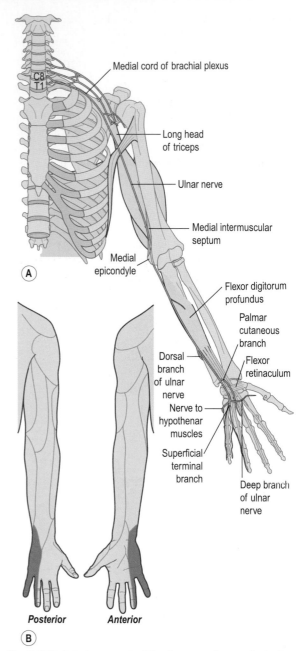

Fig. 2.138 Anterior aspect of the thorax and upper limb showing the course (A) and cutaneous distribution (B) of the ulnar nerve.

its course in the posterior compartment of the arm, it passes between the medial epicondyle of the humerus and olecranon of the ulna, lying in the ulnar groove posterior to the medial epicondyle. It enters the anterior compartment of the forearm by passing between the two heads of flexor carpi ulnaris, initially in contact with the ulnar collateral ligament of the elbow. As it descends on the medial side of the forearm, the ulnar nerve lies on flexor digitorum profundus, lateral to the ulnar artery, covered in its proximal part by the belly of flexor carpi ulnaris, but in the distal part only by its tendon. Proximal to the flexor retinaculum, it pierces the deep fascia to lie lateral to flexor carpi ulnaris passing anterior to the flexor retinaculum lateral to the pisiform, where it divides into superficial and deep branches.

During its course, the ulnar nerve gives an articular branch to the elbow joint and supplies flexor carpi ulnaris and the medial half of flexor digitorum profundus.

A palmar cutaneous branch arises from the ulnar nerve which pierces the deep fascia in the distal one-third of the forearm, descending to supply skin over the medial part of the palm (Fig. 2.138B).

The dorsal branch of the ulnar nerve also arises in the distal one-third of the forearm, and passes posteriorly deep to flexor carpi ulnaris, piercing the deep fascia on the medial side to become superficial. On the medial side of the wrist, it crosses the triquetral, against which it can be palpated, and gives branches to the dorsal surface of the wrist and hand. Here, it divides into two or three dorsal digital nerves supplying skin on the dorsum of the hand and dorsal surfaces of the medial 1½ or 2½ digits, excluding the skin over the distal phalanx. The dorsum of the distal phalanges are supplied by branches from the median or ulnar nerves derived from the palm.

The superficial branch of the ulnar nerve lies deep to palmaris brevis on the medial side of the hand where it can be compressed against the hook of the hamate. It supplies palmaris brevis, skin on the medial side of the palm of the hand and skin on the palmar surface of the little and adjacent half of the ring fingers, extending onto the dorsal surface, supplying the skin and nail bed of the distal phalanx.

The deep branch of the ulnar nerve eventually runs with the deep branch of the ulnar artery, looping across the palm from medial to lateral deep to the flexor tendons. It passes initially between abductor digiti minimi and flexor digiti minimi, and pierces opponens digiti minimi, supplying all three muscles. As it passes across the deep part of the palm, it supplies the medial two lumbricals, all dorsal and palmar interossei and adductor pollicis. Rarely, the ulnar nerve also supplies the thenar muscles. The deep branch gives articular filaments to the wrist joint.

Applied Anatomy

The ulnar nerve may be damaged in the groove posterior to the medial epicondyle either by trauma or entrapment, leading to partial or complete loss of muscular and sensory innervation; at the wrist, due to its superficial position, it can easily be cut or lacerated. The clinical picture can be complicated if the lesion occurs distal to the level where the dorsal and palmar cutaneous branches are given off as a considerable portion of skin on the ulnar side of the hand still has a sensory supply. Due to loss of power in the intrinsic muscles of the hand and unopposed actions of antagonistic muscle groups which extend the interphalangeal joints of the ring and little fingers, an ulnar nerve lesion often gives the typical 'ulnar claw-hand' deformity (Fig. 2.139A). The deformity may be corrected using a splint to counteract the pull of the unopposed muscles, which may

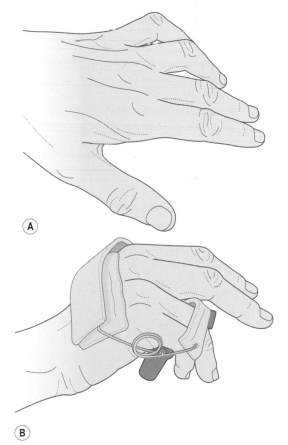

Fig. 2.139 (A) Typical ulnar nerve deformity of the hand. (B) Example of an ulnar nerve splint.

allow more functional use of the hand (Fig. 2.139B). There is 'guttering' between the metacarpals, an inability to abduct the fingers or adduct the thumb with marked wasting of adductor pollicis. The area of sensory loss usually follows the outline of the sensory map (Fig. 2.138A).

MEDIAN NERVE

Arising partly from the lateral cord (C5, C6 and C7) and partly from the medial cord (C8 and T1), the two heads of the median nerve unite around the third part of the axillary artery (Fig. 2.140). Once formed, the nerve descends deep to biceps brachii crossing anterior to the brachial artery from lateral to medial. In the distal part of the arm, the median nerve lies on brachialis; in the cubital fossa, it is protected by the bicipital aponeurosis which covers it.

The median nerve enters the forearm between the two heads of pronator teres and then passes deep to the tendinous arch connecting the heads of flexor digitorum superficialis, to access its deep surface. Closely bound

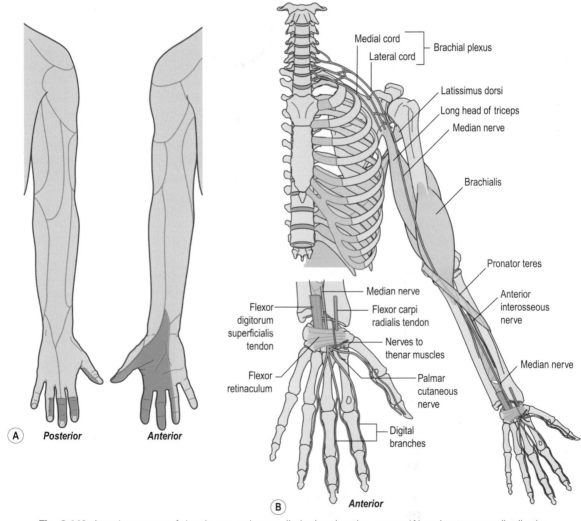

Fig. 2.140 Anterior aspect of the thorax and upper limb showing the course (A) and cutaneous distribution (B) of the median nerve.

to the deep surface of flexor digitorum superficialis, it descends on flexor digitorum profundus until just proximal to the wrist where it becomes superficial between the tendons of flexors digitorum superficialis and carpi radialis, deep to palmaris longus. The median nerve enters the hand deep to the flexor retinaculum, anterior to the long flexor tendons. It is one of the structures within the carpal tunnel.

During its course, the median nerve gives articular branches to the elbow joint and supplies pronator teres, flexor carpi radialis, palmaris longus and flexor digitorum superficialis.

The palmar cutaneous nerve arises in the distal one-third of the forearm piercing the deep fascia to enter the palm superficial to the flexor retinaculum; it supplies a small area of skin on the lateral side of the palm and thenar eminence.

The anterior interosseous nerve arises from the median nerve in the cubital fossa and descends with the anterior interosseous artery on the anterior surface of the interosseous membrane between flexors pollicis longus and digitorum profundus. It then passes deep to pronator quadratus to end at the wrist by giving articular branches to the radiocarpal and intercarpal joints. The anterior interosseous nerve supplies flexor pollicis longus, lateral half of flexor digitorum profundus and pronator quadratus.

Once through the carpal tunnel, it enters the hand where it divides into lateral and medial terminal branches. The lateral branch passes laterally and proximally to enter the thenar eminence supplying abductor pollicis brevis, flexor pollicis brevis, opponens pollicis and the 1st lumbrical; it gives sensory branches to adjacent sides of the thumb and index finger.

The medial branch divides into a variable number of branches (palmar digital nerves) with the most lateral supplying the 2nd lumbrical. These nerves are sensory to the palmar surface of adjacent sides of the index and middle, and middle and ring fingers (Fig. 2.140B). Each digital nerve gives a dorsal branch which passes posteriorly to supply the dorsal aspect of the distal phalanx and nail bed, and a variable amount of the middle phalanx of the same digit.

The digital nerves lie deep to the palmar aponeurosis and superficial palmar arch, but superficial to the long flexor tendons. In addition to their sensory innervation,

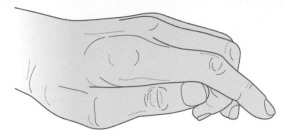

Fig. 2.141 Typical median nerve deformity.

they give articular branches to the metacarpophalangeal and interphalangeal joints.

Applied Anatomy

The median nerve can be injured in the forearm by deep cuts with a resultant loss of flexion at all interphalangeal joints, except the distal ones in the ring and little fingers (Fig. 2.141). The metacarpophalangeal joints of these same fingers can still be flexed by the lumbricals and interossei, but pronation of the forearm is severely restricted. In the hand, the thumb is extended and adducted losing its ability to oppose and abduct; combined with the sensory loss, this is a major disability. More commonly, the nerve is damaged just proximal to the flexor retinaculum by laceration or deep to it in the carpal tunnel where compression gives rise to carpal tunnel (median nerve) syndrome. In this case, only the thenar muscles, lateral two lumbricals and sensation in the hand are affected. Static splinting after a median nerve lesion often involves holding the thumb in abduction with some opposition to prevent loss of the thumb webspace.

DERMATOMES OF THE UPPER LIMB

The distribution of the cutaneous branches of the major nerves arising from the brachial plexus are shown in Fig. 2.142. During development, cells from the dermomyotome spread out to form the skin (see Figs 1.7, 1.17 and 1.18); each dermatome represents an area of skin innervated by a single nerve root. The dermatomes of the upper limb are shown in Fig. 2.142B. Branches from more than one nerve can and do contribute to an individual dermatome; however, all have the same single root value.

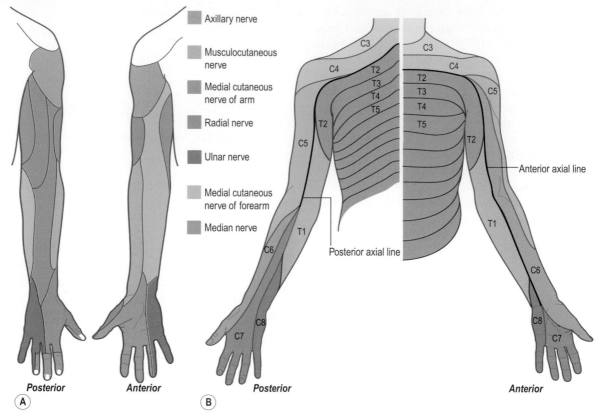

Fig. 2.142 Cutaneous innervation (A) and dermatomes (B) of the upper limb.

Section Summary

Brachial Plexus

Branches from:

Roots	Nerves to scalene muscles and longus colli (C5, C6, C7, C8)
	Contribution to phrenic nerve (C4)
	Dorsal scapular nerve (C5)
	Long thoracic nerve (C5, C6, C7)
Trunks	Nerve to subclavius ((C4), C5, C6)
	Suprascapular nerve ((C4), C5, C6)

Cords:

Medial	Medial pectoral nerve (C8, T1)
	Medial cutaneous nerve of arm (C8, T1)
	Medial cutaneous of forearm (C8, T1)
	Ulnar nerve ((C7), C8, T1)
	Medial head of median nerve (C8, T1)

Posterior	Upper subscapular nerve ((C4), C5, C6, (C7))
	Thoracodorsal nerve (C6, C7, C8)
	Lower subscapular nerve (C5, C6)
	Axillary nerve (C5, C6)
	Radial nerve (C5, C6, C7, C8, (T1))
Lateral	Lateral pectoral nerve (C5, C6, C7)
	Musculocutaneous nerve (C5, C6, C7)
	Lateral head of median nerve ((C5), C6, C7)

Musculocutaneous Nerve

From	Lateral cord
Root value	C5, C6, C7
Muscles supplied	Coracobrachialis; biceps brachii; brachialis (medial 2/3rd)
Cutaneous branch	Lateral cutaneous nerve of forearm

Section Summary—Cont'd

Axillary Nerve

From	Posterior cord
Root value	C5, C6
Muscles supplied	Deltoid; teres minor
Cutaneous branch	Upper lateral cutaneous nerve of arm

Radial Nerve

From	Posterior cord
Root value	C5, C6, C7, C8 (T1)
Muscles supplied	Triceps brachii (all three heads); anconeus; brachialis (lateral 1/3rd); brachioradialis; extensor carpi radialis longus
	From posterior interosseous nerve (deep branch): supinator; extensor carpi radialis brevis; extensor digitorum; extensor digiti minimi; extensor carpi ulnaris; extensor indicis; extensors pollicis longus and brevis; abductor pollicis longus;
Cutaneous branches	Posterior cutaneous nerve of arm; lower lateral cutaneous nerve of forearm; superficial radial

Ulnar Nerve

From	Medial cord
Root value	(C7), C8, T1
Muscles supplied	Flexor carpi ulnaris; flexor digitorum profundus (medial ½); palmaris brevis
	From deep branch: abductor, flexor and opponens digiti minimi; medial two lumbricals; palmar and dorsal interossei; adductor pollicis
Cutaneous branches	Palmar cutaneous; dorsal; superficial; digital

Median Nerve

From	Medial and lateral cords
Root value	C5, C6, C7 (lateral cord) and C8, T1 (medial cord)
Muscles supplied	Pronator teres; flexor carpi radialis; palmaris longus; flexor digitorum superficialis; abductor pollicis brevis; flexor pollicis brevis; opponens pollicis; lateral two lumbricals
	From anterior interosseous nerve: flexor pollicis longus; flexor digitorum profundus (lateral ½); pronator quadratus
Cutaneous branches	Palmar cutaneous; lateral and medial branches; digital branches

💡 SELF-ASSESSMENT QUESTIONS

139. What are the terminal branches of the medial cord?
140. What is the root value of the axillary nerve?
141. Which nerve(s) arise from the trunks of the brachial plexus?
142. Which muscle(s) is/are supplied by the lower subscapular nerve?
143. The lateral cutaneous nerve of the forearm arises from which cord of the brachial plexus?
144. The posterior interosseous nerve passes between the heads of which muscle to enter the forearm?
145. Which muscles are innervated by the axillary nerve?
146. Which nerve is sensory to the nail bed of the middle finger?
147. Which dermatome supplies skin over the thumb?
148. Which nerve gives the lower lateral cutaneous nerve of the arm?
149. What is the root value of the long thoracic nerve?
150. What is the innervation of latissimus dorsi?
151. Which nerve pierces pectoralis minor?
152. The ulnar nerve passes between the heads of which muscle to enter the forearm?
153. The skin of the lateral palm is innervated by which branch of which nerve?

BLOOD SUPPLY AND LYMPHATIC DRAINAGE

ARTERIES

The main arterial stem of the upper limb passes through the root of the neck, axilla and arm before dividing in the forearm (Fig. 2.143); its name changes in each region as it crosses specific bony or muscular landmarks.

Subclavian Artery

Arising from the brachiocephalic trunk the right subclavian artery lies entirely within the root of the neck; the left subclavian artery arises directly from the arch of the aorta in the superior mediastinum and enters the root of the neck. Each artery passes laterally over the 1st rib towards the axilla, becoming the axillary artery at its lateral border. The subclavian artery is conveniently divided into three parts by scalenus anterior, which crosses it anteriorly.

In the neck, the artery runs from the superior border of the sternoclavicular joint to the middle of the clavicle; its course is convex superiorly. The artery can be compressed against the 1st rib by posteroinferior pressure applied posterior to the clavicle, lateral to the posterior border of sternomastoid.

Branches from the subclavian artery supply structures in the neck and anterior chest wall; it provides an important supply to the brain via the vertebral artery.

Axillary Artery

Continuation of the subclavian artery at the lateral border of the 1st rib, it ends at the inferior border of teres major, becoming the brachial artery, at the level of the lateral extremity of the posterior axillary fold. For descriptive purposes, it is divided into three parts by pectoralis minor; the length of each part depending on the position of the arm. The cords of the brachial plexus are named according to their position with respect to the second part of the axillary artery.

The course of the artery is represented by a line drawn from the midpoint of the clavicle passing immediately inferior to the coracoid process to the medial lip of the intertubercular groove posterior to coracobrachialis; it describes a curve with an inferomedially facing concavity.

The axillary pulse can be palpated in the lateral wall of the axilla in the groove posterior to coracobrachialis.

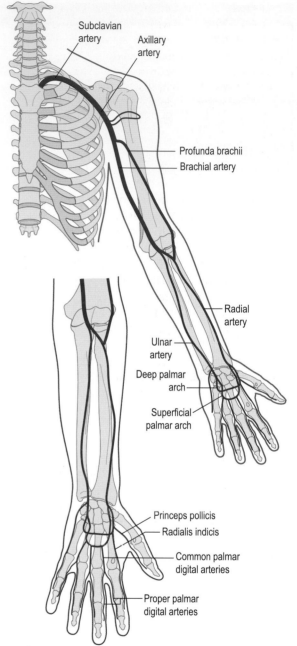

Fig. 2.143 Anterior aspect of the thorax, left upper limb and palmar aspect of the hand showing its arterial supply.

This is a useful pressure point to control distal bleeding, although paraesthesia may result from the inevitable pressure on the median, ulnar and radial nerves as they have a close relation to the artery at this point.

Branches from the axillary artery supply the shoulder and pectoral regions, as well as the lateral chest wall; they anastomose with branches from the subclavian artery and posterior intercostal arteries from the descending thoracic aorta. The vessels in these anastomoses may be enlarged in conditions where there is narrowing of the aorta beyond the origin of the left subclavian artery (coarctation of the aorta) and serve as a collateral system bypassing the restriction.

Brachial Artery

Continuation of the axillary artery at the inferior border of teres major; it bifurcates in the cubital fossa at the level of the neck of the radius into radial and ulnar arteries. It lies successively on the long and medial heads of triceps brachii, the attachment of coracobrachialis and brachialis. Anteriorly, it is covered by the medial border of biceps brachii and crossed anteriorly about halfway down the arm from lateral to medial by the median nerve. In the cubital fossa, it lies deep to the bicipital aponeurosis, separating it from the median cubital vein, with the median nerve lying medial to the artery and the tendon of biceps brachii lateral.

High division of the brachial artery can occur proximal to the cubital fossa; it can divide at any point between the axilla and cubital fossa, in which case the two arteries descend side by side following the normal course of the brachial artery.

The brachial pulse may be felt along its whole course by compressing the artery against the humerus, directing lateral pressure proximally and dorsolateral pressure distally. It is best felt just medial to the bicipital aponeurosis at the level of the medial epicondyle of the humerus; it is at this point that Korotkoff's sounds can be heard when measuring blood pressure.

A major branch of the brachial artery is the profunda brachii, which passes with the radial nerve through the triangular interval and then in the spiral groove between the lateral and medial heads of triceps brachii to enter the posterior compartment of the arm. Branches from both the brachial artery and profunda brachii supply muscles of the arm and contribute to the anastomosis around the elbow joint.

Radial Artery

Beginning in the cubital fossa at the level of the neck of the radius, the radial artery ends by completing the deep palmar arch in the hand; it is usually described as having three parts. The first part is in the forearm, the second part curves laterally around the wrist as far as the first interosseous space and the third part passes through the interosseous space into the palm.

If the arm is placed in a mid pronated position and brachioradialis tensed, the course of the first part of the radial artery follows a slightly convex line beginning at the biceps brachii tendon running along the medial side of brachioradialis to just medial to the anterior aspect of the radial styloid process. As it curves around the wrist, the second part of the artery lies within the 'anatomical snuffbox' lying on the radiocarpal ligament, scaphoid and trapezium; it is crossed by the tendons of abductor pollicis longus and extensors pollicis brevis and longus from lateral to medial.

The third part of the artery passes between the two heads of the 1st dorsal interosseous and adductor pollicis before completing the deep palmar arch.

The radial pulse may be felt against the distal border of the radius lateral to flexor carpi radialis and in the 'anatomical snuffbox' against the scaphoid.

Branches from the first part are involved in the elbow anastomosis and in supplying the muscles on the lateral side of the forearm. From the second part arise branches supplying the wrist and dorsum of the hand and thumb. Before completing the deep palmar arch, the third part gives the princeps pollicis and radialis indicis branches to the thumb and index fingers, respectively.

Ulnar Artery

Beginning in the cubital fossa as a terminal branch of the brachial artery, the ulnar artery ends at the pisiform by dividing into deep and superficial palmar arteries. It is represented by a medially convex line passing from the tendon of biceps brachii to the pisiform and, from there, to the hook of the hamate. In its course, it lies superficial to brachialis, flexor digitorum profundus and the flexor retinaculum; it is crossed anteriorly (from superior to inferior) by pronator teres, the median nerve, flexor carpi radialis, palmaris longus and flexor digitorum superficialis, and overlapped distally by flexor carpi ulnaris. Just inferior to the radial tuberosity, the common interosseous artery is given off, which almost immediately divides into anterior and posterior interosseous arteries to pass inferiorly on either side of the interosseous membrane, supplying the deep muscles of the flexor and extensor compartments. Branches from the proximal and distal aspects of the artery are involved in supplying the elbow and wrist joints, respectively.

Superficial Palmar Arch

Formed mainly by the ulnar artery, with a contribution from the superficial palmar branch of the radial artery, the superficial palmar arch lies deep to the palmar aponeurosis. The distal convexity of the arch lies level with the flexor surface of the extended thumb.

Four common palmar digital arteries arise from the superficial arch with the most medial running along the medial side of the little finger. The other three divide into two proper digital arteries, each supplying adjacent sides of the little, ring, middle and index fingers.

Deep Palmar Arch

The deep palmar arch is formed mainly by the radial artery with a contribution from the deep branch of the ulnar artery. It lies deep to the long flexor tendons and their synovial sheaths on the metacarpal bases and gives rise to the palmar metacarpal arteries. Its distal convexity is 2 cm distal to the distal crease of the wrist.

VEINS

The veins (Fig. 2.144) of the upper limb are divided into superficial, which lie in the superficial fascia, and deep, which accompany the arteries. Both sets of veins have valves which allow proximal drainage only (a fact to be borne in mind when using massage) into the axillary vein.

Deep Veins

Apart from the axillary artery, which is accompanied by a single vein, all other arteries are accompanied by two venae comitantes.

The axillary vein is the continuation of the basilic vein at the inferior border of teres major; it ends by becoming the subclavian vein at the lateral border of the 1st rib. Its course is identical to that of the axillary artery, which lies lateral to it.

Superficial Veins

These are arranged in irregular networks in the superficial fascia, connected to the deep veins by incompetent perforating veins piercing the deep fascia. The blood is drained from the superficial system principally by the basilic and cephalic veins.

Dorsal Venous Arch

Lying on the dorsum of the hand its position and pattern are highly variable; it would be better named the dorsal venous plexus as its arch-like nature is seldom apparent.

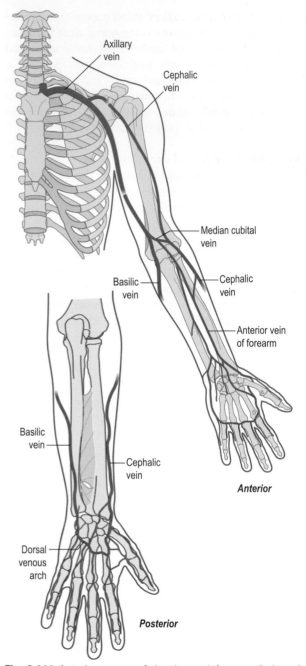

Fig. 2.144 Anterior aspect of the thorax, left upper limb and dorsum of the right hand, showing its venous drainage.

Basilic Vein

Arising from the medial side of the dorsal venous arch, the basilic vein ascends along the ulnar side of the distal half of the forearm before inclining anteriorly to pass anterior to the medial epicondyle of the humerus to enter the medial bicipital furrow. Opposite the attachment of coracobrachialis, it pierces the deep fascia to ascend along the medial side of the brachial vessels becoming the axillary vein at the inferior border of teres major. In the forearm, it can usually be clearly seen, particularly in males; it is joined by tributaries from the forearm and the median cubital vein anterior to the elbow.

Cephalic Vein

Arising from the lateral end of the dorsal venous arch the cephalic vein receives the dorsal veins of the thumb. Inclining anteriorly, it ascends on the anterolateral part of the forearm as far as the elbow and then along the lateral side of the biceps brachii tendon to the groove anterior to the shoulder between deltoid and pectoralis major (deltopectoral groove). It passes in this groove to the level of the coracoid process, where it turns medially between pectoralis major and minor, piercing the clavipectoral fascia and ending in the axillary vein just inferior to the middle of the clavicle. It receives several tributaries in the forearm; at the elbow, it is connected to the basilic vein by the median cubital vein.

Median Cubital Vein

Short wide vein useful for venepuncture, the median cubital vein usually runs superomedially across the bicipital aponeurosis, separating it from the underlying brachial artery; it joins the basilic vein just above the medial epicondyle.

Anterior Median Vein of the Forearm

When present, the anterior median vein of the forearm runs up the middle of the anterior aspect of the forearm and may join the basilic or cephalic vein, or divide at the cubital fossa into the median cephalic and median basilic veins.

LYMPHATICS

Lymphatic drainage of the upper limb is by a superficial interconnected network of vessels just below the skin and by deep lymphatic channels deep to the deep fascia. The larger lymph vessels contain numerous valves allowing lymph to move in a proximal direction only. Both groups of vessels drain proximally and end by passing through many of the 25–30 lymph nodes in the axilla. This mass of lymph nodes serves to filter the lymph, being an important defence mechanism in preventing the spread of infection.

The axillary lymph nodes are distributed in the axillary fat throughout the axilla but can be considered as being in five groups, four of which lie deep to pectoralis minor and one (apical group) superior. Ultimately, all lymph from the upper limb passes through the apical group of nodes, where the efferent lymph channels condense to form the subclavian lymph trunk. On the left-hand side, the subclavian lymph trunk joins the thoracic duct, while on the right it drains directly into the subclavian vein or via the right lymphatic duct.

Superficial Nodes and Lymph Vessels

Found in the skin they drain lymph from the superficial tissues (Fig. 2.145). In the hand, a fine network of vessels exists draining progressively into larger channels as they pass proximally. The only superficial lymph vessels that have any consistent course are the larger ones which follow the major superficial veins; they terminate in the axilla.

In the cubital fossa, one or two lymph nodes lie medial to the basilic vein, receiving lymph from the medial fingers and ulnar half of the hand and forearm. There are also one or two lymph nodes in the infraclavicular fossa associated with the cephalic vein; these receive vessels from the shoulder and breast (Fig. 2.146). A single node may be found in the deltopectoral groove.

Deep Nodes and Lymph Vessels

The deep lymph vessels are less numerous than superficial vessels with which they have many connections. Lying deep to the deep fascia, they accompany the major arteries in the upper limb, most passing directly to the lateral group of axillary nodes. Small nodes may occur along both the radial and ulnar arteries and deep within the cubital fossa. Efferents from all of these nodes pass to the lateral group of axillary nodes lying along the axillary vein, and from pectoral and subscapular nodes passing along the lateral thoracic and subscapular arteries, respectively. A central group of nodes is formed above the floor of the axilla; although it receives lymph from all areas, the main drainage of the upper limb is to the lateral group. Drainage of the breast and anterior chest wall is to the pectoral nodes and that of the scapular region and upper trunk to the subscapular nodes. Efferents from these groups pass to the central and then apical group of nodes, the latter also receiving efferents from the superficial infraclavicular nodes (Fig. 2.146).

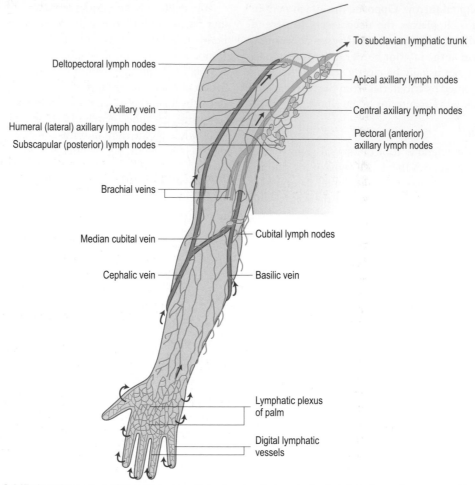

Deltopectoral lymph nodes

To subclavian lymphatic trunk

Apical axillary lymph nodes

Axillary vein

Central axillary lymph nodes

Humeral (lateral) axillary lymph nodes

Subscapular (posterior) lymph nodes

Pectoral (anterior) axillary lymph nodes

Brachial veins

Median cubital vein

Cubital lymph nodes

Cephalic vein

Basilic vein

Lymphatic plexus of palm

Digital lymphatic vessels

Fig. 2.145 Anterior aspect of the right upper limb showing its lymphatic drainage, the major groups of lymph nodes and the direction of lymph flow.

Application

The fact that larger lymph vessels contain valves is important during massage techniques aimed at reducing oedema. The massage strokes should be applied from distal to proximal towards the axilla with sufficient depth to compress the lymph vessels and encourage drainage.

Active muscle contraction also compresses the lymph vessels and encourages drainage proximally. This effect can be enhanced by placing an elastic compressive support/bandage on the upper limb and encouraging active rhythmical contraction of the muscles. Elevation of the upper limb above the level of the axilla allows gravity to assist lymphatic drainage.

Pneumatic splints which apply a rhythmically alternating compressive force to the upper limb can also increase lymphatic flow proximally, utilising the same principles as massage.

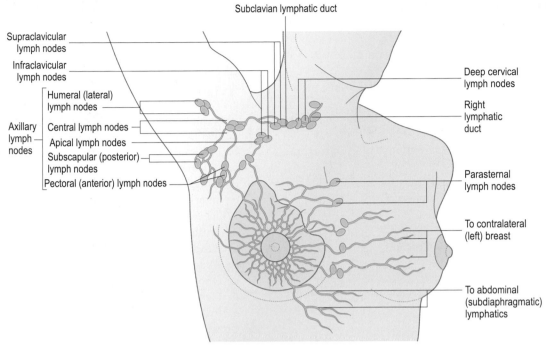

Fig. 2.146 Anterior aspect of the right thoracic wall and breast showing its lymphatic drainage to the axillary lymph nodes, subdiaphragmatic nodes and to the opposite side.

? SELF-ASSESSMENT QUESTIONS

154. Which arteries contribute to the deep and superficial palmar arches?
155. The axillary artery becomes the brachial artery after crossing which part of which muscle?
156. Does the subclavian artery pass anterior or posterior to the scalene tubercle?
157. The left subclavian artery is a branch of which vessel?
158. The cephalic vein drains into which vessel?
159. Does the median cubital vein lie deep or superficial to the bicipital aponeurosis?
160. Approximately how many lymph nodes are there in the axilla?
161. To which group of lymph nodes does the breast and anterior chest wall drain?
162. Which structure is pierced by the cephalic vein?
163. Where can the radial pulse be felt?

SELF-ASSESSMENT MULTIPLE CHOICE QUESTIONS

1. Which of the following muscles does NOT have an action at the elbow joint?
   a. Flexor carpi radialis
   b. Coracobrachialis
   c. Pronator teres
   d. Brachialis
   e. Flexor digitorum superficialis
2. Movement of the scapula forwards around the chest wall is:
   a. elevation.
   b. retraction.
   c. depression.
   d. circumduction.
   e. protraction.
3. Concerning the shoulder joint, which of the following statements is correct?
   a. Supraspinatus is an adductor.
   b. The glenoid labrum is attached to the neck of the humerus.
   c. Triceps brachii attaches to the infraglenoid tubercle.
   d. The humeral head forms two-thirds of a sphere.
   e. Downward dislocation can damage the radial nerve.

4. Which of the following statements is correct?
   a. The axillary nerve passes through the quadrangular space.
   b. The lower border of the quadrangular space is formed by teres minor.
   c. The posterior circumflex humeral artery passes through the triangular space.
   d. The circumflex scapular artery is a branch of the brachial artery.
   e. The axillary artery is a continuation of the brachial artery.

5. Which of the following muscles is NOT directly innervated by the median nerve?
   a. Flexor pollicis brevis
   b. Flexor carpi radialis
   c. Flexor digitorum superficialis
   d. Flexor pollicis longus
   e. Pronator teres

6. Which of the following do NOT articulate with the lunate?
   a. Scaphoid
   b. Ulna
   c. Triquetral
   d. Capitate
   e. Radius

7. Which of the following is NOT part of the distal row of carpal bones?
   a. Capitate
   b. Hamate
   c. Trapezium
   d. Pisiform
   e. Trapezoid

8. Which of the following is NOT a branch of the posterior cord of the brachial plexus?
   a. Thoracodorsal
   b. Radial
   c. Lower subscapular
   d. Axillary
   e. Dorsal scapular

9. Concerning the elbow joint, which of the following statements is correct?
   a. Brachioradialis is an extensor of the elbow joint.
   b. Pronator teres attaches to the medial epicondyle of the humerus.
   c. Pronation and supination are possible at the elbow joint.
   d. The elbow joint is innervated by the axillary nerve.
   e. The ulnar nerve passes anterior to the elbow joint.

10. Which of the following movements at the shoulder joint is not produced by deltoid?
    a. Adduction
    b. Flexion
    c. Lateral rotation
    d. Extension
    e. Abduction

11. Extensor carpi ulnaris is innervated by the:
    a. median nerve
    b. posterior interosseous nerve
    c. ulna nerve
    d. radial nerve
    e. anterior interosseous nerve

12. Which of the following muscles is NOT directly innervated by the ulnar nerve?
    a. Flexor carpi ulnaris
    b. Abductor digiti minimi
    c. Opponens digiti minimi
    d. Flexor digitorum profundus
    e. Palmaris longus

13. Concerning the upper limb, which of the following statements is correct?
    a. In the anatomical position the thumb is directed medially.
    b. The acromioclavicular joint is a plane synovial joint.
    c. Trapezius and serratus anterior medially rotate the scapula.
    d. In pronation of the forearm the palm of the hand faces forwards.
    e. There are 15 phalanges in the digits.

14. Concerning the brachial plexus, which of the following statements is NOT correct?
    a. The posterior cord receives contributions from the upper, middle and lower trunks.
    b. The long thoracic nerve arises from C5, C6 and C7.
    c. The ulnar nerve is a terminal branch of the medial cord.
    d. The dorsal scapular nerve arises from the upper trunk.
    e. The medial cord is a direct continuation of the upper trunk.

15. Adduction at the wrist is produced by:
    a. Flexor carpi ulnaris and extensor carpi ulnaris
    b. Flexor carpi ulnaris and flexor carpi radialis
    c. Flexor carpi radialis, extensor carpi radialis longus and extensor carpi radialis brevis
    d. Extensor carpi ulnaris, extensor carpi radialis longus and extensor carpi radialis brevis
    e. Flexor carpi radialis and flexor pollicis longus

16. What is the innervation of flexor digitorum superficialis?
    a. Median nerve
    b. Ulnar nerve
    c. Radial nerve
    d. Anterior interosseous nerve
    e. Posterior interosseous nerve

17. Concerning muscles of the upper limb, which of the following statements is NOT correct?
    a. Brachialis is innervated by the radial nerve.
    b. Pronator quadratus attaches to the anterior distal surfaces of the radius and ulna.
    c. Abductor pollicis longus is innervated by the posterior interosseous nerve.
    d. The median nerve innervates flexor carpi ulnaris.
    e. The tendons of flexor digitorum profundus pass deep to the flexor retinaculum.

18. From which cords of the brachial plexus does the median nerve receive contributions?
    a. Lateral and posterior
    b. Posterior and medial
    c. Medial and lateral
    d. Medial and posterior
    e. Lateral, medial and posterior

19. What type of synovial joint is the metacarpophalangeal joint?
    a. Ellipsoid
    b. Condyloid
    c. Hinge
    d. Ball-and-socket
    e. Plane

20. Which of the following structures pass through the shoulder joint capsule?
    a. Long head of triceps brachii
    b. Supraspinatus
    c. Teres minor
    d. Subscapularis
    e. Long head of biceps brachii

21. Abduction of the arm at the shoulder joint is produced by:
    a. teres minor
    b. pectoralis minor
    c. long head of triceps brachii
    d. trapezius
    e. supraspinatus

22. Which of the following does NOT attach to the clavicle?
    a. Costoclavicular ligament
    b. Coracoacromial ligament
    c. Trapezius

    d. Coracoclavicular ligament
    e. Subclavius

23. Which of the following does NOT pass anterior to the elbow joint?
    a. Ulnar nerve
    b. Brachialis
    c. Median nerve
    d. Brachial artery
    e. Tendon of biceps brachii

24. Which of the following muscles is NOT innervated by a branch of the posterior cord of the brachial plexus?
    a. Subscapularis
    b. Latissimus dorsi
    c. Anconeus
    d. Triceps brachii
    e. Rhomboid major

25. Which of the following muscles is NOT innervated by a branch of the lateral cord of the brachial plexus?
    a. Biceps brachii
    b. Brachioradialis
    c. Brachialis
    d. Coracobrachialis
    e. Pectoralis major

26. Which of the following is NOT part of the humerus?
    a. Trochlear notch
    b. Capitulum
    c. Medial epicondyle
    d. Deltoid tuberosity
    e. Lateral epicondyle

27. What is the root value of the musculocutaneous nerve?
    a. C5, C6
    b. C5, C6, C7
    c. C6, C7
    d. C6, C7, C8
    e. C7, C8

28. Which of the following tendons can NOT be palpated in the region of the wrist?
    a. Flexor pollicis longus
    b. Abductor pollicis longus
    c. Flexor carpi radialis
    d. Extensor pollicis longus
    e. Extensor pollicis brevis

29. Which of the following bones can NOT be palpated in the floor of the 'anatomical snuffbox'?
    a. Radial styloid process
    b. Triquetral
    c. Scaphoid
    d. Base of the 1st metacarpal
    e. Trapezium

30. Within the hand which of the following muscles is NOT innervated by the ulnar nerve?
   a. Dorsal interossei
   b. 3rd and 4th lumbricals
   c. Palmar interossei
   d. Flexor pollicis brevis
   e. Opponens digiti minimi

31. What is the action of coracobrachialis?
   a. Flexion of the forearm arm at the elbow joint
   b. Extension of the forearm at the elbow joint
   c. Abduction of the arm at the shoulder joint
   d. Extension of the arm at the shoulder joint
   e. Adduction of the arm at the shoulder joint

32. Which nerve gives sensory innervation to the anterior aspect of the index finger?
   a. Radial nerve
   b. Ulnar nerve
   c. Median nerve
   d. Anterior interosseous nerve
   e. Posterior interosseous nerve

33. Concerning movements at the shoulder joint, which of the following statements is correct?
   a. Flexion is produced by pectoralis major.
   b. Extension is produced by serratus anterior.
   c. Abduction is produced by teres minor.
   d. Adduction is produced by infraspinatus.
   e. Flexion is produced by brachioradialis.

34. Which of the following statements is correct?
   a. The ulnar artery is a branch of the axillary artery.
   b. The radial artery passes deep to the tendon of extensor pollicis longus.
   c. The axillary artery passes over the 1st rib.
   d. The brachial artery lies lateral to the biceps tendon in the cubital fossa.
   e. The subclavian artery has no branches.

35. Concerning pronation and supination of the forearm, which of the following statements is correct?
   a. Biceps brachii is a powerful pronator.
   b. In supination the palm of the hand faces posteriorly.
   c. Brachioradialis can both supinate and pronate the forearm.
   d. The posterior interosseous nerve innervates pronator quadratus.
   e. The anterior interosseous nerve innervates supinator.

36. In flexion of the elbow joint against resistance, which of the following muscles is working concentrically?
   a. Coracobrachialis
   b. Extensor carpi radialis longus
   c. Biceps brachii
   d. Anconeus
   e. Triceps brachii

37. Which of the following muscles is NOT involved in flexion of the forearm at the elbow joint?
   a. Biceps brachii
   b. Brachialis
   c. Flexor carpi radialis
   d. Coracobrachialis
   e. Pronator teres

38. Which of the following muscles is NOT innervated by the posterior interosseous nerve?
   a. Abductor pollicis brevis
   b. Abductor pollicis longus
   c. Extensor indicis
   d. Extensor digiti minimi
   e. Extensor digitorum

39. Which of the following bones does NOT articulate with the capitate?
   a. Scaphoid
   b. Lunate
   c. Trapezoid
   d. 3rd metacarpal
   e. 5th metacarpal

40. Which of the following statements is NOT correct?
   a. The princeps pollicis artery is a branch of the radial artery.
   b. The profunda brachii artery is a branch of the axillary artery.
   c. The cephalic vein arises from the lateral end of the dorsal venous arch.
   d. The basilic vein becomes the axillary vein.
   e. The superficial palmar arch lies deep to the palmar aponeurosis.

41. Which of the following groups of lymph nodes are NOT located in the axilla?
   a. Central
   b. Apical
   c. Subscapular
   d. Pectoral
   e. Infraclavicular

42. The axis of flexion/extension of the wrist passes through the:
    a. scaphoid
    b. capitate
    c. trapezium
    d. lunate
    e. hamate

43. Which of the following tendons lies over the dorsal aspect of the inferior radioulnar joint?
    a. Extensor digitorum
    b. Extensor carpi ulnaris
    c. Abductor pollicis longus
    d. Extensor digiti minimi
    e. Extensor indicis

44. Which muscle can be palpated in the web space between the thumb and index finger?
    a. 1st dorsal interosseous
    b. 1st palmar interosseous
    c. Adductor pollicis
    d. 1st lumbrical
    e. 2nd lumbrical

45. Which of the following pass deep to the flexor retinaculum?
    a. Ulnar artery
    b. Radial artery
    c. Median nerve
    d. Ulnar nerve
    e. Radial nerve

46. Which of the following muscles is NOT innervated by branches of the lateral cord of the brachial plexus?
    a. Pectoralis major
    b. Coracobrachialis
    c. Brachialis
    d. Biceps brachii
    e. Brachioradialis

47. Concerning movements at the elbow joint, which of the following statements is correct?
    a. Flexor digitorum profundus is working concentrically during flexion.
    b. Biceps brachii is working concentrically during extension against gravity.
    c. Brachioradialis is working concentrically during flexion.
    d. Triceps brachii is working eccentrically during extension against gravity.
    e. Brachialis is working concentrically during extension.

48. Concerning the wrist, which of the following statements is NOT correct?
    a. The median nerve passes deep to the flexor retinaculum.
    b. The flexor pollicis longus tendon passes through the flexor retinaculum.
    c. The ulnar artery passes deep to the flexor retinaculum.
    d. Extensors carpi radialis longus and brevis pass deep to the extensor retinaculum in the same compartment.
    e. The radial artery passes over the scaphoid in the 'anatomical snuffbox'.

49. How many bones articulate with the ulna?
    a. 1
    b. 2
    c. 3
    d. 4
    e. 5

50. Which of the following muscles does NOT attach to the medial border of the scapula?
    a. Rhomboid major
    b. Serratus anterior
    c. Rhomboid minor
    d. Trapezius
    e. Levator scapulae

51. Concerning the elbow joint, which of the following statements is correct?
    a. The medial collateral ligament attaches to the radius.
    b. The lateral collateral ligament is not attached to the radius.
    c. The ulnar nerve lies on the lateral collateral ligament.
    d. The posterior interosseous nerve enters the forearm between the two heads of pronator teres.
    e. The biceps tendon attaches to the coronoid process of the ulna.

52. Which of the following muscles is NOT considered to be part of the rotator cuff at the shoulder joint?
    a. Infraspinatus
    b. Supraspinatus
    c. Teres minor
    d. Teres major
    e. Subscapularis

53. Concerning pectoralis major, which of the following statements is NOT correct?
    a. It is innervated by the medial pectoral nerve.

b. It is a powerful adductor and medial rotator at the shoulder joint.

c. It attaches to the medial lip of the intertubercular groove.

d. It forms the anterior wall of the axilla.

e. It lies superficial to pectoralis minor.

54. Which of the following muscles does NOT have an attachment to the scapula?

   a. Serratus posterior superior
   b. Trapezius
   c. Subscapularis
   d. Teres major
   e. Omohyoid

55. Concerning muscles of the forearm, which of the following is NOT attached to the humerus?

   a. Flexor carpi ulnaris
   b. Supinator
   c. Extensor carpi radialis brevis
   d. Extensor pollicis longus
   e. Flexor carpi radialis

56. Concerning muscles of the arm, which of the following is NOT attached to the humerus?

   a. Triceps brachii
   b. Brachialis
   c. Biceps brachii
   d. Coracobrachialis
   e. Flexor digitorum superficialis

57. Which nerve supplies skin on the anterior aspect of the lateral two-thirds of the palm of the hand?

   a. Ulnar nerve
   b. Median nerve
   c. Radial nerve
   d. Musculocutaneous nerve
   e. Axillary nerve

58. What is the root value of the radial nerve?

   a. C5, C6
   b. C5, C6, C7
   c. C5, C6, C7, C8
   d. C6, C7
   e. C6, C7, C8

59. Which tendons are related to the lateral aspect of the radial styloid process?

   a. Extensor indicis and extensor digiti minimi
   b. Abductor pollicis longus and extensor pollicis brevis
   c. Abductor pollicis longus and extensor pollicis longus
   d. Extensor digitorum and extensor indicis
   e. Extensor carpi radialis longus and extensor carpi radialis brevis

60. Concerning movements of the digits, which of the following statements is NOT correct?

   a. The palmar interossei adduct the fingers.
   b. In flexion the thumb moves across the palm.
   c. The lumbricals extend the interphalangeal joints of the fingers.
   d. Passive rotation of the fingers is possible at the metacarpophalangeal joints.
   e. The axis for abduction/adduction of the fingers is along the 2nd metacarpal.

REFERENCES

American Association of Orthopaedic Surgeons. (1994) Joint Motion: Methods of Measuring and Recording (edited by WB Greene and JD Heckman). American Association of Orthopaedic Surgeons. Illinois.

Clarke, G.R., Willis, L.A., Fish, W.W., Nichols, P.J., 1975. Preliminary studies in measuring range of motion in normal and painful stiff shoulders. Rheumatol. Rehabil. 14, 39–46.

Downey, P.A., Fiebert, I., Stackpole-Brown, J.B., 1991. Shoulder range of motion in persons aged sixty and older. Phys. Ther. 71, S75.

Morrey, B.F., Chao, E.Y.S., 1981. Recurrent anterior dislocation of the shoulder. In: Black, J., Dumbleton, J.H. (Eds.), Clinical Biomechanics: A Case History Approach. Churchill Livingstone, Edinburgh, pp. 24–46.

Walker, J.M., Sue, D., Miles-Elkousy, N., Ford, G., Trevelyan, H., 1984. Active mobility of the extremities in older subjects. Phys. Ther. 64, 919–923.

Watanabe, H., Ogata, K., Amano, T., Okabe, T., 1979. The range of joint motion of the extremities in healthy Japanese people: the difference according to age. J. Jpn. Orthop. Assoc. 53, 275–281.

Lower Limb

OUTLINE

KEY CONCEPTS

- The bones of the lower limb are more robust than those of the upper limb.
- The pelvic girdle is a ring of bone providing (i) articulation of the lower limbs with the trunk and (ii) great strength for the transference of weight from the trunk to the lower limbs when standing and ischial tuberosities when sitting.
- The foot is a specialised supporting structure adapted for locomotion.
- Joint stability is maintained by the shape of articular surfaces and associated ligaments, reinforced by muscle activity.
- The articular surfaces of the joints of the lower limb are larger than their counterparts in the upper limb, reflecting the greater stresses transmitted.
- The knee is the largest joint situated between the longest bones in the body; the shape of its articular surfaces and arrangement of ligaments provide stability yet permit a wide range of motion.
- The shape of the articular surfaces of the ankle joint provides stability and support for the foot during activity.
- Innervation of the muscles of the (i) anterior, posterior and medial compartments of the thigh is by the femoral, sciatic and obturator nerves, respectively; (ii) anterior, posterior and lateral compartments of the leg/calf is by the deep fibular/peroneal, tibial and superficial fibular/peroneal)

- nerves, respectively; and (iii) dorsum and sole of the foot is by the superficial fibular/peroneal and medial and lateral plantar nerves, respectively.
- Flexor and adductor muscles are supplied by the anterior divisions of the anterior rami of the lumbar and lumbosacral plexuses by the obturator, tibial, and medial and lateral plantar nerves: extensor muscles are supplied by posterior divisions of the anterior rami of the lumbar and lumbosacral plexuses by the femoral and common, superficial and deep fibular/peroneal nerves.
- Innervation of the skin of the lower limb reflects its outpouching from the trunk: anterior thigh (L1, L2, L3), anterior leg/calf (L4, L5), dorsum of foot (L5, S1), plantar surface of foot (L4, L5, S1), posterior leg/calf (L4, L5, S2) and posterior thigh (L2, L3, S2).
- Muscles crossing more than one joint promote coordinated movement and function.
- The combination of activity in different muscles acting across a joint produces a wide range of movement in many directions.
- The role of most muscles is to stabilise the joints they cross: producing movement is a secondary function.
- The lower limb is adapted to (i) support body weight and (ii) provide restraint and propulsion during locomotion and other activities.

OVERVIEW

This part considers the anatomy, function, examination though palpation and clinical evaluation of the lower limb. It is organised into seven major sections: pelvic girdle; hip; knee; leg/calf; ankle; foot, including the toes; and nerves. In addition, there is a section on blood supply and lymphatic drainage, as well as another which considers simple activities of the lower limb.

In each section, the relevant bones are considered, including their palpation, followed by the joints between the bones, their palpation, movements possible at the joint and the muscles producing each movement. For each muscle mentioned, its attachments, innervation, action and palpation are given. Clinical examination and the evaluation of movement for each joint are presented, including

its measurement and the end feel of the movement. At the end of each section is a summary of the bones, joints and muscles (including root value of their nerve supply) involved, and the clinical examination of each movement. There is also a selection of self-assessment questions at the end of each section. At the end of this part are a series of self-assessment multiple choice questions.

INTRODUCTION

The human lower limb is adapted for weight-bearing, locomotion and maintaining the unique, erect, bipedal posture; for all of these functions, a greater degree of strength and stability are required than in the upper limb. The bones of the lower limb, therefore, are larger and more robust than their upper limb counterparts, varying in their characteristics in relation to muscular development and body build. Many bones, particularly the innominate and to a lesser extent the femur, show sexual differences (variations in the female pelvis are an adaptation for childbearing).

The form and structure of individual bones are adapted to the functions of supporting and resisting mechanical stresses; their internal architecture is organised to resist all such stresses and forces, being particularly marked in the articular regions. During growth and throughout life, continuous modifications are made to maintain the functions of support and resistance to stress as the stresses change. The attainment of a habitual erect posture and bipedal gait has resulted in a change in both the mechanical and functional requirements of all bones of the lower limb; during evolution, the lower limb has been the subject of major change.

The pelvic girdle, formed by the right and left innominates articulating anteriorly at the symphysis pubis and posteriorly with the sacrum at the sacroiliac joints, connects the lower limbs to the vertebral column. The sacroiliac joint provides great strength for weight transference from the trunk to the lower limb at the sacrifice of almost all mobility. The human ilium has developed so that it is no longer blade-like but is shortened and tightly curved posterolaterally (Fig. 3.1), changing the actions of the gluteal muscles; these pelvic changes have resulted in a shift from it lying essentially horizontal to becoming effectively

vertical. This has enabled the trunk to be held erect but has necessitated a change in the orientation of the sacrum with respect to the ilium, the result being that the axis of the pelvic canal lies almost at right angles to the vertebral column. During evolution, there has been a relative approximation of the sacral articular surface to the acetabulum providing greater stability in the transmission of the weight of the trunk to the hip joint. This increase in magnitude has resulted in an increase in contact area between the sacrum and ilium relative to the area of the ilium as a whole. For the same reason, the acetabulum and femoral head have also increased in relative size during evolution. The shortening of the ischium is an adaptation for speed and rapid movements, which is of great importance in bipeds; power has, therefore, been sacrificed for speed.

Changes have also occurred in the knee, with the femoral condyles being more parallel in humans than other primates. The major change, however, has been in bringing the knees towards the midline; this appears to be part of the overall pattern of centering body mass by reinforcing skeletal rather than muscular equilibrium.

In humans, the tibia and fibula are held tightly together, with the tibia being the weight-bearing component and the fibula mainly for muscle attachments; there has been a loss of rotation of the fibula with respect to the tibia.

It is the foot, however, which has undergone the greatest change during evolution (Fig. 3.2), reflecting not so much the evolution of a new function but more

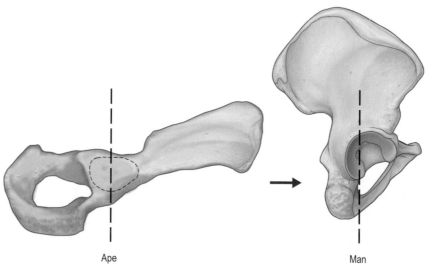

Ape   Man

Fig. 3.1 Evolutionary changes in the human pelvis as part of the adaptation to the erect posture and bipedalism.

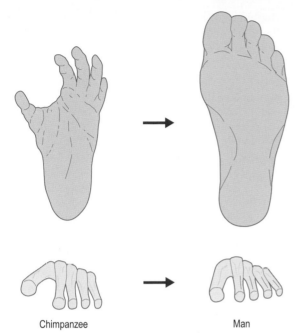

Chimpanzee   Man

Fig. 3.2 Evolutionary changes within the foot during its adaptation to bipedalism.

a reduction in the original primate functions, with the foot changing from a grasping tactile organ to a locomotor prop. Although some non-locomotor function is still possible, the foot has evolved from a generalised to a specialised organ. The joints of the human foot permit much less internal mobility as an adaptation to ground walking. In locomotion, the foot acts as a lever, adding propulsive force to that of the lower limb, with the point of pivot being the subtalar joint. The forefoot has shortened relative to the hindfoot, where the main thrust in walking is developed; the power capabilities are thus accentuated.

The shape of the bony elements of the foot has created longitudinal and transverse arches, supported by ligaments and tendons, converting it into a complex spring under tension. This enables the foot to transmit the stresses involved in walking, both when body momentum is checked at heel-strike as well as when the foot is used in propelling the body forward. The lateral arch helps steady the foot on the ground, while the medial arch transmits the main thrust in propulsion. It is the arched arrangement of the foot which is important in providing one of the major determinants of gait (minimising energy expenditure and increasing the efficiency of walking).

One important consequence of the erect bipedal posture is that the centre of gravity of the body has been brought towards the vertebral column; in humans, it lies slightly posterior to and at a similar level as the hip joint, reducing the tendency of gravity to pull the trunk forward. The centre of gravity projection then passes anterior to the knee and ankle joints; at the knee, it passes towards the lateral aspect of the joint. Because of the angulation of the femur during walking, the foot, tibia and knee joint of each leg stay close to the line followed by the centre of gravity; energy expenditure is minimal in maintaining the centre of gravity above the supporting limb. Balance is improved with more time for the free limb to swing forward, promoting an increase in stride length. The alteration in the line of weight transmission is carried into the foot, where it passes to the medial side. However, it must be remembered that weight is also transmitted through the lateral part of the foot, bringing the entire foot into use as a stabilising element.

To reduce the possibility of collapse or dislocation due to the forces they are subjected to, the joints of the lower limb are structurally more stable than those of the upper limb. This increased stability is due to either the shape of the articular surfaces, the number and strength of the associated ligaments or the size of the associated muscles; each of these factors contributes to varying extents at individual joints.

Rotation of the lower limb during development resulted in the extensor and flexor surfaces coming to lie anteriorly and posteriorly, respectively (see Fig. 1.10); this is reflected in the arrangement of its innervation. The muscles on the anterior aspect of the thigh and leg/calf are supplied by nerves from the posterior part of the lumbar and lumbosacral plexuses (femoral and common fibular/peroneal nerves), while those on the posterior aspect of the thigh and leg/calf and in the sole of the foot are from the anterior aspect of the lumbosacral plexus (tibial nerve).

As in the upper limb, many muscles cross several joints and exert their actions on each; it is unusual for one joint of the lower limb to be moved in isolation. In standing and walking, the joints and muscles of the lower limb work in coordinated patterns to produce effective movement and support.

The superior limit of the lower limb is a line joining the iliac crest, inguinal ligament, symphysis pubis, ischiopubic ramus, ischial tuberosity, sacrotuberous ligament and dorsum of the sacrum and coccyx. The bulge of tissue running between the innominate and proximal part of the femur forms the buttock but is usually referred to as gluteal after the underlying muscles. The lower limb is divided into the thigh between the hip and knee, the leg/calf between the knee and ankle, and the foot distal to the ankle joint. The foot is divided into the foot proper and the toes, and has superior (dorsal) and inferior (plantar) surfaces (Fig. 3.3); the plantar surface is the sole.

The bones of the lower limb are those of the pelvic girdle (innominate, sacrum), the femur in the thigh, the medial tibia and lateral fibula in the leg/calf, the seven tarsal bones and five metatarsals in the foot and the phalanges of the toes; two in the hallux and three in each remaining toe (Fig. 3.3).

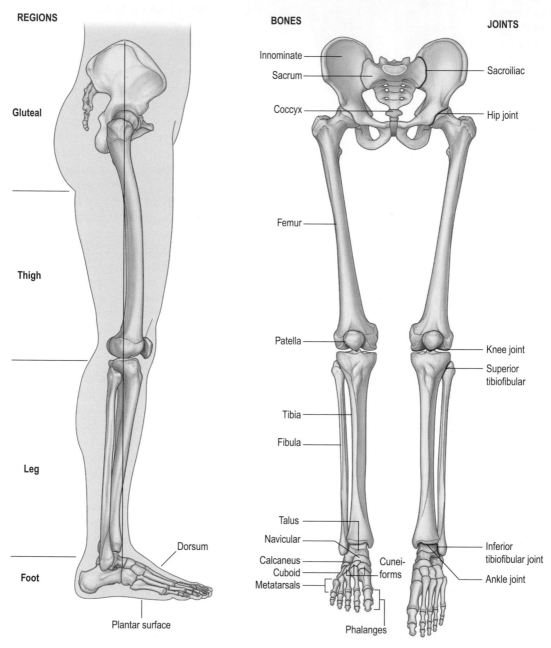

REGIONS

Gluteal

Thigh

Leg

Foot

Dorsum

Plantar surface

BONES

Innominate
Sacrum
Coccyx

Femur

Patella

Tibia
Fibula

Talus
Navicular
Calcaneus
Cuboid
Metatarsals
Cunei-forms

Phalanges

JOINTS

Sacroiliac

Hip joint

Knee joint
Superior tibiofibular

Inferior tibiofibular joint
Ankle joint

Fig. 3.3 Regions, bones and joints of the lower limb.

Fasciae of the Lower Limb
Fascial Projections from the Abdomen into the Thigh

The fascial lining of the abdomen and pelvis is a continuous membranous bag outside the peritoneum. The transversalis fascia is that part lying on the deep surface of transversus abdominis; inferiorly, it is thick and strong where it attaches to the inguinal ligament and iliac crest. From the anterior superior to posterior superior iliac spines, it becomes the iliac fascia, being reflected over the surface of iliacus. As the femoral vessels pass from the abdomen, where they are deep to the fascia, they drag with them a fascial covering (femoral sheath) with the anterior and posterior parts of the sheath derived from the transversalis and iliac parts of the fascia, respectively. The femoral sheath is divided into three compartments by septa passing between its anterior and posterior walls. About three fingers' breadth below the inguinal ligament the femoral sheath blends with the adventitia of the femoral vessels.

As the transversalis fascia passes posteriorly, it becomes continuous with the anterior layer of thoracolumbar fascia (covering quadratus lumborum) and then with the fascia over the anterior surface of psoas major. At the superior margins of quadratus lumborum and psoas major, the fascia is thickened forming the lateral and medial arcuate ligaments, respectively (p. 557). The fascia surrounding psoas major forms a sheath from its proximal attachments in the abdomen to the lesser trochanter of the femur, completely enclosing it.

Fasciae of the Thigh and Leg/Calf

Functionally, there are two types of fascia in the lower limb; the superficial fascia merges with and acts as a base for the skin enabling it to move freely over the underlying tissue, while the investing layer of the deep fascia consists of dense, tough, fibrous tissue. Where the investing layer passes over bony projections, it usually becomes attached to them. From its deep surface, sheets of similar tissue (intermuscular septa) pass between different muscle groups. The septa are usually attached to bone, serving to maintain the shape of the limb as well as exerting a compression force on the contents of the compartments formed.

Superficial fascia. Continuous with that of the abdominal wall, perineum and trunk, the two layers of superficial fascia present in the lower part of the abdominal wall and perineum continue into the proximal part of the anterior thigh. The deeper membranous layer crosses superficial to the inguinal ligament entering the thigh, fusing with the deep fascia along a line approximately one finger's breadth below and parallel to the inguinal ligament, limiting the spread of fluid into the thigh from the perineum or deep to the superficial abdominal fascia.

The superficial fascia is thick and fatty in the gluteal region, with the fat contributing to the shape of the buttock and forming the gluteal fold; there is usually a deposit of fat over the lateral part of the female thigh (secondary sexual characteristic). Over the ischial tuberosity, the fascia has many dense strands of tissue enclosing fat, helping to distribute the high pressures from the weight of the seated body, preventing tissue damage. Similarly, on the sole of the foot, the superficial fascia is characterised by its thickness and the presence of fat pads under the heel, balls and pads of the toes. These also serve to protect underlying structures from high pressures; the heel pad can be 2 cm thick. The fascia covering the rest of the leg/calf and foot has no particular features.

Deep fascia. Composed of much stronger fibres the deep fascia tends to be organised in the same direction as the applied stresses. It covers the lower limb in a similar way as the superficial fascia but attaches to the most prominent bony points, as well as all around the groin and buttocks. Further details of the deep fascia can be found in each region.

PELVIC GIRDLE

LEARNING OUTCOMES

By the end of the section, you should be able to:

1. Identify, palpate and examine the innominate and sacrum
2. Describe the bones, joints and muscles of the pelvic girdle
3. Describe and explain the movements possible, and their restraints, at the sacroiliac, symphysis pubis, lumbosacral and sacrococcygeal joints
4. Locate, palpate and examine the muscles associated with the pelvic girdle, and give their attachments, action and innervation
5. Examine and assess movements of the pelvic girdle
6. Appreciate the role of the pelvic girdle and its joints in transmitting stresses from the trunk to the lower limbs
7. Appreciate the influence of pathology and/or trauma on the function of the pelvic girdle

INTRODUCTION

The pelvic girdle is a ring of bone providing articulation for the lower limbs with the trunk (Fig. 3.4); it comprises two innominates and the sacrum, with the ring of bone formed uniting the trunk and lower limbs. Each large irregular innominate consists of two expanded triangular blades twisted 90 degrees to each other in the region of the acetabulum; each blade is also twisted within itself. The innominate is formed from three separate bones (ilium, ischium, pubis) which fuse in the region of the acetabulum; in adults, each innominate appears as a single bone. The roughly triangular sacrum consists of five fused vertebrae: the coccyx (remnant of the tail) consists of four fused coccygeal vertebrae. Each innominate articulates with the sacrum posteriorly by a synovial joint and with each other anteriorly at the symphysis pubis by a secondary cartilaginous joint; the sacroiliac joint tends to be synovial anteriorly and fibrous posteriorly. Superiorly, the sacrum articulates with the fifth lumbar vertebra at the lumbosacral junction and inferiorly with the coccyx at the sacrococcygeal joint; as part of the vertebral column, these latter two joints are both secondary cartilaginous joints. The articulation of the pelvis with the lower limb is at the acetabulum (p. 262).

The bony pelvis is arranged to provide great strength for the transference of weight from the trunk to the lower limbs when standing or to the ischial tuberosities when sitting. This major function of stability has been achieved with loss of mobility at both the sacroiliac joint and symphysis

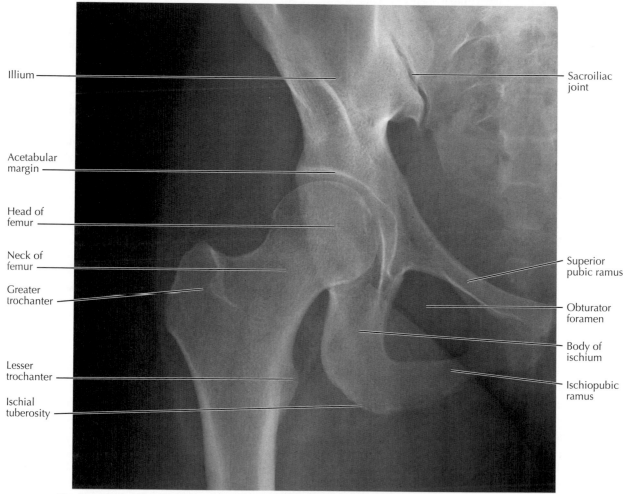

Fig. 3.4 Anteroposterior radiograph of the right hemipelvis also showing the sacroiliac joint. (From Frank, H.N., 2022. Netter Atlas of Human Anatomy: Classic Regional Approach. Elsevier.)

pubis; however, under certain conditions (childbirth) a greater degree of movement is possible at both joints.

The evolutionary development of the pelvis and its articulation with the vertebral column via the lumbosacral junction is considered by many to lag behind the adaptations of the remaining skeleton. The anatomical position of the pelvis is neither vertical, as in quadrupeds, nor horizontal; special provision has, therefore, to be made to prevent the sacrum being pushed anteroinferiorly under the superincumbent body weight. The lumbosacral junction represents the transition between the mobile and immobile portions of the vertebral column; consequently, it tends to be the least stable part of the vertebral column, being exposed to static stresses and is less well-equipped to meet them adequately than any other part of the vertebral column.

The pelvic girdle has several functions:
1. Support and protection of pelvic viscera.
2. Support body weight transmitted from the vertebral column, across the sacroiliac joints to the innominate, then to the femora when standing (Fig. 3.5) or the ischial tuberosities when sitting; the bony and associated ligamentous components reflect these functions.
3. During walking, the pelvis moves from side to side (initiated by rotation at the hip joint) accompanied by small movements at the lumbar intervertebral joints; if the hip joints become fused, pelvic rotation is taken up by the thoracic part of the vertebral column enabling the individual to walk reasonably well.
4. Gives attachment to muscles of the trunk and lower limb.
5. In females provides bony support for the birth canal.

The pelvis is essentially a basin, with the superior part being the greater (false) pelvis containing abdominal viscera, with that part inferior to the pelvic brim (pelvic inlet) being the lesser (true) pelvis. In the anatomical position, the pelvic inlet forms an angle of approximately 60 degrees with the horizontal (Fig. 3.6); the acetabulum is directed inferolaterally with the acetabular notch directed inferiorly. The anterior superior iliac spines (ASIS) and pubic tubercles lie in the same vertical coronal plane; the most inferior part of the sacrum lies above the level of the symphysis pubis.

INNOMINATE

An irregularly shaped bone (Fig. 3.7) consisting of three separate bones (ilium, pubis, ischium) fused together.

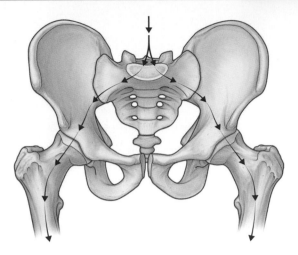

Fig. 3.5 Weight transfer from the vertebral column through the pelvis to the femur.

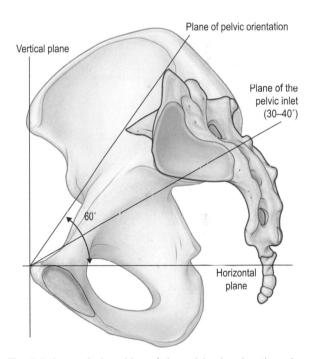

Fig. 3.6 Anatomical position of the pelvis showing the orientation of the pelvic inlet and outlet with respect to the vertical and horizontal planes.

Ilium

Forming the pelvic brim between the hip joint and articulation of the innominate with the sacrum, the superior broad blade of the ilium gives attachment to ligaments and large muscles. The anterior two-thirds form the iliac

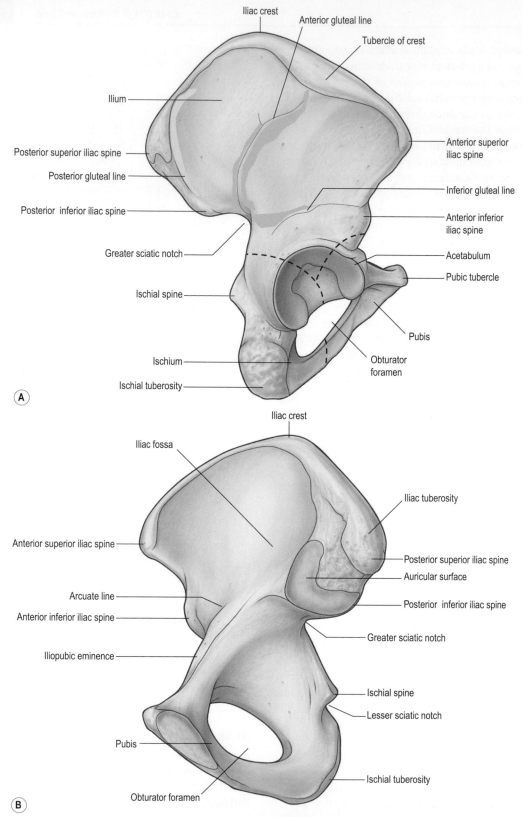

Fig. 3.7 Lateral (A) and medial (B) aspects of the right innominate; the dashed red lines represent the lines of fusion of its constituent parts.

fossa medially, part of the lateral and posterior abdominal wall, and the gluteal surface laterally for attachment of the gluteal muscles. The thicker posterior third of the medial surface carries the auricular surface for articulation with the sacrum, behind which is a prolonged rough part (iliac tuberosity) for attachment of the strong sacroiliac ligaments which bear body weight. The superior border (iliac crest) is convex superiorly and anteroposteriorly with the anterior part curved laterally. The iliac crest ends at the anterior superior iliac spine anteriorly and posterior superior iliac spine posteriorly; both spines and the whole of the crest can be palpated (p. 262). Posterior to the anterior spine on the lateral border is the prominent tubercle of the crest. Between the anterior superior and inferior iliac spines is a shallow notch, similarly between the posterior superior iliac spine and posterior inferior iliac spine is also a shallow notch; the two anterior spines are further apart than the posterior spines. Inferior to the posterior inferior iliac spine is the deep greater sciatic notch. The arcuate line (part of the pelvic brim) separates the iliac fossa from the sacropelvic surface of the ilium. The anterior part of this line has an elevation (iliopubic eminence) marking the junction of the ilium and pubis. That part participating in the formation of the acetabulum is the body of the ilium.

The lateral gluteal surface follows the curvature of the iliac crest and has three curved gluteal lines demarcating the attachments of the gluteal muscles. The most obvious (posterior gluteal line) passes from the iliac crest to anterior to the posterior inferior iliac spine. The anterior gluteal line is a series of low tubercles from the iliac crest curving superoposteriorly inferior to the iliac tubercle and then towards the greater sciatic notch. The inferior gluteal line is less prominent, curving from inferior to the anterior superior iliac spine towards the apex of the greater sciatic notch; below the inferior gluteal line is an area of multiple vascular foramina. Fusion of the ilium and ischium is marked by a rounded elevation between the acetabulum and greater sciatic notch; above this, the ilium forms the major part of the notch. The gluteal surface is succeeded inferiorly by the acetabular part of the ilium.

The iliac fossa is the smooth medial concavity of the ala of the ilium, narrowing inferiorly it ends at the roughened iliopubic eminence (line of junction between the ilium and pubis). Its deepest part, high in the fossa, consists of paper-thin translucent bone. The pelvic brim, marked by the arcuate line of the ilium, is the posteroinferior limit of the iliac fossa. Posterior and inferior to the iliac fossa and the arcuate line is the sacropelvic surface of the ilium. The

region posterior to the iliac fossa has the auricular surface for the first two segments of the sacrum and, posterosuperior to it, the iliac tuberosity. The roughened tuberosity provides attachment for the short posterior sacroiliac ligaments, together with fibres of erector spinae and multifidus. The auricular area extends from the pelvic brim to the posterior inferior iliac spine, with its surface gently undulating, convex superiorly and concave inferiorly, roughened by numerous tubercles and depressions. The surface is covered with hyaline cartilage forming an immobile synovial joint with the ala of the sacrum; in later years fibrous bands usually join the articular surfaces within the joint space.

Pubis

The quadrilateral body has a medially directed oval surface crossed by several transverse ridges giving attachment to the fibrocartilage of the symphysis pubis; the surface is covered with hyaline cartilage. The superior border of the body is the pubic crest, marked laterally by the pubic tubercle from which two ridges diverge laterally into the superior ramus. The superior of these ridges (pectineal line) is continuous with the arcuate line of the ilium, and forms part of the pelvic brim. The inferior rounded ridge (obturator crest) passes inferiorly into the anterior margin of the acetabular notch; between the two ridges is the iliopubic eminence. Below the obturator crest on the superior pubic ramus is the deep obturator groove; the superior ramus continues laterally to join the ilium and ischium at the acetabulum forming 1/5th of the acetabulum. A thin flattened inferior ramus extends inferiorly and posterolaterally from the body to fuse with the ischium inferior to the obturator foramen.

Ischium

The angulated posteroinferior part of the innominate. The angulation is in the same plane as the pubis. The blunt rounded apex of the angulation (ischial tuberosity) is divided transversely by a low ridge; the smooth oval above the ridge is further subdivided by a vertical ridge into lateral and medial areas. When seated, the weight of the body rests on the two ischial tuberosities. Anteriorly, the tuberosity passes superiorly as the ischial ramus, continuous with the inferior pubic ramus, forming the ischiopubic ramus. The body of the ischium forms 2/5th of the acetabulum. The posterior border of the body is continuous superiorly with the ilium, forming the greater sciatic notch; inferiorly it ends as the blunt medially projecting ischial spine, below which is the lesser sciatic notch. The pelvic surface of the body is continuous with the pelvic surface of the ilium and forms part of the lateral wall of the pelvis.

Acetabulum

Formed by fusion of the three components of the innominate, the ilium, ischium and pubis meet at a Y-shaped cartilage forming their epiphyseal junction; it is a hemispherical hollow on the lateral surface of the innominate facing inferoanterolaterally. The anterior 1/5th is formed by the pubis, the posterosuperior 2/5th by the body of the ilium and posteroinferior 2/5th by the body of the ischium. The prominent rim of the acetabulum is deficient inferiorly (acetabular notch); the rim gives attachment to the acetabular labrum of the hip joint, with its uneven internal edge providing attachment for the synovial membrane lining the joint capsule. The acetabular labrum continues across the acetabular notch as the transverse ligament which, together with the margins of the notch, gives attachment to the ligament of the head of the femur. The heavy acetabular wall comprises a semilunar articular portion covered with hyaline cartilage (open inferiorly) and a deep central non-articular portion (acetabular fossa); the acetabular fossa is formed mainly from the ischium and often has thin walls.

Obturator Foramen

Large opening surrounded by the sharp margins of the pubis and ischium, with those of the pubis overlapping each other in a spiral forming the obturator groove, which runs obliquely anteroinferiorly from the pelvis into the thigh; the groove is converted into a canal by a specialisation of the obturator fascia. The obturator membrane attaches to the margins of the foramen, except superiorly at the obturator groove.

Ossification

Each innominate ossifies from eight centres: three primary centres, one each for the ilium, ischium and pubis, and five secondary centres, one each for the iliac crest, anterior inferior iliac spine, ischial tuberosity, pubic symphysis and triradiate cartilage at the centre of the acetabulum. The sequence of ossification has functional significance because of the support given to the pelvic organs and its role in weight transmission. The primary ossification centres appear during the 3rd, 4th and 5th months *in utero* in the ilium, ischium and pubis, respectively. At birth, the individual bones are quite separate, with the secondary ossification centres having yet to appear. By age 13 or 14, the major parts of the ilium, ischium and pubis are completely bony, but separated by the Y-shaped triradiate cartilage in the acetabulum. At age 8 or 9, three major centres of ossification appear in the acetabular cartilage; the largest appears in the anterior wall of the acetabulum and fuses with the pubis. Further centres appear in the iliac acetabular cartilage, fusing superiorly with the ilium, and in the ischial acetabular cartilage, fusing posteriorly with the ischium. Fusion of the three bones in the acetabulum occurs between 16 and 18 years. The remaining secondary ossification centres appear around puberty and unite with the major bones between 20 and 22 years.

Palpation

The anterior superior iliac spine can easily be palpated, particularly in females, where they tend to be further apart, at the anterior end of the iliac crest in the upper part of the pocket area. Tracing posteriorly from these spines, the iliac crest is easily palpable, having a large tuberosity approximately 5 cm from its anterior end. Following the crest as far posterior as possible, the smaller posterior superior iliac spines can be palpated; they are situated in dimples in females, but in males, each appears as a small, raised tubercle.

Approximately 10 cm below the centre of the iliac crest, the greater trochanter of the femur can be clearly felt. When sitting, the body rests on the ischial tuberosity of each innominate; by placing the hands under this area the tuberosities can be readily felt. This part of the tuberosity is covered by a bursa which often becomes painful and swollen (bursitis) when sitting for too long on a hard surface.

If the hands are passed down the anterior aspect of the anterior abdominal wall, a bony ring can be felt approximately 5 cm above the genitalia which has a central depression where the pubic symphysis is situated; each pubic tubercle is approximately 1 cm superior and lateral on either side.

SACRUM

Triangular bone with an inferior apex consisting of five fused vertebrae; it is broadened by the incorporation of large costal elements and transverse processes (lateral masses), which lie lateral to the transverse tubercles on the posterior aspect of the sacrum extending between the anterior sacral foramina onto the anterior aspect of the bone; the auricular surface lies entirely on the lateral mass. The sacrum is wedged between the posterior parts of the two innominates with which it articulates at the sacroiliac joints. The pelvic (anterior) surface (Fig. 3.8A) is concave and relatively smooth, marked by four transverse ridges separating the bodies of the five sacral vertebrae. Lateral to each ridge is the anterior sacral foramen, being the anterior part of the intervertebral foramen; the foramina are directed laterally and anteriorly.

The posterior surface (Fig. 3.8B) is convex and highly irregular with posterior sacral foramina, medial to which the vertebral canal is closed over by the fused laminae;

however, the spinous processes and laminae of the fourth and fifth sacral vertebrae are usually absent, leaving an inferior entrance (sacral hiatus) into the vertebral canal, which may be used to introduce an anaesthetic agent to block the sacral nerves (during labour). Posteriorly, in the midline, the reduced spinous processes form

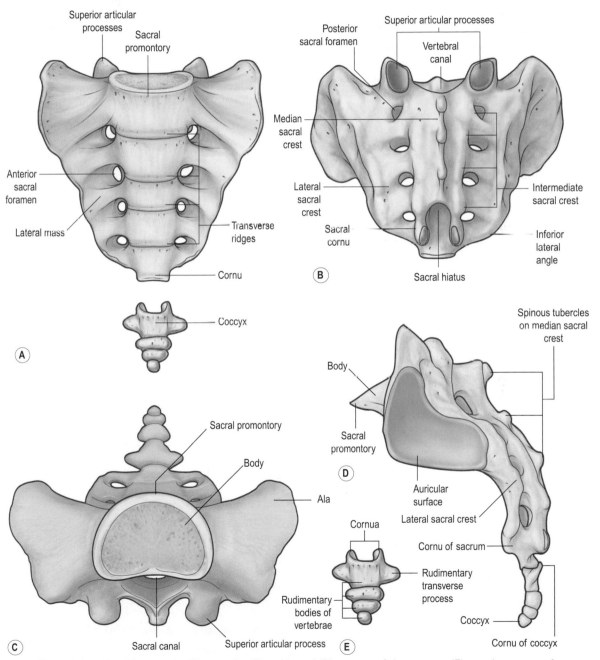

Fig. 3.8 Anterior (A), posterior (B), superior (C) and lateral (D) aspects of the sacrum; (E) anterior aspect of the coccyx.

the median sacral crest. Lateral to the posterior sacral foramina are the prominent lateral sacral crests representing the transverse processes, providing attachment for the dorsal sacroiliac ligaments, and inferiorly for the sacrotuberous and sacrospinous ligaments. Medial to the posterior sacral foramina are the indistinct intermediate sacral crests representing the fused articular processes. The superior articular processes of the first sacral vertebra are large and oval, supported by short heavy pedicles; their facets (for articulation with the inferior articular surfaces of the fifth lumbar vertebra) are concave from side to side and face posteromedially. The tubercles of the inferior articular processes of the fifth sacral vertebra (sacral cornua) articulate with the coccygeal cornua.

The triangular lateral surface (Fig. 3.8D) is narrower below; the superior part is divided into an anterior smoother pitted auricular surface covered in cartilage for articulation with a similar area on the ilium, while the rougher posterior area has three deep impressions for attachment of the powerful posterior sacroiliac ligaments. The superior surface (Fig. 3.8C) faces anterosuperiorly and has a central oval area (superior surface of the first sacral vertebra) separated from the fifth lumbar vertebra by a thick intervertebral disc; it has an anterior projecting border (sacral promontory). On each side of the body is the ala, formed by the fusion of the costal and transverse processes of the first sacral vertebra. When the sacrum articulates with the innominate, each ala of the sacrum is continuous with that of the ilium.

Ossification

Primary centres appear in the sacrum between the 3rd and 8th month *in utero*; one for each vertebral body, one for each half of each vertebral arch and one for each costal element in the upper four sacral vertebrae. The costal elements fuse with the arches by age 5, the arches with the body slightly later, with the two parts of each arch uniting between ages 7 and 10. The segments of the lateral masses fuse together during puberty, with secondary centres appearing for the vertebral bodies at about the same time. The bodies and epiphyses fuse between 18 and 25 years. Several secondary centres appear at the ends of the costal and transverse processes from which two epiphyses are formed, one of which covers the auricular surface while the other completes the inferior margin of the sacrum.

COCCYX

Usually consisting of four fused vertebrae the coccyx forms a single or two bones (Fig. 3.8E), which are mainly the bodies. The pelvic surface is concave and relatively smooth, while on the posterior surface, rudimentary articular processes are present as a row of tubercles. Superiorly, the larger pair (coccygeal cornua) articulate with the sacral cornua and enclose the fifth sacral intervertebral foramen. The posterior wall of the vertebral canal of the coccyx is absent so that the sacral hiatus continues inferiorly over the posterior aspect of the coccyx.

SACROILIAC JOINT

Articular Surfaces

Between the auricular surfaces of the ilium and ala of the sacrum (Figs 3.4 and 3.9A); the surfaces are approximately L-shaped, being broader superiorly and narrower inferiorly, and show marked reciprocal irregularities. The central part of the sacral auricular surface is concave with raised crests on either side; conversely, the ilial auricular surface has a central crest lying between two furrows. The inferior parts of the auricular surfaces are shaped so that the widest part of the sacral surface is on its pelvic side. On the sacrum, the auricular surface occupies the upper two vertebral segments in females but usually extends onto the third segment in males. The shape and degree of irregularity of the surfaces vary considerably between individuals and often between each side within the same individual. The auricular surface of the sacrum is covered with hyaline cartilage, while that on the corresponding ilial surface is usually a form of fibrocartilage. With increasing age, particularly in males, the joint cavity becomes partially (occasionally completely) obliterated by fibrous bands or fibrocartilaginous adhesions between the articular surfaces; in very old individuals, the joint may show partial bony fusion. Because the region behind the synovial joint is united by powerful interosseous ligaments, some consider it to be both a synovial (anterior) and a fibrous (posterior) joint.

Surface Marking

The line of the sacroiliac joint is too deep for it to be palpable; however, its surface marking can be estimated as follows. From the posterior superior iliac spine, an oblique line at approximately 25 degrees passing from superolateral to inferomedial and extending 2 cm in each direction represents the joint line.

Joint Capsule and Synovial Membrane

A fibrous capsule completely surrounds the joint, attaching to the articular margins on both bones. Synovial membrane lines all non-articular surfaces.

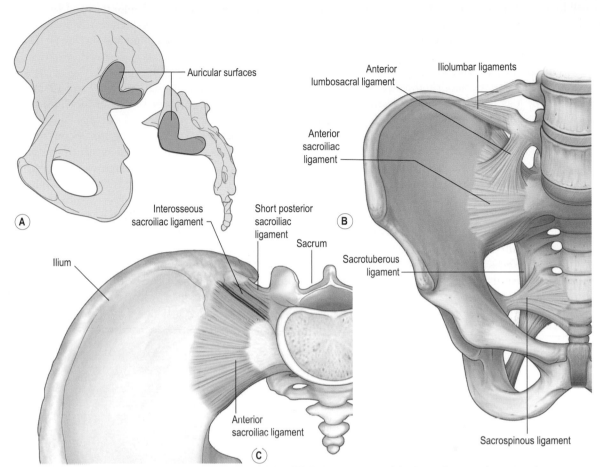

Fig. 3.9 (A) Articular surfaces of the sacroiliac joint. (B) Anterior aspect of the Innominate and sacrum showing the anterior sacroiliac, sacrotuberous and sacrospinous ligaments. (C) Superior aspect of the sacroiliac joint showing the anterior, interosseous and short posterior sacroiliac ligaments.

Ligaments

Because of the nature and position of the joint, it is richly endowed with ligaments. Extremely strong posterior and slightly weaker anterior sacroiliac ligaments surround and reinforce the joint capsule. Accessory ligaments situated some distance from the joint provide additional stability against unwanted movement.

Anterior Sacroiliac Ligament

Broad and flat, the anterior sacroiliac ligament consists of numerous thin bands on the pelvic side of the joint (Fig. 3.9B and C). It passes from the ala and pelvic surface of the sacrum, either side of the pelvic brim, to the adjoining margin of the auricular surface of the ilium. It is stronger in females, indenting a preauricular groove on the ilium just inferior to the pelvic brim.

Posterior Sacroiliac Ligaments

These lie posterior and superior to the joint and are much thicker and stronger than those anteriorly. Several distinct bands can be identified as they fill the space between the sacrum and tuberosity of the ilium.

Interosseous sacroiliac ligament. Deepest of all posterior ligaments, it is short, thick and extremely strong filling the narrow cleft between the rough areas on the bones immediately posterior and superior to the auricular surfaces (Fig. 3.9C). Small accessory joint cavities, usually no more than one or two, may sometimes be found within the ligament between facets close to the posterior superior iliac spine and transverse tubercles of the sacrum.

Long and short posterior sacroiliac ligaments. Superficial to the interosseous ligament, the posterior ligament consists of numerous bands passing between the two bones. In general, the longer fibres run obliquely inferomedially; however, within this arrangement, two sets of fibres can usually be identified. The short posterior sacroiliac ligament is found in the superior part of the cleft between the two bones passing horizontally between the first and second transverse tubercles of the sacrum and the iliac tuberosity (Figs 3.9C and 3.10A); they are arranged to resist anterior movement of the sacral promontory. The long posterior sacroiliac ligament has the longest and most superficial fibres of the posterior complex. It runs almost vertically inferiorly from the posterior superior iliac spine to the third and fourth transverse tubercles of the sacrum (Fig. 3.10A); its fibres are arranged to resist inferior movement of the sacrum with respect to the ilium.

Accessory Ligaments

In addition to the ligaments above, accessory ligaments confer added stability to the joint; the most important being the sacrotuberous and sacrospinous ligaments which help stabilise the sacrum on the innominate by preventing forward tilting of the sacral promontory. They also convert the greater and lesser sciatic notches into the greater and lesser sciatic foramina (Fig. 3.10B),

through which several important structures leave the pelvis. In addition to the sacrotuberous and sacrospinous ligaments, the iliolumbar ligament assists in strengthening the bond between the ilium and sacrum (p. 271).

Sacrotuberous Ligament

Flat, triangular band of great strength (Fig. 3.10) attaching superiorly to the posterior border of the ilium between the posterior superior and inferior iliac spines, to the posterior and lateral aspects of the sacrum inferior to the auricular surface, and the lateral aspect of the superior part of the coccyx. From this extensive attachment, the fibres pass inferolaterally towards the ischial tuberosity, converging as they do so. However, before attaching to the medial surface of the ischial tuberosity, the fibres twist upon themselves and diverge again so that the attachment is prolonged along the inferior margin of the ischial ramus. This prolongation (falciform process) lies just inferior to the pudendal canal. The ligament as a whole is narrower in its middle part than at either end.

The most superficial fibres attaching to the ischial tuberosity are closely associated with the long head of

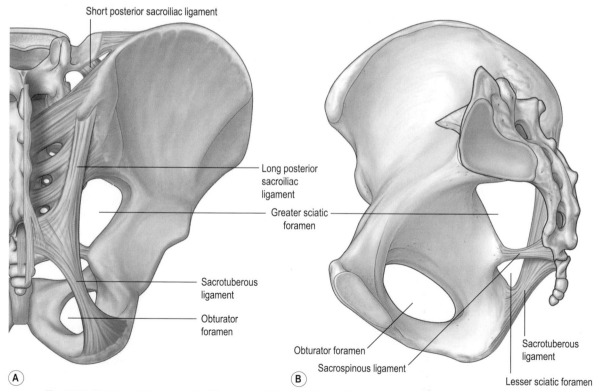

Fig. 3.10 Posterior (A) and medial (B) aspect of the right innominate and sacrum showing the sacrotuberous and sacrospinous ligaments.

biceps femoris; it is considered to be derived from biceps femoris, being the degenerated tendon of the long head. The posterior surface of the ligament gives attachment to gluteus maximus.

Sacrospinous Ligament

Lying deep to the sacrotuberous ligament (Fig. 3.10B), its broad base is attached to the lateral margin of the lower sacral and upper coccygeal segments anterior to the sacrotuberous ligament. As it passes laterally it narrows; the apex attaches to the ischial spine. Coccygus blends with it on its pelvic surface; the ligament can be considered to be a fibrous part of the muscle.

Blood Supply, Lymphatic Drainage and Innervation

The arterial supply to the joint is by branches of the iliolumbar artery anteriorly and superior gluteal artery posteriorly (Fig. 3.11), reinforced by branches from the lateral sacral arteries anteriorly and posteriorly. Venous drainage is to correspondingly named veins which eventually drain into the internal iliac vein. Lymphatic drainage of the joint follows the arteries to the internal iliac group of nodes.

The nerve supply is by direct twigs from the sacral plexus and dorsal rami of the first and second sacral nerves. In addition, it also receives branches from the superior gluteal and obturator nerves as they pass close to the joint. The joint is supplied by roots L4–S2.

Relations

At the level of the lumbosacral intervertebral disc anterior to the sacroiliac joint, the common iliac artery divides into its terminal branches (internal and external iliac arteries) (Fig. 3.11). Passing anterior to the bifurcation and in direct contact with the artery, the ureter enters the lesser pelvis on its way towards the bladder. Posterior to the joint is the erector spinae muscle mass; deep to its lateral limb tendinous fibres blend with the posterior sacroiliac, sacrotuberous and sacrococcygeal ligaments.

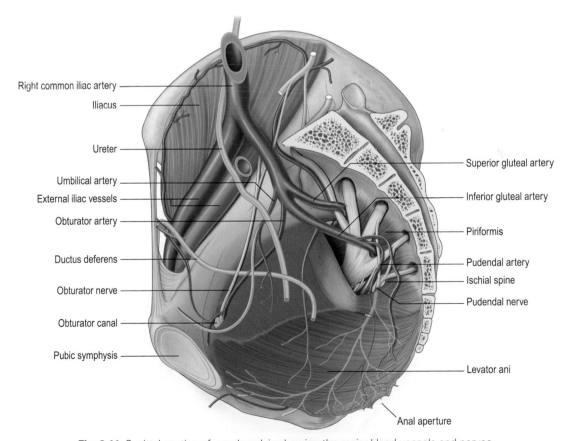

Fig. 3.11 Sagittal section of a male pelvis showing the major blood vessels and nerves.

Medial to the joint passing over the ala of the sacrum are, from lateral to medial, the obturator nerve, iliolumbar artery and lumbosacral trunk, while laterally in the iliac fossa is iliacus and its covering fascia.

Stability

The resilient support of the weight of the trunk, head and upper limbs given by curvatures of the vertebral column imposes additional stresses on the sacroiliac joints because the line of weight passes anterior to them. There is, therefore, a tendency for the sacral promontory to move antero-inferiorly into the pelvis and for the inferior part of the sacrum and coccyx to tilt superiorly. These tendencies are resisted by a number of factors, all of which are entirely dependent on ligaments associated with the joint.

Because the line of weight passes anterior to the joint, the bony surfaces are not weight-bearing *per se*; body weight is suspended by the sacroiliac ligaments supporting and holding the sacrum between the innominates. Providing the sacroiliac joints are intact, the slight wedging of the auricular surfaces, together with their reciprocal irregularities, are sufficient to help resist rotation and gliding of the sacrum with respect to the innominates; the strong interosseous and posterior sacroiliac ligaments usually maintain this relationship. Rotation of the sacrum and coccyx is also resisted by the strong sacrotuberous and sacrospinous

ligaments holding the inferior sacral segments anteriorly, preventing them from rotating posteriorly.

The iliolumbar ligaments, as well as helping oppose simple gliding movements of the joint surfaces, also help prevent the fifth lumbar vertebra from slipping anteriorly on the surface of the first sacral segment.

Movements

The arrangement of the joint surfaces and ligamentous support allow very little movement; however, there is some gliding and rotation between the two bones. Studies have shown that, when standing compared with lying supine, the sacrum moves inferiorly approximately 2 mm and undergoes anterior rotation of approximately 5 degrees; appreciable movement will clearly lead to instability in the erect posture.

During childbirth, there is a complex movement of the sacrum which has been likened to nodding of the head (nutation). This is possible because of the softening of the sacroiliac and associated ligaments during the latter part of pregnancy, leading to an increase in the diameters of the pelvic inlet and outlet facilitating the passage of the fetal head during parturition. First, the sacral promontory moves superoposteriorly, increasing the anteroposterior diameter of the pelvic inlet by between 3 and 13 mm (Fig. 3.12A). Once the fetal head has entered the pelvic canal, the sacral promontory then moves inferoanteriorly increasing

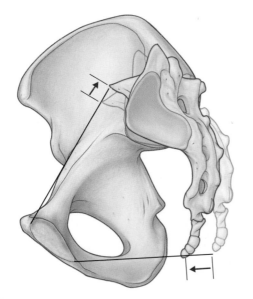
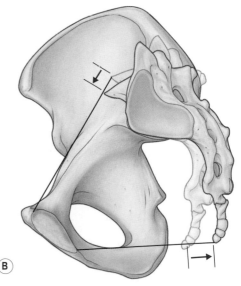

Fig. 3.12 Medial aspect of the right innominate showing movement of the sacrum at the sacroiliac joint and the resulting changes in pelvic inlet (A) and outlet (B) diameters.

the anteroposterior diameter of the pelvic outlet by 15–18 mm (Fig. 3.12B). Although the ligaments have softened, the tension developed in them still limits the degree of movement possible. The degree of the softening, together with the extent of the irregularity of the opposing joint surfaces, accounts for the variation in pelvic diameter changes.

The sacroiliac joints are important clinically as sudden bending forward can tear the posterior ligaments, possibly leading to dislocation of the joint surfaces. Both conditions are extremely painful in trunk flexion and may be disabling, with treatment in many cases being difficult; manipulation is often successful.

Accessory Movements

Ligaments associated with the sacroiliac joint are arranged to allow very little accessory movement. With the individual lying prone so that the pelvis is supported by the two anterior iliac spines and pubic region, place the heel of the hand on the apex of the sacrum and apply a downward pressure. Small rotation of the sacrum with respect to the pelvis can be elicited.

BIOMECHANICS

Trabecular Systems

Two trabecular systems arise from the auricular surface of the innominate, being continuous with those converging towards the auricular surface of the sacrum; both systems are continuous with trabeculae in the head and neck of the femur, as well as joining with other systems within the pelvis (Fig. 3.13). From the upper part of the auricular surface, trabeculae converge onto the posterior border of the greater sciatic notch, some fan out laterally towards the inferior aspect of the acetabulum, while the remainder pass into the ischium, intersecting trabeculae of the acetabular rim; the latter trabeculae resist compression as they bear body weight when sitting.

Trabeculae arising from the lower part of the auricular surface converge at the level of the pelvic brim. From here, some pass laterally towards the superior aspect of the acetabulum, with the remainder passing into the superior pubic ramus towards the body of the pubis completing a ring of trabeculae in the pelvis.

SYMPHYSIS PUBIS

Articular Surfaces

Secondary cartilaginous joint between the medial surfaces of the bodies of each pubic bone. The oval articular

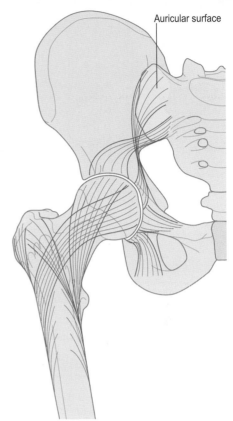

Auricular surface

Fig. 3.13 Trabeculae in the innominate and proximal femur highlighting those associated with the sacroiliac joint.

surfaces are irregularly ridged and grooved, with the irregularities fitting snugly together (Fig. 3.14A and B). The articular surface of each bone is covered with a thin layer of hyaline cartilage joined to that of the opposite side by a fibrocartilaginous interpubic disc (Fig. 3.14B), which is thicker in females than in males.

In the posterosuperior part of the interpubic disc, a small fluid-filled cavity appears in early life, which is never lined with a synovial membrane; in females, this cavity may eventually extend throughout the greater part of the disc.

Palpation

The line of the symphysis pubis can be palpated anteriorly as a groove between the bodies of the pubic bones. Joint alignment can be checked by placing the hand on the lower abdomen with the finger pointing towards the individual's feet. The index and ring fingers are then placed on the superior

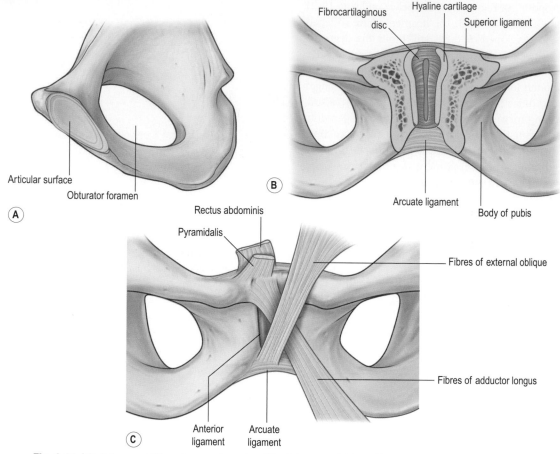

Fig. 3.14 Medial aspect (A) and coronal section (B) of the symphysis pubis; (C) anterior aspect showing the principle relations of the symphysis pubis.

surface of the pubis and the middle finger on the intervening disc.

Ligaments

Superior, inferior and anterior to the joint thickenings of fibrous tissue form ligaments.

Superior Pubic Ligament

Strengthening the anterosuperior aspect of the joint, the superior pubic ligament is attached to the pubic crest and tubercle (Fig. 3.14B).

Arcuate Pubic Ligament

The subpubic angle is smoothed and strengthened inferiorly by the arcuate pubic ligament arching between the inferior pubic rami (Fig. 3.14B). Between this thick ligamentous arch and the transverse perineal ligament of the urogenital diaphragm is a small gap through which

passes the dorsal vein of the penis or clitoris to access the pelvis.

Relations

Overlying the interpubic disc anteriorly are the decussating tendinous fibres of rectus abdominis, external oblique and adductor longus (Fig. 3.14C). These act to strengthen the joint and provide additional anterior stability; some consider this dense feltwork of fibres to constitute a thick anterior pubic ligament. The bladder lies posterior to the joint, separated from it for the most part by the retropubic fat pad.

Movements

There is normally no movement between the bones involved; however, during pregnancy the ligaments associated with the joint, as well as those of other joints, soften allowing a small degree of movement permitting some separation (~2 mm) at the symphysis pubis. Nevertheless, it increases the circumference of the pelvic inlet, probably making it easier for the fetal head to pass through the pelvic cavity. Occasionally, the bone adjacent to the joint is absorbed, again facilitating separation at the symphysis.

Pathology

Slipping of one pubic body with respect to the other occurs occasionally at the symphysis pubis (osteitis pubis). It affects some females following childbirth and, surprisingly, some professional footballers; the unevenness of the pubic arch can clearly be seen on an x-ray. Its aetiology is essentially unknown; however, it is considered to be related to abnormal stresses across the symphysis pubis. Pain associated with the condition is usually referred to the hip joint.

LUMBOSACRAL JUNCTION/JOINT

Between the last lumbar vertebra, usually the fifth, and first sacral segment (Fig. 3.15), the superior sacral surface is inclined approximately 30 degrees to the horizontal; the lumbosacral angle, formed between the axis of L5 and the sacral axis, averages 140 degrees. Being part of the vertebral column, the two bones are joined, as are all typical vertebrae, by an intervertebral disc, anterior and posterior longitudinal ligaments, ligamenta flava, interspinous and supraspinous ligaments, and by synovial joints between their adjacent articular processes. Further details of vertebral articulations can be found on pages 504 and 510.

Ligaments

In addition to the ligaments mentioned above, the iliolumbar and lateral lumbosacral ligaments help stabilise the joint.

Iliolumbar Ligament

Strong ligament passing inferolaterally from the tip of the transverse process of the fifth lumbar vertebra to the posterior part of the medial lip of the iliac crest (Fig. 3.16); it is the thickened inferior border of the anterior and middle layers of the thoracolumbar fascia. Occasionally, an additional smaller ligamentous band passes from the tip of the transverse process of the fourth lumbar vertebra to the iliac crest posterior to the main iliolumbar ligament (Fig. 3.16). A few fibrous strands pass between the transverse process of L4 and the iliac

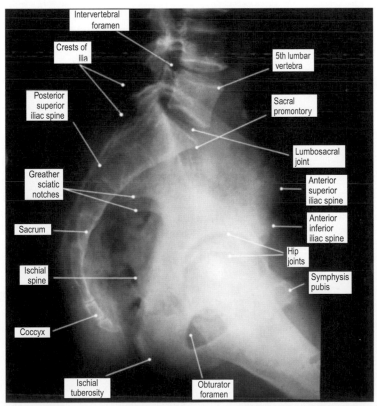

Fig. 3.15 Lateral radiograph of the sacrum and lumbar spine showing the lumbosacral junction/joint.

crest; however, only when these strands condense can they be considered to constitute a true ligament.

Lateral Lumbosacral Ligament

Partly continuous with the inferior border of the iliolumbar ligament, the lateral lumbosacral ligament passes obliquely inferiorly from the inferior border of the transverse process of the fifth lumbar vertebra to the ala of the sacrum, intermingling with the anterior sacroiliac ligament (Fig. 3.16); it contains bundles of fibres of varying strength.

Blood Supply and Innervation

The blood supply to the joint is by small branches from the median sacral and iliolumbar arteries; however, it must be remembered that the major component of the joint (intervertebral disc) is essentially avascular, obtaining its nutrients by diffusion from adjacent vertebral bodies. The nerve supply to the joint and associated ligaments is by twigs from the anterior and posterior rami of L5 and S1.

Stability

The lumbosacral junction is the weak link in the vertebral column; due to the inclination of the superior surface of the sacrum, there is a tendency for the fifth lumbar vertebra to slide anteroinferiorly, which is prevented by overlapping of the articular processes of L5 and S1. This bony arrangement, together with the supraspinous, interspinous and iliolumbar ligaments, is sufficient to prevent any abnormal movements occurring.

Pathology

Under the component of body weight acting parallel to the superior sacral surface, the inferior articular process of L5 normally fits tightly into the superior sacral facets of S1, binding the lumbar and sacral processes tightly together (Fig. 3.17A); the L5/S1 zygapophyseal joints have

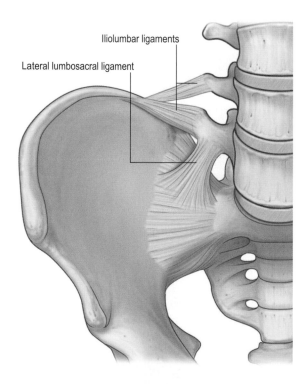

Fig. 3.16 Anterior aspect of the right innominate, sacrum and lower lumbar vertebrae showing the position and attachments of the iliolumbar and lateral lumbosacral ligaments.

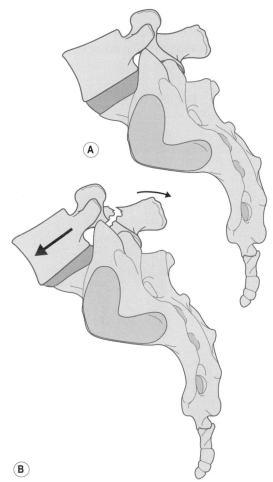

Fig. 3.17 (A) Normal anatomy of the lumbosacral junction. (B) Fracture of the vertebral arch leading to spondylolisthesis.

an important weight-bearing function. The associated forces act through the pars interarticularis, that part of the vertebral arch between the superior and inferior articular processes. Spondylolysis is the condition where the pars interarticularis is incompletely developed, becomes fractured, weakened or disrupted, with the buttressing of L5 on S1 no longer being effective; the body of the fifth lumbar vertebra slips anteroinferiorly leading to spondylolisthesis (Fig. 3.17B). The marked angulation at the lumbosacral junction assists this anteroinferior movement accentuating the lumbar curvature; extension exercises are usually extremely painful and can be dangerous because of tension on the cauda equine (p. 571), leading to motor and sensory disturbances along their distribution. The only structures supporting the joint and preventing further slippage are the lumbosacral intervertebral disc, which is put under tension, and the paravertebral muscles, which go into spasm accounting for the pain associated with the condition. The extent of anteroinferior movement of L5 relative to S1 can be assessed on oblique radiographs.

Spondylolisthesis can arise as a slowly developing fracture of the pars interarticularis, being most common in adolescents who participate in contact sports and gymnastics. The mechanism of injury is probably through impact loading accompanying repetitive flexion and extension of the lumbosacral junction. The repetitive loading is important because, unless there is some congenital anomaly, the pars interarticularis can withstand the stress induced by a single normal impact.

With frequent repetitive loading, the bending stresses eventually produce a small crack on the tensile side of the pars, which slowly extends across the bone; the bone fatigues and eventually gives way. If the fracture is incomplete when diagnosed, it may heal by avoiding repetitive bending stresses; however, once the pars interarticularis has been disrupted, the joint becomes relatively unstable. Unfortunately, conservative measures that bring about repair in a stable fracture do not appear to work, with spinal fusion then being the only option.

Movements

Movements at the lumbosacral junction are restricted to flexion and extension, together with a small degree of lateral flexion (Fig. 3.18); axial rotation is not permitted.

Flexion and Extension

Between ages 2 and 13, the lumbosacral junction is responsible for as much as 75% of the total range of flexion and extension of the lumbar spine, with the average range of movement being 18 degrees; this greatly reduces from age 35 onwards.

In flexion, the inferior articular processes of L5 glide superiorly over those on the sacrum, with movement limited by tension in the iliolumbar, interspinous and supraspinous ligaments and postvertebral muscles. Posteroinferior gliding of the L5 articular processes on those of the sacrum during extension is arrested by apposition of the spines of L5 and S1.

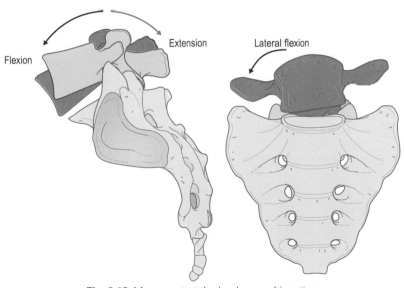

Fig. 3.18 Movement at the lumbosacral junction.

The intervertebral disc between L5 and S1 is markedly wedged (thicker anteriorly), being mainly responsible for the angulation between the lumbar and sacral parts of the vertebral column. Because the lumbosacral junction represents the transition between the mobile (lumbar) and immobile (sacral) parts of the vertebral column, it requires considerable support against potentially damaging stresses. The postvertebral muscle mass is extremely thick in this region, reinforced posteriorly by the inferior part of the strong thoracolumbar fascia. It is worth noting that between L5 and S1, the intertransverse ligaments are replaced by the much stronger iliolumbar ligaments, conferring additional stability to this region by restricting lateral flexion.

Lateral Flexion/Bending

The range of lateral flexion/bending at the lumbosacral joint is minimal, decreasing from 7 degrees in the child to 1 degree in adults and zero in the elderly. Again, the iliolumbar ligament plays an important role in limiting movement, with the contralateral ligament becoming taut and ipsilateral ligament lax. The superior band of the iliolumbar ligament restricts lateral flexion/bending of L4 with respect to the sacrum.

Accessory Movements

The movements possible at the lumbosacral junction are similar to those between adjacent lumbar vertebrae (p. 522).

SACROCOCCYGEAL JOINT

Articulation between the last sacral and first coccygeal segments (Fig. 3.19A) via an intervening interosseous ligament similar to an intervertebral disc. The articular surfaces are elliptical with their long axes lying transversely, that on the sacrum convex and that on the coccyx concave. The joint is completely surrounded and reinforced by longitudinal fibrous strands (sacrococcygeal ligaments) (Fig. 3.19B and C). The lateral parts of these strands form the lateral boundary of the foramen transmitting the anterior ramus of the fifth sacral nerve. In old age, the sacrococcygeal joint frequently becomes partially or completely obliterated.

Flexion and extension are the only movements possible at the joint, which are essentially passive occurring during defecation and labour. Increases in the anteroposterior diameter of the pelvic outlet after movement of the sacrum can be further increased by extension of the coccyx.

Palpation

The line of the sacrococcygeal joint can be felt as a horizontal groove between the apex of the sacrum and the coccyx deep within the natal cleft. By moving the palpating finger inferiorly so that it lies against the back of the coccyx, an applied anterior pressure produces a degree of rotation of the coccyx against the sacrum.

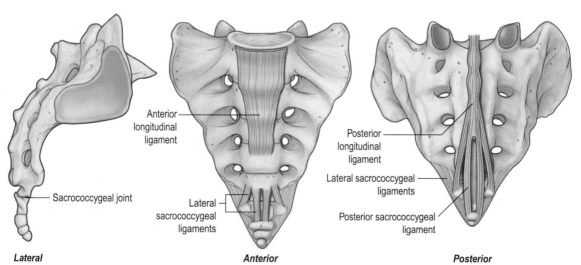

Lateral

Anterior longitudinal ligament

Sacrococcygeal joint

Lateral sacrococcygeal ligaments

Anterior

Posterior longitudinal ligament

Lateral sacrococcygeal ligaments

Posterior sacrococcygeal ligament

Posterior

Fig. 3.19 Lateral, anterior and posterior aspects of the sacrococcygeal joint and its associated ligaments.

SECTION SUMMARY

Innominate
- Comprises three bones (ilium, ischium, pubis) fused together at the acetabulum.
- Orientated so that pelvis faces superoanteriorly.
- The two innominates and sacrum form the pelvic girdle.
- Articulates with sacrum by the sacroiliac joints; pubis of other side by the symphysis pubis; head of femur by the hip joint.

Sacrum
- Curved bone (concave anteriorly) comprising five fused vertebrae.
- With the two innominates forms the pelvic girdle.
- Articulates with innominate by the sacroiliac joints; fifth lumbar vertebra by the lumbosacral joint; and the coccyx by sacrococcygeal joint.

Sacroiliac Joint

Type	Synovial plane anteriorly; fibrous posteriorly
Articular surfaces	Auricular surfaces of the ilium and sacrum
Capsule	Complete fibrous capsule surrounds the joint attaching to the articular margins
Ligaments	Anterior and posterior (interosseous, long, short) sacroiliac
	Accessory ligaments: sacrotuberous, sacrospinous

Stability	Provided by the wedge-shape of the sacrum, interlocking articular surfaces and ligaments
Movements	Slight gliding and rotation between the surfaces; during childbirth the pelvic inlet/outlet diameters increase

Symphysis Pubis

Type	Secondary cartilaginous
Articular surfaces	Medial aspects of the pubic bodies separated by a fibrocartilaginous disc
Ligaments	Superior and arcuate pubic
Movements	Normally very little movement possible; during childbirth, the joint surfaces separate slightly allowing a greater degree of movement

Lumbosacral Junction

Type	Secondary cartilaginous
Articular surfaces	Inferior surface of the body of L5 with the superior surface of the sacrum, separated by an intervertebral disc
Ligaments	Iliolumbar, lateral lumbosacral and all ligaments associated with joints between vertebrae

Sacrococcygeal Joint

Articular surfaces	Inferior surface of last sacral and first coccygeal segments
Ligaments	Sacrococcygeal
Movements	Passive flexion and extension

❓ SELF-ASSESSMENT QUESTIONS

1. What type of joint is the symphysis pubis?
2. Which ligaments are accessory to the sacroiliac joint?
3. Which of the three bones comprising the innominate forms the smallest part of the acetabulum?
4. In which plane do the anterior superior iliac spine and pubic tubercle lie?
5. What are the attachments of the iliolumbar ligament?
6. With respect to the innominate what movements of the sacrum occur to increase the diameter of the pelvic inlet?
7. What is the condition osteitis pubis?
8. What is spondylolisthesis?
9. What movements are possible at the sacrococcygeal joint?
10. Which ligament fills the narrow cleft between the roughened areas on the innominate and sacrum immediately posterosuperior to the auricular surfaces?

HIP

LEARNING OUTCOMES

By the end of the section, you should be able to:
1. Identify, palpate and examine the innominate and proximal femur
2. Describe the bones, joints and muscles of the hip
3. Describe and explain the movements possible, and their restraints, at the hip joint
4. Locate, palpate and examine the muscles associated with the hip and describe their attachments, action and innervation
5. Examine and assess movements of the hip joint
6. Appreciate the influence of pathology and/or trauma on the function of the hip

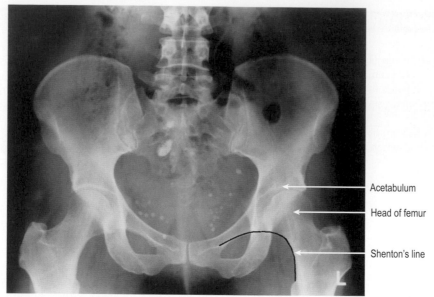

Fig. 3.20 Anteroposterior radiograph of the adult hip; also shown is Shenton's line.

INTRODUCTION

The articulation between the head of the femur and acetabulum of the innominate (Fig. 3.20), the hip joint is a synovial ball-and-socket joint permitting a wide range of movements compatible with a wide range of locomotor activities. It connects the lower limb to the trunk and is involved in the transmission of weight; the mechanical requirements of the joint are severe. It must be capable not only of supporting the entire body weight (standing on one leg) but of the stable transference of the weight, particularly during movement of the trunk on the femur when walking and running. The joint must possess great strength and stability, even at the expense of limitation of the ranges of movement. Stability of the joint is determined by the shape of the articular surfaces (deep socket securely holding the femoral head), the strength of the joint capsule and associated ligaments and the attachment of muscles crossing the joint, which tend to be some distance from the centre of movement.

Deep Fascia of the Thigh

Proximally, the deep fascia attaches to the lateral lip of the iliac crest between the anterior and posterior superior iliac spines, posterior aspect of the ilium and sacrum, sacrotuberous ligament and ischial tuberosity, anterior surfaces of the ischiopubic ramus and body of

the pubis, pubic tubercle, and inguinal ligament; it forms a complete ring of attachment around the proximal part of the thigh.

Below this attachment, it forms a strong cylinder around the thigh; it is thin medially, but extremely thick and tough laterally, consisting of two distinct layers (iliotibial tract). The iliotibial tract is attached superiorly to the tubercle of the iliac crest and inferiorly to the lateral side of the lateral tibial condyle (Fig. 3.103). The major part of gluteus maximus (p. 302) and all of tensor fascia lata (p. 369) attach between these two layers about one-third of the way down the thigh.

In the anterosuperior part of the thigh is an opening (saphenous opening) in the fascia for the long (great) saphenous vein as it passes to drain into the femoral vein; the opening (Fig. 3.187) is about three fingers' breadth inferolateral to the pubic tubercle. Fascia from the inguinal ligament passes inferolaterally forming the falciform margin of the saphenous opening. It then passes deep to the great saphenous vein, wrapping around the femoral vein to pass superiorly to attach to the superior pubic ramus. Medially, the opening has a smooth margin formed from the fascia covering pectineus (p. 301). The margins are joined by the cribriform fascia (thin perforated layer of fibrous and fatty tissue).

In the distal part of the thigh, intermuscular septa pass from the deep surface of the fascia to the femur. The lateral intermuscular septum separates the quadriceps muscles (p. 366) anteriorly from the hamstrings (p. 304) posteriorly, and the medial septum separates the adductors (p. 309) anteriorly and hamstrings posteriorly. Each septum is prolonged inferiorly onto the medial and lateral supracondylar ridges as far as the medial and lateral femoral condyles. More proximally in the thigh, a thickening of the fascial septum deep to sartorius (p. 365) forms the roof of the adductor canal.

INNOMINATE

Details of the innominate can be found on page 259.

FEMUR

Longest and strongest bone in the body (Fig. 3.21), the femur transmits body weight from the ilium to the proximal end of the tibia; it has a shaft and two extremities.

The proximal end of the femur consists of a head, neck and greater and lesser trochanters. The head is slightly more than half a sphere, entirely smooth and covered with articular cartilage except for a small hollow just inferior to its centre (fovea capitis) providing attachment for the ligament of the head of the femur. The neck connects the head to the shaft, it is approximately 5 cm long forming an angle of 125 degrees with the shaft (Fig. 3.30); the angle varies slightly with age and gender. The neck is flattened anteroposteriorly, giving superior and inferior rounded borders; the superior border is concave along its long axis and the inferior is straight. The anterior surface of the neck joins the shaft at the intertrochanteric line and posteriorly at the intertrochanteric crest, marked at its centre by the large quadrate tubercle.

The large quadrilateral greater trochanter is situated on the lateral aspect of the superior part of the shaft lateral to the neck. It has a superior border marked by a tubercle, an anterior border marked by a depression, and posterior and inferior borders both roughened for muscle attachments. Its lateral surface is crossed by a diagonal roughened line running anteroinferiorly, superior to which is a smooth area covered by a bursa. The medial surface above the neck has a deep trochanteric fossa at its centre.

The conical lesser trochanter is situated medially posteroinferior to the neck and is smaller than the greater trochanter; its tip is directed anteriorly presenting as a roughened ridge running anteroinferiorly.

The shaft is strong and, except for a prominent posterior border, almost cylindrical in cross-section. It is gently convex anteriorly, being narrowest at its centre and becoming stouter as it approaches the proximal and distal extremities. Its posterior border is rough (linea aspera) for muscle attachments and has medial and lateral lips with a flattened area between. In the superior and inferior quarters of the shaft, the two lips diverge producing a posterior surface. The superior surface is marked medially by the narrow vertical pectineal line, while the lateral truncated border is continuous superiorly with the posterior border of the greater trochanter and forms the gluteal tuberosity. The inferior surface between the supracondylar lines superiorly and the condyles inferiorly is the popliteal surface of the femur. The rest of the shaft is slightly flattened on its anterior, posteromedial and posterolateral aspects.

The distal end of the femur consists of two large condyles each projecting posteriorly beyond the shaft; the lateral is stouter than the medial. The inferior, posterior and posterosuperior surfaces of the condyles are smooth and continuous anteriorly with the triangular-shaped patellar surface, which is grooved vertically, giving larger lateral and smaller medial regions. The two condyles are separated posteriorly and inferiorly by the intercondylar notch, marked on its lateral wall posteriorly by the attachment of the anterior cruciate ligament (ACL) and on its medial wall anteriorly by the attachment of the posterior cruciate ligament (PCL). The diverging lips of the linea aspera continue inferiorly onto the superior aspects of the medial and lateral condyles (supracondylar lines), with the medial ending as the adductor tubercle.

The lateral surface of the lateral condyle is roughened, being marked just inferior to its centre by the lateral epicondyle, below which is a smooth groove for the popliteus tendon. The medial surface of the medial condyle is also roughened and marked just inferior to its centre by the medial epicondyle.

Ossification

The primary ossification centre for the shaft appears at 7 weeks *in utero*. At birth, growth plates separate the bony shaft from the proximal and distal cartilaginous epiphyses (Fig. 3.22). Secondary ossification centres appear in the distal epiphysis shortly before birth, in the proximal epiphysis for the head at 1 year, in the greater trochanter at 4 years and in the cartilaginous lesser trochanter at 12 years (Fig. 3.22). The proximal epiphysis fuses with the shaft at about age 18, the last to do so is the head; the distal epiphysis fuses with the shaft at about age 20. The

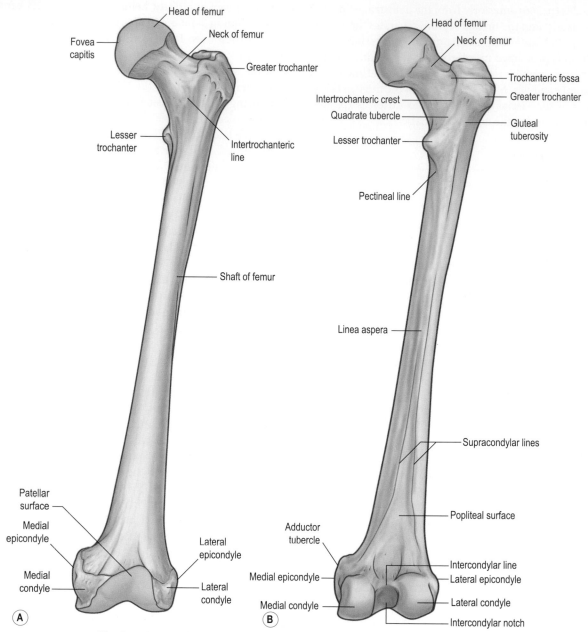

Fig. 3.21 (A) Anterior aspect of the left and (B) posterior aspect of the right femur.

neck of the femur is ossified as part of the body (shaft) and not from the proximal epiphysis.

Palpation

Being almost completely surrounded by muscles the femur is only palpable in limited areas. At the proximal end, the greater trochanter is an obvious landmark projecting more laterally than the iliac crest; it is easily located by running the hands down from the middle of the iliac crest approximately 7–10 cm. The greater trochanter is perhaps easier to feel if the fingers are brought forward from the hollows on the sides of the buttocks in the region of the back pocket; the posterior border can be palpated for approximately 5 cm running inferiorly

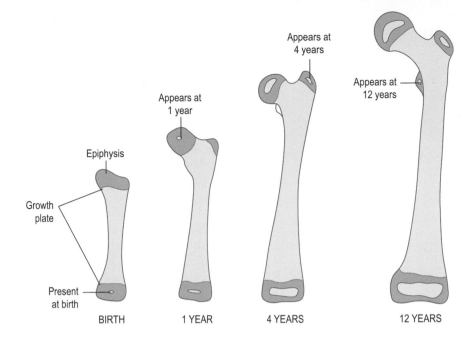

Appears at
4 years

Appears at
12 years

Appears at
1 year

Epiphysis

Growth
plate

Present
at birth

BIRTH   1 YEAR   4 YEARS   12 YEARS

Fig. 3.22 Stages in ossification of the femur.

towards the shaft, while its superior border is an important landmark in locating the level of the hip joint.

At the distal end, the femur is well covered with muscle until just above the knee joint. As the fingers pass down the medial side of the thigh, the medial condyle can be palpated. This is marked just behind its centre by the medial epicondyle, above which the adductor tubercle can be palpated with the tendinous part of adductor magnus attaching to it. On the lateral side of the knee, the lateral condyle can be palpated with the lateral epicondyle projecting from its lateral surface. At the inferior margin of each condyle, the knee joint line can be palpated, particularly as it passes anteriorly.

If the knee is fully flexed, the patella is seen to move inferiorly revealing the two femoral condyles on the anterior aspect of the knee, covered by the inferior part of quadriceps femoris and its retinaculae.

HIP JOINT

Development

For normal acetabular development to occur as the pelvis enlarges, a balance must be maintained between growth of the acetabular and triradiate cartilage and that of the adjacent bone. As the secondary centres of ossification for the acetabulum appear (8–9 years), more bone is formed at the periphery than at the medial part of the acetabulum, increasing its depth and contributing to the cuplike shape of the cavity.

The acetabular cartilage complex is composed of (i) epiphyseal growth-plate cartilage adjacent to the bones, (ii) articular cartilage around the acetabular cavity, and for the most part (iii) hyaline cartilage. Interstitial growth within the triradiate part of the cartilage complex causes the acetabular socket to expand during growth. The concavity of the acetabulum develops in response to the presence of the femoral head (Fig. 3.23A). The depth of the acetabulum increases during development as a result of (i) interstitial growth in the acetabular cartilage, (ii) appositional growth at the periphery of this cartilage and (iii) periosteal new bone formation at the acetabular margin.

Congenital displacement of the hip (CDH) is thought to be due to faulty development of the acetabulum, especially its superior rim, in addition to which the femoral head may also be poorly developed. In such hips, a cartilaginous ridge is present in the acetabulum dividing the socket into two sections; the ridge may be formed exclusively by a bulge of acetabular cartilage or by a bulge of acetabular cartilage covered by an inverted acetabular labrum. The acetabular cartilage usually shows signs of

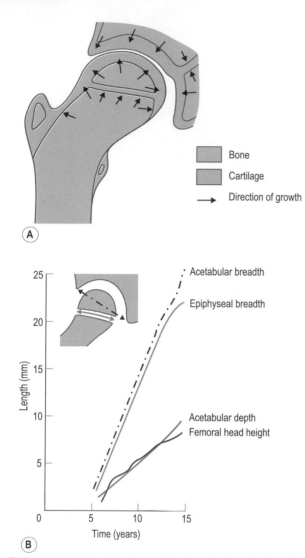

Fig. 3.23 (A) Growth in the acetabulum and proximal end of the femur; (B) growth in height of the osseous femoral head, depth of the acetabulum, and breadth of the proximal epiphysis and acetabulum. (Adapted from Meszaros, T., Kery, L., 1980. Quantitative analysis of the growth of the hip. A radiological study. Acta Orthop. Scand. 51, 275–284.)

degeneration, while the triradiate cartilage is normal. The condition is much more common in young females.

From radiographs of the developing hip, a growth quotient (acetabular index) can be determined; this shows periods of limited intensive growth of the hip, with the periods occurring in both sexes between ages 5 and 8 and again between ages 9 and 12 in females and 11 and 14 in males; in pathological hip joints, the triradiate cartilage

closes earlier. Development of the acetabular roof and closure of the triradiate cartilage are closely related.

During growth, ossification of the femoral head occurs at a faster rate in breadth than in height (Fig. 3.23B); the growth in breadth also exceeds that of the proximal metaphysis. The radiographic appearance of these two regions is, therefore, characteristic of the individual's age. Fortunately, the osseous acetabulum also grows at a faster rate in breadth than in depth (Fig. 3.23B). Up to age 15, the width of the articular space gradually decreases, approaching adult values. However, in the region of the acetabular fossa, the width of the articular space does not decrease in parallel, resulting in the appearance of a double-arched pattern of the acetabulum.

Although the hip is a ball-and-socket joint, when standing erect the femoral head is not completely covered by the acetabulum; the anterosuperior aspect is exposed. Coincidence of the articular surfaces can be achieved by flexing the hip 90 degrees, abducting 5 degrees and laterally rotating 10 degrees; this corresponds to the quadrupedal position. One consequence of attaining an erect posture and adopting bipedalism as a means of locomotion is the loss of coincidence of the articular surfaces, putting the hip in a potentially vulnerable position regarding its stability.

Articular Surfaces
Acetabulum

Hemispherical hollow on the lateral surface of the innominate formed by fusion of its three component parts (ilium, ischium, pubis) which meet at a Y-shaped cartilage, forming their epiphyseal junction (Fig. 3.24A). The anterior 1/5th is formed by the pubis, the superoposterior 2/5th by the body of the ilium and the inferoposterior 2/5th by the ischium (Fig. 3.24A); the prominent acetabular rim is deficient inferiorly (acetabular notch). The heavy wall of the acetabulum consists of a semilunar articular part covered with hyaline cartilage, open inferiorly, and a deep central non-articular part (acetabular fossa). The acetabular fossa is formed mainly from the ischium; its wall is frequently thin.

Head of the Femur

Approximately two-thirds of a sphere, the femoral head is slightly compressed anteroposteriorly: although the difference between the two principal axes is small, it is, nevertheless, best thought of as being an ellipsoid. The head is covered in articular (hyaline) cartilage, except

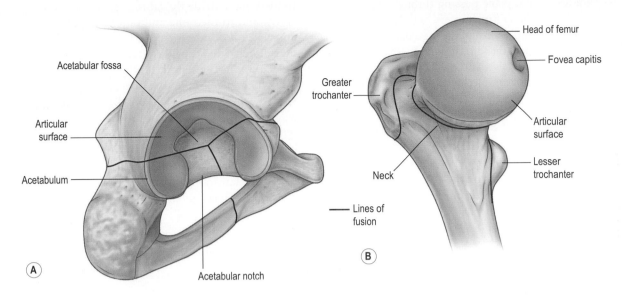

Fig. 3.24 (A) Lateral aspect of the right innominate showing the articular surface of the acetabulum and lines of fusion *(red)* of its constituent parts. (B) Anteromedial aspect of the right proximal femur showing the lines of fusion *(red)* of its constituent parts and articular surface of the femoral head.

for a small area superolaterally adjacent to the neck and at the fovea capitis. Anteriorly, the cartilage extends onto the femoral neck for a short distance (Fig. 3.24B); this is thought to be in response to pressure from the tendon of iliopsoas as it crosses the joint. Both the femoral head and acetabulum consist of cancellous bone covered by a thin layer of compact bone.

Congruence

Although the articular surfaces are reciprocally curved, the hip joint comprises two incongruent shapes, due to the arched acetabulum and the rounded femoral head. Incongruity implies limited contact between the surfaces under low loading conditions, with a gradual increase in the area of contact as load increases. It is usual, therefore, to think of the incongruity as a means of distributing load and protecting the underlying cartilage from excessive stress. An important factor in the functioning of such a mechanism is compressibility of the cartilage.

Because of the relationship between the femur and pelvis, the superior surfaces of the femoral head and acetabulum generally sustain the greatest pressures; consequently, the articular cartilage is thicker in these regions than elsewhere. In the unloaded acetabulum, the cartilage surface is almost spherical. Small deviations seen on

the cartilage surface (<150 μm) reflect the much larger deviations at the cartilage-bone interface (frequently >500 μm). Ultrasonic measurement of the acetabular region has shown that the cartilage and calcified interface surfaces are not concentric, confirming the clinical finding of thinner cartilage in the anteromedial aspect. It is only when weight is taken with the hip joints in extreme flexion, as when squatting, that this anteromedial acetabular region articulating with the inferior part of the femoral head becomes involved in weight-bearing.

Hip Joint Axis

The greater trochanters can normally be palpated; in the erect standing position, a horizontal line through their tips represents the common hip joint axis in the coronal plane. The position of the greater trochanter with respect to the hip joint varies little with flexion and extension; however, with respect to the hip joint centre, it moves superiorly in abduction and inferiorly in adduction.

Palpation

Because the joint is completely surrounded by muscles, it cannot be directly palpated. However, the approximate position of the joint centre in relation to the anterior surface can be estimated in the living. The joint centre lies in a horizontal plane passing through the superior aspect of the greater trochanters, which passes 1 cm inferior to the middle third of the inguinal ligament; this gives the position of the joint centre. Passive movement of the thigh on the pelvis and palpation in this area will improve the estimation of the centre of movement for the hip joint.

Joint Capsule and Synovial Membrane

The strong fibrous capsule is thicker anteriorly, where the head of the femur articulates, as well as superiorly enhancing stability of the joint. Proximally, the capsule surrounds the acetabulum, attaching directly to the bone outside the labrum superiorly and posteriorly, and to the bone and outer edge of the labrum anteriorly and inferiorly (Fig. 3.25A); at the acetabular notch, the capsule attaches to the transverse ligament. On the femur, it attaches anteriorly to the intertrochanteric line and the junction of the neck with the trochanters (Fig. 3.25B). Posteriorly, it has an arched free border covering the medial two-thirds only of the neck (Fig. 3.25C), approximately as far laterally as the groove formed by the tendon of obturator externus. Part of the femoral neck is, therefore, intracapsular and part extracapsular; the epiphyseal line for the head of the femur is also intracapsular,

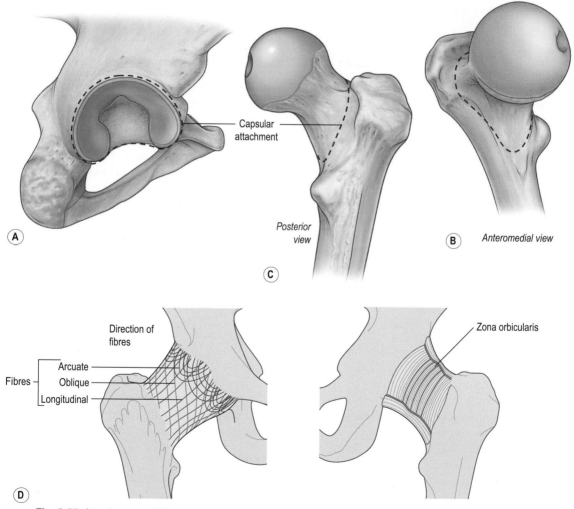

Fig. 3.25 Attachments of the hip joint capsule to the innominate (A) and femur (B and C). (D) The arrangement of capsular fibres.

while the trochanteric epiphyseal lines are extracapsular (Fig. 3.24B). The capsule may be likened to a cylindrical sleeve surrounding the joint and majority of the femoral neck. Anteromedially, the capsule is strengthened by deep fibres of the reflected head of rectus femoris and laterally by deep fibres of gluteus minimus.

Arrangement of Capsular Fibres

The majority of the capsular fibres run from the innominate to the femur in several distinct bands (Fig. 3.25D). Longitudinal fibres, running parallel to the axis of the capsule, pass between the acetabular and femoral capsular attachments. Oblique fibres, which spiral around the capsule between its attachments also unite the articular surfaces. A series of arcuate fibres arch from one part of the acetabular rim to another, helping to keep the femoral head within the acetabulum. Deeper fibres (zona orbicularis) run around the capsule having no bony attachments; these appear most marked on the posterior aspect of the capsule and are reinforced by the deep part of the ischiofemoral ligament; they can be seen on the deep surface of the capsule.

On reaching the femoral neck some deeper longitudinal fibres turn superiorly towards the articular margin (retinacular fibres); they are most marked on the superior and inferior aspects of the neck and convey blood vessels to the femoral head and neck. The main longitudinal capsular fibres form named thickened bands which resist the tensile stresses to which the capsule is subjected. The bands are named after their regional attachment around the acetabulum; they may not always be readily identifiable.

Capsular Ligaments

Iliofemoral ligament. Very strong triangular ligament of considerable thickness situated anterior to the joint (Fig. 3.26A). The apex attaches to the inferior part of the anterior inferior iliac spine and adjacent acetabular rim and base to the intertrochanteric line; because the central part is thinner the ligament is often referred to as being Y-shaped, with the stem corresponding to the apex and limbs to the base. The outer parts of the ligament attaching to the superior and inferior parts of the intertrochanteric line are the strongest, with the central area being thinner and weaker.

Pubofemoral ligament. Strengthens the anteroinferior aspect of the joint capsule (Fig. 3.26A) as it runs from the iliopubic eminence and superior pubic ramus to the inferior part of the intertrochanteric line, blending with the inferior band of the iliofemoral ligament. Between the iliofemoral and pubofemoral ligaments, the capsule is at its thinnest. The tendon of iliopsoas crosses this region, being separated from the joint capsule by the psoas bursa; the bursa usually communicates with the joint cavity through a perforation in the capsule.

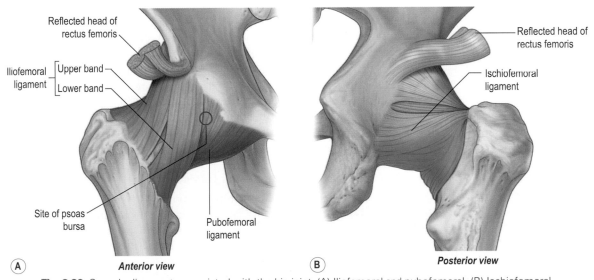

Fig. 3.26 Capsular ligaments associated with the hip joint. (A) Iliofemoral and pubofemoral. (B) Ischiofemoral.

Ischiofemoral ligament. Less well-defined than the iliofemoral and pubofemoral ligaments, the ischiofemoral ligament spirals superolaterally around the capsule. It arises from the body of the ischium posteroinferior to the acetabulum, passing to the superior aspect of the neck and root of the greater trochanter (Fig. 3.26B). Some deeper fibres are continuous with the zona orbicularis.

Role of the capsular ligaments. The capsular ligaments play important roles in limiting and controlling movements of the hip joint. When standing erect, all three ligaments are under moderate tension, while flexion of the hip relaxes all three ligaments; in hip extension, they all become taut, especially the inferior band of the iliofemoral ligament as it runs almost vertically and is responsible for checking the posterior tilt of the pelvis. The concerted action of all three ligaments seen in hip flexion/extension is not seen in abduction/adduction or medial/lateral rotation. The attachments of the ligaments demand that, during each of these latter movements, some become taut while others relax. During adduction, the superior band of the iliofemoral ligament becomes taut with the inferior band only slightly so, while the pubofemoral and ischiofemoral ligaments slacken; the opposite occurs in hip abduction. In lateral rotation, both anterior ligaments become taut, while the ischiofemoral ligament slackens; in medial rotation, the ischiofemoral ligament becomes taut, while the others slacken.

Synovial Membrane

Lining the internal surface of the fibrous joint capsule it covers the acetabular labrum; at the acetabular notch it is attached to the medial margin of the transverse ligament, almost completely covering the fatty tissue in the acetabular fossa. The synovial membrane extends around the ligament of the head of the femur like a sleeve, attaching to the margins of the fovea capitis. At the femoral attachment of the joint capsule, the synovial membrane is reflected superiorly towards the head as far as the articular margin; retinacular fibres raise this reflected part into prominent folds within which blood vessels run towards the head. An extension of the synovial membrane beyond the free margin of the capsule on the posterior aspect of the femoral neck acts as a bursa for the tendon of obturator externus. The communicating psoas bursa breaches the joint capsule between the inferior limb of the iliofemoral and pubofemoral ligaments.

Intracapsular Structures
Transverse Acetabular Ligament

The inferior deficiency in the acetabular rim is completed by the transverse acetabular ligament (Fig. 3.27A and B), creating a foramen with the acetabular notch through which vessels and nerves enter the joint. The superficial edge of the ligament is flush with the acetabular rim and consists of strong bands of fibrous tissue.

Acetabular Labrum

The acetabulum is deepened by the triangular fibrocartilaginous acetabular labrum attached to the bony rim and transverse ligament (Fig. 3.27A, B, and D); the apex of the labrum forms the thin free edge (Fig. 3.27B). The diameter of the free edge is smaller than its fixed edge and is also less than the maximum diameter of the femoral head. Extending further laterally than the equatorial region of the femoral head, the labrum cups around the head, holding it firmly in the acetabular socket (Fig. 3.27D).

Ligamentum Teres

Within the joint capsule is a weak flattened band of connective tissue (ligamentum teres/ligament of the head of the femur), attached to the adjacent margins of the acetabular notch and inferior border of the transverse ligament (Fig. 3.27A), narrowing as it passes to attach to the fovea capitis (Fig. 3.27C and D). Between these attachments, the ligament is enclosed in a sleeve of synovial membrane, so that, although it is intracapsular, it is extrasynovial; the ligament lies in the acetabular fossa inferior to the femoral head. It appears to be of little importance in strengthening and/or supporting the hip joint, being variable in size and occasionally absent. In young children, it carries the artery of the head of the femur, which becomes obliterated in late childhood; its function in adults is uncertain. It is stretched when the flexed thigh is adducted or laterally rotated; however, in many cases, it is too weak to have any definite ligamentous action. No apparent disability arises from its rupture or absence.

Acetabular Fat Pad

Lying within the acetabular fossa is the fibroelastic acetabular fat pad. It is thought to contain numerous proprioceptive nerve endings, so that, when compressed and/or partially extruded from the acetabular fossa beneath the transverse ligament, it provides additional proprioceptive information regarding hip joint movements.

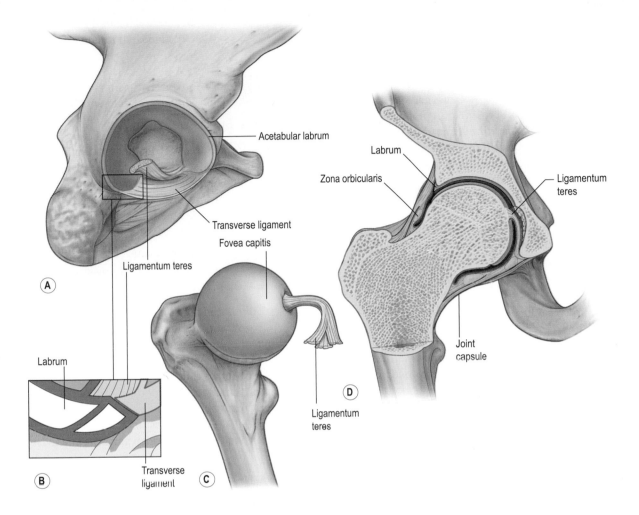

Acetabular labrum

Labrum

Zona orbicularis

Ligamentum teres

Transverse ligament

Fovea capitis

Ligamentum teres

Labrum

Joint capsule

Ligamentum teres

Transverse ligament

(A)

(B)

(C)

(D)

Fig. 3.27 (A) Lateral aspect of the acetabulum showing the position and attachments of the transverse acetabular ligament and ligamentum teres. (B) Triangular cross-section of the acetabular labrum. (C) Anteromedial aspect of the right proximal femur showing the attachment of the ligamentum teres to the fovea capitis. (D) Coronal section showing the head of the femur located in the acetabulum.

Blood Supply, Lymphatic Drainage and Innervation

The hip joint receives its blood supply from the medial and lateral circumflex femoral, obturator and superior and inferior gluteal arteries, which form a periarticular anastomosis around the joint (Fig. 3.28A and B). Within the ligamentum teres, there is a small artery in children derived from the obturator artery, gaining access to the joint by passing deep to the transverse ligament bridging the acetabular notch (Fig. 3.28B and C); however, this may only be significant before fusion of the epiphysis of the head with the femoral neck. The greatest volume of blood reaches the joint via the periarticular anastomosis, with branches piercing the joint capsule at its femoral attachment and passing in the retinaculae, between the joint capsule and synovial membrane, to reach and supply the femoral neck and head.

The patency of the periarticular arterial anastomosis is critically important for nutrition of the bone, particularly the proximal femoral epiphysis, until ossification

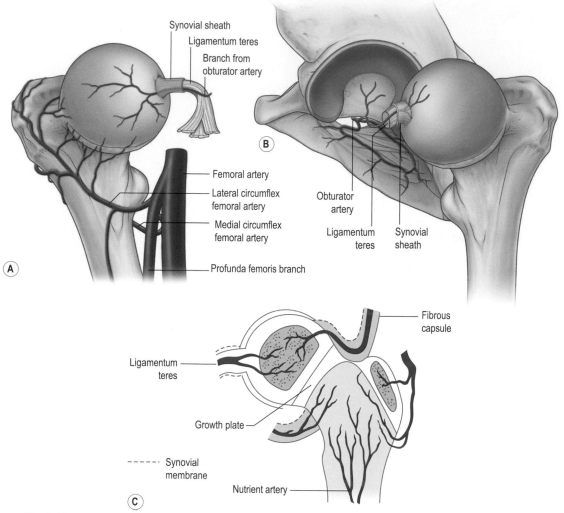

Fig. 3.28 Anteromedial aspect of the right proximal femur (A) and lateral aspect of the left acetabulum (B) showing the arterial supply to the hip joint; (C) coronal section through the proximal femur showing its blood supply prior to fusion of the proximal epiphysis with the shaft.

is completed, usually between 16 and 20 years. Similarly, following a fracture healing of the bone requires a good blood supply. Of particular concern is fracture of the femoral neck, which frequently occurs in older females; such fractures tend to be intracapsular, making realignment of the bone fragments problematic. In addition, blood vessels supplying the head and neck may also be ruptured, resulting in ischaemic degeneration of the femoral head; if present, the artery of the head of the femur provides an inadequate alternative blood supply.

For this reason, in subcapital fractures early prosthetic replacement of the femoral component or of the joint as a whole is often performed. Hip dislocation and slipping of the femoral epiphysis are both potentially damaging to the retinacular blood vessels.

Lymphatic drainage is provided by vessels accompanying the arteries supplying the joint. The lymph vessels arise primarily from the synovial membrane and drain to the deep inguinal and iliac lymph nodes, then to the common iliac group of nodes.

Innervation of the joint is from the lumbar plexus by twigs from the femoral and obturator nerves, and the lumbosacral plexus by twigs from the superior gluteal nerve and nerve to quadratus femoris, with a root value of L2–S1. This is a typical example of articular innervation where the nerve supply to the joint is derived from the same nerves supplying muscles crossing it. The articular supply consists of sensory nerve fibres, transmitting proprioceptive information, and vasomotor fibres.

In posterior dislocation of the hip, the sciatic and other posterior nerves may become stretched over the femoral head or otherwise damaged. Injury to the superior gluteal nerve on one side results in collapse of the pelvis to the opposite side as the ipsilateral leg is raised; collapse is due to paralysis of gluteus medius and minimus (positive Trendelenburg sign). Primary disease of the hip joint frequently manifests itself in pain referred to the knee because the same nerves provide branches to both joints.

Relations

Anteriorly, from inferior to superior, the hip joint is related to pectineus, tendon of psoas major, iliacus and rectus femoris (Fig. 3.29B and C); the deep part of the reflected head of rectus femoris strengthens the superior and anterior aspects of the joint capsule. Between the tendons of iliacus and psoas, separated from the joint capsule by them, is the femoral nerve, while the femoral artery and vein lie on the psoas tendon and pectineus.

Posteriorly, from superior to inferior, are piriformis, tendon of obturator internus with the two gemelli and quadratus femoris (Fig. 3.29A and C), all of which lie close to the joint capsule. The nerve to quadratus femoris is deep to obturator internus lying directly on the joint capsule. The sciatic nerve is separated from the joint capsule by obturator internus and the gemelli.

In addition to the reflected head of rectus femoris superiorly, gluteus minimus lies more laterally, part of which may blend with the joint capsule. Inferiorly, obturator externus winds posteriorly inferior to the capsule, lying between it and quadratus femoris.

The deep fascia of the thigh, of which the fascia lata is the uppermost subdivision, invests the soft tissues of the lower limb. It is a strong membranous fascia, thicker where it is reinforced by tendinous contributions and thinner in the gluteal region; it has a continuous bony and ligamentous attachment superiorly. Between the iliac crest and superior border of gluteus maximus, the fascia is thickened by vertical tendinous fibres (gluteal aponeurosis). The remaining gluteal portion and adductor part of the fascia lata are thin, except for a lateral band (iliotibial tract), which is especially strong.

An opening in the anterior aspect of the fascia lata (saphenous opening) provides passage for the long/great saphenous vein to its termination in the femoral vein. The efferent vessels from the superficial inguinal nodes also pass through this opening, mainly travelling within the femoral sheath to the external iliac nodes.

Superficial to the fascia lata, the subcutaneous connective tissue contains a considerable amount of fat over the gluteal region, hip and thigh, although it varies in different regions. In the gluteal region, the fat is deposited in a thick layer contributing to the contour of the buttock and formation of the gluteal fold. At the fold of the groin, the subcutaneous tissue can be separated into superficial fatty and deeper membranous layers, between which are subcutaneous blood vessels and nerves.

Stability

This is determined by the shape of the bones, the strong reinforced joint capsule, the acetabular labrum and muscles crossing the joint. Although the articular surfaces of the femur and acetabulum fit together well and provide a good degree of support for the joint, the periarticular muscles are essential for continued joint stability, particularly muscles crossing the joint transversely.

Bony Factors

The direction of the femoral neck in both the coronal and transverse planes is of considerable importance for stability of the hip (Fig. 3.30). During embryonic development and even after birth, the femoral shaft becomes adducted and medially rotated, resulting in the head and neck becoming angulated against the shaft in both the coronal and transverse planes. In the coronal plane, the angle between the neck and shaft (angle of inclination) is an adaptation of the femur to the parallel position of the legs in bipedalism (Fig. 3.30A); in the newborn the angle is approximately 150 degrees, decreasing in the early years to the adult value of 125 degrees. In the transverse plane, the angle between the neck and shaft (angle of anteversion) is also due to the adoption of an erect stance; the neck and head are laterally rotated

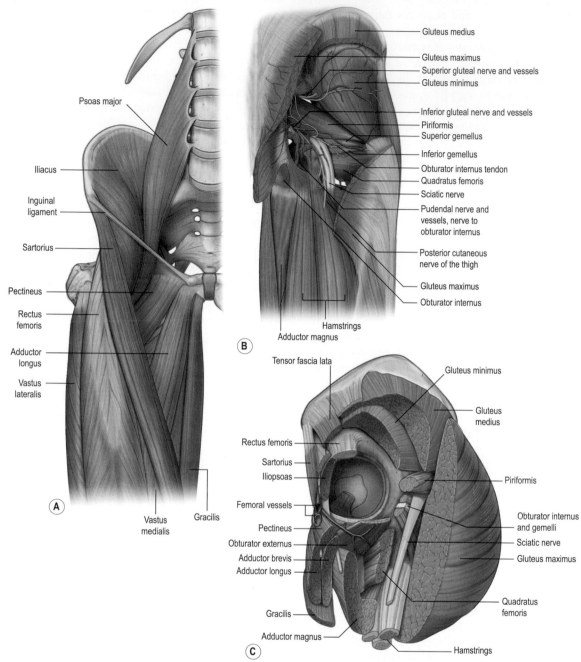

Fig. 3.29 Principle relations around the hip joint. Anterior (A) and posterior (B) aspects of the right pelvis and proximal thigh, lateral aspect (C) of the left pelvis and thigh.

against the shaft approximately 10 degrees in adults (Fig. 3.20C), having decreased from 25 degrees in infants and young children.

In some pathological conditions (congenital dysplasia of the hip (CDH)), the angle of inclination can be as much as 140 degrees, producing a coxa valga, and the

The values for the angles of inclination and anteversion given above are mean values; within a normal population, there will be considerable racial and individual variation, having important implications for joint stability. If the angle of inclination and/or the angle of anteversion are greater than 130 and 15 degrees, respectively, the coincidence and stability of the two joint surfaces are decreased.

Because of the length of the femoral neck and its angulation to the shaft, in both the coronal and transverse planes, a line joining the centre of the femoral head to the middle of the intercondylar notch mainly passes outside the bone on its medial side (Fig. 3.30A); this is the mechanical axis of the femur about which medial and lateral rotation occurs. The anatomical axis of the femur deviates approximately 3 degrees in the coronal plane from the mechanical axis, which in turn deviates approximately 3 degrees from the vertical so that its proximal end is lateral to its distal end (Fig. 3.30A).

The acetabulum faces laterally, anteriorly and inferiorly to articulate with the femoral head, which due to anteversion of the femoral neck faces medially, anteriorly and superiorly. There is, therefore, an angle of 30–40 degrees between the axes of the acetabulum and femoral neck (Fig. 3.31A), so that the anterior part of the femoral head articulates with the joint capsule. In addition, the inferolateral inclination of the acetabulum forms an angle of 30–40 degrees with the transverse plane so that the superior part of the acetabulum overhangs the femoral head laterally. An angle of 30 degrees (angle of Wiberg) is also formed between a vertical line through the centre of the femoral head and a line from this centre to the bony margin of the acetabulum (Fig. 3.31B). This angle can be measured on radiographs; decreases in the angle have implications for joint stability.

In normal individuals, a line drawn along the superior margin of the obturator foramen and inferior margin of the femoral neck to the medial side of the femoral shaft describes a smooth curve (Shenton's line) (Fig. 3.20); it is not influenced by small changes in position; however, in fractures and dislocations of the femur, it may become greatly distorted.

Muscular Factors

Muscles whose fibres run parallel to the femoral neck (psoas, iliacus, pectineus anteriorly; gluteus minimus superiorly; gluteus medius, obturator internus and externus, the gemelli, quadratus femoris, piriformis

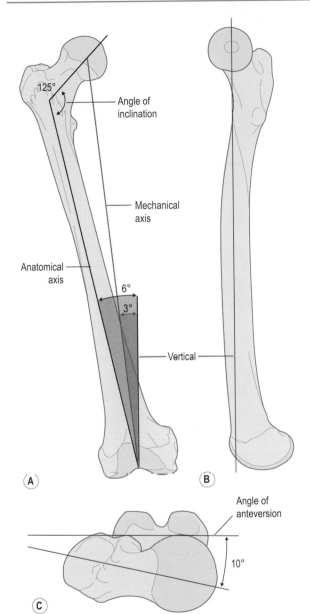

Fig. 3.30 Anterior (A), medial (B) and superior (C) aspects of the right femur showing the relationship between the mechanical and anatomical axes of the femur and the vertical, together with the angles of inclination and anteversion.

angle of anteversion as large as 40 degrees; both increase the risk of joint dislocation. In other conditions, the angle of inclination may be reduced (acquired dislocation of the hip; Fig. 3.36): in contrast, there may be a reduced or reversed angle of anteversion (the head and neck are retroverted with respect to the femoral shaft).

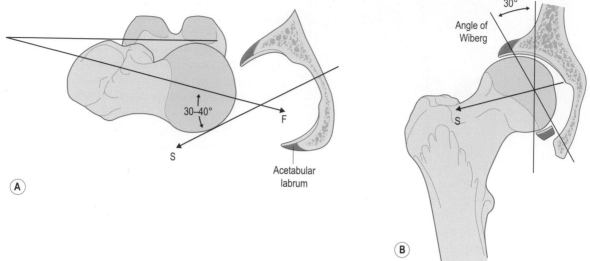

Fig. 3.31 Superior (A) and anterior (B) aspects of the right proximal femur and acetabulum showing the relationship between the axes of the femoral neck *(F)* and acetabulum *(S)*; also shown is the angle of Wiberg.

posteriorly) tend to keep the femoral head in firm contact with the acetabulum. However, muscles with fibres running parallel (longitudinal) to the femoral shaft may have a tendency to cause superior joint dislocation, particularly if the roof of the acetabulum is everted. The adductor muscles run longitudinally and, in some joint positions (attempting adduction with the thigh extended and laterally rotated) their action, without the synergistic activity of other muscles around the hip, leads to a tendency for anteromedial joint dislocation.

Pathology

It should not be inferred that the hip joint is continually liable to dislocation; in the normal joint it is not. Nevertheless, malformation of the acetabular socket (eversion of the roof) increases the probability of dislocation occurring. Eversion of the acetabular roof is present in CDH; in this case, the adductors can cause dislocation, especially when the limb is adducted. However, when the limb is abducted, the dislocating tendency of the adductors decreases until, in full abduction, the adductors eventually favour apposition of the joint surfaces.

Dislocations and Fractures

Traumatic dislocation of the hip is not common, except in car accidents; posterior dislocation is more common, favoured by the usual direction of the dislocating force in such cases. The joint capsule is ruptured, the femoral

head lies in the posterior iliac fossa and the limb is shortened, adducted and medially rotated; the knee on the affected side overlies the normal knee. The position is almost diagnostic, contrasted with the position in femoral neck fracture, in which the limb is shortened but laterally rotated.

Fracture of the proximal one-third of the femoral shaft exemplifies the effects of muscle pull. The proximal fragment has the attachment of iliopsoas to the lesser trochanter, as well as the gluteal and other posterior muscles to the greater trochanter. The proximal fragment is, therefore, flexed, abducted and laterally rotated; in contrast, the distal fragment is displaced superomedially by the adductors and hamstrings. Realignment requires traction, with surgical intervention often being necessary in adults.

MOVEMENTS OF THE THIGH AT THE HIP JOINT

The movements possible are those of a typical ball-and-socket joint; flexion and extension about a transverse axis; adduction and abduction about an anteroposterior axis; and medial and lateral rotation about a vertical axis; circumduction is also permitted. The three axes intersect at the centre of the femoral head; because the head is situated at an angle to the shaft, all movements involve conjoint rotation of the femoral head.

TABLE 3.1 Required Range of Movement at the Hip During Various Activities

Activity	Maximum range required
Walking on a level surface	30° flexion 10° extension 5° abduction 5° adduction 5° medial rotation 5° lateral rotation
Ascending/descending stairs	65° flexion 5° extension
Siting	90° flexion (minimum)
Tying shoe laces	50° flexion

Adapted from Livingston, L.A., Stevenson, J.M., Olney, S.J., 1991. Stairclimbing kinematics on stairs of differing dimensions. Arch. Phys. Med. Rehabil. 72, 398–402.

The ranges of hip joint motion associated with some common activities are given in Table 3.1.

When assessing the range of movement at the hip joint, it is important to determine that there is no movement of the pelvis or vertebral column. An apparent increase in flexion or extension may be due to flexion or extension of the vertebral column, especially in the lumbar region. Similarly, an apparent increase in abduction or adduction may be produced by a lateral flexion/bending of the trunk to the opposite or same side, respectively.

To produce movement, there is a complex arrangement of muscles around the joint which either act on the thigh with respect to the pelvis or on the pelvis with respect to the thigh. During many movements, the hip joint is weight-bearing transmitting the weight of the body above it via the lower limbs to the ground.

Muscles surrounding the joint, therefore, have a dual role; they must be capable of immediate controlled power when needed for sudden powerful activities (running uphill or upstairs), yet retain the ability to maintain a set position for long periods of time (standing, leaning forwards, sitting).

The hip joint is completely surrounded by muscles, which are thicker and stronger posteriorly and laterally; the joint, therefore, appears to be located anteriorly in the region.

Muscles anterior to the joint tend to be flexors, those posterior extensors, those medial adductors and those lateral abductors. Both medial and lateral rotation occur at the joint because of the obliquity of some of the muscle fibres. This is explained more fully under the individual muscles.

Flexion and Extension

Flexion of the hip joint is free, only limited by contact of the thigh with the anterior abdominal wall when the knee is flexed (Fig. 3.32); with the knee extended, hip flexion is limited by tension in the hamstrings. Extension of the hip beyond the vertical is limited partly by tension in the associated ligaments and partly by the shape of the articular surfaces; extension beyond 30 degrees is not normally possible (Fig. 3.32). When going from flexion to full extension, the capsular ligaments become increasingly tense, pulling the femoral head more tightly against the acetabulum. Because ligaments are slightly extensible and articular cartilage deforms slightly under compressive loads, the point at which no further extension is possible varies slightly with the magnitude of the extending force. During extension, part of the acetabular fat pad is extruded from the acetabular fossa below the transverse ligament. Flexing the joint draws the fat pad back in again to fill the potential space created by lateral movement of the femoral head, which occurs with flexion.

The total range of active flexion and extension is 135–140 degrees (Roach and Miles, 1991), with flexion being freer (120 degrees) than extension (15–20 degrees); passive movement can increase the ranges to 145 degree flexion and 30 degree extension. The ranges of both flexion and extension change with age. In neonates, flexion is 138 degrees (Watanabe et al., 1979); however, all newborns and young infants are unable to extend the hip to the neutral position from full flexion, the limitation being approximately 30 degrees (Forero et al., 1989) but may be as much as 46 degrees at birth (Waugh et al., 1983). By age 4 or 5, 30 degrees of active extension is possible (Svenningsen et al., 1989). With further increases in age, the range of flexion and extension gradually decreases to adult values, but thereafter remains relatively constant until age 70, after which a decrease in both the active and passive ranges of motion has been observed (James and Parker, 1989). Females tend to be more mobile than males at all ages (Allander et al., 1974; James and Parker, 1989).

Abduction and Adduction

These movements, some 45 degrees each (Fig. 3.33), are free in all positions of the lower limb, except of course for adduction in the anatomical position. Abduction is

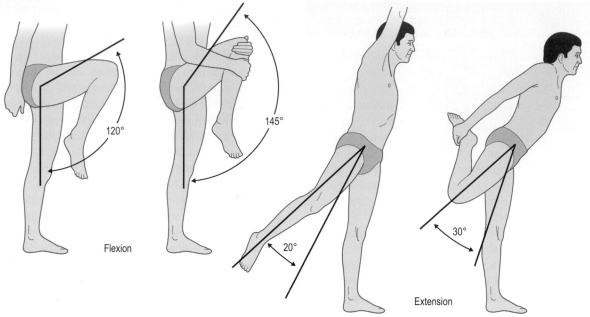

Fig. 3.32 Active and passive ranges of flexion and extension of the thigh at the hip joint.

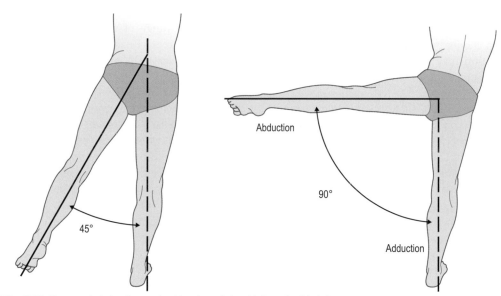

Fig. 3.33 Range of abduction and adduction of the thigh at the hip joint.

greatest when the hip is partly flexed, limited by tension in the adductors and medial part of the iliofemoral and pubofemoral ligaments. Adduction is easier with the hip flexed than extended; it is limited by the opposite limb, tension in the abductors and lateral part of the iliofemoral ligament. In young children, abduction may approach 60 degrees (Phelps et al., 1985), decreasing to adult values from age 6, while adduction, except in the newborn when it is only some 6 degrees (Drews et al., 1984), remains relatively constant. Females tend to be more mobile than males at all ages (Allander et al., 1974; James and Parker, 1989).

Medial and Lateral Rotation

Rotation occurs about the mechanical axis of the femur and not about the long axis of the shaft of the femur (Fig. 3.30). In medial rotation, the femoral shaft moves anteriorly around the mechanical axis, carrying with it the leg/calf and foot so that the toes point towards the midline; in lateral rotation, the femoral shaft moves posteriorly, with the result that the toes point away from the midline. Rotation in both directions is freer when combined with hip flexion rather than extension; of the two, lateral rotation is freer than medial rotation and is also more powerful. Lateral rotation is limited by tension in the medial rotators of the thigh and iliofemoral and pubofemoral ligaments, while medial rotation is limited by tension in the lateral rotators and ischiofemoral ligament. A small amount of hip rotation occurs automatically in association with terminal extension and the beginning of knee flexion, particularly with the foot fixed.

The total combined range of medial and lateral rotation is 90 degrees: 45 degrees medially and 45 degrees laterally (Fig. 3.34). With increasing age, the total range of movement decreases to 60 degrees (Roach and Miles, 1991), with the decrease being similar in both directions. In neonates, infants and children, the total range of rotation is much greater than in adults, with lateral rotation initially being greater, but from age 4, medial rotation is greater than that laterally. In neonates, rotation is 92 degrees laterally and 76 degrees medially (Forero et al., 1989), decreasing to 46 and 55 degrees, respectively, by age 4 (Svenningsen et al., 1989) and 43 and 48 degrees by age 11 (Svenningsen et al., 1989). Females tend to be more mobile than males at all ages (Allander et al., 1974; James and Parker, 1989).

Because the axis about which rotation occurs is mainly outside the femur, there is some confusion concerning the role of some muscles in producing medial or lateral rotation at the hip joint. In general, any muscle whose line of action passes anterior to the mechanical axis of the femur produces medial rotation, while muscles whose line of action passes posteriorly produce lateral rotation. However, the position of the line of action of a muscle with respect to the mechanical axis can change depending on the degree of flexion or extension of the joint. Consequently, in some joint positions, a muscle may medially rotate, while in others it may laterally rotate. Similarly, for large muscles crossing the hip joint, it may be more convenient to consider more than one line of action, in which case one part may medially rotate and another laterally rotate the hip joint. The line of axis through the hip joint also varies according to whether or not the foot is on the ground.

The major muscles producing movements of the thigh at the hip joint are shown in Table 3.2; further details of each muscle can be found in the following sections.

BIOMECHANICS
Joint Forces

The estimation of hip joint forces during simple activities (walking) has a long history. Such estimates are continually refined with the use of increasingly sophisticated measuring techniques and the advent of more powerful computers; the use of such estimates has been invaluable

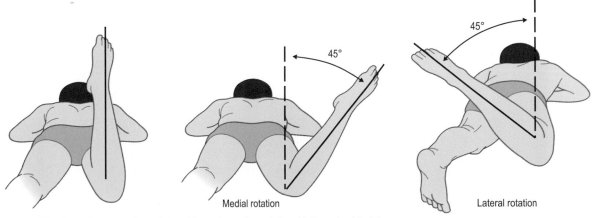

Fig. 3.34 Ranges of medial and lateral rotation of the thigh at the hip joint.

TABLE 3.2	Muscles Crossing and Producing Movement of the Thigh at the Hip Joint		
Muscle	**Attachments**	**Action**	**Innervation (root value)**
Psoas major[a]	Adjacent margins of T12–L5 bodies and medial part of transverse processes to lesser trochanter of femur	Flexor of thigh at hip joint; also flexes and laterally flexes lumbar spine if femur is fixed	(L1, L2, L3 (L4))
Iliacus[a]	Proximal posterior 2/3rd of iliac fossa, ala of sacrum and anterior sacroiliac ligament to lesser trochanter of femur	Flexor of thigh at hip joint; tilts pelvis forwards if femur is fixed	Femoral nerve (L2, L3)
Pectineus[a]	Superior ramus of pubis, iliopubic eminence and pubic tubercle to a line running from lesser trochanter to linea aspera of femur	Flexor and adductor of thigh at hip joint	Femoral nerve (L2, L3); occasionally also obturator or accessory obturator nerve (L3)
Rectus femoris[a]	Anterior inferior iliac spine (straight head) and area above acetabulum (reflected head) to superior border of patella and ligamentum patellae	Flexor of thigh at hip joint; extends leg/calf at knee joint	Femoral nerve (L2, L3, L4)
Sartorius[a]	Anterior superior iliac spine to medial aspect of tibial shaft	Flexor, lateral rotator and abductor of thigh at hip joint; flexes leg/calf at knee joint, medially rotates tibia on femur	Femoral nerve (L2, L3)
Gluteus maximus[a]	Gluteal surface of ilium medial to posterior gluteal line, posterior border of ilium, adjacent iliac crest, and superior part of sacrotuberous ligament to gluteal tuberosity of femur (25%) and iliotibial tract (75%)	Powerful extensor of thigh at hip joint (as in stepping, climbing, running) at same time laterally rotating thigh; upper fibres can adduct and lower fibres abduct thigh at hip joint; via iliotibial tract it extends leg/calf at knee joint and supports lateral aspect of knee	Inferior gluteal nerve (L5, S1, S2)
Gluteus medius[a]	Gluteal surface of ilium between posterior and anterior gluteal lines to greater trochanter of femur	With pelvis fixed it abducts thigh at hip joint; anterior fibres medially rotate thigh at hip joint; with femur fixed opposite side of pelvis is rotated forwards	Superior gluteal nerve (L4, L5, S1)
Gluteus minimus[a]	Gluteal surface of ilium between inferior and anterior gluteal lines to greater trochanter of femur	With pelvis fixed abducts thigh at hip joint; anterior fibres medially rotate thigh at hip joint; with femur fixed opposite side of pelvis is rotated forwards	Superior gluteal nerve (L4, L5, S1)
Semitendinosus[b]	Ischial tuberosity to medial surface of medial condyle of tibia	Extensor of thigh at hip joint, as well as aiding flexion of leg/calf at knee joint; with knee semiflexed it medially rotates leg/calf at knee joint; with foot fixed it laterally rotates thigh and pelvis on tibia	Sciatic nerve via its tibial part (L5, S1, S2)
Semimembranosus[b]	Ischial tuberosity to posteromedial surface of medial tibial condyle	Extensor of thigh at hip joint, as well as aiding flexion of leg/calf at knee joint; with knee semiflexed it medially rotates leg/calf at knee joint; with foot fixed it laterally rotates thigh and pelvis on tibia	Sciatic nerve via its tibial part (L5, S1, S2)

TABLE 3.2	Muscles Crossing and Producing Movement of the Thigh at the Hip Joint—cont'd		
Muscle	**Attachments**	**Action**	**Innervation (root value)**
Biceps femoris[b]	Ischial tuberosity and sacrotuberous ligament (long head), lower half of linea aspera and proximal half of lateral supracondylar ridge of femur (short head) to head of fibular	Extensor of thigh at hip joint, especially when trunk is flexed and to be raised to erect position; with knee semiflexed it laterally rotates leg/calf at knee joint; with foot fixed it medially rotates thigh and pelvis on tibia	Sciatic nerve (L5, S1, S2): *long head* by tibial part; *short head* by common fibular/peroneal part
Adductor magnus[a]	Ischiopubic ramus and ischial tuberosity to linea aspera, medial supracondylar ridge and adductor tubercle of femur	Adductor of thigh at hip joint; posterior part aids extension of thigh at hip joint	Obturator nerve (L2, L3) and sciatic nerve via its tibial part (L4)
Adductor longus[a]	Obturator crest and body of pubis to middle part of linea aspera	Adductor of thigh at hip joint; also flexor of extended thigh and extensor of flexed thigh	Obturator nerve (L2, L3, L4)
Adductor brevis[a]	Body and inferior ramus of pubis to superior half of linea aspera	Adductor of thigh at hip joint	Obturator nerve (L2, L3, L4)
Gracilis[a]	Body of pubis and its ramus to medial surface of tibial shaft	Adductor of thigh at hip joint; with knee semiflexed flexes leg/calf at knee joint; aids medial rotation of leg/calf at knee joint	Obturator nerve (L2, L3)
Piriformis[a]	Anterior aspects of S2–S4 to greater trochanter of femur	Lateral rotator of thigh at hip joint; when seated it is important when moving sideways	(L5, S1, S2)
Obturator internus[a]	Deep surface of obturator membrane and surrounding margins to greater trochanter	Lateral rotator of thigh at hip joint	Nerve to obturator internus (L5, S1, S2)
Gemellus superior[a]	Gluteal surface of ischial spine to greater trochanter	Lateral rotator of thigh at hip joint	Nerve to obturator internus (L5, S1, S2)
Gemellus inferior[a]	Ischial tuberosity to greater trochanter	Lateral rotator of thigh at hip joint	Nerve to quadratus femoris (L4, L5, S1)
Quadratus femoris[a]	Ischial tuberosity to quadrate tubercle on intertrochanteric crest of femur	Lateral rotator of thigh at hip joint; with hip flexed it can abduct thigh at hip joint	Nerve to quadratus femoris (L4, L5, S1)
Obturator externus[a]	Outer surface of obturator membrane and surrounding margins to trochanteric fossa of femur	Lateral rotator of thigh at hip joint; with hip flexed it can abduct thigh at hip joint	Obturator nerve (L3, L4)

[a]Shown in Fig. 3.29.
[b]Hamstrings.

in the design of replacement joints. The majority of studies; however, are still limited to determining joint forces during walking; in static single-leg stance, hip joint forces between 1.8 and 3 times body weight have been reported. In the stance phase of walking, hip joint forces increase to between 3.3 and 5.5 times body weight; in running, higher forces would be expected. A typical pattern of forces during walking is shown in Fig. 3.35, from which it can be seen that the resultant joint force reaches a maximum shortly after heel-strike and just before toe-off; the major component of the resultant is the vertical joint force. However, the anteroposterior force (Y in Fig. 3.35) exceeds body weight at both heel-strike and toe-off, indicating that considerable stress is placed on the joint in this direction at these times. Even during straight leg raises, when the heels are lifted 5 cm off the surface, the resultant hip joint force can be as high as two times body weight.

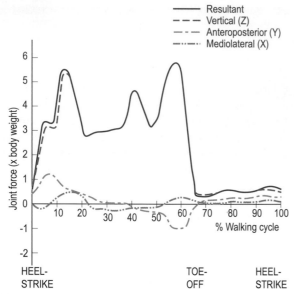

Fig. 3.35 Reaction forces at the hip joint during the stance phase of gait (walking).

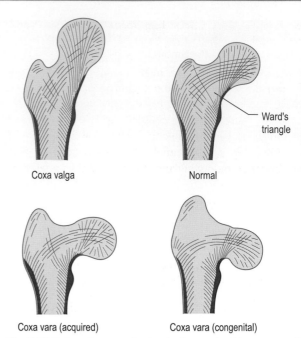

Fig. 3.36 Trabeculae organisation in the proximal femur associated with changes in the angle of inclination.

With estimates of hip joint forces in normal subjects ranging up to nearly six times body weight, the trabeculae within the acetabulum and head and neck of the femur are arranged to minimise bending and shearing stresses within the bone.

Trabecular Systems

Systems which arise in the pelvis and run towards the acetabulum are continuous with those in the femoral head and neck (Fig. 3.13), with two trabecular systems arising in the auricular surface of the innominate. From the upper part of the auricular surface, trabeculae converge onto the posterior surface of the greater sciatic notch from where they are reflected towards the inferior aspect of the acetabulum; this system lines up with one in the femur arising from the cortical layer of the lateral aspect of the shaft to the inferior aspect of the cortical layer of the neck and inferior part of the femoral head. A second system arising from the lower part of the pelvic auricular surface converges at the level of the superior gluteal line from where it is reflected laterally towards the superior aspect of the acetabulum. This system lines up with that arising from the cortical layer of the medial aspect of the femoral shaft running to the superior aspect of the femoral head; it develops in response to the compressive forces transmitted across the joint. If the pattern of stresses crossing the hip joint

changes (acquired dislocation of the hip) the two trabecular systems remodel to become realigned with the new stress patterns; the outward appearance is a change in the relationship of the head and neck of the femur with respect to the shaft (Fig. 3.36).

Within the proximal femur, there are two accessory trabecular systems. The first is a trochanteric bundle arising from the cortical layer of the medial aspect of the shaft which develops in response to the tension forces applied to the greater trochanter by muscular contraction; the second system is entirely within the greater trochanter (Figs 3.13 and 3.36).

The hip joint is the pivot upon which the body balances, especially during walking. The acetabulum and femoral head, being cancellous bone, provide some elasticity to the joint by having the ability to deform without sustaining structural damage. The presence of large quantities of relatively deformable bone suggests spreading under load; spreading does occur and is essential if the stress (force/unit area) on the articular cartilage is to be kept within tolerable limits. Because the bony portions of the hip joint deform under load, maximum contact and congruence must occur in the deformed position; such congruity should occur only with full loading. A congruous fit under no load leads to an incongruous fit under high loads when the femoral head tends to flatten.

Deformation of bone when loaded has a significant effect on protecting the overlying articular cartilage from impulsive loads. The true sparing effect of trabecular bone on the overlying cartilage involves an increase in the available potential contact area. However, excessive deformation of trabecular bone, particularly when sustained repetitively, can lead to microfracture with subsequent remodelling and stiffening of the underlying trabecular network. It has been suggested that stiffening and loss of congruence can lead to deterioration of the articular surfaces and osteoarthrosis.

Contact Area

The area of contact between the femoral head and acetabulum increases with increasing load. Under low loads, there are two distinct areas on the anterior and posterior aspects of the femoral head, which merge superiorly as load increases (Fig. 3.37A). With loads applied across the hip joint ranging from 150 to 3200 N, the contact area increases from 2470 to 2830 mm². Dividing the applied load by contact area gives the mean contact stress; it appears that during walking mean contact stress at the hip joint ranges from 2 to 3 MN/m². It is interesting to note that the measured contact areas coincide closely with regions of cartilage stiffness. The stiffest cartilage is located in bands of variable size extending over the superior aspect of the femoral head to the anterior and posterior facets; there is a relatively soft area of cartilage near the margin of the fovea capitis (Fig. 3.37B).

These observations suggest a direct link between the load or normal stress distribution and pattern of cartilage stiffness.

In situations where the load-bearing area of the femoral head is decreased or diminished (due to deformity) the stress on the remaining load-bearing cartilage is concentrated; degenerative changes frequently follow.

Both abnormally large joint incongruities and abnormally low cartilage compliance result in load shifting away from the superior weight-bearing area of the hip joint toward the periphery of the contact area. As a consequence, transverse compressive stresses, which may be of appreciable magnitude but make no contribution to weight-bearing, build up through much of the superior and central portions of the femoral head. Most small changes in overall cartilage thickness or in its distribution, when considered in isolation from hip compliance changes, have only minor effects on the internal stress distribution. However, an important exception is cartilage thinning at the superior margin of the acetabulum and femoral head, which can result in abrupt longitudinal compressive stress concentrations. Such aberrations to the normal patterns of stress transmission may contribute to sclerosis, the formation of osteophytes or cysts in osteoarthritic hips.

Joint Space

In the loaded hip, there is still a joint space, being variable in size between individuals; it changes in shape with changes in joint position in the same individual under comparable loads. The intra-articular joint space in the

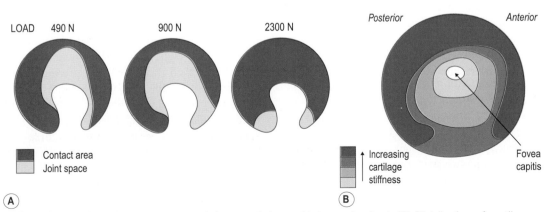

Fig. 3.37 (A) Increasing contact area of the acetabulum with increasing load. (B) Distribution of cartilage stiffness across the femoral head.

hip allows synovial fluid to access the joint providing lubrication and nutrition; the acetabular fossa acts as a fluid reservoir. Under high joint loading, movement of synovial fluid from the joint space to the reservoir occurs; when pressure in the joint space falls below that in the reservoir, flow is reversed, thus lubricating and nourishing the joint.

Limits to Mobility

In conditions other than those involving the hip, there may be some loss of hip mobility. In osteitis pubis, for example, there may be some loss of hip mobility, particularly medial rotation and, in some cases, lateral rotation, a finding typically associated with upper femoral epiphysiolysis. In situations requiring free medial rotation of the hip joint in both flexion and extension, when movement is restricted stress will be transferred across the hip joint to the pelvis. This is specifically a shearing stress causing anteroposterior movement of one side of the pelvis with respect to the other in extension or proximodistal movement in flexion. Such forces are perhaps less likely to be transferred in other instances of pathological restriction (degenerative joint disease) of hip joint movement, where soft tissue tension rather than abnormal joint shape is the restricting factor.

Pathology

Severe disruption of the blood supply can result in infarct of part of the femoral head. The viable intact bone surrounding a weakened infarct preferentially takes up additional load, with the extent of stress relief being dependent on the degree of necrotic stiffness deficit and the geometry of the infarct. Infarcted bone in the superior weight-bearing area continues to carry high stresses, even though load is progressively transferred towards the periphery of the lesion. Vulnerability to mechanical overload appears to be more pronounced superiorly than inferiorly; this could partly explain the clinically observed collapse sequence which usually begins just beneath the subchondral bone. The elastic instability at the peripheral aspects of the viable weight-bearing subchondral region suggests that the subchondral bone fractures as a result of excessive compressive hoop stresses. The increased functional demand placed upon viable bone bordering an infarct tends to enhance the sclerosing effects of hypervascularity.

Femoroacetabular impingement is a cause of early osteoarthritis of the hip resulting from abnormal hip anatomy, leading to abutment of the femoral neck against the acetabulum. Cam impingement results from an aspherical femoral head-neck junction; in contrast pincer impingement is due to acetabular overcoverage of the femoral head. Contact between the femoral neck and acetabulum damages both the articular cartilage and acetabular labrum, leading to early signs of degenerative joint disease. Patients typically present with pain around the hip and groin and may have a history of developmental hip disorders; provocation tests can be used to elicit symptoms. In the impingement test, the individual lies supine and the hip is passively internally rotated, flexed to 90 degrees and then adducted; if any pathology is present, groin pain is elicited. The Fitzgerald test is in two parts, one for anterior and one for posterior labral involvement. For anterior labral involvement, the hip is initially flexed, externally rotated and abducted, before being brought into extension, internal rotation and adduction; a positive result produces pain with or without an audible click (a strong sign of mechanical injury). To test for posterior acetabular impingement, the hip begins in extension, external rotation and abduction, and is moved through flexion, internal rotation and adduction. Treatment of femoroacetabular impingement is predominantly surgical, aiming to improve joint clearance by resecting bony prominences on the femur and/or acetabulum; it can be carried out with open surgery or arthroscopically.

Male/Female Considerations

Although the radii of the right and left femoral heads are essentially identical for any individual, the femoral head is significantly smaller in females than males in relation to pelvic dimensions; this may result in increased stress levels in females. Because of the greater breadth of the female lesser pelvis due to the adaptation for childbearing, the weight of the individual acting through the body's centre of gravity lies at a greater distance from the centre of the hip joint (Fig. 3.38). The longer resistance arm, coupled with the shorter lever arm of gluteus medius, reduces the mechanical advantage of the abductors; consequently, greater abductor force is required to control pelvic tilt. Furthermore, the greater force requirement acts over a smaller femoral head, resulting in greater femoral head pressures in females. It would appear that the adaptation to childbearing and its effects on the female pelvis is a major contributing factor to mechanical dimorphism of the human hip.

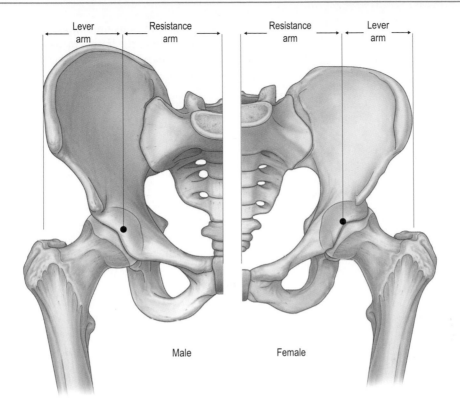

Fig. 3.38 Anterior aspect of the innominate, sacrum and proximal femur showing the lever and resistance arms acting about the hip joint in males and females.

MUSCLES FLEXING THE THIGH AT THE HIP JOINT

Psoas major
Iliacus
Pectineus
Rectus femoris (p. 366)
Sartorius (p. 365)

Psoas Major

Large, thick, powerful muscle situated mainly in the abdominal cavity (Fig. 3.39), psoas major has important relations; anteriorly at its proximal end is the diaphragm and medial arcuate ligament, while lower down the kidney, psoas minor (when present), the renal vessels and ureter all lie anterior. On the right, it is overlapped by the inferior vena cava and ileum; the ascending and descending colon lie lateral to the right and left psoas, respectively. Medially is the lumbar part of the vertebral column, while directly posterior are the transverse processes of the lumbar vertebrae. Segmental lumbar nerves emerging from the intervertebral foramina lie directly posterior to psoas major and pass anteriorly into its substance forming the lumbar plexus.

The proximal attachment of psoas major is to the adjacent margins of the vertebral bodies and intervening intervertebral discs, with the most superior attachment being to the inferior margin of T12 and the most inferior to the superior margin of L5. Psoas major also has an attachment to the anterior medial part of each transverse process and tendinous arches over the constricted part of the lumbar vertebral bodies.

The muscle fibres pass inferoanteriorly towards the pelvic brim, with the individual digitations forming a thick muscle which gradually narrows as it passes over the pelvic brim deep to the inguinal ligament. At this point, the tendon changes direction becoming more vertical before passing inferiorly, posteriorly and

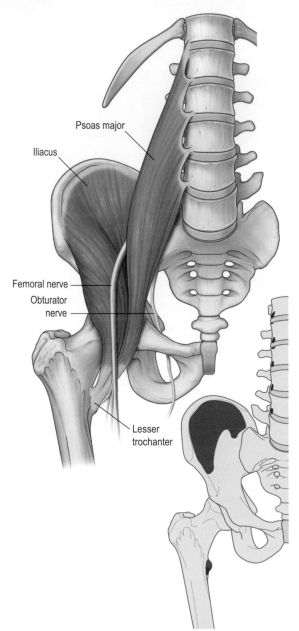

Psoas major

Iliacus

Femoral nerve

Obturator
nerve

Lesser
trochanter

Fig. 3.39 Anterior aspect of the lumbar spine, sacrum, right innominate and proximal femur showing the position and attachments of psoas major and iliacus and their relation to the femoral and obturator nerves.

laterally. It is separated from the pubis and hip joint capsule by a large bursa. Before passing over the pelvic brim, psoas is joined on its lateral side by fibres from iliacus, which continues to blend with it, even after it

becomes tendinous until it attaches to the tip and posterior aspect of the lesser trochanter of the femur. Some fibres of iliacus attach to a line on the femur running inferoanteriorly from the lesser trochanter.

Innervation

Anterior rami of L1, L2, L3 and sometimes L4. It only appears near the surface in the area of the groin; the small area of overlying skin is supplied by L1.

Action

Psoas major flexes the hip joint; because of its attachment to the lumbar spine, and using the distal attachment as the fixed point, it also flexes the lumbar spine. If psoas major of one side only acts it produces lateral flexion/bending of the lumbar spine to the same side.

There has been much discussion on the role of psoas in rotation of the hip joint; initially, because of its attachment to the posterior and medial aspects of the femur, it was thought to be a lateral rotator of the thigh. However, as rotation occurs about the anatomical axis through the femoral head and lateral tibial condyle (Fig. 3.30), it would be expected to be a medial rotator. Electromyographically, the muscle shows little activity during either medial or lateral rotation, so the question remains unanswered.

Functional Activity

The action and functional activity of psoas major are included with those of iliacus as far as hip flexion is concerned; however, it does act independently on the lumbar spine when its distal end is fixed. In sitting up from a lying position, both muscles help pull the weight of the trunk up at the same time as the abdominal muscles are working hard to flex the trunk. It is very important that the abdominal muscles are brought into action early as this prevents the lumbar spine from being drawn anteriorly before the trunk begins to rise; pulling the head up first prevents this unwanted and potentially damaging movement occurring.

Raising both lower limbs at the same time while lying supine is the cause of much back trouble; unfortunately, it can be a popular exercise with lay teachers. The mechanics of this area must be well understood before exercising as it is better to prevent back problems rather than try to treat them after they have occurred.

Each lower limb is approximately 15% of the body weight, therefore, when both legs are raised from the floor, the hip flexors are lifting approximately 30% of body weight. This initial lift involves psoas major and, for about the initial 30 degrees, the lumbar spine is pulled anteriorly. The anterior dragging of the lumbar spine can cause considerable damage to the area, particularly if some degenerative changes have already occurred. It is erroneously believed that this is a good abdominal exercise and will reduce the waistline because the abdominal muscles are working hard.

Palpation

Psoas major is almost impossible to palpate as most of its bulk lies within the abdomen. It appears near the surface in the groin, but it is still quite difficult to feel, being covered by other structures.

Iliacus

Large, fleshy, triangular muscle situated mainly in the pelvis (Fig. 3.39). The larger proximal attachment is mainly from the superior and posterior two-thirds of the iliac fossa with some fibres arising from the ala of the sacrum and anterior sacroiliac ligament (Fig. 3.9). The fibres pass inferiorly, anteriorly and medially, blending with the lateral side of psoas major. The blending continues over the pelvic brim where they change direction to pass posteroinferiorly and slightly laterally to attach to the lesser trochanter of the femur, blending with the attachment of psoas major from the tip of the lesser trochanter; a few fibres are attached to the hip joint capsule.

Innervation

By the femoral nerve (root value L2, L3). Skin covering the area where the tendon passes over the pelvic brim is supplied by L1.

Action

Its effect on the hip is similar to that of psoas major. If its proximal attachment is fixed, it pulls the thigh anteriorly as in hip flexion; if the distal attachment is fixed, it tilts the pelvis anteriorly, again as in flexion of the hip, but this time with the trunk doing the moving.

Functional Activity

Together with psoas major iliacus is used in all activities of pulling the lower limb up anterior to the trunk, as in drawing the lower limb forward in walking, running and jumping. It also helps pull the trunk anteriorly from lying supine to sitting. There is the same controversy

over its role in rotation of the femur as there is for psoas major.

Palpation

It is almost impossible to palpate (see also psoas major).

Pectineus

Quadrilateral muscle situated at the superior and medial aspect of the thigh deep in the groin (Fig. 3.40). It

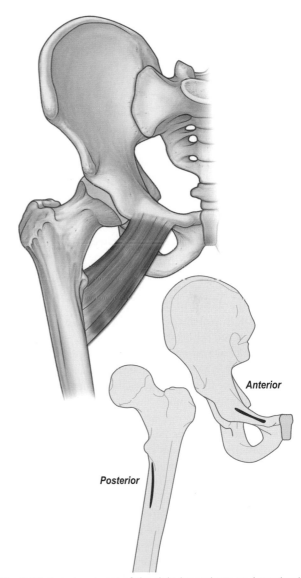

Fig. 3.40 Anterior aspect of the right innominate and proximal femur showing the position and attachments of the pectineus.

appears to consist of superficial and deep layers, which are generally supplied by different nerves.

It arises from the superior ramus (pecten) of the pubis, iliopubic eminence, pubic tubercle and covering fascia. The fibres pass inferiorly, posteriorly and laterally between psoas major and adductor longus to attach to a line running from the lesser trochanter of the femur to the proximal part of the linea aspera (pectineal line), anterior to the upper part of adductor brevis.

Innervation

By the femoral nerve (root value L2, L3) and occasionally the obturator or the accessory obturator nerve (root value L3). Skin covering this area of the groin is supplied by L1.

Action

Flexion and adduction of the thigh at the hip joint. Some also believe the muscle to be a medial rotator of the hip.

Functional Activity

It is easy to see how pectineus acts as a flexor and adductor of the thigh at the hip by considering the direction of its fibres (posteroinferolateral); contraction of the muscle draws the thigh anteromedially. Most authorities dismiss the rotation element as there is disagreement, although others feel that there must be more to the rotation than has yet been deduced.

There is no doubt that the attachment of pectineus is lateral and anterior to the mechanical axis of the femur (Fig. 3.30), in which case it would produce medial rotation. However, when the foot is off the ground, as in the swing phase of walking, the axis passes through the hip joint but now varies considerably according to the position of the thigh and pelvis, being dependent on the swing of the lower limb.

So far, the functional activity of pectineus has only been considered in the erect, standing or walking positions. Much of the time is spent sitting with the hip joint flexed at almost a right angle; the relationship between the attachments of the muscle is now reversed. To make the situation clearer, the thigh can be raised off the seat until it is at an angle of 45 degrees to the horizontal (as if the legs were going to be crossed). The muscle fibres now pass anterosuperiorly, passing posterior to the axis of the rotating thigh. The action of the muscle in this position will be adduction as before, but also extension and lateral rotation, a movement very similar to that of

crossing the legs except that the thigh is being pulled inferiorly onto the opposite thigh. This movement is comparable with the initial stages of rising from a very low chair or from squatting, especially if the movement is carried out at some speed and under load.

Taking the argument one stage further, pectineus is clearly a flexor and adductor of the thigh at the hip joint in the erect position, with perhaps some medial rotation; it is an extensor and lateral rotator in the fully flexed position, but still performs adduction. Therefore, as in the case of many muscles, pectineus can perform different actions according to its starting position and the relative position of its attachments. It is not surprising that it is supplied by nerves from both the flexor and adductor compartments of the thigh.

Remembering the dual nerve supply, dual action, closeness of the muscle to the hip joint and its important relations, it is surprising that pectineus only merits a few lines in most anatomy texts. It must have played a vital role in locomotion with a flexed hip, either in climbing or when all four limbs were on the ground. Has its role diminished that much, or are we overlooking the true action and worth of pectineus?

MUSCLES EXTENDING THE THIGH AT THE HIP JOINT

Gluteus maximus
Hamstrings:
  Semitendinosus
  Semimembranosus
  Biceps femoris

Gluteus Maximus

Largest of the gluteal muscle it is situated on the posterior aspect of the hip joint; it is very powerful. In lower primates, gluteus maximus is a hip adductor, as was the case in early primitive humans; however, with changes in the human pelvis associated with the erect posture (Fig. 3.1), gluteus maximus has mainly become a hip extensor. It is essentially responsible for the erect posture, freeing the forelimbs (upper limbs) from a weight-bearing role, enabling them to become the precision implements they are today.

Gluteus maximus (Fig. 3.41) is a thick quadrilateral muscle arranged in two layers as it passes to its distal attachment; it comprises bundles of muscle fibres arranged in the line of pull of the muscle, giving its

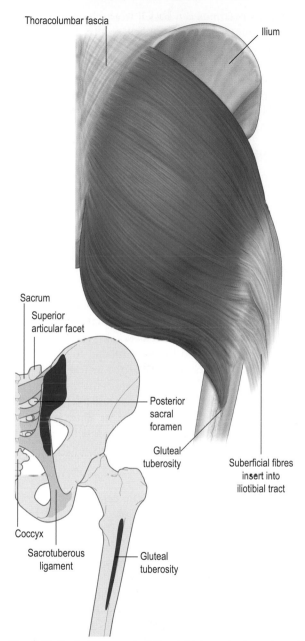

Fig. 3.41 Posterior aspect of the right innominate and proximal femur showing the position and attachments of gluteus maximus.

Thoracolumbar fascia

Ilium

Sacrum

Superior articular facet

Posterior sacral foramen

Gluteal tuberosity

Coccyx

Sacrotuberous ligament

Gluteal tuberosity

Superficial fibres insert into iliotibial tract

superior part of the sacrotuberous ligament. Its upper fibres attach to the aponeurosis of sacrospinalis while its deep anterior fibres come from the fascia covering gluteus medius.

The fibres pass anteroinferiorly towards the proximal end of the femur. The most superficial 75% of fibres form a separate lamina which narrows to attach between the two layers of the fascia lata, helping form the iliotibial tract. The remaining deeper fibres form a broad aponeurosis attaching to the gluteal tuberosity of the femur.

Innervation

By the inferior gluteal nerve (root value L5, S1, S2). Skin covering the muscle is mainly supplied by branches from L2 and S3.

Action

When acting from above, the muscle pulls the shaft of the femur posteriorly, producing extension of the flexed hip joint. As its distal attachment is nearer to the lateral side of the thigh, it also tends to rotate the thigh laterally during extension. The lower fibres can adduct the thigh, while the upper fibres may help in abduction.

Those fibres attaching to the iliotibial tract can extend the knee joint because the distal end of the tract attaches to the lateral tibial condyle anterior to the axis of movement. Through the iliotibial tract, gluteus maximus also provides powerful support to the lateral side of the knee. If the femur is fixed, contraction of gluteus maximus pulls the ilium and pelvis posteriorly around the hip joint, but this time the pelvis and trunk are the moving parts, and lifting the trunk from a flexed position occurs.

Functional Activity

As a powerful extensor of the thigh, especially when the hip joint has been flexed, means that gluteus maximus is ideally suited for fulfilling its role in powerful movements (stepping up onto a stool, climbing, running); however, it is not used to any great extent as an extensor in ordinary walking.

With the hamstrings, it participates in raising the trunk from a flexed position (standing erect from a forward flexed position). Indeed, gluteus maximus and the hamstrings provide the main control in flexion of the trunk as the movement primarily occurs at the hip joint.

surface a coarse appearance. Superiorly, it attaches to the gluteal surface of the ilium posterior to the posterior gluteal line, posterior border of the ilium and adjacent part of the iliac crest, as well as from the side of the coccyx and posterior aspect of the sacrum, including the

Gluteus maximus plays an important role in balancing the pelvis on the femoral heads, helping maintain the erect posture; its ability to aid lateral rotation of the thigh when standing assists in raising the medial longitudinal arch of the foot.

The role of gluteus maximus during sitting should not be dismissed. Although the ischial tuberosities support the majority of the weight of the trunk when sitting, pressure is regularly relieved from these bony points by static or sometimes dynamic contractions of the muscle raising the ischial tuberosities from the supporting surfaces; it then relaxes and weight is lowered. Sometimes, the weight is shifted from side to side with the alternate use of gluteus maximus of each side.

Paralysis of gluteus maximus leads to flattening of the buttock and an inability to climb stairs or run. However, other muscles can be brought into action to extend the hip, although it is a weaker movement. Gluteus maximus can be developed to produce functional extension of the knee in individuals where the quadriceps femoris is either very weak or paralysed. This is not a powerful movement but may be sufficient to enable the individual to extend the knee and the lower limb to become weight-bearing during walking or standing.

Palpation

First, locate the iliac crest approximately at the belt level; moving the hand posteriorly along the crest, a small bony process can be felt (posterior superior iliac spine). With the fingers running inferomedially, place the centre of the palm over this point. The hand now just about covers the proximal attachment of gluteus maximus; the palm is over the posterior part of the ilium, sacrum and sacroiliac joint, while the fingertips are on the edge of the coccyx and upper part of the sacrotuberous ligament. The bulk of the muscle is now under the palm; follow this to the greater trochanter of the femur. Now try the following:

1. Extend the lower limb while standing, keeping the hand over the muscle; the muscle goes hard producing a much clearer shape.
2. Place the foot on a stool and put the hand in the same position as before and step up; again, the muscle can be felt coming into action very strongly.
3. When standing, place the hands on each gluteus maximus as if they were in the back pocket. Raise the medial borders of the feet as if to shorten the medial longitudinal arch of the foot; as the arch is raised,

gluteus maximus can be felt working quite strongly, the femur also tends to rotate laterally.

4. Finally, when sitting, place a hand under each buttock so that the ischial tuberosity rests on it. Now move the weight from side to side as if getting tired of sitting; gluteus maximus can be felt to contract alternately taking the weight off the tuberosity and then lowering it down again.

Hamstrings

Semitendinosus, semimembranosus and biceps femoris are collectively known as the hamstrings.

Semitendinosus

Arising from the lower medial facet of the lateral section of the ischial tuberosity, the tendon of semitendinosus is combined with that of the long head of biceps femoris (Fig. 3.42); the two muscles run together for a short distance. It then forms a fusiform muscle belly, quickly giving way to a long tendon, hence its name. The tendon passes inferomedially posterior to the medial condyle of the femur, separated from the medial collateral ligament by a small bursa, to attach to a vertical line on the medial aspect of the medial condyle of the tibia just posterior to the attachment of sartorius and posteroinferior to the attachment of gracilis. Near its attachment, it is separated from gracilis by a bursa and, with gracilis, is separated from sartorius by another bursa.

Innervation

By the tibial division of the sciatic nerve (root value L5, S1, S2). Skin covering the muscle is supplied mainly by S2.

Action

Working with the distal attachment fixed, semitendinosus helps extend the hip joint when the trunk is flexed. Working with the proximal attachment fixed, it aids flexion of the knee joint; if the knee is semiflexed, it produces medial rotation of the knee. If the foot is fixed, semitendinosus acts as a lateral rotator of the femur and pelvis on the tibia.

Semimembranosus

Situated on the posteromedial side of the thigh in its distal part, deep to semitendinosus, semimembranosus attaches by a strong membranous tendon to the upper lateral facet on the rough part of the ischial tuberosity (Fig. 3.43) and passes inferomedially. It becomes fleshy

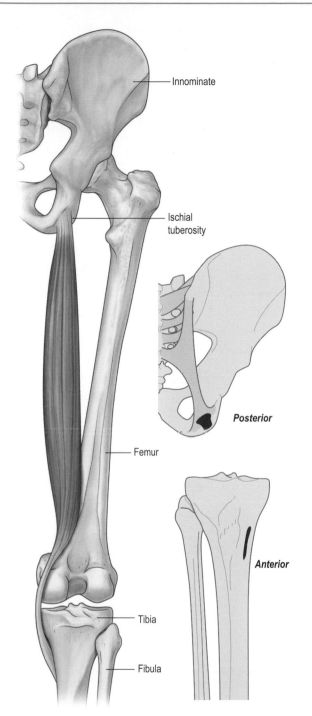

Fig. 3.42 Posterior aspect of the right innominate, femur and proximal tibia and fibula showing the position and attachments of semitendinosus.

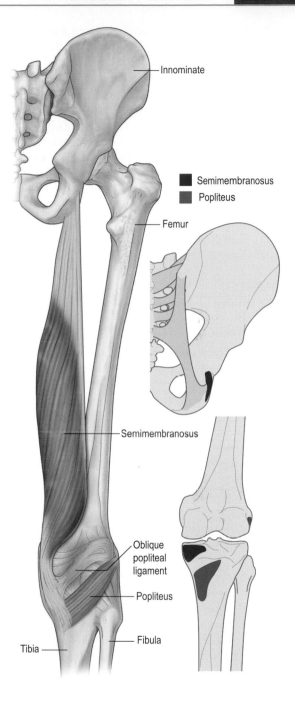

Fig. 3.43 Posterior aspect of the right innominate, femur and proximal tibia and fibula showing the position and attachments of semimembranosus and popliteus.

on the medial side of the tendon, being deep to semi-tendinosus and biceps femoris. From the distal part of the muscle, a second aponeurotic tendon arises, narrowing towards its distal attachment to a horizontal groove on the posteromedial aspect of the medial tibial condyle. From here, its fibres spread in all directions, but especially superolaterally, forming the oblique popliteal ligament. Bursae separate the muscle from the medial head of gastrocnemius and the tibia near its attachment.

Innervation

By the tibial division of the sciatic nerve (root value L5, S1, S2). Skin covering the muscle is the same as that for semitendinosus, being mainly from S2.

Action

As for semitendinosus.

Biceps Femoris

Situated on the posterolateral aspect of the thigh, biceps femoris (Fig. 3.44) arises by two heads separated by a considerable distance.

The long head attaches to the lower medial facet on the ischial tuberosity, together with the tendon of semitendinosus, spreading onto the sacrotuberous ligament. The two tendons descend together for a short distance and then separate into the two individual muscles; the long head of biceps femoris forms a fusiform muscle running inferolaterally across the posterior aspect of the thigh superficial to the sciatic nerve. In the distal one-third of the thigh, the long head narrows and is joined on its deep aspect by the short head of biceps femoris.

The short head arises from the distal half of the lateral lip of the linea aspera, reaching almost as far as the attachment of gluteus maximus and running inferiorly to the proximal half of the lateral supracondylar line of the femur; some fibres arise from the lateral intermuscular septum. The fibres of the short head gradually blend with the narrowing tendon of the long head superficial to it.

Before its attachment to the head of the fibula, the tendon of biceps femoris is split in two by the fibular (lateral) collateral ligament. Some tendon fibres join the ligament, a few attach to the lateral tibial condyle and some to the posterior aspect of the lateral intermuscular septum lying anterior to it. A bursa separates the tendon from the lateral collateral ligament.

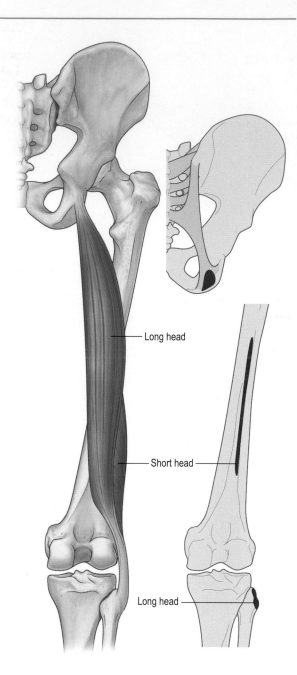

Long head

Short head

Long head

Fig. 3.44 Posterior aspect of the right innominate, femur and proximal tibia and fibula showing the position and attachments of biceps femoris.

Innervation

The long head is supplied by the tibial division of the sciatic nerve, and the short head by the common fibular/peroneal division (the root value of both is L5, S1, S2). Skin covering the muscle is supplied mainly by S2.

Action

Biceps femoris helps the other hamstrings extend the hip joint, particularly when the trunk is flexed and is to be raised to the erect position. All three hamstrings control forward flexion of the trunk; however, in this case, they are working eccentrically. Biceps femoris aids semimembranosus and semitendinosus in flexing the knee joint. With the knee semiflexed it laterally rotates the leg/calf on the thigh or, if the foot is fixed, medially rotates the thigh and pelvis on the leg/calf.

Palpation

On approaching the knee, the tendon can be felt crossing its posterolateral aspect as it passes towards the head of the fibula.

Functional Activity of the Hamstrings

The hamstrings make up the large muscle mass which can be palpated on the posterior aspect of the thigh; all three muscles cross the posterior aspects of both the hip and knee joints. The stabilising effect in flexion of the knee is a very important function of these muscles, although, for this action, a much smaller muscle bulk would be sufficient. Extension of the hip joint when the thigh is moving would also require a smaller group of muscles, especially when gluteus maximus is better situated to do this. Raising the trunk from a flexed position on the other hand requires a great deal more power as the muscles are working with a very short lever arm (the ischium and its ramus); the weight of the trunk acting on the other side of the hip joint is considerable.

The mode of action of this group of muscles may well be the reason it is injured so frequently during sporting activities. The most common cause of a sports injury appears in running, being more common in the first 10 to 20 m of a sprint. This is often blamed on inadequate preparation and warm-up before the start, and to some extent, this may be true; however, it is at this stage in a race that the hamstrings are contracting strongly across two joints.

At the start of a race, the athlete is in a forward-lean position to gain as much forward motion as possible; starting blocks serve to increase the degree of forward leaning. The hamstrings are, therefore, working to their maximum, either to raise the trunk into an erect position or to hold the trunk in such a position that forward collapse of the body as a whole is imminent. At the same time, the lower limb is thrust forward to gain as much ground as possible, with flexion of the knee preventing the foot from touching the ground. The hamstrings are under immense strain in this position, and it is not surprising that they may tear.

The hamstrings also play an important role in the fine balance of the pelvis when standing, particularly when the upper trunk moves from the vertical. Working in conjunction with the abdominal muscles anterosuperiorly and gluteus maximus posteroinferiorly, the anteroposterior tilt of the pelvis can be altered; this has an effect on lumbar lordosis.

Finally, the hamstrings have a role in decelerating the forward motion of the tibia when the free-swinging leg is extended during walking, preventing the knee from snapping into extension.

MUSCLES ABDUCTING THE THIGH AT THE HIP JOINT

Gluteus maximus (p. 302)
Gluteus medius
Gluteus minimus
Tensor fascia lata (p. 369)

Gluteus Medius

Fan-shaped muscle situated on the superolateral part of the buttock just inferior to the iliac crest, gluteus medius (Fig. 3.45) is broader superiorly, narrowing to its tendon inferiorly. Filling the space between the iliac crest and greater trochanter of the femur, it is overlapped posteriorly by gluteus maximus.

It arises from the gluteal (lateral) surface of the ilium between the posterior and anterior gluteal lines (Fig. 3.7); this is an extensive area, reaching to the iliac crest superiorly and almost as far as the sciatic notch inferiorly. Gluteus medius is covered by a strong layer of fascia from the deep surface of which it has a firm attachment; it shares the posterior part of the fascia with gluteus maximus.

The posterior fibres pass inferoanteriorly, middle fibres inferiorly and anterior fibres posteroinferiorly. The fibres come together to form a flattened tendon attaching to a roughened area running anteroinferiorly on the superolateral aspect of the greater trochanter of the femur. The tendon is separated from the trochanter by a bursa; its position is given by a smooth area anterior to the tendon's attachment.

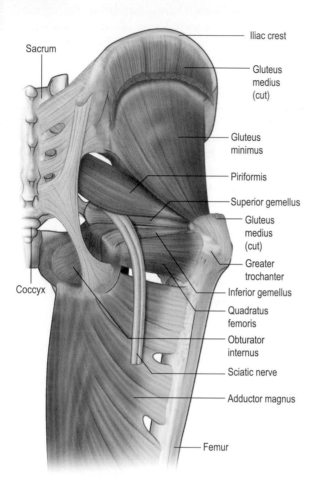

Fig. 3.45 Posterior view of the right gluteal region.

Innervation

By the superior gluteal nerve (root value L4, L5, S1). Skin covering the muscle is mainly supplied from L1 and L2.

Action

With the pelvis fixed, gluteus medius pulls the greater trochanter of the femur superiorly; however, as the fulcrum of movement is at the hip joint, this causes the femoral shaft to move laterally producing abduction.

If the distal muscle attachment is fixed, it pulls the wing of the ilium inferiorly, producing a downward tilting of the pelvis to the same side and raising the pelvis on the opposite side. In addition, acting from a fixed pelvis, the anterior fibres help medially rotate the femur;

with the femur fixed, these same fibres rotate the opposite side of the pelvis forwards.

Functional Activity

Gluteus medius plays a vital role in walking, running and single limb weight-bearing. With the opposite limb off the ground, the pelvis on that side would tend to drop through loss of support from below. Gluteus medius on the supporting side works hard to maintain, or even raise, the opposite side of the pelvis, allowing the raised limb to be brought forward for the next step during walking. Paralysis of the muscle results in dropping of the pelvis on the opposite side during this manoeuvre.

In walking or running, not only is gluteus medius important for support, but with the help of other muscles (gluteus minimus, tensor fascia lata) it produces rotation of the hip joint. This time with the femur as the more fixed point, it controls pelvic rotation on the same side. If it is unable to work efficiently due to paralysis or poor mechanics of the hip joint, the pelvis will drop on the opposite side (Trendelenburg sign); in this case, walking is awkward and difficult, and running virtually impossible.

Palpation

The bulk of the muscle is two finger's breadth below the middle of the iliac crest, which itself is directly above the greater trochanter of the femur. When standing alternately on one limb and then the other, the muscle becomes hard as the weight is borne on the same limb. Place the fingers of the other hand on the opposite side and walk slowly around the room, the two muscles can be felt alternately coming into action.

An individual with a Trendelenburg gait, either on one or both sides, compensates for the lack of support of the swinging limb by throwing the trunk over the supporting limb so that the weight is balanced over the hip, giving time to swing the limb through.

Gluteus Minimus

Although the smallest of the gluteal muscles, gluteus minimus has the largest attachment from the gluteal surface of the ilium; it is triangular in shape, wider superiorly, narrowing to a tendon inferiorly (Fig. 3.45).

Arising from the gluteal surface of the ilium anterior to the anterior and superior to the inferior gluteal lines (Fig. 3.7), reaching as far anteriorly as the anterior border of the ilium anteriorly and almost to the sciatic notch posteriorly. Its fibres pass inferiorly, posteriorly and slightly laterally, forming a tendon which attaches to a small depression on the anterosuperior aspect of the greater trochanter of the femur.

Innervation

By the superior gluteal nerve (root value L4, L5, S1). Skin overlying the muscle is mainly supplied by L1.

Action

If the proximal attachment is fixed, contraction of its anterior fibres medially rotates the femur; this is because the femoral attachment lies lateral to the fulcrum of the movement (hip joint). If the distal attachment is fixed, it raises the opposite side of the pelvis in a similar way to gluteus medius. It will also, by pulling the anterior part of the ilium laterally, swing the opposite side of the pelvis forwards.

Functional Activity

Gluteus minimus appears to play its most important role in supporting and controlling pelvic movements. It is a well-developed and powerful muscle, using its power to a maximum in walking and running when the opposite limb is off the ground. As the limb is swung forward, the pelvis on the same side also swings forward. This uses the hip of the weight-bearing limb as the fulcrum of the movement, with gluteus medius and minimus both supporting the pelvis and swinging it forward on the opposite side.

Palpation

Find the anterior superior iliac spine on the iliac crest. Allow the pads of the fingers to slip inferoposteriorly towards the greater trochanter of the femur; within two fingers' breadth they will be on the muscle bulk. Keeping the hand in this position while medially rotating the lower limb the muscle belly can be felt contracting hard. Do the same on the opposite side of the body and then begin to walk forward; the muscles can be felt contracting alternately as each limb assumes weight-bearing.

MUSCLES ADDUCTING THE THIGH AT THE HIP JOINT

Adductor magnus
Adductor longus
Adductor brevis
Gracilis (p. 364)
Pectineus (p. 301)

These muscles are situated on the medial aspect of the hip joint and pass inferiorly to the medial side of the thigh.

Adductor Magnus

Largest and most posterior of adductor muscles, adductor magnus (Fig. 3.46) lies posterior to adductors brevis and longus (Fig. 3.47) and anterior to semimembranosus and semitendinosus. Consisting of two parts (adductor, hamstring) it forms a large triangular sheet of muscle with a thickened medial margin.

Arising from the outer surface of the ischiopubic ramus and lateral part of the inferior surface of the ischial tuberosity (Fig. 3.48), the part of the muscle attaching anteriorly to the ischiopubic ramus (adductor part) represents a sheet of muscle which twists before attaching to the femur, while the posterior fibres from the ischial tuberosity (hamstring part) pass vertically inferiorly as a thickened cord.

The ischiopubic fibres fan out forming a large triangular muscular sheet, with the most anterior fibres passing laterally and slightly posteriorly to attach to the proximal part of the linea aspera, continuing superiorly as far as the greater trochanter medial to the attachment of gluteus maximus; these superior fibres may fuse with quadratus femoris. Fibres from the posterior part of the ischiopubic ramus attach to the whole length of the linea aspera and medial supracondylar ridge; the attachment is not continuous as there are small fibrous arches close to the bone allowing vessels and nerves to pass from the medial (adductor) to posterior compartments of the thigh. The posterior ischial fibres pass inferiorly, attaching mainly to the adductor tubercle situated on the medial condyle of the femur at the distal end of the medial supracondylar ridge; some fibres continue inferiorly fusing with the medial collateral ligament of the knee.

Innervation

Because of its two parts, adductor magnus has a dual nerve supply; the adductor part is supplied by the posterior division of the obturator nerve (root value L2, L3), and the hamstring part by the tibial division of the sciatic nerve (root value L4). Skin covering the medial aspect of the thigh being mainly supplied from L3.

Action

Working as a whole, the muscle adducts the thigh at the hip joint, although the posterior portion aids in hip

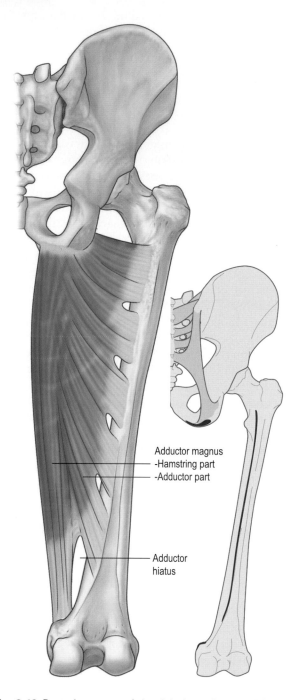

Adductor magnus
-Hamstring part
-Adductor part

Adductor
hiatus

Fig. 3.46 Posterior aspect of the right innominate and femur showing the position and attachments of adductor magnus.

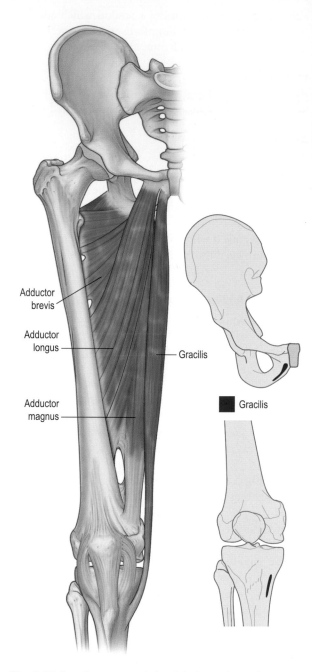

Adductor
brevis

Adductor
longus

Gracilis

Adductor
magnus

Gracilis

Fig. 3.47 Anterior aspect of the right innominate, femur and proximal tibia and fibula showing the position and attachments of the adductor muscles and gracilis.

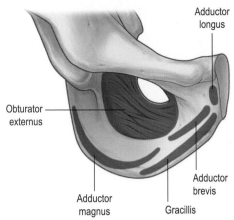

Fig. 3.48 Outer aspect of the inferior lateral right innominate and obturator membrane showing the attachments of the adductors, gracilis and obturator externus.

extension. Some consider that adductor magnus, together with adductor longus, medially rotates the thigh at the hip joint, although it has previously been thought that they also act as lateral rotators. Whether the muscle acts as a medial or lateral rotator depends on the position of the thigh and the line of action of the muscle with respect to the mechanical axis of the femur (Fig. 3.30). All adductor muscles are important in preventing lateral overbalancing during the support phase of walking.

It is worth noting that the medial collateral ligament of the knee joint appears to be an inferior continuation of the tendon of adductor magnus and, as such, it may at some time have crossed the knee joint and, therefore, have been a flexor of the knee in a similar manner to gracilis.

Palpation

Adductor magnus is a deep muscle and difficult to palpate; nevertheless, if the fingers are pushed in just above the medial femoral condyle, the adductor tubercle can be identified (Fig. 3.21). If the medial side of the foot of the same limb is now pressed against a stationary obstacle, the vertical part of the muscle can be felt contracting. The muscle can be traced about a third of the way up the thigh until it becomes hidden by other muscles.

Adductor Longus

Long, slender, triangular muscle, adductor longus (Fig. 3.49) lies in the medial aspect of the thigh overlying the middle part of adductor magnus. It has a narrower

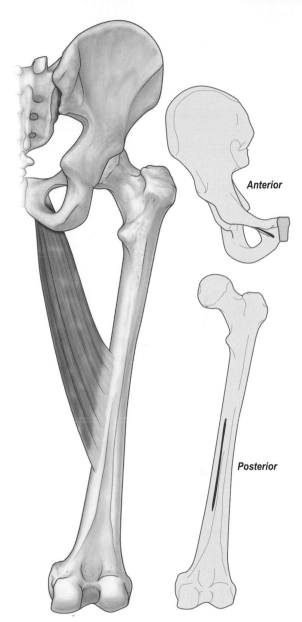

Fig. 3.49 Posterior aspect of the right innominate and femur showing the position and attachments of adductor longus.

superior attachment from a small, roughened area just inferior to the medial end of the obturator crest on the anterior aspect of the body of the pubis (Fig. 3.48).

Its fibres pass inferolaterally, spreading out as they attach to the middle two-quarters of the linea aspera, anterior to adductor magnus inferiorly and adductor brevis superiorly, and posterior to vastus medialis.

Innervation

By the anterior division of the obturator nerve (root value L2, L3, L4). Skin covering overlying adductor longus is supplied by L3.

Action

Adductor longus adducts the thigh at the hip joint, but as a rotator of the thigh, there is some doubt (see also adductor magnus). It can also flex the extended thigh and extend the flexed thigh.

Adductor Brevis

Triangular muscle situated on the medial aspect of the thigh (Fig. 3.50), it arises from the lateral part of the anterior aspect of the body and inferior ramus of the pubis (Fig. 3.48). Its fibres pass inferiorly, laterally and posteriorly to attach to the proximal half of the linea aspera anterior to adductor magnus. Its proximal part is posterior to pectineus and the distal part posterior to adductor longus.

Innervation

By the anterior division of the obturator nerve (root value L2, L3, L4). Skin covering the area of adductor brevis is supplied by L2.

Action

Adducts the thigh at the hip joint.

Palpation

If the fingers are placed high up on the medial aspect of the thigh and the lower limb is adducted against resistance, a mass of muscle can be palpated running towards the thigh. These are the adductors; however, it is difficult to distinguish between individual muscles.

Functional Activity of the Adductors

Although it is clear that these muscles adduct the thigh, they appear to work most strongly with the hip joint in neutral (anatomical position). They certainly work strongly and synergistically when the knee and hip joints are flexed and extended when weight-bearing. However, there is still some confusion over whether the muscles are involved in either medial or lateral rotation of the thigh. They work strongly during walking as they pull the supporting limb into adduction, moving the line of gravity over the supporting foot. They also contribute to the delicate balancing of the pelvis on the hip joint. The adductors

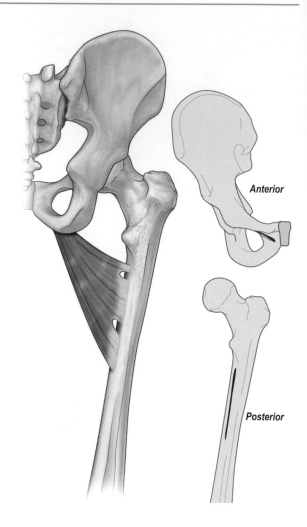

Fig. 3.50 Posterior aspect of the right innominate and proximal femur showing the position and attachments of adductor brevis.

as a group work very strongly when an object is being held between the knees when sitting (riding a horse).

MUSCLES MEDIALLY ROTATING THE THIGH AT THE HIP JOINT

Anterior part of gluteus medius (p. 307)
Anterior part of gluteus minimus (p. 308)
Tensor fascia lata (p. 369)
Psoas major (p. 299)
Iliacus (p. 301)

MUSCLES LATERALLY ROTATING THE THIGH AT THE HIP JOINT

Gluteus maximus (p. 302)
Piriformis
Obturator internus
Gemellus superior
Gemellus inferior
Quadratus femoris
Obturator externus

Piriformis

Located posterior to the hip joint in the same plane as the gluteus medius, piriformis (Fig. 3.51) is a triangular muscle with its base in the pelvis and apex in the gluteal region.

It arises from the anterior aspect of the second to fourth sacral segments between and lateral to the anterior sacral foramina. As it passes out of the pelvis through the greater sciatic foramen into the gluteal region, it gains an additional attachment to the gluteal surface of the ilium and pelvic surface of the sacrotuberous ligament. The fibres continue to pass inferiorly, laterally and anteriorly, narrowing to a tendon attaching to the superior border and medial aspect of the greater trochanter of the femur. The fibres run in a straight line between the attachments through the greater sciatic foramen.

Innervation

By the anterior rami of the lumbosacral plexus (L5, S1, S2; mainly S1). Skin covering this area is supplied by the same nerve roots.

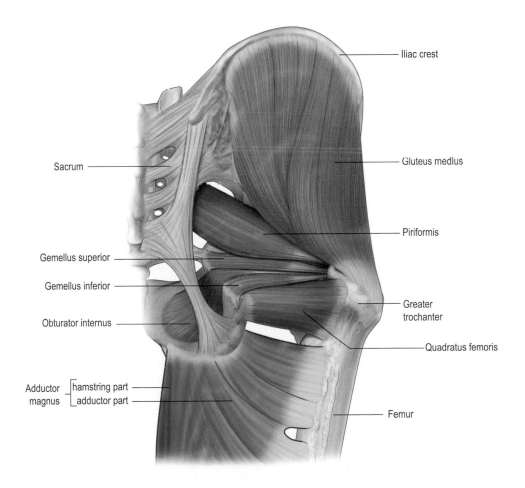

Fig. 3.51 Posterior aspect of the right innominate and proximal femur showing the muscles responsible for lateral rotation of the thigh at the hip joint.

Action

In the anatomical position, piriformis is a lateral rotator of the thigh at the hip joint, even though it is situated a little high. However, when seated, it is important in abduction, being well positioned for this action. It is an important muscle holding the femoral head in the acetabulum.

Functional Activity

It must be remembered that muscle action is often only considered in the anatomical position. When seated, the line of action of muscles changes and the movement produced may bear little or no relation to the former action. Piriformis is particularly important in the following activities; abduction when seated (moving from one chair to another without standing up), moving the legs to the outside of a car in preparation for standing up, stabilising the pelvis when the trunk is rotated, controlling the balance of the pelvis when standing on a moving bus. It is not surprising that strain of this muscle is fairly common, but unfortunately easily overlooked.

Palpation

A deep muscle with gluteus maximus intervening between it and the skin, palpation is not easy. Dig your fingers into the buttock just lateral to the sacrum and then push the outside of the thigh up against the leg of a table or some suitable resistance; the muscle can then be felt to contract even though a large part of it is in the pelvis.

Obturator Internus

A triangular-shaped muscle, obturator internus (Fig. 3.51) is situated partly in the pelvis and partly in the gluteal region posterior to the hip joint. It arises from the deep surface of the obturator membrane and surrounding bony margin, except at the obturator canal; this bony attachment extends as far posteriorly as the pelvic surface of the ilium. The muscle fibres pass laterally, but mainly posteriorly towards the lesser sciatic foramen, through which they pass, narrowing and becoming tendinous as they do so.

As the tendon passes through the lesser sciatic foramen deep to the sacrotuberous ligament, it changes direction to pass anterolaterally, to attach to the medial surface of the greater trochanter of the femur anterior and superior to the trochanteric fossa. Before attaching to the femur, the tendon is commonly joined by those of gemellus superior superiorly and gemellus inferior inferiorly. Occasionally, the two gemelli tendons attach to the greater trochanter superior and inferior to the tendon of obturator internus.

The deep (pelvic) surface of obturator internus is covered by the obturator fascia, from which arises part of levator ani. As the tendon passes around the lesser sciatic notch, the surface of the bone in this region is grooved and covered with cartilage; a bursa intervenes between the tendon and cartilage.

Innervation

By the nerve to obturator internus (root value L5, S1, S2). Skin covering this area is mainly supplied by S3.

Action

In the anatomical position, obturator internus laterally rotates the thigh at the hip joint pulling the greater trochanter posteriorly using the hip joint as the fulcrum. However, when the hip is flexed to 90 degrees, it pulls the proximal end of the femur medially; the distal end moves laterally as in abduction.

Functional Activity

As with piriformis (p. 313), obturator internus is used when moving sideways when seated, in swinging the lower limb sideways as in placing the limb outside a car, and in balancing and controlling the stability of the trunk when being rocked from side to side when seated. For the same reasons, moving around on the floor or on a platform, either sitting or crawling, requires considerable activity in the muscle.

Gemellus Superior

As obturator internus passes out of the pelvis around the lesser sciatic notch, it is joined by gemellus superior and inferior. Gemellus superior (Fig. 3.51) arises from the gluteal surface of the ischial spine. It runs laterally and slightly inferiorly to blend with the superior aspect of the tendon of obturator internus. Sometimes its fibres are prolonged onto the medial surface of the greater trochanter of the femur.

Innervation

By the nerve to obturator internus (root value L5, S1, S2).

Gemellus Inferior

Gemellus inferior (Fig. 3.51) arises from the superior part of the ischial tuberosity. It runs laterally and slightly superiorly to blend with the inferior aspect of the tendon of obturator internus.

Innervation

By the nerve to quadratus femoris (root value L4, L5, S1).

Action

The gemelli aid obturator internus in its action; as obturator internus winds around the lesser sciatic notch, it loses some of its power, the gemelli compensates for this loss.

Quadratus Femoris

A flat quadrilateral muscle, quadratus femoris is situated inferior to gemellus inferior and superior to the proximal margin of adductor magnus (Fig. 3.51); it is separated from the hip joint by obturator externus. It attaches to the ischial tuberosity just inferior to the inferior acetabular rim, the fibres then pass laterally to attach to the quadrate tubercle halfway along the intertrochanteric crest of the femur and area of bone surrounding it.

Innervation

By the nerve to quadratus femoris (root value L4, L5, S1).

Action

In the anatomical position, quadratus femoris laterally rotates the thigh at the hip joint, but with the hip flexed, it acts as an abductor.

Obturator Externus

Triangular muscle with its muscular base attached to the outer surface of obturator membrane and surrounding margins of the pubis and ischium, excluding the area superiorly around obturator canal (Fig. 3.48). The muscle fibres converge onto a tendon which runs in a groove inferior to the acetabulum across the posterior aspect of the femoral neck, which it grooves, to attach to the trochanteric fossa of the femur. The muscle lies deep to the quadratus femoris.

Innervation

By the posterior branch of obturator nerve (root value L3, L4).

Action

In the anatomical position, obturator externus laterally rotates the thigh at the hip joint. However, when the hip is flexed, it pulls the proximal part of the femur medially so that the distal part moves laterally, as in abduction.

Functional Activity

The functional activities of the lateral rotators must be considered together. Piriformis, the gemelli, obturators internus and externus, and quadratus femoris are always considered in the anatomical position, in which they perform an important role in controlling the pelvis, particularly when only one foot is on the ground and even more so in walking. They are responsible, together with gluteus maximus and the posterior part of gluteus medius, for producing lateral rotation of the lower limb in the forward swing phase of gait. However, when sitting, crawling and turning over when lying down, they have a completely different role producing abduction of the thigh at the hip joint and controlling movement of the pelvis on the flexed thigh.

Palpation

The lateral rotators are situated deep to gluteus maximus so that it is almost impossible to distinguish their individual contractions through the overlying muscle, especially as gluteus maximus is usually contracting at the same time. However, overactivity or strain of these muscles may result in acute tenderness deep to the posterior aspect of the hip joint; pain can then be elicited with the relevant movement.

It is difficult to precisely determine the actions of the lateral rotators, primarily because of their depth in the gluteal region, but also because much of their action is concerned with controlling movement at the hip joint and pelvis. They may be in a state of contraction even when movement opposite to their primary action is occurring. The muscles are arranged sequentially, often being referred to as the ladder of muscles (Fig. 3.51).

CLINICAL EXAMINATION AND EVALUATION

Flexion

With the individual lying supine:
- Place the hip in neutral abduction/adduction and rotation.
- Flex the opposite hip sufficiently to flatten the lumbar spine.

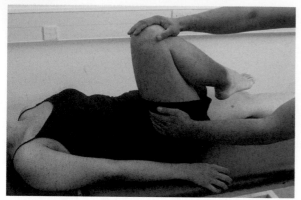

Fig. 3.52 Evaluation of the range of flexion at the hip joint with the individual lying supine.

- Extend the knee.
- Then flex the hip while stabilising the pelvis (Fig. 3.52).
- As flexion approaches its maximum, allow the knee to flex to prevent tension in the hamstrings limiting the movement.

Maximum active flexion is reached when the pelvis begins to rotate; maximum passive flexion occurs when the anterior thigh makes contact with the lower abdominal wall. The end feel to flexion is usually soft due to soft tissue contact; however, it may be firm due to tension in the posterior joint capsule and gluteus maximus.

To measure hip flexion, the centre of the goniometer is placed over the lateral aspect of the greater trochanter, with the proximal arm aligned over the lateral midline of the pelvis and distal arm in line with the lateral femoral epicondyle.

Extension

With the individual prone:
- Place the hip in neutral abduction/adduction and rotation.
- Extend the knee.
- Then extend the hip (Fig. 3.53A).

Maximum extension is taken when the pelvis begins to rotate. The end feel to extension is firm due to tension developed in the anterior joint capsule and the iliofemoral, pubofemoral and ischiofemoral ligaments; there may also be tension in the hip flexors.

To measure hip extension, the centre of the goniometer is placed over the lateral aspect of the greater trochanter, with the proximal arm aligned over the lateral midline of the pelvis and the distal arm in line with the lateral femoral epicondyle.

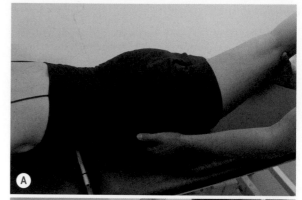

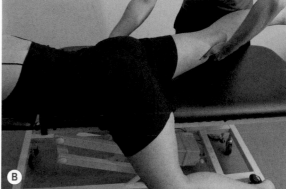

Fig. 3.53 Evaluation of the range of extension at the hip joint with the individual (A) lying prone and (B) with the opposite hip flexed and foot on the ground.

Alternatively, the individual supports the trunk on the examination table with the opposite hip flexed and foot on the ground (Fig. 3.53B). Movement of the pelvis is more easily determined; however, this method can be awkward in adults, although it easier to perform in children.

Abduction

With the individual lying supine:
- Place the hip in neutral flexion/extension and rotation.
- Extend the knee.
- Then abduct the hip while stabilising the pelvis to prevent rotation and lateral tilting (Fig. 3.54A).
- During movement, the ankle is held to prevent lateral rotation of the hip.

Maximum abduction is reached when the pelvis starts to tilt, determined by (i) placing the hand over the opposite anterior superior iliac spine or (ii) when there is lateral flexion/bending of the trunk. The end feel to hip abduction is firm due to tension in the joint capsule,

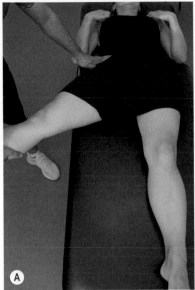

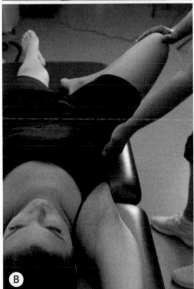

Fig. 3.54 Evaluation of the range of abduction at the hip joint with the individual (A) lying supine and hip in neutral flexion/extension and (B) with the hip flexed to 90 degrees.

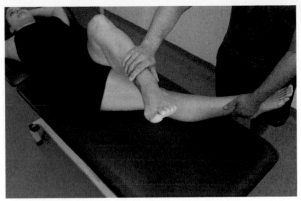

Fig. 3.55 Evaluation of the range of adduction at the hip joint with the individual lying supine with the opposite hip flexed and the limb supported.

the flexed hip and not laterally rotate it. Measuring abduction in flexion is useful in neonates and young infants.

Adduction

With the individual lying supine:
- Place the hip in neutral rotation.
- Flex the opposite hip sufficiently to enable the lower limb to move under it during the movement.
- Extend the knee.
- Then adduct the hip while stabilising the pelvis to prevent rotation and lateral tilting (Fig. 3.55).
- During movement, the ankle is held to prevent lateral rotation of the hip.

Maximum adduction is reached when the pelvis starts to tilt, determined by (i) placing the hand over the opposite anterior superior iliac spine or (ii) when there is lateral flexion/bending of the trunk. The end feel to hip adduction is firm due to tension in the joint capsule, ischiofemoral and lateral band of the iliofemoral ligaments, as well as the hip abductors.

To measure adduction, place the centre of the goniometer over the anterior superior iliac spine, with the proximal arm aligned with the opposite anterior superior iliac spine and the distal arm in line with the midline of the patella.

Medial Rotation

With the individual seated and legs hanging freely over the side of the supporting surface:
- Place the hip in neutral abduction/adduction and 90 degree flexion.
- Medially rotate the hip by moving the leg away from the midline while stabilising the distal end of the

pubofemoral and medial band of the iliofemoral ligaments, as well as in the hip adductors.

To measure hip abduction, the centre of the goniometer is placed over the anterior superior iliac spine, with the proximal arm aligned with the opposite anterior superior iliac spine and the distal arm in line with the midline of the patella.

Abduction can also be measured with the hip flexed at 90 degrees (Fig. 3.54B); however, care must taken to abduct femur to prevent adduction and further flexion at the hip (Fig. 3.56A); a rolled towel placed under the distal femur helps maintain the femur horizontal.

- During movement, rotation and lateral tilting of the pelvis must also be prevented.

Maximum medial rotation is reached when the pelvis begins to lift off the supporting surface. The end feel to medial rotation is firm due to tension in the joint capsule and ischiofemoral ligament, as well as the lateral rotators of the hip.

To measure medial rotation, the centre of the goniometer is placed over the anterior aspect of the patella, with one arm aligned perpendicular to the floor or supporting surface and the other in line with the tibial tuberosity and midway between the malleoli.

Medial rotation may also be measured with the individual lying supine or prone. With the individual supine:

- Place the hip in neutral flexion/extension and abduction/adduction.
- Extend the knee.
- Place the ankle in neutral plantarflexion/dorsiflexion.
- Medially rotate the hip by moving the foot towards the midline (Fig. 3.56B).

To measure medial rotation, place the centre of the goniometer over the centre of the heel, with one arm perpendicular to the supporting surface and the other in line with the second toe.

With the individual prone:

- Place the hip in neutral flexion/extension and abduction/adduction.
- Flex the knee 90 degrees.
- Medially rotate the hip by moving the leg away from the midline (Fig. 3.56C).

To measure medial rotation, place the centre of the goniometer over the anterior aspect of the patella, with one arm aligned perpendicular to the supporting surface and the other in line with the tibial tuberosity and midway between the malleoli.

Lateral Rotation

The testing positions and goniometer placements are similar to those outlined for medial rotation. With the individual seated and legs hanging freely over the side of the supporting surface, the hip is laterally rotated by moving the leg towards the midline (Fig. 3.57A). Maximum lateral rotation is reached when the pelvis begins to lift off the supporting surface. The end feel to lateral rotation is firm due to tension in the joint capsule, and iliofemoral and pubofemoral ligaments, as well as in the medial rotators of the hip.

With the individual lying supine, lateral rotation is measured by rotating the foot away from the midline (Fig. 3.57B), and with the individual prone, it is determined by rotating the leg/calf towards the midline (Fig. 3.57C).

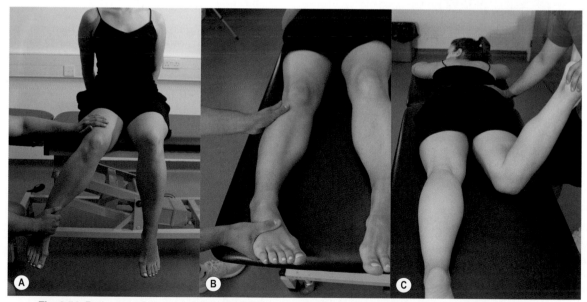

Fig. 3.56 Evaluation of the range of medial rotation at the hip with the individual (A) seated, (B) lying supine or (C) prone with the knee flexed to 90 degrees.

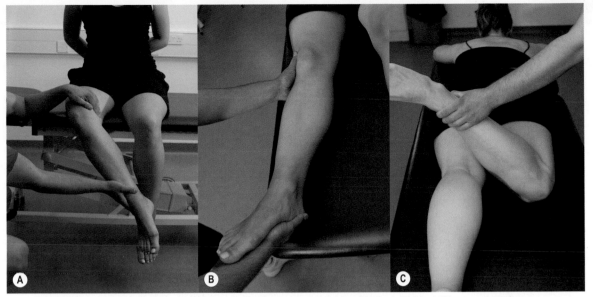

Fig. 3.57 Evaluation of the range of lateral rotation at the hip joint with the individual (A) seated, (B) lying supine and (C) prone with the knee flexed to 90 degrees.

SECTION SUMMARY

Innominate
- Consists of three bones (ilium, ischium, pubis) fused together at the acetabulum.
- Articulates with head of femur at the hip joint.

Femur
- Long bone of the thigh having a proximal head, neck, greater and lesser trochanters; shaft with linea aspera posteriorly; distal end with medial and lateral condyles.
- Head articulates with acetabulum of innominate forming the hip joint.
- Condyles articulate with tibia and patella forming the tibiofemoral and patellofemoral joints, respectively; both are part of the knee joint.

Hip Joint

Type	Synovial Ball-and-Socket
Articular surfaces	Head of the femur with the acetabulum of the innominate and acetabular labrum
Capsule	Strong fibrous capsule attaching to the margins of the acetabulum and intertrochanteric line (anterior) and neck of the femur (posterior); has longitudinal, oblique, arcuate and zona orbicularis fibres
Ligaments	Iliofemoral; pubofemoral; ischiofemoral; ligamentum teres; transverse ligament of acetabulum
Stability	Shape of articular surfaces; associated muscles and ligaments
Movements	Flexion and extension; abduction and adduction; medial and lateral rotation

Movements at Hip Joint
The hip joint consists of the head of the femur and acetabulum of the innominate; it is capable of a wide range of movement produced by the following muscles:

Movement	Muscles (Root Value of Nerve Supply)
Extension	Gluteus maximus (L5, S1, S2)
	Hamstrings
	Semitendinosus (L5, S1, S2)
	Semimembranosus (L5, S1, S2)
	Biceps femoris (L5, S1, S2)
Abduction	Gluteus maximus (L4, L5, S1)
	Gluteus medius (L4, L5, S1)
	Gluteus minimus (L4, L5, S1)
	Tensor fascia lata (L4, L5)

SECTION SUMMARY—cont'd

Movement	Muscles (Root Value of Nerve Supply)
Adduction	Adductors magnus (L2, L3, L4)
	Adductor longus (L2, L3, L4)
	Adductor brevis (L2, L3, L4)
	Gracilis (L2, L3)
	Pectineus (L2, L3)
Flexion	Psoas major (L1, L2, L3, (L4))
	Iliacus (L2, L3)
	Pectineus (L2, L3)
	Rectus femoris (L2, L3, L4)
	Sartorius (L2, L3)
Lateral rotation	Gluteus maximus (L5, S1, S2)
	Piriformis (L5, S1, S2)
	Obturator internus (L5, S1, S2)
	Obturator externus (L5, S1, S2)
	Gemellus superior (L5, S1, S2)
	Gemellus inferior (L4, L5, S1)
	Quadratus femoris (L4, L5, S1)
Medial rotation	Gluteus medius (L4, L5, S1)
	Gluteus minimus (L4, L5, S1)
	Tensor fascia lata (L4, L5)

- All of these muscles contribute to the stability of the hip joint.
- Long muscles acting across two joints (hamstrings, rectus femoris) can only work efficiently across one joint at a time (hamstrings can only extend the hip strongly with the knee extended).
- The hip abductors and adductors have an important function during gait when they work with their distal (femoral) attachments fixed to stabilise the pelvis.
- Some muscles attaching to the pelvis and lumbar spine are important in producing movements of the trunk (gluteus maximus, psoas major).

Clinical Examination

1. Movement and Maximum Range	2. End Feel to Movement
Flexion 120° (active)/145° (passive)	Soft
Extension 20° (active)/30° (passive)	Firm
Abduction 45°	Firm
Adduction 45°	Firm
Medial rotation 45°	Firm
Lateral rotation 45°	Firm

⑨ SELF-ASSESSMENT QUESTIONS

11. Which part of the innominate contributes to the hip joint?
12. Which muscle(s) attach to the lesser trochanter?
13. What type of tissue is the acetabular labrum?
14. Which muscle(s) flex the hip joint?
15. What is the root value of the nerve supplying rectus femoris?
16. Which parts of the innominate contribute to the acetabulum?
17. Which structure completes the inferior part of the acetabular rim?
18. To which part of the femoral head does the ligamentum teres attach?
19. What is the role of the ischiofemoral ligament?
20. What is the angle of anteversion of the femur; give its value in degrees?
21. Through which parts of the femur does the mechanical axis pass?
22. Which muscle(s) attach to the trochanteric fossa?
23. Is the adductor tubercle associated with the medial or lateral epicondyle?
24. What is the nerve supply, including root value, of gluteus maximus?
25. To which part of the femur does gluteus minimus attach?
26. What are the attachments of semitendinosus?
27. What are the actions of gracilis?
28. Adductor longus forms the medial border of which region in the thigh?
29. What is the nerve supply of gluteus medius, give its root value?
30. What are the attachments of quadratus femoris?
31. Which muscle(s) accompany obturator internus to its femoral attachment?
32. Which muscle(s) attach to the obturator membrane?
33. What are the active and passive ranges of hip extension?
34. What and where is the acetabular fat pad?
35. How many sets of fibres are associated with the hip joint capsule and what are they?
36. What is Shenton's line?
37. In which position of the hip are the articular surfaces most congruent?
38. Which muscle(s) abduct the hip joint?
39. What is the nerve supply, including its root value, of adductor brevis?
40. What is the nerve supply to psoas major?

KNEE

LEARNING OUTCOMES

By the end of the section, you should be able to:

1. Identify, palpate and examine the distal femur, proximal tibia and fibula and patella
2. Describe the bones, joints and muscles involved at the knee joint
3. Describe and explain the movements possible, and their restraints, at the knee joint
4. Locate, palpate and examine the muscles associated with the knee and know their attachments, action and innervation
5. Examine and assess movements of the knee joint
6. Appreciate the influence of pathology and/or trauma on the function of the knee joint

INTRODUCTION

The largest and one of the most complex joints of the body, the knee is a synovial bicondylar hinge joint between the condyles of the femur and those of the tibia and the patella anteriorly (Fig. 3.58). Three separate articulations can be identified: two femorotibial joints and the femoropatellar articulation. The arrangement of the synovial membrane suggests that these three articulations were separate at some stage in human evolution; however, in *Homo sapiens* the three joint cavities are connected by restricted openings forming a large single joint cavity.

The knee joint satisfies the requirements of a weight-bearing joint by allowing free movement in one plane only, combined with considerable stability, particularly in extension. Usually, stability and mobility are incompatible functions of a joint, with the majority of joints sacrificing one for the other. However, at the knee, both functions are secured by the interaction of ligaments and muscles, together with complex gliding and rolling movements at the articular surfaces (p. 345). Nevertheless, the relatively poor degree of interlocking of the articular surfaces, which is essential for great mobility, renders it liable to strains and dislocations. Although functionally the knee is a hinge joint, allowing flexion and extension in the sagittal plane, it also permits

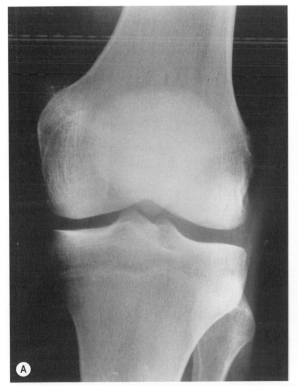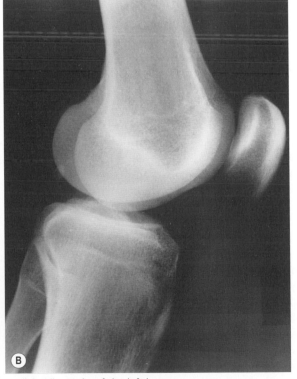

Fig. 3.58 (A) Anteroposterior and (B) medial radiographs of the left knee.

a small amount of rotation of the leg/calf, particularly when the knee is flexed and the foot is off the ground.

Supporting body weight on the vertically opposed ends of the two largest bones in the body is clearly an unstable arrangement; stability at the knee is ensured by a number of compensating mechanisms. Among these are (i) an expansion of the weight-bearing surfaces of both femur and tibia; (ii) the presence of strong collateral and intracapsular ligaments; (iii) a strong joint capsule; and (iv) the reinforcing effects of aponeuroses and tendons crossing the joint.

The knee joint plays an important role in locomotion, being the shortener and lengthener of the lower limb; it can also be considered to work by axial compression under the action of gravity. Endowed with powerful muscles, it acts with the ankle joint as a strong forward propeller of the body. It receives and absorbs vigorous stresses that lateral body movements in the coronal plane and axial rotations in the transverse plane impart to it.

Around the knee, the deep fascia is continuous with that of the leg/calf, attaching to the medial and lateral condyles of the tibia, head of the fibula and anteriorly to the patella. The patella is held to the tibial condyle by thickened bands of the deep fascia (medial and lateral patellar retinaculae). Posterior to the knee, over the popliteal fossa, the fascia is reinforced by transverse fibres.

FEMUR

Details of the femur can be found on page 277.

PATELLA

Triangular sesamoid bone (Fig. 3.59) formed in the tendon of quadriceps femoris, with its apex inferior and base superior; it is flattened anteroposteriorly, having anterior and posterior surfaces and superior, lateral and medial borders.

The anterior surface is marked by a series of roughened vertical ridges produced by the fibres of quadriceps femoris as they pass over it; it is slightly convex anteriorly with its shape varying according to the habitual pull of the muscle.

The posterior surface has a large, smooth, oval facet covered with hyaline cartilage for articulation with the patellar surface of the femur: the facet is divided by a broad vertical ridge into smaller medial and larger lateral parts. The cartilage on each facet is marked by two horizontal lines dividing each surface into upper, middle

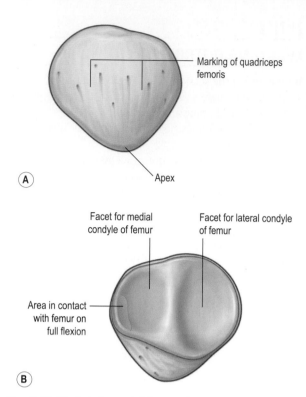

Fig. 3.59 (A) Anterior and (B) posterior aspects of the right patella.

and lower sections. Inferiorly is a roughened area on the posterior aspect of the apex for the proximal attachment of the ligamentum patellae.

The base of the patella is roughened for the attachment of rectus femoris and vastus intermedius; the medial and lateral borders are rounded, but also roughened, receiving attachments of vastus medialis and lateralis, respectively.

Ossification

At birth, the patella is cartilaginous, ossifying from a single centre or several centres between 3 years and puberty; occasionally, the patella may be absent.

Palpation

As the patella lies subcutaneously, the whole margin and its anterior surface can be palpated.

TIBIA

Long bone (Fig. 3.60) transmitting body weight from the medial and lateral femoral condyles to the foot via

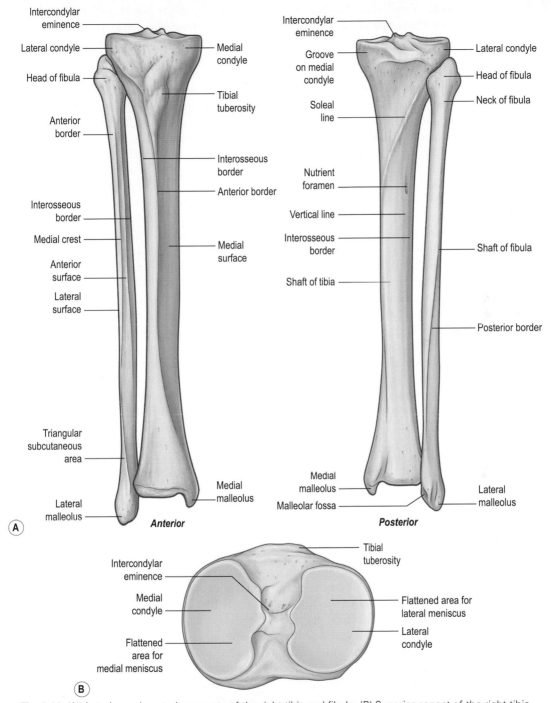

Fig. 3.60 (A) Anterior and posterior aspects of the right tibia and fibula. (B) Superior aspect of the right tibia.

the ankle joint; the tibia is the larger of the two bones of the leg, lying medial to the fibula. It consists of a shaft and two extremities, with the proximal being larger than the distal.

The proximal end is expanded in all directions, particularly posteriorly where it projects beyond the shaft. It consists of two condyles, between which is a large, truncated area anteriorly elongated in its vertical axis (tibial tuberosity), roughened proximally and smooth distally; the roughened area is for attachment of the ligamentum patellae. The lateral condyle projects further laterally than the shaft and has a round articular facet on its posterolateral aspect for articulation with the head of the fibula. Posteriorly, the space between the condyles is smooth. On the superior condylar surfaces are two areas for articulation with the femoral condyles separated by two raised tubercles (medial and lateral intercondylar tubercles) situated close together (intercondylar eminence). Anterior and posterior to the eminence are uneven non-articular areas, narrow close to the eminence becoming wider as they pass anteriorly and posteriorly; these areas give attachment to important structures associated with the knee joint. Anterior to the intercondylar eminence, three structures are attached: anterior horn of the medial meniscus most anteriorly; anterior horn of the lateral meniscus closest to the eminence; with the ACL between. The area behind the intercondylar eminence also gives attachment to three structures: PCL most posteriorly; posterior horn of the lateral meniscus closest to the eminence; with the posterior horn of the medial meniscus between.

The tibial shaft is triangular in cross-section, tapering slightly from the condyles for about two-thirds of its length then widening again distally. It has an anterior border running from the distal aspect of the tibial tuberosity inferiorly to the anterior part of the medial malleolus. The medial border begins just inferior to the posterior aspect of the medial condyle; although not always easy to see, it can be traced to the posterior part of the medial malleolus. The interosseous border begins just inferior to the articular facet on the lateral condyle, running in a curved line (concave forwards) to the roughened triangular area on the lateral side at the distal end of the tibia.

The shaft, therefore, has three surfaces: medial, posterior and lateral. The smooth medial surface slopes posteriorly from the anterior border below the medial condyle superiorly to the medial malleolus inferiorly; it is subcutaneous for its whole length and commonly called the shin. The lateral surface lies between the anterior and interosseous borders and is slightly concave, particularly in its proximal two-thirds, and gives attachment to tibialis anterior; inferiorly, it becomes continuous with the anterior surface of the distal end of the tibia. The posterior surface lies between the interosseous and medial borders and is crossed by two raised lines, one running obliquely from just inferior to the lateral condyle inferomedially to join the posterior border about halfway down (soleal line). The area superior to it is roughened for the attachment of popliteus; inferior to the soleal line is a vertical line to which the fascia covering tibialis posterior attaches. The inferior part of the posterior surface is divided into two roughened areas for muscle attachment; tibialis posterior laterally and flexor digitorum longus medially.

The distal end is expanded, but to a lesser extent than that proximally; it has a prominent medial malleolus continuous with the medial surface of the shaft which projects inferiorly from its medial side. The inferior surface is smooth for articulation with the superior surface of the body of the talus; it is continuous medially with the malleolar articular surface and then usually turns superiorly on the lateral surface where it becomes concave anteriorly for articulation with the fibula, superior to which it continues superiorly as a rough triangular area for attachment of the interosseous ligament. The posterior surface is coarse and grooved by tendons passing into the foot. The anterior surface is smooth and slightly convex.

Ossification

The primary ossification centre for the tibia appears in the shaft during the 7th week *in utero*, spreading so that only the ends are cartilaginous at birth. The secondary centre for the proximal end, including the tibial tuberosity, appears at birth spreading into the tuberosity after the 10th year. There may be an independent centre for the tuberosity; if so, it appears at 11 years. The secondary centre for the distal end appears during the 2nd year. Fusion of the proximal epiphysis with the shaft occurs between 19 and 21 years, and of the distal epiphysis with the shaft a few years earlier, between ages 17 and 19.

Palpation

The tibial tuberosity is easily recognisable at the superior end of the anterior tibial border (shin), with the ligamentum patellae attaching to its upper part. The medial and lateral condyles can be palpated about 2 cm higher, being subcutaneous as far as the hamstring muscles on either side. The superior margins of the condyles indicate the knee joint line.

Just inferior and posterior to the midpoint on the lateral side, the head of the fibula stands out clearly. Running down the whole length of the tibia from the medial surface of the medial condyle is the medial surface of the shaft, being subcutaneous as far as the medial malleolus; both anterior and posterior borders are palpable at their edges. The medial malleolus is subcutaneous and its medial surface, borders and tip are easily palpable.

Applied Anatomy

Because the medial surface of the tibia is subcutaneous, the risks of damage to and fracture of the bone are increased; the likelihood of infection and delayed/non-union are very high and a common complication. The most common area of damage is at the junction between the superior two-thirds and inferior one-third of the shaft, its thinnest part and unfortunately the area with the poorest blood supply.

FIBULA

Long slender bone (Fig. 3.60A) expanded both at its proximal and distal ends. The proximal end (head) is expanded in all directions, having on its superomedial aspect a facet for articulation with the lateral condyle of the tibia; lateral to the facet is the apex of the head projecting superiorly. The remainder of the proximal end is roughened for attachment of the tendon of biceps femoris. Just below the head is the neck around which runs the common fibular/peroneal nerve.

The shaft varies considerably between individuals with its features often being difficult to recognise; it has three borders and three surfaces. The anterior border is more prominent inferiorly where it widens into a smooth, triangular, subcutaneous area continuous with the lateral surface of the malleolus; it runs from inferior to the anterior aspect of the head vertically down to the triangular subcutaneous area. Medial to the anterior border is the often poorly marked interosseous border; extending from the neck, it lies close to the anterior border in its proximal one-third, then passes posteromedially to join the apex of the roughened triangular area superior to the malleolar articular surface. The posterior border begins below the lateral aspect of the head and neck and passes inferiorly to the medial margin of the posterior surface of the lateral malleolus; it is rounded and more difficult to trace. The lateral surface is concave and posterolateral to the anterior border, becoming convex as it winds posterior to the triangular subcutaneous area to the posterior surface of the malleolus; it is roughened for attachment of the fibularis/peroneal muscles. The anterior surface is a narrow strip between the anterior and interosseous borders proximally, expanding as it continues distally. The posterior surface is more expanded than the anterior and lateral surfaces, being divided by a vertical ridge (crest) into medial and lateral parts similar to the tibia. The region between the crest and interosseous border is concave, usually divided by an oblique line, while the region between the crest and posterior border is flat and roughened in its proximal part by the attachment of soleus.

The distal end can be readily recognised, being flattened medially and laterally with a deep malleolar fossa posteriorly. On its medial side, above the fossa, is a smooth triangular area for articulation with the lateral surface of the body of the talus. Just above this medial articular area is an elongated roughened area for attachment of the interosseous ligament of the inferior tibiofibular joint, below which is the malleolar fossa. The fibula varies in shape according to the muscles attaching to it and their strength; it carries no weight but contributes to the lateral stability of the ankle joint.

Ossification

The primary centre appears in the shaft during the 7th week *in utero*, spreading so that, at birth, only the ends are cartilaginous. The secondary centre for the distal end appears during the 2nd year and fuses with the body between 17 and 19 years. The secondary centre for the proximal end appears during the 3rd or 4th year, fusing with the body between 19 and 21 years.

At birth, the fibula is relatively thick, about half as thick as the tibia in the 3rd postnatal month. As development and growth continue, the thicknesses of the fibula and tibia progressively change, approaching adult proportions. The distal end of the fibula does not extend below the medial malleolus until after its ossification has begun (after the 2nd year); it is only after this time that the adult relations of the malleoli can be seen.

Palpation

The head of the fibula can be readily palpated on the posterolateral aspect below the knee joint. If the hand is placed on the lateral side of the leg/calf and moved superiorly towards the knee, the bony head can be felt projecting laterally. The head can also be easily palpated if the fingers are placed in the hollow on the lateral side of the knee when it is flexed 90 degrees. Little of the shaft can be palpated as it is surrounded by muscles; however, in its distal one-third an elongated triangular area can be palpated, the lateral aspect of which can be traced inferiorly to the lateral malleolus. The lateral malleolus is easily palpated on the lateral side of the ankle, projecting to a point 2.5 cm below the level of the ankle joint.

KNEE JOINT

Articular Surfaces

Femur

The articular surfaces of the femur are the two condyles, which rest on the tibia, and the patellar surface, which unites the condyles anteriorly and is opposed to the deep surface of the patella (Fig. 3.61A). At the junction of the condylar and patellar surfaces are two faint grooves. Laterally, these are almost transverse, emphasised at each end, while on the medial condyle, the medial end of the grooves begin further anteriorly, passing obliquely posteriorly then disappearing before reaching the lateral edge. In this region, there is a narrow crescentic area marked off where the patella articulates in acute flexion. The medial condylar area can be divided into two parts; a posterior part parallel to the lateral condyle and equal in extent, and an anterior triangular extension passing obliquely laterally. The patellar surface is divided by a well-marked groove into smaller medial and larger more prominent lateral parts.

Viewed inferiorly, the femoral condyles form two prominences convex in both planes, longer anteroposteriorly than

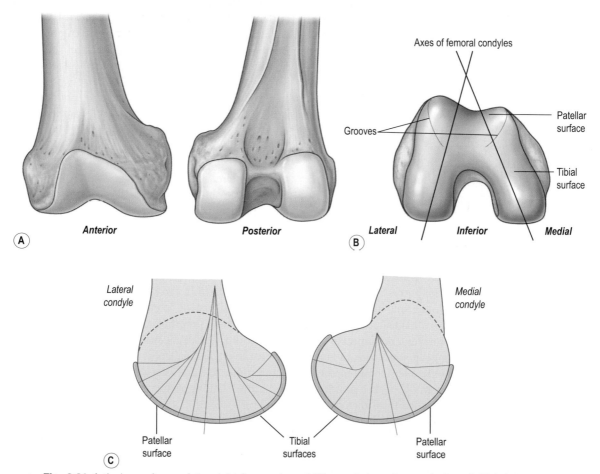

Fig. 3.61 Articular surfaces of the right femur viewed (A) anteriorly and posteriorly and (B) inferiorly. (C) Schematic paramedian sections of the femoral articular condyles indicating the spiral nature of their profiles.

transversely; they are not identical as the medial condyle juts out further from the median plane than the lateral and is also narrower. In addition, their long axes are not parallel but diverge posteriorly (Fig. 3.61B); the intercondylar notch continues the line of the groove of the patellar surface. In a coronal plane, the convexity of the femoral condyles corresponds more or less to the concavity of the tibial condyles, while in the sagittal plane, the radius of curvature of the condyles varies as a spiral. The manner in which the condyles become increasingly flatter from anterior to posterior is particularly significant in the mechanics of the joint.

Even though their radii of curvature increase regularly, the spirals of the femoral condyle are not simple spirals because they do not have a single centre of rotation, but rather a series of centres themselves lying on a spiral; the curve of the condyles represents a spiral of a spiral (Fig. 3.61C). The groove separating the condylar and patellar surface areas can be identified on each condyle, anterior and posterior to which the radius of curvature decreases. It must be remembered that the two

condyles do not show the same curvature; their radii of curvature differ. The internal architecture of the femoral condyles reflects their geometry and the stresses to which they are subjected (see Fig. 3.91).

Tibia

The tibial articular surfaces are cartilage-covered areas on the superior surface of each condyle, separated from each other by the intercondylar eminence and triangular intercondylar areas anteriorly and posteriorly (Fig. 3.62A). The articular areas are comparatively flat following the slight (3–5 degrees) posteroinferior inclination of the tibial condyles with respect to the horizontal. The medial articular surface is larger, oval and slightly concave, while the lateral articular surface is smaller, rounded and concave from side to side but concavoconvex anteroposteriorly (Fig. 3.62B). Posteriorly, the lateral surface extends inferiorly over the condyle in relation to the tendon of popliteus. The fossae of the articular surfaces of the tibia are deepened by the menisci,

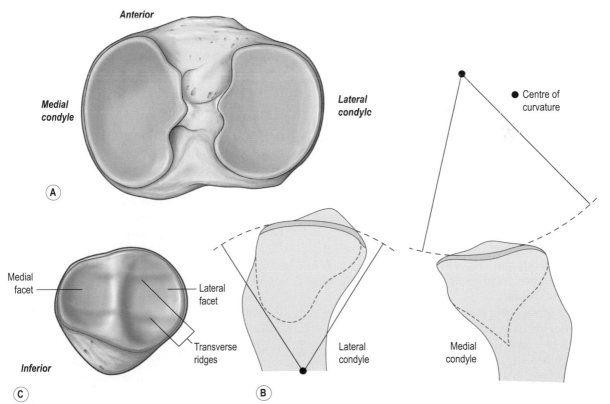

Fig. 3.62 (A) Superior aspect of the right tibia showing the articular surfaces. (B) Schematic representation of the anteroposterior condylar curvatures. (C) Articular surface of the right patella.

intervening between the femur and tibia, resting on a flattened strip at the periphery of each tibial condyle. Again, the internal architecture reflects the shape of the proximal end of the tibia and the stresses to which it is subjected (see Fig. 3.91).

The basic shapes of the femoral and tibial articular surfaces essentially only allow movement in one plane (flexion/extension). Axial rotation involves twisting of the femur against the tibia or vice versa, during which the intercondylar eminence of the tibia lodging in the intercondylar notch of the femur acts as a pivot. The pivot consists of the intercondylar tubercles which form the lateral border of the medial condyle and medial border of the lateral condyle; it is through this latter point that the vertical axis about which axial rotation occurs passes.

Patella

The articular surface of the patella is oval and divided into larger lateral and smaller medial areas by a vertical ridge for corresponding areas on the femur. Two faint transverse ridges separate three facets on each side; a further faint vertical ridge separates a medial perpendicular facet from the main medial area (Fig. 3.62C). In acute flexion, this medial facet articulates with the crescentic facet of the medial femoral condyle. The remaining facets articulate in succession from superior to inferior with the patellar surface of the femur as the joint goes from flexion to full extension. Because of the stresses to which the patella is subjected, particularly during walking and running, the cartilage on its deep surface is extremely thick; it may be the thickest anywhere in the body.

Palpation

Several parts of the knee joint can be readily palpated, especially laterally and anteriorly, confirming its superficial position within the lower limb. Although many musculotendinous structures cross the joint, they tend to do so posteriorly, together with the major blood vessels and nerves. The following parts of the joint can be palpated:

1. Whole of the circumference of the patella, especially its medial border
2. Articular margin of each femoral condyle
3. Anterior articular margin of each tibial condyle
4. Joint line medially, anteriorly and laterally
5. Tibial tuberosity together with the ligamentum patellae attaching to it
6. Adductor tubercle, medial and lateral epicondyles of the femur

No part of the joint can be identified posteriorly; however, the tendons of semitendinosus and semimembranosus medially and that of biceps femoris laterally stand out and can be easily identified as the knee is flexed against resistance (see Figs 3.74 and 3.75).

Joint Capsule

The knee joint is surrounded by a thick ligamentous sheath composed mainly of muscle tendons and their expansions (Fig. 3.63). There is no complete, independent, fibrous capsule uniting the two bones; only occasionally are there true capsular fibres running between them. The capsular attachment to the femur is deficient anteriorly where it blends with the fused tendons of the quadriceps muscles. Its attachment to the tibia is more complete, being deficient only in the region of the tibial tuberosity, which gives attachment to the ligamentum patellae. Despite its composite nature, it is, nevertheless, convenient to think of the joint capsule as a cylindrical sleeve passing between the femur and tibia, with a deficiency anteriorly lodging the patella.

Posteriorly, true capsular fibres arise from the femoral condyles, just above the articular surfaces, and intercondylar line passing vertically inferiorly, attaching to the posterior border of the proximal end of the tibia. At the sides of the joint, capsular fibres pass between the femoral and tibial condyles, blending posteriorly with a ligamentous network and anteriorly with the various tendinous expansions of the quadriceps muscles.

Capsular Strengthening

The majority of what is seen and taken for as the knee joint capsule is the ligamentous feltwork associated with the joint. This feltwork is extremely important, providing the capsule with its strength, as well as the necessary control and restriction to movement required at the knee.

Oblique popliteal ligament. The central region of the posterior part of the capsule is strengthened by the oblique popliteal ligament (Fig. 3.63A), an expansion of the semimembranosus tendon. It passes superolaterally, attaching to the intercondylar line of the femur; it has large foramina to accommodate the vessels and nerves which perforate it.

Arcuate popliteal ligament. The inferolateral part of the capsule is strengthened by the arcuate popliteal ligament (Fig. 3.63A) passing from the posterior aspect of the fibular head, arching superomedially over the popliteal tendon and then spreading out over the posterior surface. The most medial part of the ligament passes inferiorly to the posterior part of the intercondylar area of the tibia, while the most lateral fibres appear as a

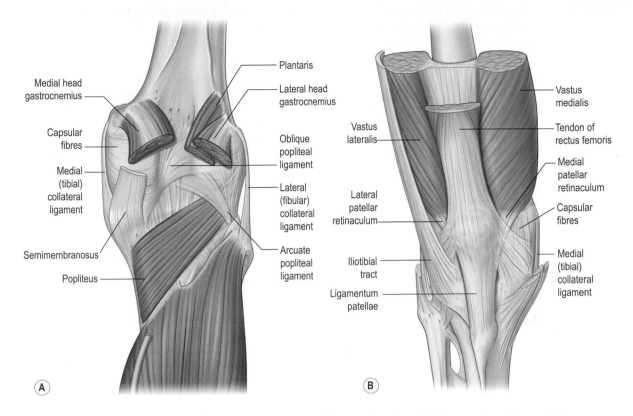

Fig. 3.63 (A) Posterior and (B) anterior aspects of the right knee showing the joint capsule and the contributions from various muscles and ligaments crossing the joint.

separate band running to the posterior aspect of the lateral femoral condyle.

On the lateral side of the joint, true capsular fibres are short and weak, bridging only the interval between the femoral and tibial condyles; some are separated from the lateral meniscus by the passage of the popliteal tendon.

On the anterior aspect of the joint, the ligamentous sheath consists of the fused tendons of the quadriceps muscles (Fig. 3.63B). Their fibres descend from above and each side to attach to the margins of the patella as far to the attachment of the ligamentum patellae; superficial tendinous fibres pass inferiorly over the patella into the ligamentum patellae. The aponeurotic tendons of vastus medialis and lateralis expand over the sides of the joint capsule as the medial and lateral patellar retinacula, respectively, attaching to the anterior aspect and oblique lines of the tibial condyles as far to the sides as the collateral ligaments. Medially, the retinaculum blends with the periosteum of the tibial shaft, and laterally with the overlying iliotibial tract. Some tendinous

fibres of the vastus muscles pass obliquely inferiorly across the patella into the opposite retinaculum, while deeper fibres from each side of the patella pass across to the anterior aspect of each femoral epicondyle.

Ligamentum Patellae

Continuation of the tendon of quadriceps femoris (Fig. 3.63B), the ligamentum patellae is a strong flat band attaching around the apex of the patella, continuous over its anterior surface with fibres of the quadriceps tendon. It extends to the tibial tuberosity, ending obliquely but prolonged further inferiorly laterally than medially. Between the ligament and bone, immediately proximal to its attachment, is the deep infrapatellar bursa, while in the subcutaneous tissue over the ligament is the large subcutaneous infrapatellar bursa.

Superficial to the fibrous bands associated with the quadriceps complex are strong expansions of the fascia lata covering the anterior and lateral aspects of the joint.

As it descends to attach to the tibial tuberosity and oblique lines of the condyles, the ligamentum patellae overlies and blends with the patellar retinaculae. The strong, thickened iliotibial tract passes inferiorly across the anterolateral aspect of the joint, attaching to the lateral tibial condyle after blending with the joint capsule (Fig. 3.63B). A strong band passes anteriorly from the iliotibial tract attaching to the superior aspect of the lateral edge of the patella (superior patellar retinaculum). On the thinner medial side of the patella, the fascia lata gives a few fibres inferiorly which blend with the expansion of sartorius.

The whole anterior covering of the knee joint, together with the patella, is kept tense by the tone of the extensor muscles (quadriceps femoris), tightly braced when they are active in extension. This appears to contradict the philosophy of hinge joints in that the extensor part of joint capsules should be loose in the extended position to permit free flexion. At the knee, the extensor part of the capsule is continued into the extensor muscles superiorly rather than being attached directly to bone; consequently, it is kept relatively taut in all joint positions.

Ligaments

As is characteristic of all hinge joints, collateral ligaments are found at the sides of the knee joint, although their form differs greatly.

Medial (Tibial) Collateral Ligament

Strong flat band extending from the medial epicondyle of the femur, passing inferiorly and slightly anteriorly, to attach to the medial tibial condyle and medial side of the shaft (Fig. 3.64). A few fibres at the femoral attachment can usually be traced superiorly into adductor magnus; consequently, it has been regarded as having been formed, in part at least, from an original tibial attachment of adductor magnus. The most superficial fibres descend inferiorly to the level of the tibial tuberosity; deeper fibres have a shorter course from femur to tibia, with the deepest spreading triangularly to attach to the medial meniscus (Fig. 3.64). The medial collateral ligament is 8 cm to 9 cm long and well-defined anteriorly where it blends with the medial patellar retinaculum; bursae may partially separate them. Deep to the ligament's posterior border, an inferior expansion from semimembranosus reaches the tibial shaft, strengthening this aspect of the joint capsule. The inferior medial genicular vessels and nerve pass between the semimembranosus expansion and ligament.

Lateral (Fibular) Collateral Ligament

Rounded cord some 5 cm long, standing clear of the thin lateral part of fibrous capsule (Fig. 3.64), attaching to the lateral epicondyle of the femur superiorly and posterior to the groove for popliteus, passing inferiorly to the

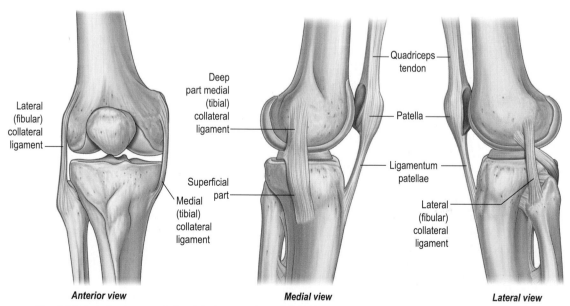

Fig. 3.64 Anterior aspect of the right knee and medial and lateral aspects of the left knee showing the position and attachments of the medial (tibial) and lateral (fibular) collateral ligaments.

lateral surface of the head of the fibula anterior to the apex, splitting the tendon of biceps femoris as it does so. Occasionally, the lateral collateral ligament continues into the proximal part of fibularis/peroneus longus and can be thought of as a femoral attachment of the muscle. Passing deep to the ligament is the tendon of popliteus, together with the inferior lateral genicular vessels and nerve as they pass anteriorly.

Because the points of attachment of both collateral ligaments lie behind the vertical axes of the bones, they are most tightly stretched in extension and prevent hyperextension; they also prevent abduction or adduction of the femur or tibia. In extension, the lateral collateral ligament is directed inferiorly, while the medial collateral ligament runs inferoanteriorly. This relationship prevents medial rotation of the femur or lateral rotation of the tibia. With the knee flexed, the ligaments become relaxed, allowing rotation to occur.

Synovial Membrane and Bursae

The knee joint cavity is the largest within the body, having an irregular shape with identifiable regions in free communication with each other. Synovial membrane lines the joint capsule, being reflected onto the bone as far as the margins of the articular cartilage. The central part of the joint space lies between the deep surface of the patella anteriorly and patellar surface of the femur

and cruciate ligaments posteriorly; it extends outwards between the femoral and tibial condyles, as well as above and below the menisci. From the articular margins of the patella, the synovial membrane passes in all directions onto the deep surface of the anterior joint capsule. Inferior to the patella, the synovial membrane is pushed posteriorly into the joint space by the infrapatellar fat pad lying on the deep surface of the ligamentum patellae and extending towards the intercondylar notch. The synovial reflections over this fat pad are thrown into a series of folds (Fig. 3.65). A vertical crescentic fold (infrapatellar fold) passes in the median plane towards the cruciate ligaments attaching to the intercondylar fossa anterior to the ACL and lateral to the PCL. The infrapatellar fat pad is the remnant of a septum dividing the embryonic knee into two compartments; the attachment of the synovium to the intercondylar fossa are the infrapatellar plicae. From the edges of the patella, double horizontal folds of synovial membrane (alar folds) project into the interior of the joint; they also cover collections of fat. Two further reflections (plicae) of synovium have been consistently observed in arthroscopy. The infrapatellar plica extends posteriorly from the infrapatellar fat pad; the suprapatellar plica is a horizontal fold level with the superior border of the patella, while the mediopatellar plica forms a shelf-like fold partway between the femur and patella. The significance of these plicae is that, if they

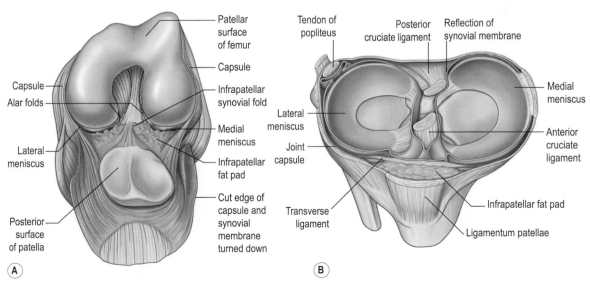

Fig. 3.65 (A) Right knee joint opened anteriorly showing the infrapatellar fat pad and synovial folds. (B) Intracapsular reflections of the synovial membrane on the tibia.

become trapped between the joint surfaces, they can become inflamed, causing pain on certain movements or in certain positions of the knee; arthroscopic removal of an inflamed plica usually resolves this problem.

Several recesses extend from the central part of the joint cavity. The suprapatellar bursa extends approximately 6 cm superior to the patella between the femoral shaft and quadriceps femoris; initially, it develops as a separate bursa but soon communicates freely with the joint space. Bundles of muscle fibres (articularis genu) from the deep surface of vastus intermedius attach to the superior aspect of the suprapatellar bursa (Fig. 3.66A); they maintain the bursa during extension of the knee. There are also recesses behind the posterior part of each femoral condyle. In this region, the two heads of gastrocnemius overlie the joint capsule; there is usually a bursa between each head and the joint capsule (Fig. 3.66B). The bursa under the medial head of gastrocnemius occasionally communicates with the joint cavity; it may also enlarge presenting as a cyst behind the knee

joint. The recesses posterior to the femoral condyles are separated by the intracapsular, but extrasynovial, cruciate ligaments. A vertical fold of synovial membrane covers the cruciate ligaments anteriorly and laterally, but not posteriorly where the tibial attachment of the PCL blends with the joint capsule (Fig. 3.65B).

The remaining recess of the joint cavity is associated with the tendon of popliteus (Fig. 3.66B). As the tendon passes from its intracapsular femoral attachment, the synovial membrane invests its medial side, separating it from the lateral meniscus, except where the tendon is attached to the meniscus. As the popliteal tendon emerges through the posterior aspect of the joint capsule, it takes with it a synovial extension associated with its deep surface which lies between the tendon and superior tibiofibular joint. Occasionally, the superior tibiofibular joint cavity communicates with the subpopliteal bursa and, therefore, with the knee joint itself.

Because all tendons and muscles which cross the knee run parallel to the bones involved, and therefore

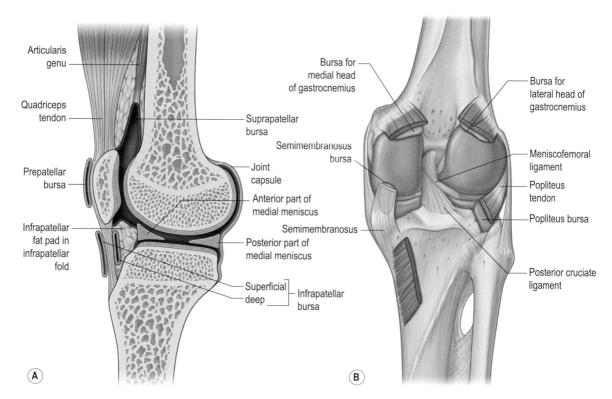

Fig. 3.66 (A) Paramedian section and (B) posterior aspect of the left knee showing synovial membrane reflections and bursae of the knee.

pull lengthwise across the joint, numerous other bursae are associated with it. The subcutaneous prepatellar bursa (Fig. 3.66A) lies between the skin and distal part of the patella, while the subcutaneous infrapatellar bursa overlies the patellar tendon; the subfascial prepatellar bursa lies between the tendinous and fascial expansions that pass over the patella, while the subtendinous prepatellar bursa separates the deep and superficial tendinous fibres; finally, the deep infrapatellar bursa lies between the patellar tendon and proximal tibia separated from the knee joint by the infrapatellar fat pad (Fig. 3.66A). On the lateral side of the joint, the subtendinous bursa of biceps femoris lies between the lateral collateral ligament and the tendon. In addition to the subpopliteal bursa, a further bursa may intervene between the popliteus tendon and lateral collateral ligament. Medially, the bursa anserina separates the tendons of sartorius, gracilis and semitendinosus from the medial collateral ligament; additional

bursae may be present between the individual tendons. The semimembranosus bursa (Fig. 3.66B) lies between the muscle and the tibia and medial collateral ligament.

Intra-Articular Structures

Within the knee joint capsule are two sets of structures which play an important part in knee joint function, both anatomically and mechanically. These are the anterior (ACL) and posterior (PCL) cruciate ligaments, and the medial and lateral menisci; the cruciate ligaments are extrasynovial.

Cruciate Ligaments

The cruciate ligaments are so called because they cross each other between their attachments; they are named according to their tibial attachment.

Anterior cruciate ligament. Attached to the tibia immediately anterolateral to the anterior tibial spine

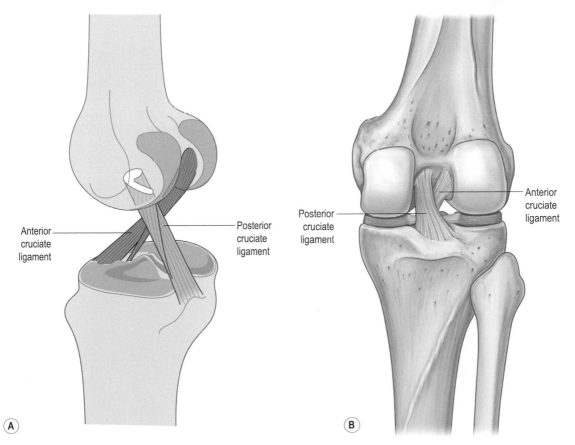

Anterior cruciate ligament

Posterior cruciate ligament

Posterior cruciate ligament

Anterior cruciate ligament

(A)

(B)

Fig. 3.67 (A) Oblique and (B) posterior aspects of the right knee showing the position, attachments and relationship of the anterior and posterior cruciate ligaments.

(Figs 3.65B, 3.67 and 3.69), the ACL passes inferior to the transverse ligament blending with the anterior horn of the lateral meniscus. It runs posteriorly, laterally and proximally attaching to the posterior aspect of the medial surface of the lateral femoral condyle (Figs 3.67 and 3.69). The femoral attachment is not as strong as the tibial, taking the form of a segment of a circle; in its course from tibia to femur, the ACL undergoes a medial spiral of approximately 110 degrees. The ligament can be anatomically divided into two parts: an anteromedial band attaching to the anteromedial region of the tibial attachment and a posterolateral band constituting the remainder. The posterolateral band tends to be taut in extension and the anteromedial band lax; the reverse is the case in flexion. Functionally, the ACL should be considered as a continuum, with some part being taut throughout the whole range of movement at the knee, thereby having a restraining influence in all joint positions.

Posterior cruciate ligament. Attaching to a depression in the posterior intercondylar area of the tibia (Figs 3.65B, 3.67 and 3.69), the PCL runs anteriorly, medially and proximally medial to the ACL to attach to the anterior part of the lateral surface of the medial femoral condyle (Fig. 3.67). The PCL is shorter and less oblique in its course, as well as being almost twice as strong in tension, than the ACL. It is closely aligned to the centre of knee joint rotation and, as such, may be its principal

stabiliser. Like the ACL, the PCL can be divided into two parts: anterolateral and posteromedial bands. The more superficial posteromedial band also has an attachment to the posterior horn of the lateral meniscus constituting the meniscofemoral ligament. Functionally, the PCL is also best considered as a continuum.

The crossing and twisting of the cruciate ligaments as they pass between the tibia and femur arise because the attachments on the tibia are more or less in a sagittal plane, while those on the femur are almost in a coronal plane. The cruciate ligaments are said to have a constant length ratio of 5:3 (ACL:PCL); however, this varies between individuals. Nevertheless, this ratio, together with their sites of attachment, is a primary factor in controlling the type of movement possible at the knee joint (Fig. 3.68). Almost exclusively they provide resistance to anterior and posterior displacements of the tibia with respect to the femur, with the ACL providing approximately 86% of the restraint to anterior displacement and the PCL approximately 94% of the restraint to posterior displacement of the tibia on the femur. Rupture of the ACL results in very little increase in anterior draw (anterior tibial displacement at 90 degree knee flexion); however, rupture of the PCL results in a posterior draw up to 25 mm. The latter is probably due to lack of collateral resistance to posterior displacement, as well as a lax joint capsule posteriorly. In addition to their role

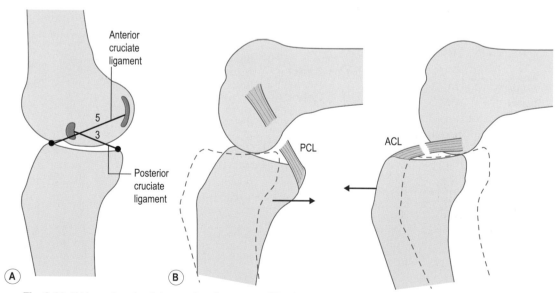

Fig. 3.68 (A) Length ratio of the cruciate ligaments; (B) schematic representation showing tibial displacement following posterior *(PCL)* and anterior *(ACL)* cruciate ligament rupture.

in maintaining anteroposterior stability, the cruciate ligaments also contribute to mediolateral stability, with the PCL providing 36% of the resistance to lateral tibial displacement, and ACL 30% of the resistance to medial tibial displacement.

Microscopically, the cruciate ligaments are mainly composed of collagen fibres with a small proportion (10%) of elastic fibres, giving them high tensile strength; the fibres are arranged in fasciculi a few millimetres in diameter. In the ACL, two types of fasciculi can be identified; those running directly between the tibial and femoral attachments, and those spiralling around the longitudinal axis of the ligament with a helical axis of 25 degrees. The helical arrangement of many of the fibres has important consequences; when lightly loaded, only a few fibres are put under tension, but as load increases the ligament unwinds bringing more fibres into play, effectively increasing its strength. Two phases of loading can be identified; before the yield point, the deformation is elastic due to stretching and unwinding of the ligament – further loading, however, disrupts the cross-links between fibres resulting in permanent deformation. Although gross damage may not be apparent until this later phase, microfailure can occur at stresses below the yield point. The strength of the ligaments is influenced by several factors:

1. Tensile strength, but not stiffness, decreases significantly with age.
2. Cyclical loading, as in walking and running, softens the ligaments, decreasing the yield point; however, recovery usually occurs within a few hours.
3. Immobilisation may decrease tensile strength by up to 60%, even in otherwise healthy ligaments. This is probably due to disuse atrophy; recovery does occur, but it may take many months.
4. Internal rotation reduces tensile strength by as much as 6%; consequently, torsional forces tend to be potentially much more damaging.
5. Exercise may slightly increase strength.

The ligament's bony attachments show a complex interdigitation of collagen fibres from the bone and the ligament, between which is a transitional zone of fibrocartilage; this allows a gradual change in stiffness preventing stress concentrations in this region.

The cruciate ligaments possess a fairly good blood supply mainly derived from the middle genicular artery, with a small contribution from the inferior lateral genicular artery. The blood vessels form a periligamentous sheath around the ligaments from which small penetrating vessels arise.

Mechanoreceptors resembling Golgi tendon organs (p. 32) are situated near the femoral attachments of both ligaments, located around the periphery where maximum bending occurs, running parallel to the long axis of the ligament. These probably convey information regarding angular acceleration and may also be involved in reflexes protecting the knee joint from potential injury. The nerve supply enters and leaves via the femoral attachments of each ligament.

Menisci

So called because of their 'half-moon' or 'meniscal' configuration, the menisci are also referred to as semilunar cartilages. Intra-articular discs are found where three conditions exist: (i) in joints with large degrees of rotation about an axis perpendicular to the articular surface; (ii) in joints with flat articular surfaces; and (iii) where forces across a joint tend to bring the two surfaces together in a rotatory movement. The menisci in the knee are slightly inclined to the tibial surface enabling a viscous lubricating film to be set up in the region of the loadline of the joint. Joints without menisci (surgically removed) show increased mechanical curvature. The function of the menisci is to:

1. Increase the congruence between the tibial and femoral articular surfaces
2. Participate in weight-bearing across the joint
3. Act as shock absorbers
4. Aid lubrication
5. Participate in the locking mechanism at the knee joint

The menisci are first recognisable as regions of closely packed cells with a long axis transverse to that of the limb at about 8 weeks in utero. By week 19, both menisci are well developed with well-defined collagen arrangements. During the next 4 weeks, extensive collagenous rearrangement occurs so that, at week 23, the collagen bundles lie parallel to one another and show the adult meniscal morphology even though there is no fibrocartilage present. However, the fetal meniscus has a high cellular content and is well vascularised. Postnatal changes in the menisci are:

1. Gradually decreasing cellularity
2. Decreasing vascularity from centrally outwards
3. Growth matching enlargement of the femoral and tibial condyles
4. Configurational changes accommodating changing contact areas, with growth of the menisci being linearly related to that of the tibial condyles
5. Increasing collagen content

The higher vascularity of young menisci results in increased efficiency of repair and reduced tendency to injury. With increasing age, the ratio of collagenous to non-collagenous proteins increases, leading to a lower tensile strength; the changing biochemical balance is an important determinant of collagen fibre arrangement. The histological arrangement is accounted for by adaptation of the menisci to weight-bearing, with the collagen fibres becoming more circumferentially arranged. This latter refinement occurs at about 3 years of age after the attainment of an erect posture and a more or less adult pattern of gait in infants; this change in fibrillar arrangement is an important factor confirming the role of the menisci in weight-bearing.

The menisci are crescent-shaped structures, triangular in cross-section, interposed between the femoral and tibial condyles (Fig. 3.69); they are normally composed of fibrocartilage. The thick peripheral borders are convex attaching to the deep surface of the joint capsule; capsular fibres attaching the menisci to the tibial condyles constitute the medial and lateral coronary ligaments. Through its capsular attachment, the medial meniscus is anchored to the medial collateral ligament, while the lateral meniscus is attached only by weak fibres of the lateral joint capsule and not the lateral collateral ligament. Furthermore,

where the lateral meniscus is crossed by the popliteal tendon, its periphery is not attached to the joint capsule; the lateral meniscus is, therefore, much more mobile than the medial. The inner border of each meniscus is thin and concave, forming the free inner edge. Superiorly, the meniscal surface is smooth and concave, articulating with the femoral condyles. The horns of the menisci are the sites of attachment to the tibia, regions where fibrocartilage gives way to bands of fibrous tissue.

Medial meniscus. Larger of the two menisci, the medial meniscus is semicircular, with its posterior part being broader than that anteriorly (Fig. 3.69A). The anterior horn attaches to the anterior part of the intercondylar area on the tibia immediately anterior to the ACL; the most posterior fibres are continuous with the transverse ligament of the knee. The posterior horn attaches to the posterior intercondylar area between the PCL posteriorly and posterior horn of the lateral meniscus anteriorly (Fig. 3.70); its entire periphery attaches to the joint capsule.

Lateral meniscus. This forms about four-fifths of a circle of uniform breadth throughout (Fig. 3.69A), with the two horns attached close together. The anterior horn attaches anterior to the intercondylar eminence, posterolateral to the ACL, with which it partially blends; in this region, it is twisted superoposteriorly as it rests on

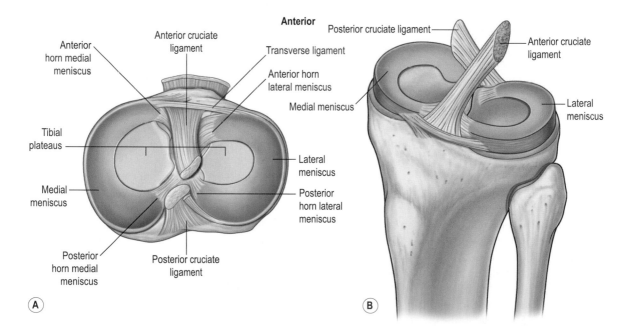

Fig. 3.69 (A) Superior aspect of the right knee and (B) oblique aspect of the left knee showing the medial and lateral menisci and their relationship to the cruciate ligaments.

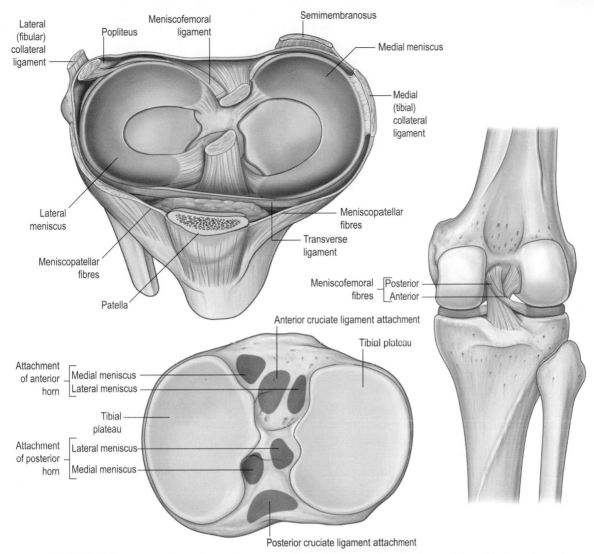

Fig. 3.70 Oblique, posterior and superior aspects of the right knee showing the position, attachments and relations of the medial and lateral menisci.

the sloping tibial condyle. The posterior horn attaches posterior to the intercondylar eminence anterior to the posterior horn of the medial meniscus (Fig. 3.70); posterolaterally it is grooved by the tendon of popliteus, from which it receives a few fibres.

Meniscal attachments. In addition to their capsular attachments, the menisci are attached anteriorly by a fibrous band of variable thickness (transverse ligament of the knee); a posterior transverse ligament is present in 20% of knees. The posterior part of the lateral meniscus usually gives a ligamentous slip to the PCL, which splits on the lateral side of the ligament to run both anterior

and posterior to the PCL (Fig. 3.70). That part running anteriorly is the anterior meniscofemoral ligament and that posteriorly the posterior meniscofemoral ligament; the posterior is the more constant. When present, both attach to the medial femoral condyle in association with the PCL. Some fibres from the anterior horn of the medial meniscus may run with the ACL.

The connection between the lateral meniscus and PCL is in keeping with the typical lower mammalian arrangement in which the lateral meniscus is attached posteriorly to the medial femoral condyle posterior to the PCL rather than to the tibia.

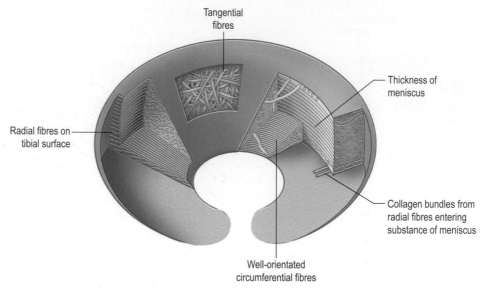

Tangential fibres

Thickness of meniscus

Radial fibres on tibial surface

Collagen bundles from radial fibres entering substance of meniscus

Well-orientated circumferential fibres

Fig. 3.71 Organisation of collagen bundles within a meniscus.

Posteriorly, the lateral meniscus gives rise to some fibres of popliteus, while the medial meniscus is attached via the joint capsule to the oblique popliteal ligament (expansion of semimembranosus).

Structure. Histologically, the fibrocartilaginous menisci are between dense fibrous cartilage and hyaline cartilage containing large collagen bundles embedded in a matrix. The fibrocartilage retains the ability to become either hyaline or fibrous cartilage, as seen in regenerating menisci where the hypertrophic cells form a purely fibrous structure.

Microscopically, the collagen fibres are arranged circumferentially (passing between the tibial attachments) and radially, being determined by meniscal age and functional requirements (Fig. 3.71). Radially arranged fibres are primarily associated with the femoral and tibial surfaces, many curving to run perpendicular to the meniscal surface; the orientation of the collagen fibres is closely related to the direction of stresses during weight-bearing. Under compression, the major force is directed outwards, this is resisted by the circumferential fibres; the radial fibres probably act as ties preventing longitudinal splitting.

Severe strain applied to a meniscus, usually involving rotation at the knee joint, can lead to longitudinal and occasionally transverse splitting of the fibrocartilage (Fig. 3.72). Because of its attachment to the medial collateral ligament, the medial meniscus is more frequently injured, with the inner thinner portion separating from the thicker outer part (bucket-handle rupture). The

detached part may move into the centre of the joint preventing full extension of the knee.

The menisci receive a blood supply from the middle, medial and lateral inferior genicular arteries; a peripheral perimeniscal plexus gives rise to small penetrating branches reaching the menisci via the coronary ligaments. In the fetus and young child, the entire meniscus is vascularised, but with increasing age the central regions become avascular; by age 11 only the peripheral 20% and horns are vascular (adult pattern). The vessels themselves are located mainly within the deep part of the meniscus, with the various surfaces receiving only a limited blood supply; the main source of nutrition of the menisci is by diffusion from the synovial fluid. The outer one-third of the menisci may be innervated by a few myelinated and non-myelinated fibres; no specialised nerve endings have been found, so their precise role is not understood, although some will undoubtedly be vasomotor.

Blood Supply, Lymphatic Drainage and Innervation

At the knee, there is an important genicular anastomosis consisting of a superficial plexus proximal and distal to the patella, and a deep plexus on the joint capsule and adjacent condylar surfaces of the femur and tibia. Ten vessels are involved in the anastomosis: two from above (descending branch of the lateral circumflex femoral artery and descending genicular branch of the femoral artery), three from below (circumflex fibular artery from the posterior tibial artery, and anterior and posterior

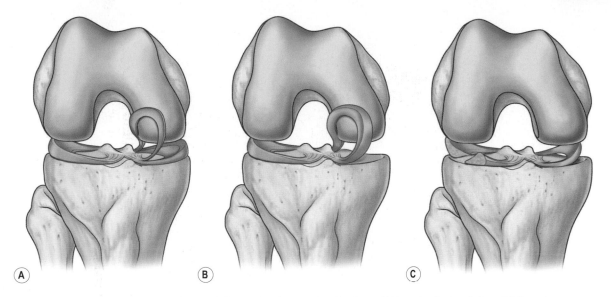

Fig. 3.72 Anterior aspect of the right knee showing meniscal lesions. (A) Longitudinal splitting. (B) Complete detachment. (C) Transverse tear and detachment of the anterior horn.

tibial recurrent branches from the anterior tibial artery) and the remainder branches of the popliteal artery (lateral superior and inferior, medial superior and inferior and middle genicular arteries) (Fig. 3.73). The popliteal artery lies deep within the popliteal fossa lying on (superior to inferior) fat covering the popliteal surface of the femur, posterior knee joint capsule and fascia covering popliteus.

Venous drainage is by corresponding veins accompanying the arteries; venostasis is a major contributory factor in degenerative changes of the knee joint. Lymphatics drain to the popliteal and inguinal lymph nodes.

The nerve supply to the joint is from many sources; the articular cartilage has no direct nerve supply. Proprioceptive information is conveyed via nerve endings located in bone, periosteum and the cruciate ligaments, while pain and pressure sensitivity come from endings in the collateral ligaments and joint capsule. The root values of the branches supplying the knee joint are L2–S3. From the femoral nerve, articular branches travel via the nerves to vastus medialis and the saphenous nerve. After supplying adductor magnus, the posterior division of obturator nerve ends in the knee joint; both the tibial and common fibular/peroneal nerves also send articular branches to the joint. Those from the tibial nerve follow the medial genicular arteries and middle genicular artery, and those from the common fibular/peroneal nerve follow the lateral genicular arteries and anterior tibial recurrent artery.

Relations

Muscles crossing the lateral and medial aspects of the joint are shown in Fig. 3.74.

Popliteal Fossa

Located on the posterior aspect of the joint is the popliteal fossa containing, from superficial to deep, the major nerves, veins and arteries passing between the thigh and leg/calf. It is diamond-shaped, bound superiorly by the diverging hamstring tendons and inferiorly by the medial and lateral heads of gastrocnemius (Fig. 3.75); laterally, the tendon of biceps femoris crosses the lateral head of gastrocnemius, and medially, the superimposed tendons of semitendinosus and semimembranosus cross the medial head of gastrocnemius. The floor of the popliteal fossa is formed from superior to inferior by the popliteal surface of the femur, posterior part of the knee joint capsule reinforced by the oblique popliteal ligament, and popliteus with its covering fascia.

The whole fossa is covered by dense popliteal fascia continuous with the fascia of the thigh and that of the leg/calf; it is strengthened by transverse fibres and by expansions from the tendons of sartorius, gracilis, semitendinosus and biceps femoris (Fig. 3.75). Directly under the fascia are the tibial and common fibular/peroneal divisions of the sciatic nerve, together with the posterior cutaneous nerve of the thigh. Within the fossa, the tibial nerve emerges from deep to semimembranosus, passing obliquely posterior to the popliteal vessels to lie medial to them on popliteus, deep to

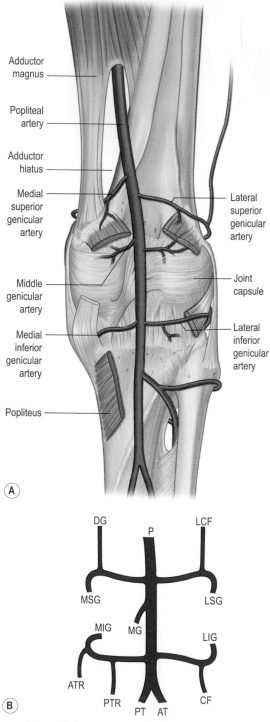

Fig. 3.73 (A) Posterior aspect of the right knee showing its blood supply. (B) Schematic representation of the vessels involved in the genicular anastomosis. *AT*, Anterior tibial; *ATR*, anterior tibial recurrent; *CF*, circumflex fibular; *DG*, descending genicular; *LCF*, lateral circumflex femoral; *LIG*, lateral inferior genicular; *LSG*, lateral superior genicular; *MG*, middle genicular; *MIG*, medial inferior genicular; *MSG*, medial superior genicular; *P*, popliteal; *PT*, posterior tibial; *PTR*, posterior tibial recurrent.

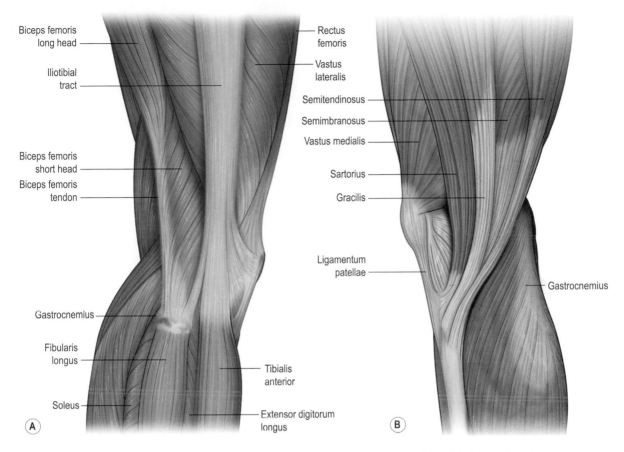

Fig. 3.74 Muscles crossing the (A) lateral and (B) medial aspects of the right knee joint.

gastrocnemius and plantaris. The tibial nerve gives muscular branches to gastrocnemius, plantaris and popliteus, genicular branches to the knee joint and the cutaneous sural nerve which eventually pierces the deep fascia in the middle one-third of the posterior surface of the leg/calf. The common fibular/peroneal nerve passes deep to biceps femoris and its tendon, passing inferiorly along the lateral margin of the fossa to reach the posterior aspect of the head of the fibula. It passes subfascially into the leg/calf by curving around the neck of the fibula where it can be readily palpated. Within the popliteal fossa, the common fibular/peroneal nerve gives genicular branches to the knee joint and two cutaneous branches (lateral cutaneous nerve of the leg, fibular/peroneal communicating branch which joins the sural nerve).

Immediately superior to the popliteal fossa, the femoral vessels lie opposite the posterior border of the femur and distal end of the adductor canal against the tendon of adductor magnus. Continuing their posterior inclination,

they pass through the adductor hiatus into the popliteal fossa becoming the popliteal vessels. The popliteal artery is the deepest of the major structures within the popliteal fossa, lying adjacent to the bone where it is protected from external trauma but vulnerable to supracondylar fractures of the femur. It ends at the distal border of popliteus, level with the distal part of the tibial tuberosity, by dividing into anterior and posterior tibial arteries. With the knee flexed, the popliteal pulse can be felt. Within the fossa, the artery gives off five genicular branches supplying the knee joint and participating in the genicular anastomosis.

The popliteal vein is formed by the anterior and posterior tibial veins at the distal border of popliteus. Ascending through the fossa, it crosses from medial to lateral posterior to the artery, bound to it by a dense fascial sheath. In addition to receiving the genicular veins, the popliteal vein also receives the small (lesser) saphenous vein, which pierces the fascial roof of the fossa.

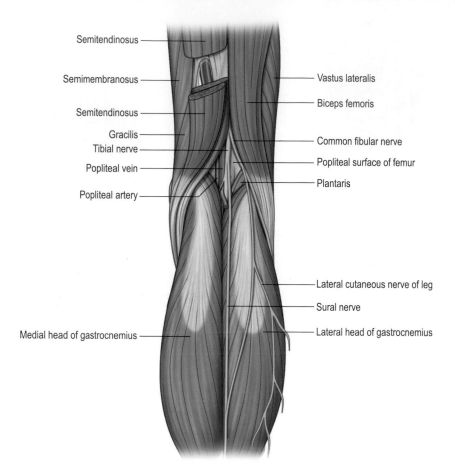

Semitendinosus

Semimembranosus

Semitendinosus

Gracilis

Tibial nerve

Popliteal vein

Popliteal artery

Medial head of gastrocnemius

Vastus lateralis

Biceps femoris

Common fibular nerve

Popliteal surface of femur

Plantaris

Lateral cutaneous nerve of leg

Sural nerve

Lateral head of gastrocnemius

Fig. 3.75 Posterior aspect of the right knee showing the boundaries and contents of the popliteal fossa.

Both the popliteal artery and vein are embedded in a considerable amount of fat and areolar connective tissue, which also lodges the popliteal lymph nodes.

Palpation

The medial collateral ligament can be palpated medially and tested for laxity by applying a laterally directed force to the medial side of the ankle with the knee extended. The lateral collateral ligament can be palpated as a rounded cord above the head of the fibula laterally and tested for laxity by applying a medially directed force to the lateral side of the ankle. The ligamentum patellae can be palpated running between the apex of the patella and tibial tuberosity.

The cruciate ligaments are placed deep within the joint and cannot be palpated. However, they can be tested for laxity by placing the knee, with the individual supine, at 90 degrees with the foot flat on the bed and applying alternative anterior and posterior pressure on

the proximal end of the tibia. Pressure directed posteriorly tests the PCL and anteriorly the ACL.

When sitting with the knees flexed at 90 degrees, place the fingers of both hands on the anterior surface of the right patella. The skin and fascia can be moved from side to side against the prepatellar bursa; the vertical ridges on the patella produced by the fibres of quadriceps femoris can be felt. Moving either side of the patella, trace down to the apex and locate the ligamentum patellae. This broad strong tendon of quadriceps femoris, approximately 4 cm long and 2 cm wide, joins the patella to the superior part of the tibial tuberosity; its distal half is prominent, covered by the superficial infrapatellar bursa. The surface marking of the knee joint is represented by a horizontal line bisecting this tendon.

On each side of the ligamentum patellae is a triangular depression bounded superiorly by the appropriate femoral condyle and inferiorly by the tibia and margin of the ligamentum patellae. Deep within each hollow, the broad horizontal anterior margin of the knee joint can be palpated. On medial tibial rotation, the medial meniscus protrudes anteriorly, while on lateral rotation, the lateral meniscus can be felt, but to a lesser extent; movement of the tibia beneath the femur is quite clear.

On the medial side, the joint line becomes difficult to palpate just posterior to the midpoint, where the broad medial collateral ligament crosses the joint. Similarly, on the lateral side, the joint line becomes difficult to palpate where the thickened articular capsule and lateral collateral ligament cross the joint. The lateral collateral ligament can be traced inferiorly to the head of the fibula lying just inferior and posterior to the joint line, with the tendon of biceps femoris attaching to its proximal posterior part.

On the medial side, both the tibial and femoral condyles are easily palpable with the tendons of gracilis and semitendinosus approximately 5 cm posteroinferior to the medial collateral ligament. These become distinct if the knee is flexed against resistance; gracilis is the more medial tendon.

Posteriorly is the popliteal fossa (p. 339) containing several structures and a variable amount of fat; it does not permit knee joint palpation.

From the anterior surface of the patella, draw your fingers up to its base; on either side is a narrow groove between the patella and femoral condyles. On extending the knee, the patella can be felt gliding superiorly against the femoral condyles, with the superior part coming clear of the patellar surface of the femur. The tendon of quadriceps femoris lies between your hands, while the belly of vastus medialis lies under the left or right hand depending on which knee is being palpated. Flexing the knee, the patella can be felt gliding down the patellar surface of the femur, coming to lie on the distal part of the femoral condyles in full flexion. The whole of the patellar surface of the femur can now be palpated, even though it is covered by the tendon of quadriceps femoris.

Stability

Knee joint stability is primarily maintained by the collateral and cruciate ligaments reinforced by the musculotendinous ties crossing the joint; it is the interaction between the two sets of ligaments which provides the all-around stability of the joint.

Because the anatomical axis of the femur runs inferiorly and medially, the force (F) applied to the tibia can be resolved into vertical (V) and horizontal (T) components (Fig. 3.76A). The horizontal component tends to tilt the

joint, widening the medial joint interspace; this potential disruption is normally resisted by the medial collateral ligament. The greater the degree of genu valgus, the greater the demands made upon the medial collateral ligament.

During walking and running, the knee is continually exposed to side-to-side stresses; there is no danger of tearing the collateral ligaments during such activities unless accompanied by a violent transverse force. However, when the knee is severely sprained, abnormal side-to-side movements can be demonstrated about an anteroposterior axis. Such movements are best seen with the knee fully extended or hyperextended; in such a position, displacement of the leg/calf laterally indicates disruption of the medial collateral ligament (Fig. 3.76D). Similarly, medial displacement of the leg/calf indicates disruption of the lateral collateral ligament (Fig. 3.76E).

In addition to the collateral and cruciate ligaments, musculotendinous ties are also important in providing joint stability. Laterally, the lateral collateral ligament is aided by the iliotibial tract, which can be tightened by tensor fascia lata and/or gluteus maximus. Medially, the medial collateral ligament is assisted by sartorius, semitendinosus and gracilis. The collateral ligaments are further aided by the retinacular fibres of quadriceps femoris; fibres which do not cross the midline prevent opening out of the joint space on the same side, while those crossing the midline prevent it opening out on the opposite side. Consequently, each vastus muscle contributes to joint stability on both its medial and lateral aspects. Not surprisingly, atrophy of quadriceps femoris may decrease knee joint stability so that it tends to 'give way'.

The structures involved in maintaining anteroposterior stability of the knee are position dependent. If the knee is flexed, even slightly, the projection of the line of gravity falls posterior to the knee joint axis and acts to cause further flexion; this is resisted by quadriceps femoris. If the knee is hyperextended, the centre of gravity projection falls anterior to the joint axis with a natural tendency for hyperextension to increase. In this position, the cruciate ligaments have both become taut, which, with the arcuate, oblique popliteal and collateral ligaments, act to limit further hyperextension. Although the ligaments are sufficiently strong to limit hyperextension, their action is reinforced by the flexor muscles crossing the joint. Without this active component, the ligaments would become lax through stretching, eventually leading to decreased stability at the joint.

In individuals with paralysis of quadriceps femoris, an exaggerated hyperextension of the knee (genu

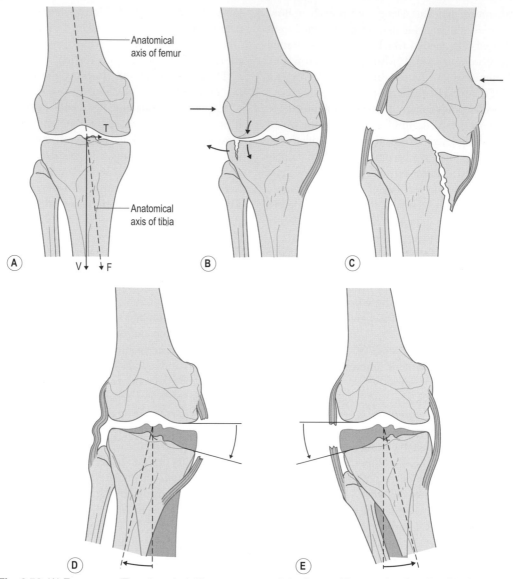

Fig. 3.76 (A) Transverse (T) and vertical (V) components of the forces (F) transmitted to the tibia from the femur. (B) Impact-dislocation of the lateral tibial condyle. (C) Fracture-dislocation of the medial tibial condyle. (D) Rupture of the medial collateral ligament. (E) Rupture of the lateral collateral ligament.

recurvatum) is often seen. This allows the individual to stand erect and even to walk; however, when the knee is hyperextended the mechanical axis of the femur runs obliquely inferolaterally. The resultant force vector can be resolved into vertical and horizontal components; the posteriorly directed horizontal component acts to accentuate hyperextension. If the genu recurvatum is too severe, the cruciate, collateral and posterior ligaments become stretched, creating a vicious circle resulting in accentuation of hyperextension.

Rotational stability at the knee is provided by the collateral and cruciate ligaments. Axial rotation can only occur with the knee flexed; in the extended knee, it is prevented by tension in both the cruciate and collateral ligaments. In the flexed knee, lateral tibial rotation with respect to the femur causes the cruciate ligaments to become more vertical and separated, becoming relaxed. However, at the same time, the collateral ligaments become more oblique with a corresponding increase in their tension. Lateral tibial rotation with respect to the

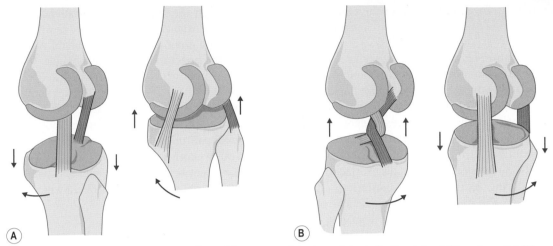

Fig. 3.77 Role of the cruciate and collateral ligaments of the knee joint in limiting lateral (A) and medial (B) axial rotation.

femur is resisted by the collateral ligaments, especially the lateral (Fig. 3.77A).

When the tibia medially rotates with respect to the femur, the collateral ligaments become more vertical and relaxed, particularly the lateral collateral ligament, while the cruciate ligaments become twisted around each other, effectively shortening and tightening them. The most effective elements in resisting tibial rotation are the PCL, as it twists around the ACL, and the medial collateral ligament (Fig. 3.77B).

It is clear that the cruciate and collateral ligaments work together providing three-dimensional stability of the knee joint. However, the menisci, by their movements accompanying those of the femur and tibia, interact with the ligaments in providing stability at the joint. Disruption of the ACL leads to decreased stability and increased movement in all actions in which it is put under tension, as well as in movements limited by the PCL twisting around the ACL. Experiment has shown that isolated ACL section significantly increases anterior displacement of the tibia (Fig. 3.78), with a loss of the coupled tibial rotation accompanying this displacement. By itself, medial meniscectomy does not influence anterior displacement at the joint, but when associated with ACL section, it is significantly greater than in isolated ACL section, highlighting that, although it is possible to assign specific roles to individual stabilising structures in the knee joint, there is considerable interaction between them which may not always be fully appreciated.

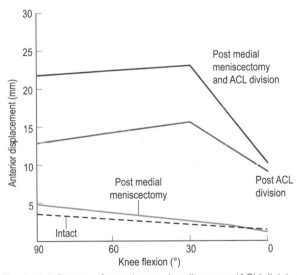

Fig. 3.78 Influence of anterior cruciate ligament *(ACL)* division and medial meniscectomy on anterior displacement of the tibia. (Adapted from Levy, I.M., Torzilli, P.A., Warren, R.F., 1982. The effect of medial meniscectomy on anterior-posterior motion of the knee. J. Bone Joint Surg. 64A, 883–887.)

MOVEMENTS OF THE LEG/CALF AT THE KNEE JOINT

When considering movements at the knee, two separate articulations have to be considered; that between the femur and tibia is the most important, controlling lengthening and shortening of the lower limb, and that between the patella and femur, with the patella acting as a pulley for the quadriceps tendon changing its line of action.

The main movements occurring at the knee joint are flexion and extension, together with a limited amount of active rotation when the joint is flexed; the knee can, therefore, be thought of as a modified hinge joint. It differs from a typical hinge joint (interphalangeal joints) not only because there is rotation, but also because the axis about which movement occurs, together with the contact area between the articular surfaces, moves anteriorly during extension and posteriorly during flexion. The change in the position of the axis of flexion/extension is due to the constantly changing radius of curvature of the femoral condyles; there is also an accompanying passive rotation of the joint towards the end of extension.

The ranges of knee joint flexion associated with some common activities are shown in Table 3.3, from which it can be seen that a range of at least 105 degrees appears to be required to carry out everyday activities. No difference has been reported between men and women in the range of knee joint flexion during these activities.

TABLE 3.3 Knee Flexion Range of Movement Required in Various Activities

Activity	Maximum flexion required (°)
Walking	65
Slow (stance phase)	5
Free (stance phase)	15
Fast (stance phase)	20
Running (stance phase)	30
Ascending and descending stairs	105
Rising from a chair	90
Sitting down	95
Tying shoe laces	105

Adapted from (i) Laubenthal, K.N., Smidt, G.I., Kettelkamp, D.B., 1972. A quantitative analysis of knee motion during activities of daily living. Phys. Ther. 52, 34–43; (ii) Livingston, L.A., Stevenson, J.M., Olney, S.J., 1991. Stairclimbing kinematics on stairs of different dimensions. Arch. Phys. Med. Rehabil. 72, 398–402; (iii) Jevsevar, D.S., Riley, P.O., Hodge, W.A., et al., 1991. Knee kinematics and kinetics during locomotion activities of daily living in subjects with knee arthroplasty and in healthy control subjects. Phys. Ther. 73, 229–239.

Although the main movement at the knee joint is flexion and extension, with the knee semiflexed and the foot off the ground, medial and lateral rotation of the tibia with respect to the femur is possible. If the feet are on the ground when the knees are flexed, the rotation is taken up by the femur, which rotates about a vertical axis running approximately through the intercondylar eminence. This allows mediolateral movement of the proximal part of the femur as in moving sideways from one seat to another.

Movement between the patella and patellar surface of the femur must also be considered when considering movements of the knee.

Flexion and Extension

Flexion is movement of the leg/calf so that its posterior aspect moves towards the posterior aspect of the thigh; extension being the opposite movement. Some movement, usually passive, of the tibia beyond the position of alignment of the long axis of the leg/calf and thigh may be possible (hyperextension).

The range of flexion achieved is dependent on the position of the hip and also whether the movement is performed actively or passively; maximum flexion is achieved when the movement is carried out passively.

The total range of active movement from full flexion to full extension is approximately 140 degrees with the hip flexed (Fig. 3.79A) (Boone and Azen, 1979; Roaas and Anderson, 1982) and 120 degrees with the hip extended (Fig. 3.79A); the difference being due to the hamstrings losing some of their efficiency with hip extension. Passive movement at the joint can increase the total range to 160 degrees allowing the heel to touch the buttock (Fig. 3.79A). According to Roach and Miles (1991), beyond age 40 active knee flexion decreases to 130 degrees, with a loss of motion of more than 10% considered abnormal. Normally, knee flexion is only limited by contact of the thigh and leg/calf muscles; however, if movement is arrested before this occurs, it may be due to contraction of the quadriceps muscles or shortening of the capsular ligaments. In such circumstances, the effectiveness of intervention procedures can be assessed in terms of the distance between the heel and buttock.

Newborn children lack approximately 15–20 degrees of knee extension (Drews et al., 1984; Waugh et al., 1983). By age 2, full extension is possible (Watanabe et al., 1979) and by age 10 there is 7 degree hyperextension (Cheng et al., 1991). During the remainder of

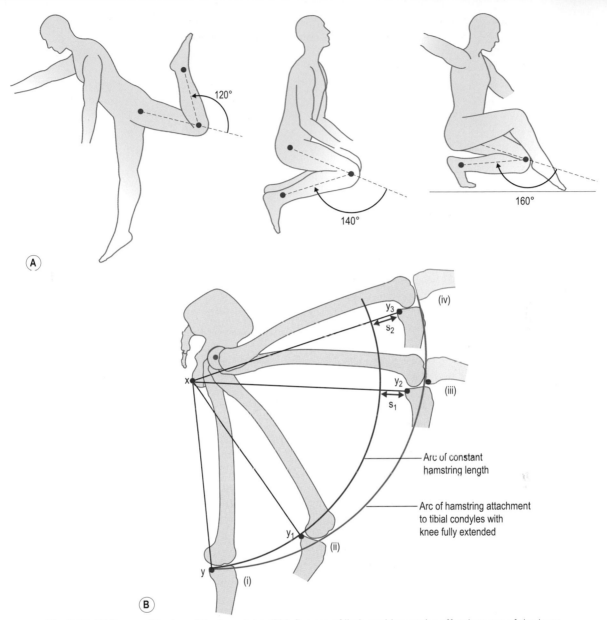

Fig. 3.79 (A) Range of flexion of the knee joint. (B) Influence of limb position on the effectiveness of the hamstrings in flexing the knee. *S*, Extent of lengthening; *x* and *y*, hamstring attachment to the ischium and tibia.

childhood and throughout most of adulthood, hyperextension, when present, is usually of the order of only a few degrees.

Because the hamstrings are extensors of the hip and flexors of the knee, their action on the knee depends on the position of the hip. As the hip flexes, the distance between the hamstring attachments increases as they wrap around the ischial tuberosity (Fig. 3.79B); the greater the degree of flexion, the greater the relative shortening of the hamstrings, and the more stretched they become. With hip flexion greater than 90 degrees, it becomes increasingly difficult to keep the knee fully extended because of stretching of the hamstrings (Fig. 3.79B(iii)); however, with stretching, their efficiency as

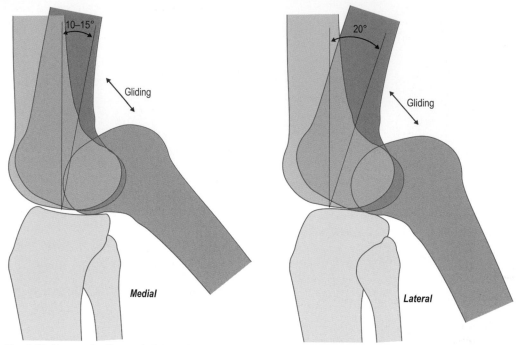

Fig. 3.80 Extent of rolling and gliding of the femoral condyles over the tibial plateaux during flexion and extension of the knee joint. —, Limit of pure rolling.

knee flexors increases. Similarly, knee extension also increases the efficiency of the hamstrings as hip extensors. It might appear that the efficiency of knee flexion is subject to modification according to the position of the hip; this is not necessarily the case as both the short head of biceps femoris and popliteus, crossing only the knee joint, have the same efficiency irrespective of hip joint position.

Movement of the femoral condyles over the tibial plateaux is achieved by a combination of rolling and gliding, with the ratio of rolling to gliding changing during flexion and extension (Fig. 3.80). Beginning with full extension, the femoral condyles roll without gliding, after which gliding becomes progressively more important so that, towards the end of flexion, the condyles glide without rolling. For the medial condyle, pure rolling occurs for the initial 10–15 degrees of flexion, while for the lateral condyle, it may continue until 20 degrees of flexion. This initial 15–20 degrees of pure rolling corresponds to the normal range of movement at the knee during the support phase of gait when stability is the prime requirement.

The change from rolling to gliding is very significant for knee joint function in which both stability and mobility are required. Beyond 20 degree flexion, the knee becomes looser as the radius of the femoral condyles becomes smaller. The tibia moves closer to the axis of movement in the femur; consequently, the ligaments passing between the two bones become relaxed; this loosening up prepares the joint for axial rotation.

During the last 10–15 degrees of active extension, an automatic rotation of the knee occurs in which, if the foot is fixed, the femur medially rotates on the tibia; alternatively, if the foot is free the tibia laterally rotates on the femur. Therefore, to enable flexion to begin, the knee must undergo some degree of rotation opposite in direction to that which occurred in extension. The rotation accompanying full extension or the initial phase of flexion is not under voluntary control; it is entirely automatic. The Helfet test can be used to determine whether lateral rotation of the tibia occurs during knee extension (Helfet, 1974), confirming whether the screw-home mechanism is intact. The test is performed with the individual seated with the hip and knee each flexed 90 degrees and the leg/calf hanging freely over the side of the supporting surface. The medial and lateral borders of the patella are marked on the skin, lines are drawn on the middle of the patella and tibial tuberosity (Fig. 3.81)

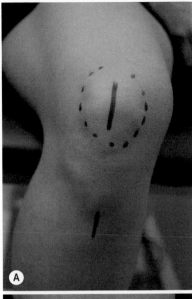

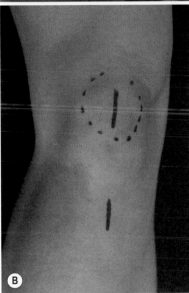

Fig. 3.81 Helfet test: knee (A) flexed and (B) extended.

and the alignment of the tuberosity with the patella are checked. The knee is then extended, and movement of the tibial tuberosity is observed; in a normal knee the tibial tuberosity moves laterally during extension, becoming aligned with the lateral half of the patella in full extension.

Not only do the relative positions of the femur and tibia change during flexion and extension, with the contact area increasing and moving anteriorly with

extension promoting greater stability of the joint, the two menisci also move (Fig. 3.82). If this were not so, then the range of movement possible at the joint would be severely impaired. In addition to following movement of the femur with respect to the tibia, the menisci also undergo considerable distortion. When going from extension to flexion, both menisci move posteriorly, with the lateral receding twice as far as the medial, approximately 12 and 6 mm, respectively. The lateral meniscus undergoes greater distortion than the medial, primarily because its anterior and posterior horns are attached closer together.

Only one passive element is involved in displacement of the menisci during flexion and extension; they are pushed posteriorly in flexion by the femoral condyles and anteriorly in extension. In contrast, a number of active elements are involved in meniscal movements. During extension, both menisci are pulled anteriorly by the meniscopatellar fibres stretching and pulling the transverse ligament anteriorly. In addition, the posterior horn of the lateral meniscus is pulled anteriorly by the meniscofemoral ligament as the PCL becomes taut. During flexion, the lateral meniscus is pulled posteriorly by its attachment to popliteus. At the same time, the medial meniscus is drawn posteriorly by the semimembranosus expansion attached to its posterior edge, while the anterior horn is pulled posterosuperiorly by ACL fibres attached to it.

While movements of the femur, tibia and menisci are occurring, the patella also changes its relationship to the femur as the meniscopatellar fibres attaching to its margins become stretched, pulling the menisci anteriorly during extension. Movement of the patella during flexion occurs along the groove of the patellar surface of the femur as far as the intercondylar notch. This almost vertical displacement over a distance of twice its length is accompanied by a turning movement of the patella about a transverse axis (Fig. 3.83A). Considering the tibia as the moving bone, when going from extension to flexion the deep surface of the patella initially faces posteriorly then superiorly. However, if the tibia is fixed with the femur moving, the patella tilts on itself approximately 35 degrees so that its deep surface, which initially faced posteriorly, now faces posteroinferiorly in full flexion (Fig. 3.83B).

It is the capsular recesses in relation to the patella which facilitate these movements (suprapatellar bursa superiorly, parapatellar recesses either side).

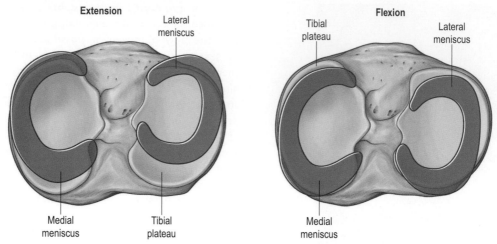

Fig. 3.82 Movements of the menisci of the right knee joint with respect to the tibial plateaux during flexion and extension.

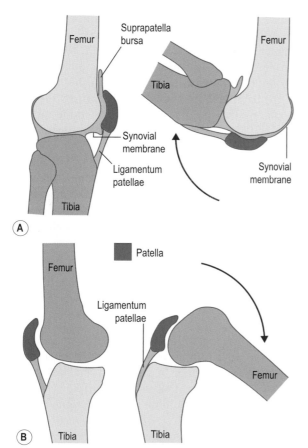

Fig. 3.83 Movements of the patella with the femur (A) and tibia (B) fixed.

Inflammatory adhesions develop in these recesses, obliterating their cavities, resulting in the patella being held firmly against the femur so that it cannot move inferior to the intercondylar notch; this is one of the causes of post-traumatic or post-infective 'stiff knee'.

Normally, there is no transverse movement of the patella as it is held against the femur by the quadriceps tendon, increasingly more firmly as flexion increases. In full extension, the appositional force is diminished, there may even be separation of the femur and patella in hyperextension. If this occurs, there is a tendency for the patella to move laterally due to the pull of quadriceps femoris. Lateral displacement is prevented by the lateral lip of the patellar surface of the femur projecting further anteriorly than the medial lip, as well as the horizontal fibres of vastus medialis attaching to the medial patellar border. With underdevelopment of the lateral lip or weakness of vastus medialis, the patella is no longer held firmly in place and may dislocate laterally in extension. A severely underdeveloped lateral lip may lead to lateral patellar dislocation during flexion; this is the mechanism underlying recurrent dislocation of the patella.

Lateral displacement or patella misalignment can cause knee pain as the articular surfaces are subjected to increased compressive forces over a smaller area. Lateral movement of the patella may be due to abnormal patella tracking associated with a tight patellofemoral retinaculum, which is often combined with a tight iliotibial tract. The resulting pain has led to a number of surgical procedures including lateral release techniques and transposition of the tibial tuberosity. However, conservative treatment of the patellar tracking mechanism is increasingly used to reduce the pain associated with patellar misalignment. The treatment involves taping techniques combined with specific isometric and eccentric re-education of the oblique fibres of vastus medialis. By selectively training this part of the quadriceps, lateral tracking of the patella may be minimised.

It has been suggested that the previously discussed technique also corrects soft tissue abnormalities around the knee, decreasing the effect of abnormal foot mechanics.

Axial Rotation

Rotation of the leg/calf about its long axis occurs in a transverse plane and is influenced by the degree of flexion of the joint; medial and lateral rotations bring the toes to face medially or laterally, respectively (Fig. 3.84).

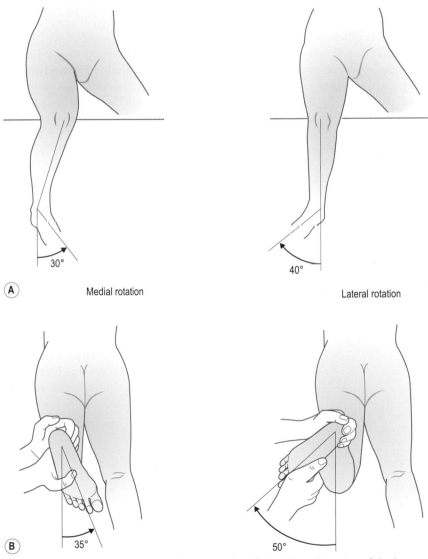

Fig. 3.84 Active (A) and passive (B) ranges of medial and lateral rotation of the knee.

The ranges of rotation are influenced by the degree of knee flexion, and, therefore, the efficiency of the appropriate part of the hamstrings. With the knee flexed to 90 degrees, active medial and lateral rotation are 30 and 40 degrees, respectively; this may be increased to 35 and 50 degrees if the movement is performed passively. Beyond 90 degrees of knee flexion, the total range of rotation decreases due to restrictions imposed by the soft tissues.

In lateral rotation of the tibia on the femur, the lateral femoral condyle moves anteriorly over the lateral tibial condyle while the medial femoral condyle moves posteriorly over the medial tibial condyle; the reverse occurs in medial rotation. The extent of anteroposterior movement of the femoral condyles differs for the medial and lateral condyles; the medial condyle moves hardly at all, while the lateral moves an appreciable amount and, in so doing, comes to lie slightly higher than the medial condyle; although small the height difference is real. The shape difference between the tibial condyles is reflected in the configuration of the intercondylar tubercles. The medial tubercle acts as a shoulder against which the medial femoral condyle rests, while the lateral femoral condyle moves easily past its respective tubercle. The axis of rotation, therefore, passes through the medial tubercle and not between the two tubercles.

As expected, the menisci follow the movements of the femoral condyles during axial rotation (Fig. 3.85). During lateral femoral rotation, the medial meniscus moves anteriorly over the tibia while the lateral meniscus

is drawn posteriorly; in medial rotation, the reverse occurs. During these movements, both menisci undergo distortion. Meniscal displacements during axial rotation are mainly passive due to movement of the femoral condyles; however, the meniscopatellar fibres become taut as a result of patella movement with respect to the tibia, drawing the menisci anteriorly. Failure of the menisci to follow movements of the femoral condyles can lead to transverse tears, longitudinal splitting, detachment of the anterior horn or complete detachment of the meniscus from the joint capsule (Fig. 3.72). Once a meniscus is damaged, the injured part fails to follow the normal movements and may become wedged between the femoral and tibial condyles, with the knee 'locking' in a position of flexion; locking becomes more marked the more posterior the damage, with full extension being impossible.

During axial rotation, the patella moves in a coronal plane with respect to the tibia. In medial tibial rotation with respect to the femur, the patella is dragged laterally so that the ligamentum patellae run obliquely inferiorly and medially; the opposite occurs in lateral tibial rotation (Fig. 3.86).

There is also an automatic involuntary rotation at the knee associated with the terminal part of extension and beginning of flexion; it can be described with respect to either the femur or tibia, depending on whether the thigh or leg/calf is fixed. With the tibia fixed, the femur undergoes medial rotation in the terminal stages of

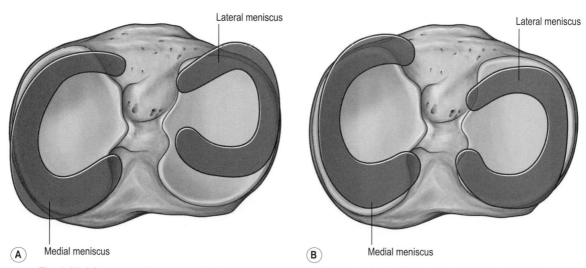

Fig. 3.85 Movement of the menisci with respect to the tibial plateaux during (A) medial and (B) lateral rotation of the femur on the tibia.

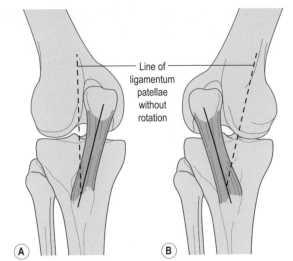

Fig. 3.86 Movement of the patella during (A) lateral and (B) medial rotation of the tibia with respect to the femur.

extension; during the initial part of flexion the femur is laterally rotated by popliteus. When the knee is fully extended it is in the close-packed position, denoting maximum contact between the femoral and tibial articular surfaces, with all the ligaments under tension; the joint is at its most stable. The rotation that occurs is due to three independent mechanisms:

1. The unequal lengths of the articular profiles of the femoral condyles, with the lateral condyle rolling over a greater distance than the medial
2. The shape of the tibial condyles, with the medial femoral condyle being more or less contained within the concave medial tibial condyle, while the lateral femoral condyle glides more freely over the convex lateral tibial condyle
3. The direction of the collateral ligaments, with the medial collateral ligament becoming stretched less rapidly than the lateral

In addition to these mechanisms, there are two force couples acting to produce rotation. At the beginning of flexion, lateral femoral rotation with respect to the tibia is brought about by gracilis, sartorius, semitendinosus and popliteus, while towards the end of extension it is the tension developed in the ACL which produces medial femoral rotation, again with respect to the tibia.

Abduction and Adduction

Abduction and adduction in the coronal plane, although limited, are again influenced by the degree of knee flexion. In full extension no motion is possible, but passive abduction and adduction both increase up to 30 degree knee flexion; beyond 30 degree knee flexion, coronal plane motion decreases due to soft tissue limitations.

Accessory Movements

The extent of accessory movement possible at the knee joint is determined by its position and the degree of tension in the ligaments; in the close-packed position no accessory movements are possible. However, with the knee flexed to 25 degrees, a number of accessory movements can be demonstrated. The tibia can be moved anteriorly and posteriorly on the femur by applying forces in the appropriate directions. Also in this position, tibial rotation on the femur can be taken further than the available range by applying a firm rotatory force to the tibia; in this position the tibia can also be rocked medially and laterally. Finally, it is possible to distract the tibia from the femur if a longitudinal force is applied across the joint.

The major muscles producing movements of the leg/calf at the knee joint are shown in Table 3.4; further details of each muscle can be found in following sections.

BIOMECHANICS

Because the femoral neck overhangs the shaft medially, the anatomical axes of the femur and tibia do not coincide; they form an outward (lateral) opening angle between 170 and 175 degrees (femorotibial angle). However, the joint centres of the hip, knee and ankle all lie on a straight line; the mechanical axis of the lower limb (Fig. 3.87). In the leg/calf, the axis coincides with the anatomical axis of the tibia, while in the thigh it forms an angle of approximately 6 degrees with the axis of the femoral shaft. Because the hip joints are further apart than the ankle joints, the mechanical axis of the lower limb runs obliquely inferomedially forming an angle of 3 degrees with the vertical; the wider the pelvis the larger this angle (as in females). In some pathological conditions, the femorotibial angle may be increased or decreased giving the appearance of 'bowlegs' (genu varus) or 'knock-knees' (genu valgus) (Fig. 3.88); genu valgus is common in toddlers, generally disappearing with growth.

The transverse axis of the knee joint is horizontal, with the common axis of both joints lying in a coronal plane; this axis does not bisect the femorotibial angle, the angle between it and the tibia being larger

354 Anatomy and Human Movement

TABLE 3.4 Muscles Crossing and Producing Movement of the Leg/Calf at the Knee Joint

Muscle	Attachments	Action	Innervation (root value)
Semitendinosus[a,b]	Ischial tuberosity to medial surface of medial condyle of tibia	Flexor of leg/calf at knee joint; with knee semiflexed it medially rotates leg/calf at knee joint; with foot fixed it laterally rotates thigh on tibia; also extends thigh at hip joint	Sciatic nerve via its tibial part (L5, S1, S2)
Semimembranosus[a,b]	Ischial tuberosity to posteromedial surface of medial tibial condyle	Flexor of leg/calf at knee joint; with knee semiflexed it medially rotates leg/calf at knee joint; with foot fixed it laterally rotates thigh on tibia; also extends thigh at hip joint	Sciatic nerve via its tibial part (L5, S1, S2)
Biceps femoris[a–c]	Ischial tuberosity and sacrotuberous ligament (long head), distal $1/2$ of linea aspera and proximal $1/2$ of lateral supracondylar ridge of femur (short head) to head of fibular	Flexor of leg/calf at knee joint; with knee semiflexed it laterally rotates leg/calf at knee joint; with foot fixed it medially rotates thigh on tibia; also extends thigh at hip joint, especially when trunk is to be raised to erect position	Sciatic nerve (L5, S1, S2): *long head* by tibial part; *short head* by common fibular/peroneal part
Gastrocnemius[b,c]	Medial supracondylar ridge, adductor tubercle, popliteal surface of femur (medial head) and lateral surface of lateral femoral condyle (lateral head) to posterior surface of calcaneus via tendocalcaneus (Achilles tendon)	Powerful flexor of leg/calf at knee joint; also plantarflexes foot at ankle joint	Tibial nerve (S1, S2)
Plantaris[b]	Lateral supracondylar ridge, popliteal surface of tibia and knee joint capsule to posterior surface of calcaneus	Weak flexor of leg/calf at knee joint; weak plantarflexor of foot at ankle joint	Tibial nerve (S1, S2)
Popliteus	Lateral femoral epicondyle deep to the joint capsule to posterior surface of tibia proximal to soleal line	Lateral rotator of femur on tibia with foot fixed; flexor of leg/calf at knee joint	Tibial nerve (L5)
Gracilis	Body of the pubis and its ramus to medial surface of shaft of tibia	With knee semiflexed flexes leg/calf at knee joint; aids medial rotation of leg/calf at knee joint; also contributes to adduction of thigh at hip joint	Obturator nerve (L2, L3)
Sartorius	Anterior superior iliac spine to medial side of tibial shaft	Flexor of leg/calf at knee joint, medially rotates tibia on femur; also flexes, laterally rotates and abducts thigh at hip joint	Femoral nerve (L2, L3)
Rectus femoris[c,d]	Anterior inferior iliac spine (straight head) and area superior to acetabulum (reflected head) to superior border of patella and ligamentum patellae	Extensor of leg/calf at knee joint; flexor of thigh at hip joint	Femoral nerve (L2, L3, L4)

TABLE 3.4 **Muscles Crossing and Producing Movement of the Leg/Calf at the Knee Joint—cont'd**

Muscle	Attachments	Action	Innervation (root value)
Vastus lateralis[b,d]	Intertrochanteric line, greater trochanter, gluteal tuberosity, proximal $1/2$ of lateral lip of linea aspera and lateral intermuscular septum to base and lateral border of patella and ligamentum patellae	Extensor of leg/calf at knee joint	Femoral nerve (L2, L3, L4)
Vastus intermedius[d]	Anterior and lateral surfaces of proximal 2/3rd of femur to base of patella; articularis genu fibres arise from distal 1/3rd of anterior surface of femur to suprapatellar bursa	Extensor of leg/calf at knee joint; articularis genu prevents synovial membrane lining suprapatellar bursa becoming trapped between articulating bones during movement	Femoral nerve (L2, L3, L4)
Vastus medialis[d]	Intertrochanteric line, medial aspect of proximal end of femoral shaft, medial lip of linea aspera, medial supracondylar line and medial intermuscular septum to medial patella border, medial tibial condyle and ligamentum patellae	Extensor of leg/calf at knee joint; oblique medial fibres help prevent lateral displacement of patella	Femoral nerve (L2, L3, L4)
Tensor fascia lata	Iliac crest between iliac tubercle and anterior superior iliac spine to lateral tibial condyle via iliotibial tract	Extensor of leg/calf at knee joint; helps flex, abduct and medially rotate thigh at hip joint	Superior gluteal nerve (L4, L5)

[a]Part of quadriceps femoris.
[b]Can be seen in Fig. 3.75.
[c]Can be seen in Fig. 3.63.
[d]Part of the hamstrings.

(~93 degrees) than that with the femur (~84 degrees; Fig. 3.87). Comparing the axes of the hip, knee and ankle joints in erect standing, the knee maintains a position of medial rotation with respect to both the femoral head and neck and the distal end of the tibia.

Joint Forces

When considering knee joint forces, those acting on both joint compartments (femorotibial, femoropatellar) must be taken into account. During level walking, the force across the femorotibial joint can reach five times body weight, although, for most of the gait cycle, it is usually between two and four times body weight (Fig. 3.89); the force across the femoropatellar joint in similar circumstances is approximately half body weight. The precise level of loading depends on internal (alignment

between the femur and tibia, any residual deformity) and external (speed of walking, environmental conditions) factors. Ascending or descending ramps and stairs appear to have little influence on femorotibial forces; in contrast, femoropatellar forces increase significantly to between one-and-a-half and two times body weight when ascending and to between two-and-a-half and three times body weight when descending ramps and stairs. However, in everyday as opposed to vigorous activities, the greatest forces across the femoropatellar joint are found when getting out of a chair without using the arms. In such an activity, femoropatellar forces reach three-and-a-half times body weight, while the corresponding femorotibial forces are four times body weight.

Activities such as running and jumping significantly increase the magnitude of all forces acting across the

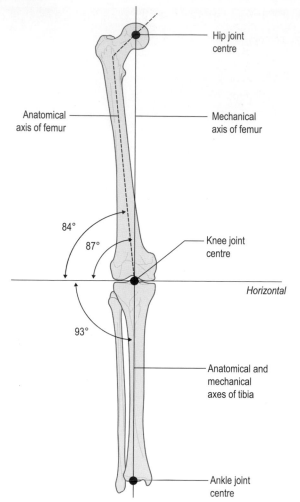

Fig. 3.87 Relationship between the anatomical and mechanical axes of the right femur and tibia.

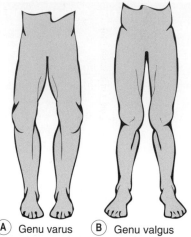

Fig. 3.88 (A) Genu varus and (B) genu valgus.

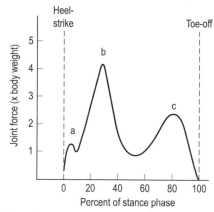

Fig. 3.89 Loading profile in normal knees during the stance phase of gait; peaks a, b and c correspond to hamstring, quadriceps and gastrocnemius contraction. (From Banasik, J.l., 2018. Pathophysiology. Elsevier.)

joint. In jumping, femorotibial joint forces may reach 24 times body weight and femoropatellar joint forces reach 20 times body weight; the articular cartilage of the joints is, therefore, subjected to extremely high stresses. It is not surprising that gymnasts present with articular cartilage degeneration of the knee, accompanied by significant bone buttressing of the femoral and tibial condyles. The pattern and magnitude of the forces in level walking is shown in Fig. 3.89; the joint force increases rapidly after heel-strike reaching a peak value as the foot makes full contact with the ground. The peak magnitude depends on two factors: acceptance of full body weight onto the supporting limb and the effect of muscle activity across the joint preventing collapse. The

second force peak is associated with the propulsive part of the stance phase of gait, its magnitude being primarily determined by the level of muscle activity across the joint, with quadriceps femoris extending the knee and gastrocnemius plantarflexing the foot to propel the body forwards. When walking up and down stairs, increased activity in quadriceps femoris is responsible for the three to sixfold increase in femoropatellar joint forces.

In contrast to the high vertical forces across the joint, mediolateral joint forces are low, being approximately one-quarter body weight.

Because of the angulation (varus or valgus) between the femur and tibia, the medial and lateral parts of the femorotibial joint are not equally loaded; the degree

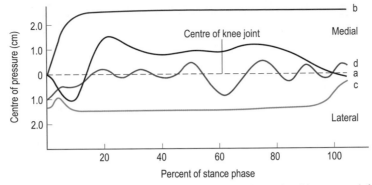

Fig. 3.90 Centre of joint pressure during level walking. *a*, Normal knee; *b*, with a varus deformity; *c* and *d*, with a valgus deformity.

of angulation has a profound influence on the loading pattern. During gait in normal individuals, the centre of force is located just medial to the midline of the joint for the majority of the stance phase (Fig. 3.90, line a). This does not necessarily mean that the contact stresses are greater on the medial side; because of the shape of the femoral and tibial condyles it is likely that contact stresses on the lateral side of the joint are greater. In varus deformities, the medial contact forces increase dramatically; in 2.5 degree varus, the medial forces increase by 70% and in 5 degrees varus by 95%. Consequently, the centre of force location throughout the stance phase lies medial to the midline of the joint (Fig. 3.90, line b). Similarly, in valgus deformities there is an increase in contact forces on the lateral side of the joint; in 2.5 degree valgus the lateral forces increase by 50% and in 5 degrees valgus by 75%. In such conditions, the centre of force location is now on the lateral side of the joint midline (Fig. 3.90, line d). However, when the valgus deformity reaches 15 degrees the centre of force location fluctuates on either side of the midline of the joint (Fig. 3.90, line c). This is achieved by the individual compensating for the valgus load to reduce lateral compartment loading. One compensatory mechanism individuals adopt is to use the hip abductors during the stance phase to produce a large lateral horizontal force at the foot; this necessitates an abduction movement on the tibia, loading the knee medially. Alternatively, and perhaps more commonly, the hip may be abducted during the swing phase, placing the foot medially at heel-strike; this also requires similarly large lateral forces at the foot during stance to maintain equilibrium, resulting in increased loading of the medial compartment of the knee.

It appears that individuals can modify force transmission by adopting compensatory mechanisms resulting in the unloading of a particular compartment of the knee; studies suggest it is easier to compensate for a valgus than for a varus deformity. Whether femoropatellar joint forces increase with a valgus or varus deformity is not known; however, it is likely that the pattern of loading at this joint changes.

Trabecular Arrangement

In addition to being subject to high contact forces during activity, the knee joint is also subjected to considerable side-to-side stresses. This is reflected in the internal architecture of the articulating bones where the trabeculae are arranged along the lines of mechanical stress, either tension or compression (Fig. 3.91).

The distal end of the femur shows two main sets of trabeculae arising from the cortex of the shaft, with a transverse set uniting the two condyles (Fig. 3.91). From the cortical region of the shaft medially and laterally, trabeculae fan out into both condyles; the system running to the ipsilateral condyle resists compression forces, and that to the contralateral condyle tensile forces. The proximal end of the tibia has similarly arranged trabecular systems (Fig. 3.91). From the cortex of the shaft, trabeculae radiate into both tibial condyles; ipsilaterally they resist compression forces and contralaterally tensile forces; a transverse system unites the two tibial condyles. As in the femur, trabecular systems arising from the medial and lateral sides of the tibial shaft cross each other approximately at right angles. An important set of trabeculae run into the tibial tuberosity from the anterior aspect of the shaft; this system has developed in response to the tensile stresses to which the tuberosity is subject by the pull of quadriceps femoris and the ligamentum patellae.

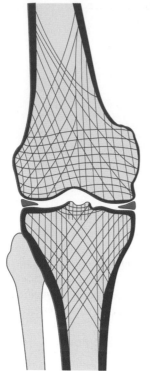

Fig. 3.91 Trabecular arrangement in the distal femur and proximal tibia.

Contact Areas
Femorotibial Joint

Because the radius of curvature of the femoral condyles increases anteriorly, the greatest area of contact between the femur and tibia is in full extension; however, not only is the contact area position-dependent, it is also load-dependent. At low loading levels (<500 N) the joint (including menisci) is not congruous, but with loads greater than 1500 N, it becomes markedly congruous. The menisci play a very important role in load transmission across the joint, with the total contact area doubling with the menisci present (Fig. 3.92A); with the knee fully extended and an applied load of 1000 N, the contact area is approximately 11.5×10^2 mm² with the menisci present and only 5.2×10^2 mm² without menisci. This suggests that in removing the menisci the average stress across the joint doubles compared with that of the intact knee. Peak pressure at 1000 N loading on the intact knee is approximately 3 MPa, while without menisci it is closer to 6 MPa. The highest pressure areas are on the lateral meniscus and the uncovered part of the articular cartilage of the lateral compartment.

The menisci actually account for about 70% of the total contact area at 1000 N loading; at lower loads, they account for a greater proportion of the total contact

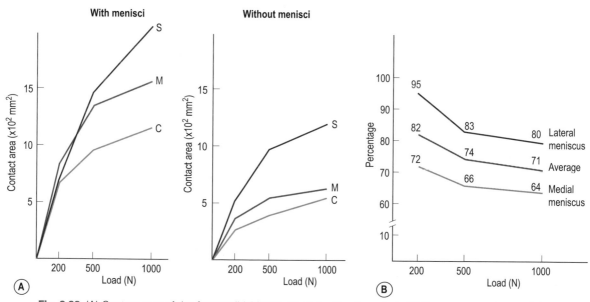

Fig. 3.92 (A) Contact area of the femorotibial joint with and without menisci. (B) Percent contact area of the menisci compared with total contact area. C, Control; M, mild osteoarthritis; S, severe osteoarthritis. (Adapted from Fukubayashi, T., Kurosawa, H., 1980. The contact area and pressure distribution pattern of the knee. A study of normal and osteoarthritic knee joints. Acta Orthop. Scand. 51, 871–880.)

area (Fig. 3.92B). The two menisci do not contribute the same percentage of contact areas in the medial and lateral compartments (Fig. 3.92B); this is due to their different shapes, as well as the relative positions of their attachments to the intercondylar eminence. Somewhat surprisingly, contact areas in osteoarthritic knees are significantly larger than in normal knees, both with and without menisci (Fig. 3.92A), suggesting that the menisci play a less significant role in osteoarthritic knees.

It is clear that the menisci give elastic stability to the joint, having both load-bearing and load-spreading functions. They provide surface compliance serving to transmit stresses across a wider area to the periphery of the joint. The menisci help avoid stress concentrations both in the articular cartilage and the subchondral bone.

Femoropatellar Joint

This has two complex mechanisms for ameliorating the forces transmitted across it. With increasing flexion, the lever arm of the extensors is lengthened as the axis of rotation moves posteriorly, particularly between 30 and 70 degree flexion; in addition, there is increasing contact between the patella and femur. Within the 30–70 degree range of knee flexion, the patella is solely responsible for transmitting the quadriceps force to the femur. The deep surface of the patella is covered by the thickest cartilage in the body and, not surprisingly, is the most frequent

site of cartilage degeneration. Stresses applied to the cartilage of between 2 MN/m^2 and 4 MN/m^2 have been calculated for level walking and ascending/descending steps, respectively.

Between 30 and 90 degree knee flexion the contact area almost triples (Fig. 3.93A), achieved by an increasingly larger proportion of the patella coming into contact with the femur (Fig. 3.93B). By 135 degree flexion, this contact area has decreased (Fig. 3.93C), being limited to the superior part of the lateral and the odd facets.

The Q-angle and valgus vector explain the predominance of pathological lesions on the lateral side of the joint, as well as the associated dislocations, subluxations, lateral pressure syndromes and patellofemoral arthrosis. (The Q-angle is the angle between the anatomical axis of the femur and that of the tibia (Fig. 3.87), determined on the lateral side of the leg/calf.) A number of anatomical factors affect patella tracking as it moves in the groove on the femur. Physiotherapy techniques involving specific exercises for parts of vastus medialis, together with carefully applied skin taping, are used in some cases to improve tracking, helping reduce anterior knee pain.

Mechanical Role of the Menisci

The average pressure in the articular cartilage of the femorotibial joints is much less with load-bearing menisci

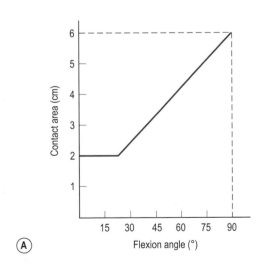

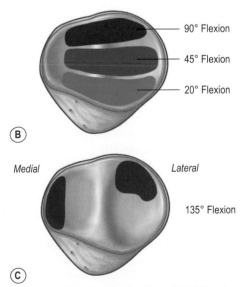

Fig. 3.93 Contact area between the patella and femur increasing up to 90 degree flexion (A and B) following which it decreases (C).

than without. With loads distributed over a larger contact area, not only is the average pressure lower, but the pressure gradients are also lower; cartilage deformation is, therefore, small. Following meniscectomy, the pressure distribution becomes non-uniform with a higher average pressure, higher stress gradients and large cartilage deformations. As articular cartilage contains 65%–85% water, the less uniform the pressure distribution, the greater the loss of fluid from high-pressure zones, and the greater the rate of increase in cartilage deformation. With several thousand stress reversals within the course of a single day, cartilage degeneration often ensues.

Failure or removal of a meniscus usually has detrimental effects on the adjacent articular cartilage. The area of cartilage most frequently affected following meniscectomy is that on the tibial condyle originally enclosed by the meniscus because it is unavoidably subjected to increased pressure each time the joint is loaded. There may also be modification in the shapes of the femoral and tibial condyles, as a response of the bone to the changes in pressure distribution. The articular cartilage on the tibial condyle within the embrace of the meniscus is an area of non-habitual contact; it is said to be functionally different from the cartilage in other areas of the joint. Age-dependent surface degeneration is commonly encountered at these sites. The menisci should be regarded as an important and integral part of the articular surfaces of the tibia, with their function being to distribute load over a large area of the articular surfaces at pressures that the cartilage can tolerate.

The importance of the menisci in lubricating and providing nutrients for the articular surfaces should not be underestimated. A specific pattern of articular degeneration can be seen in many knees in the form of a triangle of erosion or osteophyte formation on the medial femoral condyle, often associated with a strip on the lateral condyle (Fig. 3.94); the base of the triangle on the medial condyle is where rotation occurs with full extension. The regions of degeneration are those normally in contact with the anterior horns of the menisci in full extension and are only found in association with flexion contractures. In other words, the lesion arises in areas which have no opposing articular surface because of the inability to fully extend the joint.

The menisci also play an important role in absorbing shock transmitted across the knee joint; meniscectomy reduces the knee's shock-absorbing capacity by some 20%.

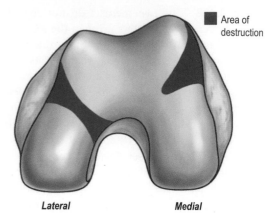

Area of destruction

Lateral   Medial

Fig. 3.94 Commonly observed pattern of articular cartilage damage on the femoral condyles associated with flexion deformities.

Patella Pathology

Stress analysis of the normal patella suggests that areas of high tensile stress on its medial aspect may exist during knee flexion. The high tensile stress is a function of Q-angle, a reduction of which dramatically reduces the values of combined stresses within the cartilage, reducing the possibility of fatigue failure of the cartilage collagen.

Vertical tensile stresses can occur over the medial aspect of the lateral facet, which when combined with high contact stresses applied perpendicular to the surface, a situation exists of very high shear stresses which may fatigue the deeper layers of articular cartilage (Fig. 3.95). If the combination of stresses persists, it may lead to a closed type of chondromalacic lesion centred on the medial region commonly extending onto the lateral surface.

Chondrosclerotic lesions, which are rare, are caused by an extreme compression phenomenon, being the result of high bending stresses combined with high contact stresses over the lateral facet.

To some extent, high stresses within the patella articular cartilage may be relieved by anterior or anteromedial displacement of the tibial tuberosity. More recently, the problem has been approached using osteochondral grafts to replace the damaged area, followed by rehabilitation aimed at correcting patellar glide.

Cruciate Ligament Replacement

Injuries to the knee joint are rarely isolated; other damage is frequently obscured at the time of injury due to swelling, only becoming apparent later. Secondary

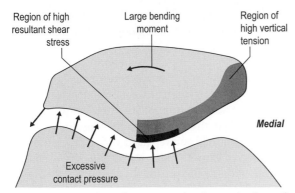

Region of high resultant shear stress

Large bending moment

Region of high vertical tension

Medial

Excessive contact pressure

Fig. 3.95 Pattern of patellar stresses leading to the formation of closed chondromalacic lesions of the patella.

injury may develop from abnormal forces acting across the joint. The cruciate ligaments, because of their blood supply, are capable of a certain amount of repair; however, severe ruptures have to be dealt with surgically. The primary aim of cruciate ligament repair is restoration of static and dynamic stability of the flexed knee as this is the usual position of function. It is vital that any reparative measures restore normal biomechanical functioning of the joint. If this fails to happen, the altered force patterns transmitted across the joint may lead to secondary changes, both at the knee and other joints similar to that occurring in the absence of surgical intervention.

The complexity of the cruciate ligaments with their spiralling fibres and intracapsular position makes reconstruction difficult. Surgical repair with sutures has not, in general, been very successful. Ligament replacements are now more common and successful as new surgical techniques continue to be developed. There are two broad categories of cruciate ligament replacement: single- and double-strand autologous tendon grafts.

Synthetic prostheses are still used but have two major disadvantages: (i) they cannot withstand the forces generated at the joint and often break; and (ii) they can induce foreign body change (fibrosis) within the joint. The latter can lead to compromised joint function.

One way of avoiding implant rejection is to use the individual's own tendons as the graft; by preserving the graft's original blood supply, the success of the procedure is enhanced as the tendon is capable of repair and remodelling. Nevertheless, the strength of tendon grafts is still less than that of the original cruciate ligament, with rupture occasionally occurring. Tendon grafts are essentially of two types (static or dynamic stabilisers); static stabilisers attempt to mimic the course of the

original ligament with the ends of the graft secured to the tibia and femur, often in specially prepared tunnels.

Commonly used tendons in autologous grafts are those of semitendinosus, gracilis and part of the patellar tendon (ligamentum patellae); although initially quite effective, the grafts often stretch with recurrence of the original problems. To counter this, the graft is often plaited using three or four strands to increase its strength. The fixation sites are also prone to rarefication and may become loose.

In contrast to static tendon grafts, dynamic tendon grafts preserve the muscular attachment of the tendon. In these situations, the tendon attachment is detached and passed through the joint capsule and a tunnel in one bone and secured to the other by staples or a bone plug; the course of the tendon mimics the original ligament. The ACL may be replaced by the iliotibial tract, semitendinosus, gracilis, sartorius or by a middle patellar tendon (ligamentum patellae) graft. Dynamic tendon grafts give little passive resistance to movement, with the 'drawer sign' usually persisting, although it may be slightly decreased. During use, subluxing forces are resisted by active contraction of the muscle. Such grafts may also provide protection against excessive movements by initiating muscle stretch reflexes to oppose the movement.

Advances in cruciate ligament repair have been such that dynamic tendon grafts are only used when other procedures have failed. Very often, the type of 'salvage' operation gives good results, allowing moderate functional activity but precluding high-impact sports. Although the extremes of the range of movement may be protected using knee braces, early mobilisation, particularly weight-bearing, improves the effectiveness of ligament reconstruction.

Replacement of the Menisci

The treatment of meniscal injuries includes complete or partial meniscectomy, repair and prosthetic replacement; however, complete meniscectomy can lead to instability and osteoarthritic changes at the knee and other joints. Loss of the shock-absorbing capacity of the meniscus may lead to back pain and headaches. Partial meniscectomy with a peripheral rim being preserved has two functional consequences: (i) it maintains some stability and prevents high-stress concentrations; (ii) because the periphery is vascular it facilitates meniscal regeneration. The new meniscus is formed from the synovial membrane and resembles the original, except that its attachments are usually thicker and it projects less into the centre of the joint cavity. The success of regeneration is age-dependent, being more successful in younger patients.

Meniscal repair is an important consideration for competitive athletes who want to return to training as soon as possible. Meniscal repair by suturing is considered if the tear is in the peripheral vascular part of the meniscus. While meniscal repair is taking place, rehabilitation progresses slowly in the early stages. If the procedure is successful, the long-term results are claimed to be better than partial or complete meniscectomy.

Knee Joint Replacement

Because of the complex nature of the knee, it presents many problems in designing a suitable prosthesis. The purpose of total knee replacement is to restore normal function and range of movement by relieving pain and disability, as well as restoring normal limb alignment. The common indications for total knee replacement include severe and unremitting degenerative bone disease, osteoarthritis and inflammatory arthritis which conservative medical treatment has failed to manage. Extreme deformity and structural damage are also frequent reasons for replacement, particularly in rheumatoid arthritis and other inflammatory joint conditions.

Early designs were simple hinge devices which had a high rate of loosening because they did not allow the normal rotatory movements of the knee to occur. Nevertheless, hinge replacements are still used in individuals with badly deformed or unstable knees; they are only suitable for sedentary individuals who will not make great demands on the prosthesis. There are a large range of prostheses now available, all attempting to mimic, to a greater or lesser extent, knee joint movement. The particular prosthesis implanted depends on several factors, including the adequacy of the collateral and cruciate ligaments and amount of bone stock available. Many devices provide a series of options depending on the prevailing anatomy; all modern devices allow at least 110 degrees of movement, the range required for normal functional activities. Of interest and debate is whether the PCL should be retained, sacrificed or substituted as part of the replacement. Anatomical designs aim to retain as much normal joint anatomy as possible, especially the PCL and occasionally the ACL. They rely on the remaining soft tissues of the joint to provide stability

and adequate support; however, PCL substituting models are available. Functional designs often ignore knee joint anatomy and do not rely on any remaining soft tissues to operate efficiently. Non-anatomical joint surfaces have been created to improve congruence and reduce complications (polyethylene wear). Some prostheses use mobile joint surface components that can be manipulated to preserve the PCL, but more commonly the PCL is removed entirely and replaced with a cruciate substituting mechanism.

Irrespective of the prosthetic design or whether the PCL has been retained, sacrificed or substituted, correct alignment of the implant is important in the transmission of forces across the joint and the possibility of loosening. Loosening, particularly of the tibial component, is a fairly common problem. As the knee extends, the anterior part of the tibial implant is pushed inferiorly tending to raise the posterior part; the bone resection required greatly reduces the amount of bony buttress at the posterior aspect of the tibia, which, coupled with the cement's inability to resist tensile stresses, promotes prosthesis loosening.

To give the implant some shock-absorbing features and reduce the transmission of high-frequency, high-magnitude forces across the joint, the tibial component is usually polyethylene. A few prostheses have attempted to insert artificial menisci between the replacement joint surfaces in an attempt to (i) improve stability, (ii) increase the area of contact and spread the load more evenly and (iii) improve the shock-absorbing capacity of the joint.

Even if the replacement has been clinically successful in reducing or removing pain on movement and a more or less full range of movement has been achieved, abnormalities of gait and difficulty in negotiating stairs may still be present. Total knee arthroplasty is not advised for young active individuals unless deterioration in joint function is so severe that it limits normal functional activities. If only one knee is involved, every effort should be made through medical treatment to restore function. In some osteoarthroses, only the medial, or less commonly, the lateral half of the joint is involved. In these cases, it may be possible to avoid joint replacement and provide adequate relief by realigning the axis of the knee so that most of the forces are redirected through the less affected part of the joint. This procedure (tibial osteotomy) is useful in young patients with high levels of activity and a long life expectancy. As an alternative to tibial osteotomy, a unicondylar replacement preserving more of the undamaged parts of the knee joint can be inserted.

MUSCLES FLEXING THE LEG/CALF AT THE KNEE JOINT

Hamstrings (semitendinosus, semimembranosus and biceps femoris; p. 304)
Gastrocnemius (p. 397)
Gracilis
Sartorius
Popliteus (p. 370)

Hamstrings
Functional Activity
With the exception of the short head of biceps femoris, the hamstrings cross and act upon both the hip and knee joints; their action is extremely complex. Although details of their attachments and much of their action are covered on page 307, the functional activities of these muscles with respect to the knee joint have yet to be considered. Their relationship with one to another in the posterior thigh, together with their relationship to the gluteal muscles, is shown in Fig. 3.96.

Rotation of the knee joint by the hamstrings is usually considered to take place when the foot is off the ground; however, this is not entirely true. It is certainly easier to describe when the foot is off the ground, but in practice, it occurs when the feet are firmly on the ground (when moving sideways from seat to seat). The feet are fixed and they assume body weight, the individual remains in the seated position just allowing the buttock to come clear of the seat. The trunk is then moved to one side by rotating the femur on the superior surface of the tibia; this is achieved by the combined action of medial rotation of one knee and lateral rotation of the other.

The simultaneous action of the hamstrings on both the hip and knee joints also has to be considered; this occurs in athletes accelerating towards a bend. Here the hamstrings function to lift the trunk into a more erect

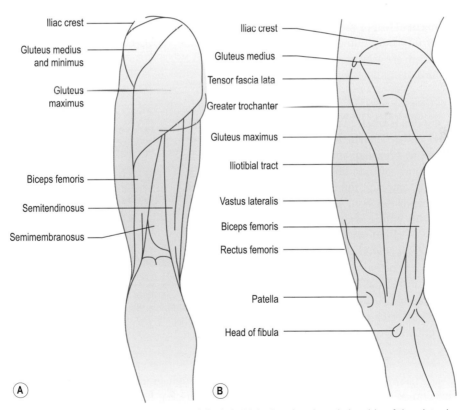

Fig. 3.96 (A) Posterior and (B) lateral aspects of the left thigh showing the relationship of the gluteal muscles and hamstrings.

position, as well as flex the knee of the limb being swung-through ready for the next stride. As the body is moving around the bend, the hamstrings have to produce knee rotation to produce this turning force. It is thought that they act as a tie between the posterior aspect of the pelvis and the tibia and can, therefore, adjust the relationship between them. This is particularly important when the body is changing posture during active movement as there are additional forces due to the acceleration of body segments. This concept goes some way to explain why there are so many hamstring injuries in athletes.

Gastrocnemius
Functional Activity
Gastrocnemius (Fig. 3.127A) is mainly a strong plantar-flexor of the foot at the ankle joint and is dealt with in that section; however, it is also a strong flexor of the leg/calf at the knee.

The medial and lateral heads of gastrocnemius cross the knee joint on their respective sides. It appears to come into action when the foot is fixed and the body is pulled anteriorly over the feet. This is best seen when pulling forwards on the slide of a rowing boat seat or manoeuvring the fully reclined body. The turning and pulling down of the body when in bed or on a plinth are very important considering that we spend one-third of our lives lying down.

Gracilis
Long thin muscle, gracilis is situated on the medial side of the thigh (Figs 3.47 and 3.97); it is the most superficial of the adductor group. Its proximal attachment is to the anterior aspect of the body of the pubis and its inferior ramus just encroaching onto the ramus of the ischium (Fig. 3.48). As it descends between semimembranosus posteriorly and sartorius anteriorly, gracilis develops a fusiform-shaped belly at about its middle. It becomes tendinous superior to the knee crossing the joint before expanding to attach to a short vertical line on the superior aspect of the medial surface of the shaft of the tibia. The attachment is proximal to that of semitendinosus, blending with that of sartorius posteriorly. Bursae separate the tendon of gracilis from those of sartorius and semitendinosus.

Innervation
By the anterior division of obturator nerve (root value L2, L3). Skin covering this area is innervated by roots L2 and L3, the superior part by obturator nerve and inferior part by the femoral nerve.

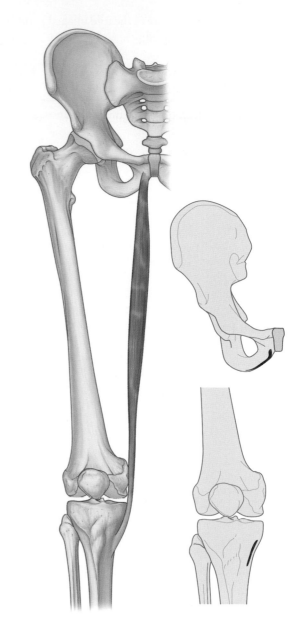

Fig. 3.97 Anterior aspect of the right innominate, femur and proximal tibia and fibula showing the position and attachments of gracilis.

Action
Although gracilis is situated with the adductor group of muscles, its action of adduction of the thigh at the hip joint is not as important as its action on the knee, where it is mainly a flexor; with the knee semiflexed it aids medial rotation of the leg/calf on the thigh.

Functional Activity

As a flexor of the knee, gracilis helps the hamstrings in simple flexion activities, such as the beginning of the swing phase in walking when the knee needs to be flexed. It also helps when strong flexion is required, as when pulling the body forward on the sliding seat of a rowing boat. In horse riding, gracilis is used in all its actions; when the rider is gripping the horse it helps the adductor muscles, while at the same time helping control the flexed knee.

Palpation

In the seated position with the medial aspect of the foot against a solid object (table leg) or when the toes are pointing towards the midline, the tendon can be felt on the posteromedial aspect of the knee joint, being the proximal of the two obvious tendons. If traced superiorly, the muscle belly can be palpated and traced to its attachment on the anterior aspect of the pubic body.

Sartorius

Long strap-like muscle with flattened tendons at each end, sartorius is the most superficial muscle in the anterior compartment of the thigh (Figs 3.98 and 3.102); its distal part lies on the medial side anterior to gracilis. It is renowned as the longest muscle in the body, getting its name from its action, which is to produce most of the actions needed in the lower limb to produce cross-legged sitting, the traditional position used by tailors when making clothes.

Its proximal attachment is to the anterior superior iliac spine and area just inferior. From here, it passes inferomedially attaching to a vertical line on the medial side of the shaft of the tibia anterior to both semitendinosus and gracilis, partly blending with the latter. A bursa separates sartorius from gracilis at its distal end. A few fibres from the distal tendon go to the medial collateral ligament of the knee joint and fascia of the leg/calf. The medial border of the proximal one-third forms the lateral boundary of the femoral triangle, while the middle one-third forms the roof of the adductor canal.

Innervation

By the femoral nerve (root value L2, L3). Skin covering the muscle is also supplied by L2 and L3.

Action

Sartorius produces many of the movements which combine to produce cross-legged sitting: flexion of the hip

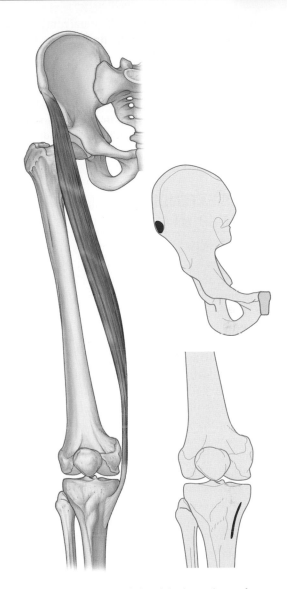

Fig. 3.98 Anterior aspect of the right innominate, femur and proximal tibia and fibula showing the position and attachments of sartorius.

and knee, lateral rotation and abduction of the thigh and medial rotation of the tibia on the femur. These actions can be summarised by placing the heel on the medial side of the opposite knee.

Functional Activity

Going into the cross-legged or the tailor sitting position is a functional activity; however, sartorius also helps produce any activity involving flexion of the knee and hip joints together, combined with lateral rotation of the thigh, as in drawing up the lower limbs when using the breaststroke in swimming.

Palpation

It is most easily palpated at its proximal end just inferior to the anterior superior iliac spine. Here, its strap-like shape can be easily palpated, particularly when the leg/calf, with the knee slightly flexed, is raised some 15 cm from the floor when lying supine.

MUSCLES EXTENDING THE LEG/CALF AT THE KNEE JOINT

Quadriceps femoris
    Rectus femoris
    Vastus lateralis
    Vastus medialis
    Vastus intermedius
Tensor fascia lata

Rectus Femoris

A spindle-shaped bipennate muscle, rectus femoris (Figs 3.99 and 3.102) stands out on the anterior aspect of the thigh. Its proximal attachment is by two heads continuous with each other, one to the anterior inferior iliac spine (straight head) and the other to a rough area immediately superior to the acetabulum (reflected head); it is thought that the straight head is a human acquisition associated with evolution of the erect posture. From this continuous attachment, a single tendon passes inferiorly from which arises the fleshy muscle. About two-thirds the way down the thigh, the muscle narrows to a thick tendon attaching to the proximal border of the patella; some fibres pass around the patella, helping form the ligamentum patellae. The deep surface of the muscle is tendinous and smooth, allowing free movement over a similar surface on vastus intermedius, permitting its independent action on the hip joint.

Vastus Lateralis

Situated on the anterolateral aspect of the thigh lateral to rectus femoris, vastus lateralis (Figs 3.100 and 3.102) has an extensive linear attachment from the superolateral part of the intertrochanteric line, inferior border of the greater trochanter, lateral side of the gluteal tuberosity and proximal half of the lateral lip of the linea aspera; it also attaches to the fascia lata and lateral intermuscular

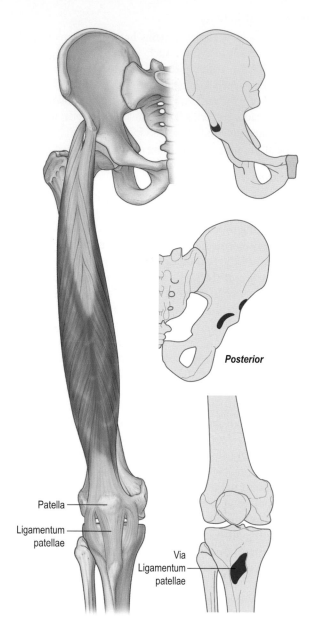

Posterior

Patella

Ligamentum patellae

Via Ligamentum patellae

Fig. 3.99 Anterior aspect of the right innominate, femur and proximal tibia and fibula showing the position and attachments of rectus femoris.

septum. From here the muscle fibres run inferoanteriorly, with those most superficial passing almost vertically inferiorly.

The muscle bulk is mainly situated in the proximal half of the lateral side of the thigh, from which a broad

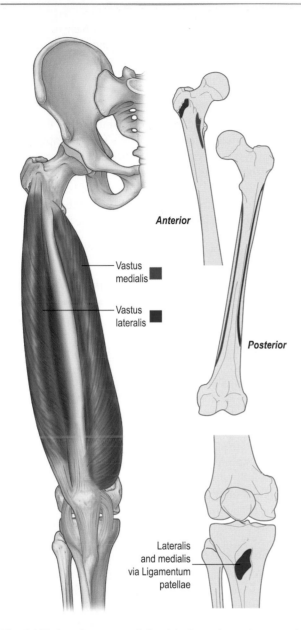

Fig. 3.100 Anterior aspect of the right innominate, femur and proximal tibia and fibula showing the position and attachments of vastus lateralis and vastus medialis.

tendon arises, narrowing as it approaches the lateral side of the patella. The tendon attaches to the tendon of rectus femoris and base and lateral border of the patella. Some fibres pass anterior to the lateral tibial condyle, blending with the iliotibial tract, helping to form the expansion that finally attaches to the line running towards the tibial tuberosity; to some extent this part of its attachment replaces the knee joint capsule in this region.

Vastus Medialis

Situated on the anteromedial aspect of the thigh medial to rectus femoris (Figs 3.100 and 3.102), with most of its bulk showing at the distal one-third just superior to the patella. It has an extensive linear attachment from a line beginning at the distal medial end of the intertrochanteric line, running inferiorly around the medial aspect of the proximal end of the shaft on the spiral line, medial lip of the linea aspera, continuing on to the proximal two-thirds of the medial supracondylar line, medial intermuscular septum and tendon of adductor magnus.

Its proximal fibres mainly pass inferiorly, while its distal fibres pass almost horizontally laterally. The two sets of fibres making up vastus medialis are considered by some to be anatomically and functionally distinct, with the oblique fibres being known as vastus medialis obliquus. The muscle attaches to the tendon of rectus femoris, medial border of the patella and anterior aspect of the medial condyle of the tibia. The expansions passing across the knee joint attaching to the tibia replace the joint capsule in this region, becoming fused with the deep fascia; this attachment also runs to the tibial tuberosity.

Vastus Intermedius

The deepest part of quadriceps femoris, vastus intermedius lies between vastus lateralis and medialis deep to rectus femoris (Fig. 3.101). It arises by fleshy fibres from the proximal two-thirds of the anterior and lateral surfaces of the femur, the fibres passing inferiorly forming a broad tendon on its more superficial aspect; this part attaches to the deep surface of the tendon of rectus femoris, the other vastus muscles and the base of the patella. In the middle of the thigh, vastus intermedius is difficult to separate from vastus lateralis, while inferiorly it is impossible to separate it from vastus medialis.

Articularis Genu

Some deep fibres of vastus intermedius, arising from a small area on the distal one-third of the anterior surface of the femur, pass inferiorly to attach to the proximal part of the suprapatellar bursa of the knee joint, lying deep to vastus intermedius; this is articularis genu. Its main function is to prevent the synovial membrane from becoming trapped and interfering with normal movements of the knee joint.

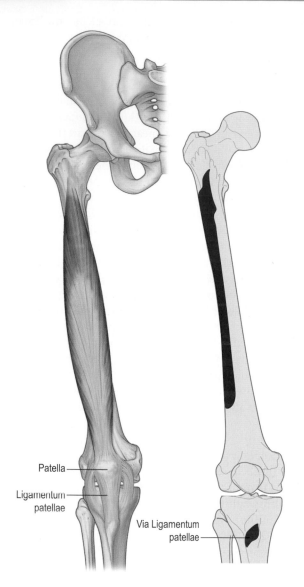

Patella

Ligamentum
patellae

Via Ligamentum
patellae

Fig. 3.101 Anterior aspect of the right innominate, femur and proximal tibia and fibula showing the position and attachments of vastus intermedius.

Innervation

By the femoral nerve (root value L2, L3, L4), including articularis genu. Skin covering the quadriceps is supplied by L2 and L3.

Quadriceps Femoris

The large muscle bulk on the anterior surface of the thigh. As its name implies it consists of four main parts: one part (rectus femoris) has its attachment superior to the hip joint, while the other three attach to the shaft of the femur. All four parts join together around the patella, forming a thick strong tendon (ligamentum patellae) attaching to the tibial tuberosity.

Ligamentum Patellae

All four quadriceps tendons contribute to the formation of the ligamentum patellae; it runs from the apex of the patella to the proximal part of the tibial tuberosity acting as the tendon of quadriceps femoris. The patella is really a sesamoid bone in the tendon of rectus femoris and vastus intermedius, helping to relay the pull of the quadriceps over the anterior aspect of the femur.

Action

Although part of quadriceps femoris, by crossing anterior to the hip joint, rectus femoris also flexes the thigh.

Quadriceps femoris is the main extensor of the knee joint; each muscle appears to have a particular role often becoming active at different parts of the range of the movement. Vastus medialis is more obviously active in the final part of extension and is believed to resist the tendency of the patella to move laterally, due to the angulation of the femur. Specific exercises designed to strengthen the oblique fibres of vastus medialis are advocated by some practitioners to affect tracking of the patella, resisting dislocation and possibly helping reduce anterior knee pain in some cases. Rectus femoris works particularly strongly in straight leg raising or in the combined movement of hip flexion and knee extension.

The relationship between quadriceps femoris and sartorius on the anterior aspect of the thigh is shown in Fig. 3.102.

Functional Activity

Quadriceps femoris is used strongly in stepping activities (stair climbing, squats). Rectus femoris performs its function particularly in the swing phase of walking when the lower limb is carried forward and the knee is extended. In the final stages of knee extension, vastus medialis helps in the locking mechanism of the joint when the femur is allowed to rotate medially.

Surprisingly, when standing, there is very little or no action in the quadriceps as, in this position, the knees are in the close-packed position. It is at these times that, if the knees are knocked from behind, collapse almost certainly occurs; however, when standing on a moving vehicle, the quadriceps are active. When standing on one leg, all muscles around the knee work isometrically providing stability at the joint.

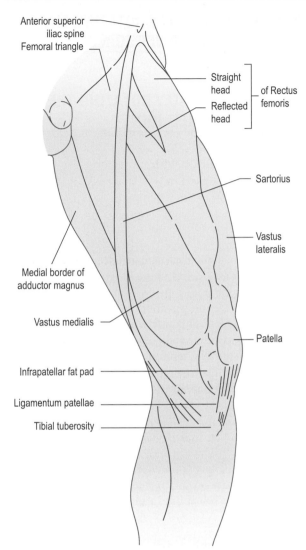

Fig. 3.102 Anteromedial aspect of the left thigh showing the relationship between muscles on the anterior aspect of the thigh.

Labels: Anterior superior iliac spine; Femoral triangle; Straight head / Reflected head of Rectus femoris; Sartorius; Vastus lateralis; Medial border of adductor magnus; Vastus medialis; Infrapatellar fat pad; Ligamentum patellae; Tibial tuberosity; Patella.

place your hands on the front of each thigh; the three parts of the muscle (as previously described) can be readily palpated.

In straight leg raising, the muscle should be able to extend the knee into a few degrees of hyperextension; this is the extra range required for the knee to lock. Individuals not able to do this often complain of the knee giving way during walking.

Tensor Fascia Lata

Situated anterolateral to the hip joint, tensor fascia lata (Fig. 3.103) lies superficial to gluteus minimus. It attaches proximally to the anterior part of the lateral lip of the iliac crest, between and including the iliac tubercle and anterior superior iliac spine, the area of the gluteal surface just inferior to it, the fascia between it and gluteus minimus and that covering its superficial surface. Inferiorly, it attaches between the two layers of the iliotibial tract inferior to the level of the greater trochanter.

Innervation

By the superior gluteal nerve (root value L4, L5), skin overlying the muscle is supplied by L1.

Action

Tensor fascia lata overlies gluteus minimus helping in flexion, abduction and medial rotation of the thigh at the hip joint; it also straightens out the posterior pull of gluteus maximus on the iliotibial tract.

Acting with the superficial fibres of gluteus maximus, it tightens the iliotibial tract and, through its attachment to the lateral tibial condyle, extends the leg/calf at the knee joint. Acting with gluteus minimus, it medially rotates the thigh at the hip joint; its posterior fibres may aid abduction of the thigh.

Functional Activity

As tensor fascia lata, with gluteus maximus, links the pelvis and tibia, it helps steady and control movements of the pelvis and femur on the tibia when the limb is weight-bearing. It produces strong medial rotation of the thigh when the hip is extended and the lower limb, pelvis and trunk are preparing to take the thrust relayed through the lower limb by the leg/calf muscles during the 'toe-off' phase of walking.

When quadriceps femoris is paralysed, tensor fascia lata can be developed to produce sufficient knee extension to enable the individual to walk, but its action is weak and limited in range.

Quadriceps femoris is a powerful and important muscle working strongly throughout its full range. It loses strength and bulk rapidly following injury to it or the knee joint; it may take months to regain power, but only days to lose it.

Palpation

When seated on a chair with the knee extended, particularly against resistance, the separate parts of quadriceps femoris, except vastus intermedius, can easily be palpated; medialis on the distal medial aspect, lateralis in the proximal lateral aspect and rectus femoris running down the centre. Standing with the knees semiflexed,

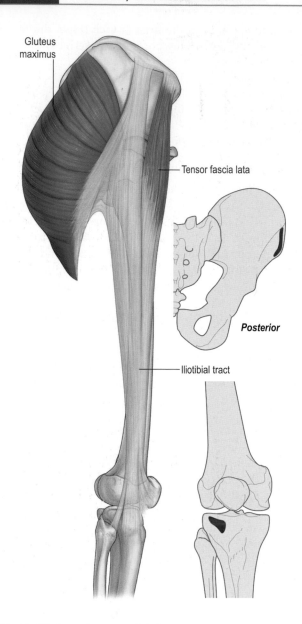

Gluteus maximus

Tensor fascia lata

Posterior

Iliotibial tract

Fig. 3.103 Lateral aspect of the right innominate, femur and proximal tibia and fibula showing the position and attachments of tensor fascia lata and the iliotibial tract. Also shown is gluteus maximus.

Palpation

Place the fingers halfway between the anterior superior iliac spine and greater trochanter of the femur. When the lower limb is medially rotated, the muscle can be felt powerfully contracting. If the weight is taken on the limb and the pelvis rotated to the same side, a similar contraction of the muscle is observed.

MUSCLES LATERALLY ROTATING THE LEG/CALF AT THE KNEE JOINT

Biceps femoris (p. 306)

MUSCLES MEDIALLY ROTATING THE LEG/CALF AT THE KNEE JOINT

Semitendinosus (p. 304)
Semimembranosus (p. 304)
Gracilis (p. 364)
Sartorius (p. 365)
Popliteus

Popliteus

Triangular-shaped muscle situated deep in the popliteal fossa inferior and lateral to the knee joint (Fig. 3.43). It arises within the joint capsule from a tendinous attachment to the anterior aspect of the groove on the lateral surface of the lateral condyle of the femur inferior to the lateral epicondyle and attachment of the lateral collateral ligament. The tendon passes posteriorly, inferiorly and medially crossing the joint line over the outer border of the lateral meniscus, to which it is attached. The proximal part within the joint capsule of the knee joint is enclosed in a double layer of synovial membrane until it leaves the capsule deep to the arcuate popliteal ligament, from which it has a fleshy origin. Continuing inferomedially, popliteus attaches by fleshy fibres to a triangular area on the posterior surface of the tibia, superior to the soleal line, and the fascia covering the muscle.

Innervation

By a branch from the tibial division of the sciatic nerve (root value L5) entering the muscle on its anterior surface after winding around its inferolateral border. Skin covering the area is supplied mainly by S2.

Action

Popliteus laterally rotates the femur on the tibia when the foot is on the ground releasing the knee from its close-packed (locked) position enabling it to flex. By exerting a posterior pull on the lateral surface of the lateral condyle of the femur it is rotated laterally about a vertical axis running through it just medial to its centre. This allows the medial condyle of the femur to glide anteriorly releasing the ligaments and muscles involved in maintaining its close-packed position.

When strong knee flexion is required, popliteus comes into action, drawing the tibia posteriorly on the femoral condyles; if the foot is off the ground, it also aids the medial hamstrings in medial tibial rotation.

Through its attachments to the lateral meniscus, popliteus pulls the meniscus posteriorly during lateral rotation of the femur preventing it from becoming trapped between the moving bones. This is believed by some to be why the lateral meniscus is damaged much less frequently than the medial.

Muscles crossing the knee joint medially and laterally are shown in Fig. 3.104.

CLINICAL EXAMINATION AND EVALUATION

Flexion

With the individual lying supine:
- Place the hip in neutral and extend the knee.
- Flex the hip and the knee (Fig. 3.105A).

The end feel to movement is usually soft due to contact of the soft tissues of the leg/calf or heel and thigh; however, the end feel may be firm due to tension in the vastus muscles. At approximately 90 degrees of hip flexion, the femur is stabilised to prevent further hip flexion.

To measure knee flexion, the centre of the goniometer is placed over the lateral epicondyle of the femur, with the proximal arm pointing towards the greater trochanter and the distal arm pointing towards the lateral malleolus.

Alternatively, have the individual lying prone with the foot hanging over the end of the supporting surface so that the hip is in neutral (Fig. 3.105B). The end feel to movement, if not soft, is firm due to tension in rectus femoris. The goniometer is aligned for the supine position.

In both positions, care should be taken to stabilise the femur to prevent unwanted movements.

Extension

The initial testing positions and goniometer alignment are the same as when measuring flexion (Fig. 3.105C). The end feel is firm due to tension in the posterior joint capsule, the oblique and arcuate popliteal, collateral and cruciate ligaments.

Rotation

With the individual seated with the leg/calf hanging freely over the side of the supporting surface:
- Hold the sole of the foot horizontally and move the foot so that the toes point medially (medial rotation) (Fig. 3.106A) or laterally (lateral rotation) (Fig. 3.106B).

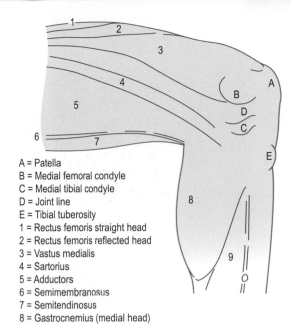

A = Patella
B = Medial femoral condyle
C = Medial tibial condyle
D = Joint line
E = Tibial tuberosity
1 = Rectus femoris straight head
2 = Rectus femoris reflected head
3 = Vastus medialis
4 = Sartorius
5 = Adductors
6 = Semimembranosus
7 = Semitendinosus
8 = Gastrocnemius (medial head)
9 = Soleus

(A)

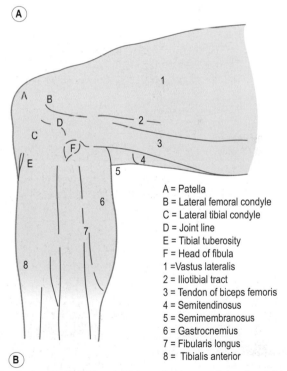

A = Patella
B = Lateral femoral condyle
C = Lateral tibial condyle
D = Joint line
E = Tibial tuberosity
F = Head of fibula
1 = Vastus lateralis
2 = Iliotibial tract
3 = Tendon of biceps femoris
4 = Semitendinosus
5 = Semimembranosus
6 = Gastrocnemius
7 = Fibularis longus
8 = Tibialis anterior

(B)

Fig. 3.104 (A) Medial and (B) lateral aspects of the distal thigh and proximal leg/calf with the knee flexed showing the muscles crossing the knee.

The end feel to movement is firm due to tension in the collateral (lateral rotation) or cruciate (medial rotation) ligaments.

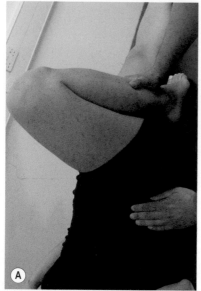

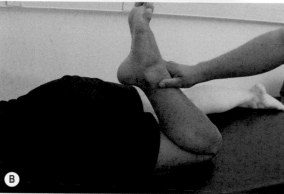

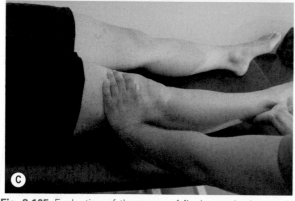

Fig. 3.105 Evaluation of the range of flexion at the knee with the individual (A) lying supine and (B) prone; (C) evaluation of the range of extension at the knee joint with the individual lying supine.

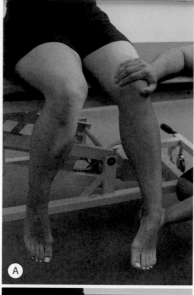

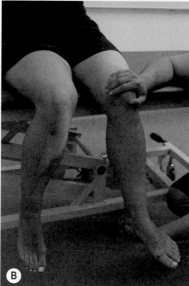

Fig. 3.106 Evaluation of the range of (A) medial and (B) lateral rotation of the leg/calf at the knee joint with the individual seated.

The centre of the goniometer is placed over the centre of the heel with one arm in line with the long axis of the thigh and the other in line with the long axis of the foot.

Alternatively, the individual can lie prone with the knee flexed to 90 degrees:

- Hold the foot horizontally while moving it so that the toes point medially (medial rotation) (Fig. 3.107A) or laterally (lateral rotation) (Fig. 3.107B).

The goniometer placement is as before.

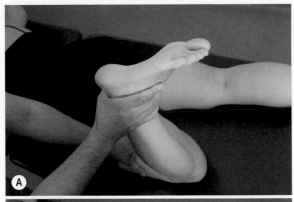

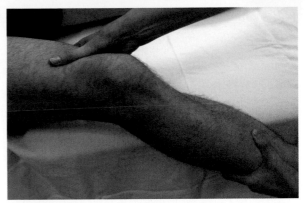

Fig. 3.108 Determination of knee joint laxity using the Drop Leg Lachman test.

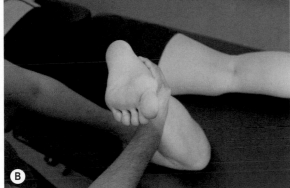

Fig. 3.107 Evaluation of the range of (A) medial and (B) lateral rotation of the leg/calf at the knee joint with the individual lying prone and knee flexed to 90 degrees.

Abduction and Adduction

In a normal joint, it is not possible to measure these movements.

Joint Laxity

Given the importance of the cruciate ligaments in providing anteroposterior stability at the knee joint, injury to them can have a major influence on joint laxity. ACL injury can have a profound effect on stability, while PCL injury may have minimal effect due to the action of the hamstrings. It is very important to have an accurate assessment of laxity so that appropriate recommendations can be made for treatment. Females tend to have a greater degree of joint laxity than males at all ages; this should be borne in mind when evaluating joint laxity after potential injury.

The classic sign of a ruptured ACL is an anterior drawer sign with excessive mobility of the tibia on the femur at 90 degree knee flexion. A normal knee shows 2–3 mm of movement, yet a knee with a completely ruptured ACL might show up to 25 mm of movement.

Unfortunately, the anterior drawer test often shows very little abnormal movement. If the test is performed with the knee flexed 10 degrees, an abnormal movement in the anterior direction is seen with ACL damage; this is the Lachman test. Several factors can influence the Lachman test, including knee flexion angle, joint rotation, muscle tone, displacement force and soft tissue restraints. Medial tibial rotation tightens the PCL, limiting the anterior draw effect; conversely, lateral tibial rotation increases anterior displacement.

A modified method of evaluating ACL integrity is the Drop Leg Lachman test (Fig. 3.108).

With the individual lying supine:

- Abduct the leg to be tested so that the leg/calf lies over the side of the supporting surface.
- Flex the knee to 25 degrees.
- Hold the foot between the examiner's lower limbs to maintain flexion and rotation of the leg/calf.
- Hold the thigh steady on the table using one hand.
- Extend and abduct the leg/calf to relax the hamstrings and tensor fascia lata.
- Place the free hand behind the individual's leg/calf and apply an anterior force as in the Lachman test.

The test must be conducted with the individual relaxed or, if necessary, anaesthetised.

The Drop Leg Lachman test has several advantages over the Lachman test: (i) it is easier to perform; (ii) is highly reproducible; (iii) allows bulky legs/calves to be handled easily; and (iv) is more sensitive. It is also easier to appreciate and visualise anterior movement of the tibia; the end point is easier to detect, nevertheless, it may still be influenced by muscle tone and soft tissue restraints.

SECTION SUMMARY

Femur
- Long bone of the thigh having a proximal head, neck, greater and lesser trochanters; shaft with linea aspera posteriorly; distal end with medial and lateral condyles.
- Head articulates with acetabulum of innominate forming the hip joint.
- Condyles articulate with tibia and patella forming tibiofemoral and patellofemoral joints respectively; both are part of the knee joint.

Patella
- Sesamoid bone in the tendon of quadriceps femoris.
- Deep surface articulates with anterior aspects of lateral and medial femoral condyles forming the patellofemoral joint.

Tibia
- Medial bone of leg/calf having proximal expanded end (tibial condyles); shaft with tibial tuberosity anteriorly and sharp, lateral facing interosseous border; slightly expanded distal end with medial malleolus.
- Proximally, the medial and lateral tibial condyles articulate with the medial and lateral femoral condyles forming the knee joint; the facet below the lateral condyle articulates with the head of the fibula forming the superior tibiofibular joint.
- Distally it articulates with the fibula forming the inferior tibiofibular joint; the talus forming the ankle joint.

Fibula
- Lateral bone of leg/calf having proximal head; irregular shaft with sharp medial facing interosseous border; expanded distal end with lateral malleolus projecting inferiorly.
- Articulates with the tibia superiorly and inferiorly forming the superior and inferior tibiofibular joints; the talus inferiorly forming part of the ankle joint.

Knee Joint

Type	Synovial bicondylar hinge joint
Articular surfaces	Condyles of femur with condyles of tibia; posterior surface of patella with patellar surface of femoral condyles
Capsule	Thick ligamentous sheath mainly composed of tendinous expansions; attached to articular margins of femoral condyle (except anterosuperiorly) and medial and lateral margins of tibial condyles
Ligaments	Oblique popliteal and arcuate popliteal; ligamentum patellae; tibial and fibular collateral
Intra-articular structures	Anterior and posterior cruciate ligaments; medial and lateral menisci; transverse ligament; coronary ligaments
Stability	Provided by collateral and cruciate ligaments (most stable in full extension – 'close-packed' position); muscles crossing the joint
Movements	Flexion and extension; medial and lateral rotation

Movements at Knee Joint
The knee joint consists of the distal end of the femur and proximal end of the tibia with the patella anterior. It primarily flexes and extends but is also capable of rotation when the knee is flexed.

Movement	Muscles (Root Value of Nerve Supply)

Flexion	Hamstrings:
	    Semitendinosus (L5, S1, S2)
	    Semimembranosus (L5, S1, S2)
	    Biceps femoris (L5, S1, S2)
	Gastrocnemius (S1, S2)
	Gracilis (L2, L3)
	Sartorius (L2, L3)
	Popliteus (L5)

Extension	Quadriceps femoris:
	    Rectus femoris (L2, L3, L4)
	    Vastus lateralis (L2, L3, L4)
	    Vastus medialis (L2, L3, 4L)
	    Vastus intermedius (L2, L3, L4)
	Tensor fascia lata (L4, L5)

Lateral rotation	Biceps femoris (L5, S1, S2)
Medial rotation	Semitendinosus (L5, S1, S2) Semimembranosus (L5, S1, S2) Gracilis (L2, L3) Sartorius (L2, L3) Popliteus (L5)

- The knee extensors are important 'antigravity' muscles as they frequently extend the knee (working concentrically) and control knee flexion (working eccentrically).
- Rotational movements of the knee are complex, involving interaction between muscles and ligaments.

Continued

SECTION SUMMARY—cont'd

Clinical Evaluation

Movement and Maximum Range	End Feel to Movement
Active flexion 140° (hip flexed)/120° (hip extended): passive flexion 160°	Soft: firm due to tension in the vastus muscles
Extension ~5°	Firm

Movement and Maximum Range	End Feel to Movement
Medial rotation 30° (active)/35° (passive)	Firm
Lateral rotation 40° (active)/50° (passive)	Firm

Medial and lateral rotation is with the knee flexed 90 degrees.

? SELF-ASSESSMENT QUESTIONS

41. Which structure forms the superolateral border of the popliteal fossa?
42. The oblique popliteal ligament is derived from which muscle?
43. Which muscles comprise the quadriceps femoris group?
44. From anterior to posterior, what attaches to the intercondylar eminence?
45. Which meniscus is the more mobile during movements at the knee joint?
46. Are the cruciate ligaments (A) intracapsular and intrasynovial, (B) intracapsular and extrasynovial, (C) extracapsular and intrasynovial or (D) extracapsular and extrasynovial?
47. Which muscle is responsible for lateral rotation of the femur on the tibia during the initial part of flexion?
48. The patella is a sesamoid bone situated within the tendon(s) of which group of muscles?
49. What is the nerve supply, including root value, of the short head of biceps femoris?
50. What attaches to the tibial tuberosity?
51. What are the attachments of the lateral collateral ligament?
52. Which muscle(s) produce medial rotation of the tibia on the femur at the knee joint?
53. What is the role of the anterior cruciate ligament (ACL)?
54. What are the functions of the menisci?
55. Which structure pulls the lateral meniscus posteriorly during the initial part of knee flexion?
56. Which artery lies immediately posterior to the knee joint?
57. What is the nerve supply, including root value, of sartorius?
58. What happens to the menisci during lateral rotation at the knee?
59. At 90 degree knee flexion, how much of the deep surface of the patella is in contact with the patella surface of the femur?
60. What are the attachments of gracilis?

| LEG/CALF

LEARNING OUTCOMES

By the end of the section, you should be able to:
1. Describe, identify and palpate the bones and joints of the leg/calf
2. Describe and explain the movements possible at the superior and inferior tibiofibular joints
3. Locate, palpate and examine the muscles associated with the leg/calf and to know their attachments, action and innervation
4. Examine and assess movements of the leg/calf
5. Appreciate the influence of pathology and/or trauma on the function of the leg/calf

INTRODUCTION

Although the tibia and fibula articulate together, there is no active movement between them; however, there is slight movement between the two bones which is mechanically linked to movement at the ankle joint. The two bones are united by a synovial joint at their proximal ends, a fibrous joint at their distal ends and an interosseous membrane connecting their shafts.

Inferior to the knee, the deep fascia encloses the leg/calf attaching mainly to the anterior and medial borders of the tibia and the medial and lateral malleoli; where the tibia and fibula are subcutaneous the deep fascia blends with the periosteum of the bone. Intermuscular septa pass to the fibula, separating the fibularis/peroneal muscles from the extensors anteriorly and flexors posteriorly; a further septum passes across the posterior aspect of the leg/calf, separating the superficial and deep flexor muscles. Around the ankle the fascia is thickened by numerous transverse fibres, forming retaining bands (retinaculae) for the tendons of the muscles which pass across the ankle.

TIBIA AND FIBULA

Details of the tibia and fibula can be found on pages 322 and 325, respectively.

SUPERIOR TIBIOFIBULAR JOINT

Plane synovial joint between the circular/oval facet on the head of the fibula and a similar facet on the posterolateral aspect of the inferior surface of the lateral tibial condyle (Figs 3.58A and 3.109); the fibular articular facet faces anteriorly, superiorly and medially, while that on the tibia faces posteriorly, inferiorly and laterally. A fibrous capsule attaches to the margins of the facets on both tibia and fibula, strengthened anteriorly and posteriorly by accessory ligaments.

The fibrous bands of the short, thick anterior ligament of the head of the fibula pass obliquely superomedially from the anterior aspect of the head of the fibula to the anterior aspect of the lateral tibial condyle. Posteriorly, a single band (posterior ligament of the head of the fibula) runs in a similar direction between the head of the fibula and posterior aspect of the lateral tibial condyle. The tendon of popliteus is intimately related to the posterosuperior aspect of the joint crossing the posterior ligament (Fig. 3.109C). The popliteal bursa, prolonged under the tendon from the knee joint, occasionally communicates with the joint cavity through an opening in the proximal part of the capsule.

The blood supply to the joint is from the lateral inferior genicular and anterior tibial recurrent arteries; lymphatic drainage is to the popliteal nodes. The nerve supply to the joint is by twigs from the recurrent branch of the common fibular/peroneal nerve, and the branch to popliteus is from the tibial nerve; the root value is L5.

The joint is overhung by the apex of the head of the fibula, to which attaches part of the tendon of biceps femoris, the remainder going to the lateral aspect of the head inferior to the apex. The lateral collateral ligament attaches between biceps femoris attachment and the joint.

There is slight movement at the superior tibiofibular joint giving a small degree of flexibility to the relationship between the tibia and fibula during movements of the ankle joint, as well as in response to the pull of the muscles attached to the fibula.

INFERIOR TIBIOFIBULAR JOINT

Fibrous joint (syndesmosis) between the rough triangular convex surface of the medial aspect of the distal end of the fibula superior to the articular facet and a

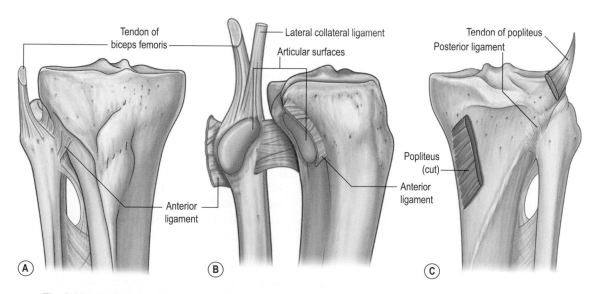

Fig. 3.109 (A) Anterior, (B) lateral and (C) posterior aspects of the right superior tibiofibular joint showing the articular surfaces and associated structures.

corresponding rough triangular concave surface (fibular notch) on the lateral side of the tibia (Fig. 3.110). Uniting the two bones is the strong interosseous ligament, continuous with the interosseous membrane superiorly, consisting of short fibrous bands; it forms the principal connection between the two bones. The joint is

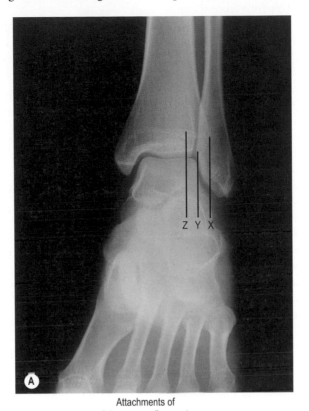

Attachments of
interosseous ligament

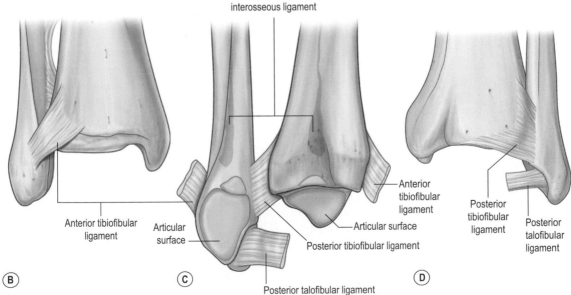

Anterior tibiofibular
ligament

Articular
surface

Anterior
tibiofibular
ligament

Articular surface

Posterior tibiofibular ligament

Posterior talofibular ligament

Posterior
tibiofibular
ligament

Posterior
talofibular
ligament

(B)   (C)   (D)

Fig. 3.110 (A) Anteroposterior radiograph of the left inferior tibiofibular joint; (B) anterior, (C) lateral and (D) posterior aspects of the right tibiofibular joint showing the articular surfaces and supporting ligaments.

supported by anterior, posterior and transverse tibiofibular ligaments.

The anterior and posterior tibiofibular ligaments are longer, more superficial bands stretching from the borders of the fibular notch of the tibia to the anterior and posterior surfaces of the lateral malleolus of the fibula; the posterior ligament is thicker and broader. The inferior edge of both ligaments covers the lateral ridge of the trochlear surface of the talus, the anterior during flexion of the ankle joint and posterior during extension; both ligaments run inferolaterally. Under cover of the posterior ligament is the transverse tibiofibular ligament attaching along the whole length of the inferior border of the posterior surface of the tibia and proximal part of the malleolar fossa of the fibula. This strong thick ligament projects inferior to the margin of the bones, closing the posterior angle between the tibia and fibula; it forms part of the articular surface for the posterior part of the trochlear surface of the talus.

A synovial-lined recess of the ankle joint cavity usually extends superiorly approximately 1 cm between the tibia and fibula, blocked superiorly by the distal end of the interosseous membrane. Occasionally, the articular cartilage on the distal ends of the tibia and fibula extends superiorly for a short distance on the walls of the recess.

The blood supply to the joint is from the fibular/peroneal and anterior tibial arteries. The nerve supply is by twigs from the deep fibular/peroneal and tibial nerves, with root value L4–S2.

Anterior to the inferior tibiofibular joint is the tendon of fibularis/peroneus tertius, with that of extensor digitorum longus lying medially together with the anterior tibial artery and deep fibular/peroneal nerve. Posteriorly, the tendons of fibularis/peroneus longus and brevis lie lateral to the joint, with brevis overlying it slightly.

The inferior tibiofibular joint provides a firm union between the tibia and fibula making a significant contribution to the integrity of the malleolar mortise of the ankle joint. The fibrous tissue of the joint allows slight movement of the bones accommodating the talus in movements of the ankle joint. In radiographs centred on the ankle, the fibula shadow encroaches upon the anterior border of the fibular notch (Fig. 3.110A); if distance YZ is greater than XY, then there is diastasis of the ankle joint.

Interosseous Membrane

Often regarded as a form of fibrous joint uniting the tibia and fibula, the interosseous membrane is stretched

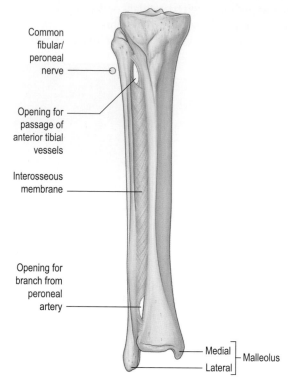

Common fibular/peroneal nerve

Opening for passage of anterior tibial vessels

Interosseous membrane

Opening for branch from peroneal artery

Medial — Lateral } Malleolus

Fig. 3.111 Anterior aspect of the right tibia and fibula showing the interosseous membrane.

tightly between the interosseous borders of the two bones; it predominantly consists of fibres passing inferolaterally from the tibia to fibula (Fig. 3.111). The proximal margin of the membrane does not reach as far as the superior tibiofibular joint allowing the anterior tibial vessels to gain access to the anterior compartment of the leg/calf. The membrane is, however, continuous inferiorly with the interosseous ligament of the inferior tibiofibular joint. Distally, there is a small opening for the passage of a branch from the fibular/peroneal artery.

The interosseous membrane separates muscles of the anterior and posterior compartments of the leg/calf, as well as giving attachment to some muscles of each group (Fig. 3.112).

Palpation

The head of the fibula can be palpated inferior to the posterior part of the lateral condyle of the tibia at approximately the same horizontal level as the tibial tuberosity;

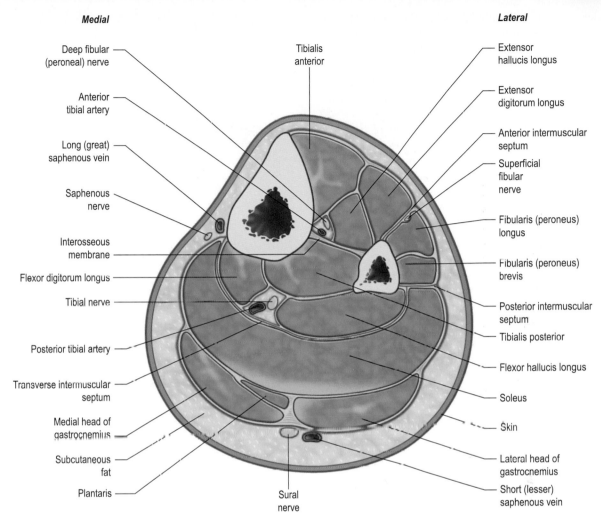

Fig. 3.112 Transverse section through the middle of the right leg/calf showing the relative positions of the tibia, fibula, interosseous membrane and muscles of the leg/calf.

the tendon of biceps femoris can be felt and seen passing to its attachment on the head of the fibula. Immediately inferior to the head is the narrower neck, around which passes laterally the common fibular (peroneal) nerve (Fig. 3.111).

In the region of the ankle, both malleoli can be palpated, the lateral extending further distally and lying more posterior than the medial. Various tendons pass behind both malleoli on their way to the foot; passing anterior to the ankle joint to the dorsum of the foot are the extensor tendons. All tendons are enclosed within synovial sheaths and bound down by thickenings of the deep fascia (retinaculae).

MOVEMENTS OF THE FIBULA

Plantarflexion and dorsiflexion of the foot at the ankle joint automatically cause passive movements at both tibiofibular joints; although the magnitude of these movements is small, they are real.

In dorsiflexion, the broader anterior part of the trochlear surface of the talus is forced into the narrower posterior part of the tibiofibular socket, causing separation of the tibia and fibula, increasing tension in the interosseous and transverse tibiofibular ligaments; the talus is held securely between the two malleoli. In plantarflexion the narrower part of the talus moves into the broader part of the tibiofibular socket; the malleoli come together again retaining their grip on the talus; however, in full plantarflexion, some side-to-side movement can be demonstrated. The grip of the malleoli on the talus is a function of the inferior tibiofibular joint, the strong ligaments of which provide the spring mechanism involved.

The moving apart and coming together of the two malleoli during ankle movements impart a complex movement to the fibula, partly guided by the shape and orientation of the lateral surface of the talus and partly by tension developed in various ligaments associated with the inferior tibiofibular joint. When the malleoli are separated, as in dorsiflexion of the foot at the ankle joint, both the anterior and posterior tibiofibular ligaments are put under tension; because their fibres run inferolaterally there is a tendency for the fibula to be lifted superiorly in an attempt to maintain the integrity of the ligaments. There are no bony constraints to this movement as the lateral articular surface of the talus is convex anteroposteriorly and concave superoinferiorly. At the same time as the lateral malleolus is moving superolaterally, the fibula undergoes a small degree of axial rotation (Fig. 3.113A). The direction of rotation depends upon the shape of the lateral talar surface; if it is convex anteroposteriorly, there is slight medial rotation and if plane slight lateral rotation of the fibula occurs.

With plantarflexion of the foot at the ankle joint, the two malleoli come together again, partly because of tension developed in the anterior, posterior and interosseous tibiofibular ligaments, but also under the action of tibialis posterior, especially in full plantarflexion. As the lateral malleolus moves medially, it also moves inferiorly with the fibula undergoing axial rotation in the opposite direction to that experienced in dorsiflexion (Fig. 3.113B).

Movement of the fibula at the inferior tibiofibular joint is transmitted to the synovial superior tibiofibular joint, which has plane articular surfaces and offers no resistance to movement.

Accessory Movements

Superior tibiofibular joint. An anteroposterior gliding of the fibula on the tibia can be produced by pressure in the appropriate direction when the head of the fibula is gripped between thumb and index finger.

Inferior tibiofibular joint. Accessory movements are difficult to produce at the inferior tibiofibular joint, but a slight anteroposterior movement can be felt if the lateral malleolus is gripped between thumb and index finger and pressed anteriorly then posteriorly.

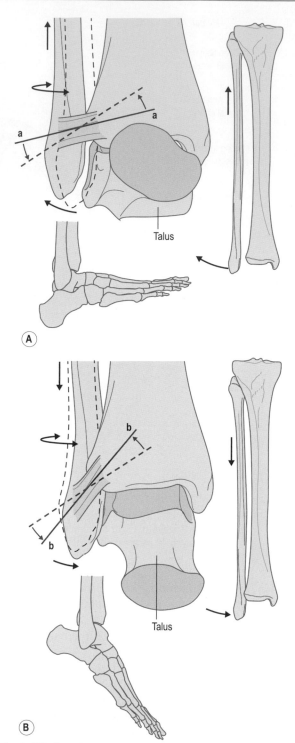

Fig. 3.113 Anterior aspect of the right tibia, fibula and talus showing movements of the fibula during (A) dorsiflexion and (B) plantarflexion of the foot at the ankle joint. Red arrows indicate movement of the fibula. Changes in the direction of fibres in the tibiofibular and interosseous ligaments from the neutral position in either full dorsiflexion (aa) or full plantarflexion (bb).

SECTION SUMMARY

Tibia

- Medial bone of leg/calf having proximal expanded end (tibial condyles); shaft with tibial tuberosity anteriorly and sharp, lateral facing interosseous border; slightly expanded distal end with medial malleolus.
- Proximally, the medial and lateral tibial condyles articulate with the medial and lateral femoral condyles forming the knee joint; the facet inferior to the lateral condyle articulates with the head of the fibula forming the superior tibiofibular joint.
- Distally articulates with the fibula forming the inferior tibiofibular joint; the talus forming part of the ankle.

Fibula

- Lateral bone of leg/calf having proximal head; irregular shaft with sharp medial facing interosseous border; expanded distal end with lateral malleolus projecting inferiorly.

- Articulates with the tibia superiorly and inferiorly forming the superior and inferior tibiofibular joints; the talus inferiorly forming part of the ankle joint.

Tibiofibular Articulations

Superior Tibiofibular Joint

Type	Synovial plane joint
Articular surfaces	Head of fibula with inferior surface lateral tibial condyle
Capsule	Attaches to articular margins
Ligaments	Anterior and posterior
Interosseous membrane	Attaches to the interosseous borders of tibia and fibula

Inferior Tibiofibular Joint

Type	Syndesmosis
Articular surfaces	Distal ends of fibula and tibia
Ligaments	Interosseous; anterior, posterior and transverse tibiofibular
Movements	Slight accessory rotation accompanying movement at ankle joint

❓ SELF-ASSESSMENT QUESTIONS

61. What type of joint is the inferior tibiofibular joint?
62. Where are the articular surfaces of the superior tibiofibular joint?
63. In which direction do the majority of fibres of the interosseous membrane run?
64. What happens to the distal end of the fibula during dorsiflexion of the foot at the ankle joint?
65. Which ligaments are associated with the inferior tibiofibular joint?
66. Which structure passes around the lateral aspect of the neck of the fibula?
67. Which vessels pass through the opening in the superior part of the interosseous membrane?
68. Does the fibula lie medial or lateral to the tibia in the leg/calf?
69. Which bone of the leg/calf bears the majority of the weight transmitted to the talus?
70. In which direction do fibres in the posterior tibiofibular ligament run?

ANKLE

LEARNING OUTCOMES

By the end of the section, you should be able to:
1. Identify, palpate and examine the talus and distal ends of the tibia and fibula
2. Describe the bones forming the ankle joint
3. Describe the retinaculae associated with the ankle joint, including their attachments, function and structures passing through or deep to them
4. Describe and explain the movements possible, and their restraints, at the ankle joint
5. Locate, palpate and examine the muscles moving the foot at the ankle joint and know their attachments, action and innervation
6. Examine and assess movements of the ankle joint
7. Appreciate the influence of pathology and/or trauma on the function of the ankle joint

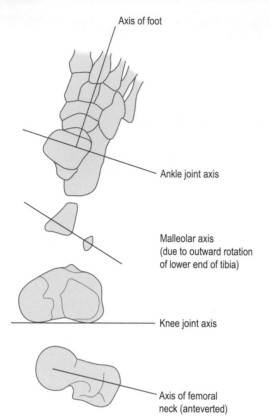

Fig. 3.114 Relationship between the ankle joint, malleolar, knee joint and femoral neck axes of the right lower limb.

INTRODUCTION

A synovial hinge joint with one degree of freedom of movement allowing only plantarflexion (flexion) and dorsiflexion (extension). The anterior and posterior fluctuation of the line of gravity in erect standing falls anterior to the joint; it is regulated at the ankle to keep it within the limits of the supporting surface. The ankle joint has the appearance of a mortise and tenon, with the boxlike mortise formed by the distal ends of the tibia and fibula, and the tenon by the body of the talus (Fig. 3.110A).

In the anatomical position, the ankle joint axis lies in a horizontal plane but is set obliquely to the coronal plane 20–25 degrees so that it passes posterolaterally (Fig. 3.114). Although both the knee and ankle joint axes lie in a horizontal plane, simultaneous movement at both joints can only be achieved if movement is allowed at other joints to compensate for the obliquity of the ankle joint axis; this compensation is essentially provided at the subtalar joint. Movement of the foot at the ankle

joint is rarely performed alone, it is usually combined with movements at the subtalar and midtarsal joints so that plantarflexion is associated with adduction and supination of the foot, and dorsiflexion with abduction and pronation of the foot. The combined movements at the subtalar and midtarsal joints are usually referred to as inversion and eversion of the foot, respectively.

The ankle and foot provide the restraint and propulsion at each step during locomotion so that equilibrium is maintained while the body is in motion. To achieve this, there have been changes in some tarsal bones and the establishment of interrelated articulations. A single joint (ankle joint) has been established between the leg/calf and foot controlling the foot in the sagittal plane; it is responsible for adjusting the line of gravity during standing and providing the propulsion and restraint required during gait. A second articulation (subtalar joint: p. 412) has been established between the talus and calcaneus. Lastly, a joint (midtarsal joint: p. 418) has been established interrupting the structure of the foot in the middle of the tarsus.

This series of joints, assisted by axial rotation at the knee, is equivalent to a single joint with three degrees of freedom of movement allowing the foot to take up any position in space and adapt to any irregularities in the supporting surface during walking. However, unlike a single joint, these separate articulations provide a high degree of stability without sacrificing mobility.

Deep Fascia Around the Ankle
Retinaculae

Around the ankle the deep fascia is thickened by transversely orientated bands forming retinaculae serving to hold the tendons passing across the ankle joint in position and preventing bowstringing; they are named according to the tendons they restrain (flexor, extensor, fibular/peroneal).

The flexor retinaculum passes from the posterior aspect of the medial malleolus to the medial tubercle of the calcaneus. From its deep surface, septa pass to the tibia and ankle joint capsule forming four compartments; from medial to lateral, these compartments transmit the tendons of tibialis posterior, flexor digitorum longus, the posterior tibial vessels and tibial nerve, and the tendon of flexor hallucis longus, with each tendon enclosed in its own synovial sheath.

The extensor retinaculae are the most extensive. The superior extensor retinaculum (Fig. 3.115) runs

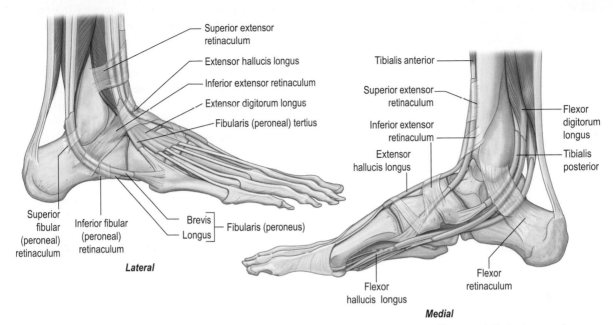

Superior extensor retinaculum
Extensor hallucis longus
Inferior extensor retinaculum
Extensor digitorum longus
Fibularis (peroneal) tertius

Tibialis anterior
Superior extensor retinaculum
Inferior extensor retinaculum
Extensor hallucis longus

Flexor digitorum longus
Tibialis posterior

Superior fibular (peroneal) retinaculum
Inferior fibular (peroneal) retinaculum
Brevis
Longus
Fibularis (peroneus)

Lateral

Flexor hallucis longus
Flexor retinaculum

Medial

Fig. 3.115 Lateral and medial relations of the ankle joint showing the extensor, flexor and fibular/peroneal retinaculae.

horizontally across all the extensor tendons between the tibia and fibula just superior to the ankle joint. The inferior extensor retinaculum is a Y-shaped thickening on the dorsum of the foot (Fig. 3.115): the stem attaches to the superior surface of the calcaneus anteriorly and floor of the sinus tarsi, with the upper band passing to the medial malleolus and lower band blending with the deep fascia on the medial side of the foot. The lower band splits into superficial and deep layers with a septum passing between them, forming two compartments. In the most medial compartment is the tendon of tibialis anterior with that of extensor hallucis longus in the other; each tendon is enclosed within its own synovial sheath. Passing deep to the stem laterally are the tendons of extensor digitorum longus and fibularis/peroneus tertius in a common synovial sheath. The tendons of the tibialis anterior and extensor hallucis longus usually pass deep to the upper band, each in its own synovial sheath, although tibialis anterior may pierce it. The anterior tibial vessels and deep fibular/peroneal nerve pass deep to both extensor retinaculae.

The fibular/peroneal retinaculae are also in two parts (Fig. 3.115). The superior attaches to the lateral side of the calcaneus passing over the tendons of fibularis/peroneus longus and brevis to the posterior border of the

lateral malleolus; the two tendons are enclosed within a single synovial sheath. The inferior retinaculum binds the two fibular/peroneal tendons to the lateral side of the calcaneus. A septum passing from its deep surface to the fibular/peroneal tubercle forms two separate compartments, one above the tubercle for the tendon of fibularis/peroneus brevis and one below for that of fibularis/peroneus longus; at this point, each tendon is enclosed in its own synovial sheath.

Synovial Sheaths

As the various tendons pass deep to the retinaculae, they are invaginated from the lateral side into a double layer of synovial membrane lining the compartments formed, protruding approximately 1 cm above each retinaculum. The sheath of tibialis posterior continues to its attachment, while those of the tendons of flexors digitorum longus and hallucis longus continue as far as the base of the metatarsals.

Laterally, the tendons of fibularis/peroneus longus and brevis initially share the same sheath, after passing around the lateral malleolus they occupy separate compartments, each lined by a separate synovial sheath continuing as far as the lateral side of the cuboid. Fibularis/peroneus longus is surrounded by another synovial sheath as it passes through a fibrous tunnel formed on the plantar surface of the cuboid.

Anteriorly, both tibialis anterior and extensor hallucis longus are surrounded by separate synovial sheaths; the former reaches almost to the attachment of the tendon, while the latter passes as far as the mid-metatarsal region. The tendons of extensor digitorum longus and fibularis/peroneus tertius share the same sheath; it is only present as the tendons pass deep to the extensor retinacula (Fig. 3.115).

The sheaths facilitate sliding of the tendons deep to the retinaculae and normally are not evident; when damaged (trauma, infection, overactivity) they become inflamed and swollen presenting as a 'sausage-like' swelling along the length of the sheath around the tendon; this is often acutely painful and incapacitating. The condition is referred to as tenosynovitis and can occur around any tendon surrounded by a synovial sheath. It is one of the conditions commonly labelled repetitive strain injury (RSI) and may occur anywhere in the body where tendons pass through sheaths in confined spaces.

TIBIA AND FIBULA

Details of the tibia and fibula can be found on pages 322 and 325, respectively.

TALUS

Transmitting body weight from the tibia to the calcaneus and navicular, the talus (Figs 3.116, 3.131, 3.133 and 3.135B) has a head and neck directed anteromedially. The body is wedge-shaped from anterior to posterior, being wider anteriorly, lying between the malleoli of the tibia and fibula. Its superior surface is convex from anterior to posterior and slightly concave (pulley-shaped) from side-to-side articulating with the trochlear surface of the tibia. The lateral surface is triangular with its apex pointing inferiorly and articulates with the medial surface of the lateral malleolus. The medial surface is partly articular; the superior articular part is comma shaped. The medial and lateral articular surfaces are continuous with the superior surface of the talus. Below the medial articular surface is a depressed roughened area for attachment of the deep part of the deltoid ligament. The inferior surface of the body is also articular, concave from anterior to posterior, articulating with the posterior facet on the superior surface of the calcaneus.

On its posterior aspect is a groove running inferomedially for the tendon of flexor hallucis longus; lateral and medial to the groove are the lateral and medial talar tubercles.

From the anteromedial aspect of the body, the neck projects anteromedially; its superior, medial and lateral surfaces are roughened, and its inferior surface has an area for articulation with the calcaneus on the superior surface of the sustentaculum tali. Posterior to this articular surface is a deep groove (sulcus tali) lying immediately superior to the sulcus calcanei forming the sinus tarsi.

The head of the talus is slightly flattened anteriorly articulating with the posterior surface of the navicular. Below this main articulation are two smaller articular areas, one for the superior surface of the plantar calcaneonavicular ('spring') ligament (p. 415) and the other, continuing onto the inferior surface of the neck, for the anterior articular area of the calcaneus.

ANKLE JOINT

Articular Surfaces

These are at the distal ends of the tibia and fibula proximally and body of the talus distally; the stabilising surfaces are those of the medial and lateral malleoli gripping the body of the talus. The weight-bearing surfaces are the trochlear surfaces of the tibia and talus.

Tibia

The distal end of the tibia provides a continuous articular surface receiving the trochlear surface and medial edge of the body of the talus (Fig. 3.116). The trochlear surface is concave anteroposteriorly and slightly convex transversely, with a blunt sagittal ridge fitting into a corresponding groove on the talus; it is slightly wider anteriorly than posteriorly. On either side of the ridge are medial and lateral gutters for the corresponding lips of the talar trochlear surface. The posterior part of this surface projects slightly inferiorly; it is occasionally known as the posterior malleolus.

The cartilage on the trochlear surface of the tibia is continuous medially with that on the lateral surface of the medial malleolus; the junction is a rounded angle.

Fibula

The medial surface of the lateral malleolus of the fibula forms the lateral surface of the mortise of the joint. The

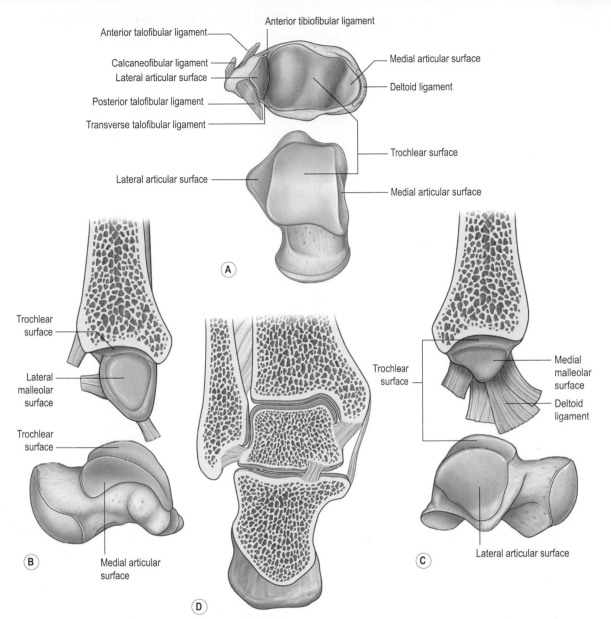

Fig. 3.116 Articular surfaces of the ankle joint. (A) Trochlear surfaces of the tibia and talus. (B) Medial and (C) lateral aspects. (D) Coronal section.

articular surface is approximately triangular with the inferior apex slightly convex (Fig. 3.116). The base of the triangle extends superiorly as far as the tibial articular surface, with the joint cavity extending between the two bones. In the angle between the lateral malleolus and trochlear surface of the tibia is a narrow cleft distal to the interosseous ligament; it disappears posteriorly being filled by the transverse tibiofibular ligament.

Talus

The body of the talus forms the whole of the distal surface of the ankle joint, articulating superiorly and medially with the tibia and laterally with the fibula (Fig. 3.116). The trochlear surface is convex anteroposteriorly with a central longitudinal groove bound by medial and lateral lips; it is slightly broader anteriorly than posteriorly. The groove and lips make the trochlear surface slightly concave transversely. The cartilage covering the trochlear surface is continuous with that on the sides of the body.

The medial surface is nearly plane, except anteriorly where it inclines medially, and can be likened to a comma placed on its side with the tail pointing posteriorly; it lies in a parasagittal plane articulating with the lateral surface of the medial malleolus. The lateral articular surface runs obliquely anterolaterally; it is concave superoinferiorly and anteroposteriorly. The lateral surface is triangular and much larger than the medial, curving inferiorly to a laterally projecting apex. It articulates with the medial surface of the lateral malleolus and deep surface of the transverse tibiofibular ligament posterosuperiorly at the angle between the trochlear and lateral surfaces. The interval between the tibia, fibula and transverse tibiofibular ligament posteriorly is padded by a synovial fold.

Palpation

The anterior and posterior borders, as well as the tips, of both malleoli can be readily palpated. The two malleoli are, however, basically different. The lateral malleolus is larger, extends further distally and lies more posteriorly than the medial. The fibularis/peroneal tendons can be palpated posterior to the lateral malleolus (Figs 3.115 and 3.120) and those of tibialis posterior and flexor digitorum longus posterior to the medial malleolus (Figs 3.115 and 3.120). All tendons crossing anterior to the joint can be identified and palpated.

Pulsations of the anterior tibial artery can be felt between the tendons of extensor hallucis longus and extensor digitorum, while those of the posterior tibial artery can be felt posterior to the medial malleolus posterior to the tendon of flexor digitorum longus.

The ankle joint, which lies horizontally 1 cm above the tip of the medial malleolus and 2 cm above the tip of the lateral malleolus, can be palpated on the dorsal surface. Starting medially, the joint can be identified by applying firm pressure along the lateral border of the medial malleolus. If the extensor tendons are moved aside, the distal end of the tibia can be palpated, as well as the medial edge of the lateral malleolus.

Joint Capsule and Synovial Membrane

A fibrous capsule completely surrounds the joint, attaching superiorly to the articular margins of the tibia and fibula, and inferiorly to just outside the edges of the corresponding articular areas of the talus, except anteriorly where it attaches to the neck of the talus. The capsule is thin and weak anteriorly and posteriorly to accommodate plantarflexion and dorsiflexion, but it is strengthened laterally and medially by collateral ligaments. Posteriorly, the capsule is attached to the posterior tibiofibular ligament.

The synovial membrane lining the joint capsule is loose and capacious; it is reflected anteriorly onto the neck of the talus before attaching to the articular margins and covers well-marked fatty pads lying in relation to its anterior and posterior parts. The synovial membrane extends superiorly between the tibia and fibula as far as the interosseous ligament of the inferior tibiofibular joint; it may be partly covered by an extension of the articular cartilage on the tibia and fibula.

Ligaments

As with all hinge joints, there is an extremely strong set of collateral ligaments associated with the ankle joint; medially is the deltoid ligament and laterally three separate ligaments. Each set of ligaments radiate inferiorly from the respective malleolus; both have a middle band attached to the calcaneus, and anterior and posterior bands attached to the talus. The deltoid and anterior and posterior lateral ligaments blend with the ankle joint capsule.

Deltoid Ligament

Strong, roughly triangular ligament composed of several bands of fibres fused together; the various bands are differentiated by their distal attachments (Fig. 3.117A). It can be considered as having deep and superficial parts attaching by its apex to the anterior and posterior borders and fossa at the tip of the medial malleolus. The thick base forms a continuous attachment from the navicular anteriorly to the body of the talus posteriorly.

The deeper parts of the ligament are the anterior and posterior tibiotalar bands. The anterior band is the most anterior, running obliquely anteroinferiorly to attach to the medial part of the neck of the talus. The posterior band is the most posterior and thickest part; its fibres run posterolaterally to the medial side of the talus under the tail of the comma-shaped articular facet and the medial tubercle of its posterior process.

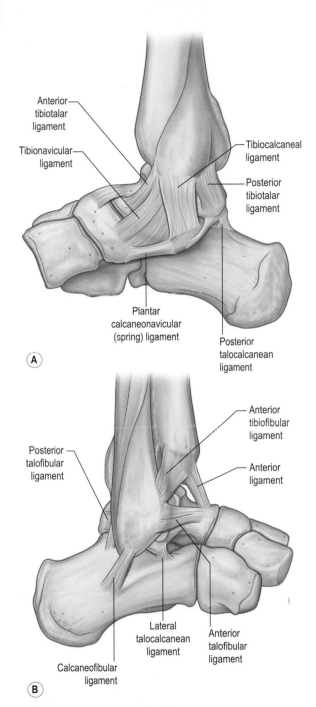

The more superficial parts have a continuous attachment from the navicular to the sustentaculum tali of the calcaneus (p. 408), partly overlying the anterior tibiotalar band. The tibionavicular band runs anteroinferiorly towards the tuberosity on the navicular attaching to its superior and medial parts (p. 409). Continuing posteriorly, this band blends inferiorly with the superior medial border of the plantar calcaneonavicular ('spring') ligament (p. 415). It is succeeded by the tibiocalcaneal band whose fibres pass almost vertically to attach to the whole length of the sustentaculum tali.

Lateral Ligaments

The lateral collateral ligament consists of three separate parts: anterior and posterior talofibular, and calcaneofibular ligaments (Fig. 3.117B). These separate ligaments are not as strong as the deltoid ligament, as evidenced by the fact that most ankle sprains involve the lateral ligaments. The anterior talofibular ligament is a flat band stretching between the anterior border and tip of the lateral malleolus to the neck of the talus; its fibres run anteromedially. The posterior talofibular ligament is a strong thick ligament running almost horizontally, arising from the malleolar fossa of the lateral malleolus, passing posteromedially to the lateral tubercle of the posterior process of the talus. Superior to it lies the posterior tibiofibular ligament. In plantarflexion, the two ligaments lie edge-to-edge, while in dorsiflexion they diverge medially.

Between the two talofibular ligaments is the narrow, rounded cord of the calcaneofibular ligament; although it is free from the fibrous capsule, its superior part fuses with the talofibular ligaments. It arises from the anterior aspect and tip of the lateral malleolus, passing inferiorly and slightly posteriorly, attaching superior and posterior to the fibular/peroneal tubercle on the middle of the lateral calcaneal surface.

Role of the collateral ligaments. Laxity of the ankle joint is dependent on its position, with full dorsiflexion being the position of least laxity, reflecting talar geometry and the inferior tibiofibular syndesmosis. The collateral ligaments are primarily responsible for maintaining its stability and controlling its movements. Damage to some or all of the collateral ligaments seriously impairs the integrity of the joint (Fig. 3.118).

Fig. 3.117 (A) Medial and (B) lateral aspects of the right tibia, fibular, talus and calcaneus showing the position and attachments of the medial (deltoid) and lateral collateral ligaments of the ankle joint.

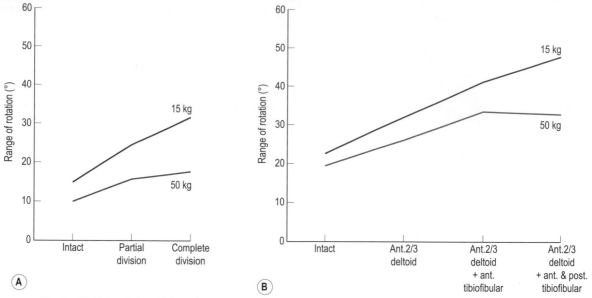

Fig. 3.118 Role of the (A) lateral and (B) medial collateral ligaments in providing rotational stability of the ankle joint. (Adapted from McCullough, C.J., Burge, P.D., 1980. Rotatory stability of the load-bearing ankle. An experimental study. J. Bone Joint Surg. 62B, 460–464.)

Sectioning the lateral ligaments is associated with an increased range of dorsiflexion, but not plantarflexion, as well as increased internal rotation of the talus, particularly when the ankle is plantarflexed. Only when all collateral ligaments have been severed is an increase in external talar rotation observed, being more marked in dorsiflexion. Talar tilt also increases with gradually increasing injury. Before complete severing of all collateral ligaments, talar tilt is maximum in plantarflexion, but after total ligament disruption, it is most marked in dorsiflexion.

The role of the various parts of the collateral ligaments in maintaining stability can be summarised as follows:

- The tibiocalcaneal and tibionavicular bands limit and control abduction of the talus
- The calcaneofibular ligament limits and controls adduction.
- The anterior tibiotalar band and anterior talofibular ligament limit and control plantarflexion.
- The posterior tibiotalar band and posterior talofibular ligament limit and control dorsiflexion.
- In combination, both the anterior tibiotalar and tibionavicular bands limit control external (lateral) rotation of the talus (Fig. 3.118).

- The anterior talofibular ligament limits and controls internal (medial) rotation of the talus (Fig. 3.118).
- In isolation, neither the anterior nor the posterior tibiotalar ligaments appear to play any major role in ankle stability.

From the above it appears that the anterior talofibular ligament is an extremely important structure, probably being the primary stabiliser of the ankle joint, and providing significant resistance to varus talar tilt in all positions of plantarflexion.

Apart from the pain involved in an ankle sprain, the accompanying instability is probably due to involvement of the anterior talofibular ligament; most sprains are due to turning the ankle outwards (foot inwards) with an associated straining of the lateral ligaments (inversion stress).

Anterior and Posterior Ligaments

Localised thickenings of the joint capsule (Fig. 3.119). The anterior ligament runs obliquely from the anterior margin of the distal end of the tibia to the superior surface of the anterior aspect of the neck of the talus. The posterior ligament has fibres arising from both the tibia and fibula converging to attach to the medial tubercle of the posterior surface of the talus.

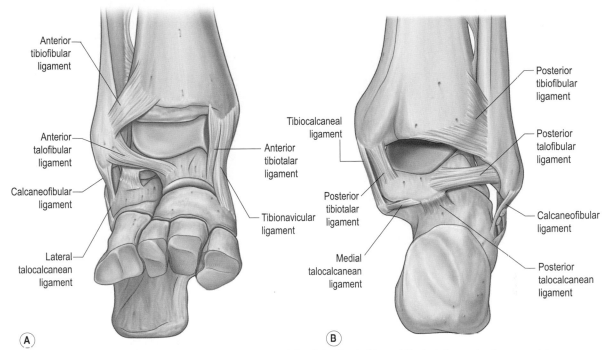

Fig. 3.119 (A) Anterior and (B) posterior aspects of the right distal tibia and fibula, talus and calcaneus showing thickenings of the ankle joint capsule (capsule removed).

Blood Supply, Lymphatic Drainage and Innervation

The blood supply of the joint is from the malleolar branches of the anterior tibial, fibular/peroneal and posterior tibial arteries forming an anastomosis around the malleoli. Venous drainage is by corresponding venae comitantes accompanying the arteries. The lymphatics drain into the deep system of vessels, again accompanying the arteries.

The nerve supply to the joint is from roots L4–S2 by articular branches from the tibial nerve and lateral branch of the deep fibular/peroneal nerve.

Relations

All of the muscles, vessels and nerves entering the foot cross the ankle joint. Anteriorly, from medial to lateral, are the tendons of tibialis anterior, extensor hallucis longus, extensor digitorum longus and fibularis/peroneus tertius as they pass through the inferior extensor retinaculum (Figs 3.115 and 3.120). The first two tendons lie within separate compartments surrounded by their own synovial sheaths, while the latter two share a compartment and synovial sheath. Deep to the extensor retinaculum behind the middle compartment, the anterior tibial artery passes (becoming the dorsalis pedis artery at the inferior border of the retinaculum) and deep fibular/peroneal nerve. Anterior to the extensor retinaculum is the superficial fibular/peroneal nerve, while anterior to the medial malleolus is the long (great) saphenous vein arising from the medial side of the dorsal venous plexus and the saphenous branch of the femoral nerve (Fig. 3.120).

Posterior to the medial malleolus and bound down by the flexor retinaculum are, from anteromedial to posterolateral, the tendons of tibialis posterior and flexor digitorum longus, the posterior tibial artery, tibial nerve and tendon of flexor hallucis longus (Figs 3.115 and 3.120). The latter tendon passes in a groove on the posterior aspect of the talus between the medial and lateral tubercles and enters the foot by passing inferior to the sustentaculum tali. As they pass posterior to the medial malleolus, the posterior tibial artery and tibial nerve divide into their terminal medial and lateral plantar branches. All tendons are surrounded by individual synovial sheaths.

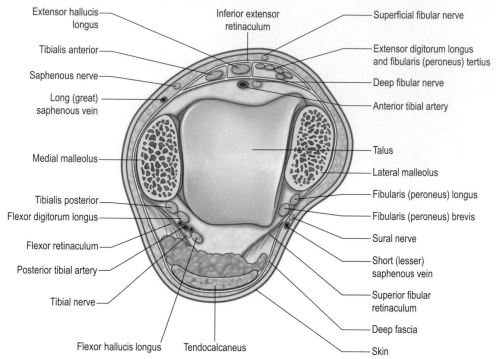

Fig. 3.120 Transverse section through the right ankle showing the relationship of structures crossing the joint.

The tendons of fibularis/peroneus longus (anterolateral) and fibularis/peroneus brevis (posteromedial) pass in a common synovial sheath posterior to the lateral malleolus, bound down by the superior fibular/peroneal retinaculum (Figs 3.115 and 3.120). Inferior to the level of the joint, the tendons diverge passing either side of the fibular/peroneal tubercle of the calcaneus (longus below, brevis above); at this point, each tendon is enclosed within its own synovial sheath. Posterior to the two tendons as they pass posterolateral to the ankle joint are the sural nerve and short (lesser) saphenous vein, which arises from the lateral side of the dorsal venous network.

Posterior to the joint, but separated from it by an extensive fat pad, is the tendocalcaneus (Achilles tendon) passing to attach to the posterior tubercle of the calcaneus.

Stability

Anteroposterior stability of the ankle joint and coaptation of its articular surfaces depend upon the effect of gravity keeping the distal tibia pressed against the superior surface of the talus. Due to its concave shape, the anterior and posterior margins of the tibial surface form bony spurs which help prevent the talus from escaping anteriorly or posteriorly, respectively. Provided that the joint is intact, the collateral ligaments are passively responsible for coaptation of the articular surfaces, being assisted by muscles crossing the joint. In a subluxed or dislocated joint, the ligaments and muscles may cause further joint distraction.

By virtue of its structure, the ankle joint should not exhibit movements other than plantarflexion and dorsiflexion; transverse stability depends on the interlocking of its articular surfaces (Fig. 3.121A). Provided the distance between the malleoli remains relatively unchanged they grip the talus on each side; this can only be achieved when the malleoli and ligaments of the inferior tibiofibular joint are intact. Furthermore, the collateral ligaments prevent rolling movements of the talus about its long axis.

When the foot is forcibly moved laterally (violent abduction) the lateral surface of the talus knocks against the lateral malleolus. The sequence of events which follow depends on the severity of the movement, state of the bone and integrity of the various ligaments of the

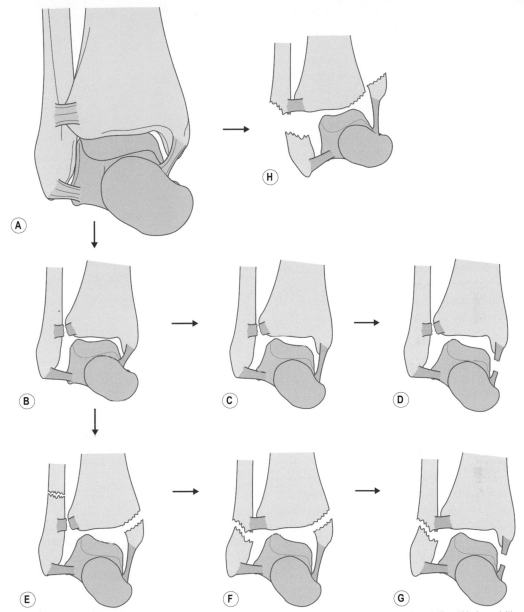

Fig. 3.121 Anterior aspect of the distal right tibia, fibula and talus showing the normal stability (A), instability due to ligament rupture (B)–(D) and combined ligament rupture and malleolar fracture (E)–(H).

joint. After rupture of the inferior tibiofibular ligaments the grip of the malleoli on the talus is disrupted, leading to a widening of the mortise (diastasis of the ankle). The talus is no longer held tightly and can move from side to side (rattling of the talus) (Fig. 3.121B and C). It is also able to rotate about its long axis (tilting of the talus), made easier if the deltoid ligament is disrupted

(Fig. 3.121D), and rotate about its vertical axis so that the posterior part of the talar body abuts against the posterior margin of the tibia, possibly fracturing it. If abduction continues, both the medial and lateral malleoli may become fractured, the lateral superior to the inferior tibiofibular joint (Fig. 3.121E), one form of Pott's fracture. Occasionally, the lateral malleolus does not fracture, instead, fibular fracture occurs at the level of the neck.

Both inferior tibiofibular ligaments do not always rupture, often the anterior tibiofibular ligament resists tearing; there may still be fracture of both malleoli, with the lateral malleolus fracturing through the inferior tibiofibular joint (Fig. 3.121F), another form of Pott's fracture. Instead of the medial malleolus fracturing, the deltoid ligament may be ruptured; again the lateral malleolus fractures through the inferior tibiofibular joint (Fig. 3.121G).

In all fractures, a chip of bone is often broken off the posterior margin of the tibia, which can present as a separate fragment of bone or form a single unit with the malleolar fragment.

In violent adduction of the foot, the talus is forced to rotate about its vertical axis fracturing both malleoli, the lateral inferior to the inferior tibiofibular joint. In these bimalleolar adduction fractures the inferior tibiofibular joint and both collateral ligaments remain intact (Fig. 3.121H).

Clearly, these lesions require proper treatment if full structural and functional integrity of the ankle joint is to be restored. If the bony and soft tissue damage is excessive, then joint fusion may be the only practical way of restoring stability.

MOVEMENTS OF THE FOOT AT THE ANKLE JOINT

The only movements possible at the ankle joint are plantarflexion (flexion) and dorsiflexion (extension) about a transverse axis level with the tip of the lateral malleolus and slightly inferior to the level of the medial malleolus. Strictly speaking, the axis is not horizontal but slopes slightly inferolaterally, passing through the lateral surface of the talus just inferior to the apex of the articular triangle and through the medial surface at a higher level just inferior to the concavity of the comma-shaped articular area. The axis also changes slightly during movement because the superior surface of the talus is elliptical rather than being an arc of a circle; however, this change is of no practical significance. Because of the obliquity of the joint axis, there is slight movement resembling inversion on full plantarflexion and eversion on full dorsiflexion; these 'inversion/eversion' movements are not true inversion and eversion.

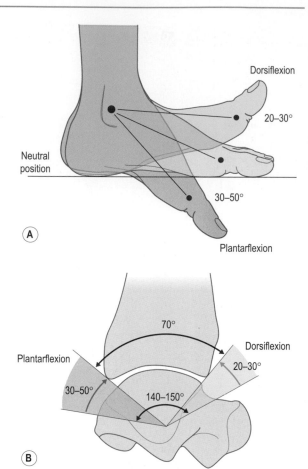

Fig. 3.122 (A) Range of dorsiflexion and plantarflexion at the ankle joint and (B) how these are determined by the profiles of the tibial and talar articular surfaces.

In normal standing, the foot makes a right angle with the leg; this is the neutral position of the joint (Fig. 3.122A). In dorsiflexion, the foot is drawn towards the anterior aspect of the leg/calf; plantarflexion is movement in the opposite direction from the neutral position. The ranges of dorsiflexion and plantarflexion are essentially determined by the profiles of the articular surfaces. Dorsiflexion has a maximum range of 30 degrees and plantarflexion of 50 degrees (Fig. 3.122B); however, Boone and Azen (1979) report a range of plantarflexion of 56 degrees. Neonates have 59 degree dorsiflexion and 26 degree plantarflexion (Waugh et al., 1983), while at age 2, the values are 41 and 26 degrees, respectively (Watanabe et al., 1979). With increasing age, the range of motion gradually decreases, with females having a greater range of both plantarflexion and dorsiflexion

TABLE 3.5 Range of Movement at the Ankle Joint Required for Various Activities

Activity	Maximum range required
Walking on a level surface	15° dorsiflexion, 30° plantarflexion
Ascending stairs	25° dorsiflexion, 30° plantarflexion
Descending stairs	35° dorsiflexion, 30° plantarflexion
Putting on shoes	25° plantarflexion
Tying shoe laces	15° dorsiflexion

than males (Bell and Hoshizaki, 1981; Walker et al., 1984). There is, however, considerable individual variation in the extent of these movements.

The ranges of ankle motion associated with some common everyday activities are given in Table 3.5.

In dorsiflexion, the broader anterior part of the trochlear surface of the talus is forced between the narrower posterior part of the tibiofibular mortise, causing slight separation of the tibia and fibula and increased tension in the interosseous and transverse tibiofibular ligaments; it is in this close-packed position that stability of the ankle joint is greatest. Movement of the fibula away from the tibia during dorsiflexion causes rotation about its long axis and superior movement (see tibiofibular joints, p. 379). Dorsiflexion is produced by tibialis anterior, extensors hallucis longus and digitorum longus and fibularis/peroneus tertius crossing the joint anteriorly. It is limited by tension in gastrocnemius and soleus, the posterior part of the deltoid ligament, the calcaneofibular ligament and posterior joint capsule, as well as wedging of the talus between the malleoli. Should dorsiflexion continue, the anterior margin of the tibia can come into contact with the superior surface of the neck of the talus; if sufficient force is behind the movement, the neck of the talus, the anterior tibial margin or both can be fractured. The anterior joint capsule is prevented from being trapped between the tibia and talus by the extensor muscles, whose sheaths attach to the capsule (Fig. 3.123A), pulling it superiorly.

Gastrocnemius and soleus shortening may check dorsiflexion prematurely, if shortening is severe the ankle may be permanently fixed in plantarflexion (talipes equinus); lengthening of the tendocalcaneus by surgical intervention may be required to restore full function.

In plantarflexion, the narrower posterior part of the trochlea of the talus moves anteriorly into the broader part of the tibiofibular mortise; the malleoli tend to come together again, retaining their grip upon the talus. In full plantarflexion, some rotation, abduction/adduction and side-to-side movement of the talus is possible; this is the position of least stability of the ankle joint. Approximation of the medial and lateral malleoli during plantarflexion is partly passive (recoil of the stretched interosseous and transverse tibiofibular ligaments) and partly active under the action of tibialis posterior attaching to both the tibia and fibula. The accessory movements of the fibula are the reverse of those seen during dorsiflexion (p. 379).

Plantarflexion is brought about mainly by soleus and gastrocnemius; however, all muscles entering the foot posterior to the malleoli produce plantarflexion (tibialis posterior, flexor digitorum longus, flexor hallucis longus, fibularii/peronei longus and brevis). Movement is checked by tension in the anterior muscles, anterior part of the deltoid ligament, the anterior talofibular ligament and anterior joint capsule. If these fail to arrest a forceful plantarflexion, the posterior margin of the tibia may come into contact with the tubercles on the posterior surface of the talus, especially the lateral; rarely does the posterior tubercle fracture. The posterior joint capsule avoids becoming trapped between the bones by the posterior talofibular ligament and its attachment to the sheath of flexor hallucis longus medially and fibularii/peronei laterally (Fig. 3.123B).

The wedge-shaped form of the joint surfaces helps prevent posterior displacement of the foot on the leg/calf when coming to a sudden stop in jumping or running. Maintenance of this positive grip on the talus is the function of the inferior tibiofibular joint.

When the body is erect, muscular effort (mainly soleus and gastrocnemius) is necessary to prevent forward collapse. The destabilising effect of gravity can be and usually is minimised by turning the feet out a little laterally so that the inclination between the two ankle joint axes is increased.

Accessory Movements

Two accessory movements are possible at the ankle joint. The first is a longitudinal distraction pulling the talus away from the tibia and malleoli; it is undertaken with the individual lying supine. The calcaneus at the heel and head of the talus on the dorsum of the foot are gripped and a longitudinal pull exerted along the line of the tibia.

The second movement is in an anteroposterior direction undertaken with the individual lying supine. The knee is flexed to 90 degrees, keeping the sole of the foot firmly pressed against the table and the ankle joint partly plantarflexed. Gripping the distal ends of the tibia

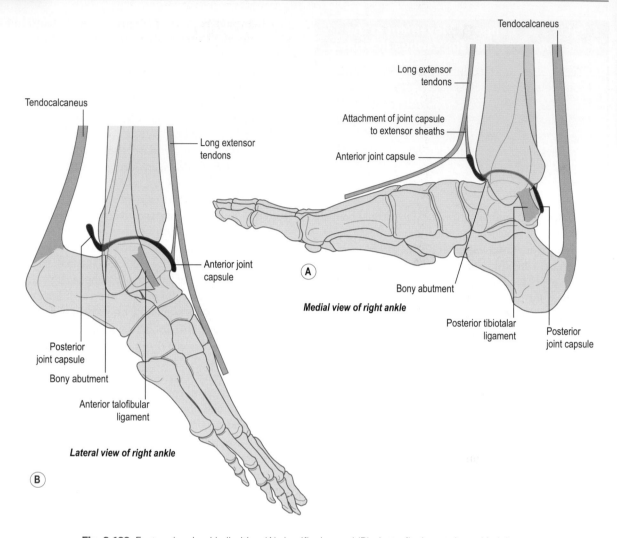

Fig. 3.123 Factors involved in limiting (A) dorsiflexion and (B) plantarflexion at the ankle joint.

and fibula, they can be moved anteriorly and posteriorly by applying pressure in the appropriate direction.

Muscles crossing the ankle joint and producing movement are shown in Table 3.6. Further details of each muscle can be found in following sections.

BIOMECHANICS

Although the total range of ankle joint motion approaches 80 degrees, a much smaller range is used during gait (Table 3.5); however, with the increasing speed of walking, ankle joint motion decreases, being mainly a decrease in plantarflexion (Fig. 3.124).

At heel-strike, the ankle is slightly plantarflexed, immediately after which plantarflexion increases and then decreases when full foot contact is made with the supporting surface. As the body moves over the supporting foot, the ankle goes into dorsiflexion, reaching a maximum just prior to the heel leaving the ground, after which it decreases again; just before toe-off the ankle once again plantarflexes. During the swing phase, there is a second wave of dorsiflexion which, together with a second wave of knee flexion, ensures clearance of the toes with the ground. Towards the end of the swing phase, the ankle becomes plantarflexed before heel-strike. Not only does increasing cadence decrease the range of motion during the stance phase, it also brings

TABLE 3.6   Muscles Crossing and Producing Movement at the Ankle Joint

Muscle	Attachments	Action	Innervation (root value)
Tibialis anterior	Proximal 2/3rd of lateral surface of tibia and adjacent interosseous membrane to medial side of medial cuneiform and base of 1st metatarsal	Dorsiflexor of foot at ankle joint; with tibialis posterior it inverts foot at subtalar and midtarsal joints	Deep fibular (peroneal) nerve (L4, L5)
Fibularis/peroneus tertius	Anterior aspect of distal 1/4 of fibula to medial and dorsal aspects of base of 5th metatarsal	Weak dorsiflexor and evertor of foot at ankle joint	Deep fibular (peroneal) nerve (L5, S1)
Gastrocnemius	Medial supracondylar ridge, adductor tubercle, popliteal surface of femur (medial head) and lateral surface of lateral femoral condyle (lateral head) to posterior surface of calcaneus via tendocalcaneus (Achilles tendon)	Plantarflexor of foot at ankle joint; powerful flexor of the leg/calf at knee joint	Tibial nerve (S1, S2)
Soleus	Posterior surfaces of tibia and proximal 1/3rd of fibula to posterior surface of calcaneus via tendocalcaneus (Achilles tendon)	Plantarflexor of foot at ankle joint	Tibial nerve (S1, S2)
Plantaris	Lateral supracondylar ridge, popliteal surface of tibia and knee joint capsule to posterior surface of calcaneus	Weak plantarflexor of foot at ankle joint; weak flexor of the leg/calf at knee joint	Tibial nerve (S1, S2)
Tibialis posterior	Proximal 1/2 of posterior surface of tibia inferior to soleal line, interosseous membrane and posterior surface of fibula to medial side of navicular and plantar surfaces of all tarsal bones	Aids plantarflexion of foot at ankle joint; main evertor of foot at subtalar and midtarsal joints	Tibial nerve (L4, L5)

forward peak dorsiflexion before the heel leaves the ground (Fig. 3.124).

Joint Forces

During the gait cycle, both tangential shear forces and compressive forces act across the ankle joint. Tangential shear forces are in an anteroposterior direction, being the result of a combination of internal musculotendinous forces and external forces as the body moves over the foot. The force is biphasic being mainly directed posteriorly during the stance phase, reaching 80% body weight as the heel leaves the ground (Fig. 3.125). During the last 15% of the stance phase, as the ankle goes into plantarflexion, the shear force is directed anteriorly reaching 20% of body weight before toe-off.

Compressive forces across the ankle joint rise to three times body weight between heel-strike and full foot contact. After heel-lift, these forces rise to five times body weight and then decreases to toe-off (Fig. 3.126). With increasing speed, the relatively smooth pattern of compressive forces becomes markedly biphasic. Although the absolute force magnitudes after heel-strike and

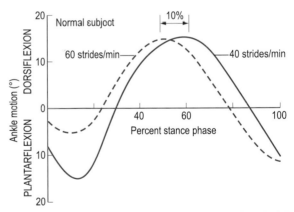

Fig. 3.124 Effect of walking speed on the range of ankle joint motion. (Adapted from Stauffer, R.N., Chao, E.Y.S., Brewster, R.C., 1977. Force and motion analysis of the normal, diseased, and prosthetic ankle joint. Clin. Orthop. Relat. Res. 127, 189–196.)

before toe-off are not much greater than at lower speeds, the relative unloading of the cartilage between the two peaks effectively means that the articular cartilage undergoes two loading cycles per gait cycle. This rapid alternating pattern of loading of the articular cartilage

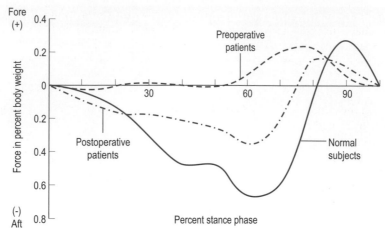

Fig. 3.125 Pattern of tangential force transmitted across the ankle joint during the stance phase of gait. (Adapted from Stauffer, R.N., Chao, E.Y.S., Brewster, R.C., 1977. Force and motion analysis of the normal, diseased, and prosthetic ankle joint. Clin. Orthop. Relat. Res. 127, 189–196.)

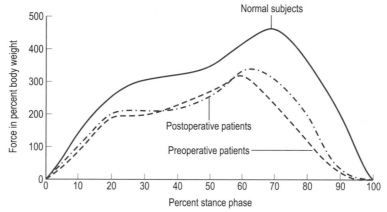

Fig. 3.126 Pattern of compressive forces transmitted across the ankle joint during the stance phase of gait. (Adapted from Stauffer, R.N., Chao, E.Y.S., Brewster, R.C., 1977. Force and motion analysis of the normal, diseased, and prosthetic ankle joint. Clin. Orthop. Relat. Res. 127, 189–196.)

during fast walking may, over a long period of time, be responsible for some cartilage degeneration.

It appears that individuals with ankle joint disease have poor tolerance to both compressive and shear forces transmitted across the joint (dashed lines in Figs 3.125 and 3.126). Consequently, individuals modify their gait patterns in an attempt to reduce the magnitude of these forces.

Contact Area and Contact Stresses

The occurrence of osteoarthrosis of the ankle joint is small compared with other joints of the lower limb. If degenerative disease results from a fatigue process, it becomes important to know the magnitude of the contact stresses and the loading cycle; to determine contact stresses the joint contact area needs to be known. Studies suggest that the mean ankle joint contact area is between 1000 and 1500 mm², giving compressive forces across the joint of between three and five times body weight for the majority of the stance phase, giving compressive contact stresses of 1.4–3.5 MN/m². These values are similar to those calculated for the hip joint, which shows a much higher incidence of osteoarthrosis. The difference in the incidence of pathology under similar contact stresses can probably be accounted for by the much more complex loading patterns at the hip.

Trabecular Arrangement

The transmission of mechanical forces across the joint is reflected in the arrangement and direction of the trabeculae within the associated bones. Two sets of trabeculae cross the ankle joint (Fig. 3.158A and B): one arising from the cortex on the anterior tibial surface passes posteroinferiorly through the talus to the calcaneus; the other, beginning in the cortex on the posterior tibial surface, passes anteroinferiorly through the talus. Medially, this system can be traced to the 1st metatarsal head (Fig. 3.156A and B), and laterally to the 5th metatarsal head. The trabecular systems within the bones of the foot are considered in more detail on page 437.

Joint Replacement/Fusion

With total replacement of the ankle joint, the range of motion during gait is generally within normal limits; however, the patterns are often abnormal. In normal gait, initial foot contact is with the heel, with the ankle slightly plantarflexed. In contrast, in individuals with total joint replacement, initial foot-floor contact tends to be with the entire foot, with the ankle in maximum available passive plantarflexion. At the end of the stance phase, the normal change from dorsiflexion to plantarflexion is not seen. Such alterations in the pattern of motion do not appear to be related to ligament instability, stiffness or pain in the ankle or foot. Consequently, ankle fusion remains the procedure of choice for many painful ankle conditions, particularly if the subtalar and midtarsal joints are not involved and the individual subjects the lower limb to high levels of activity. Arthrodesis should be performed in a neutral position; an equinus position is unfavourable as it prevents an effective heel-strike occurring at the beginning of the stance phase of gait.

Total joint replacement has been and continues to be limited to a select group of individuals in whom only a few degrees of motion allow a degree of independence that would otherwise not be achieved. The use of ankle prostheses in single joint involvement (after severe trauma, joint degeneration, osteochondritic damage to the articular surface) results in early breakdown of the prosthesis and later conversion to an arthrodesis. In general, ankle prostheses do not tolerate a normal degree of activity, even in individuals leading a relatively sedentary life.

First-generation designs of ankle prostheses were not very successful, with many individuals experiencing loosening; consequently, many were removed and the ankle fused. However, total joint replacement is becoming more common with the advent of later generations of designs, which have paid attention to reproducing normal ankle anatomy, joint kinematics, ligament stability and mechanical alignment. Two- and three-component designs are currently available, with the latest designs improving fixation, allowing increased bone ingrowth. With improvements in surgical techniques, instrumentation, implant design and patient selection, total ankle arthroplasty is becoming more successful.

MUSCLES PLANTARFLEXING THE FOOT AT THE ANKLE JOINT

Gastrocnemius
Soleus
Plantaris
Fibularis/peroneus longus (p. 423)
Fibularis/peroneus brevis (p. 425)
Tibialis posterior (p. 422)
Flexor digitorum longus (p. 445)
Flexor hallucis longus (p. 447)

Gastrocnemius

The shape of the calf is mainly due to the two fleshy bellies of gastrocnemius (Fig. 3.127A) situated on the posterior aspect of the leg/calf, with its muscle bulk mainly in the proximal half; together with soleus it forms a composite muscle (triceps surae). The two heads form the distal boundaries of the popliteal fossa (p. 339), which can only be readily seen when the knee is flexed. The heads arise from the medial and lateral condyles of the femur; the medial head from posterior to the medial supracondylar ridge and adductor tubercle on the popliteal surface of the femur, the lateral head from the lateral surface of the lateral condyle of the femur superoposterior to the lateral epicondyle. Each has an additional attachment from the capsule of the knee joint and the oblique popliteal ligament, below which each is separated from the joint capsule by a bursa. The bursa associated with the medial head often communicates with the knee joint, that under the lateral head rarely does. There is often a sesamoid bone (fabella) in the lateral head as it crosses the lateral femoral condyle; less commonly there may be one associated with the medial head.

From each head, a fleshy bulk of muscle fibres arise gradually coming together, although not blending with each other, to attach to the posterior surface of a broad membranous tendon which fuses with the tendon of soleus, forming the proximal part of the tendocalcaneus. This broad tendon gradually narrows, becoming more

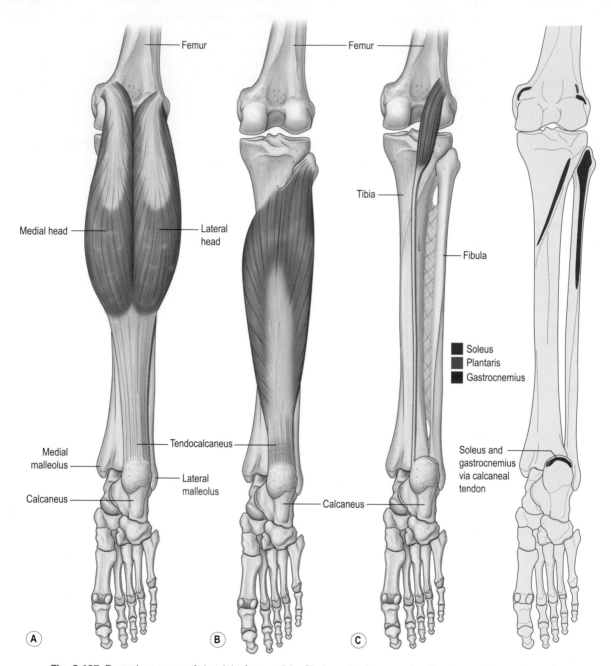

Fig. 3.127 Posterior aspect of the right femur, tibia, fibula and calcaneus showing the position and attachments of (A) gastrocnemius, (B) soleus and (C) plantaris.

rounded, until it reaches about three fingers' breadth above the calcaneus, where it expands again continuing to do so until its attachment into the middle part of the posterior surface of the calcaneus. The tendon fibres spiral as they pass from the myotendinous junction to their attachment so that the most medial fibres superiorly become posterior. This helical arrangement results in less buckling when the tendon is lax and less deformity of individual strands when under tension. A bursa lies between the tendon and proximal part of the calcaneus, while a fat pad lies between the tendon and posterior aspect of the ankle joint; inferior to the attachment is the fat pad of the heel.

Innervation

Each head is innervated by a branch from the tibial nerve (root value S1, S2). Skin covering the muscle is supplied by roots L4, 5 and S2.

Action

Gastrocnemius, together with soleus, is the main plantarflexor of the foot at the ankle joint providing the propelling force for locomotion. As it crosses the knee joint, it is also a powerful flexor of that joint; however, it is not able to exert its full power on both joints simultaneously; if the knee is flexed gastrocnemius cannot exert maximum power at the ankle joint and vice versa.

Functional Activity

In running, walking and jumping, gastrocnemius provides a considerable amount of the propulsive force. Considering the power needed to launch the body into the air, triceps surae must be one of the most powerful muscle groups in the body.

The habitual wearing of shoes with high heels can cause considerable shortening of the fibres of gastrocnemius as the muscle attachments are brought closer together. With shortening, difficulty in walking in flat shoes or bare feet may be experienced due to limited ankle dorsiflexion.

Soleus

Situated deep to the gastrocnemius, soleus is a broad flat muscle wider in its middle section and narrower distally (Fig. 3.127B). It arises from the soleal line on the posterior surface of the tibia, posterior surface of the proximal one-third of the fibula (including the head) and a fibrous arch between them. The fibres pass inferiorly forming a belly about halfway down the leg/calf to the deep surface of a membranous tendon, which faces posteriorly. The tendon glides over a similar one on the deep surface of gastrocnemius enabling independent movement of the two muscles. Inferiorly, the tendons fuse forming the proximal part of the tendocalcaneus passing posterior to the ankle joint to attach to the middle part of the posterior surface of the calcaneus.

Innervation

By two branches from the tibial nerve (root value S1, S2), one arising in the popliteal fossa entering the superficial surface of the muscle, the other arising in the leg/calf entering the deep surface. Skin over the region of the muscle is predominantly supplied by root S2.

Action

Soleus is one of the two main plantarflexors of the ankle joint. Situated to prevent the body falling forwards at the ankle joint during standing, it is an important postural muscle. Intermittent contraction during standing aids venous return (soleal pump) due to communicating vessels joining the deep and superficial venous systems passing through its substance.

Tendocalcaneus (Achilles Tendon)

Considered to be the thickest and strongest tendon in the body, the tendocalcaneus is the tendon by which gastrocnemius and soleus exert their force on the posterior part of the foot during the propulsive phase of many activities (walking, running, jumping); it has been suggested that it is able to withstand strains of up to 10 tonnes. As its fibres pass inferiorly, they spiral through 90 degrees with the medial fibres passing posteriorly; this arrangement is thought to explain the apparent elastic qualities of the tendon. When jumping, the body lands in an erect position with the foot plantarflexed by the action of triceps surae; the strain is taken by the tendocalcaneus producing a recoil effect.

Plantaris

Long slender muscle variable in composition (Fig. 3.127C); it may have one muscle belly high in the leg/calf or two smaller bellies separated by a tendon. It arises from the most distal part of the lateral supracondylar ridge, adjacent part of the popliteal surface of the femur and knee joint capsule. The tendon passes obliquely inferiorly between gastrocnemius and soleus, emerging on the medial side of the tendocalcaneus. It may attach to the tendocalcaneus or to the medial side of the posterior surface of the calcaneus.

Innervation

By the tibial nerve (root value S1, S2).

Action

Plantaris is a weak flexor of the leg/calf at the knee joint and plantarflexor of the foot at the ankle joint.

Functional Activity of the Leg/Calf Muscles

The leg/calf muscles plantarflex the foot at the ankle joint. Gastrocnemius acts as the propelling force, working mainly on the ankle joint, but also producing knee flexion if working strongly enough. Soleus is better situated to act more as a postural muscle because its distal attachment is the fixed point preventing the leg/calf from moving forwards under the influence of body weight; the vertical projection from the centre of gravity of the body falls anterior to the ankle joint.

Gastrocnemius is composed of muscle fibres giving it a pale appearance; consequently, it is often referred to as a 'white' muscle, while soleus has fibres giving it a red appearance and is termed a 'red' muscle.

Plantaris plays very little part in ankle plantarflexion; it can cause pain and disability when torn. This condition ('tennis leg') occurs during a game of tennis when the player believes that they have been struck on the back of the leg/calf by a tennis ball: the tendon is often completely ruptured and may have to be surgically removed.

Palpation of the Leg/Calf Muscles

When standing, draw your hand down the back of the knee. The two large muscular bellies of gastrocnemius can be felt on either side in the proximal part of the calf; the medial head projecting slightly higher and lower than the lateral. Both can be felt joining a broad flattened tendon just over halfway down the leg/calf. The junction between the muscle fibres and tendon is clear; it is along this line that many leg/calf injuries occur.

Being deep to gastrocnemius, soleus is not quite so easy to palpate. Its lateral boundary appears as a flattened elevation inferolateral to the lateral head of gastrocnemius when the foot is plantarflexed. When standing on tiptoe, soleus can be seen and felt bulging on either side of gastrocnemius. Passing the hand further down the leg/calf, it encounters the flattened tendocalcaneus, which is felt to narrow becoming rounded at the level of the ankle joint; it then expands slightly to its attachment to the middle part of the posterior surface of the calcaneus.

MUSCLES DORSIFLEXING THE FOOT AT THE ANKLE JOINT

Tibialis anterior
Extensor digitorum longus (p. 442)
Extensor hallucis longus (p. 440)
Fibularis/peroneus tertius (p. 426)

Tibialis Anterior

Long fusiform muscle situated on the anterior aspect of the leg/calf lateral to the anterior border of the tibia (Fig.

3.128). It is covered by strong fascia, gaining its proximal attachment from the deep surface of this fascia, the proximal two-thirds of the lateral surface of the tibia and adjoining part of the interosseous membrane. It becomes tendinous in its distal one-third, passing inferomedially over the distal end of the tibia. The tendon continues

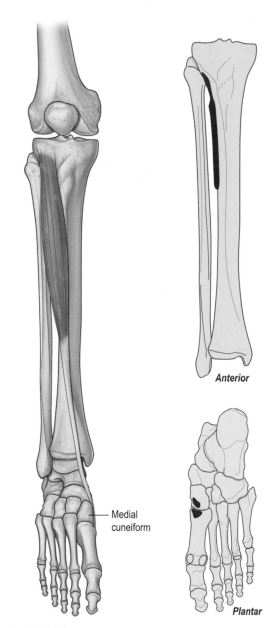

Anterior

— Medial cuneiform

Plantar

Fig. 3.128 Anterior aspect of the right distal femur, tibia, fibula and dorsum of the foot showing the position and attachments of tibialis anterior.

through both the superior and inferior extensor retinaculae to attach to the medial side of the medial cuneiform and base of the 1st metatarsal, reaching the inferior surface of both bones, blending with that of fibularis/peroneus longus.

Innervation

By the deep fibular/peroneal nerve (root value L4, L5). Skin covering the muscle is also supplied by roots L4 and 5.

Action

Tibialis anterior dorsiflexes the foot at the ankle joint. Working with tibialis posterior, it acts to invert the foot in which the sole is turned to face medially.

Functional Activity

As with other muscles in the leg/calf, tibialis anterior is concerned with balancing the body over the foot. It works with the surrounding muscles to maintain balance during activities of the upper part of the body which change its weight distribution.

Not only is tibialis anterior responsible for dorsiflexing the foot as the lower limb is carried forward during the swing-through phase of walking, preventing the toes catching the ground, it also controls the placement of the foot on the ground after initial ground contact by the heel. On close observation, the heel does not strike the ground, remaining immobile at the initiation of the stance phase, but glides onto the surface, acting as the first braking force of the lower limb's forward movement. Overactivity of tibialis anterior accounts for the wear pattern seen on the posterolateral aspect of the heel due to frictional forces between the shoe and ground. The rest of the foot is gradually lowered to the ground in a controlled manner taking up the undulations of the surface. The landing of the foot on the ground is similar to the landing of an aeroplane; the main wheels touch down first, applying the initial braking force, followed by a controlled lowering of the front of the aircraft as speed decreases.

Tibialis anterior, in association with other dorsiflexors, plays an important part in lowering the forefoot to the ground in walking or running and is put under stress in extended activities, particularly over rough terrain. The anterior calf muscles are enclosed in a particularly tight fascia, allowing very little expansion of the tissues, resulting in compression of the muscle during activity and a pulling on the surrounding fascial attachments, particularly those to bone, leading to a painful condition ('shin splints').

Paralysis of tibialis anterior causes footdrop because the remaining dorsiflexors are not strong enough to raise the toes and prevent them from dragging along the ground. The individual may overcome this by flexing the leg/calf at the knee joint more than normal while walking; alternatively, a 'toe-raise' orthosis may be fitted to the individual or their shoe.

Palpation

Both the muscle belly and tendon can be seen and felt when the foot is dorsiflexed against resistance; the tendon is the most medial at the ankle joint.

CLINICAL EXAMINATION AND EVALUATION

Plantarflexion

With the individual seated:
- Flex the knee 90 degrees.
- Put the foot in neutral abduction/adduction and pronation/supination.
- Stabilise the tibia and fibula to prevent knee movement and hip rotation.
- Then plantarflex the foot (Fig. 3.129A).

The end feel to movement is firm due to tension in the anterior joint capsule, the anterior components of the medial and lateral collateral ligaments and the extensor muscles crossing the joint; contact between the posterior talar tubercle and posterior tibial margin may give a hard feel to the end point.

To measure plantarflexion, the centre of the goniometer is placed over the lateral aspect of the lateral malleolus, with the proximal arm pointing towards the head of the fibula and the distal arm aligned with the 5th metatarsal.

Dorsiflexion

The individual positioning and goniometer placement are the same as for plantarflexion, but the foot is dorsiflexed (Fig. 3.129B). The end feel to movement is firm due to tension in the posterior joint capsule, Achilles tendon and posterior components of the medial and lateral collateral ligaments.

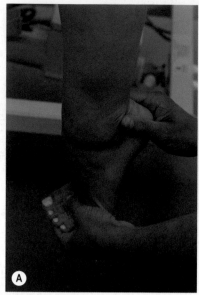 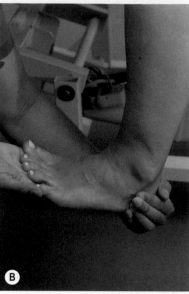

Fig. 3.129 Determination of the range of (A) plantarflexion and (B) dorsiflexion of the foot at the ankle joint with the individual seated.

SECTION SUMMARY

Tibia

- Medial bone of leg/calf having proximal expanded end (tibial condyles); shaft with tibial tuberosity anteriorly and sharp, lateral facing interosseous border; slightly expanded distal end with the medial malleolus projecting inferiorly.
- Proximally, the medial and lateral tibial condyles articulate with the medial and lateral femoral condyles forming the knee joint; the facet below the lateral condyle articulates with the head of the fibula forming the superior tibiofibular joint.
- Distally articulates with fibula forming the inferior tibiofibular joint; the talus forming the ankle.

Fibula

- Lateral bone of the leg/calf having proximal head; irregular shaft with sharp medial facing interosseous border; expanded distal end with lateral malleolus projecting inferiorly.
- Articulates with the tibia superiorly and inferiorly forming the superior and inferior tibiofibular joints; the talus inferiorly forming part of the ankle joint.

Talus

- Irregular bone of the hindfoot with a wedge-shaped body anteroposteriorly, medial and lateral articular surface, and medial projecting neck and head.
- Articulates with tibia and fibula forming the ankle joint.

Ankle Joint

Type	Synovial hinge joint
Articular surfaces	Distal end of tibia and inner surfaces of medial and lateral malleoli with trochlear surface and sides of talus
Capsule	Thin, loose capsule attaching to articular margins, except for attachment to neck of talus anteriorly
Ligaments	Medial collateral (deltoid); lateral collateral (anterior and posterior talofibular, calcaneofibular); anterior and posterior capsular
Stability	Provided by coaptation of articular surfaces, collateral ligaments and muscles
Movements	Dorsiflexion (extension) and plantarflexion (flexion)

Movements at the Ankle Joint

The ankle joint is only capable of dorsiflexion and plantarflexion; inversion and eversion occur at the subtalar and transverse (mid) tarsal joints. In addition to the major muscles working on the ankle joint, other muscles crossing the ankle to reach more distal attachments on the toes can contribute to these movements.

SECTION SUMMARY—cont'd

Movement	Muscles (root value of nerve supply)
Dorsiflexion	Tibialis anterior (L4, L5)
	Fibularis/peroneal tertius (L5, S1)
	Extensor digitorum longus (L5, S1)
	Extensor hallucis longus (L5, S1)
Plantarflexion	Gastrocnemius (S1, S2)
	Soleus (S1, S2)
	Plantaris (S1, S2)
	Fibularis/peroneus longus (L5, S1)
	Fibularis/peroneus brevis (L5, S1)
	Tibialis posterior (L4, L5)
	Flexor digitorum longus (L5, S1, S2)
	Flexor hallucis longus (S1, S2)

- Muscles in italics have their primary function in plantarflexing (flexing) or dorsiflexing (extending) the toes; once this has been achieved, they can aid movement at the ankle in continued action.
- All of the muscles crossing the ankle have an important *role* in *the maintenance of* balance.

Clinical Evaluation

Movement and Maximum Range	End Feel to Movement
Plantarflexion 50°	Firm
Dorsiflexion 30°	Firm

❓ SELF-ASSESSMENT QUESTIONS

71. In which direction does the head of the talus point?
72. Which malleolus projects further distally?
73. Is the body of the talus broader anteriorly or posteriorly?
74. What are the attachments of gastrocnemius?
75. What is the nerve supply, including root value, of soleus?
76. What are the actions of tibialis anterior?
77. Where does tibialis posterior cross the ankle joint?
78. What shape is the inferior extensor retinaculum and what are its attachments?
79. Which muscles contribute to the tendocalcaneus (Achilles tendon)?
80. What shape is the trochlear surface of the talus?
81. Which parts of the deltoid ligament are deepest?
82. Name the individual parts of the lateral collateral ligament of the ankle.
83. Which of the tendons crossing the ankle joint anteriorly is most medial?
84. What are the attachments of tibialis posterior?
85. What are the actions of gastrocnemius?
86. What is the nerve supply, including root value, of tibialis anterior?
87. In which position of the ankle joint are the collateral ligaments most lax?
88. What type of joint is the ankle joint?
89. The ankle joint is said to have the appearance of a 'mortise and tenon'; which parts of the joint form the mortise and which the tenon?
90. What and where is the malleolar fossa?

▌FOOT

LEARNING OUTCOMES

By the end of the section, you should be able to;
1. Identify, palpate and examine the tarsal bones, metatarsals and phalanges
2. Describe the bones, joints and muscles of the foot
3. Describe and explain the movements possible, and their restraints, at the subtalar, midtarsal, metatarsophalangeal and interphalangeal joints of the toes
4. Locate, palpate and examine the muscles associated with the toes and know their attachments, action, function and innervation
5. Examine and assess movements at the subtalar, midtarsal, metatarsophalangeal and interphalangeal joints of the foot
6. Appreciate the influence of pathology and/or trauma on the function of the foot

INTRODUCTION

It is widely believed that the human foot has evolved from the mobile prehensile organ seen in many primates to the specialised supporting structure necessary for bipedal locomotion. In contrast to the anthropoid foot, the human foot is characterised by a reduced ability to oppose the hallux (Fig. 3.130A). The ability is not completely lost as the requisite musculature is still present; under some circumstances (congenital absence of

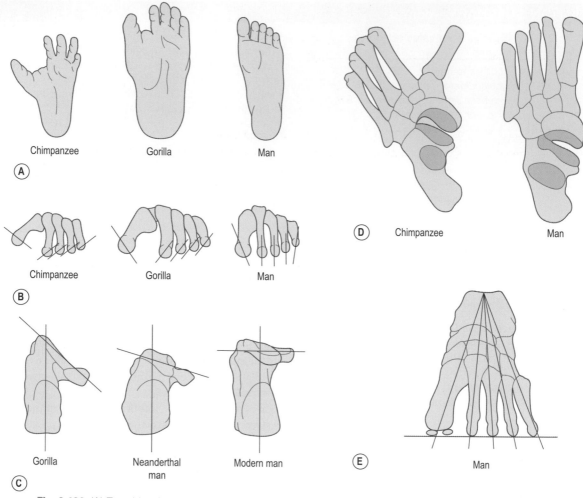

Fig. 3.130 (A) Transition from an anthropoid to a human foot. (B) Loss of rotation of the metatarsals during evolution. (C) Changes in the obliquity of the sustentaculum tali. (D) Reduction in angulation of the hallux (E) Anterior support of the foot indicating that all metatarsals participate.

the upper limbs), opposition of the hallux can become remarkably well developed, to the extent of holding a pen or fork. With the general reduction in opposability, the metatarsal heads are no longer rotated towards each other as the gripping function of the toes require but are directed anteroposteriorly (Fig. 3.130B). With this, the axis of leverage of the foot has shifted from between the 2nd and 3rd metatarsals to between the first and second metatarsals. Correspondingly, the axis of abduction/adduction of the toes is through the second digit compared with the third in the hand.

With the adoption of bipedal locomotion, important changes occurred within the calcaneus; the sustentaculum tali has become more massive, as has the calcancus as a whole, and assumed a more horizontal position (Fig. 3.130C) to support the body of the talus and superincumbent body weight. The calcaneus as a whole has changed its relative position within the foot from an inferiorly directed to a superiorly directed upward one.

In primates, adduction of the hallux gives the forefoot a medial direction; in the human foot, this angulation disappears so that the axis of the foot follows a straight line (Fig. 3.130D). Consequently, the first and second metatarsals lie more parallel to each other. With the medial shift of the axis of leverage, the medial border of the foot became flattened and depressed; a transverse arch developed so that the supporting ball occupies the entire width of the foot (Fig. 3.130E).

These developmental changes are essentially based upon the requirements to adjust the centre and line of gravity to a small supporting surface area. Having achieved this and adjusted the gravitational stresses to the area of support for bipedal gait, further changes enabling bipedal gait to be adopted had to be undertaken. An alternating bipedal gait has been the stimulus for the development of certain articulations providing for static balance during standing and dynamic propulsion during walking and running.

The ankle and foot provide propulsion and restraint at each step. A single joint (ankle joint: p. 384) has been established between the leg/calf and foot, controlling the foot in the sagittal plane. A second articulation allowing side-to-side adjustment of the line of gravity in standing, as well as participating in restraint and propulsion, has been established between the talus and calcaneus (subtalar joint). Lastly, a composite functional joint interrupting the structure of the foot in the middle of the tarsus (transverse (mid) tarsal joint) has been established. The latter joint plays an important role by providing spring to the propulsive phase of gait by allowing the anterior part of the foot to adjust itself against the posterior. By doing so, the anterior footplate is able to maintain full contact with the supporting surface independent of the posterior part of the foot.

Besides forcing the foot into a right-angled relationship with the leg/calf, bipedal gait has also produced changes in the arrangement of musculature around the ankle and within the foot. In humans, tibialis anterior has lost its attachment to the hallux. Both extensors digitorum longus and hallucis longus split from the primitive extensor plate as separate units and a new unit (fibularis/peroneus tertius) is formed; fibularis/peroneus tertius is an important muscle aiding pronation of the formerly supinated foot. Fibularis/peroneus longus and brevis run posterior to the ankle joint axis and become plantarflexors as opposed to their previous role as dorsiflexors. In addition, because of the increased stress on the anterior part of the foot in bipedal locomotion, the attachment of fibularis/peroneus longus has migrated across the sole of the foot; it now helps maintain the arches of the foot against depression. Finally, tibialis posterior has developed a fan-shaped attachment to all tarsal bones, except the talus, providing one of the principal supports of the longitudinal arches of the foot.

The human foot is strong enough to support the weight of the body, but also flexible and resilient enough to absorb the shocks transmitted to it and provide spring and lift during activity. These properties are achieved by a series of arches (convex above) composed of a number of bones and their interconnecting joints. The joints and ligaments, together with muscle action, provide spring as they yield when weight is applied and recoil when the weight is removed.

The bones of the foot are arranged in longitudinal and transverse arches (Fig. 3.131). The longitudinal arch, sometimes regarded as having two parts (lateral, medial), is supported posteriorly on the tuberosity of the calcaneus and anteriorly on the metatarsal heads. The talus is at the summit of this arch, primarily related to the navicular, cuneiforms and medial three metatarsals (medial longitudinal arch), while the calcaneus is directly related to the cuboid and lateral two metatarsals (lateral longitudinal arch). These differences appear in the function of the foot, with the medial longitudinal arch having a greater curvature and being more elastic than the lateral. The flatter, more rigid lateral arch makes contact with the ground, providing a firm base for support. The transverse arch results from the (i) shape of the distal row of tarsal bones and (ii) metatarsal bases; being broader dorsally, the bones articulate in a domed curve forming a transverse arch.

Maintenance of these arches depends on the integrity of the tarsal, tarsometatarsal and intermetatarsal joints as it is here that the bones are held in their proper relationships as segments of the arches. Some ligaments are more important than others, as they are extremely strong to resist undue yielding of the joints and collapse of the arches; these are on the plantar aspect of the joints and are themselves supported by the plantar aponeurosis and intervening musculature.

In addition to plantarflexion and dorsiflexion of the foot, both of which occur at the ankle joint, the foot can be adducted/abducted about the long axis of the leg/calf (Fig. 3.132A) and pronated/supinated about its own longitudinal axis (Fig. 3.132B). Adduction (toes pointing towards the midline) and abduction (toes pointing away from the midline) take place in a transverse plane; they are only possible when the knee is flexed, when axial rotation of the tibia at the knee is possible. The total range of abduction and adduction when they occur exclusively in the foot is 35–45 degrees. However, contributions from the leg/calf (with the knee flexed) or

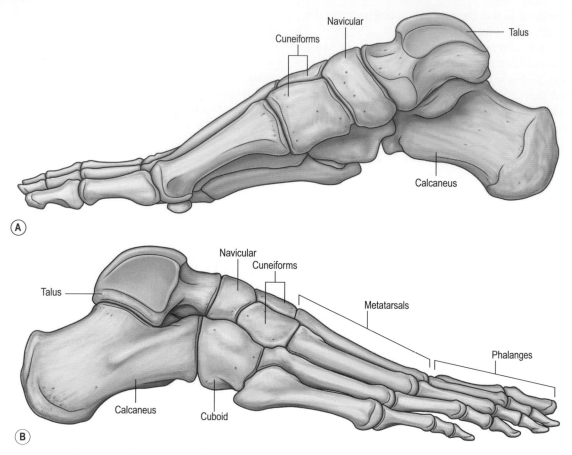

Fig. 3.131 Medial (A) and lateral (B) aspects of the right foot showing the medial and lateral longitudinal arches.

whole limb (at the hip joint) can increase this range to 90 degrees in each direction, as seen in ballerinas. Movement of the foot about its long axis causes the sole to face medially (supination) or laterally (pronation); the range of supination is about 50 degrees and that of pronation 25–30 degrees.

Due to the arrangement of the joints within the foot, neither adduction/abduction nor supination/pronation occur as pure movements; adduction is always accompanied by supination, giving inversion, and abduction by pronation, giving eversion; adding plantarflexion and dorsiflexion respectively increases their range. An apparent pure supination movement can be achieved by laterally rotating the leg/calf at the knee to compensate for the accompanying adduction. Similarly, medial rotation of the leg/calf at the knee can compensate for the linked abduction producing an apparent pure pronation

movement. When balancing on one lower limb, lateral rotation of the leg/calf (relative adduction of the foot) is accompanied by pronation of the forefoot while attempting to maintain full foot contact with the supporting surface. Supination of the forefoot accompanies medial rotation of the leg/calf under similar circumstances.

Deep Fascia of the Foot

The fascia of the foot is continuous with that of the leg/calf. On the dorsum, it is thin, wrapping around either side of the foot, becoming continuous with the plantar aponeurosis; anteriorly, it splits covering the dorsum of the toes.

Plantar Aponeurosis

This comprises some of the thickest fascia in the body (up to 80 layers thick); it is continuous with the fascia

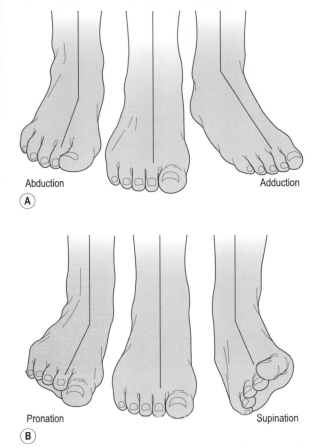

Abduction   Adduction

(A)

Pronation   Supination

(B)

Fig. 3.132 (A) Abduction and adduction of the foot about the longitudinal axis of the leg/calf. (B) Pronation and supination about the longitudinal axis of the foot.

over the heel and with the dorsal fascia over the sides of the foot. Triangular in shape with the apex at the heel attaching to the inferior aspect of the calcaneus posterior to the medial tubercle, it spreads out anteriorly into five slips, becoming continuous with the fibrous flexor sheaths of the toes. Most of its fibres run longitudinally, except anteriorly where it splits, with transverse fibres binding the five slips together. As each slip approaches the metatarsal head, it splits into superficial and deep layers; the superficial layer attaches to the superficial fascia, producing a deep cleft under the base of the toe. The deeper layer splits again into medial and lateral parts, attaching either side of the base of the proximal phalanx of each toe and deep transverse metatarsal ligament; this is the start of the fibro-osseous tunnel containing the flexor tendons of the toes.

The central part of the aponeurosis gives partial attachment to the muscles lying deep to it. At its edges,

strong septa pass superiorly separating abductor hallucis, flexor digitorum brevis and abductor digiti minimi. Between the five slips, close to the base of the toes, is a space giving access to the nerves and vessels supplying them.

The plantar aponeurosis is extremely important in maintaining the longitudinal arches of the foot. With the toes dorsiflexed, the proximal phalanx winds its slip of aponeurosis around the metatarsal head ('windlass' effect) tightening the aponeurosis and raising the longitudinal arches.

Fibro-Osseous Tunnels

Where the anterior attachment of the plantar aponeurosis splits, attaching to either side of the proximal phalanx, it forms the beginning of a fibro-osseous tunnel running under the toe accommodating the flexor tendons. It is composed of arching fibres passing over the tendons, attaching to the flat plantar surface of each phalanx. At the interphalangeal joints, the fibres criss-cross from the medial side of the head of one phalanx to the lateral side of the base of the adjacent phalanx and vice versa. Each tunnel is lined with a double layer of synovial membrane facilitating movement of the tendons in the tunnel.

BONY STRUCTURE OF THE FOOT

The foot (Figs 3.133 and 3.134) consists of many small bones, posteriorly are the tarsus and anteriorly the metatarsals and phalanges; the tarsus (talus, calcaneus, navicular, cuboid, cuneiforms) and metatarsals comprise the foot proper and the phalanges the toes. The largest bone in the foot is the calcaneus, and the largest metatarsal is the most medial having anterior to it the two phalanges of the hallux (big toe); the other metatarsals each have three phalanges distal to them. Along the medial longitudinal arch, from posterior to anterior, are the calcaneus, talus (situated more on top of the calcaneus), navicular, three cuneiform bones, first, second and third metatarsals and their associated phalanges. Along the lateral longitudinal arch of the foot, from posterior to anterior, are the calcaneus, cuboid, fourth and fifth metatarsals and their associated phalanges.

TARSUS

Talus

Details of the talus can be found on page 384.

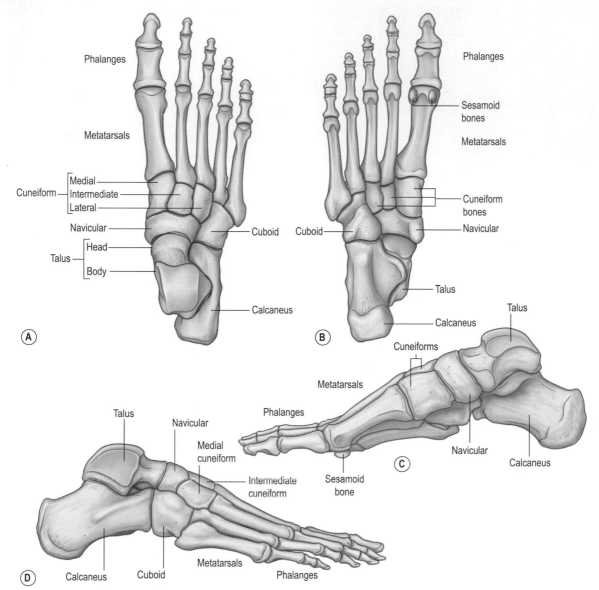

Fig. 3.133 Superior (A), inferior (B), medial (C) and lateral (D) aspects of the right foot.

Calcaneus

Lying inferior to the talus and projecting posteriorly forming the prominence of the heel (Fig. 3.133), the calcaneus is strongly bound to all tarsal bones by ligaments; it is the largest bone in the foot, being oblong with six surfaces. The anterior surface faces anteriorly articulating with the cuboid; it is slightly convex from superior to inferior and more or less flat from side to side, the medial part of the surface extends onto the medial side of the calcaneus accommodating a posterior projection of the cuboid. The posterior surface is rounded having three areas: the upper area is smooth where a bursa lies between it and the tendocalcaneus; the middle area is smooth and convex except at its lower margin where it ends as a jagged rough edge receiving the attachment of the tendocalcaneus; the lowest subcutaneous area is roughened and covered by the strong fibrous tissue and fat of the heel pad. The lowest area transmits body

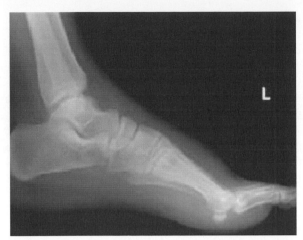

Fig. 3.134 Mediolateral radiograph of the left foot showing the medial aspect.

weight from the heel to the ground during heel-strike in walking, curving anteriorly onto the inferior surface with the larger medial and smaller lateral tubercles projecting anteriorly.

The inferior surface continues anteriorly as a rough area terminating as the anterior tubercle; the long plantar ligament attaches to the rough area. The lateral surface is slightly roughened and nearly flat, and has two tubercles, one for attachment of part of the lateral ligament of the ankle joint, and the other slightly inferoanterior providing attachment for the inferior fibular/peroneal retinaculum; the fibular/peroneal tubercle is elongated with grooves superior and inferior. The medial surface is smooth and hollowed, overhung anteriorly by the sustentaculum tali, inferior to which is the groove for the tendon of flexor hallucis longus. On the superior surface of the sustentaculum tali is the middle articular surface for the head of the talus, posterior to which is a deep groove (sulcus calcanei) continuing across the superior surface in a posteromedial direction. Anterior to the sinus calcanei is a roughened area for muscle and ligament attachments; posterior is the posterior articular surface, convex from anterior to posterior and flat from side to side for articulation with the inferior surface of the body of the talus. Behind this articular surface is a further roughened area, concave superiorly from anterior to posterior and convex from side to side.

The trabeculae of the calcaneus (Fig. 3.158) have a particular arrangement due to its weight-bearing nature. From the posterior articular surface, supporting trabeculae pass inferoposteriorly to the heel and

inferoanteriorly to the articular area for the cuboid. Running from the heel to the anterior surface are superior and inferior arcuate systems uniting the anterior and posterior parts of the bone; between these systems is an area of less dense weaker bone.

Navicular

Lies anterior to the head of the talus (Fig. 3.133). The posterior surface is concave, articulating with the head of the talus. The anterior surface is subdivided into three triangular areas by two faint ridges for articulation with the three cuneiforms: the small, lateral, subcutaneous anterior surfaces, together forming a curve, are rough near their edges for attachment of interosseous ligaments. The inferior surface is narrow and roughened for ligament and muscle attachments; on its inferomedial side is a large tuberosity.

Cuboid

Situated lateral to the navicular, anterior to the calcaneus and posterior to the fourth and fifth metatarsals (Fig. 3.133), the cuboid has six surfaces; in reality, it is a cube flattened superoinferiorly. The posterior surface is slightly concave from superior to inferior, but flat from side to side articulating with the anterior surface of the calcaneus. The medial surface is smooth on its anterior two-thirds articulating with the lateral cuneiform and occasionally the navicular, while the posterior one-third is usually roughened for ligament attachments. Anteriorly, it is nearly flat, divided by a slight ridge into two facets articulating with the bases of the fourth and fifth metatarsals.

The lateral surface is the smallest due to the convergence of the anterior and posterior surfaces passing laterally. Nearly the entire surface is taken up by a deep groove passing inferoanteriorly, through which the tendon of fibularis/peroneus longus passes; the groove continues on the inferior surface of the bone crossing anteromedially towards the medial cuneiform. The groove is very close to the anterior border of the cuboid, limited by a prominent ridge posterior to it; the remainder of the inferior surface is rough for attachment of the long and short (calcaneocuboid) plantar ligaments. The dorsal surface is roughened and, with the dorsal surfaces of the cuneiforms and navicular, is subcutaneous.

Cuneiforms

There are three cuneiforms (medial, intermediate, lateral) (Fig. 3.133); each is wedge-shaped, triangular at their anterior and posterior ends with three rectangular surfaces along their length.

Medial Cuneiform

Largest of the cuneiforms it has the apex projecting superiorly and base inferiorly. The anterior and posterior surfaces are smooth articulating with the first metatarsal and anterior surface of the navicular, respectively. The smooth lateral surface articulates with the intermediate cuneiform on its posterior two-thirds and the base of the second metatarsal on its anterior one-third. The superior, medial and inferior surfaces form a continuous surface on the medial side of the foot, which is roughened by ligament attachments. It has a smooth impression at the anteroinferior part of its medial aspect over which the tendon of tibialis anterior passes.

Intermediate Cuneiform

Its base is superior and apex inferior; it is shorter than the other two cuneiforms and is only non-articular on its dorsal surface. It articulates medially with the medial cuneiform, laterally with the lateral cuneiform, anteriorly with the second metatarsal and posteriorly with the navicular. Part of the medial surface is roughened for attachment of ligaments.

Lateral Cuneiform

The apex of the lateral cuneiform projects inferiorly and its base superiorly. The medial surface articulates mainly with the intermediate cuneiform, having a small facet anteriorly for the second metatarsal. The lateral surface articulates with the medial surface of the cuboid, the posterior surface with the navicular and the anterior surface with the third metatarsal. The non-articular parts of the medial and lateral surfaces are roughened for attachment of ligaments.

That the medial cuneiform has its base projecting inferiorly while the other two have their bases superior contributes to the arch shape across the foot from medial to lateral. With the addition of the cuboid laterally, the cuneiforms make up part of the transverse tarsal arch.

Ossification of the Tarsus

Each tarsal bone ossifies from a primary centre appearing in the cartilaginous precursor; only the calcaneus has a secondary centre. Primary centres for the calcaneus and talus appear before birth in the 6th and 8th months *in utero*, respectively. That for the cuboid

appears at 9 months *in utero* and may be present at birth; if not, it appears soon afterwards. The centres of ossification for the remaining bones appear at the end of the 1st year for the lateral cuneiform, during the third year for the medial cuneiform and navicular, and during the 4th year for the intermediate cuneiform. Ossification is completed shortly after puberty.

The secondary centre for the calcaneus appears at about 9 years in its posterior end, extending to include the medial and lateral tubercles; occasionally the lateral tubercle ossifies separately. Fusion occurs between 15 and 20 years.

Because the ossification centres for the calcaneus, talus and cuboid are usually present before birth, they can be used to assess the skeletal maturity of a newborn child. They may be used in conjunction with the secondary centres in the distal end of the femur and the proximal end of the tibia.

Palpation

Posteriorly, the calcaneus can be clearly identified, being subcutaneous on its lateral, posterior and medial aspects. The inferior surface is covered with thick fascia, but the medial and lateral tubercles are identifiable on deep palpation posteriorly. Medially 1 cm inferior to the tip of the medial malleolus, the sustentaculum tali appears as a horizontal ridge, while on the lateral aspect, the fibular/peroneal tubercle lies approximately 2 cm inferior to the tip of the lateral malleolus, with the lateral tubercle (attachment of the calcaneofibular ligament) being slightly posterior.

The head and neck of the talus can be gripped between the finger and thumb in the two hollows anteroinferior to the medial malleolus, the tubercle of the navicular forming a clear landmark anterior to the medial hollow. Midway along the lateral border of the foot, the base of the fifth metatarsal, with its tubercle directed posteriorly, is prominent. The bases of the fourth to first metatarsals can be identified across the dorsum of the foot, the base of the first being 1 cm anterior to the tubercle of the navicular with the cuneiforms between.

METATARSALS

There are five metatarsals in each foot, the most medial of which is the stoutest, although it is also the shortest; the second is the longest, and the fifth can be recognised by the large tubercle projecting posterolaterally from its base. All five metatarsals have certain features in common (proximal base, shaft, distal head); the bases articulate with the tarsus and heads with the proximal phalanx of each toe (Fig. 3.133A and B).

The base of the first metatarsal is concave from side to side and flat from superior to inferior, articulating with the anterior surface of the medial cuneiform. Its lateral surface has a facet for articulation with the base of the second metatarsal; its inferior surface projects inferiorly, ending as a tuberosity. The base of the second metatarsal articulates with the intermediate cuneiform posteriorly; medially, it articulates with the medial cuneiform and first metatarsal; laterally, it articulates with the lateral cuneiform and third metatarsal. The base of the third metatarsal is flat, articulating with the lateral cuneiform and with adjacent metatarsals on either side; it is roughened on its superior and inferior surfaces. The fourth and fifth metatarsal bases articulate with the anterior surface of the cuboid; the fourth has a small facet on either side for articulation with adjacent metatarsals, while the base of the fifth is more expanded, having a large tubercle on its lateral side. The superior and inferior surfaces of each are roughened.

All the shafts are more or less cylindrical, the first being the thickest and second usually the thinnest; all narrow as they pass anteriorly towards their heads.

The heads are smooth and convex from superior to inferior, as well as from side to side. Immediately posterior to the head on either side is a tubercle, anterior to which is a small depression for the attachment of ligaments. The superior non-articular surface is roughened, while the inferior surface is marked by a groove passing anteriorly, giving passage to the long and short flexor tendons. The head of the first metatarsal is large and wide, forming the ball of the hallux, articulating with the base of its proximal phalanx and two sesamoid bones; the plantar surface is grooved on each side of a prominent central ridge by sesamoid bones in the tendons of the short muscles passing inferior to it.

Ossification

A primary centre appears in the body of each metatarsal at 9 weeks *in utero* so that, at birth, they are well-ossified. Secondary centres appear in the base of the first metatarsal and heads of the remaining metatarsals during the second and third years, with the medial ones appearing earlier. Fusion of the epiphyses with the bodies occurs between 15 and 18 years. In the lateral metatarsals, the epiphyses may occasionally be found in the bases rather than the heads.

It is interesting to note that the first metatarsal has an ossification pattern similar to that of the phalanges. It could be argued that, instead of the middle phalanx in the hallux being missing, it is the metatarsal that is missing, so that what is now referred to as the first metatarsal is in fact an enlarged proximal phalanx.

Palpation

The shafts and heads of the metatarsals can be readily palpated on the dorsum of the foot with the bases proximal and heads towards the toes. If the toes are extended, the metatarsal heads, especially the 1st, become palpable under the forefoot; the heads are less obvious on the dorsum of the foot when the metatarsophalangeal joints are flexed.

PHALANGES

There are two phalanges in the hallux and three in each of the other toes (Fig. 3.133): each is a miniature long bone having a shaft and two extremities and have certain features in common. Each base of the proximal phalanges has a smooth, concave, proximal surface articulating with the head of its metatarsal; the remaining phalanges have a proximal surface divided by a vertical ridge. Each phalanx is flattened on its plantar surface and rounded on its dorsum. The head of each phalanx, except the terminal phalanges, is divided into two condyles by a vertical groove giving it a pulley shape. The articular surface tends to be more extensive on the plantar surface of the head where it joins the flattened surface of the shaft. The sides of the heads are roughened and marked by a small tubercle at the centre.

The head of each distal phalanx is flattened on its dorsum and has no articular area; this surface is the nail bed.

Ossification

Primary centres for the distal and proximal phalanges appear during the fourth month *in utero*, with the distal ones appearing first; the primary centre for the middle phalanx appears between 6 months and birth. Secondary centres for the bases of all phalanges appear during the second and third years, fusing with the bodies between 15 and 20 years.

Palpation

The proximal phalanx of each toe is easily recognised, being the longest of the three; the rest are hidden to a certain extent by the pulp of the toe.

JOINTS OF THE FOOT

These can be divided into four groups: (i) intertarsal; (ii) tarsometatarsal and intermetatarsal; (iii) metatarsophalangeal; and (iv) interphalangeal.

INTERTARSAL JOINTS

The intertarsal joints are the subtalar, talocalcaneonavicular, calcaneocuboid, transverse (mid) tarsal, cuneonavicular, intercuneiform and cuneocuboid joints. The transverse tarsal joint is a functional description comprising the talocalcaneonavicular joint medially and calcaneocuboid joint laterally. The most important joints are those between the talus, calcaneus and navicular, and between the calcaneus and cuboid. All joints are characterised by interosseous, dorsal and plantar ligaments, of which the plantar ligaments are stronger. The bones and ligaments receive their blood supply from branches of the dorsalis pedis and medial and lateral plantar arteries. They are supplied on the dorsal aspect by the deep fibular/peroneal nerve and on their plantar aspect by the medial and lateral plantar nerves.

SUBTALAR JOINT

Articular Surfaces

Synovial joint between the concave facet on the inferior surface of the body of the talus and the convex posterior facet on the superior surface of the calcaneus (Fig. 3.135). The articular facet on the calcaneus is roughly oval with its long axis running anterolaterally; it is about this axis that the facet is convex, being plane or concave about the other axis. The joint surface can, therefore, be considered to be cylindrical with the long axis of the cylinder running obliquely from anterior, lateral and superior to posterior, medial and inferior.

The corresponding surface of the talus also has a cylindrical shape with a similar radius and axis.

Palpation

The depth and complex articulations involved at the subtalar joint make surface marking and palpation impractical.

Joint Capsule and Synovial Membrane

A thin loose fibrous capsule surrounds the joint, attaching close to the margins of the articular surfaces; it is

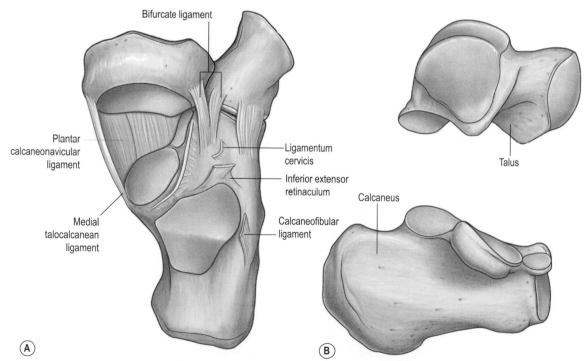

Fig. 3.135 Articular surfaces of the right subtalar joint with (A) the talus removed and (B) the bones separated.

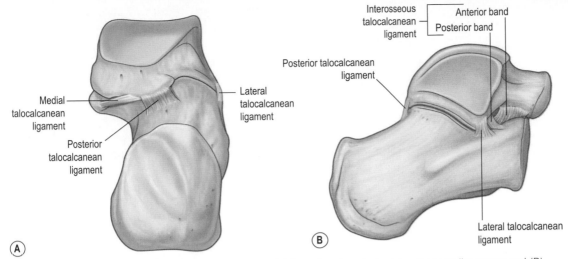

Fig. 3.136 Right subtalar joint showing (A) the medial, lateral and posterior talocalcanean ligaments and (B) lateral aspect showing the interosseous talocalcanean ligament.

thickened medially, posteriorly and laterally forming the medial, posterior and lateral talocalcanean ligaments. The capsule is lined with synovial membrane; the joint cavity does not communicate with that of any other joint.

The anterior part of the capsule is thin, attaching to the floor and roof of the sinus tarsi. (The sinus tarsi is a narrow tunnel running obliquely anterolaterally between the talus and calcaneus anterior to the subtalar joint; its anterolateral end opens onto the dorsum of the foot.) Also attaching within the sinus tarsi is the posterior part of the talocalcaneonavicular joint capsule; where the two joint capsules are adjacent to each other, they are thickened, forming the interosseous (talocalcanean) ligament.

Ligaments

Interosseous (Talocalcanean) Ligament

Strong band consisting of several laminae of fibres with fatty tissue in between, the interosseous ligament (Fig. 3.136B) is best thought of as two thick quadrilateral bands (anterior, posterior). The dense fibres of the anterior band pass obliquely superiorly, anteriorly and medially from the floor of the sinus tarsi to the inferior surface of the neck of the talus, just posterior to the articular surface of the head. The thick fibres of the posterior band run from the floor of the sinus tarsi obliquely superiorly, posteriorly and medially to just anterior to the posterior articular facet of the talus.

Between the two bands lies the deep extension of the lateral limb of the inferior extensor retinaculum attaching to the floor of the sinus tarsi (Fig. 3.135A).

Medial Talocalcanean Ligament

Runs from the medial tubercle of the posterior talar process to the posterior border of the sustentaculum tali (Fig. 3.136A).

Posterior Talocalcanean Ligament

Short band with fibres radiating out from a narrow attachment on the lateral talar tubercle to the superior and medial surfaces of the calcaneus (Fig. 3.136).

Lateral Talocalcanean Ligament

Lying parallel and deep to the calcaneofibular ligament, the lateral talocalcanean ligament runs obliquely posteroinferiorly from the lateral talar tubercle to the lateral surface of the calcaneus (Fig. 3.136).

Ligamentum Cervicis

At the lateral end of the sinus tarsi is the strong discrete band of the ligamentum cervicis (Fig. 3.135A), attaching to the neck of the talus superiorly and calcaneus inferiorly. It forms a strong ligamentous connection between the two bones, becoming taut in inversion.

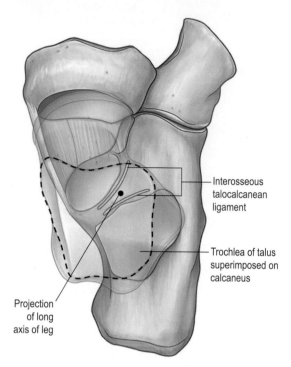

Fig. 3.137 Long axis of the right leg/calf projected onto the foot showing its relationship to the interosseous talocalcanean ligament.

Accessory Ligaments

The calcaneofibular ligament and talocalcaneal part of the deltoid ligament of the ankle joint act as accessory ligaments for the subtalar joint, providing additional support.

Stability

The interosseous talocalcanean ligament plays an essential role in maintaining stability at the subtalar joint, both at rest and during activity. It occupies a central position between the subtalar and talocalcaneonavicular joints, lying directly below the long axis of the leg/calf (Fig. 3.137). Acting as the fulcrum around which movements of the leg/calf and foot occur, the interosseous talocalcanean ligament is continually subjected to twisting and stretching.

The calcaneal parts of the medial and lateral ankle ligaments confer a considerable degree of stability to the subtalar joint by holding the talus between the leg/calf and calcaneus. In addition, the fibularis/peroneal muscles laterally and flexor hallucis longus medially reinforce the ligamentous support; without active muscle

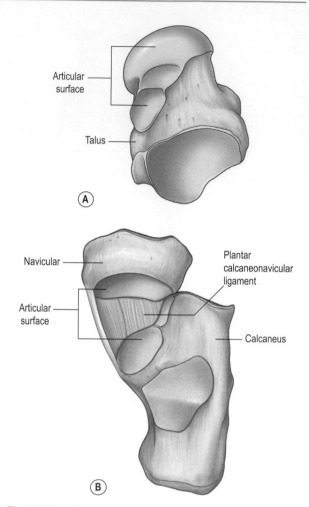

Fig. 3.138 Articular surfaces of the inferior aspect of the (A) talus and (B) articular surfaces of the calcaneus, navicular and plantar calcaneonavicular ligament involved in the talocalcaneonavicular joint.

support, the ligaments around the joint, as well as the joint capsule, would stretch under continuous strain.

TALOCALCANEONAVICULAR JOINT

Articular Surfaces

Synovial joint of the ball-and-socket variety, the ball being formed by a large continuous facet on the head and inferior surface of the neck of the talus (Fig. 3.138A). The articular surface conforms in shape to the socket marked by faint ridges into a facet for the navicular anteriorly, for the sustentaculum tali posteroinferiorly with an anterolateral facet for the anterior part of the calcaneus, and a facet inferomedially for the plantar calcaneonavicular ligament.

The deep extensive socket is formed partly by bone and partly by ligaments (Fig. 3.138B); anteriorly, by the concave articular surface of the navicular and posteriorly the concave superior aspect of the sustentaculum tali, and a concave facet on the anterior end of the superior surface of the calcaneus; the latter two facets may be fused into a single concavity. Between the articular surfaces on the calcaneus and navicular, the head of the talus articulates with the deep surfaces of two ligaments; medially, the plantar calcaneonavicular ligament; laterally, the calcaneonavicular fibres of the bifurcate ligament.

Joint Capsule and Synovial Membrane

A thin joint capsule encloses the common articular cavity; because of the nature of the bony and ligamentous socket, a true fibrous capsule is only present on the posterior and dorsal aspects of the joint. One end of the capsular sleeve attaches to the neck of the talus around the articular margin of the head, extending anteriorly so that the other end of the sleeve attaches to the superior margin of the navicular, medially with the anterior fibres of the deltoid ligament that go to the navicular, superior medial edge of the plantar calcaneonavicular ligament, floor of the sinus tarsi, the medial limb of the bifurcate ligament and back to the superior surface of the navicular. The posterior part within the sinus tarsi blends with the anterior part of the subtalar joint capsule forming the interosseous (talocalcanean) ligament (p. 413).

Synovial membrane lines all non-articular surfaces, including the fat pad lying between the bifurcate and plantar calcaneonavicular ligaments on the plantar aspect of the joint. It is thought that the fat pad helps spread synovial fluid over the moving head of the talus.

Ligaments

Two ligaments are intimately associated with the joint; their deep parts participate in forming the articular surfaces.

Plantar Calcaneonavicular Ligament

Thick, dense, fibroelastic ligament of considerable strength extending from the anterior end and medial border of the sustentaculum tali posteriorly, spreading out to attach to the entire width of the inferior surface of the navicular and its medial surface posterior to the tuberosity (Figs 3.138B and 3.139A). The inferior fibres

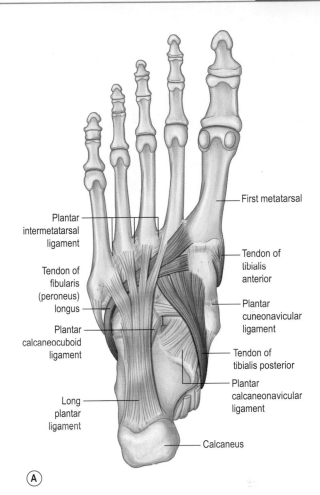

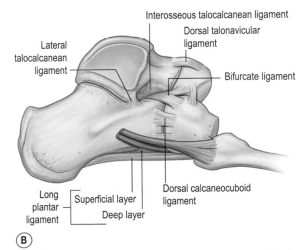

Fig. 3.139 (A) Plantar and (B) lateral aspects of the right foot showing ligaments associated with the talocalcaneonavicular joint.

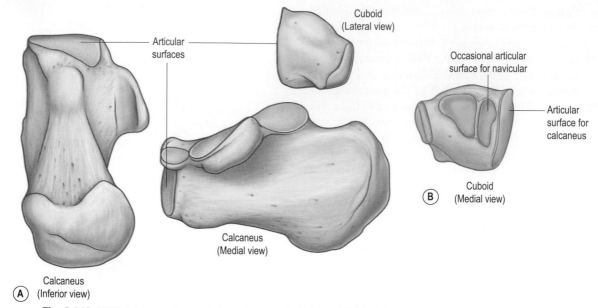

Fig. 3.140 (A) Articular surfaces of the calcaneocuboid joint. (B) Medial aspect of the cuboid showing the occasional articular surface for the navicular.

lie almost transversely across the foot; the ligament blends with and is supported by the deltoid ligament medially. The superior surface of the ligament is smooth and faceted, containing a fibrocartilaginous plate which articulates with the head of the talus (Fig. 3.138B). Because of its elasticity, it is also known and referred to as the 'spring' ligament.

Bifurcate Ligament

The calcaneonavicular part of the bifurcate ligament (completing the socket laterally) is composed of short fibres passing from the superior surface of the anterior aspect of the calcaneus to the adjacent lateral surface of the navicular (Fig. 3.139B). See also page 417.

Dorsal Talonavicular Ligament

Running from the neck of the talus to the dorsal surface of the navicular (Fig. 3.139B), the dorsal talonavicular ligament reinforces the joint capsule dorsally between the bifurcate and plantar calcaneonavicular ligaments.

Stability

The major elements contributing to stability of the joint are the plantar calcaneonavicular and bifurcate ligaments, together with the tendon of tibialis posterior. The latter turns into the sole of the foot inferior to the

plantar calcaneonavicular ligament, which acts as a sling for both the ligament and head of the talus. Tension within the plantar calcaneonavicular ligament, supported by tibialis posterior, resists the tendency of body weight to push the head of the talus inferiorly between the bones with which it articulates.

CALCANEOCUBOID JOINT

Articular Surfaces

Between facets on the anterior surface of the calcaneus and posterior surface of the cuboid (Fig. 3.140); the articular surfaces of both bones are quadrilateral and gently undulating. The superior part of the calcaneal facet is concave transversely and vertically, while the inferior part is convex both transversely and vertically; the articular surface of the cuboid is reciprocally concavoconvex. There may be a medial extension of the cuboid facet for articulation with the navicular (Fig. 3.140B); if present, it is a plane surface.

Palpation

The line of the calcaneocuboid joint can be determined by applying pressure to the dorsal surface of the lateral border of the foot proximal to the tubercle of the fifth metatarsal.

Joint Capsule and Synovial Membrane

A simple fibrous capsule completely surrounds the joint separating the joint cavity from those adjacent; it is thickened superiorly and inferiorly by the dorsal and plantar calcaneocuboid ligaments, respectively. Synovial membrane lines the joint capsule attaching to the margins of the articular surfaces.

Ligaments

Dorsal Calcaneocuboid Ligament

A relatively thin broad band strengthening the dorsal aspect of the capsule (Fig. 3.141A).

Bifurcate Ligament

On the dorsomedial aspect of the joint is the calcaneocuboid part of the bifurcate ligament (Fig. 3.141A). It arises with the calcaneonavicular part from the deep hollow on the superior surface of the calcaneus, lateral to the anterior articular surface, anterior to the sinus tarsi deep to extensor digitorum brevis, attaching to the adjacent dorsomedial angle of the cuboid. This part of the ligament is one of the main connections between the first and second row of tarsal bones.

Plantar Calcaneocuboid Ligament

On the plantar aspect of the joint are two special ligaments separated by areolar tissue; the deeper plantar calcaneocuboid ligament (short plantar ligament) blends with and reinforces the joint capsule (Fig. 3.141B). It is a strong broad band of short fibres passing anteriorly from a rounded eminence at the anterior aspect of the inferior calcaneal surface to the plantar surface of the cuboid posterior to the ridge bounding the fibular/peroneal groove.

Long Plantar Ligament

Superficial to the plantar calcaneocuboid ligament is the long plantar ligament covering the plantar surface of the calcaneus (Fig. 3.141B). Posteriorly, it attaches between the anterior and posterior tubercles of the calcaneus. Passing anteriorly, the deeper fibres attach to the ridge on the cuboid, with intermediate fibres bridging the groove on the cuboid, attaching to its tuberosity, forming a fibrous roof over the tendon of fibularis/peroneus longus. The most superficial fibres pass anteriorly attaching to the bases of the lateral four metatarsals. Most of the ligament is covered by flexor accessorius (quadratus plantae), so that only its posterior part may

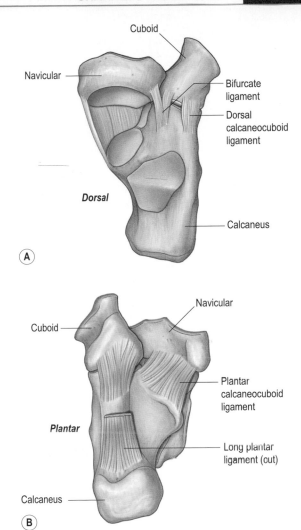

Fig. 3.141 Dorsal (A) and plantar (B) aspects of the right foot showing ligaments associated with the calcaneocuboid joint.

be visible in the gap between the medial fleshy and lateral tendinous parts of the muscle. The long plantar ligament stretches nearly the whole length of the lateral part of the foot strengthening the plantar aspect of all joints in the region.

Stability

The calcaneocuboid joint receives body weight transmitted to the lateral part of the longitudinal arch of the foot; stability is provided by the plantar calcaneocuboid and long plantar ligaments. The tendon of fibularis/peroneus longus passing anteromedially across the cuboid is an important tie reinforcing the ligaments.

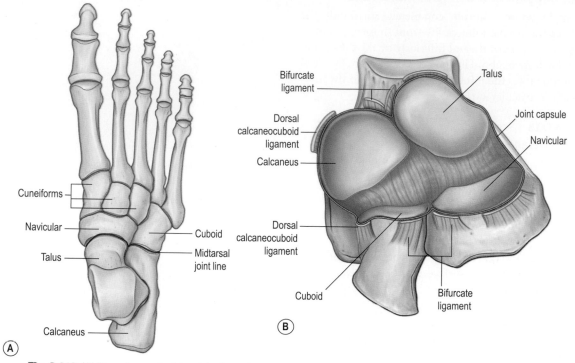

Fig. 3.142 (A) Dorsal aspect of the right foot showing the line of the mid-tarsal joint. (B) Articular surfaces of the mid-tarsal joint (opened).

TRANSVERSE (MID) TARSAL JOINT

The combined talocalcaneonavicular and calcaneocuboid joints, it provides an irregular plane from medial to lateral across the foot with the talus and calcaneus posterior and navicular and cuboid anterior (Figs 3.142 and 3.143). Although the joints do not communicate, they combine in a distinctive pattern of movement providing an important contribution to the action of the foot. A small joint cavity frequently exists between the posteromedial angle of the cuboid and lateral margin of the navicular. When present, the articulation is continuous anteriorly with the cuneonavicular joint.

Ligaments

In addition to the ligaments associated with the component parts of the joint, additional ligaments unite the cuboid and navicular.

Dorsal and Plantar Cuboideonavicular Ligaments

These pass between adjacent parts of the corresponding surfaces of the two bones.

Interosseous Cuboideonavicular Ligament

Strong ligament connecting the rough non-articular portions of their adjacent surfaces.

MOVEMENTS OF THE SUBTALAR AND TRANSVERSE (MID) TARSAL JOINTS

In dorsiflexion and plantarflexion, the talus moves within the tibiofibular mortise enabling the foot to move as a single unit. In other movements of the foot, the calcaneus and navicular move on the talus, carrying with them the distal tarsus and metatarsals. Movements occurring at the subtalar and transverse tarsal joints produce inversion and eversion of the foot, allowing it to be placed firmly on slanting or irregular surfaces, yet still providing a firm base of support. When walking across sloping surfaces one foot is everted and the other inverted. Furthermore, when turning at speed, inversion and eversion are essential to enable leaning sideways on a foot whose sole is flat on the ground. Most inversion/eversion movements are consequently performed on a foot anchored to the ground with the leg/calf and body inverting and everting above it.

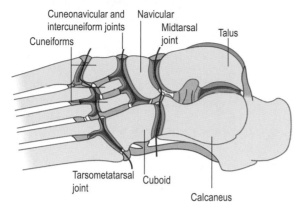

Cuneonavicular and   Navicular
intercuneiform joints
Cuneiforms   Midtarsal   Talus
                         joint

Tarsometatarsal Cuboid
joint
                    Calcaneus

Fig. 3.143 Oblique view of the left foot showing the mid-tarsal and tarsometatarsal joint lines.

In inversion, the foot is twisted raising the medial border and depressing the lateral border until the sole faces medially. Inversion is the combined movement of adduction and supination of the foot, often accompanied by plantarflexion of the foot at the ankle joint; adduction and supination cannot occur as pure movements, one always accompanies the other. Eversion is the opposite of inversion so that the lateral border of the foot is raised and the medial lowered, turning the sole to face laterally. Similarly, eversion is the combined movement of abduction and pronation of the foot, usually accompanied by dorsiflexion of the foot at the ankle joint; abduction and pronation cannot occur as pure movements, one always accompanies the other.

Inversion and eversion occur principally at the subtalar and transverse tarsal joints, although movement does occur at other tarsal and the tarsometatarsal joints, with the amount of movement diminishing the further distal the joint. The composite movements of the calcaneus, navicular and cuboid, with respect to the fixed talus, are complex. Nevertheless, inversion and eversion can be considered to occur around a single axis running obliquely superiorly, anteriorly and medially from the posterolateral tubercle of the calcaneus, through the sinus tarsi in the region of the ligamentum cervicis, emerging at the superomedial aspect of the neck of the talus. The subtalar and transverse tarsal joints are thus mechanically linked.

Inversion is produced by tibialis anterior and tibialis posterior assisted occasionally by extensor and flexor hallucis longus; the dorsiflexing and plantarflexing effects of tibialis muscles cancel out, producing inversion. Under the action of tibialis posterior, the navicular and cuboid are pulled medially (adducted) moving the forefoot anteromedially (Fig. 3.144A); the movement is checked by tension in the dorsal talonavicular ligament. At the same time the two bones rotate about an anteroposterior axis passing through the bifurcate ligament, which actively resists torsion and traction stresses. The rotation produces supination because the navicular is raised while the cuboid is lowered (Fig. 3.144A). Elevation and depression of the medial and lateral longitudinal arches, respectively, cause the sole to face medially.

Eversion is produced by fibularis/peroneus longus, brevis and tertius; the plantarflexing action of fibularis/peroneus longus and brevis are offset by the dorsiflexing action of fibularis/peroneus tertius and extensor digitorum longus. Under the action of the fibularis/peroneal muscles, the navicular and cuboid are pulled laterally (abducted) moving the forefoot anterolaterally (Fig. 3.144B). Rotation of the two bones about the same anteroposterior axis produces pronation by raising the cuboid and lowering the navicular (Fig. 3.144B). The effect on the lateral and medial longitudinal arches is to turn the sole to face laterally. Eversion is checked by impact of the talus on the floor of the sinus tarsi, closing it down. Superior movement of the cuboid on the calcaneus is limited by the anterior process of the calcaneus and tension in the powerful plantar calcaneocuboid ligament, which rapidly stops the joint interspace opening out inferiorly.

During inversion/eversion movements, the calcaneus does not remain immobile below the talus; in inversion, it is pulled anteriorly by the cuboid, while during eversion, it moves posteriorly.

The muscles involved in producing inversion and eversion of the foot are shown Table 3.7. Further details of each muscle can be found in following sections.

Accessory Movements of the Subtalar Joint

With the individual lying prone with the foot overhanging the end of the bed, the talus can be gripped and stabilised by hooking one hand in front of its anterior surface. Firm pressure applied to the back of the heel with the other hand causes the calcaneus to slide forward on the talus.

Accessory Movements of the Calcaneocuboid Joint

With the joint line identified, grip the calcaneus firmly between thumb and index finger of one hand and cuboid with the other; holding the calcaneus still, the cuboid can slide up and down against it.

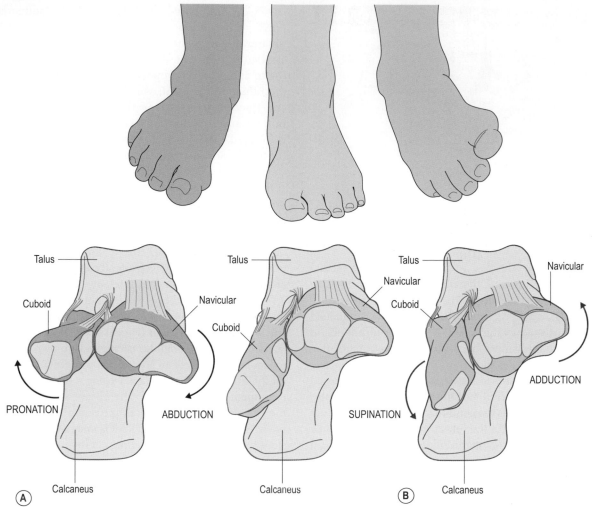

Fig. 3.144 Changing relationship between the talus, calcaneus, cuboid and navicular of the right foot during inversion (A) and eversion (B).

CUNEONAVICULAR JOINT

Articular Surfaces

The anterior surface of the navicular is generally convex but has three distinct articular facets (Fig. 3.145A) separated by more or less vertical ridges for the concave posterior ends of the three cuneiforms. The articular surfaces glide against each other and move apart so that the joint interspaces gape slightly.

Joint Capsule

A distinct fibrous capsule surrounds the joint, except laterally where it may communicate with the cuneocuboid joint and always with the cuboideonavicular joint when present. Anteriorly, the joint cavity forms recesses between the cuneiforms (Fig. 3.143), which may communicate with the tarsometatarsal joint between the intermediate cuneiform and second and third metatarsals, and with the intermetatarsal joints between the second and third, and third and fourth metatarsals.

Ligaments
Dorsal Cuneonavicular Ligaments

Relatively weak short bands in the superior and medial parts of the capsule passing from the navicular to each cuneiform (Fig. 3.145C).

TABLE 3.7   Muscles Involved in Producing Inversion and Eversion of the Foot

Muscle	Attachments	Action	Innervation (root value)
Tibialis anterior	Proximal 2/3rd of lateral surface of tibia and adjacent interosseous membrane to medial aspect of medial cuneiform and base of 1st metatarsal	Invertor of foot at subtalar and mid-tarsal joints; also dorsiflexes foot and ankle joint	Deep fibular (peroneal) nerve (L4, L5)
Tibialis posterior	Proximal 1/2 of posterior surface of tibia below soleal line, interosseous membrane and posterior surface of fibula to medial aspect of navicular and plantar surfaces of all tarsal bones	Main evertor of foot at subtalar and mid-tarsal joints; also aids plantarflexion of foot at ankle joint	Tibial nerve (L4, L5)
Fibularis/ peroneus tertius	Front of distal 1/4 of fibula to medial and dorsal aspects of base of 5th metatarsal	Weak evertor at subtalar and mid-tarsal joints; weak dorsiflexor of foot at ankle joint	Deep fibular (peroneal) nerve (L5, S1)
Fibularis/ peroneus longus	Lateral tibial condyle and proximal 2/3rd of lateral surface of fibula to plantar and lateral surfaces of medial cuneiform and base of 1st metatarsal	Evertor of foot at subtalar and mid-tarsal joints; it also aids plantarflexion of foot at ankle joint	Superficial fibular (peroneal) nerve (L5, S1)
Fibularis/ peroneus brevis	Distal 1/3rd of lateral surface of fibula to tubercle and lateral side of 5th metatarsal	Evertor of foot at subtalar and mid-tarsal joints; also contributes to plantarflexion of foot at ankle joint	Superficial fibular (peroneal) nerve (L5, S1)

Plantar Cuneonavicular Ligaments

Stronger bands on the plantar surface of the joint that blend with and are inseparable from the slips of attachment of the tendon of tibialis posterior.

INTERCUNEIFORM JOINTS

The cuneiforms articulate by plane synovial joints on the posterior aspect of their adjacent surfaces (Fig. 3.143). The three cuneiforms are bound together by relatively weak transverse dorsal intercuneiform ligaments and much stronger interosseous and plantar intercuneiform ligaments; the latter two usually form the anterior boundary of the joint cavities.

CUNEOCUBOID JOINT

Articular Surfaces

Between a round facet on the posterosuperior surface of the cuboid and a large round articular surface on the posterolateral aspect of the lateral cuneiform (Fig. 3.145B).

Palpation

The tuberosity of the navicular can be readily palpated distal to the head of the talus on the medial border of the foot. With careful and fairly deep palpation, the transverse running joint lines of the cuneonavicular joints and anteroposterior joint lines of the intercuneiform joints can be identified on the dorsum of the foot.

Ligaments
Dorsal Cuneocuboid Ligament
Weak band blending with the capsule passing between the dorsal surfaces of the two bones (Fig. 3.145C).

Plantar Cuneocuboid Ligament

Weak ligament attaching to adjacent surfaces of the bones blending with the joint capsule.

Interosseous Cuneocuboid Ligament

Stronger than the dorsal and plantar ligaments, the interosseous cuneocuboid ligament unites adjacent bony surfaces, limiting the joint cavity anteriorly.

Stability

The cuboid and cuneiforms form the tarsal part of the transverse arch. Stability and integrity of the joints are maintained by strong interosseous and plantar intercuneiform and cuneocuboid ligaments; the tendon of fibularis/peroneus longus passing transversely across the foot provides additional support.

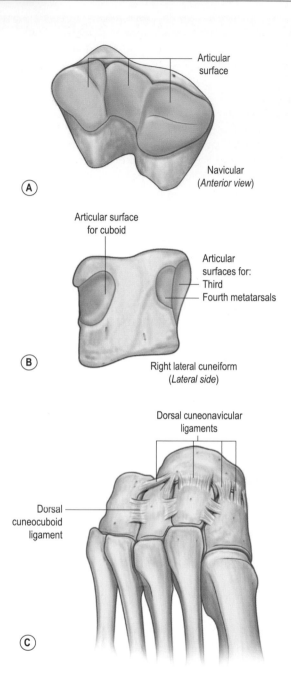

Articular surface

Navicular
(*Anterior view*)

(A)

Articular surface
for cuboid

Articular
surfaces for:
Third
Fourth metatarsals

(B)

Right lateral cuneiform
(*Lateral side*)

Dorsal cuneonavicular
ligaments

Dorsal
cuneocuboid
ligament

(C)

Fig. 3.145 (A) Articular surface of the navicular for the cune-iforms. (B) Articular surface on the lateral cuneiform for the cuboid. (C) Dorsal aspect of the right foot showing the position and attachments of the dorsal cuneonavicular and cuneocuboid ligaments.

Movements

The cuneonavicular, intercuneiform and cuneocuboid joints permit slight gliding between adjacent bones contributing to the flexibility and adaptability of the foot.

Accessory Movements

The basic principle of demonstrating accessory movements at the cuneonavicular, intercuneiform and cuneocuboid joints is the same; one bone is held steady while the other is moved against it. This is achieved by gripping both bones between the thumb and index finger of each hand; gliding of one bone against the other is produced by holding one steady and applying pressure to the other (if the navicular is held steady the medial cuneiform can be moved superiorly and inferiorly against it).

MUSCLES INVERTING THE FOOT

Tibialis posterior
Tibialis anterior (p. 400)

Tibialis Posterior

Deepest muscle in the posterior compartment of the leg/calf (Fig. 3.146), tibialis posterior arises from the proximal half of the lateral aspect of the posterior surface of the tibia (inferior to the soleal line), interosseous membrane, posterior surface of the fibula between the medial crest and interosseous border, and fascia covering it posteriorly. Enclosed in its own synovial sheath, the tendon passes posterior to the medial malleolus grooving it; it lies medial to flexors hallucis longus and digitorum longus, superficial to the deltoid ligament. Lying superficial to the plantar calcaneonavicular ligament, the tendon passes inferiorly attaching principally to the tubercle on the medial side of the navicular and plantar surface of the medial cuneiform (Figs 3.115 and 3.146). Tendinous expansions pass to the plantar surfaces of all tarsal bones except the talus, although a strip passes posteriorly to the tip of the sustentaculum tali, and the bases of the middle three metatarsals.

Innervation

By a branch of the tibial nerve (root value L4, L5). Skin over the area on the posterior aspect of the leg/calf is supplied by root S2.

Action

With tibialis anterior, tibialis posterior is the main invertor of the foot. By its attachment to the tubercle of the

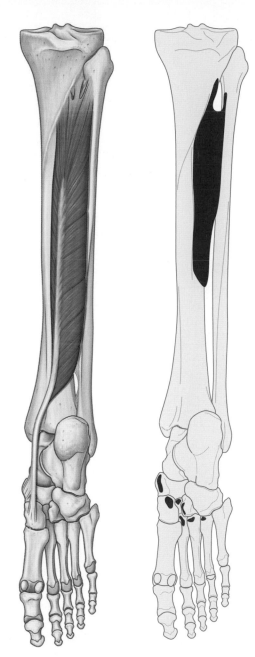

Fig. 3.146 Posterior aspect of the right tibia, fibula and plantar surface of the foot showing the position and attachments of tibialis posterior.

navicular, it pulls superomedially, rotating the forefoot so that the plantar surface faces medially. Inversion and eversion of the foot involve movement at the mid-tarsal joint, with the navicular and cuboid moving against the head of the talus and the calcaneus, respectively (Fig. 3.144).

Tibialis posterior also plantarflexes the foot at the ankle joint, but its contribution is small; gastrocnemius and soleus are better situated having a more direct line of action. If the tendocalcaneus is ruptured, it can produce plantarflexion. Because of its attachments to both the tibia and fibula, contraction of tibialis posterior also tends to bring the two bones closer together. During plantarflexion, the malleoli are approximated maintaining their grip on the narrower posterior part of the trochlear surface of the talus.

Functional Activity

Tibialis posterior helps maintain the balance of the tibia on the foot, particularly when body weight is tending to move laterally. Being a strong invertor of the foot, it controls the forefoot in walking and running by positioning the foot so that the medial arch is not completely flattened. Its many tendinous expansions help maintain the various arches of the foot.

Palpation

It is not possible to palpate the muscle belly as it lies deep to other muscles; it is quite easy to feel the tendon as it passes posterior to the medial malleolus and particularly as it attaches to the tubercle of the navicular. When lying supine, the tendon can be felt and seen behind the medial malleolus when inversion of the plantarflexed foot against resistance is attempted. From just proximal to the flexor retinaculum to its attachment, it is surrounded by a synovial sheath. It is in this area that the tendon becomes painful if the muscle has been overactive; the pain is sharp and knifelike (tenosynovitis).

MUSCLES EVERTING THE FOOT

Fibularis/peroneus longus
Fibularis/peroneus brevis
Fibularis/peroneus tertius

Fibularis/Peroneus Longus

Long thin fusiform muscle (Figs 3.147A and 3.161B) situated on the lateral side of the leg/calf, fibularis/peroneus longus has a long belly and even longer tendon. It is unique in that the tendon changes direction three times on its way to attach to the medial aspect of the sole of the foot.

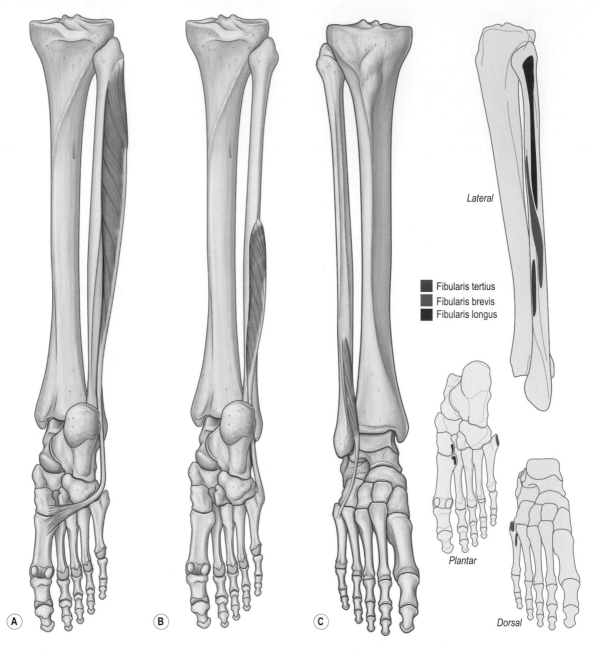

Lateral

Fibularis tertius
Fibularis brevis
Fibularis longus

Plantar

Dorsal

Fig. 3.147 Posterior aspect of the right tibia, fibula and plantar surface of the foot showing the position and attachments of fibularis/peroneus longus (A) and fibularis/peroneus brevis (B). (C) Anterior aspect of the right tibia, fibula and dorsum of the foot showing the position and attachments of fibularis/peroneus tertius.

It arises from a small area on the lateral condyle of the tibia (with extensor digitorum longus) and proximal two-thirds of the lateral surface of the fibula, its distal half lying posterior to the proximal part of the attachment of fibularis/peroneus brevis. It also has an attachment to the lateral side of the head of the fibula, leaving a small area around the neck for the passage of the common fibular/peroneal nerve anteriorly. It has an attachment to the intermuscular septa and fascia surrounding the muscle, both anteriorly and posteriorly.

The tendon forms about a hand's breadth above the lateral malleolus, lying superficial to that of fibularis/peroneus brevis, sharing the same synovial sheath. It runs in a shallow groove posterior to the lateral malleolus, passing deep to the superior fibular/peroneal retinaculum. From here, the tendon passes inferiorly and slightly anteriorly inferior to the fibular/peroneal tubercle on the calcaneus, being held in position by the inferior band of the inferior fibular/peroneal retinaculum; here the tendon is enclosed in a separate synovial sheath. Reaching the inferolateral side of the cuboid, grooving it, the tendon turns, entering the groove on its inferior aspect. The groove is converted into a tunnel by fibres from the long plantar ligament and tibialis posterior tendon; in the tunnel the tendon is still surrounded by a synovial sheath. The tunnel conveys the tendon anteromedially across the foot to attach to the plantar and lateral surfaces of the medial cuneiform and base of the first metatarsal.

Innervation

By the superficial fibular/peroneal nerve (root value L5, S1). Skin covering the muscle is supplied by roots L5 and S1.

Action

Because it arises from the lateral side of the leg/calf and passes around the lateral side of the foot fibularis/peroneus longus is an evertor of the foot. Passing from posterior to the lateral malleolus to the medial cuneiform and first metatarsal, it produces plantarflexion of the foot, with the medial side of the foot drawn inferiorly as in pronation.

It is worth noting that the distal attachment is to the same two bones as tibialis anterior, although the latter approaches from the medial side of the foot; this provides a stirrup for the arches of the foot, helping control their height during activity. The attachment of both muscles to the medial cuneiform and base of the first metatarsal emphasises the importance of the control of the medial side of the foot during activity, particularly on uneven terrain.

Functional Activity

In standing, fibularis/peroneus longus, together with surrounding muscles, helps maintain the erect position controlling mediolateral sway by pressing the medial side of the foot to the ground. This function is better seen and appreciated when standing on one lower limb when fibularis/peroneus longus works hard maintaining the leg/calf over the foot, preventing the body from falling to the opposite side. Its main functional activity, however, is during powerful action of the foot (running, especially over rough ground) where its control, together with that of tibialis anterior, over the medial side of the foot and first metatarsal (carrying the hallux) is vital.

Palpation

When seated, place the fingers on the lateral side of the knee and locate the head of the fibula just below the level of the knee joint; the tendon of biceps femoris can be identified coming from the posterior thigh. Run the fingers inferiorly, keeping the tip of the index finger on the head of the fibula, and spread the remaining fingertips down the lateral side of the fibula. Keeping the fingers in this position, raise the lateral side of the foot; the long vertical muscle belly can be felt contracting. If the fingers are placed below and behind the lateral malleolus and the same manoeuvre is performed, the tendons of fibularis/peroneus longus and brevis can be palpated and traced to the fibular/peroneal tubercle where they part, longus passing below and brevis above.

Fibularis/Peroneus Brevis

Situated on the lateral side of the leg/calf, enclosed in the same osseofascial compartment as fibularis/peroneus longus (Figs 3.147B and 3.161B). It arises from the distal two-thirds of the lateral surface of the fibula, the proximal half anterior to fibularis/peroneus longus; it also attaches to the intermuscular septa at its sides.

The muscle belly is fusiform and short, soon becoming a tendon accompanying that of fibularis/peroneus longus passing posterior to the lateral malleolus in a common synovial sheath. The tendon passes anteroinferiorly into a groove superior to the fibular/peroneal tubercle on the calcaneus, which is converted into a tunnel by the superior band of the inferior fibular/peroneal retinaculum; superior to the tubercle, the tendon is surrounded by a synovial sheath separate from that of fibularis/peroneus longus. It then passes anteriorly to its attachment to the tubercle on the lateral side of the base of the fifth metatarsal. A slip from the tendon usually joins the long extensor tendon to the little toe; other separate slips may join fibularis/peroneus longus or pass to the calcaneus or cuboid.

Innervation

By the superficial fibular/peroneal nerve (root value L5, S1). Skin covering the muscle is innervated by roots L5, S1 and S2.

Action

Fibularis/peroneus brevis is an evertor of the foot. Because of its course and attachments, the pull of its tendon produces plantarflexion of the ankle at the same time.

Functional Activity

The muscle is well positioned to prevent mediolateral sway when standing; when standing on one lower limb, it helps prevent the body falling to the opposite side. In walking or running, especially over rough ground, it plays an important role in controlling foot position, preventing it from becoming too inverted. In many cases, however, this mechanism does not always appear to work correctly with the foot often overinverting, causing the weight to come down on the lateral side of the foot, forcing it into further inversion. This can severely damage or even snap the tendon and, often, the anterior talofibular ligament of the ankle joint.

Palpation

With the fingers placed over the belly of fibularis/peroneus longus, move inferiorly to the distal half of the fibula (but in the same vertical line), the muscle can be palpated when the foot is everted and plantarflexed. Its tendon can be traced to the groove just above the fibular/peroneal tubercle and then anteriorly to its attachment to the tubercle of the fifth metatarsal.

Fibularis/Peroneus Tertius

Situated on the distal lateral aspect of the leg/calf fibularis/peroneus tertius (Figs 3.147C and 3.161B) appears to have been part of extensor digitorum longus. It arises from the anterior aspect of the lower quarter of the fibula in continuation with the attachment of extensor digitorum longus (with no gap between them), the intermuscular septum and adjoining fascia. Its fibres pass inferolaterally to a tendon passing deep to the superior and through the inferior extensor retinaculum to attach to the medial and dorsal aspect of the base of the fifth metatarsal.

Innervation

By the deep fibular (peroneal) nerve (root value L5, S1). Skin covering the muscle is also supplied by roots L5 and S1.

Action

Weak evertor and dorsiflexor of the foot at the ankle joint.

Functional Activity

It is difficult to assess the importance of this small muscle as its actions appear to be covered by other muscles having a much better mechanical leverage; in some individuals it is absent. It does, however, pass superficial to the anterior talofibular ligament of the ankle joint and is often damaged in inversion injuries. It is well placed to help prevent excessive inversion during sporting activities and may be responsible for reducing the number of injuries. Unfortunately, it is often torn and may be completely ruptured during violent inversion, resulting in considerable pain and swelling. It is possible that, with the attainment of bipedalism, fibularis/peroneus tertius has assumed a more important role as eversion of the foot is a peculiarly human characteristic.

Palpation

Fibularis/peroneus tertius is very difficult to palpate. However, by drawing the fingers inferiorly from the anterior part of the lateral malleolus into the small hollow found there, the tendon can be felt crossing the lateral part of the hollow to its attachment to the medial side of the base of the fifth metatarsal. Care should be taken not to confuse the tendon of fibularis/peroneus tertius with that of fibularis/peroneus brevis, which lies lateral as it passes anteriorly to attach to the tubercle on the lateral side of the fifth metatarsal.

TARSOMETATARSAL JOINTS

These are between the four anterior tarsal bones (cuboid, cuneiforms) and bases of all five metatarsals (Fig. 3.148A); the 'joint line' is irregular and arched, yet remains fairly mobile.

Articular Surfaces

The plane synovial tarsometatarsal joints overlap one another. The first metatarsal articulates only with the medial cuneiform; the base of the second metatarsal is

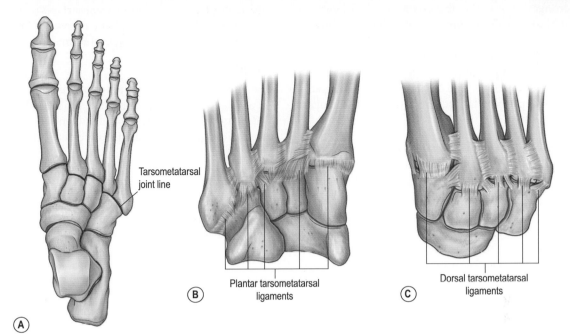

Fig. 3.148 (A) Tarsometatarsal joint line seen on the dorsum of the right foot. (B) Plantar and (C) dorsal tarsometatarsal ligaments.

held in a mortise formed by the three cuneiforms articulating with all of them (lateral side of the medial, anterior end of the intermediate, medial side of the lateral) (Fig. 3.148A); because of this deep mortise, the second metatarsal is the least mobile. The third metatarsal articulates with the lateral cuneiform only; the fourth mainly with the cuboid, but also to a small extent with the lateral cuneiform; and the fifth only with the cuboid.

Palpation

The transverse joint line between the base of the first metatarsal and medial cuneiform is palpable on the medial side of the foot. Similarly, on the lateral side, the joint line between the base of the fifth metatarsal and cuboid is also easily recognised. However, the joint lines of the second, third and fourth tarsometatarsal joints are not so easy to determine.

Joint Cavities, Capsule and Synovial Membrane

The presence of two strong interosseous tarsometatarsal ligaments divides the joint cavity into three separate parts (Fig. 3.143). The medial cavity is confined to the articulation between the first metatarsal and medial cuneiform. The intermediate cavity includes the articulations between the second and third metatarsals with the intermediate and lateral cuneiforms, respectively; it is usually prolonged anteriorly between the bases of the two metatarsals and may also communicate posteriorly with the cuneonavicular joint between the intermediate and medial cuneiforms. The lateral cavity is the articulation between the fourth and fifth metatarsals and cuboid extending anteriorly between the bases of the two metatarsals.

The joint capsules surrounding the tarsometatarsal joints attach to the articular margins of the various bones. In practice, there are very few true capsular fibres as the interosseous, plantar and dorsal tarsometatarsal ligaments close the joints.

Synovial membrane lines the non-articular joint surfaces attaching to the articular margins.

Ligaments
Plantar Tarsometatarsal Ligaments
Similar bands on the plantar surface of the joints but generally less well organised, consisting of both longitudinal and oblique fibres (Fig. 3.148B). The ligaments associated with the medial two metatarsals are

the strongest; the remaining tarsometatarsal joints are strengthened by fibres from the long plantar ligament.

Dorsal Tarsometatarsal Ligaments

Weak short slips passing between adjacent dorsal surfaces of the tarsal bones and metatarsals; each metatarsal receives a slip from the tarsal bones that it articulates with (Fig. 3.148C).

Interosseous Tarsometatarsal Ligaments

Two interosseous tarsometatarsal ligaments are always present; there may occasionally be a third. The first interosseous ligament passes from the anterolateral surface of the medial cuneiform to the medial side of the base of the second metatarsal. The second interosseous ligament passes from the anterolateral angle of the lateral cuneiform to the medial surface of the base of the fourth metatarsal. Between them is found the third inconstant interosseous ligament; when present, it passes from the lateral side of the second metatarsal to the lateral cuneiform.

Stability

The various ligaments associated with the joints convey a certain degree of stability, especially medially. Stability is reinforced on the plantar surface medially by the attachment of muscles. Slips from tibialis posterior tendon reinforce the plantar aspects of the joints of the medial three metatarsals. The attachment of tibialis anterior to the medial sides of the first metatarsal and medial cuneiform, and of fibularis/peroneus longus laterally, further strengthens and stabilises the tarsometatarsal joint of the hallux.

INTERMETATARSAL JOINTS

The bases of the lateral four metatarsals articulate by small synovial joints between facets on their adjacent sides (Fig. 3.143); there is no joint between the bases of the first and second metatarsals as they are united by interosseous fibres only. The joint spaces between the second and third, and third and fourth metatarsals are anterior extensions of the intermediate tarsometatarsal joint cavity, while that between the fourth and fifth metatarsals is continuous with the lateral tarsometatarsal joint cavity.

The joint spaces are closed on their dorsal and plantar aspects by transverse running dorsal and plantar ligaments passing between adjacent surfaces of the metatarsal bases. Anteriorly, the joint spaces are limited by the strong interosseous metatarsal ligaments.

Palpation

The lines of the metatarsal joints between the first and second, and fourth and fifth metatarsals can be identified running anteroposteriorly between the bones; the intervening joint lines are difficult to determine.

Stability

This is due to the dorsal, plantar and interosseous metatarsal ligaments. The strong bands of the interosseous ligaments help maintain the transverse arch of the foot by holding together the metatarsal bases as segments of that arch.

Blood Supply and Innervation

The blood supply to the tarsometatarsal and intertarsal joints is from branches of the dorsalis pedis on their dorsal aspects and medial and lateral plantar arteries of their plantar aspect.

Similarly, the nerve supply is by twigs from the deep fibular/peroneal nerve dorsally and medial and lateral plantar nerves on their plantar aspect.

MOVEMENTS OF THE TARSOMETATARSAL JOINTS

Except for the first tarsometatarsal joint, interlocking of the bones and strong intermetatarsal ligaments permits only a small degree of movement; nevertheless, the joints contribute to the flexibility of the foot, particularly inversion and eversion.

As a whole, the line of the tarsometatarsal joints runs obliquely from medial, superior and anterior to lateral, inferior and posterior so that its medial end lies approximately 2 cm anterior to the lateral end (Fig. 3.149A). Although the joint line as a whole is oblique, the ends have opposite obliquity; the medial joint space runs anterolaterally and the lateral anteromedially. The obliquity of the axis essentially only allowing flexion and extension is a contributory factor to inversion and eversion. Consequently, the axis of flexion and extension of the lateral tarsometatarsal joints is oblique to the long axis of the metatarsals, so that during plantarflexion, the metatarsals move towards the axis of the foot (flexion of the metatarsals is accompanied by adduction). Similarly,

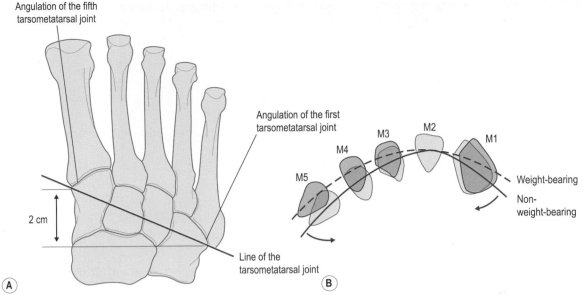

Fig. 3.149 (A) Obliquity of the tarsometatarsal joint axis, with the medial end being some 2 cm anterior to the lateral end. (B) Change in transverse metatarsal arch height upon weight-bearing.

because of the obliquity of the first tarsometatarsal joint, plantarflexion of the first metatarsal is accompanied by about 15 degrees of adduction (Fig. 3.149B).

Plantarflexion and adduction of the first metatarsal are accompanied by slight rotation; adduction of the metatarsals is assisted by the shapes of the articular surfaces of the cuboid and cuneiforms.

As the heads of the metatarsals move inferiorly and towards the axis of the foot in plantarflexion, this increases the curvature of the transverse arch with a hollowing of the anterior part of the foot (Fig. 3.149B). Conversely, dorsiflexion at the tarsometatarsal joint in which the metatarsals move superiorly and away from the axis of the foot causes a flattening of the transverse arch.

The mobility of the first metatarsal compared with the remaining ones is necessary during adaptation of the foot to the ground in inversion and eversion, as when walking over rough terrain. In contrast, the immobility of the second metatarsal wedged between the medial and lateral cuneiforms, together with the slenderness of its shaft, is a contributory factor in its 'spontaneous' fracture (also referred to as a 'March' fracture).

Accessory Movements

Accessory movements between adjacent bones can be demonstrated by holding one bone steady and moving the other. The most impressive movement in this region is that between the base of the fifth metatarsal and cuboid.

METATARSOPHALANGEAL JOINTS

Articular Surfaces

Synovial condyloid joints between the rounded head of the metatarsal and cupped base of the proximal phalanx (Fig. 3.150). The convex metatarsal articular surfaces cover the dorsal, distal and plantar surfaces, with the plantar surface being more extensive facilitating plantarflexion at the joint.

Palpation

With the metatarsophalangeal joints flexed the metatarsal heads stand out and can be palpated on the dorsum of the foot. If the toes are moved slowly back to the neutral position the line of each metatarsophalangeal joints can be identified of the dorsum of the foot.

Joint Capsule

The joint capsule is loose attaching close to the articular margins of the bones (Fig. 3.151A); it is lined by synovial membrane, which also attaches to the articular margins. The capsule is reinforced laterally by strong collateral ligaments, on its plantar surface by the plantar ligament and dorsally by fibres from the extensor tendons.

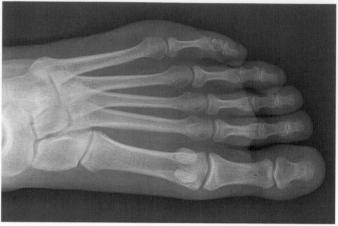

Fig. 3.150 Radiograph showing the tarsometatarsal, metatarsophalangeal and interphalangeal joints of the right foot. (From Herring, W., 2023. Learning radiology: recognizing the basics. Elsevier.)

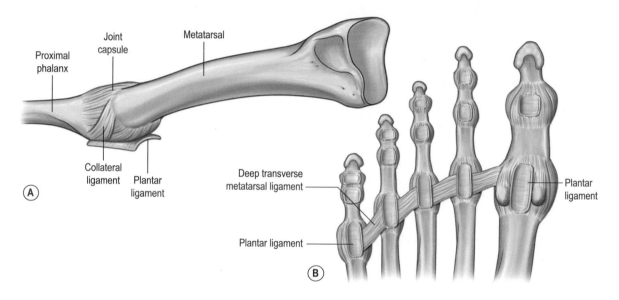

Fig. 3.151 (A) Metatarsophalangeal joint showing the arrangement of the collateral and plantar ligaments. (B) Plantar aspect of the right forefoot showing the relation of the plantar ligaments to the deep transverse metatarsal ligament.

Ligaments
Collateral Ligaments

Strong collateral ligaments associated with each joint pass from the tubercles on each side of the metatarsal head, fanning out to attach to the sides of the base of the phalanx and sides of the plantar ligament (Fig. 3.151A). Passing obliquely anteroinferiorly, they become tense during flexion restricting this movement.

Plantar Ligament

Dense fibrocartilaginous plate firmly attached to the plantar border of the base of the proximal phalanx, forming part of the articular surface for the metatarsal head, attaching at the sides to the collateral and deep transverse metatarsal ligaments. In the hallux, sesamoid bones and their interconnecting ligamentous band almost completely replace the plantar ligament. The sesamoid bones

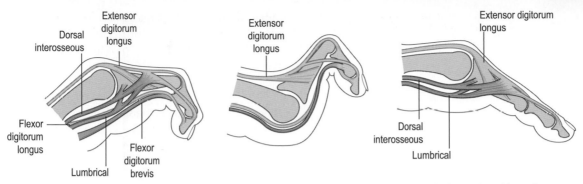

Fig. 3.152 Medial aspect of the second toe showing movements at the metatarsophalangeal and interphalangeal joints.

are cartilage covered on their superior surface articulating with grooves on the inferior surface of the head of the first metatarsal. The plantar ligaments are grooved by the long flexor tendons passing to the toes.

Deep Transverse Metatarsal Ligament

The plantar ligaments of all joints are interconnected by the deep transverse metatarsal ligament, which connects the heads and joint capsules of all metatarsals (Fig. 3.151B). It is crossed on its plantar surface by the tendons of the lumbrical muscles and on its dorsal surface by the tendons of the interossei.

Stability

The metatarsophalangeal joints have the long extensor and flexor tendons crossing their dorsal and plantar surfaces, respectively. In the lateral four toes, these provide some stability for the joints; however, the hallux has no extensor expansion or flexor sheath, the long tendons being held in place by strands of deep fascia. If the phalanges of the hallux become displaced laterally and the fibrous sheaths give way, the pull of extensor hallucis longus, like that of extensor hallucis brevis, becomes oblique to the long axis of the toe, tending to increase the hallux valgus deformity.

In rheumatoid arthritis, the metatarsophalangeal joints often assume a dorsiflexed position due to imbalance in muscle tension across the joint. There may be dislocation of the sesamoid bones, becoming repositioned in the first web space. In association with the dorsiflexed position of the joint, the metatarsal heads become depressed and subcutaneous; if the depression is severe, it produces a plantarward convex arch.

MOVEMENTS AT THE METATARSOPHALANGEAL JOINTS

The metatarsophalangeal joints permit dorsiflexion, plantarflexion, abduction, adduction and circumduction. Dorsiflexion is by the extensors such that the proximal phalanx can be carried beyond the line of the metatarsal (Fig. 3.152). During dorsiflexion, the toes tend to be spread apart, becoming slightly inclined laterally. The total range of movement for the hallux is 110 degrees, of which the majority is dorsiflexion (Shereff et al., 1986). Observation suggests that the remaining toes have a total range of movement between 80 degrees medially and 40 degrees laterally, again with the majority of movement being dorsiflexion.

Plantarflexion is performed by the flexor tendons passing to the digits (Fig. 3.152), during which the toes tend to be pulled together.

Because of the arrangement of the interosseous muscles and immobility of the second metatarsal, abduction and adduction take place about the second toe. Abduction is produced by the dorsal interossei and abductors hallucis and digiti minimi, adduction by the plantar interossei and adductor hallucis.

Accessory Movements

With the head of the metatarsal gripped and stabilised between the thumb and index finger of one hand and the adjacent phalanx held with the other, the phalanx can be slid up and down, as well as rotated with respect to the metatarsal.

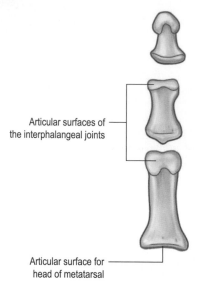

Articular surfaces of
the interphalangeal joints

Articular surface for
head of metatarsal

Fig. 3.153 Plantar aspect of the phalanges showing the articular surfaces of the interphalangeal joints.

INTERPHALANGEAL JOINTS

Articular Surfaces

The head of the more proximal phalanx articulates with the base of the next distal phalanx (Figs 3.148A and 3.150). The heads of the phalanges have a pulley-shaped articular surface, which appears as a double convexity, articulating with a double concavity on the base of the more distal phalanx (Fig. 3.153).

Palpation

The larger interphalangeal joints can be palpated on the dorsal surface of the toes; the joint lines run transversely between the bones.

Joint Capsule

As with the metatarsophalangeal joints, the joint capsule attaches close to the articular margins, reinforced or often replaced by collateral ligaments at the sides, the thick plantar ligament and the expansion of the extensor tendon, where appropriate, dorsally. The joint capsule is lined by synovial membrane attaching to the articular margins. The distal interphalangeal joint of the little toe is often obliterated.

Ligaments
Collateral Ligaments

Strong collateral ligaments of each joint pass inferoanteriorly from the sides of the head of each phalanx adjacent to the articular surface to the base of the more distal phalanx, attaching adjacent to the articular surface (Fig. 3.151A); they also pass to the sides of the plantar ligaments.

Plantar Ligaments

Like those of the metatarsophalangeal joints, the plantar ligaments are fibrocartilaginous pads forming part of the articular surface for the phalangeal head.

Blood Supply and Innervation

The blood and nerve supply to both metatarsophalangeal and interphalangeal joints are from branches of the dorsal and plantar digital vessels and nerves.

MOVEMENTS AT THE INTERPHALANGEAL JOINTS

Due to the shape of the articular surfaces, the interphalangeal joints are hinge joints, permitting dorsiflexion and plantarflexion only (Fig. 3.152). Plantarflexion towards the sole of the foot is produced by flexors digitorum longus and brevis at the distal and proximal interphalangeal joints, respectively. Dorsiflexion away from the sole is produced by the extensor muscles, as well as the lumbricals and interossei. The range of motion for the hallux is 45 degree plantarflexion and 70 degree dorsiflexion (American Association of Orthopaedic Surgeons, 1994). For the lesser toes, the ranges of plantarflexion and dorsiflexion at the proximal interphalangeal joint are 35 and 40 degrees, and 60 and 40 degrees for the distal interphalangeal joint.

Accessory Movement

Similar to those for the metatarsophalangeal joints, except that there is little rotation.

Muscles crossing and producing movement at the metatarsophalangeal and interphalangeal joints are given in Table 3.8. Further details of each muscle can be found in following sections.

BIOMECHANICS

Owing to its wide variety of functions, the foot may be considered one of the most dynamic structures within the body, providing physical contact with the environment. It is strong enough to support the weight of the body, yet also flexible and resilient to absorb shocks transmitted to it while providing the spring and lift for

TABLE 3.8 **Muscles Crossing and Producing Movement at the Metatarsophalangeal and Interphalangeal Joints**

Muscle	Attachments	Action	Innervation (root value)
Extensor hallucis longus	Middle 1/2 of anterior surface of fibula and adjacent interosseous membrane to base of distal phalanx of hallux	Extensor of all joints of the hallux; also a powerful dorsiflexor of foot at ankle joint	Deep fibular (peroneal) nerve (L5, S1)
Extensor digitorum longus	Lateral condyle of tibia, anterior surface of fibula and proximal part of interosseous membrane, dividing into four tendons (at level of ankle joint) to base of middle phalanx of each toe	Extensor of metatarsophalangeal joints of lateral four toes and assists extension at the interphalangeal joints; also aids dorsiflexion of foot at ankle joint	Deep fibular (peroneal) nerve (L5, S1)
Flexor hallucis longus	Distal 2/3rd of posterior surface of fibula to base of distal phalanx of hallux	Flexor of all joints of hallux; also aids plantarflexion of foot at ankle joint	Tibial nerve (S1, S2)
Flexor digitorum longus	Posterior surface of tibia (dividing into four tendons in sole of foot) to base of distal phalanx of lateral four toes	Flexor of all joints of lateral four toes; also aids plantarflexion of foot at ankle joint; with ankle plantarflexed its action on toes is diminished	Tibial nerve (L5, S1, S2)
Extensor digitorum brevis	Superior surface of calcaneus to extensor expansion of second, third and fourth toes	Aids extensor digitorum longus dorsiflex second, third and fourth toes at metatarsophalangeal joints; also helps lumbricals dorsiflex interphalangeal joints	Deep fibular (peroneal) nerve (L5, S1)
Extensor hallucis brevis	Superior surface of calcaneus to base of proximal phalanx of hallux	Aids extensor hallucis longus dorsiflex hallux at metatarsophalangeal joint	Deep fibular (peroneal) nerve (L5, S1)
Lumbricals	Medial sides of tendons of flexor digitorum longus to medial side of extensor expansion and base of proximal phalanx of same toe	Plantarflexor of toes at metatarsophalangeal joints and dorsiflexor of interphalangeal joints	1st (medial) medial plantar nerve (S1, S2); 2nd, 3rd, 4th (lateral 3) lateral plantar nerve (S2, S3)
Flexor accessorius (quadratus plantae)	Calcaneus and long plantar ligament to tendon of flexor digitorum longus proximal to attachment of lumbricals	Aids long flexor tendons plantarflex all joints of lateral four toes; is important during walking when flexor digitorum longus is already shortened	Lateral plantar nerve (S2, S3)
Flexor digitorum brevis	Calcaneus and plantar aponeurosis splitting into separate tendons to lateral four toes	Plantarflexor of proximal interphalangeal joints followed by plantarflexion of metatarsophalangeal joints	Medial plantar nerve (S1, S2)
Flexor hallucis brevis	Cuboid, lateral cuneiform and tendon of tibialis posterior to base of proximal phalanx of hallux	Plantarflexor of metatarsophalangeal joint of hallux	Medial plantar nerve (S1, S2)
Flexor digiti minimi brevis	Plantar surface of base of 5th metatarsal to plantar surface of proximal phalanx of fifth toe	Plantarflexor of metatarsophalangeal joint of fifth toe; also helps support lateral longitudinal arch of foot	Lateral plantar nerve (S2, S3)

Continued

TABLE 3.8   Muscles Crossing and Producing Movement at the Metatarsophalangeal and Interphalangeal Joints—cont'd

Muscle	Attachments	Action	Innervation (root value)
Abductor hallucis	Plantar aspect of calcaneus to medial side of base of proximal phalanx of hallux	Abducts and helps plantarflex hallux at metatarsophalangeal joint	Medial plantar nerve (S1, S2)
Abductor digiti minimi	Calcaneus to base of proximal phalanx of fifth toe	Abducts and helps plantarflex fifth toe at metatarsophalangeal joint	Lateral plantar nerve (S2, S3)
Adductor hallucis	Bases of 2nd, 3rd and 4th metatarsals (oblique head) and plantar surfaces of lateral 3 metatarsophalangeal joints (transverse head) to lateral side of base of proximal phalanx of hallux	Adducts hallux towards second toe and plantarflexes metatarsophalangeal joint of hallux	Lateral plantar nerve (S2, S3)
Dorsal interossei	Sides of adjacent metatarsals to side of proximal phalanx and capsule of metatarsophalangeal joint	Abductor of toes at metatarsophalangeal joint; with plantar interossei plantarflex metatarsophalangeal joint	Lateral plantar nerve (S2, S3)
Plantar interossei	Medial side of base of metatarsal to medial side of base of proximal phalanx	Adducts third, fourth and fifth toes second: with dorsal interossei plantarflex metatarsophalangeal joint of lateral 3 toes	Lateral plantar nerve (S2, S3)

many activities. Changes in its structure and/or flexibility modify its function, resulting in changes in the way the foot is used during activity.

The arched structure of the foot involves a number of bones and their interconnecting joints, together with numerous ligaments and muscle action, giving it the stability and flexibility necessary for function. Of the longitudinal arches, the medial has a greater curvature and is characterised by its remarkable elasticity. The more rigid and flatter lateral arch makes contact with the ground, providing a firm base of support in the erect position. The factors maintaining the integrity of the arches of the foot are the same as those in any joint of the body (ligaments, muscles); however, their relative importance differs for each of the three arches of the foot.

In the medial longitudinal arch, ligaments are important but, by themselves, are incapable of maintaining the arch. The plantar aponeurosis is the most important ligament stretching between the supporting pillars of the arch (Fig. 3.154); extension of the toes tightens the aponeurosis, bringing the pillars closer together and increasing the concavity of the arch. The

plantar calcaneonavicular ('spring') ligament supports the head of the talus, preventing it from sinking between the navicular and calcaneus (Fig. 3.154); when stretched the medial arch decreases in height. In addition to these two major ligamentous components, all the interosseous ligaments assist in maintaining the medial arch; however, muscles are indispensable as, if they are paralysed or weakened, the ligaments alone cannot cope.

In a living foot, the medial arch cannot be flattened because the ligaments are too strong. In static standing, the ligaments are the primary support; the muscles are relaxed. Muscular support of the foot only becomes significant in the larger movements of shifting the weight in the erect posture and in more extensive body movements. If the muscles weaken, the ligaments progressively stretch resulting in flat foot, which is usually accompanied by eversion and adduction of the forefoot.

The most important and efficient muscular supports are those running longitudinally beneath the medial arch (Fig. 3.154). Of these, flexor hallucis longus is the most efficient, being the largest of the deep leg/calf

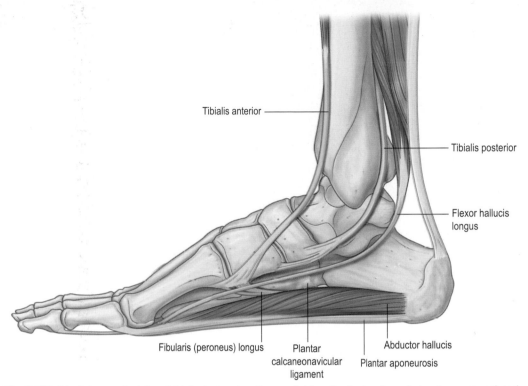

Tibialis anterior

Tibialis posterior

Flexor hallucis longus

Fibularis (peroneus) longus

Plantar calcaneonavicular ligament

Abductor hallucis

Plantar aponeurosis

Fig. 3.154 Medial aspect of the right foot showing the medial longitudinal arch and structures associated with its maintenance.

muscles; as well as running to the hallux, it also gives a slip to the tendons of flexor digitorum longus passing to the second and third toes. During short periods of standing, flexor hallucis longus is not active because body weight is supported towards the posterior aspect of the foot with the pads of the toe off the ground. However, in prolonged standing flexor hallucis longus contracts, pressing the toe pads against the ground, relieving the ligaments. It is during the toe-off phase of gait, and when landing on the feet, that flexor hallucis longus contracts strongly, taking the greater strain placed on the medial arch. Abductor hallucis and the medial part of flexor digitorum brevis also assist in maintaining the arch.

Both tibialis anterior and posterior significantly influence the medial arch (Fig. 3.154), but in a different way to the muscles already mentioned, as they have no direct action on the pillars of the arch; their action of inverting and adducting the foot raises the medial border from the ground. Although of functional

importance, these two muscles are less important factors in maintaining arch integrity. Finally, fibularis/peroneus longus accentuates the medial arch by pulling it towards the ground during eversion (Fig. 3.154); fibularis/peroneal spasm in young children is usually seen as an everted flat-foot.

In the lateral longitudinal arch, ligaments play a relatively more important role than medially, with the lateral part of the plantar aponeurosis and various plantar ligaments being significant in their action. The thick short plantar ligament joins the calcaneus and cuboid, while the thinner long plantar ligament helps maintain the concavity of the arch (Fig. 3.155). Several muscles provide support for the lateral arch. Fibularis/peroneus longus pulls it superiorly as its tendon passes under the foot, also providing elastic support for the calcaneus as it passes inferior to the fibular/peroneal tubercle (Fig. 3.155); it is the single most important factor maintaining the integrity of the lateral arch. Fibularis/peroneus brevis and tertius

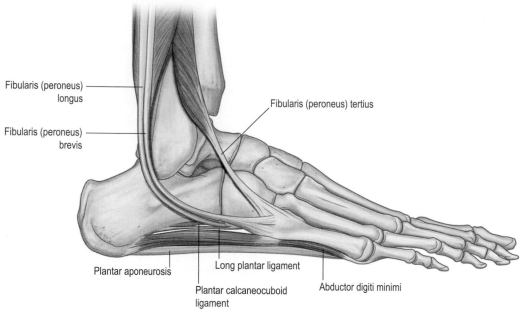

Fibularis (peroneus) longus

Fibularis (peroneus) brevis

Fibularis (peroneus) tertius

Plantar aponeurosis

Long plantar ligament

Plantar calcaneocuboid ligament

Abductor digiti minimi

Fig. 3.155 Lateral aspect of the right foot showing the lateral longitudinal arch and the structures associated with its maintenance.

prevent the arch opening out inferiorly. The tendons of flexor digitorum longus to the fourth and fifth toes, assisted by flexor accessorius (quadratus plantae), together with the lateral half of flexor digitorum brevis and abductor digiti minimi help maintain the lateral arch by preventing separation of the supporting pillars.

Although the wedge-shaped cuneiforms and, to some extent, the cuboid suggest that integrity of the transverse arch is maintained by bony factors, because of the shape of the medial cuneiform, it is clear that bony factors play only a small part. Ligaments binding together the cuneiforms and bases of the metatarsals are more important; however, the most important factor appears to be fibularis/peroneus longus pulling the medial and lateral borders of the foot together (Fig. 3.156). At the level of the metatarsal heads, a shallow arch is maintained by the deep transverse ligament uniting the metatarsal heads, by transverse fibres binding together digital slips of the plantar aponeurosis, and by the relatively weak transverse head of adductor hallucis (Fig. 3.156). This shallow arch rests on the ground via soft tissues; the head of the second metatarsal, the highest from the ground, is the keystone of this arch. The second and third metatarsal heads occupy intermediate positions above the ground, while the first and fifth lie at approximately the same level on the ground. The arch of the metatarsal heads is the area of culmination of the metatarsal rays of the foot. Because of the nature of the arch involving the cuneiforms and cuboid, each metatarsal makes a different angle with the ground as it passes distally (Fig. 3.157). The first (medial) ray forms an angle between 18 and 25 degrees with the ground; passing laterally, the angle gradually decreases, being approximately 15 degrees for the second ray, 10 degrees for the third, 8 degrees for the fourth and only 5 degrees for the fifth (lateral) ray.

Having considered the factors contributing to the integrity of the foot and its arched structure, it is possible to understand how they work to enable the foot to act in propulsion of the body, as well as a shock absorber. A rigid foot could act as a propulsive mechanism because the main factor responsible for propulsion during walking, running and jumping is contraction of gastrocnemius and soleus, with plantarflexion of the foot at the ankle joint; this mechanism is greatly enhanced and made more efficient by having a flexible foot.

During walking, body weight is taken successively on the heel, lateral border and then ball of the foot, with the

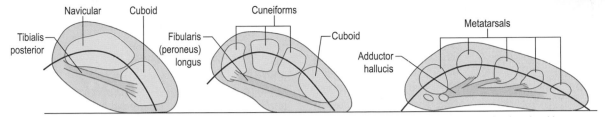

Fig. 3.156 Transverse arches of the right foot at different levels, together with important muscles involved in their maintenance at each level.

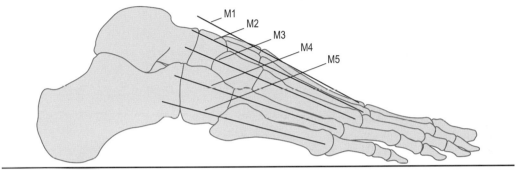

Fig. 3.157 Lateral aspect of the right foot showing decreasing angulation of each metatarsal with respect to the horizontal.

anterior pillar of the medial longitudinal arch the last part to leave the ground. In contrast, in sprinting, the heel does not make contact with the ground; the anterior pillar is still the last to leave. As the heel leaves the ground during walking, the medial toes are extended. Extension of the hallux pulls the plantar aponeurosis around the head of the first metatarsal, increasing the height of the medial longitudinal arch. In addition, flexors hallucis longus and digitorum longus are stretched, increasing the force of their subsequent contraction. Contraction of the long and short toe flexors presses the toes against the ground, increasing the force of toe-off; the most powerful muscle acting this way is flexor hallucis longus. The toes are prevented from buckling under by the lumbricals.

When landing from a jump, the toes and then the forefoot take the strain before the heel touches the ground. In this way, much of the damaging high energy and high frequency components associated with ground impact are dissipated. Muscles and ligaments are put under tension and stretched, absorbing as much as 50% of the energy. Even in quiet walking, the muscles and ligaments play an essential role in absorbing the shock of foot contact with the ground. Stretching of the ligaments and muscles stores energy which is released

towards the end of the stance phase of gait, contributing to propulsion and reducing the overall energy cost of walking.

Trabecular Arrangement Within the Foot

The transmission of mechanical forces within and through the foot is reflected, as in other regions, in the arrangement of bony trabeculae. On the medial side of the foot, following the medial longitudinal arch, trabeculae in the distal tibia can be traced posteriorly and anteriorly (Fig. 3.158A). Trabeculae arising from the cortex of the anterior tibial surface pass obliquely inferoposteriorly through the body of the talus to the calcaneus, where they spread out, reaching the posterior tubercle of the calcaneus. From the cortex of the posterior tibial surface, trabeculae run inferoanteriorly through the neck and head of the talus, navicular and medial cuneiform to the first metatarsal.

On the lateral side of the foot, transmission of mechanical forces occurs through the talus and underlying calcaneus; two sets of trabeculae can be identified (Fig. 3.158B). Arising from the cortex of the anterior tibial surface, trabeculae pass inferiorly through the posterior part of the body of the talus fanning out into the calcaneus. Trabeculae from the posterior tibial shaft

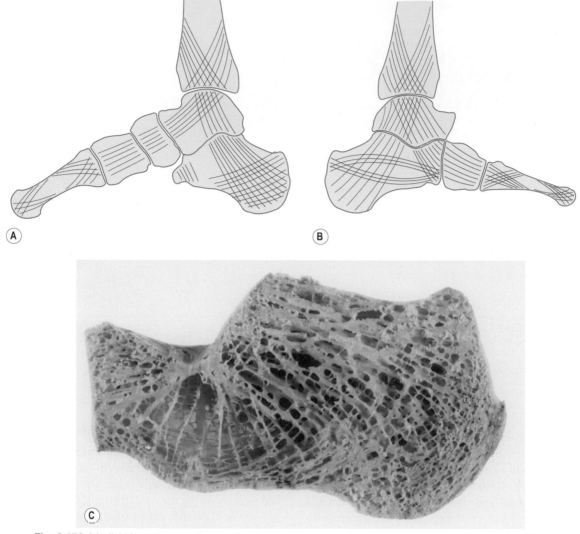

Fig. 3.158 Medial (A) and lateral (B) aspects of the left foot showing the trabecular arrangement within the tarsus and metatarsals. (C) Sagittal section through the calcaneus showing the trabecular arrangement.

pass initially through the neck of the talus, where it rests on the sustentaculum tali, then run forwards through the cuboid and fifth metatarsal to the anterior part of the lateral longitudinal arch.

Because of the stresses imparted to the calcaneus, two additional trabecular systems are seen within it (Fig. 3.158B and C). A superior arcuate system (concave inferiorly) converges into a dense lamella at the floor of the sinus tarsi; these trabeculae resist compressive stresses. The inferior arcuate system (concave superiorly) converges towards the cortical bone of the inferior surface of the calcaneus; this system resists tension forces.

Between these two systems lies an area with relatively few trabeculae and thus an area of weakness; if a sufficiently violent stress is applied vertically through the talus, injury involving this weaker region may result. The long plantar ligament may be able to resist the shock, but the lateral arch gives way at the anterior process of the calcaneus (keystone of the arch), with the sustentaculum tali broken off along a vertical line passing through the weaker area. The medial calcaneal tubercle may also be detached along a line running sagittally. Such fractures may prove difficult to reduce as not only does the superior articular surface of the calcaneus have to be

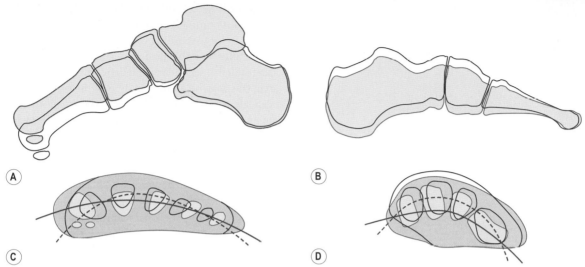

Fig. 3.159 Influence of weight-bearing on the medial (A) and lateral (B) longitudinal arches, and the anterior (C) and midfoot (D) transverse arches of the foot. (*Red* outlines of the bones show the non-weight-bearing relationships and solid bones the weight-bearing relationships. In 'C' and 'D' *solid lines* represent the relationship between segments on weight-bearing; *dotted lines* show the non-weight-bearing relationships.)

restored, but also the sustentaculum tali, otherwise the medial arch remains collapsed.

Distribution of Stresses During Static Loading

On weight-bearing, the forces are distributed in three directions towards the supports of the plantar vault, with the result that each arch of the foot is flattened and lengthened.

In the medial arch, the soft tissue under the posterior calcaneal tubercle becomes compressed and the arch comes to lie closer to the ground; the sustentaculum tali moves inferiorly, with the talus moving posteriorly on the calcaneus. As the talus moves closer to the ground, the navicular rises on the talar head. Both the cuneonavicular and medial tarsometatarsal joints gape inferiorly, while the angle that the first metatarsal makes with the ground reduces. The arch is lengthened by posterior displacement of the heel and slight anterior displacement of the sesamoid bones under the head of the first metatarsal (Fig. 3.159A).

In the lateral arch, movements of the calcaneus are the same; both the cuboid and lateral tubercle of the fifth metatarsal move inferiorly by similar amounts. The calcaneocuboid and lateral tarsometatarsal joints gape inferiorly so that the head of the fifth metatarsal is displaced anteriorly, which, together with recession of the calcaneus, lengthens the lateral arch (Fig. 3.159B).

The anterior arch flattens so that the foot becomes splayed out either side of the second metatarsal (Fig. 3.159C); the transverse arch involving the cuneiforms and cuboid is also flattened (Fig. 3.159D).

Flattening the arches results in the head of the talus and lateral calcaneal tubercle becoming displaced medially, leading to twisting of the foot at the mid-tarsal joint. The hindfoot becomes slightly adducted, pronated and extended, while the forefoot undergoes a relative movement of flexion, abduction and supination.

Because each heel receives approximately one quarter of body weight when standing erect and more momentarily when walking, wearing shoes with a small heel area results in indentations on floors with a plastic covering.

Foot Pathology

The curvature of the various arches of the foot, as well as the orientation of their components, depends upon a delicate balance between the muscles and ligaments involved. An insufficiency or contracture of even a single muscle disrupts the overall equilibrium of the foot, leading to some form of deformity. The process may be gradual with progressively more muscles becoming involved until the foot assumes an unnatural shape and position. Simple footprints may provide a useful aid to diagnosis (compared with a normal footprint); the various stages

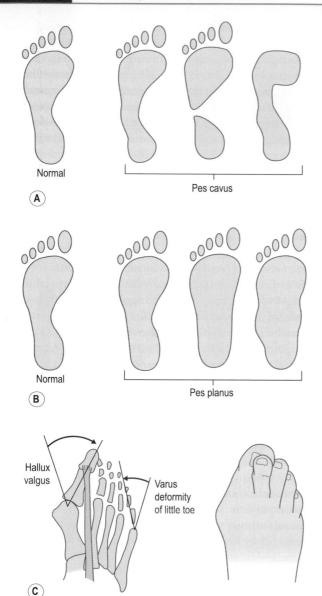

Normal

Pes cavus

(A)

Normal

Pes planus

(B)

Hallux valgus

Varus deformity of little toe

(C)

Fig. 3.160 Progressive change in the footprint in pes cavus (A) and pes planus (B). (C) Outward appearance of the foot in hallux valgus with an associated varus of the little toe.

in the development of clawfoot (pes cavus) can be identified (Fig. 3.160A). In the first stage, the footprint shows a lateral projection on its lateral border with a deepening concavity medially; the next stage shows a divided footprint; and finally the toe prints disappear due to a secondary clawtoe deformity.

In a similar manner, the progression of flat foot (pes planus) can be seen when compared with a normal

footprint (Fig. 3.160B). In this case, the medial border of the foot gradually becomes filled in and may become convex in long-standing cases.

The muscle imbalance associated with pes cavus may also result in a secondary imbalance involving the anterior arch; this may be an overloading of the medial, lateral or both supports of the anterior arch, with callosities forming under the appropriate metatarsal heads. Occasionally, the anterior arch may become flattened and splayed with the formation of callosities under each metatarsal head.

If a widely splayed foot is confined within a pointed shoe, the hallux becomes displaced laterally (Fig. 3.160C). With time, the imbalance becomes permanent due to shortening of the capsular ligaments of the joints, lateral dislocation of the sesamoid bones and tendon, and formation of an exostosis on the medial side of the first metatarsal head (hallux valgus); the intermediate metatarsals are displaced by the hallux, exaggerating the deformity. The fifth toe may undergo a converse deformity, further enhancing the deformity of the intermediate toes (Fig. 3.160C); if the deformity is severe, the anterior arch may become convex.

Both normal and pathologic foot function may be assessed clinically by observation of the individual's gait and the pattern of wear on the soles of shoes; callosities on the sole of the foot can indicate areas of excessive loading. The magnitude and duration of such loading can be assessed using suitable forms of instrumentation; from such techniques both minor and major changes in foot function can be determined and evaluated.

MUSCLES EXTENDING (DORSIFLEXING) THE TOES

Extensor hallucis longus
Extensor digitorum longus
Extensor digitorum brevis
Lumbricals

Extensor Hallucis Longus

Unipennate muscle deep to and between tibialis anterior and extensor digitorum longus on the anterior aspect of the leg/calf (Figs 3.161 and 3.162). Arising from the middle half of the anterior surface of the fibula and adjacent interosseous membrane, the muscle fibres pass inferomedially to the tendon which forms on its anterior surface. The tendon passes deep to the superior extensor retinaculum, through the proximal part of the inferior extensor

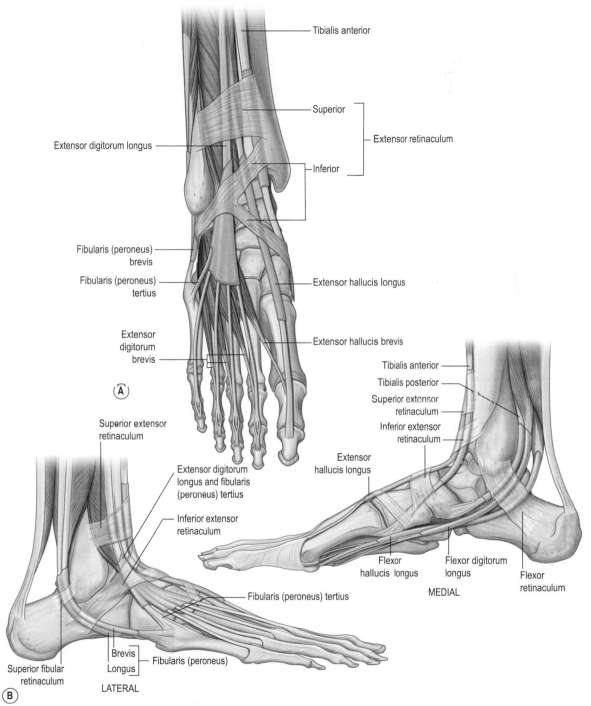

Fig. 3.161 (A) Tendons passing onto the dorsum of the foot. (B) Tendons on the lateral and medial aspects of the foot. (The extent of the associated synovial sheaths is also shown.)

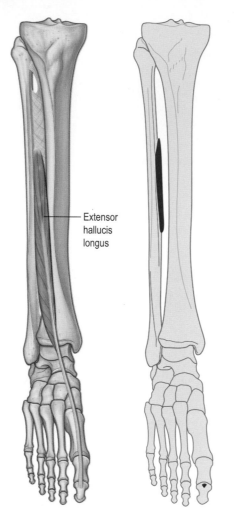

Extensor
hallucis
longus

Fig. 3.162 Anterior aspect of the right tibia, fibula and dorsum of the foot showing the position and attachments of extensor hallucis longus.

retinaculum in a separate compartment enclosed in its own synovial sheath and then deep to the distal band of the inferior extensor retinaculum on its way to the base of the hallux. Generally, the tendon does not form a fully developed extensor expansion but attaches to the base of the distal phalanx on its dorsal surface. Tendinous slips may be given off to the dorsal aspect of the base of the proximal phalanx and first metatarsal.

Innervation

By the deep fibular/peroneal nerve (root value L5, S1). Skin covering this area is supplied by roots L4 and L5.

Action

As its name implies, extensor hallucis longus extends all joints of the hallux, but mainly the metatarsophalangeal joint; it is also a powerful dorsiflexor of the foot at the ankle joint.

Functional Activity

In running, the hallux is the last part of the foot to leave the ground, therefore the final thrust comes from the long flexors of the toes. After this, the hallux must be extended at the same time as the foot is dorsiflexed and slightly inverted, ready for the heel to be placed on the ground for the next weight-bearing phase; by extending the hallux and dorsiflexing the foot, clearance of the surface is achieved. The hallux does not have a lumbrical or interossei associated with it, consequently, extension of the interphalangeal joint depends entirely on extensor hallucis longus. Paralysis of the muscle results in flexion of the joint and buckling of the hallux during the last phase of gait due to the unopposed action of the flexor muscles.

Palpation

If the hallux is extended, the tendon is clearly visible as it crosses the first metatarsophalangeal joint to its attachment to the base of the distal phalanx. Trace the fingers up the tendon; it can be felt and seen crossing the anterior aspect of the ankle joint lateral to the tendon of tibialis anterior. From here, the tendon can be felt passing superolaterally before passing deep to the surrounding muscles. Continue to move the fingers superiorly another 12 cm, allowing them to pass a little laterally; when the hallux is rhythmically extended and flexed the muscle can be felt contracting under the fingers.

Extensor Digitorum Longus

Unipennate muscle situated on the anterior aspect of the leg lateral to tibialis anterior and overlying extensor hallucis longus (Fig. 3.163). It has a linear attachment from the proximal two-thirds of the anterior surface of the fibula, deep fascia and proximal part of the interosseous membrane with its proximal fibres reaching across to the lateral condyle of the tibia in conjunction with those of fibularis/peroneus longus. Its tendon appears on the medial side with the muscle fibres passing inferomedially to reach it. The tendon passes anterior to the ankle joint deep to the superior extensor retinaculum and then through the inferior extensor retinaculum, accompanied by fibularis/peroneus tertius. At the level of the

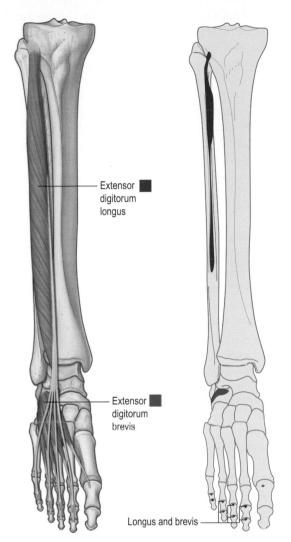

Extensor
digitorum
longus

Extensor
digitorum
brevis

Longus and brevis

Fig. 3.163 Anterior aspect of the right tibia, fibula and dorsum of the foot showing the position and attachments of extensor digitorum longus and extensor digitorum brevis.

inferior extensor retinaculum, or immediately distal, it gives four tendons passing to the lateral four toes; the four separate tendons are enclosed in a common synovial sheath at the level of the inferior extensor retinaculum. On the dorsal surface of the proximal phalanx, each tendon forms a triangular membranous expansion (extensor expansion). Each expansion is joined on its medial side by the tendon of the lumbrical and on the lateral side for the second to fourth toes by the tendons of extensor digitorum brevis. The interossei of the foot do not attach to the extensor expansion.

As the extensor expansion passes over the proximal phalanx, it divides into three parts before reaching the dorsum of the proximal interphalangeal joint. The central part attaches to the base of the middle phalanx, while the two outer parts unite before attaching to the base of the distal phalanx. An attachment of the extensor expansion to the dorsal aspect of the proximal phalanx has also been noted.

Innervation

By the deep fibular/peroneal nerve (root value L5, S1). Skin covering the muscle is supplied by root L5.

Action

As its name implies, extensor digitorum longus is an extensor of the lateral four toes at the metatarsophalangeal joints; it also assists extension at the interphalangeal joints. However, it is unable to perform the latter action unaided, which is primarily performed by the lumbricals. If the lumbricals are paralysed, extensor digitorum longus produces hyperextension of the metatarsophalangeal joint, with the interphalangeal joints becoming flexed. As the muscle passes anterior to the ankle joint, it also aids dorsiflexion of the foot.

Functional Activity

During walking and running, extensor digitorum longus pulls the toes superiorly after they have been flexed before toe-off, keeping them clear of the ground until the heel and foot make contact again. Unfortunately, the lateral four toes in most individuals tend to be flexed at the proximal interphalangeal joint and extended at the distal interphalangeal joint; consequently, extensor digitorum longus lifts the toes in this adapted position.

Palpation

The muscle belly is easily palpated on the anterolateral aspect of the leg/calf. From the head of the fibula just below the knee joint, run the fingers inferomedially for about 2 cm; when raising the toes off the floor, the muscle can be felt contracting. Now place the fingers over the anterior aspect of the ankle joint; the tendon can be identified standing out clearly, lateral to those of tibialis anterior and extensor hallucis longus. From here, it can now either be traced superiorly, deep to the superior part of the extensor retinaculum to join the muscle belly, or inferiorly, where it divides into four tendons running towards each of the lateral four toes. Each tendon stands clear of the metatarsophalangeal joint as it passes towards the dorsum of the toe.

Extensor Digitorum Brevis

Thin muscle on the dorsum of the foot beyond the inferior part of the extensor retinaculum (Fig. 3.163), lateral to and partly covered by the tendons of fibularis/peroneus tertius and extensor digitorum longus. It arises from the anterior roughened part of the superior surface of the calcaneus and deep fascia covering the muscle, including the stem of the inferior extensor retinaculum. From the small belly, short tendons pass anteromedially, the most medial of which crosses the dorsalis pedis artery to attach separately onto the dorsal aspect of the base of the proximal phalanx of the hallux. The remaining three tendons join the lateral side of the extensor expansion of the second, third and fourth toes. The most medial part of the muscle may develop a separate belly (extensor hallucis brevis).

Innervation

By the deep fibular/peroneal nerve (root value L5, S1). Skin covering the muscle is supplied by roots L5 and S1.

Action

The medial part of the muscle aids extensor hallucis longus extend the hallux at the metatarsophalangeal joint; the other three tendons aid extensor digitorum longus. As with the long extensor tendons, extensor digitorum brevis helps the lumbricals extend the interphalangeal joints; however, it is unable to do this independently.

Functional Activity

Extensor digitorum brevis helps extensor digitorum longus and extensor hallucis longus raise the toes clear of the ground in running and walking.

Palpation

Place the fingers on the tendon of extensor digitorum longus as it splits into its four parts. When the toes are extended, extensor digitorum brevis can be felt just lateral and deep to the tendons; the tendons are difficult to trace distally as they become inseparable from those of extensor digitorum longus.

Lumbricals

Four small muscles associated with the tendons of flexor digitorum longus passing from the flexor to extensor compartment of the foot (Fig. 3.165B). The most medial lumbrical arises from the medial side of the tendon to the second toe, adjacent to the attachment of flexor accessorius (quadratus plantae) to the main longus tendon. The remaining lumbricals arise by two heads from adjacent sides of two tendons (second from the tendons to the second and third toes; third from the tendons to the third and fourth toes; fourth from the tendons to the fourth and fifth toes). Each muscle then passes anteriorly superficial to the deep transverse metatarsal ligament on the medial side of the toe, winding obliquely superiorly to attach to the medial side of the extensor expansion and base of the proximal phalanx.

Innervation

The first (most medial) lumbrical is supplied by the medial plantar nerve (root value S1, S2) and the lateral three by the lateral plantar nerve (root value S2, 3), both being terminal branches of the tibial nerve. Skin on the dorsum of the foot at the point of attachment is supplied by roots L5 and S1; skin of the plantar aspect of the foot overlying the muscles is supplied by the medial and lateral plantar nerves, which have the same root values as the supply to the muscles. It should be noted that only the most lateral lumbrical has skin over its plantar aspect.

Action

There has been much discussion over the role of these small almost insignificant muscles; they have a long muscle belly compared with their tendon and link the flexors and extensors of the toes. By their attachment to the proximal phalanx, contraction produces flexion of the toes at the metatarsophalangeal joint. However, because they also attach to the extensor expansion, they extend the interphalangeal joints; this action is primarily due to the lumbricals and not the long and short extensor tendons.

Functional Activity

The action of the lumbricals prevents clawing of the toes during the propulsive phase of gait. Their paralysis results in the extensor muscles pulling the toes into hyperextension at the metatarsophalangeal joints; even at rest, the toes become clawed.

The nerves supplying the muscles appear to have many more fibres than would be necessary for such a small muscle; many are sensory, leading to the conclusion that they may have an important role in providing

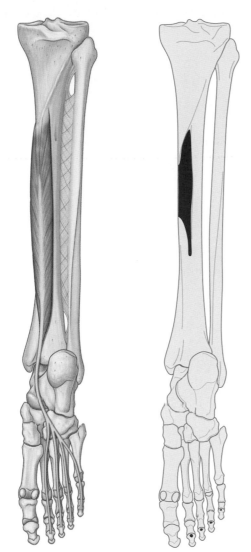

Fig. 3.164 Posterior aspect of the right tibia, fibula and plantar surface of the foot showing the position and attachments of flexor digitorum longus.

information regarding tension developed between the long flexor and extensor muscles. This sort of information is of great importance in locomotion, especially as their point of attachment is a long way from the muscle bellies of the extensor and flexor muscles.

Palpation

It is not possible to palpate the lumbricals as they lie deep in the sole of the foot covered by many small muscles of the sole, as well as the long flexor tendons.

MUSCLES FLEXING (PLANTARFLEXING) THE TOES

Flexor digitorum longus
Flexor accessorius (quadratus plantae)
Flexor digitorum brevis
Flexor hallucis longus
Flexor hallucis brevis
Flexor digiti minimi brevis
Interossei (pp. 451 and 452)
Lumbricals (p. 444)

Flexor Digitorum Longus

Situated on the posterior aspect of the leg/calf for most of its course (Fig. 3.164), flexor digitorum longus arises from the medial part of the posterior surface of the tibia inferior to the soleal line and deep transverse fascia surrounding it. The tendon forms about three fingers' breadth superior to the medial malleolus, lying next to that of tibialis posterior which has crossed anterior to it to come to lie on its medial side, and medial to the tendon of extensor hallucis longus. Passing deep to the flexor retinaculum, the tendon lies in its own synovial sheath along the medial aspect of the sustentaculum tali, sometimes grooving it, entering the sole of the foot deep to abductor hallucis. Passing anterolaterally, it crosses the tendon of flexor hallucis longus (on its plantar aspect), usually receiving a slip from it which passes into the medial two of its four digitations. About halfway along the sole on its lateral side, the tendon is joined by flexor accessorius (quadratus plantae, Fig. 3.165B). At this point, it divides into four individual tendons, one for each of the lateral four toes. Just distal to the attachment of flexor accessorius (quadratus plantae), the lumbrical muscles arise.

Distal to the metatarsophalangeal joint, the tendons enter their respective fibrous sheaths, together with the appropriate tendon of flexor digitorum brevis lying superficial to it. The tendon of brevis splits, enabling that of longus to pass through and reach the plantar surface of the base of the distal phalanx where it attaches. Both tendons share a common synovial sheath.

Innervation

By the tibial nerve (root value L5, S1, S2). Skin covering this area on the posteromedial aspect of the leg/calf and sole is supplied by roots L4, L5 and S1.

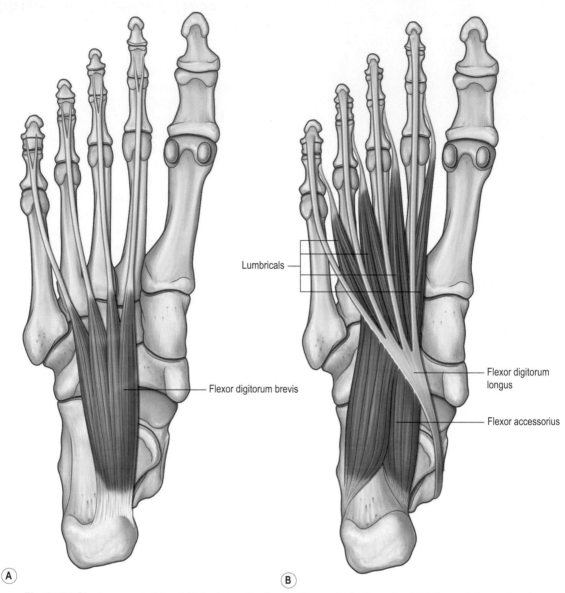

Fig. 3.165 Plantar aspect of the right foot showing the position and attachments of (A) flexor digitorum brevis and (B) the lumbricals and flexor accessorius (quadratus plantae).

Lumbricals

Flexor digitorum brevis

Flexor digitorum longus

Flexor accessorius

A   B

Action

Flexor digitorum longus flexes the lateral four toes, flexing the distal interphalangeal joints first, then the proximal interphalangeal joints and finally the metatarsophalangeal joints. Its course posterior to the medial malleolus means that it also helps plantarflex the foot at the ankle joint. With the ankle plantarflexed, its action on the toes is diminished.

Functional Activity

In the propulsive phase of running, jumping and walking, flexor digitorum longus pulls the toes firmly towards the ground to get the maximum grip and thrust during the toe-off phase. When standing, the toes tend to grip the ground to improve balance.

Palpation

Flexor digitorum longus is very difficult to distinguish as its proximal attachment is deep to soleus, while its tendons in the foot, with the lumbricals, lie deeply. However, with care, the tendon can just be identified as it passes alongside the sustentaculum tali.

Flexor Accessorius (Quadratus Plantae)

Lying deep to flexor digitorum brevis, flexor accessorius (Fig. 3.165B) arises by two heads from the medial and lateral tubercles of the calcaneus and adjacent long plantar ligament. A flattened muscular band is formed by merging of the two heads which attach to the tendon of flexor digitorum longus in the midpart of the sole, proximal to the attachment of the lumbricals.

Innervation

By the lateral plantar nerve (root value S2, S3). Skin over the region is supplied by root S1.

Action

Flexor accessorius helps the long flexor tendons flex all joints of the lateral four toes. By pulling on the lateral side of the tendon of flexor digitorum longus, it changes the direction of pull so that the toes flex towards the heel and not towards the medial malleolus.

Functional Activity

It plays an important role in gait when flexor digitorum longus is already shortened due to plantarflexion of the ankle joint. It exerts its action on the long flexor tendons so that the toes can be flexed to grip the ground, giving support and thrust during the propulsive phase of gait. This action essentially means that flexor digitorum longus can be considered to act powerfully across two joints at the same time, an unusual phenomenon.

Palpation

Lying deep in the sole of the foot, flexor accessorius cannot be palpated.

Flexor Digitorum Brevis

Situated in the sole of the foot deep to the central part of the plantar aponeurosis, flexor digitorum brevis (Fig. 3.165A) lies between abductor hallucis medially and abductor digiti minimi laterally. Arising from the medial tubercle of the calcaneus, deep surface of the central portion of the plantar aponeurosis and muscular septa on either side, the fibres pass anteriorly in the middle of the sole, separating into four tendons passing to the lateral four toes. Just distal to the metatarsophalangeal joint, within their respective fibrous flexor sheaths, each tendon splits into two to allow the tendon of flexor digitorum longus to pass from deep to superficial. After rotating through almost 180 degrees, the outer margins of the slips of each tendon rejoin, leaving a shallow groove along which the flexor digitorum longus tendon slides. After passing over the proximal interphalangeal joint, the tendon again splits to attach to the sides of the base of the middle phalanx.

Innervation

By the medial plantar nerve (root value S2, S3). Skin covering this area is supplied by roots L5 and S1.

Action

Flexor digitorum brevis primarily flexes the proximal interphalangeal joint of the lateral four toes followed by flexion of the metatarsophalangeal joints.

Functional Activity

Together with flexor digitorum longus, flexor digitorum brevis produces thrust from the toes when the demand arises.

Palpation

It is almost impossible to palpate as it is covered by some of the thickest fascia in the body and its tendons lie deep within the foot.

Flexor Hallucis Longus

Powerful unipennate muscle (Fig. 3.166) situated deep to triceps surae deep to the deep fascia of the leg/calf. It arises from the distal two-thirds of the posterior surface of the fibula and adjacent fascia.

The muscle fibres pass to a central tendon on its superficial surface, with those on the lateral side extending more distally. The tendon passes distally, deep to the flexor retinaculum in its own synovial sheath, crossing the posterior aspect of the ankle joint lateral to flexor digitorum longus. During its course, it grooves the distal end of the tibia, posterior aspect of the talus (between the medial and posterior tubercles) and inferior surface

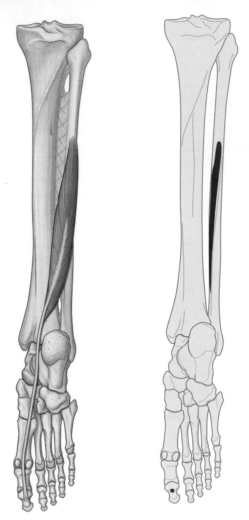

Fig. 3.166 Posterior aspect of the right tibia, fibula and plantar surface of the foot showing the position and attachments of flexor hallucis longus.

of the sustentaculum tali, where it is held in position by a synovial-lined fibrous sheath forming a tunnel through which it passes.

In the sole of the foot, the tendon lies superficial to the plantar calcaneonavicular ligament, lateral to the tendon of flexor digitorum longus. As it passes anteriorly, the tendon crosses deep to that of flexor digitorum longus; in doing so, it usually gives a slip to its medial two tendons. It then enters the fibrous digital sheath of the hallux between the two sesamoid bones situated on either side of the base of the proximal phalanx to attach to the plantar surface of the base of the distal phalanx.

Innervation

By a branch of the tibial nerve (root value S1, S2). Skin covering this area is supplied by root S2.

Action

Flexor hallucis longus flexes all joints of the hallux, acting initially on the interphalangeal joint and then the metatarsophalangeal joint. As it crosses the ankle joint, it helps plantarflex the foot.

Functional Activity

Flexor hallucis longus is of great importance, producing much of the final thrust from the foot during walking. At this point in the gait cycle, the leg/calf muscles have already produced their maximum power and the flexors of the lateral four toes are just completing their maximum contraction. Flexion of the hallux is thus the final act before the foot is lifted from the ground ready for the next step. It also plays an important role in maintaining the medial longitudinal arch.

Palpation

Flexor hallucis longus is almost impossible to palpate as it lies deep within the leg/calf, and deep to the flexor retinaculum, plantar aponeurosis and muscles in the foot. Its tendon is set deep within both the leg/calf and plantar aspect of the foot.

Flexor Hallucis Brevis

Short muscle (Fig. 3.167) situated deep in the sole of the foot between abductor hallucis medially and flexor digitorum brevis laterally. It arises from the medial side of the plantar surface of the cuboid, posterior to the groove for fibularis/peroneus longus, and adjacent surface of the lateral cuneiform and from the tendon of tibialis posterior.

The muscle fibres run anteromedially towards the hallux separating into two fleshy bellies lying on either side deep to the tendon of flexor hallucis longus. The tendon from each belly attaches to the appropriate side of the base of the proximal phalanx; the medial tendon joins that of abductor hallucis and the lateral tendon that of adductor hallucis, giving common attachments. Small sesamoid bones running in shallow grooves on the head of the first metatarsal develop in each tendon.

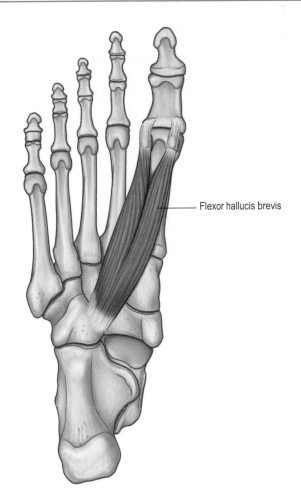

Flexor hallucis brevis

Fig. 3.167 Plantar aspect of the right foot showing the position and attachments of flexor hallucis brevis.

Innervation

By the medial plantar nerve (root value S1, S2). Skin covering the area is supplied by root L5.

Action

Flexor hallucis brevis flexes the metatarsophalangeal joint of the hallux.

Functional Activity

Flexor hallucis brevis aids flexor hallucis longus in the final push-off from the ground during activity. Being accompanied at its distal attachment by abductor and adductor hallucis suggests that steadying the hallux during propulsion is of great importance ensuring generation of maximum force. When the hallux is deformed

(hallux valgus, where the tip of the toe points laterally and base medially), this thrust is lost and the individual finds it difficult to run or sometimes walk, even at slow speeds.

It is not uncommon for injuries to occur to the sesamoid bones, particularly in individuals who put considerable strain on the hallux. Such injuries produce an inflamed region where the sesamoid bone slides against the metatarsal; this can cause considerable pain and altered function.

Palpation

The muscle is set so deep within the plantar surface of the foot that it is not possible to palpate. Only the sesamoid bones within its tendons can be felt and then only with considerable practice.

Flexor Digiti Minimi Brevis

Small muscle (Fig. 3.168) situated on the lateral side of the plantar surface of the foot, flexor digiti minimi brevis arises from the plantar aspect of the base of the fifth metatarsal and sheath of the tendon of fibularis/peroneus longus. It attaches to the lateral side of the plantar surface of the proximal phalanx of the little toe in conjunction with abductor digiti minimi.

Innervation

By the lateral plantar nerve (root value S2, S3). Skin covering the muscle is supplied by root S1.

Action and Functional Activity

Flexor digiti minimi brevis flexes the metatarsophalangeal joint; it also helps support the lateral longitudinal arch of the foot.

Palpation

By applying deep pressure, flexor digiti minimi brevis can be felt contracting in the middle part of the lateral plantar aspect of the foot when the little toe is flexed.

ABDUCTION AND ADDUCTION OF THE TOES

In the hand, the middle finger is regarded as the central digit when considering abduction and adduction; in the foot, the central digit for these movements is the second toe. If the hallux is drawn medially, it is said to be abducted, while if all other toes are drawn laterally (away from the second toe) this is also termed abduction. If all

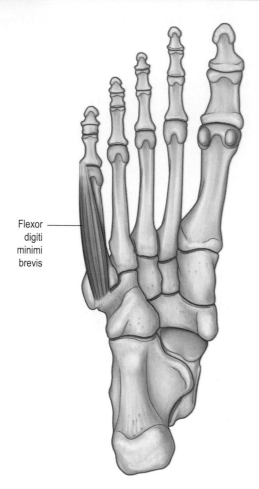

Flexor
digiti
minimi
brevis

Fig. 3.168 Plantar aspect of the right foot showing the position and attachments of flexor digiti minimi brevis.

the toes are drawn towards the second toe, they are said to be adducted.

MUSCLES ABDUCTING THE TOES

Abductor hallucis
Abductor digiti minimi
Dorsal interossei

Abductor Hallucis

Powerful and important muscle (Fig. 3.169A) located superficially on the medial side of the plantar aspect of the foot deep to the medial part of the plantar aponeurosis, abductor hallucis arises from the plantar aponeurosis, plantar aspect of the medial tubercle of the calcaneus, flexor retinaculum and intermuscular septum, separating

it from flexor digitorum brevis. The fibres pass distally forming a tendon passing over the medial side of the metatarsophalangeal joint of the hallux, attaching to the medial side of the base of the proximal phalanx in conjunction with the tendon of flexor hallucis brevis.

Innervation

By the medial plantar nerve (root value S1, S2), with skin covering the muscle supplied by root L5.

Action

Abductor hallucis abducts, and helps flex, the hallux at the metatarsophalangeal joint.

Functional Activity

Abduction of the hallux is not of importance as such, except perhaps as a party trick and then very few people are able to perform the action easily! However, it is strong and bulky, and must, therefore, be assumed to have an important role in specific activities.

Due to its position along the medial side of the foot, together with its attachment to either end of the medial longitudinal arch, it can act as a bowstring to the arch when the foot is propelling the body forwards. Its attachment to the medial side of the hallux also helps control its central position when it is flexed.

When it contracts hard, the hallux moves medially, but more importantly the foot is positioned laterally, improving the relationship between the hallux and medial side of the foot. If this alignment of the foot and toes was encouraged from an early age, many deformities of the toes might be prevented.

Palpation

Place the fingers on the medial plantar aspect of the foot under the medial longitudinal arch. On flexing the toes, the muscle belly can be palpated towards the heel. Tracing forwards from the heel, the tendon can also be felt.

Abductor Digiti Minimi

Situated on the lateral side of the plantar aspect of the foot (Fig. 3.169A) deep to the plantar aponeurosis from which it gains part of its attachment. It also arises from the medial and lateral tubercles of the calcaneus and intervening area, as well as the intermuscular septum separating it from flexor digitorum brevis. The fibres pass distally forming a tendon which attaches to the lateral side of the base of the proximal phalanx of the fifth toe.

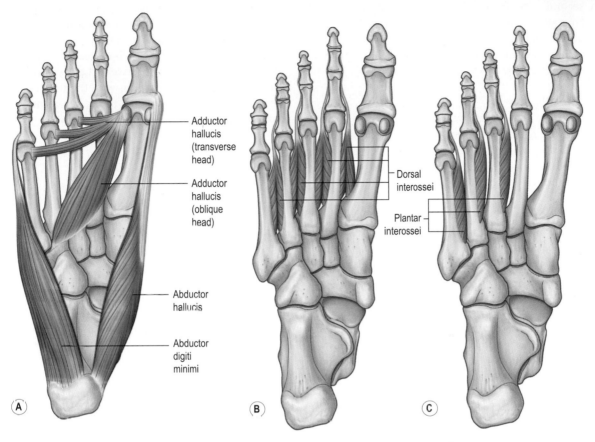

Fig. 3.169 Plantar aspect of the right foot showing the position and attachments of (A) abductor and adductor hallucis and abductor digiti minimi, the (B) dorsal and (C) plantar interossei.

Innervation

By the lateral plantar nerve (root value S2, S3), with skin covering the muscle supplied by root S1.

Action

Abductor digiti minimi abducts, and helps flex, the fifth toe at the metatarsophalangeal joint.

Functional Activity

Because the muscle runs from the posterior to anterior parts of the lateral longitudinal arch, it acts as a bowstring to the arch similar to abductor hallucis on the medial side of the foot, except that the lateral arch can hardly be called a true arch. Nevertheless, it comes into action in running and jumping activities ensuring that the arch is maintained under stress.

Palpation

Unless a subject can abduct the fifth toe easily, the muscle is difficult to palpate.

Dorsal Interossei

Four small bipennate muscles (Fig. 3.169B) situated between the metatarsals. Each arises from the proximal half of the sides of adjacent metatarsals, forming a central tendon passing anteriorly deep to the deep transverse metatarsal ligament. It passes between the metatarsal heads, attaching to the side of the proximal phalanx and capsule of the metatarsophalangeal joint; the tendons do not attach to the extensor expansion.

The first (most medial) arises from adjacent sides of the first and second metatarsals attaching to the medial side of the base of the proximal phalanx of the second toe.

The second arises from adjacent sides of the second and third metatarsals attaching to the proximal phalanx of the second toe, but to the lateral side. The third and fourth dorsal interossei attach to the lateral side of the proximal phalanx of the third and fourth toes, respectively.

Innervation

By the lateral plantar nerve (root value S2, S3), with those in the fourth interosseous space being from the superficial branch and remainder from the deep branch. Skin covering this area on the dorsum of the foot is supplied by root L5 medially and S1 laterally.

Action

The dorsal interossei abduct the toes at the metatarsophalangeal joint; however, as an action, it is of little importance in the foot. Acting with the plantar interossei, they flex the metatarsophalangeal joint.

Functional Activity

The dorsal interossei are powerful muscles; their activity in combination with the plantar interossei controls the direction of the toes during violent activity enabling the long and short flexors to perform their appropriate actions.

Because of their relationship to the metatarsophalangeal joint, they can flex these joints and so raise the heads of the second, third and fourth metatarsals, helping maintain the anterior metatarsal arch. They also help, to a limited extent, with maintaining the medial and lateral longitudinal arches of the foot.

Palpation

Place the fingertips between the proximal parts of the metatarsals on the dorsum of the foot; when the toes are abducted, they can be felt contracting.

MUSCLES ADDUCTING THE TOES

Adductor hallucis
Plantar interossei

Adductor Hallucis

Situated deep within the plantar aspect of the foot (Fig. 3.169A), adductor hallucis arises by two heads (oblique, transverse). The oblique head arises from the plantar surface of the bases of the second, third and fourth metatarsals and tendon sheath of fibularis/peroneus longus. The transverse head arises from the plantar surface of the lateral three metatarsophalangeal joints and deep transverse metatarsal ligament.

The muscle fibres of the oblique head pass anteromedially while those of the transverse head pass medially. The two heads unite blending with the medial part of flexor hallucis brevis to attach to the lateral side of the base of the proximal phalanx of the hallux.

Innervation

By the lateral plantar nerve (root value S2, S3), skin covering this area is supplied by root S1.

Action

It adducts the hallux towards the second toe and flexes the first metatarsophalangeal joint.

Functional Activity

Working with abductor hallucis, adductor hallucis helps control the position of the hallux so that active flexion can be produced and provide the final thrust needed in walking, running and jumping. Due to its transverse position across the forefoot, it also helps maintain the anterior metatarsal arch of the foot.

The pull of adductor hallucis is almost at right angles to the phalanx and therefore has a better mechanical advantage than abductor hallucis. If the medial longitudinal arch is allowed to fall, allowing the foot to drift medially and toes laterally, the pull of adductor hallucis overcomes that of abductor hallucis, adding to the deformity often seen in the hallux.

Palpation

It is too deep to be palpated.

Plantar Interossei

Smaller than their dorsal counterparts and fusiform in shape (Fig. 3.169C), the plantar interossei are found in the lateral three interosseous spaces. Each arises from the plantar and medial aspect of the base and proximal end of the shaft of the metatarsal. The tendon passes anteriorly deep to the deep transverse metatarsal ligament attaching to the medial side of the base of the proximal phalanx of the same toe.

Innervation

By the lateral plantar nerve (root value S2, S3), with that in the fourth interosseous space supplied by the superficial

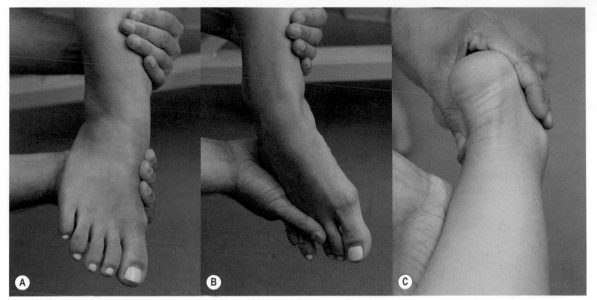

Fig. 3.170 Evaluation of the range of (A) abduction and (B) adduction at the subtalar joint with the individual seated, (C) evaluation of the range of abduction with the individual lying prone.

branch of the nerve. Skin covering the area is supplied on the lateral side by root S1 and medially by root L5.

Action

The plantar interossei adduct the third, fourth and fifth toes towards the second. In conjunction with the dorsal interossei, they flex the metatarsophalangeal joints of the lateral three toes.

Functional Activity

With the help of the dorsal interossei and abductor digiti minimi, the plantar interossei help control the position of the third, fourth and fifth toes during the push-off phase of walking and running. They also help prevent splaying of the toes when weight is suddenly applied to the forefoot.

Palpation

The muscles are too deep to be palpated.

CLINICAL EXAMINATION AND EVALUATION

Abduction and Adduction at the Subtalar Joint

With the individual seated:

- Place the hip in neutral flexion/extension, abduction/adduction and medial/lateral rotation.
- Extend the knee.
- Place the foot over the edge of the supporting surface.
- Stabilise the tibia and fibula to prevent movement at the hip and knee.
- Then turn the heel laterally for abduction (Fig. 3.170A) or medially for adduction (Fig. 3.170B).

The end feel to movement for abduction is firm due to tension in the medial ligaments and tibialis posterior, or hard due to contact between the calcaneus and floor of the sinus tarsi. The end feel to movement for adduction is firm due to tension in the lateral, posterior and interosseous talocalcanean ligaments.

Alternatively, for abduction, with the individual lying prone:

- Flex the knee 90 degrees.
- Dorsiflex the ankle until the soft tissues become taut.
- Then move the heel laterally (Fig. 3.170C).

The end feel to movement is as before.

To measure both abduction and adduction, the centre of the goniometer is placed over the posterior aspect of the ankle midway between the two malleoli, with the proximal arm aligned with the midline of the posterior aspect of the distal leg/calf and the distal arm in line with midline of the posterior aspect of the calcaneus.

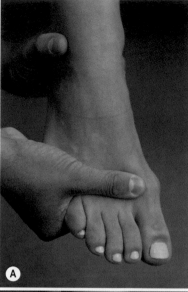

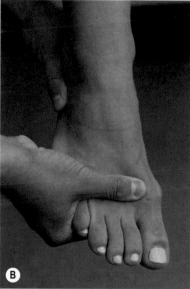

Fig. 3.171 Evaluation of the range of (A) pronation and (B) supination at the mid-tarsal joint with the individual seated.

Pronation and Supination at the Transverse (Mid) Tarsal Joint

With the individual seated:

- Flex the knee 90 degrees so that the leg/calf hangs over the edge of the supporting surface.
- Place the hip in neutral abduction/adduction and medial/lateral rotation.

- Stabilise the calcaneus and talus to prevent ankle plantarflexion and supination at the subtalar joint.
- Then turn the forefoot laterally for pronation (Fig. 3.171A) or medially for supination (Fig. 3.171B).

For pronation, the end feel to movement is firm due to tension in the medial, dorsal and plantar ligaments and tibialis posterior. For supination, the end feel is also firm due to tension in the lateral, dorsal and plantar ligaments, and fibularis/peroneus longus and brevis.

To measure both pronation and supination, the centre of the goniometer is placed over the anterior aspect of the ankle just distal to a point midway between the malleoli, with the proximal arm aligned with the anterior midline of the leg/calf and the distal arm aligned with the second metatarsal. Alternatively, the centre of the goniometer can be placed at the lateral aspect of the fifth metatarsal head for pronation or medial aspect of the first metatarsal head for supination, with the proximal arm parallel with the anterior midline of the leg/calf and the distal arm aligned with the plantar surface of the metatarsal heads.

Eversion and Inversion at the Subtalar and Transverse (Mid) Tarsal Joints

With the individual seated:

- Flex the knee 90 degrees so that the leg/calf overhangs the edge of the supporting surface.
- Place the hip in neutral abduction/adduction and medial/lateral rotation.
- Stabilise the tibia and fibula to prevent lateral flexion and rotation at the knee and medial rotation and abduction at the hip.
- Then evert (Fig. 3.172A) or invert (Fig. 3.172B) the foot.

The end feel to movement for eversion is firm due to tension in the medial, dorsal and plantar ligaments and tibialis posterior; if there is contact between the calcaneus and floor of the sinus tarsi, the end feel will be hard. The end feel to movement for supination is firm due to tension in the anterior, posterior, lateral, dorsal and plantar ligaments, and fibularis/peroneus longus and brevis.

To measure both eversion and inversion, the centre of the goniometer is placed over the anterior aspect of the ankle midway between the malleoli, with the proximal arm directed towards the tibial tuberosity and the distal arm aligned along the second metatarsal.

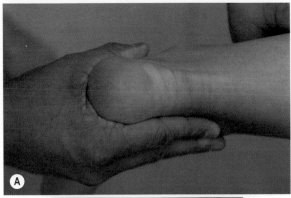

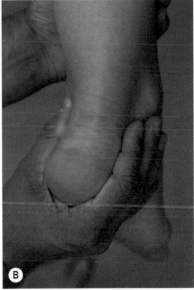

Fig. 3.172 Evaluation of the range of (A) eversion and (B) inversion of the foot at the mid-tarsal and subtalar joints with the individual seated.

Plantarflexion and Dorsiflexion at the Metatarsophalangeal Joints

With the individual seated or lying supine with the foot extending over the edge of the supporting surface:

- Place the ankle in neutral dorsiflexion/plantarflexion.
- Place the foot in neutral eversion/inversion.
- Place the metatarsophalangeal joint in neutral abduction/adduction.
- Place the interphalangeal joint in neutral dorsiflexion/plantarflexion.
- Stabilise the metatarsal to prevent ankle plantarflexion and inversion or eversion of the foot.

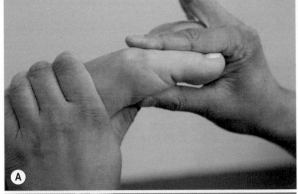

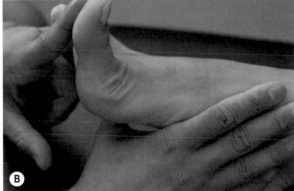

Fig. 3.173 Evaluation of the range of (A) plantarflexion and (B) dorsiflexion at the first metatarsophalangeal joint.

- Then plantarflex (Fig. 3.173A) or dorsiflex (Fig. 3.173B) the joint.

If the ankle and interphalangeal joints are plantarflexed, movement is restricted due to tension in the extensor muscles. The remaining toes should not be held in extension as tension in the deep transverse metatarsal ligament will also restrict movement. The end feel for plantarflexion is firm due to tension in the dorsal joint capsule and collateral ligaments. The end feel for dorsiflexion is firm due to tension in the plantar joint capsule and plantar ligaments.

To measure plantarflexion and dorsiflexion of the hallux, the centre of the goniometer is placed over the medial aspect of the metatarsophalangeal joint, with the proximal arm along the medial midline of the first metatarsal and the distal arm aligned with the medial midline of the proximal phalanx. For the lateral four toes, the centre of the goniometer is placed over the dorsal aspect of the metatarsophalangeal joint, with the proximal arm over the dorsal midline of the metatarsal and the distal arm aligned with the dorsal midline of the proximal phalanx.

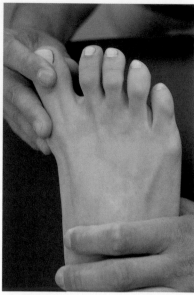

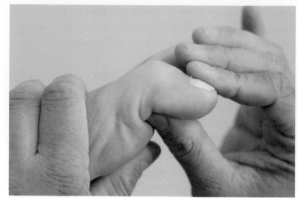

Fig. 3.175 Evaluation of the range of plantarflexion at the inter-phalangeal joint of the hallux.

Fig. 3.174 Evaluation of the range of abduction at the first metatarsophalangeal joint.

Abduction at the Metatarsophalangeal Joints

With the individual seated or lying supine:
- Place the foot in neutral inversion/eversion.
- Place the metatarsophalangeal and interphalangeal joints in neutral dorsiflexion/plantarflexion.
- Stabilise the metatarsal to prevent inversion or eversion.
- Then move the hallux (Fig. 3.174), third, fourth and fifth toes away from the second.

The end feel to movement is firm due to tension in the joint capsule, collateral ligaments and fascia in the web spaces.

To measure abduction, the centre of the goniometer is placed over the dorsal aspect of the metatarsophalangeal joint, with the proximal arm along the dorsal midline of the metatarsal and the dorsal arm aligned with the dorsal midline of the proximal phalanx.

Dorsiflexion and Plantarflexion at the Proximal Interphalangeal Joint

With the individual seated or lying supine:
- Place the ankle in neutral dorsiflexion/plantarflexion.
- Place the foot in neutral inversion/eversion.
- Place the metatarsophalangeal joint in neutral dorsiflexion/plantarflexion and abduction/adduction.

- Stabilise the metatarsal and proximal phalanx to prevent movement at the ankle or inversion/eversion of the foot.
- While avoiding movement at the metatarsophalangeal joint, plantarflex (Fig. 3.175) or dorsiflex the proximal interphalangeal joint.

If the ankle and metatarsophalangeal joints are plantarflexed, movement is restricted due to tension in the extensor muscles; if the metatarsophalangeal joint is fully dorsiflexed, tension in the lumbricals and interosseii may also limit movement. The end feel to dorsiflexion is soft due to compression of the soft tissues between the plantar surfaces; however, it may be firm due to tension in the dorsal joint capsule and collateral ligaments. The end feel to plantarflexion is also firm due to tension in the plantar joint capsule and plantar ligaments.

To measure dorsiflexion and plantarflexion of the hallux, place the centre of the goniometer over the medial aspect of the interphalangeal joint, with the proximal arm along the medial midline of the proximal phalanx and the distal arm aligned along the medial midline of the distal phalanx. For the lateral four toes, place the centre of the goniometer over the dorsal aspect of the joint being examined, with the proximal arm over the dorsal midline of the proximal phalanx and the distal arm over the dorsal midline of the middle phalanx.

Dorsiflexion and Plantarflexion at the Distal Interphalangeal Joint

With the individual seated or lying supine:
- Place the ankle in neutral dorsiflexion/plantarflexion.

- Place the foot in neutral inversion/eversion.
- Place the metatarsophalangeal and proximal interphalangeal joints in neutral.
- Stabilise the metatarsal, proximal and middle phalanx to prevent movement at the ankle and inversion/eversion of the foot.
- Stabilise the metatarsophalangeal and proximal interphalangeal joints to prevent their movement.
- Then dorsiflex or plantarflex the distal interphalangeal joint.

For dorsiflexion, if the ankle, metatarsophalangeal and proximal interphalangeal joints are dorsiflexed, movement is restricted by tension in the flexor muscles, lumbricals and interosseii. For plantarflexion, if the ankle, metatarsophalangeal and proximal interphalangeal joints are plantarflexed, movement is restricted by tension in the extensor muscles; if the metatarsophalangeal and proximal interphalangeal joints are fully extended, additional tension in the oblique retinacular ligament also restricts movement. The end feel for dorsiflexion is firm due to tension in the plantar joint capsule and plantar ligaments; for plantarflexion, the end feel is also firm due to tension in the dorsal joint capsule, collateral and oblique retinacular ligaments.

To measure both dorsiflexion and plantarflexion, the centre of the goniometer is placed over the dorsal aspect of the joint, with the proximal arm along the dorsal

---

SECTION SUMMARY

Tarsus

- Seven irregular bones (talus, calcaneus, navicular, cuboid, medial/intermediate/lateral cuneiform) located in the hindfoot and midfoot.
- Talus articulates with tibia and fibula forming the ankle joint; calcaneus forming the subtalar joint; navicular as part of the talocalcaneonavicular joint.
- Calcaneus articulates with talus forming the subtalar joint; cuboid forming the calcaneocuboid joint.
- Navicular articulates with talus as part of the talocalcaneonavicular joint; cuneiforms forming the cuneonavicular joints.
- Cuneiforms (medial, intermediate, lateral) articulate with navicular forming the cuneonavicular joints; bases of medial three metatarsals forming the tarsometatarsal joints.
- Cuboid articulates with calcaneus forming the calcaneocuboid joint; bases of the lateral two metatarsals forming tarsometatarsal joints.

Metatarsals

- Five long bones in the foot, each with a proximal quadrilateral base, shaft, distal rounded head.
- Bases articulate with the cuneiforms, cuboid and adjacent metatarsals.
- Heads articulate with base of corresponding proximal phalanx forming metatarsophalangeal joints.

Phalanges

- Fourteen individual bones with two in the hallux (proximal, distal) and three in the remaining toes (proximal, middle, distal); each has a base, shaft and head.
- Bases of proximal phalanx articulate with heads of corresponding metatarsal.
- Heads of phalanges articulate with base of next (middle or distal) phalanx forming interphalangeal joints

Subtalar Joint

Type	Synovial plane joint
Articular surfaces	Concave facet on inferior surface of talus; convex facet on superior surface of calcaneus
Capsule	Thin and loose attaching to articular margins
Ligaments	Interosseous (talocalcanean); ligamentum cervicis; medial, lateral and posterior talocalcanean
Stability	Maintained by ligaments especially the interosseous ligaments
Movements	Adduction and abduction of the foot contributing to inversion and eversion, respectively

Talocalcaneonavicular Joint

Type	Synovial ball-and-socket joint
Articular surfaces	Head and inferior surface of neck of talus with posterior concave surface of navicular, anterior calcaneus, plantar calcaneonavicular ligament
Capsule	Attaches to articular margins
Ligaments	Plantar calcaneonavicular ('spring'); calcaneonavicular part of bifurcate; dorsal talonavicular

Continued

SECTION SUMMARY—CONT'D

Stability	Maintained by 'spring' and bifurcate ligaments, tibialis posterior
Movements	Inversion and eversion of the foot

Calcaneocuboid Joint

Type	Synovial plane joint
Articular surfaces	Anterior surface of calcaneus with posterior surface of cuboid
Capsule	Surrounds the joint, thick inferiorly and superiorly
Ligaments	Dorsal and plantar calcaneocuboid (short plantar); calcaneocuboid part of bifurcate; long plantar
Stability	Maintained by plantar ligaments and fibularis/peroneus longus
Movements	Pronation and supination of forefoot

Transverse (Mid) Tarsal Joint

Comprises the talocalcaneonavicular and calcaneocuboid joints, acting as a single functional unit.

Ligaments	Dorsal, plantar and interosseous cuboideonavicular
Movements	Movement at this joint is always accompanied by movement at the subtalar joint and vice versa; inversion of forefoot achieved by adduction at the subtalar joint and supination of the forefoot at the mid-tarsal joint, plantarflexion at the ankle increases inversion; eversion of forefoot achieved by abduction of the foot at the subtalar joint and pronation of the forefoot at the mid-tarsal joint, dorsiflexion at the ankle increases eversion

Movements at Transverse (Md) Tarsal Joint

Movement	Muscles
Inversion	Tibialis posterior
	Tibialis anterior
Eversion	Fibularis/peroneus longus
	Fibularis/peroneus brevis
	Fibularis/peroneus tertius

Joints of the Forefoot

Cuneonavicular Joint

Type	Synovial plane joint
Articular surfaces	Facets on anterior surface of the navicular with concave posterior surfaces of cuneiforms
Capsule	Surrounds the joint
Ligaments	Dorsal and plantar cuneonavicular

Intercuneiform Joints

Type	Synovial plane joints

Cuneocuboid Joint

Type	Synovial plane joint
Articular surfaces	Posterosuperior surface of cuboid; posterolateral surface of lateral cuneiform
Ligaments	Dorsal, plantar and interosseous cuneocuboid
Stability	Maintained by associated ligaments

Tarsometatarsal Joints

Type	Synovial plane joints
Articular surfaces	Anterior surfaces of cuboid and cuneiforms with bases of metatarsals
Capsule	Attached to articular margins
Ligaments	Dorsal, plantar and interosseous tarsometatarsal
Stability	Maintained by ligaments and muscles crossing and/or attaching to the bones
Movements	Dorsiflexion and plantarflexion of toes

Intermetatarsal Joints

Type	Synovial plane joints between adjacent surfaces of metatarsal bases

Metatarsophalangeal Joints

Type	Synovial condyloid joints
Articular surfaces	Rounded head of metatarsal; base of proximal phalanx
Capsule	Loose, replaced by plantar ligament on plantar surface
Ligaments	Collateral, plantar and deep transverse metatarsal
Movements	Plantarflexion and dorsiflexion of toes

Interphalangeal Joints

Type	Synovial hinge joint
Articular surfaces	Head of proximal phalanx with base of next distal phalanx
Capsule	Completely encloses joint; reinforced by collateral ligaments; replaced by plantar ligament on plantar surface
Ligaments	Collateral, plantar
Stability	By ligaments and tendons crossing joint
Movements	Plantarflexion and dorsiflexion of toes

SECTION SUMMARY—CONT'D

Movements of the Foot as a Whole
These movements mainly occur at the subtalar and transverse (mid) tarsal joints, although other joints within the foot may also contribute.

Movement	Muscles (root value of nerve supply)
Inversion	Tibialis anterior (L4, L5)
	Tibialis posterior (L4, L5)
Eversion	Fibularis/peroneus longus (L5, S1)
	Fibularis/peroneus brevis (L5, S1)
	Fibularis/peroneus tertius (L5, S1)

Movements at the Joints of the Toes
The (hallux) has two joints: interphalangeal (IP) and metatarsophalangeal (MTP). Each of the remaining four toes has distal interphalangeal (DIP), proximal interphalangeal (PIP) and MTP joints. As in the hand, the muscles are capable of moving one or more of these joints. The joints that the muscle acts on are given for each muscle.

Movement	Muscles (root value of nerve supply)
Hallux	
Extension	Extensor hallucis longus at IP, MTP (L5, S1)
	Extensor digitorum brevis (medial tendon) at IP, MTP (L5, S1)
Flexion	Flexor hallucis longus at IP, MTP (S1, S2)
	Flexor hallucis brevis at IP, MTP (S1, S2)
Abduction	Abductor hallucis at MTP (S1, S2)
Adduction	Adductor hallucis at MTP (S1, S2)

Movement	Muscles (root value of nerve supply)
Remaining Toes	
Extension	Extensor digitorum longus at DIP, PIP, MTP (L5, S1)
	Extensor digitorum brevis (lateral 3 tendons) at DIP, PIP, MTP (L5, S1)
Flexion	Flexor digitorum longus at DIP, PIP, MTP (L5, S1, S2)
	Flexor digitorum brevis at PIP, MTP (S2, S3)
	Flexor accessories at DIP, PIP, MTP (S2, S3)
	Flexor digiti minimi brevis (little toe only) at MTP (S2, S3)
	Dorsal and plantar interossei at MTP (S2, S3)
	Lumbricals at MTP (S1, S2, S3)
Abduction	Abductor digiti minimi (little toe only) at MTP (S2, S3)

Movement	Muscles (root value of nerve supply)
	Dorsal interossei at MTP (S2, S3)
Adduction	Plantar interossei at MTP (S2, S3)

- Interaction between the extrinsic and intrinsic muscles allows the various arches of the foot to be formed and maintained.
- Variation in the shape and size of the arches allows the foot to function both as a rigid lever and as a pliable platform.

Clinical Evaluation

Movement and Maximum Range (where values exist)	End Feel to Movement
Subtalar Joint	
Abduction	Firm (may be hard due to contact between calcaneus and floor of sinus tarsi)
Adduction	Firm
Transverse (Mid) Tarsal Joint	
Pronation	Firm
Supination	Firm
Eversion	Firm (may be hard due to contact between calcaneus and floor of sinus tarsi)
Inversion	Firm
Metatarsophalangeal Joints	
Plantarflexion	Firm
Dorsiflexion	Firm
(maximum total range for hallux is 110°; for lesser toes is 80°–40° from medial to lateral)	
Abduction	Firm
Proximal Interphalangeal Joints	
Plantarflexion 45° for hallux, 35° for lateral four toes	Firm
Dorsiflexion 70° for hallux, 40° for lateral four toes	Soft (may be firm due to tension in dorsal joint capsule and collateral ligaments)
Distal Interphalangeal Joints	
Plantarflexion 60°	Firm
Dorsiflexion 40°	Firm

❓ SELF-ASSESSMENT QUESTIONS

91. How many tarsal bones are there and what are they called?
92. What type of joint is an intertarsal joint?
93. To which bones is the bifurcate ligament attached?
94. To which bones in the foot does the tendon of extensor hallucis longus attach?
95. What is the nerve supply, including root value, of flexor accessories (quadratus plantae)?
96. What is the action of the plantar interossei?
97. What and where is the plantar fascia?
98. Which muscles pass superior and inferior to the fibular/peroneal tubercle on the lateral side of the calcaneus?
99. Which muscles produce inversion of the foot?
100. What is the nerve supply, including root value, of abductor hallucis?
101. What are the attachments of abductor digiti minimi?
102. Which joint is the interosseous talocalcanean ligament associated with?
103. Which bones articulate at the transverse (mid) tarsal joint?
104. What are the attachments of the long plantar ligament?
105. Which joints are involved in everting the foot?
106. Which is the most robust metatarsal?
107. Which muscles help maintain the transverse arches of the foot?
108. Which ligament attaches to all metatarsal heads?
109. What movements are possible at the metatarsophalangeal joints?
110. Which bones articulate with the navicular?
111. Which tendon passes inferior to the sustentaculum tali of the calcaneus?
112. Which bone forms the heel?
113. Which muscle(s) attach(es) to the tubercle of the fifth metatarsal?
114. What is the nerve supply, including root value, of flexor digitorum longus?
115. What is the action of flexor hallucis brevis?
116. Which longitudinal arch of the foot is closer to the supporting surface?
117. With which bones does the second metatarsal articulate?
118. What movements occur at the tarsometatarsal joints?
119. What is hallux valgus?
120. Which part of the calcaneus is the weakest?

midline of the middle phalanx and the distal arm over the dorsal midline of the distal phalanx.

SIMPLE ACTIVITIES OF THE LOWER LIMB

INTRODUCTION

It is only possible to give a basic outline of the following activities as each differs considerably according to the individual's height, weight and build. An additional problem is that everyone has their own characteristic pattern, which may be so clearly individual that they can be recognised by their movements. Many activities can be influenced by the clothing worn (high heels, tight jeans, trousers, skirts). The muscular work involved and joint activity also varies depending on the speed at which the activity is performed and the surrounding environment. Nevertheless, certain factors tend to be common to most individuals; it is these which are considered here.

Walking

Walking involves the whole of the body; consequently, a change in the pattern of movement of the upper body will affect the walking pattern. This section only considers the lower limbs and lower trunk in any detail, with the upper body referred to in outline only.

Each lower limb performs a cycle of similar events but performed half a cycle out of phase with each other. The left limb will be weight-bearing while the right is off the ground; as the toes are pushing off in one limb, the heel of the other limb is making contact with the ground, and as one limb is moving forward the other is drawn backwards.

By examining the cycle of events associated with one limb, an understanding of the composite movement of both limbs can be obtained. Movements of the right lower limb are presented in the following account; any reference to the other limb is clearly distinguished. When considering walking, it is often easier to break up the pattern observed into different phases; this should not detract from the fact that this is a continuous cycle of events performed smoothly, precisely and efficiently.

Toe-off phase. This account begins when the foot is powerfully plantarflexed at the ankle joint, pushing the body forward. At this point, the trunk becomes flexed, abducted and rotated at the supporting hip; the rotation is equivalent to medial rotation of the femur. At the hip joint, the hip is extended, adducted and medially rotated, the knee extended and the ankle dorsiflexed. Although the toes are in a neutral position, they are gripping the supporting surface.

Powerful ankle plantarflexion is achieved by the calf muscles (gastrocnemius, soleus). As the movement progresses, the toes are forced into extension; after receiving this initial stretch, the toe flexors also work powerfully, the lateral four toes first, closely followed by the hallux. Because quadriceps femoris is holding the knee almost fully extended, the powerful thrust from the foot is transmitted to the hip, pelvis and trunk, which, due to their forward inclination, are pushed anterosuperiorly.

Carry-through phase. As the hallux leaves the ground, the first part of the carry-through phase begins. There is extension of the toes, brought about by extensors hallucis longus and digitorum longus; ankle dorsiflexion by tibialis anterior and extensor digitorum longus; knee flexion by the hamstrings; and hip flexion by psoas major, iliacus, rectus femoris, sartorius and pectineus. The hip is laterally rotated by piriformis, obturators internus and externus, quadratus femoris and the gemelli; this continues until the foot passes a point immediately below the hip joint. During this phase, the unsupported side of the pelvis is moving forward, initially because of the thrust it receives at toe-off, and secondly because it is pivoting about the opposite hip joint. The upper trunk tends to rotate in the opposite direction so that the same side shoulder carrying the arm with it moves backwards. To maintain the head facing forwards, the neck rotates towards the opposite side.

After the foot passes below the hip joint, the limb begins to extend again. The dorsiflexors allow the ankle and toes to assume a neutral (or slightly flexed) position, with the foot slightly inverted by tibialis anterior and posterior. Contraction of quadriceps femoris extends the knee to just short of full extension. The hip is still flexed by the same group of muscles, and the pelvis is still pivoting forwards under the action of gluteus medius and minimus, and tensor fascia lata of the supporting limb. The carry-through phase terminates when the foot makes contact with the ground again; the support phase begins once more.

Heel-strike phase. Because the foot is slightly inverted, the heel comes into contact with the ground on its lateral side. The frictional forces generated have a dragging effect which slows the foot, allowing it to land and make full contact with the supporting surface. As the foot takes the full weight of the body, the heel is compressed and its intrinsic musculature contracts, supporting the arches of the foot. The weight is then relayed via the lateral side of the foot forwards to the forefoot. The intrinsic muscles of the foot convert it into a semi-rigid lever, enabling it to absorb the stresses associated with foot contact, yet preparing it for the next propulsive phase preceding toe-off.

Support phase. As body weight is taken onto the foot, the body is moving forward, the ankle is dorsiflexed, the knee undergoes a small flexion wave and the hip is extended by the momentum of the body aided, particularly when walking fast, by gluteus maximus and the hamstrings. The pelvis is maintained in a more or less level position by the abductors of the right hip (gluteus medius, gluteus minimus) allowing the opposite foot to be raised from the ground.

After the foot passes behind the line of the hip joint, the calf muscles contract strongly, completing the cycle mentioned earlier. From the point where the weight is borne on the heel to where the toes push the body anterosuperiorly, the other limb is lifted from the ground to undergo the carry-through phase previously described.

Standing Up from the Sitting Position

There are many ways in which to stand up from a seated position. In addition to the factors listed earlier, the height and type of chair may have a profound effect on the pattern of movement. Nevertheless, the fundamentals of rising from a seated position will be outlined; bear in mind there are many variations.

Sitting. The starting position is sitting erect on a wooden chair with a firm seat but no arm rests. The feet are both on the floor, parallel to one another, about 10 cm apart; the ankles are at right angles to the leg/calf, as are the knees and hips. The arms are by the sides and give no assistance to the movement, except as a mechanism to aid balance. The line of gravity through the trunk and upper limbs falls through the seat between, but anterior to, the ischial tuberosities. During movement, the base is changed from the seat to the feet; consequently, some readjustment of body weight and foot position must be carried out.

Preparation for standing. The first phase in preparation for standing is to move the trunk forwards and feet backwards so that the centre of gravity of the upper body is brought as far forward as possible. The feet are drawn backwards by the hamstrings of both limbs; knee flexion and ankle dorsiflexion are both increased. However, full contact is still maintained between the feet and ground. At the same time, the trunk is flexed forward by the abdominal muscles, the pectoral girdle is protracted by serratus anterior and pectoralis minor, the neck is flexed by the prevertebral muscles, while the head is extended by rectus capitis posterior major and minor. (Extension of the head is not a natural movement when standing from the seated position.) If leaning forwards does not bring the centre of gravity of the upper body sufficiently over the feet to allow the transfer of weight, then the whole trunk must be shifted forwards.

The next phase is to transfer the weight of the body over the new base (feet). This is brought about by additional contraction of the abdominal muscles bringing the upper part of the body forward. The weight is now taken by the feet; the intrinsic foot muscles contract to maintain the various arches.

Standing. There is now ankle plantarflexion, bringing the foot back to just short of a right angle with the leg/calf; plantarflexion is brought about mainly by soleus while the knee is extended by quadriceps femoris. Extension at the hip is brought about by a combination of the hamstrings (acting as a tie-mechanism) drawn down by the tibia as it moves forwards in relation to the femur, and gluteus maximus, which, as well as its effect on the hip, pulls on the iliotibial tract, aiding extension of the knee. At the same time, the hip and knee joints are being extended, the back is extended by the long back muscles (sacrospinalis). The pectoral girdle is retracted by the rhomboids and middle fibres of trapezius, while the neck is extended by the upper fibres of trapezius and splenius cervicis. The head is brought to the neutral position by contraction of longus capitis.

All of these movements occur simultaneously until the erect standing position is achieved.

Climbing Steps

Variations in this activity are again so wide that description is difficult. There are many combinations of step height and tread which can modify the pattern of movement. The example given here is with a step height of 25 cm, with the movement being performed fairly slowly.

Toe-off phase. The starting position is with the left foot already up one step and the right about to push off. Each limb performs a complete cycle of movement, with the limbs being out of phase, so that as the left limb is weight-bearing, the right is being carried through. The right foot pushes off with strong plantarflexion of the ankle brought about by the leg/calf muscles producing a passive extension of the toes, stretching the flexors. The latter respond immediately by flexing the toes, producing the final thrust from the right foot. It is at this point that the whole body is inclined forward; however, the knee and hip are maintained in an extended position, while the trunk flexes to bring body weight forwards. At the same time, the left quadriceps femoris is working maximally to extend the left knee and raise the body to the next step.

Carry-through phase. The right limb now begins its carry-through phase. This involves extension of the toes by extensors digitorum longus and hallucis longus; ankle dorsiflexion by tibialis anterior and the long toe extensors; knee flexion by the hamstrings; hip flexion by psoas major and iliacus and raising and forward rotation of the pelvis on the same side by gluteus medius and minimus of the weight-bearing side. This movement continues until the foot has passed the left leg and comes to lies just above the next step.

Foot down and step-up phase. The foot is then lowered onto the step by the eccentric contraction of the hip flexors, and weight is transferred to it, beginning the next weight-bearing phase. The intrinsic muscles of the right foot contract to stabilise the arches while the long flexors pull the toes towards the supporting surface. The ankle, which was in slight dorsiflexion because of the forward inclination of the tibia, now comes into a neutral position brought about partly by soleus and partly by extension of the knee. The movements at both the ankle and knee contribute to the extension force at the hip which, aided by gluteus maximus and the hamstrings, produces a backward tilting of the pelvis. The back muscles use this firm base to extend the trunk into an erect position.

The carry-through phase of the limb is augmented by forward rotation of the pelvis at the hip of the supporting side by the action of gluteus medius and minimus of the weight-bearing limb.

When the hip and knee are fully extended, the other foot is placed onto the step above. The ankle of the supporting lower limb is plantarflexed, throwing the body forward onto the left limb to complete the cycle.

Cycling

Cycling is a popular activity either as a pleasurable pastime, a means of transport or a form of keeping fit. It is important to understand the movements of the joints involved and the muscles producing the movements. The activity varies according to both the type and size of machine used and the stature and ability of the individual. Although only the activity of the lower limbs is considered, cycling exercises the body as a whole; muscles of the trunk and upper limbs contribute to the stability, control, balance and counter pressure needed for efficient and effective power to be applied by the lower limbs.

The following analysis considers an individual using a mountain bike with straight handlebars and a fairly low saddle. The trunk is inclined slightly forwards with some body weight transferred through the arms to the handlebars.

Each lower limb performs a similar action but 180 degrees out of phase with each other. As one lower limb is pushing hard against the pedal, the other is passing through a recovery phase; consequently, only one limb needs to be considered.

Thrust phase. The thrust phase begins immediately after the pedal has reached its highest point. Although the power generated is usually the same throughout the downward thrust, maximum work is produced when the crank shaft of the pedal is at right angles to the leg/calf. Experienced cyclists learn to apply the maximum pressure to the pedal, approximately 45 degrees either side of this point, easing off near the top and bottom of the thrust phase.

At the beginning of this phase, the hip is flexed to almost 90 degrees and the ankle is fully dorsiflexed. From this position to the mid-thrust position, the hip extends some 70 degrees, brought about by the concentric and isotonic action of gluteus maximus and the hamstrings. Slight abduction of the weight-bearing hip is brought about by powerful concentric contraction of gluteus medius assisted by the anterior fibres of gluteus maximus and posterior fibres of gluteus minimus.

A small degree of medial rotation of the working hip occurs at the lower part of the thrust phase as the pelvis rotates forward in preparation for the equivalent phase in the opposite limb. This is brought about by gluteus minimus and tensor fascia lata, aided by the anterior fibres of gluteus medius, all working concentrically.

Powerful extension at the knee is brought about by the concentric action of quadriceps femoris, the knee joint moving through approximately 90 degrees to reach almost full extension. There is also powerful ankle plantarflexion due to the concentric action of the leg/calf (triceps surae) and posterior tibial muscles.

The toes, particularly the hallux, are flexed at their metatarsophalangeal and interphalangeal joints by flexor digitorum longus, with quadratus plantae and flexor hallucis longus, aided by flexor digitorum brevis, flexor hallucis brevis and the interossei.

The height of the saddle considerably influences the range of joint movement, as well as the extent of muscle activity, critically affecting the efficiency of the downward thrust. For professional cyclists, the saddle height can dramatically affect their performance.

Recovery phase. The recovery phase produces elevation of the opposite side of the pelvis. In this phase, the upward-moving pedal pushes the foot upwards as it rises. Weight is reduced on the pedal maintaining contact, so the foot is positioned ready for the next thrust phase.

There is extension of the toes and ankle dorsiflexion, both through almost their full range brought about by the upward movement of the pedal, controlled by eccentric work of the toe flexors and ankle plantarflexors, respectively. At the same time, there is knee and hip flexion due to the same upthrust of the pedal, controlled by quadriceps femoris and by gluteus maximus and the hamstrings, respectively, all working minimally but eccentrically. In addition, the hip abductors are working to maintain the position of the lower limb, although the pelvis is raised by the flexors of the same side. As the foot passes the highest point of the cycle, the thrust phase begins again.

If the pedal is fitted with a toe clip, the recovery phase becomes a dynamic 'pulling-up' phase involving active toe extension, ankle dorsiflexion and knee and hip flexion, with the appropriate muscles all working concentrically to augment the thrust phase of the opposite limb.

Stationary (exercise) cycles have become extremely popular; joint movement and muscle analysis is essentially the same as previously described. The power of the thrust phase, however, is normally controlled by friction applied to a flywheel driven by the pedals. Cycling is a good way of improving and maintaining cardiovascular fitness.

Squats

Explanation of movement. Squats are a common form of physical activity, particularly advantageous for building up the leg/calf muscles, quadriceps femoris, the glutei and extensor muscles of the back. They are convenient, require no apparatus and can be performed in a limited space. Performance can be assessed by numerical progression; they are frequently used to enhance stamina. There is a full range of activity at the ankle and knee joints and, except for the last few degrees of extension, at the hip and trunk. As in other activities, the lower limbs are dealt with in detail. Small variations in the performance of squats can be included; the subject can rise onto the toes or leave the feet flat on the floor; the trunk can be bent over the knees or remain vertical when reaching the fully squat position. In the following description, the heels are raised and the trunk is allowed to bend forward over the knees.

Starting position. The activity begins from the standing position. The ankles are slightly dorsiflexed; the knees fully extended with quadriceps femoris relaxed; the hips are in neutral maintained by slight contraction of gluteus maximus and the hamstrings and slightly laterally rotated; the trunk is erect.

Heel raise phase. There is plantarflexion of the ankle joints brought about by concentric contraction of gastrocnemius, soleus and plantaris. The longitudinal and transverse arches of the feet are raised by the extrinsic and intrinsic muscles of the foot.

Body weight is then transferred to the metatarsal heads, particularly the first and fifth, and to all toes, the latter being passively forced into extension by raising the heel. The long (flexors digitorum longus and hallucis longus) and short (flexors hallucis brevis, digitorum brevis and accessorius) flexors of the toes initially contract concentrically and then statically to maintain balance.

The knees remain in their close-packed position, with quadriceps femoris contracting strongly to maintain this position. The hips become slightly extended with the glutei acting statically to maintain balance. The flexor, extensor and lateral flexor muscles of the trunk all contract statically to maintain the trunk position and balance.

Knees bend phase. The knees are 'unlocked' by the action of popliteus pulling on the lateral side of the lateral femoral condyle, rotating the femur laterally and sliding the medial condyle slightly forwards. The knee then flexes under the action of body weight, controlled by the eccentric action of quadriceps femoris; the power needed to control the movement increases as the knee flexes. Movement is arrested as the buttocks and posterior thigh make contact with the heels and leg/calf.

The ankles become dorsiflexed under both the action of body weight and change in position of the tibia; however, the posterior leg/calf muscles act powerfully, eccentrically controlling the movement. The feet maintain their high arches as weight is still borne on the metatarsal heads and pads of the toes. All muscles crossing the ankle joint and those of the feet interact to maintain balance.

The hips are flexed because the trunk bends forward to maintain equilibrium, the movement is controlled by powerful eccentric activity of gluteus maximus and the hamstrings. There is interplay between the abductors (gluteus medius and minimus) and adductors (longus, brevis, magnus) to maintain balance.

Rising phase. The knees are extended by powerful concentric contraction of quadriceps femoris, with maximum force applied when the knees are fully flexed, decreasing as they become more extended. At full extension, the knees move into a 'close-packed' position as the femur rotates medially with respect to the tibia, and the medial femoral condyle slides posteriorly on the tibial plateau. As the knees extend, the ankles plantarflex, and the hip and vertebral column both extend. The ankles are plantarflexed by the concentric action of the posterior leg/calf muscles; the hips are extended by the concentric contraction of gluteus maximus and the hamstrings, while the trunk is extended by the concentric contraction of the postvertebral muscles.

Rowing

The joint movement and muscle work of the lower limbs in rowing is intimately related with the timing of the movements of the upper limb (p. 224). It is this timing, power and balance combined with other factors which determines the efficiency of the rower and the speed of movement through the water.

Outline of activity. The description begins from the fully forward position, as in the upper limb (p. 224). The seat is fully forward on the runners. The whole body is then pushed backwards by extension of the lower limbs, the trunk extended and the oars drawn backwards by the upper limbs.

Starting position. The feet are usually strapped to the stretcher, the ankles are fully dorsiflexed and held at this point by the dorsiflexors (tibialis anterior, extensors hallucis longus and digitorum longus), also producing extension of the toes. The knees are fully flexed and held by the hamstrings working statically. The hips are fully flexed and held by the hip flexors (psoas major, pectineus, rectus femoris). The trunk is also flexed (p. 224).

Sequence of movement

Stroke phase. At the beginning of this phase, the lower limbs are forcefully extended. There is ankle plantarflexion to the neutral position partly brought about by concentric contraction of the leg/calf muscles (gastrocnemius, soleus) and partly due to changes in knee position. The toes are thrust against the stretcher mainly by static work of flexors digitorum longus and brevis and hallucis longus. There is vigorous and full knee extension brought about by strong concentric contrac-

tion of quadriceps femoris, and there is hip extension from the flexed position to just short of neutral, brought about by powerful concentric contraction of gluteus maximus and the hamstrings. This is one occasion when the hamstrings act as a tie between the knee and hip. As the knees are extended, the distal hamstring attachments move downwards while its fibres are contracting concentrically extending the hip joints.

The trunk and neck are extended while the head is stabilised in a neutral position (see upper limb and trunk action, p. 224).

Recovery phase. At the end of the stroke phase when the hands and oar reach the abdomen, the wrists are extended, the oars are removed from the water and begin their movement backwards, parallel with the water. The rower on the seat now begins to move forwards. The ankles are dorsiflexed by concentric action of tibialis anterior, extensor digitorum longus, extensor hallucis longus and fibularis/peroneus tertius.

The knees are flexed by the concentric action of the hamstrings (semitendinosus, semimembranosus, biceps femoris). The hips are flexed by the concentric action of psoas major, iliacus, pectineus and rectus femoris. The trunk is flexed by the abdominal muscles working concentrically (p. 224).

When the forward position is reached, the wrists are flexed to the neutral position, the oar is placed in the water (p. 224) and the full cycle begins again.

LUMBAR, LUMBOSACRAL AND SACRAL PLEXUSES AND NERVES OF THE LOWER LIMB

LEARNING OUTCOMES

By the end of the section, you should be able to:
1. Describe the formation of the lumbar, lumbosacral and sacral plexuses from their roots to their terminal branches
2. Give the root value of each terminal branch
3. State the muscles supplied by each branch
4. Describe the course and distribution of each branch
5. Describe the sensory innervation of the lower limb
6. Appreciate the influence of pathology and/or trauma to the lumbar, lumbosacral and sacral plexuses and their terminal branches

INTRODUCTION

The nerve supply to the lower limb is from the ventral rami of the first lumbar to fourth sacral spinal nerves (Fig. 3.176). Before emerging from their appropriate intervertebral foramina, the spinal nerve roots have travelled some distance in the vertebral canal. The first lumbar nerve roots separate from the spinal cord about two vertebrae above their exit, while those of the fourth sacral nerve separate from the cord at its termination between the first and second lumbar vertebrae.

As each nerve passes out of the intervertebral foramen, it receives a grey ramus communicans connecting it to the sympathetic trunk; the first and second lumbar roots are also connected to the sympathetic trunk by a white ramus communicans.

The ventral rami of the first three and upper part of the fourth lumbar nerves form the lumbar plexus within the substance of psoas major. The remainder of the fourth lumbar and ventral ramus of the fifth lumbar nerve form the lumbosacral trunk, passing over the ala of the sacrum to join the ventral rami of the first, second, third and upper part of the fourth sacral nerves to form the lumbosacral plexus. The fourth and fifth sacral nerves form the sacral plexus.

LUMBAR PLEXUS

The lumbar plexus is formed by the ventral rami of the first, second, third and part of the fourth lumbar nerves; occasionally, there is a contribution from the subcostal nerve (T12). The plexus forms within the substance of psoas major with the rami entering between its attachments to the body and transverse process of each vertebra.

The most common arrangement is that the first lumbar nerve, with the communication from T12 if present, divides into upper and lower branches. The upper branch divides into the iliohypogastric and ilioinguinal nerves; the lower part joins the upper part of the second lumbar nerve forming the genitofemoral nerve (Fig. 3.176A).

The lower part of the second, third and upper part of the fourth nerves divide into smaller anterior and larger posterior divisions. The anterior divisions join forming obturator nerve; branches from the third and fourth divisions may occasionally unite forming an accessory obturator nerve. The posterior divisions join forming

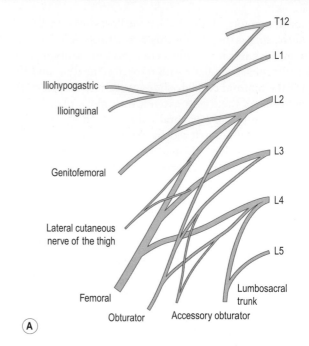

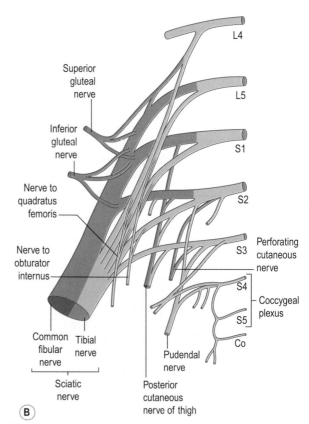

Fig. 3.176 Formation of the lumbar (A) and lumbosacral (B) plexuses.

the femoral nerve, with branches from the second and third only forming the lateral cutaneous nerve of the thigh (Fig. 3.176A).

Direct muscular branches to psoas major (L1, L2, L3) and quadratus lumborum (L1–L4) arise separately from the ventral rami.

Iliohypogastric Nerve

The nerve fibres arise from the L1 and occasionally T12 nerves; it emerges from the proximal lateral border of psoas major (Fig. 3.177A) passing anterior to quadratus lumborum and posterior to the kidney. Close to the mid-axillary line, it pierces the deep surface of transversus abdominis, gives a lateral cutaneous branch, before continuing forwards in the neurovascular plane between transversus abdominis and internal oblique, which it usually pierces 2 cm medial to the anterior superior iliac spine. It passes medially deep to

the external oblique aponeurosis, becoming cutaneous approximately 4 cm above the superficial inguinal ring (p. 542). The iliohypogastric nerve supplies the muscles of the lateral abdominal wall and a strip of skin running from the proximal lateral gluteal region to just superior to the pubis (Figs 3.177B and 3.182).

Ilioinguinal Nerve

The nerve fibres arise from L1 and occasionally the T12 nerves; it emerges from the lateral border of psoas major just inferior to the iliohypogastric nerve passing obliquely inferiorly around the deep aspect of the abdominal wall deep to quadratus lumborum (Fig. 3.177A). It pierces internal oblique, passing deep to the external oblique aponeurosis, entering the inguinal canal (p. 542) to reach the skin through the superficial inguinal ring and external spermatic fascia. The ilioinguinal nerve gives branches to internal and external

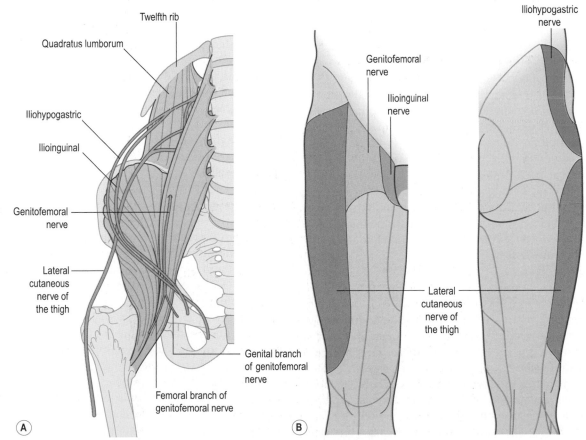

Fig. 3.177 Nerves arising from the lumbar plexus (A) and their cutaneous distribution (B).

5

oblique as it passes between them and is sensory to skin over the pubic symphysis and proximal medial part of the femoral triangle, as well as to part of the genitalia (Figs 3.177B and 3.182).

Genitofemoral Nerve

Formed within the substance of psoas major from the L1 and L2 nerves, it emerges from its anterior surface close to its medial border (Fig. 3.177A), piercing the fascia as it does so. It descends inferoanteriorly on the fascia, passing posterior to the ureter towards the inguinal ligament, where it divides into genital and femoral branches.

The genital branch enters the deep inguinal ring (p. 542), passing into the inguinal canal, supplying cremaster, and is then sensory to skin of the scrotum (or labia major) and adjacent part of the thigh (Figs 3.177B and 3.182).

The femoral branch passes deep to the inguinal ligament lateral to the femoral artery, becoming superficial by passing through the saphenous opening (p. 276), supplying skin over the proximal part of the femoral triangle (Figs 3.177B and 3.182).

Lateral Cutaneous Nerve of the Thigh

Formed from the posterior divisions of the L2 and L3 nerves, it emerges from the lateral border of psoas major (Fig. 3.177A). Passing inferoanteriorly onto the pelvic surface of iliacus, it leaves the pelvis just medial to the anterior superior iliac spine, either deep to or through the inguinal ligament. It passes laterally through or deep to sartorius and then the fascia lata to become superficial. The nerve then divides into two branches passing distally on the lateral surface of the thigh. The anterior branch supplies the anterolateral surface of the thigh as far as the knee, and the posterior branch the lateral proximal two-thirds of the thigh inferior to the greater trochanter (Figs 3.177B and 3.182).

Accessory Obturator Nerve

When present, it arises from the anterior divisions of the L3 and L4 nerves (Fig. 3.176A) between obturator and femoral nerves. It emerges from the medial border of psoas major descending between the pelvic brim and external iliac vessels entering the thigh between the pubic bone and femoral vessels. Here it usually splits into three branches: one to pectineus, one to the hip joint and one communicating with the anterior branch of obturator nerve.

OBTURATOR NERVE

Formed by the anterior divisions of the L2, L3 and L4 nerves, which unite within the substance of psoas major, it emerges from its medial border on the lateral part of the sacrum (Fig. 3.178A). The obturator nerve crosses the sacroiliac joint and obturator internus to enter obturator canal between the superior pubic ramus and obturator membrane. On leaving the canal, it lies superior to obturator externus and divides into anterior and posterior branches. The anterior branch descends into the thigh anterior to obturator externus and adductor brevis, and posterior to pectineus and adductor longus, with its terminal twigs lying between adductor magnus and the medial intermuscular septum.

The anterior branch supplies adductor longus, gracilis, adductor brevis (usually) and pectineus (occasionally); it is sensory to skin on the medial side of the thigh (Figs 3.178B and 3.182), the distal one-third of which is via the subsartorial plexus. In addition, an articular branch reaches the hip joint via the acetabular notch.

The posterior branch pierces obturator externus and descends between adductors brevis anteriorly and magnus posteriorly; it passes obliquely through adductor magnus to enter the popliteal fossa. It ends by piercing the oblique popliteal ligament supplying the posterior part of the knee joint including the cruciate ligaments.

The posterior branch supplies obturator externus and adductor magnus.

FEMORAL NERVE

Formed from the posterior divisions of the L2, L3 and L4 nerves, it emerges from the lateral border of psoas major, running in the groove between it and iliacus deep to the iliac fascia (Fig. 3.178A). It passes into the thigh deep to the inguinal ligament lateral to the femoral sheath (p. 257), entering the femoral triangle where it almost immediately divides into a number of branches loosely grouped into anterior and posterior divisions passing anterior or posterior to the lateral circumflex femoral artery. The anterior division supplies sartorius and gives the medial and lateral branches of the anterior cutaneous nerve of the thigh (Figs 3.178B and 3.182). The posterior division supplies quadriceps femoris and gives articular branches to the hip and knee joints, as well as giving the

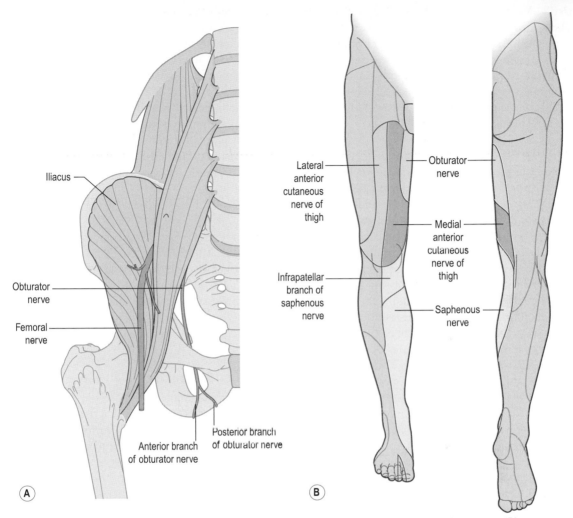

Iliacus

Obturator
nerve

Femoral
nerve

Anterior branch
of obturator nerve

Posterior branch
of obturator nerve

Ⓐ

Lateral
anterior
cutaneous
nerve of
thigh

Infrapatellar
branch of
saphenous
nerve

Obturator
nerve

Medial
anterior
cutaneous
nerve of
thigh

Saphenous
nerve

Ⓑ

Fig. 3.178 Femoral and obturator nerves within the pelvis (A) and their cutaneous distribution (B).

saphenous nerve (Figs 3.178B and 3.182). While in the abdomen, the main nerve supplies the iliacus.

Nerves to Sartorius

These arise from the anterior division of the femoral nerve entering the deep surface of the muscle by long and short fibres.

Nerves to Quadriceps Femoris

These pass to all four parts of quadriceps femoris: those to rectus femoris and vastus lateralis pass with branches of the lateral circumflex femoral artery entering the deep surfaces of the muscles. Vastus medialis is supplied by two branches, one entering proximally which also

supplies vastus intermedius; the other accompanies the saphenous nerve in the adductor canal to about halfway down the thigh, entering the medial surface of the muscle. The nerve to vastus intermedius enters the superficial surface of the muscle passing through it to supply articularis genus. All branches to the vastus muscles also supply the knee joint; the nerve to rectus femoris sends a branch to the hip joint.

Anterior Cutaneous Nerves of the Thigh

These arise as lateral and medial branches from the lateral side of the femoral nerve in the proximal part of the femoral triangle. After entering the adductor canal and crossing to the medial side of the artery, the medial branch divides into anterior and posterior parts, becoming subcutaneous anterior and posterior to sartorius to supply an area of skin over the distal part of the medial side of the thigh, knee and proximal leg/calf. The two lateral branches pass directly inferiorly in the thigh, becoming superficial by piercing the fascia covering sartorius to supply skin on the anterior aspect of the thigh as far as the knee joint (Fig 3.178B).

Saphenous Nerve

The longest branch of the femoral nerve beginning about 3 cm inferior to the inguinal ligament, it passes through the femoral triangle to enter the adductor canal on the lateral side of the femoral vessels; it gives a branch to the subsartorial plexus. The saphenous nerve pierces the roof of the adductor canal, becoming cutaneous between sartorius and gracilis posteromedial to the knee joint, to which it sends a branch. Passing posterior to the medial condyles of the femur and tibia, it descends along the medial side of the leg/calf with the long/great saphenous vein lying anterior to the medial malleolus. It then passes to the medial side of the foot as far as the head of the first metatarsal; branches supply skin and fascia on the anterior and medial aspects of the knee, leg/calf and foot as far as the base of the hallux (Figs 3.178B and 3.182).

LUMBOSACRAL PLEXUS

Lying on the posterior wall of the pelvis between piriformis and its fascia, the lumbosacral plexus (Fig. 3.176B) is formed from the ventral rami of the fourth lumbar to fourth sacral nerves. The lower part of the fourth and fifth lumbar nerves forms the lumbosacral trunk, passing over the ala of the sacrum, joining the laterally running ventral rami of the first to fourth sacral nerves. A grey ramus communicans joins each ramus, while from the second, third and fourth sacral ventral rami, preganglionic parasympathetic fibres (pelvic splanchnic nerves) pass, joining the autonomic plexuses of the pelvis, supplying the urogenital organs and distal one-third of the gastrointestinal tract.

Each ventral ramus divides into anterior and posterior divisions which converge on the greater sciatic foramen. The following nerves are formed by the union of various anterior divisions: nerve to quadratus femoris; nerve to obturator internus; pelvic splanchnic nerves; posterior femoral cutaneous nerve; and pudendal nerve. Similarly, from the posterior divisions arise the following: branches to piriformis, coccygeus and levator ani; superior and inferior gluteal nerves; posterior femoral cutaneous nerve; perforating cutaneous nerve; and perineal branch of the fourth sacral nerve. The sciatic nerve consists of the medially placed tibial nerve (anterior divisions of the L4–S3 nerves) and the laterally placed common fibular/peroneal nerve (posterior divisions of the L4–S2 nerves), bound together in a common sheath.

Nerves to Piriformis, Coccygeus and Levator Ani

The nerve to piriformis arises from the posterior division of S2 with an occasional contribution from S1. It passes directly posteriorly, entering the anterior surface of the muscle; twigs from S3 and S4 descend, supplying coccygeus and levator ani. The perineal branch of S4 also supplies coccygeus and levator ani, as well as the external anal sphincter, and the overlying skin and fascia (Fig. 3.183).

Superior Gluteal Nerve

Formed by the union of the posterior divisions of the L4, L5 and S1 nerves (Fig. 3.176B), it passes posterolaterally leaving the pelvis superior to piriformis with the superior gluteal vessels. It divides into superior and inferior branches which pass anteriorly between gluteus medius and minimus; the superior branch supplies gluteus medius and the inferior gluteus medius and minimus and tensor fascia lata.

Inferior Gluteal Nerve

From the posterior divisions of the L5, S1 and S2 nerves (Fig. 3.176B), it leaves the pelvis inferior to piriformis superficial to the sciatic nerve, passing directly into the deep surface of gluteus maximus supplying it.

Nerve to Quadratus Femoris

From the anterior divisions of the L4, L5 and S1 nerves (Fig. 3.176B), it enters the gluteal region through the inferior part of the greater sciatic foramen anterior to the sciatic nerve on the posterior surface of the ischium. It supplies quadratus femoris and inferior gemellus and gives an articular branch to the hip joint.

Posterior Cutaneous Nerve of the Thigh

Formed from the posterior divisions of the S1 and S2 nerves, and the anterior divisions of the S2 and S3 nerves, the posterior cutaneous nerve of the thigh leaves the pelvis through the greater sciatic foramen on the posterior surface of the sciatic nerve inferior to piriformis, descending inferiorly on the posterior aspect of the thigh as far as the posterior aspect of the knee joint deep to the fascia lata, which it pierces. Branches are given off supplying skin over the distal part of the buttock, posterior aspect of the thigh, popliteal fossa and proximal part of the leg/calf (Figs 3.179 and 3.182).

Perforating Cutaneous Nerve

From the posterior divisions of the S2 and S3 nerves, it leaves the pelvis by piercing the sacrotuberous ligament or by passing directly posteriorly through the medial side of gluteus maximus becoming cutaneous. It supplies skin covering the distal part of the buttock and medial part of the gluteal fold (Figs 3.179 and 3.182).

Pudendal Nerve

The principal nerve of the perineum it is usually formed from the anterior divisions of the S2, S3 and S4 nerves (Fig. 3.176B). It leaves the pelvis through the inferomedial part of the greater sciatic foramen with the pudendal vessels and nerve to obturator internus. Passing superficial to the sacrospinous ligament, it gains the lesser sciatic foramen entering the pudendal canal on the deep surface of obturator fascia. In addition to supplying the genitalia, the pudendal nerve also supplies levator ani and is cutaneous to skin around the anus.

SCIATIC NERVE

Formed by the ventral rami of the L4, L5, S1, S2 and S3 nerves (Fig. 3.176B), the sciatic nerve leaves the pelvis entering the gluteal region through the greater sciatic foramen inferior to piriformis (Fig. 3.180A). Passing down the posterior aspect of the thigh deep to biceps femoris it lies on, from superior to inferior: superior gemellus, obturator internus, inferior gemellus, quadratus femoris and adductor magnus. At a point usually about two-thirds of the way down the thigh, it divides into its terminal branches (common fibular/peroneal and tibial nerves). However, division of the nerve may occur at a higher level in the thigh, or the two components may be separate as they leave the pelvis. In the

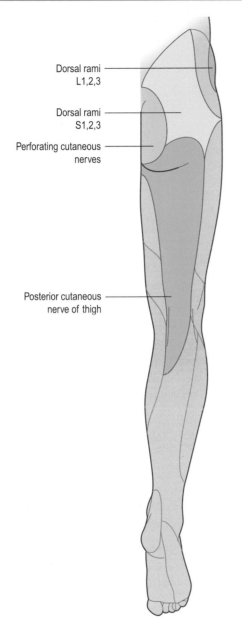

Fig. 3.179 Posterior aspect of the right lower limb showing the distribution of the cutaneous branches of the lumbosacral plexus in the gluteal region and thigh.

Labels on figure:
Dorsal rami L1,2,3
Dorsal rami S1,2,3
Perforating cutaneous nerves
Posterior cutaneous nerve of thigh

Nerve to Obturator Internus

From the anterior divisions of the L5, S1 and S2 nerves (Fig. 3.176B), the nerve passes around the ischial spine between the sciatic nerve and pudendal vessels leaving the greater sciatic foramen to enter the lesser sciatic foramen. It supplies obturator internus and superior gemellus, the former from its deep medial surface.

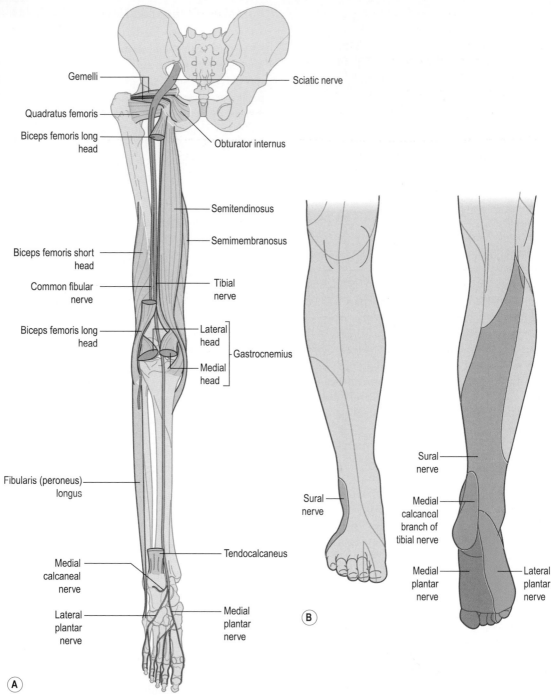

Fig. 3.180 (A) Posterior aspect of the pelvis and left lower limb and plantar surface of the foot showing the course and distribution of the sciatic and tibial nerves. (B) Cutaneous distribution of the tibial nerve and its branches on the posterior aspect of the leg/calf and plantar surface of the foot.

latter case, the tibial nerve leaves inferior to piriformis, while the common fibular/peroneal may leave superior to piriformis or pierce it. The nerve can be marked on the surface by a line drawn from a point midway between the ischial tuberosity and greater trochanter of the femur to a point two-thirds of the way down the posterior aspect of the thigh where the medial and lateral hamstrings part.

The sciatic nerve gives articular branches to the knee joint and muscular branches to semitendinosus, semimembranosus, biceps femoris and the hamstring part of adductor magnus. The short head of biceps femoris is supplied by the common fibular/peroneal part of the nerve, while the others are supplied by the tibial part.

TIBIAL NERVE

Medial terminal branch of the sciatic nerve, formed by the anterior divisions of the ventral rami of L4, L5, S1, S2 and S3, it continues the course of the sciatic nerve through the popliteal fossa (Fig. 3.180A), lying at first lateral to the popliteal vessels crossing superficially to the medial side entering the leg/calf deep to the tendinous arch of soleus. It descends obliquely inferomedially between flexors digitorum longus and hallucis longus, passing posterior to the medial malleolus deep to the flexor retinaculum between the muscle tendons. Entering the plantar aspect of the foot, the tibial nerve divides into its terminal branches (medial and lateral plantar nerves).

In the popliteal fossa, it gives muscular branches to both heads of gastrocnemius, soleus, plantaris, popliteus and tibialis posterior. Gastrocnemius is supplied from its deep surface, while soleus and plantaris are supplied from their superficial surfaces. The nerve to popliteus descends over its superficial surface, passing around its inferior border, to enter its deep surface. Articular branches are given to the knee, superior tibiofibular and ankle joints, and cutaneous branches through the sural nerve. The sural nerve descends between the two heads of gastrocnemius, piercing the deep fascia in the middle of the leg/calf, where it is joined by the fibular/peroneal communicating nerve, and passes posterior to the lateral malleolus, running anteriorly along the lateral side of the foot. The sural nerve is sensory to skin over the posterior and lateral aspects of the distal one-third of the leg/calf, lateral border of the foot and fifth toe except the distal phalanx (Figs 3.180B and 3.182).

In the leg/calf, the tibial nerve gives muscular branches to the deep surface of soleus, flexor digitorum longus, flexor hallucis longus and tibialis posterior. It also gives articular branches to the ankle joint and a cutaneous branch to the heel and posterior part of the foot.

MEDIAL PLANTAR NERVE

Passing distally deep to abductor hallucis accompanied on its medial side by the medial plantar artery to the interval between the muscle and flexor digitorum brevis, the medial plantar nerve supplies abductor hallucis, flexor digitorum brevis, flexor hallucis brevis and the first lumbrical. At the base of the metatarsals, it passes transversely across the foot giving cutaneous branches to the medial side of the sole and hallux, and adjacent sides of the first, second, third and fourth toes, including the dorsal surface of the distal phalanx and nail bed (Figs 3.180A and 3.182). Articular branches are given to the tarsal and tarsometatarsal joints.

LATERAL PLANTAR NERVE

Passing anterolaterally towards the base of the fifth metatarsal (Fig. 3.180A) between flexor digitorum brevis and flexor accessorius (quadratus plantae), the lateral plantar nerve then divides into superficial and deep branches. The superficial branch runs distally between flexor digitorum brevis and abductor digiti minimi, while the deep branch passes medially with the plantar arch on the plantar surface of the metatarsal bases. The lateral plantar nerve gives muscular branches to flexor accessorius (quadratus plantae), flexor digiti minimi brevis, abductor digiti minimi, adductor hallucis, lateral three lumbricals and all interossei. It also gives cutaneous branches to the lateral aspect of the sole and fifth toe, and to adjacent sides of the fourth and fifth toes, including the nail beds and dorsum of the distal phalanx (Figs 3.180B and 3.182). Articular branches are given to the tarsal and tarsometatarsal joints.

It is worth noting the similarity in the distribution of the lateral plantar nerve in the foot with the ulnar nerve in the hand, and of the medial plantar nerve of the foot with the median nerve in the hand.

COMMON FIBULAR/PERONEAL NERVE

Lateral terminal branch of the sciatic nerve, the common fibular/peroneal nerve contains the posterior divisions

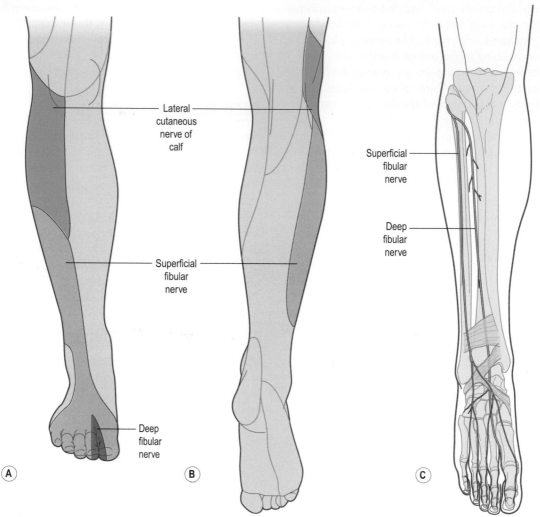

Fig. 3.181 Anterior (A) and posterior (B) aspects of the right leg/calf showing the distribution of the cutaneous branches of the fibular/peroneal nerves. (C) The course of the superficial and deep fibular/peroneal nerves on the anterior aspect of the leg/calf and dorsum of the foot.

of L4, L5, S1 and S2. It passes along the proximal lateral aspect of the popliteal fossa deep to biceps femoris and its tendon, reaching the posterior aspect of the head of the fibula (Fig. 3.180A). It then passes anteriorly around the neck of the fibula within the substance of fibularis/peroneus longus and ends by dividing into the superficial and deep fibular/peroneal nerves. The nerve can be palpated posterior to the head of the fibula and as it winds around the neck of the fibula. The common fibular/peroneal nerve gives articular branches to the knee and superior tibiofibular joints. The lateral cutaneous nerve of the calf (Figs 3.181A and B and 3.182) supplies the posterolateral aspect of the proximal two-thirds of the leg/calf. It usually arises in common with the fibular/peroneal communicating branch which joins the sural nerve in the middle one-third of the leg/calf.

Applied Anatomy

The common fibular/peroneal nerve is vulnerable to injury at the neck of the fibula where it may be crushed by direct trauma (kick, car bumper) or pressure (tight immobilising cast, bandage). This affects both the superficial and deep fibular/peroneal nerves, resulting in paralysis of the dorsiflexors ('foot drop'). This

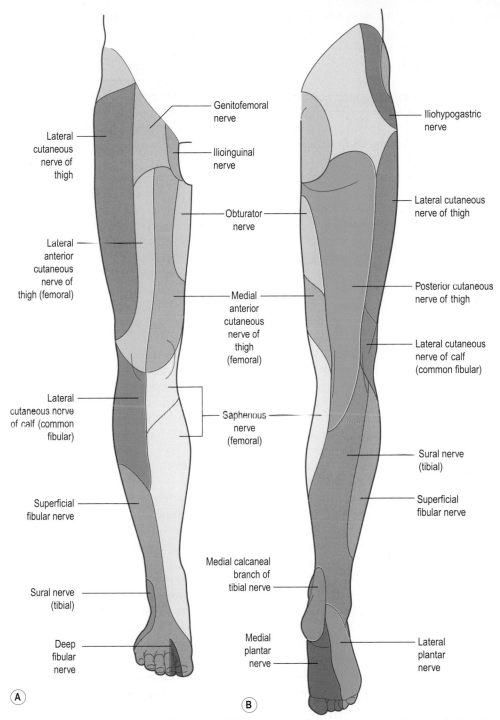

Fig. 3.182 Cutaneous innervation of the anterior (A) and posterior (B) aspects of the right lower limb and foot.

has a profound effect on gait and may require splinting to allow the foot to clear the ground during the swing phase of gait. While extensive, the sensory loss is of less significance.

SUPERFICIAL FIBULAR/PERONEAL NERVE

It descends almost vertically between extensor digitorum longus and fibularis/peroneus longus anterior to the fibula. About halfway down the leg, it becomes superficial piercing the deep fascia on the anterior surface, dividing into its terminal branches (medial and intermediate dorsal cutaneous nerves) passing over the anterolateral aspect of the ankle joint to enter the foot (Fig. 3.181).

The superficial fibular/peroneal nerve gives muscular branches to fibularis/peroneus longus and brevis and cutaneous branches to the anterolateral aspect of the leg/calf and around the lateral malleolus (Figs 3.181A and B and 3.182). The medial dorsal cutaneous branch supplies the medial aspect of the dorsum of the foot, hallux and adjacent sides of the second and third toes. The intermediate dorsal branch supplies the dorsum of the foot and adjacent sides of the third, fourth and fifth toes (Figs 3.181A and B and 3.182). Skin over the distal phalanx is supplied by branches from the plantar nerves.

DEEP FIBULAR/PERONEAL NERVE

Passing inferomedially into the anterior compartment of the leg/calf deep to extensor digitorum longus to join the anterior tibial vessels on the anterior surface of the interosseous membrane, the deep fibular/peroneal nerve descends on the interosseous membrane deep to extensor hallucis longus and the superior extensor retinaculum. At the ankle joint, it lies deep to the inferior extensor retinaculum and tendon of extensor hallucis longus, which crosses it. Entering the dorsum of the foot, the nerve lies superficially between the tendons of extensors hallucis and digitorum longus, dividing into medial and lateral branches. The medial branch passes to the cleft between the first and second toes, supplying the skin on the adjacent sides as far as the distal interphalangeal joint (Figs 3.181A and 3.182). The lateral branch supplies extensor digitorum brevis and many small joints of the foot, particularly on the lateral side.

In the leg/calf, the nerve gives muscular branches to extensor digitorum longus, tibialis anterior, extensor hallucis longus and fibularis/peroneus tertius, and gives

articular branches to the inferior tibiofibular and ankle joints.

SACRAL PLEXUS

This is formed from the ventral rami of S4 and S5; muscular branches pass to both coccygeus and levator ani. The plexus is cutaneous to the region next to the coccyx and posterior to the anus.

DERMATOMES OF THE LOWER LIMB

Throughout the previous account of the lumbar and lumbosacral plexuses, cutaneous nerves supplying particular areas of the lower limb have been described; gradually, the whole skin surface has been covered (Fig. 3.182). The various cutaneous nerves derive their fibres from the rami of their parent nerves; described this way, they appear to have no particular pattern to them.

A dermatome is an area of skin supplied by one spinal nerve through both its dorsal and ventral rami; the overlap of these areas is considerable, particularly with immediately adjacent nerves. In some areas, the main supply of the nerves is located some distance from those above and below, in which case overlap is minimal. If these regions are now traced onto the surface of the limb, paying little regard to the actual nerve through which the fibres reach the surface, a clearer pattern of innervation emerges (Fig. 3.183). In development of the lower limb, the part inferior to the knee has completely reversed so that what was the anterior surface of the leg/calf has become medial and then posterior, and what was posterior has become lateral and anterior. Consequently, the tibial nerve, deriving its fibres from the anterior divisions of the ventral rami, lies on the posterior aspect of the limb, supplying this area and the plantar aspect of the foot, while the common fibular/peroneal nerve, deriving its fibres from the posterior divisions of the ventral rami, passes anterolaterally to supply the areas on the anterior and lateral aspects of the lower limb.

The dermatomes form bands running from posterior to anterior around the lateral side of the lower limb, displaying a simpler distribution than at first imagined. When the cutaneous supply from the posterior primary rami is included, most roots supply a strip of skin varying in width from the spinal region to the lower limb. Some strips are so narrow proximally that they are merely a line, their main distribution being further distally.

SECTION SUMMARY

Nerves of the Lumbar Plexus

Obturator Nerve

From	Anterior divisions of lumbar plexus
Root value	L2, L3, L4
Muscles supplied	Adductors longus, brevis, magnus; gracilis; pectineus (occasionally)

Femoral Nerve

From	Posterior divisions of lumbar plexus
Root value	L2, L3, L4
Muscles supplied	Iliacus; sartorius; quadriceps femoris (rectus femoris, vastus medialis, vastus lateralis, vastus intermedius)
Cutaneous branches	Anterior cutaneous nerve of thigh; saphenous nerve

Nerves of the Lumbosacral Plexus

Superior Gluteal Nerve

From	Lumbosacral plexus
Root value	L4, L5, S1
Muscles supplied	Gluteus medius, minimus; tensor fascia lata

Inferior Gluteal Nerve

From	Lumbosacral plexus
Root value	L5, S1, S2
Muscles supplied	Gluteus maximus

Sciatic Nerve

From	Lumbosacral plexus
Root value	L4, L5, S1, S2, S3
Muscles supplied	Hamstrings (semitendinosus, semimembranosus, biceps femoris); hamstring part of adductor magnus

Tibial Nerve

From	Terminal branch of sciatic nerve
Root value	L4, L5, S1, S2, S3
Muscles supplied	Gastrocnemius; soleus; plantaris; popliteus; tibialis posterior; flexor digitorum longus; flexor hallucis longus
Cutaneous branches	Sural nerve; fibular/peroneal communicating nerve

Medial Plantar Nerve

From	Terminal branch of tibial nerve
Muscles supplied	Abductor hallucis; flexor digitorum brevis; first lumbrical; flexor hallucis brevis

Lateral Plantar Nerve

From	Terminal branch of tibial nerve
Muscles supplied	Flexor accessorius; flexor digiti minimi brevis; abductor digiti minimi; adductor hallucis; lateral three lumbricals; plantar interossei; dorsal interossei

Common Fibular (Peroneal) Nerve

From	Terminal branch of sciatic nerve
Root value	L4, L5, S1, S2
Cutaneous branches	Lateral cutaneous nerve of calf; fibular/peroneal communicating nerve

Superficial Fibular/Peroneal Nerve

From	Terminal branch of common fibular/peroneal nerve
Muscles supplied	Fibularis/peroneus longus, brevis

Deep Fibular/Peroneal Nerve

From	Terminal branch of common fibular/peroneal nerve
Muscles supplied	Extensor digitorum longus; tibialis anterior; extensor hallucis longus; fibularis (peroneus) tertius; extensor digitorum brevis

⁇ SELF-ASSESSMENT QUESTIONS

121. What is the root value of the sciatic nerve?
122. Which muscles are supplied by the medial plantar nerve?
123. What are the terminal branches of the common fibular/peroneal nerve?
124. What is the root value of the lateral cutaneous nerve of the thigh?
125. Which muscles are supplied by the superior gluteal nerve?
126. Which nerve supplies skin in the cleft between the first and second toes?
127. Which muscles are supplied by the nerve to obturator internus?
128. Which muscle in the abdomen is supplied by the femoral nerve?
129. What is the difference in nerve supply between the long and short heads of biceps femoris?
130. Which muscles are supplied by the superficial fibular/peroneal nerve?
131. What is the root value of the nerve supply to the majority of skin of the anterior and lateral aspects of the thigh?
132. What is the root value of the inferior gluteal nerve?
133. Which nerve supplies the dorsal and plantar interossei?
134. The saphenous nerve is a cutaneous branch of which nerve?
135. Where within the lower limb is the common fibular/peroneal nerve most vulnerable?

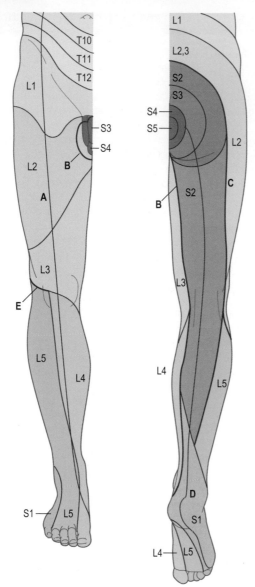

Fig. 3.183 Dermatomes of the right lower limb and foot. *A*, Preaxial border; *B*, ventral axial line; *C*, dorsal axial line; *D*, postaxial border; *E*, extension from dorsal axial line.

BLOOD SUPPLY AND LYMPHATIC DRAINAGE

ARTERIES

The main arterial supply to the lower limb is by the femoral artery, although there is sufficient collateral circulation to maintain tissues of the resting limb for a period of several hours. The collateral circulation is invaluable when there is blockage of the femoral artery if surgery needs to be performed on the major vessels.

Femoral Artery

The femoral artery is the continuation of the external iliac artery, itself arising from the abdominal aorta via the common iliac artery. It enters the thigh deep to the inguinal ligament (Fig. 3.184) contained in a funnel-shaped prolongation of the abdominal fascia (femoral sheath: p. 257). The femoral vein lies medially within a separate compartment of the sheath, with the femoral nerve lateral and outside the sheath. Psoas major lies deep to the artery, which can be palpated just inferior to the fold of the groin, halfway between the anterior superior iliac spine and pubic tubercle (femoral pulse). Within the femoral triangle, the artery passes medially anterior to the femoral vein, entering the adductor canal, which continues from the apex of the femoral triangle. It leaves the anterior compartment of the thigh by passing deep to a fibrous arch in adductor magnus (adductor hiatus) to enter the popliteal fossa and become the popliteal artery.

The femoral artery gives branches to the lateral iliac and gluteal region through the superficial circumflex iliac artery. It supplies the genital region through the superficial and deep external pudendal arteries; a descending genicular branch participates in the anastomosis around the knee, muscular branches to the surrounding muscles and through the profunda femoris to most deep structures in the thigh.

Profunda Femoris

Largest branch of the femoral artery with a similar diameter, arising from its lateral side approximately 5 cm inferior to the inguinal ligament (Fig. 3.184), passing posterior to the femoral artery to leave the femoral triangle between pectineus and adductor longus, to gain access to the anterior surface of adductors brevis and magnus. In the distal part of the thigh, it passes through adductor magnus as the fourth perforating artery contributing to the anastomosis around the knee joint. The profunda femoris gives several branches soon after its origin: the lateral circumflex femoral artery which gives ascending, transverse and descending branches supplying the gluteal region and hip joint, the quadriceps and knee joint, respectively; and the medial circumflex femoral artery which anastomoses with the lateral circumflex femoral giving branches supplying similar areas.

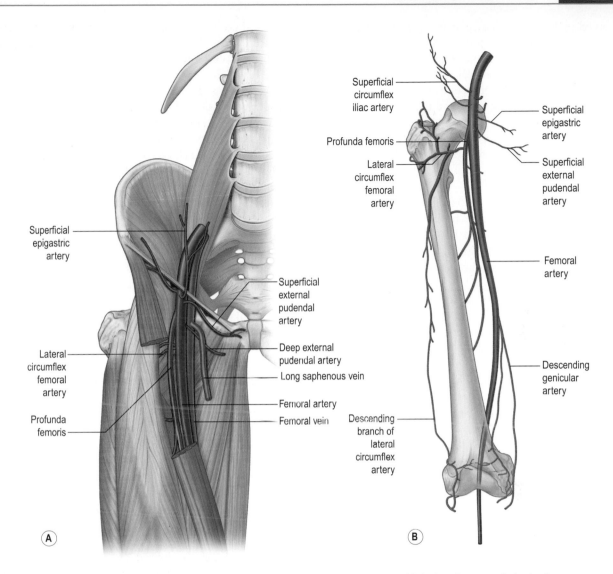

Fig. 3.184 (A) Anteromedial aspect of the right pelvic region and proximal thigh showing vessels in the femoral triangle. (B) Major arteries of the thigh.

In addition to giving numerous muscular branches, the profunda femoris also gives the perforating arteries passing either superior to or through small openings in adductor magnus linking the descending branch of the lateral circumflex femoral artery (Fig. 3.184B).

Popliteal Artery

Continuation of the femoral artery as it emerges through the adductor hiatus (Fig. 3.185). Within the popliteal fossa, it runs vertically from its proximal medial border

and ends by dividing into anterior and posterior tibial arteries at the level of the tibial tuberosity.

The popliteal artery is the deepest structure within the popliteal fossa, giving cutaneous branches to the posterior aspect of the leg/calf, muscular branches to adductor magnus and the hamstrings, and articular branches to anastomose around the knee joint. The latter are given off in three groups: the superior group being the medial and lateral superior genicular arteries encircling the distal part of the femur just superior to the condyles; the middle genicular artery is smaller, piercing the posterior part of the joint capsule supplying the cruciate ligaments; and the inferior group being the medial and lateral inferior genicular arteries encircling the proximal part of the tibial condyles just inferior to the knee joint line. The superior and inferior arteries communicate via vertical arteries passing either side of the patella (Fig. 3.185B). Further details of the blood supply to the knee joint can be found on page 338.

Anterior Tibial Artery

Beginning at the distal border of popliteus and ending anterior to the ankle joint by becoming the dorsalis pedis artery (Figs 3.185 and 3.186A), the anterior tibial artery passes anteriorly through an opening superior to the interosseous membrane between the tibia and fibula. As it passes anteriorly recurrent branches are given off passing superiorly, joining the anastomosis around the knee joint. Running inferiorly on the anterior surface of the interosseous membrane, it becomes superficial crossing the ankle joint deep to the extensor retinaculum between the tendons of extensor hallucis longus and extensor digitorum longus; here it can be palpated (anterior tibial pulse). It enters the dorsum of the foot as the dorsalis pedis artery running distally towards the first interosseous space through which it passes to the plantar aspect of the foot (Fig. 3.186A). In this region, the pulse may again be palpated (dorsalis pedis pulse).

Before leaving the dorsum of the foot, the dorsalis pedis gives a large branch (arcuate artery) passing across the metatarsal bases, becoming continuous laterally with the fibular/peroneal artery. From the arcuate artery arise dorsal metatarsal arteries which, when they reach the cleft of the toe, divide into two dorsal digital arteries supplying adjacent sides of the toes. The medial side of the first toe and lateral side of the fifth are usually supplied by separate branches from the arcuate artery.

Posterior Tibial Artery

Larger of the two terminal branches of the popliteal artery, the posterior tibial artery begins at the distal border of popliteus (Fig. 3.185A). It passes inferiorly on the posterior aspect of the leg/calf deep to soleus and gastrocnemius, lying on flexor digitorum longus and flexor hallucis longus. About two-thirds of the way down the leg/calf, it is only covered by deep fascia and skin; it

crosses the ankle joint posterior to the medial malleolus deep to the flexor retinaculum with the tendon of flexor digitorum longus anterolaterally and tibial nerve posteromedially. It immediately divides into medial and lateral plantar arteries; in this region the posterior tibial pulse may be palpated.

As the posterior tibial artery passes inferiorly on the posterior aspect of the leg/calf, it gives the large fibular/peroneal artery (Fig. 3.185A) descending between tibialis posterior and flexor hallucis longus. During its course, it gives malleolar branches and a perforating branch crossing the ankle joint to anastomose with branches of the anterior tibial and dorsalis pedis arteries.

Medial and Lateral Plantar Arteries

The smaller medial plantar artery passes distally along the medial aspect of the foot (Fig. 3.186B) medial to the medial plantar nerve between abductor hallucis and flexor digitorum brevis; it gives three digital branches passing distally to join the medial plantar metatarsal arteries.

The lateral plantar artery passes anteriorly and laterally between flexor digitorum brevis and flexor accessorius (quadratus plantae) on the lateral aspect of the lateral plantar nerve. At the base of the fifth metatarsal, it passes medially and deep, arching across the foot on the metatarsals as the plantar arch, becoming continuous with the dorsalis pedis artery on the lateral side of the first metatarsal. The arch gives the plantar metatarsal arteries, each dividing when it reaches the cleft of the toes after being joined by the digital arteries from the medial plantar artery.

The arteries on the dorsum of the foot communicate with those on the plantar aspect by perforating arteries passing between the metatarsals.

VEINS

Venous drainage of the lower limb varies considerably from individual to individual and even from limb to limb; the following description is that most commonly found. The veins are usually described as being superficial and deep; superficial veins are larger with fewer valves and situated in the superficial fascia; deep veins are normally two small vessels (venae comitantes) accompanying the arteries and situated deep in the limb, they possess many valves.

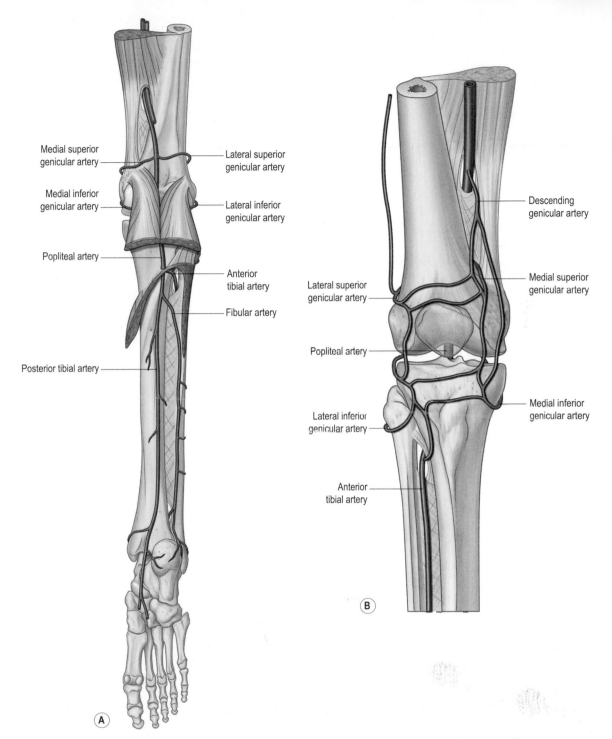

Medial superior genicular artery

Lateral superior genicular artery

Medial inferior genicular artery

Lateral inferior genicular artery

Popliteal artery

Anterior tibial artery

Fibular artery

Posterior tibial artery

Descending genicular artery

Lateral superior genicular artery

Medial superior genicular artery

Popliteal artery

Lateral inferior genicular artery

Medial inferior genicular artery

Anterior tibial artery

(A)

(B)

Fig. 3.185 (A) Arteries of the posterior aspect of the right knee, leg/calf and dorsum of the foot. (B) Anterior aspect of the right distal femur and proximal tibia, fibula and patella showing the vessels involved in the anastomosis around the knee.

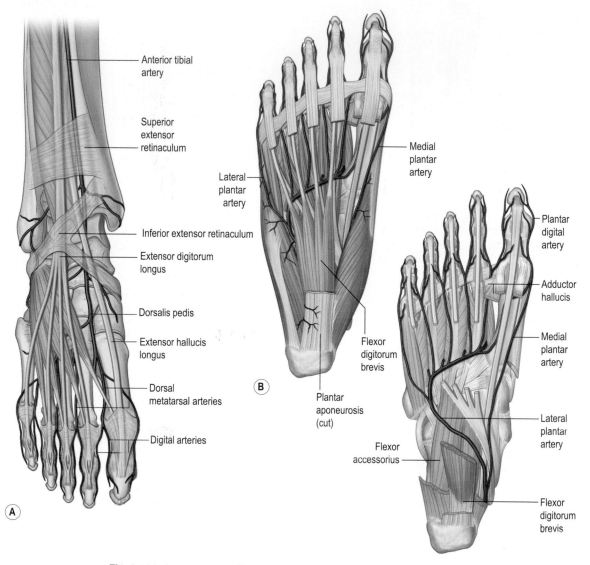

Fig. 3.186 Arteries on the dorsal (A) and plantar (B) aspects of the right foot.

Superficial Veins

On the dorsum of the foot, the superficial veins can be easily seen (Fig. 3.187A) forming a network receiving venous blood from the dorsal and plantar aspects of the toes, either side of the foot, and deep plantar areas via perforating veins passing between the metatarsals. The dorsal venous network is drained on either side by the medial and lateral marginal veins; the medial continuing as the long/great saphenous vein and lateral as the short/lesser saphenous vein.

Long/Great Saphenous Vein

Passing anterior to the medial malleolus, it ascends obliquely superiorly on the posteromedial aspect of the leg/calf towards the knee (Fig. 3.187A) lying posteromedial to the femoral and tibial condyles, continuing superiorly and anterolaterally in the thigh. It then passes through the cribriform fascia of the saphenous opening situated just inferior to the centre of the inguinal ligament joining the femoral vein deep in the groin. During its course, the long/great saphenous vein has between 8 and 20 bicuspid valves.

draining the medial side of the leg/calf and thigh. In the leg/calf, it communicates freely with the short/lesser saphenous vein and through the deep fascia with deep intermuscular veins, particularly near the knee and ankle joints. Before passing through the saphenous opening, it receives drainage laterally from the iliac region through the circumflex iliac vein, from the genital area through the superficial external pudendal vein and from the lower abdominal area through the superficial epigastric vein.

Short/Lesser Saphenous Vein

Passing posterior to the lateral malleolus along the lateral side of the tendocalcaneus to the posterior aspect of the leg/calf (Fig. 3.187B), it enters the popliteal fossa between the two heads of gastrocnemius by piercing the deep fascia forming the roof of the fossa to drain into the popliteal vein posterior to the knee joint. In its course, it contains between 6 and 12 bicuspid valves and is accompanied by the sural nerve. The short/lesser saphenous vein receives tributaries from the lateral side of the ankle and leg/calf.

Deep Veins

Two veins (venae comitantes) accompany the smaller arteries of the lower limb and are similarly named; only the popliteal, femoral and profunda femoris veins are single vessels. The veins possess numerous valves.

Popliteal Vein

Formed at the inferior border of popliteus by the union of the anterior and posterior tibial veins, the popliteal vein receives the genicular and short/lesser saphenous veins. In its course through the popliteal fossa, it passes from medial to lateral crossing anterior to the artery. It passes through the adductor hiatus to become the femoral vein.

Femoral Vein

Ascending in the adductor canal to enter the femoral triangle, the femoral vein ends by becoming the external iliac vein as it passes deep to the medial part of the inguinal ligament within the femoral sheath. In its course from the adductor hiatus to the inguinal ligament, it passes posterior to the femoral artery from lateral to medial. During its course, it receives the profunda femoris and long/great saphenous veins. The long/great saphenous vein enters some 3 cm below the

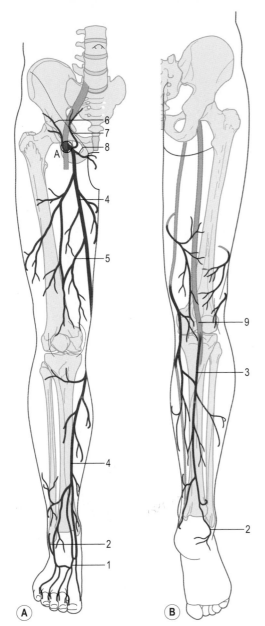

Fig. 3.187 Anterior (A) and posterior (B) aspects of the right lower limb showing the position of the superficial veins. *1,* Dorsal venous arch; *2,* lateral marginal vein; *3,* short/lesser saphenous vein; *4,* long/great saphenous vein; *5,* lateral accessory vein; *6,* superficial circumflex iliac vein; *7,* superficial epigastric vein; *8,* superficial external pudendal vein; *9,* popliteal vein; *A,* saphenous opening.

The long/great saphenous vein receives many tributaries as it passes proximally up the limb, mainly inguinal ligament just before the femoral vein enters the femoral sheath.

Application

There is abundant communication between the superficial and deep venous systems. The veins deep within the foot tend to drain into the dorsal venous network, while in the leg/calf drainage is from the superficial to the deep veins via perforating veins. Contraction of the leg/calf muscles compresses the local veins within the surrounding fascial compartments, pumping blood into the deep system because of the arrangement and direction of the valves within the perforating vessels.

Commonly, valves in the perforating veins become incompetent allowing blood to flow back into the superficial system, the veins of which then become engorged, swollen and tortuous. In such situations, the veins appear as large, ugly and often blue swellings (varicose veins) on the posteromedial aspect of the leg/calf and medial side of the thigh.

LYMPHATIC DRAINAGE

Lymphatic vessels begin in the tissues as a series of blind-ended tubules composed of a single cell layer; they exist between most tissues gradually becoming larger in diameter as they pass proximally. In their course, lymph vessels are interrupted by lymph nodes serving partly as filters and partly as a source of lymphocytes. The superficial vessels lie in skin and subcutaneous tissues, and frequently accompany the superficial veins joining deep vessels at constant sites in the lower limb. The deep vessels draining areas deep to the fascia accompany blood vessels of the region.

Superficial Drainage

The superficial drainage of the lower limb follows the long/great saphenous vein on the medial side and short/lesser saphenous vein on the lateral side (Fig. 3.188). The vessels on the medial side of the limb converge to the vertical group of superficial inguinal nodes around the long/great saphenous vein near the saphenous opening. The horizontal group of superficial inguinal nodes receives lymph from skin below the level of the umbilicus, as well as from the distal part of the anal canal and external genitalia (excluding the testes in males). The efferent vessels from both groups of superficial nodes

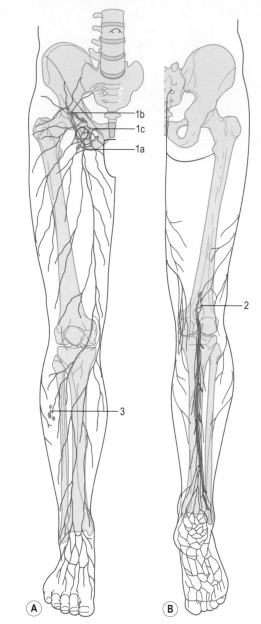

Fig. 3.188 Anterior (A) and posterior (B) aspects of the right lower limb showing the major lymphatics and groups of lymph nodes. *1*, Superficial inguinal lymph nodes (*1a*, vertical group; *1b*, lateral group; *1c*, medial group); *2*, popliteal nodes; *3*, anterior tibial nodes; *A*, saphenous opening.

pass through the cribriform fascia of the saphenous opening, ending mainly in the external iliac nodes with some passing to deep inguinal nodes.

The superficial vessels associated with the short/lesser saphenous vein pierce the deep fascial roof of the popliteal fossa to drain into the popliteal nodes.

Deep Drainage

The deep lymph vessels accompany the arteries and venae comitantes, following the same route back to the femoral triangle as the deep veins, gradually growing larger in diameter as they pass proximally. The few nodes associated with the deep vessels are usually small. An anterior tibial node is situated on the proximal part of the interosseous membrane. The popliteal nodes receive the anterior and posterior tibial vessels and lymphatic drainage from the knee, as well as the vessels accompanying the short/lesser saphenous vein. Efferents from the popliteal nodes pass to deep inguinal nodes lying on the medial side of the femoral vein. They receive some vessels from the superficial inguinal nodes and all deep vessels from the territory of the femoral artery.

From the deep and superficial inguinal nodes, lymphatics leave the lower limb by passing deep to the inguinal ligament through the femoral canal (most medial compartment of the femoral sheath) to reach the external iliac nodes. A deep inguinal node may be situated within the femoral canal.

❓ SELF-ASSESSMENT QUESTIONS

136. When does the femoral artery become the popliteal artery?
137. What are the terminal branches of the posterior tibial artery?
138. The horizontal group of superficial inguinal lymph nodes drain which regions?
139. Where can the posterior tibial pulse be felt?
140. What is the major branch of the femoral artery?
141. Into which vessel does the long/great saphenous vein drain?
142. How does the short/lesser saphenous vein enter the popliteal fossa?
143. How many genicular arteries arise from the popliteal artery and what are they?
144. Within the femoral sheath does the femoral vein lie lateral or medial to the femoral artery?
145. What does the femoral canal contain?

■ SELF-ASSESSMENT MULTIPLE CHOICE QUESTIONS

1. Concerning the innominate, which of the following statements is NOT correct?
   a. It articulates with the sacrum at the sacroiliac joint.
   b. The symphysis pubis is a secondary cartilaginous joint.
   c. The posterior inferior iliac spine can be palpated.
   d. The gluteal muscles attach to the lateral surface of the ilium.
   e. Semitendinosus attaches to the ischial tuberosity.
2. Which of the following is NOT a function of the pelvis?
   a. It contributes to kyphosis of the thoracic part of the vertebral column.
   b. It supports and protects the pelvic viscera.
   c. It provides bony support for the birth canal in females.
   d. It transmits superincumbent body weight to the lower limbs.
   e. It gives attachment to muscles of the trunk and lower limbs.
3. Concerning the sacroiliac joint, which of the following statements is correct?
   a. It is supported anteriorly by the iliolumbar ligaments.
   b. It is supported anteriorly by the interosseous sacroiliac ligament.
   c. It has the sacral auricular surface lying entirely on the lateral mass.
   d. It allows no movement.
   e. It is between the auricular surfaces of the sacrum and ischium.
4. Concerning the symphysis pubis, which of the following statements in NOT correct?
   a. The articular surfaces are covered in hyaline cartilage.
   b. The interpubic fibrocartilaginous disc is thicker in females than males.

c. The line of the joint can be palpated anteriorly.
d. Decussating fibres of adductor longus cross the joint anteriorly.
e. The arcuate pubic ligament strengthens the joint superiorly.

5. Concerning the femur, which of the following statement is NOT correct?
   a. It articulates with the patella.
   b. The lesser trochanter projects posterolaterally.
   c. Gluteus medius attaches to the greater trochanter.
   d. The hip joint capsule attaches to the intertrochanteric line.
   e. The quadrate tubercle lies at the centre of the intertrochanteric crest.

6. Concerning the hip joint, which of the following statement is NOT correct?
   a. The acetabular labrum deepens the acetabulum.
   b. The ligamentum teres attaches to the fovea capitis on the femoral head.
   c. The zona orbicularis contributes to the narrowest part of the joint capsule.
   d. All ligaments associated with the joint are relaxed in flexion of the joint.
   e. The joint capsule is reinforced posteriorly by the iliofemoral ligament.

7. Concerning movements at the hip joint, which of the following statements is correct?
   a. Vastus lateralis contributes to extension at the joint.
   b. Pectineus contributes to flexion at the joint.
   c. The hamstrings contribute to flexion at the joint.
   d. Gluteus maximus is a powerful adductor at the joint.
   e. Medial and lateral rotations occur about the anatomical axis of the femur.

8. Concerning muscles of the thigh, which of the following statements is NOT correct?
   a. The hamstring part of adductor magus attaches to the adductor tubercle of the femur.
   b. Gluteus medius is innervated by the superior gluteal nerve.
   c. Biceps femoris has long and short heads.
   d. Semimembranosus attaches to the medial epicondyle of the femur.
   e. Gracilis adducts the thigh at the hip joint.

9. Concerning muscles of the leg/calf, which of the following statements is correct?
   a. Tibialis anterior is innervated by the superficial fibular/peroneal nerve.

b. Flexor hallucis longus passes directly posterior to the lateral malleolus.
c. Tibialis posterior lies deep to gastrocnemius.
d. Fibularis/peroneus longus passes posterior to the medial malleolus.
e. Plantaris lies deep to soleus.

10. Concerning muscles of the foot, which of the following statements is correct?
    a. Abductor hallucis is innervated by the lateral plantar nerve.
    b. Flexor accessorius (quadratus plantae) attaches to the tendon of flexor digitorum longus.
    c. Flexor digiti minimi brevis flexes the metatarsophalangeal joint of the hallux.
    d. Fibularis/peroneus longus attaches to the tubercle of the fifth metatarsal.
    e. Flexor digitorum brevis attaches to the lateral tubercle of the calcaneus.

11. Concerning the knee joint, which of the following statements is NOT correct?
    a. The medial meniscus is of constant width.
    b. Flexion is produced by the hamstrings.
    c. The tendon of popliteus has an attachment to the lateral meniscus.
    d. The menisci move anteriorly and posteriorly during extension and flexion of the joint.
    e. The oblique popliteal ligament reinforces the joint capsule posteriorly.

12. Concerning the ankle joint, which of the following statements is correct?
    a. It is between the talus and calcaneus.
    b. It permits inversion and eversion.
    c. The anterior part of the trochlear surface of the talus is wider than the posterior part.
    d. Flexion is produced by tibialis anterior.
    e. The deltoid ligament lies laterally.

13. The lateral cutaneous nerve of the thigh has root value:
    a. L1
    b. L1, L2
    c. L1, L2, L3
    d. L2, L3
    e. L2, L3, L4

14. Concerning obturator nerve, which of the following statements is NOT correct?
    a. It is formed by the anterior divisions of L2, L3 and L4.
    b. It innervates gracilis.

c. It leaves the pelvis by passing deep to the inguinal ligament.

d. It innervates adductor magnus.

e. Its terminal part innervates the cruciate ligaments.

15. Rectus femoris:

a. is part of the hamstring group of muscles.

b. is innervated by the tibial division of the sciatic nerve.

c. has a direct attachment to the femur.

d. produces medial rotation of the femur on the tibia.

e. crosses both the hip and knee joints.

16. Concerning muscles of the leg/calf, which of the following statements is NOT correct?

a. Tibialis posterior passes posterior to the lateral malleolus.

b. Fibularis/peroneus tertius extends the foot at the ankle joint.

c. Soleus lies deep to gastrocnemius.

d. The tendon of flexor hallucis longus runs inferior to the sustentaculum tali.

e. Plantaris, when present, lies between soleus and gastrocnemius.

17. Which of the following nerves arises from the lumbar plexus?

a. Superior gluteal nerve.

b. Genitofemoral nerve.

c. Nerve to obturator internus.

d. Medial cutaneous nerve of the thigh

e. Nerve to piriformis.

18. Which of the following muscles does NOT laterally rotate the thigh at the hip joint?

a. Obturator internus

b. Gemellus superior

c. Gluteus maximus

d. Piriformis

e. Gluteus medius

19. Which of the following muscles produces lateral rotation of the tibia against the femur?

a. Semimembranosus

b. Gracilis

c. Gastrocnemius

d. Biceps femoris

e. Semitendinosus

20. The base of which metatarsal is held in a mortise formed by the cuneiform bones?

a. First

b. Second

c. Third

d. Fourth

e. Fifth

21. Concerning inversion and eversion, which of the following statements is correct?

a. Tibialis anterior everts the foot.

b. It occurs at the ankle joint.

c. It is a combined movement at the subtalar and transverse (mid) tarsal joints.

d. During inversion the sole of the foot is turned to face laterally.

e. It involves the metatarsophalangeal joints.

22. Concerning the knee joint, which of the following statements is NOT correct?

a. Popliteus produces medial rotation of the femur on the tibia.

b. The patella is a sesamoid bone in the tendon of quadriceps femoris.

c. The anterior cruciate ligament prevents anterior movement of the tibia on the femur.

d. It is a modified hinge joint.

e. The cruciate ligaments are extrasynovial.

23. Concerning the tibiofibular joints, which of the following statements is correct?

a. Both tibiofibular joints are plane synovial joints.

b. The superior joint is crossed anteriorly by popliteus.

c. An interosseous membrane is only present between the proximal ends of the tibia and fibula.

d. During extension of the foot at the ankle joint the distal end of the fibula moves laterally.

e. The tibiofibular joints are both weight bearing.

24. Concerning arteries of the lower limb, which of the following statements is correct?

a. The dorsalis pedis is a continuation of the posterior tibial artery.

b. The popliteal artery is a direct continuation of the profunda femoris artery.

c. The femoral artery is a direct continuation of the internal iliac artery.

d. The obturator artery is a branch of the external iliac artery.

e. The dorsalis pedis pulse can be felt lateral to the tendon of extensor hallucis longus.

25. Concerning the gluteal muscles, which of the following statements is NOT correct?

a. Gluteus maximus is innervated by the inferior gluteal nerve.

b. Gluteus minimis attaches to the lateral surface of the ilium.
c. Gluteus medius extends the thigh at the hip joint.
d. Gluteus maximus attaches to the fascia lata.
e. Gluteus minimis abducts the thigh at the hip joint.

26. Concerning venous drainage of the lower limb, which of the following statements is NOT correct?
    a. The femoral vein becomes the external iliac vein.
    b. The small/lesser saphenous vein drains into the popliteal vein.
    c. The long/great saphenous vein passes anterior to the medial malleolus.
    d. The popliteal vein is formed by the union of the anterior and posterior tibial veins.
    e. The long/great saphenous vein pierces the posterior part of the deep fascia of the thigh.

27. Gastrocnemius is innervated by a nerve with root value:
    a. L4, L5, S1
    b. L5, S1
    c. L5, S1, S2
    d. S1, S2
    e. S1, S2, S3

28. Vastus medialis is innervated by a nerve with root value:
    a. L1, L2, L3
    b. L2, L3, L4
    c. L3, L4, L5
    d. L4, L5, S1
    e. L5, S1, S2

29. Concerning sartorius, which of the following statements is NOT correct?
    a. It attaches just inferior to the anterior superior iliac spine.
    b. It is innervated by the femoral nerve.
    c. It helps produce any activity involving flexion of the hip and knee joints together.
    d. It medially rotates the thigh at the hip joint.
    e. It can be palpated proximally.

30. Which of the following features is NOT associated with the femur?
    a. Adductor tubercle
    b. Greater trochanter
    c. Quadriceps tubercle
    d. Gluteal tuberosity
    e. Linea aspera

31. Which of the following features is NOT associated with the tibia?
    a. Intercondylar eminence
    b. Lateral malleolus
    c. Soleal line
    d. Interosseous border
    e. Trochlear surface

32. Which of the following features is NOT associated with the fibula?
    a. Head
    b. Neck
    c. Malleolar fossa
    d. Lateral crest
    e. Anterior border

33. Concerning the bones of the foot, which of the following statements is NOT correct?
    a. The cuboid articulates with the fourth and fifth metatarsals.
    b. The calcaneus articulates with the lateral cuneiform.
    c. The joint between the talus and navicular is part of the transverse (mid) tarsal joint.
    d. The posteroinferior surface of the calcaneus has medial and lateral tubercles.
    e. The medial cuneiform articulates with the first metatarsal.

34. Concerning the muscles of the leg/calf, which of the following statements is NOT correct?
    a. Tibialis posterior attaches to the navicular and medial cuneiform.
    b. Tibialis anterior attaches to both the tibia and fibula.
    c. Fibularis/peroneus longus attaches to the medial cuneiform and base of the first metatarsal.
    d. Tibialis anterior extends the foot at the ankle joint.
    e. Soleus attaches to the tibia.

35. Concerning the gluteal region, which of the following statements is correct?
    a. The sciatic nerve leaves the pelvis superior to piriformis.
    b. The pudendal nerve and vessels enter the gluteal region via the lesser sciatic foramen.
    c. Obturator externus lies deep to quadratus femoris.
    d. Obturator externus is attached to the lesser trochanter of the femur.
    e. The gemelli muscles lie either side of piriformis.

36. Which of the following arteries is NOT a branch of the femoral artery?
    a. Profunda femoris
    b. Medial circumflex femoral artery
    c. Lateral circumflex femoral artery
    d. Deep external pudendal artery
    e. Ascending genicular artery
37. Which of the following arteries is NOT involved in the anastomosis around the knee?
    a. Medial inferior genicular artery
    b. Medial superior genicular artery
    c. Middle genicular artery
    d. Lateral inferior genicular artery
    e. Lateral superior genicular artery
38. Which of the following muscles is NOT innervated by the femoral nerve?
    a. Rectus femoris
    b. Sartorius
    c. Vastus intermedius
    d. Gracilis
    e. Iliacus
39. Which of the following muscles is NOT innervated by the deep fibular/peroneal nerve?
    a. Extensor digitorum longus
    b. Extensor hallucis longus
    c. Tibialis anterior
    d. Fibularis/peroneus tertius
    e. Abductor hallucis
40. Which of the following muscles is NOT innervated by the lateral plantar nerve?
    a. Adductor hallucis
    b. First lumbrical
    c. Plantar interossei
    d. Flexor digiti minimi brevis
    e. Abductor digiti minimi
41. Concerning the femoral nerve, which of the following statements is NOT correct?
    a. It leaves the pelvis outside the femoral sheath.
    b. It innervates the quadriceps group of muscles.
    c. The saphenous nerve is a cutaneous branch.
    d. It arises from the anterior divisions of L2, L3, L4.
    e. It emerges from the lateral side of psoas major within the pelvis.
42. Which of the following statements is NOT correct?
    a. The axis of the ankle joint runs from anteromedial to posterolateral.
    b. The long axis of the foot is along the third metatarsal.

c. The femoral neck is anteverted with respect to the femoral shaft.
d. The angle of inclination of the femur decreases from childhood to adulthood.
e. The anatomical axis of the femur lies entirely within the femoral shaft.
43. Concerning muscles of the thigh, which of the following statements is correct?
    a. Adductor brevis forms the medial border of the femoral triangle.
    b. The femoral artery becomes the popliteal artery after passing through an opening in adductor longus.
    c. Semimembranosus attaches to the ischial tuberosity.
    d. Biceps femoris attaches to the lateral tibial condyle.
    e. Adductor magnus forms the roof of the adductor canal.
44. Which of the following muscles only crosses one joint?
    a. Soleus
    b. Rectus femoris
    c. Biceps femoris
    d. Gastrocnemius
    e. Semitendinosus
45. Which of the following muscles has a bipennate arrangement of its fibres?
    a. Tibialis anterior
    b. Biceps femoris
    c. Rectus femoris
    d. Fibularis/peroneus longus
    e. Semimembranosus
46. What is the root value of the inferior gluteal nerve?
    a. L2, L3, L5
    b. L3, L4, L5
    c. L4, L5, S1
    d. L5, S1, S2
    e. S1, S2, S3
47. Which of the following structures does NOT pass through the superior extensor retinaculum?
    a. Saphenous nerve
    b. Fibularis/peroneus tertius
    c. Extensor hallucis longus
    d. Tibialis anterior
    e. Extensor digitorum longus
48. Which of the following structures does NOT pass posterior to the medial malleolus?

a. Flexor digitorum longus
b. Tibialis posterior
c. Posterior tibial artery
d. Tibial nerve
e. Sural nerve.

49. Which of the following is NOT a synovial joint?
a. Subtalar joint
b. Talonavicular joint
c. Tarsometatarsal joints
d. Inferior tibiofibular joint
e. Calcaneocuboid joint

50. How many phalanges are there in each foot?
a. 15
b. 14
c. 13
d. 12
e. 11

51. Which of the metatarsals is the least mobile?
a. First
b. Second
c. Third
d. Fourth
e. Fifth

52. Which of the following ligaments is NOT associated with the knee joint?
a. Arcuate ligament
b. Oblique popliteal ligament
c. Medial collateral ligament
d. Bifurcate ligament
e. Lateral collateral ligament

53. Which is the freest movement at the hip joint?
a. Extension
b. Abduction
c. Adduction
d. Flexion
e. Medial rotation

54. Which movement(s) at the hip joint are restricted by the superior band of the iliofemoral ligament?
a. Extension only
b. Extension and medial rotation
c. Lateral and medial rotation
d. Abduction
e. Adduction and lateral rotation

55. Concerning the femoral triangle, which of the following statements is NOT correct?
a. The lateral border is formed by the medial border of sartorius.
b. The femoral canal is the most medial compartment of the femoral sheath.

c. The obturator nerve divides into anterior and posterior divisions within the triangle.
d. Iliopsoas forms part of the floor.
e. The long/great saphenous vein pierces the roof.

56. Concerning the popliteal fossa, which of the following statements is NOT correct?
a. The inferior boundaries are formed by the two heads of gastrocnemius.
b. The popliteal artery lies directly against the distal shaft of the femur.
c. The most superficial structure is the tibial nerve.
d. The roof is pierced by the small/lesser saphenous vein.
e. The floor is partly formed by soleus.

57. Concerning the lymphatic drainage of the lower limb, which of the following statements is NOT correct?
a. The lateral group of superficial horizontal inguinal nodes also drains the lower part of the trunk.
b. The medial group of superficial horizontal inguinal nodes also drains the distal part of the anal canal.
c. The vertical group of inguinal nodes drains superficial structures of the lower limb.
d. The deep inguinal nodes receives lymphatic drainage directly from the superficial groups of nodes.
e. There are no lymph nodes within the popliteal fossa.

58. Concerning the sciatic nerve, which of the following statements is NOT correct?
a. It usually divides into its tibial and common fibular/peroneal components in the proximal third of the thigh.
b. The common fibular/peroneal component innervates the short head of biceps femoris.
c. The common fibular/peroneal component may leave the pelvis by passing through piriformis.
d. The tibial component has a root value of L4, L5, S1, S2, S3.
e. The tibial component divides into medial and lateral plantar nerves.

59. Concerning the foot, which of the following statements is NOT correct?
a. The plantar interossei adduct the toes.
b. The bifurcate ligament is attached to the calcaneus, navicular and cuboid.
c. Adductor hallucis has oblique and transverse heads.

d. Extensor digitorum brevis is innervated by the superficial fibular/peroneal nerve.

e. Apart from skin, the plantar fascia is the most superficial structure within the sole.

60. Concerning joints of the lower limb, which of the following statements is NOT correct?

a. The range of movement at the ankle joint is determined by the extent of the trochlear surface of the talus.

b. During flexion of the leg/calf at the knee joint the initial movement of the femur against the tibia is one of gliding.

c. In the hip joint, the ligamentum teres attaches to the fovea capitis.

d. The subtalar joint is between the talus, calcaneus and navicular.

e. Movement at the ankle joint is accompanied by movement at the tibiofibular joints.

REFERENCES

Allander, E., Bjornsson, O.J., Olafsson, O., et al., 1974. Normal range of joint movement in shoulder, hip, wrist and thumb with special reference to side: a comparison between two populations. Int. J. Epidemiol. 3, 253–261.

American Association of Orthopaedic Surgeons (1994) Joint Motion: Methods of Measuring and Recording (edited by WB Greene and JD Heckman). American Association of Orthopaedic Surgeons. Illinois.

Bell, R.D., Hoshizaki, T.B., 1981. Relationships of age and sex with range of motion in seventeen joint actions in humans. Can. J. Appl. Sport. Sci. 6, 202–206.

Boone, D.C., Azen, S.P., 1979. Normal range of motion of joints in male subjects. J. Bone Joint Surg. 61A, 756–759.

Cheng, J.C., Chan, P.S., Hui, P.W., 1991. Joint laxity in children. J. Pediatr. Orthop. 11, 752–756.

Drews, J.E., Vraciu, J.K., Pellino, G., 1984. Range of motion of the lower extremities of newborns. Phys. Occup. Ther. Pediatr. 4, 49–62.

Forero, N., Okamura, L.A., Larson, M.A., 1989. Normal range of hip motion in neonates. J. Pediatr. Orthop. 9, 391–395.

Helfet, A.J., 1974. Anatomy and biomechanics of movement of the knee joint. In: Helfet, A.J. (Ed.), Disorders of the Knee. JB Lippincott, Philadelphia, pp. 1–17.

James, B., Parker, A.W., 1989. Active and passive mobility of lower limb joint in elderly men and women. Am. J. Phys. Med. Rehab. 68, 162–167.

Phelps, E., Smith, L.J., Hallum, A., 1985. Normal range of hip motion of infants between nine and 24 months of age. Dev. Med. Child Neurol. 27, 785–792.

Roaas, A., Anderson, G.B., 1982. Normal range of motion of the hip, knee and ankle joint in male subjects, 30–40 years of age. Acta Orthop. Scand. 53, 205–208.

Roach, K.E., Miles, T.P., 1991. Normal hip and knee active range of motion: the relationship to age. Phys. Ther. 71, 656–665.

Shereff, M.J., Bejjani, F.J., Kummer, F.J., 1986. Kinematics of the first metatarsophalangeal joint. J. Bone Joint Surg. 68A, 392–398.

Svenningsen, S., Terjesen, T., Auflem, M., et al., 1989. Hip motion related to age and sex. Acta Orthop. Scand. 60, 97–100.

Walker, J.M., Sue, D., Miles-Elkousy, N., et al., 1984. Active mobility of the extremities in older subjects. Phys. Ther. 64, 919–923.

Watanabe, H., Ogata, K., Amano, T., et al., 1979. The range of joint motions of the extremities in healthy Japanese people: the difference according to age. J. Jpn. Orthop. Assoc. 53, 275–281.

Waugh, K.G., Minkel, J.L., Parker, R., et al., 1983. Measurement of selected hip, knee and ankle joint motion in newborns. Phys. Ther. 63, 1616–1621.

4

Trunk

KEY CONCEPTS

- The trunk comprises the lumbar and thoracic regions of the vertebral column.
- The vertebrae articulate with each other by joints between the bodies (secondary cartilaginous) and between the vertebral arches (synovial).
- Summation of the small amount of movement between adjacent vertebrae gives the vertebral column a wide range of movement in flexion/extension, lateral flexion/bending and rotation.
- The intervertebral disc and ligaments associated with the vertebral column give it a high degree of stability despite its wide range of movement.
- The spinal cord is the part of the central nervous system housed within the vertebral canal; it is continuous with the peripheral nervous system via the spinal nerves.
- The spinal cord comprises peripheral white and central grey matter, with the grey matter having a characteristic butterfly shape.
- Spinal nerves attach to the spinal cord by ventral (motor) and dorsal (sensory) roots.
- Each spinal nerve divides into ventral and dorsal rami containing both motor and sensory fibres.

- Dorsal rami innervate the muscles of the back and are sensory to skin as far as the mid-axillary line. Ventral rami form plexuses (cervical in the neck; brachial for the upper limb; lumbar and lumbosacral for the lower limb) or continue as individual nerves (intercostal) and are distributed throughout the body.
- The autonomic nervous system has sympathetic and parasympathetic parts: the sympathetic part arises between spinal cord segments T1 and L2, and the parasympathetic from cranial nerves III (oculomotor), VII (facial), IX (glossopharyngeal) and X (vagus), as well as from spinal cord segments S2–S4.
- The components of the cardiovascular system are located in the thorax, while those of the respiratory system are located in the neck and thorax.
- The components of the digestive and urogenital systems are located in the abdomen and pelvis.
- The endocrine system (major communication system in the body) is a collection of ductless glands which, with the nervous system, regulate and coordinate numerous body functions.

OVERVIEW

This chapter considers the anatomy and function of the trunk: it is organised into four major sections: trunk; thorax; spinal cord and autonomic nervous system (ANS); and body systems.

In the trunk section, the organisation of the vertebrae is considered, including their ossification and palpation, then the articulations between vertebrae are discussed, followed by a discussion of the muscles of the trunk, including their function. The thorax section covers the bones, joints, muscles and movements of the thoracic cage during respiration. In each of the above sections for each muscle mentioned, its attachments, innervation, action and palpation are presented. Finally, the clinical examination and evaluation of movement of the trunk, including its measurement, are considered.

In the spinal cord and ANS section, the major features of both are outlined. In the body systems section, the development and major features of the cardiovascular, respiratory, digestive, urogenital and endocrine systems within the thorax, abdomen and pelvis are presented.

At the end of each section is a summary of the main points covered. There is also a selection of self-assessment questions at the end of each section, together with a selection of self-assessment multiple choice questions at the end of the chapter.

INTRODUCTION

One of the major features distinguishing human beings from other animals is their bipedal posture and gait. As the hindlimbs progressively took over the locomotor function, the vertebral column assumed a new role. No longer is it held horizontally (Fig. 4.1A), where it is under compression, but it has become a vertical weight-bearing rod (Fig. 4.1B) held erect by ligaments and muscles. This change in function has been accompanied by changes in its form, as well as by changes in its relationship to the skull (see Fig. 5.1) and pelvic girdle (see Fig. 3.3).

Major differences in the form of the vertebral column are evident among quadrupeds, where it depends mainly on the distribution of mass in the animal. The so-called centre of gravity moves forwards or backwards along the vertebral column in relation to more weight in the head and forelimbs or in the hindlimbs and tail, respectively. In the evolution of primates, the centre of gravity moved backwards towards the hindlimbs because both the length and musculature of the hindlimbs increased, in addition to enlargement of the tail. The first of these changes gave additional power to leaping and grasping, while the latter provided balance when jumping. An important factor in locomotion is that the forward-propelling force should pass through the centre of gravity, otherwise the body tends to rotate about the centre of gravity.

The early changes in body form during primate evolution made the sitting position possible, freeing the forelimbs for manipulative activities. It also made the later stages of human evolution possible with the adoption of a bipedal gait. Although the human tail has been lost, the low position of the body's centre of gravity has been maintained because of further development of the hindlimbs, a slightly reduced muscle mass in the forelimbs and changes in the form and position of the trunk and abdomen.

A prerequisite for efficient arboreal locomotion was the evolution of an extremely flexible vertebral column. The increased range of flexion, together with that of the lower limbs, gave additional propulsion in jumping, as well as the ability to absorb the shock of impact on landing. However, in brachiating primates, some flexibility of the vertebral column has been lost due to it not having such an important role in locomotion. It seems that human beings could have evolved from a brachiating primate because of the relative stiffness of the vertebral column, as well as other morphological features. In addition, four other fundamental changes have occurred in both the vertebral column and thorax during human evolution, all of which are adaptations to a fully erect posture.

First, the vertebral bodies increase in size towards the lumbar region (Fig. 4.1B) because the compression forces along the trunk are no longer constant, but increase progressively from superior to inferior: the proportions of the vertebral bodies also change from superior to

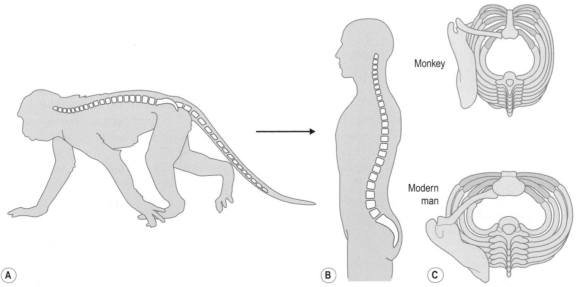

(A) (B) (C)

Fig. 4.1 Orientation of the vertebral column in a (A) quadrupedal monkey and (B) modern humans; (C) changes in the anteroposterior dimensions of the thoracic cage.

inferior. Second, the spinous processes are more or less equally developed along the length of the vertebral column because the tendency to bend is no longer restricted to the points of support (limb girdles) but is more evenly distributed. This is perhaps most clearly seen in the neck because the human head is more or less balanced on the vertebral column. Third, the stiffening effect of the sternum and abdominal muscles on the vertebral column has become less important. The sternum has come to lie nearer to the vertebral column so that the thorax is wider and less deep anteroposteriorly (Fig. 4.1C). This has resulted in a less abrupt change in direction of the ribs at their angles. Finally, the increased weight transmission through the pelvis and legs has brought about an enlargement of the sacrum, which in humans is usually composed of five fused segments: it is also relatively wide and more convex on its pelvic surface.

In humans, the tail is reduced to between two and four fused coccygeal vertebrae, which curve ventrally and help form the pelvic cavity. Ligaments running from the coccyx to the ischium play an important role in maintaining this relationship and, in so doing, contribute to supporting the abdominal and pelvic viscera. The abdominal viscera are carried in a saclike cavity, supported posteriorly by the vertebral column, inferiorly by the pelvis and anterolaterally by the abdominal muscles (rectus abdominis, external and internal abdominal oblique, transversus abdominis).

Although the vertebral column has changed in form and orientation during human evolution, it still has to fulfil the same functional requirements as in quadrupedal animals:

1. Carry and support the thoracic cage, maintaining the balance between it and the abdominal cavity.
2. Give attachment to many muscles of the pectoral and pelvic girdles.
3. Provide anchorage for many powerful muscles which move the vertebral column: these same muscles maintain the balance and erectness of the trunk.
4. Surround and protect the spinal cord against mechanical injury.
5. Act as a shock absorber by virtue of its curvatures and the intervertebral discs, receiving and distributing the impacts associated with the dynamic functioning of the body.
6. By virtue of its flexibility, it is capable of producing and accumulating moments of force, as well as concentrating and transmitting forces received from other parts of the body.

The erect posture and independent functioning of the upper limbs have greatly increased the dynamic demands made on the vertebral column. Nevertheless, the adaptation has been reasonably, although not altogether, successful: the vertebral column has become a complicated and delicate mechanical unit. That the transition from quadrupedal to bipedal has not been entirely successful is witnessed by the fact that low back pain and its associated problems take a heavy toll.

The vertebral column comprises a series of mobile segments held together by ligaments and muscles, each separated from adjacent segments by an intervertebral disc. There are usually 33 bony segments, of which 24 present as separate bones; the lower 9 are fused (5 form the sacrum and 4 the coccyx). The 24 presacral vertebrae are designated cervical, thoracic and lumbar according to their features and position within the trunk: there are 7 cervical, 12 thoracic and 5 lumbar vertebrae (Fig. 4.2). The length of the vertebral column is between 72 and 75 cm in the majority of individuals, of which approximately one-quarter is from the intervertebral discs: approximately 40% of an individual's height is due to the length of the vertebral column. Variations in height between individuals mainly reflect differences in lower limb length rather than differences in vertebral column length. However, diurnal variations in height (up to 2 cm between early morning and late evening) are due to compression and loss of thickness of the individual intervertebral discs: this should be borne in mind when charting the change in height of an individual. Loss of height in elderly individuals is associated with thinning of the discs as a result of age-related changes.

The adult vertebral column has four curvatures (Fig. 4.2A): anterior convexities in the cervical and lumbar regions; anterior concavities in the thoracic and sacrococcygeal regions. Both the cervical and lumbar curvatures are acquired in the sense that they are not present in early foetal development. Until late in foetal development, the vertebral column shows a single curvature concave anteriorly (Fig. 4.2B(i)). Late in foetal life, the secondary cervical curvature (Fig. 4.2B(ii)) begins to appear, becoming more accentuated between 6 and 12 weeks after birth as the infant begins to hold up its head to enlarge its visual environment. The secondary lumbar curvature (Fig. 4.2B(iii)) appears when the child begins to sit up at around 6 months, becoming more marked with standing and the onset of walking. Extension of the hip accompanying standing and walking tilts the pelvis forwards so that the axis of the pelvic cavity is no longer

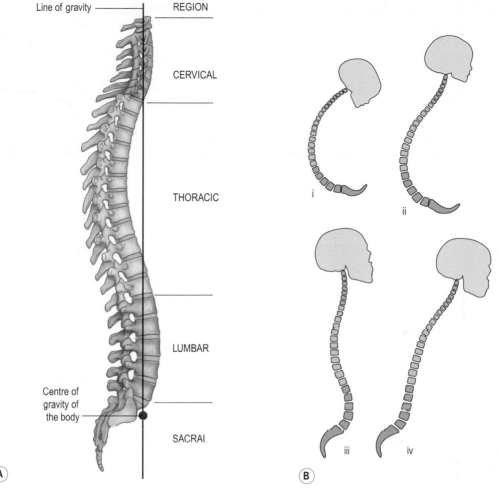

Fig. 4.2 (A) Lateral aspect of the adult vertebral column; (B) changing curvatures of the human vertebral column: (i) at birth, (ii) at 6 months, (iii) adult and (iv) in old age.

in line with that of the abdominal cavity. The lumbar curvature develops to keep the trunk erect when standing: it is not fully developed until after the age of 2 years, when a more or less adult pattern of walking is established. Sadly, in old age, the vertebral column tends to assume a gentle C-shaped curve (Fig. 4.2B(iv)) reminiscent of the early foetal curve. This change is due to the shape of the vertebral column being largely determined by the intervertebral discs and, to a much lesser extent, the vertebrae. Consequently, as the discs degenerate and thin with increasing age, the secondary curvatures gradually disappear.

The relatively shallow cervical curvature begins in the dens of the axis and ends at the level of the second thoracic vertebra: it can be reduced or obliterated by flexing the neck and head. The permanent thoracic curve is due in part to the shape of the thoracic vertebral bodies, being

higher posteriorly than anteriorly: it ends at the 12th thoracic vertebra (kyphosis is an increase in curvature). The lumbar curvature, which tends to be deeper and more prominent in females, ends at the lumbosacral junction. Changes in orientation of the pelvis (pelvic tilt) are accompanied by changes in lumbar curvature in an attempt to keep the trunk erect: wearing high-heeled shoes throws the pelvis forwards, resulting in an increase in the lumbar curvature. A similar situation arises during pregnancy in an attempt to move the centre of gravity posteriorly to prevent overbalancing. An increase in lumbar curvature is a lordosis, although the normal lumbar curve is often referred to as a lumbar lordosis. The curvature of the sacrum is permanent because of its fused constituent parts. The lumbosacral angle is not a part of the vertebral curvatures; however, because it is where the mobile and immobile parts of the vertebral column meet, the structures associated with it (intervening intervertebral disc and ligaments) are put under considerable stress.

The normal curvatures of the vertebral column make it a flexible support, imparting resilience to axial compressive forces which are absorbed by the giving way and recovery of the various curves.

Viewed anteriorly, the vertebral column appears almost straight and symmetrical with perhaps a very slight right thoracic curve (probably due to the presence of the aortic arch). A large lateral curvature (scoliosis) is abnormal (Fig. 4.31): scoliosis also involves rotation of the vertebrae so that their spinous processes turn towards the concavity of the curvature. Compensatory curves in the reverse direction occur to keep the head facing forwards and over the feet. The condition is extremely complex, often appearing in childhood during periods of increased growth (between 6 and 8 years; during early puberty).

The vertebral curves pass anterior and posterior to the line of gravity along which the weight of the head, upper limbs and trunk is projected to the lower limbs. This line is said to pass progressively through the dens, bodies of the 2nd and 12th thoracic vertebrae and promontory of the sacrum (Fig. 4.2A), with the centre of gravity of the body located just anterior to the sacral promontory. However, it must be remembered that the line of gravity is not constant: it is continually changing, both as the body moves and also when standing still. Nevertheless, it is a useful concept in reminding us of the natural balance and beauty of the body. By visualising changes in the projection of this line, it may be possible to determine the structures put under increased strain in certain postures and pathologies.

Fasciae of the Trunk
Superficial Fascia

Over the back, the superficial fascia is thick and contains a large amount of fat held within a meshwork of fibres, while anteriorly and laterally it contains a variable amount of fat. Laterally, it is loosely connected to the skin, but in the midline, particularly in the neck, it holds the skin more firmly to the deep fascia. In the superficial fascia of the anterior abdominal wall, fat is commonly deposited in middle age: the upper part of the abdomen in males and lower part in females.

As the superficial fascia of the trunk passes inferiorly towards the thigh, it divides into two layers between which are found the superficial vessels and nerves: it is continuous with the superficial fascia of the thigh. The deeper of these layers is a thin elastic membrane, which, in the lower part of the abdominal wall, is loosely attached to the external oblique aponeurosis and more firmly to the linea alba and symphysis pubis. In the lower abdomen, this deeper membranous layer is a substitute for the deep fascia proper, which is very scant: it passes superficial to the inguinal ligament and attaches to the deep fascia of the thigh (fascia lata) some 2 cm distal and parallel to the inguinal ligament.

Deep Fascia

Over the anterior and lateral parts of the chest and trunk, the deep fascia has no special features: it is relatively thin and elastic to allow both the thorax and abdomen to expand. In the lower part of the abdomen, it may be replaced by the external oblique aponeurosis and membranous layer of the superficial fascia: it is attached superiorly to the clavicle and lateral margins of the sternum, and inferiorly to the iliac crest.

The back, however, is covered by a layer of deep fascia of variable thickness and strength. In the neck, it is dense and strong becoming relatively thin inferiorly: it covers and encloses the superficial muscles connecting the upper limb to the trunk, being attached to the spine and acromion process of the scapula, the spines of the thoracic and lumbar vertebrae, the iliac crest and posterior aspect of the sacrum. Laterally, it is continuous with the deep fascia of the axilla, thorax and abdomen: it also blends with the deep investing fascia of the arm.

Thoracolumbar Fascia

Deep to the superficial muscles of the back is an extremely strong layer of the deep fascia (thoracolumbar fascia); however, it is really only well developed in the lower thoracic and lumbar regions, where it consists of three separate layers (see Fig. 4.35C).

The posterior layer is superficial to erector spinae, attaching medially to the spinous processes of the thoracic, lumbar and sacral vertebrae and associated supraspinous ligaments. It extends from the sacrum and iliac crest to the angles of the ribs, lateral to iliocostalis: latissimus dorsi partly arises from the strong membranous part of this layer in the lower part of the back.

The middle layer attaches medially to the tips of the lumbar transverse processes and the intertransverse ligaments, extending from the inferior border of the 12th rib and lumbocostal ligament superiorly to the iliac crest and iliolumbar ligament inferiorly. It is sandwiched between the erector spinae and quadratus lumborum, joining the posterior layer at the lateral border of the erector spinae.

The anterior layer lies anterior to the quadratus lumborum, attaching to the anterior aspect of the lumbar transverse processes medially: laterally, it fuses with the middle layer at the lateral border of the quadratus lumborum. It extends from the iliac crest and iliolumbar ligament inferiorly to the inferior border of the 12th rib. Superiorly, it is thickened between the 12th rib and the transverse process of L1, forming the lateral arcuate ligament; it is the thinnest of the three layers.

The single sheet of fascia formed laterally acts as the point of attachment for the transversus abdominis and internal oblique. In the lumbar region, the thick sheet of fascia is important in filling the gap between the 12th rib and iliac crest, acting as a protective membrane: it is considered by some to function as a large ligament. In the thoracic region, the fascia is thinner, sandwiched between the erector spinae and latissimus dorsi, and the rhomboids.

TRUNK

LEARNING OUTCOMES

By the end of the section, you should be able to:
1. Identify, palpate and examine lumbar and thoracic vertebrae
2. Describe the joints of the vertebral column
3. Describe and explain the movements possible, and their restraints, in the lumbar and thoracic regions of the vertebral column
4. Locate, palpate and examine the muscles associated with the trunk and give their attachments, action and innervation
5. Examine and assess movements of the lumbar and thoracic regions of the vertebral column
6. Appreciate the influence of pathology and/or trauma on the function of the trunk

VERTEBRAL COLUMN

Extending from the base of the skull to the pelvis, the vertebral column consists of a series of irregularly shaped bones which increase in size from superior to inferior: the vertebrae are bound together by ligaments and have intervertebral discs between their bodies. In young children, 33 separate vertebrae can be identified; however, by the time adulthood is reached, five have fused to form the sacrum and four the coccyx. Of the remaining 24, 7 are found in the neck (cervical vertebrae), 12 articulate with the ribs (thoracic vertebrae) and 5 are found in the lower back (lumbar vertebrae). Within each group, the vertebrae have similar features, some of which are distinctive regarding their shape and orientation of the articular processes.

With the exception of the first and second cervical vertebrae, all vertebrae possess a large weight-bearing body anteriorly and a vertebral arch posteriorly, which consists of a series of bony processes (Fig. 4.3A). The body varies in shape and size depending on its location in the vertebral column, but is roughly cylindrical with flattened superior and inferior surfaces. On these surfaces, markings for attachment of the intervertebral disc around the periphery can be seen surrounding a roughened central area. The anterior and lateral aspects of the bodies are roughened, particularly at their superior and

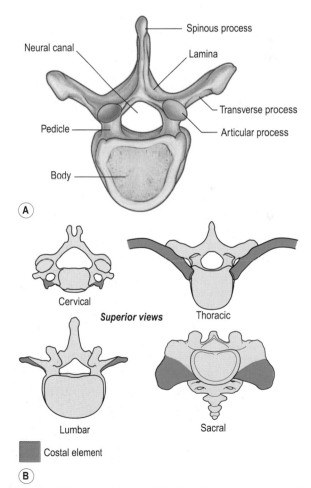

Fig. 4.3 (A) Typical vertebra; (B) fate of the costal element in each region.

inferior margins, and concave from superior to inferior: the posterior surface is fairly smooth with a large foramen for the passage of the basivertebral vein. The vertebral arch arises from the posterolateral aspect of the body, with which it surrounds the vertebral foramen. *In situ* adjacent vertebral foramina, together with the intervertebral discs and ligamenta flava, form the vertebral canal which houses the spinal cord and its various coverings.

The vertebral arch consists of two pedicles and two laminae. Each pedicle passes from the superior part of the posterolateral aspect of the vertebral body to join with the anterolateral extremity of the corresponding lamina: the laminae slope posteriorly to meet in the midline where they are continuous with the posterior projecting spinous process. Because the pedicles are not as deep as the vertebral bodies, the opening formed between them (intervertebral foramen) enables the spinal nerves and supporting blood vessels to leave or enter the vertebral canal. The intervertebral foramen is closed anteroinferiorly by the intervertebral disc, an important relation to note in some pathologies of the vertebral column and spinal nerves.

Arising from the junction of each pedicle and lamina are three processes: transverse process projecting laterally and articular processes, one directed superiorly and one inferiorly. In adjacent vertebrae, superior and inferior articular processes articulate with each other by small synovial joints (zygapophyseal joints). It is the shape and orientation of the articular facets on these processes which largely determine the range and type of movement possible between adjacent vertebrae.

With some exceptions, each part of a vertebra is potentially present in every other vertebra, the main features of which are shown in Fig. 4.3A. The body is the only part of a vertebra represented throughout the whole series of vertebrae, with that of the atlas having been displaced as the dens of the axis. The major difference between cervical, thoracic, lumbar and sacral vertebrae is related to the size and fate of their costal elements (Fig. 4.3B).

In the thoracic region, the costal element remains separate giving rise to the rib, which articulates directly with the body and transverse process of its corresponding vertebra.

In the lumbar region, the costal element has again been incorporated into the vertebra, which is so complete that, apart from the root of the transverse (lateral) process, the remainder is composed of costal element. The true transverse process in the lumbar region gives rise to the accessory and superior processes as well as the lateral process.

Even in the sacrum, the costal elements have been incorporated and form the major part of the lateral masses.

Details of cervical vertebrae can be found on page 628 and of the sacrum and coccyx on pages 262 and 264.

Lumbar Vertebrae

The five lumbar vertebrae are much stouter and stronger than those in either the thoracic or cervical regions (Fig. 4.4): they have neither foramina transversaria nor articular facets for the ribs. Each has a large, kidney-shaped

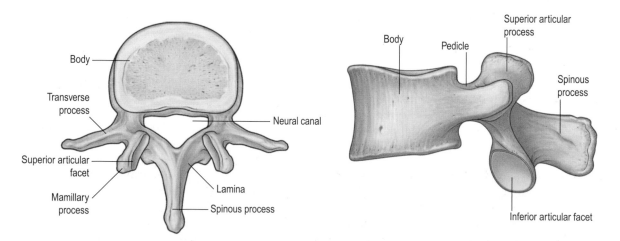

Fig. 4.4 Superior and lateral aspects of a lumbar vertebra.

body with almost parallel superior and inferior surfaces, except for L5 which is deeper anteriorly than posteriorly. The short strong pedicles pass almost directly posteriorly to join the narrow laminae which pass posteromedially towards the spine. Adjacent laminae are widely separated from each other, leaving diamond-shaped spaces containing the ligamenta flava.

The spinous processes of lumbar vertebrae project almost horizontally posteriorly level with the distal half of the body: they are wider from superior to inferior with a thickened posterior edge, with that of L5 being frequently rounded.

The articular processes project superiorly and inferiorly from the region where the pedicle joins the lamina. The articular facets on the superior process are concave transversely, flat vertically and face posteromedially: on the posterior edge of the superior articular process is the rounded mamillary process. The inferior articular processes are set closer together than the superior and have reciprocally curved facets which face anterolaterally. The superior facets articulate with the inferior facets of the vertebra immediately above. The inferior articular processes of the fifth lumbar vertebra are more widely set apart and flatter than those of other lumbar vertebrae: their articular facets face anterolaterally to meet the superior articular facets of the sacrum.

The triangular vertebral (neural) canal is larger than that in the thoracic region, but slightly smaller than in the cervical region.

With the exception of the fifth lumbar vertebra, the transverse processes are short and thin, projecting laterally and slightly posteriorly from the lateral aspects of the vertebral body and base of the pedicles: the third is the longest, with the fourth and fifth being inclined superiorly. The transverse processes of L5 are short and stout, and may be fused with the lateral part of the sacrum. From the root of each transverse process, a small tubercle (accessory process) projects posteriorly: the root of the transverse process is the lateral tubercle.

Thoracic Vertebrae

The distinctive feature of thoracic vertebrae is the presence of articular (costal) facets on the sides of the vertebral body for articulation with the heads of at least one pair of ribs (Fig. 4.5). Viewed from above, the bodies of thoracic vertebrae are typically heart-shaped and bear articular facets on their lateral aspects. The body

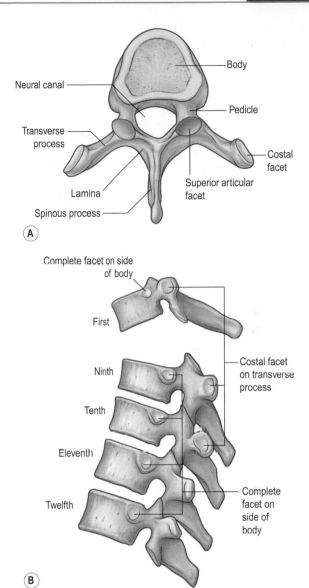

Fig. 4.5 (A) Superior aspect of a typical thoracic vertebra; (B) lateral aspects of the 1st, 9th, 10th, 11th and 12th thoracic vertebrae.

of T1 has a complete oval facet near its superior edge and a demifacet at its inferior edge. The bodies of the second to eighth vertebrae have large, almost complete oval facets near their superior borders and smaller demifacets near their inferior borders. Although similar in basic arrangement, the superior facet of the ninth thoracic vertebra is situated at the base of the pedicle. The 10th, 11th and 12th vertebrae have single complete facets located at the junction of the body and pedicle: between T10 and T12, the facets gradually move from the superior to inferior region of the junction (Fig. 4.5B).

The short pedicles project almost directly posteriorly from the superoposterior part of the body, gradually becoming larger and stronger from superior to inferior. The laminae are inclined towards the midline and, although they are narrow from side to side, they overlap one another from above.

The spinous processes are long and slope inferiorly, with those in the middle being almost vertical: the superior and inferior spinous processes are shorter and generally less sloping. The 12th is almost horizontal, resembling a typical lumbar vertebra.

The long, thick, rounded transverse processes project laterally, posteriorly and slightly superiorly from the junction of the pedicle and lamina. They have an oval facet on the anterior surface near the tip, which faces anterolaterally, for the tubercle of the corresponding rib. In upper thoracic vertebrae, these facets are concave but gradually become flatter from superior to inferior: the transverse processes of the 11th and 12th thoracic vertebrae have no facets. The transverse process of the 12th thoracic vertebra is very short and has features similar to lumbar vertebrae.

From just medial to the base of the transverse process, the articular processes project almost vertically: the superior superiorly and the inferior inferiorly. The articular facets on the superior process are slightly concave transversely, flat from superior to inferior and face posteriorly but also slightly superolaterally. The facets on the shorter inferior articular processes are reciprocally curved and face in the opposite direction. The superior articular facets of one vertebra articulate with the inferior facets of the vertebra above. The joints so formed lie on the arc of a circle whose centre lies within or just anterior to the body of the vertebra. Consequently, rotation as well as flexion and extension are possible in the thoracic region (p. 517).

The inferior articular processes of T12, although they project vertically, do not lie in the same general plane as other thoracic articular processes: they are lumbar in type, being markedly convex transversely and face anterolaterally.

The vertebral (neural) canal is smaller than that in either the cervical or lumbar region, being nearly circular in appearance.

Cervical Vertebrae

Details of cervical vertebrae can be found on page 628.

Ossification

A typical vertebra ossifies in cartilage from three primary and five secondary ossification centres.

The primary centres appear in the vertebral body and in each half of the vertebral arch. That for the centrum, the larger median part of the body, appears between the second and fifth month *in utero*, appearing first in the lower thoracic region and then spreading sequentially up and down the column. The centres for the coccygeal vertebrae appear between birth and puberty, with ossification spreading without the formation of secondary centres. Because each centrum is usually ossified from two centres, anomalies may arise if they fail to unite and remain as two separate parts, or only one may ossify giving rise to a hemivertebra.

The primary centre in each half of the vertebral arch appears at the junction of the pedicle and lamina at 2 months *in utero* in the upper cervical region, spreading inferiorly to the sacrum by the fifth month. From each centre, ossification spreads into the lamina and pedicle, where it extends into the centrum to complete the body and into the root of the transverse process.

At birth, the centrum and each part of the vertebral arch are separated by cartilage. That between the centrum and each arch begins to ossify in the cervical region during the third year, extending to other regions by the seventh year. The laminae begin to unite soon after birth in the lumbar region, spreading to the cervical region by the 2nd year: this process is not complete in the sacrum until the 7th–10th year. Once the laminae have fused, ossification spreads into the root of the spinous process.

Multiple secondary centres for the superior and inferior surfaces of the bodies appear during the ninth year, fusing to form flat rings of bone around the periphery of the surfaces. Secondary centres appear in the tips of the transverse processes during the 18th year. Fusion of all secondary epiphyses with the rest of the vertebra begins at 18 for the bodies and is complete by age 25.

The lumbar vertebrae also have secondary centres for the mamillary processes. In addition, the first lumbar vertebra may have separate primary centres for its transverse processes, which may remain separate forming a lumbar rib. In the fifth lumbar vertebra, there may be two primary centres in each half of the vertebral arch united by cartilage between the superior and inferior articular processes: there is a temporary risk of separation between the two parts.

With so many ossification processes and patterns occurring simultaneously, it is not surprising to find some variations in the total number of vertebrae present. This is usually due to a reduction, or more rarely, an increase in the number of coccygeal vertebrae.

The number of cervical vertebrae is constant at seven. However, the number of thoracic vertebrae may be increased by the presence of ribs associated with L1: similarly, the number of lumbar vertebrae may be reduced as described earlier or by incorporation of L5 into the sacrum. Such sacralisation may be partial or complete: the sacrum may gain or lose additional segments.

Many congenital conditions of the vertebral column are due to incomplete fusion of its constituent parts. Hemivertebrae can cause an abnormal lateral curvature (scoliosis) of the vertebral column. The laminae may fail to fuse or meet in any region, but most commonly in the lumbosacral region (spina bifida). The spinous process, laminae and inferior articular processes of L4 and L5 may be joined to the rest of the vertebrae by cartilage and not completely fused. Under certain loading conditions, this can lead to a separation in which the vertebral body, most commonly L5, slides forwards (spondylolisthesis: p. 273).

Palpation

Unfortunately, there is considerable variation in the location of bony points between individuals and even from side to side within the same individual. This is particularly apparent in the trunk, where the length of the spines can vary considerably, be angled differently or occasionally be absent. The best way of identifying vertebral spines is, therefore, to count downwards or upwards from known bony landmarks and cross-check with other surface markings. Considerable time and practice are involved in developing palpation techniques, but once mastered, it will prove to be an invaluable asset in the future.

The most obvious surface markings are the posteriorly directed spines; however, their palpation can vary considerably due to lordosis (convexity forwards) in the cervical and lumbar regions and kyphosis (concavity forwards) in the thoracic and sacral regions of the vertebral column.

Lumbar region. This has a lordosis similar to that of the cervical region: identification of the spinous processes may not be easy. With the individual lying prone and with sufficient support under the abdomen to raise the lumbar region so that it is level, the whole lumbar region can be examined. The spinous processes of the lumbar vertebrae can be palpated in a central cleft in the midline. Approximately 3 cm each side of the midline, a small dimple can be seen on the posterosuperior aspect of the buttock: this marks the location of the posterior superior iliac spine, which can be easily palpated and acts as an important landmark for the identification of other structures. From these spines, the crests of the ilium can be traced superiorly and anteriorly. The spinous process of L5 can be felt in a deep hollow, just proximal to the sacrum, approximately 2 cm above a line drawn between the posterior superior iliac spines. From here, the spinous process of L4 is easily recognisable superior to that of L5. With care, the small gaps between the spinous processes of L4–T12 can be palpated and each process identified. The centre of the spinous process of each vertebra, unlike that in the thoracic region, lies just inferior to the centre of the body of its corresponding vertebra. On either side of the midline is a powerful column of muscle (erector spinae) running from the posterior aspect of the sacrum superiorly towards the thoracic region.

On deep palpation, lateral to this muscle bulk small pointed tubercles can be felt running inferiorly either side. These are the tips of the transverse processes, each being located just superior to the level of the centre of its corresponding spinous process. Higher up, level with the spinous process of L1, the tip of the 12th rib can be palpated, level with the ninth costal cartilage anteriorly lying in the transpyloric plane.

Thoracic region. The spinous processes are much easier to identify, particularly if the individual is sitting with the trunk flexed. The spines of the seventh cervical and first thoracic vertebrae are even more prominent than when lying prone: it is now easy to identify the spines of individual thoracic vertebrae. Identification is made easier, however, if one finger is placed on the spine above to mark it while that below is determined. Each spinous process appears to be quite pointed as far as T11. That of the 12th thoracic vertebra on the other hand is flattened and similar to that of a lumbar vertebra.

With the individual lying prone, a line of smaller tubercles can be felt approximately 2 cm either side of the spines: these are the posterior aspects of the transverse processes and, as they are usually covered by the long back muscles, are less easy to palpate. The transverse processes pass slightly superolaterally, in line with the superior part of the body of the corresponding vertebra. The spinous processes, however, pass inferoposteriorly up to a maximum of 3 cm below the transverse process of the same vertebra. This is important to remember when palpation is being used for diagnostic purposes.

Just lateral to the transverse process, each rib can be felt passing inferolaterally around the chest wall.

Cervical region. Details can be found on page 631.

ARTICULATIONS OF THE VERTEBRAL COLUMN

Introduction

The function of the human vertebral column, together with a consideration of the adaptations that have occurred, in assuming a bipedal posture and gait has been mentioned in the introductory section to this chapter (p. 495). Nevertheless, it is worth restating that there are 24 free vertebrae in the vertebral column, with the 5 fused sacral and 4 fused coccygeal vertebrae forming the sacrum and coccyx, respectively: these have already been considered (pp. 262, 264). Of the free vertebrae, 7 are cervical, 12 thoracic and 5 lumbar (Fig. 4.6): there are specific differences between the vertebrae in each region. Although in adults the vertebrae are arranged to give specific curvatures to the column (Fig. 4.6), the joints between adjacent vertebrae have a common plan, with the exception of the specialised joints between the atlas (C1) and axis (C2), which are considered on pages 637 and 639.

Anteriorly, the bodies of adjacent vertebrae are principally bound together by the strong and important intervertebral discs. The more posterior parts of the vertebral arches are united by synovial joints (zygapophyseal joints) between the articular processes as well as by ligaments. The joints between the vertebral bodies and the vertebral arches are separated by the intervertebral foramina, through which the spinal nerves pass. The superior and inferior boundaries of these foramina are formed by the pedicles of the arches.

The joints between the vertebral bodies and those between the vertebral arches are considered separately; however, functionally they are both concerned with the structure of the vertebral column, interacting to give it a controlled flexibility.

JOINTS BETWEEN VERTEBRAL BODIES

Between the second cervical and first sacral vertebrae, the articulations of adjacent vertebral bodies are cartilaginous joints of the symphysis type: the intervening intervertebral discs are composed of fibrocartilage separated from the vertebral bodies by a thin layer of hyaline cartilage.

Intervertebral Discs

There are at least 24 intervertebral discs interposed between the vertebral bodies: 6 in the cervical, 12 in the thoracic and 5 in the lumbar region, with 1 between the sacrum and coccyx: additional discs may be present between fused sacral segments. The discs account for approximately one-quarter of the length of the vertebral column and are primarily responsible for the presence of the various curvatures. On descending the vertebral column the discs increase in thickness, being thinnest in the upper cervical and thickest in the lower lumbar regions (Fig. 4.6): in the upper thoracic region the discs appear to narrow slightly. In the cervical region, the disc is about two-fifths the height of the vertebrae, being approximately 5 mm thick; in the thoracic region, they average 7 mm in thickness, being one-quarter of vertebral body height; discs in the lumbar regions are at least 10 mm thick, being equivalent to one-third of the vertebral body height. The relative height of the disc to the vertebral body is an important factor in determining the mobility of the vertebral column in each region. Individual discs are not of uniform thickness: they are slightly wedge-shaped in conformity with the curvature of the vertebral column in the region of the disc. The curvatures in the cervical and lumbar regions are primarily due to the greater anterior thickness of the discs in these regions.

The overall shape of the discs also varies from one region to another, being similar to the shape of adjacent vertebral bodies: in the cervical region they tend to be oval; in the thoracic region almost heart-shaped; and in the lumbar region kidney-shaped.

It is of considerable practical importance to remember that the intervertebral disc forms one of the anterior boundaries of the intervertebral foramen: as the spinal nerves pass through the foramina they lie directly posterior to the corresponding discs. In addition, the discs also form part of the anterior wall of the vertebral canal. Consequently, any posterior bulging of the disc may compress the spinal cord, as well as individual spinal nerves.

Structure

Each disc is structurally characterised by three integrated tissues: the central nucleus pulposus, the surrounding

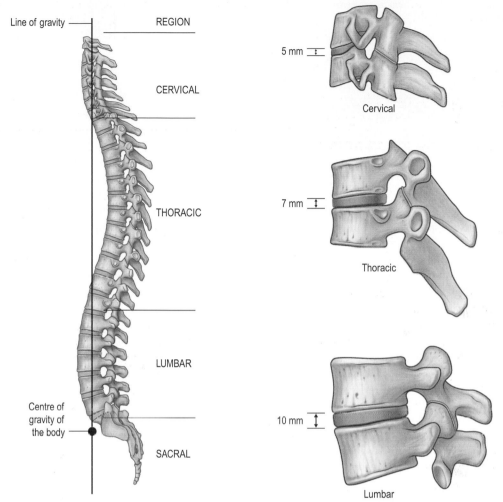

Fig. 4.6 Lateral aspect of the adult vertebral column and typical vertebrae in each region giving the mean thickness of the intervertebral disc in each region.

annulus fibrosus and the limiting cartilage end plates (Fig. 4.7A). It is anchored to the vertebral body by fibres of the annulus fibrosus and by the cartilage end plate.

Nucleus pulposus. Contained within the centre of the disc is the soft highly hydrophilic nucleus pulposus. There appears to be no clear division between the nucleus pulposus and surrounding annulus fibrosus, the main difference being the density of the fibres each contains: the nucleus has large extrafibrillar spaces containing glycosaminoglycans, enabling it to retain fluid. The classical idea of a distinct division between the two regions is, therefore, not true: nor is the concept of the

nucleus being round or oval, discography has shown it to be more rectangular in infants and young children, and anything from oval to multilobed in adults. (Discography is a radiographic technique allowing visualisation of the disc in living individuals: clinically, it enables the disc's health to be assessed.) The region between the nucleus and annulus fibrosus is an area of maximum metabolic activity: it is also sensitive to physical forces, as well as to chemical and hormonal regulation of growth processes. Consequently, it can be considered to represent the growth plate of the nucleus pulposus (similar to epiphyseal growth plates) because the nucleus can only increase in size and remodel itself at the expense

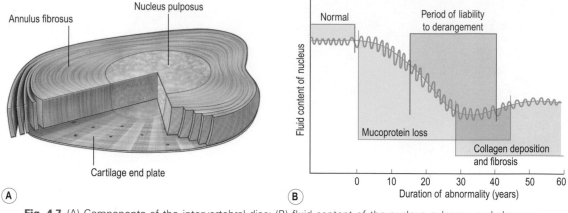

Fig. 4.7 (A) Components of the intervertebral disc; (B) fluid content of the nucleus pulposus and changes with trauma. (Adapted from Hendry, N., 1958. The hydration of the nucleus pulposus and its relation to the intervertebral disc derangement. J. Bone Joint Surg. 40B, 132–144.)

of the deep part of the annulus fibrosus. In contrast, the annulus increases its horizontal diameter by the addition of new lamellae at the periphery.

The position of the nucleus pulposus within the disc varies regionally, being more centrally located in cervical and thoracic discs and posteriorly in lumbar discs (Fig. 4.8): see also page 632. The position of the nucleus is related to certain aspects of function.

The nucleus pulposus consists of a three-dimensional lattice of collagen fibres, in which a proteoglycan gel is enmeshed which is responsible for its hydrophilic nature. Patchy loss and disappearance of this gel occurs with ageing, lowering the water content until, in advanced degeneration, the collagen may be almost devoid of proteoglycan material (Fig. 4.7B). This is the major change underlying dehydration of the nucleus in later life. In early life, a water content of 80%–88% is usual; however, from about the fourth decade onwards, this decreases to 70%. These proteoglycan changes in the nucleus, both in terms of their loss and composition, influence the mechanical behaviour of the disc.

Studies suggest that the nucleus pulposus represents the functional centre of the disc: systemic changes within it may be important as a primary cause of pathological change within the disc and consequently of all pathological change within the intervertebral space. There is, however, the view that, in disc degeneration, the first morphological change observed is separation of part of the cartilage end plate from the adjacent vertebral body.

Annulus fibrosis. A series of annular bands whose geometry varies as a function of vertebral level and

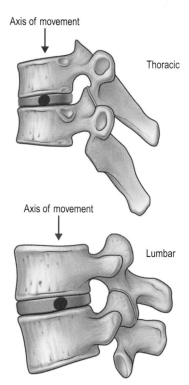

Fig. 4.8 Relative positions of the nucleus pulposus within the intervertebral disc and its relation to the axis about which movement occurs in the thoracic and lumbar regions.

intradiscal region. Each annular band has a roughly parallel course, with the directional arrangement of fibres alternating in adjacent bands (Fig. 4.7A): the obliquity of these bands is greatest in the innermost layer of any given disc. The number of lamellae, as well as their size, thickness and obliquity, shows large variations for any given band within different parts of the same disc, for any particular vertebral level, and between individuals. Nevertheless, the average number of lamellae is 20 and their thickness generally varies from 200 to 400 μm, increasing from deep to superficial. Within each lamella, the fibrils (0.1–0.2 μm) are uniformly arranged, but their orientation varies considerably from lamella to lamella.

Each lamella is composed of obliquely arranged bundles of fibrils, varying in size between 10 and 50 μm. Except for thin fibrils, there is little interconnection between adjacent lamellar sheets, providing only limited restriction to movement during compression and tension. The question arises as to whether the orientation of the collagen bundles is predetermined or mechanically induced when movement occurs. There are considerable differences in fibril thickness and lamellar organisation in the foetus: it is likely, therefore, that mechanical phenomena (especially torsion) are responsible for the adult arrangement.

The density of the fibrocartilaginous lamellae is a function of the annular region, being more closely packed anteriorly and posteriorly than laterally. Lamellar bands do not form complete rings, but split intricately or merge to interlock with other bands, with the posterolateral regions appearing to have marked irregularities and be much less orderly. With ageing, the annulus becomes weakest in these posterolateral regions, predisposing to nucleus herniation.

Elastic fibres are present within both the annulus fibrosus and nucleus pulposus. In the annulus, they are arranged circularly, obliquely and vertically, although they are not distributed throughout, being restricted to the lamellae at the vertebral epiphysis and disc interface. Interlamellar elastic fibres branch and join, freely imparting a dynamic flexibility to the tissue, with obvious implications for function. Intralamellar elastic fibres penetrate the bony vertebrae as perforating fibres.

Within the annulus, the total collagen content is not constant, decreasing from the outer layers towards the nucleus. However, the proportion of type I to type II collagen (principal collagen types within the disc) decreases from the outer layer of the annulus to the nucleus, as well as varying from region to region (Fig. 4.9). Type I collagen predominates in the outermost regions of the annulus and type II the innermost: the nucleus contains type II only. As type I collagen is typical of tendons

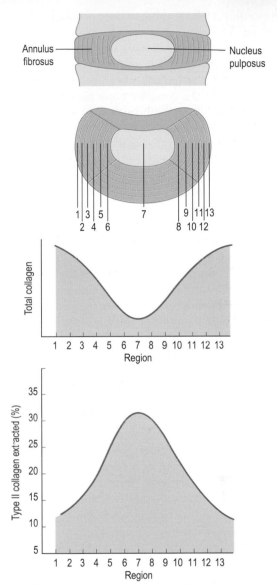

Fig. 4.9 Type and ratio of collagen within the intervertebral disc. (Adapted from Taylor, T.K.F., Ghosh, P., Bushel, G.R., 1981. The contribution of the intervertebral disc to scoliotic deformity. Clinical Orthopaedics and Related Research 156, 79–90.)

and type II of articular cartilage, where large transient compressive forces are generated, the tensile strength of the annulus is probably provided by type I collagen, while the compressive component involves type II. With increasing age, the collagen content of the annulus increases from deep to superficial in the disc and also inferiorly from cervical to lumbar regions; however, the proportion of type II collagen does not appear to change with age.

Attachment of the annulus fibrosus to the vertebrae is fairly complicated. The annulus fibres pass over the edges of the cartilage end plate anchoring themselves to and beyond the compact bony zone that forms the periphery of the vertebral rim, as well as to the margins of the adjacent vertebral body and its periosteum, forming stable connections between adjacent vertebral bodies. These perforating fibres become interwoven with fibrillar lamellae of the bony trabeculae: the fibrillar anchorage is already present at birth, even though the vertebral rim is not ossified.

Cartilage end plate. Located on each surface of the vertebral body, the cartilage end plate represents the anatomical limit of the disc (Fig. 4.7A): it is approximately 1 mm thick at the periphery, decreasing towards the centre. It can be considered to have three main functions: (1) protect the vertebral body from pressure atrophy; (2) confine the annulus fibrosus and nucleus pulposus within their anatomical boundaries; and (3) act as a semipermeable membrane to facilitate fluid exchanges between the annulus, nucleus and vertebral body via osmotic action. Regarding the last function, studies suggest that only the central part of the end plate is permeable.

In the first few years of life, the end plates are loosely attached by a thin layer of calcified material to irregular, radiating, fan-shaped ridges and furrows on the vertebral bodies. Later, a thin layer of calcified material on the end plate firmly adheres to the trabeculae of the porous surface of the vertebral body. It is thought that the end plate is in contact with the bone marrow, through which it receives its nutrients.

In early life, numerous minute vascular channels (cartilage canals) penetrate deeply into the end plate from the vertebral side; however, they disappear with increasing age so that, by the third decade, they are largely obliterated. Following the third decade, retrogressive changes occur in the end plate: it begins to show signs of ossification and there is an increase in calcification. It becomes more brittle, with fimbriation becoming more evident, ranging from thinning to complete destruction of the central end plate zone.

Development

The vertebral column begins to develop in the embryonic mesoderm at about 4 weeks, with individual vertebrae developing under the combined inductive influence of the notochord and neural tube: ablation of either at an early stage results in failure of sclerotomal and myotomal segmentation. The segmental vessels of aortic origin pass between two sclerotomal zones, which then fuse to form the mesenchymal body of the vertebra (Fig. 4.10). The intervertebral disc develops initially in an environment containing few blood vessels and is surrounded

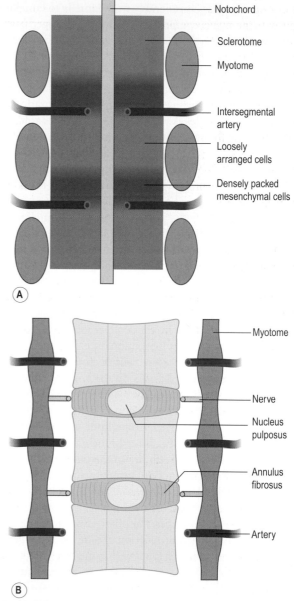

Fig. 4.10 (A) Development of the intervertebral disc at 4 weeks showing sclerotome cells around the notochord; (B) the adult arrangement.

by a perichondral layer, whose continuity foreshadows the longitudinal vertebral ligaments. The nerves come to lie close to the discs, while the intersegmental arteries come to lie either side of the vertebral bodies.

In regions where the notochord is surrounded by the developing vertebral body, it degenerates and disappears. Between vertebrae, however, the notochord expands as local aggregations of cells within a proteoglycan matrix, forming the gelatinous centre of the disc (nucleus pulposus). The nucleus is later surrounded by the circularly arranged fibres of the annulus fibrosus, derived from the perichordal mesenchyme: the nucleus pulposus and annulus fibrosus constitute the embryonic intervertebral disc. Remnants of notochord may persist in any part of the axial skeleton and give rise to a chordoma: this slow-growing neoplasm occurs most frequently at the base of the skull and in the lumbosacral region.

Following proliferation and later degeneration of notochordal cells, there is fibrocartilaginous invasion of the nucleus pulposus by the original mesenchymal intervertebral cells: the invasion occurs at about 6 months in utero.

Intervertebral discs lose their embryonic integrity with time, with structural changes occurring in the nucleus throughout adulthood. These normal processes are often considered to be signs of degeneration: they are merely stages in the natural evolution of connective tissue subjected to mechanical stress in the form of combined shear and compression forces. Growth of the intervertebral disc, together with microscopic changes within it, has been correlated with changes associated with weight-bearing in the erect posture. This may be a similar mechanism to that associated with the formation of subcutaneous connective tissue bursae (housemaid's knee) in which the alternate action of compression forces at right angles to the skin surface and tangential shear stresses induce thickening and delamination of the connective tissue.

Intervertebral discs are subjected to compression, torsion and shear: the shear stresses are constantly changing, being dependent on the instantaneous centre of rotation between adjacent vertebrae. This could explain mechanical delamination of the central region of the disc at different vertebral levels: the appearance of an irregular cavity in the central region being mechanically induced.

The cartilage end plate also appears to follow this mechanical induction. It is thought to be derived not from the vertebra, but from undifferentiated cells which accumulate in early embryonic life: it develops as an organised structure under mechanical influences. The annular epiphysis of the vertebral body develops in the marginal part of this thin plate of hyaline cartilage and can, therefore, be considered to be either part of the disc or part of the vertebral body.

Ligaments

The bodies of the vertebrae are further held together by longitudinal ligaments extending along the whole length of the vertebral column.

Anterior Longitudinal Ligament

Supporting the anterior aspect of the vertebral column, including the intervertebral discs (Fig. 4.11A), the anterior longitudinal ligament is between 1 and 2 mm thick. It consists of three dense layers of collagen fibres: superficial layers extend across several vertebrae, while deeper fibres pass between adjacent vertebrae. Superiorly, it has a narrow attachment to the anterior tubercle of the atlas: as it passes inferiorly it becomes wider, terminating by spreading over the pelvic surface of the proximal aspect of the sacrum. In the lumbar region, the anterior longitudinal ligament is between 20 and 25 mm wide, giving it a cross-sectional area between 20 and 50 mm^2.

Above the level of the atlas, the anterior longitudinal ligament is continuous with the anterior atlanto-occipital membrane (p. 641).

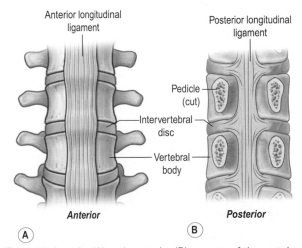

Fig. 4.11 Anterior (A) and posterior (B) aspects of the vertebral column showing the position and attachments of the anterior and posterior longitudinal ligaments.

Posterior Longitudinal Ligament

Providing the posterior support to the vertebral bodies, the posterior longitudinal ligament forms part of the anterior wall of the vertebral canal. It is between 1 and 1.4 mm thick, being broader superiorly than inferiorly and consists of two dense layers of collagen fibres: again, superficial fibres cross several vertebrae, while deeper fibres pass between adjacent vertebrae.

Unlike the anterior longitudinal ligament, the posterior longitudinal ligament is attached only to the intervertebral discs and adjacent margins of the vertebral bodies (Figs 4.11B and 4.13). Opposite the middle of each vertebra, it is separated from the bone by an interval into which the basivertebral vein passes from the vertebral body. As the ligament narrows in the thoracic and lumbar regions, its edges appear serrated (Fig. 4.11B). In the lower thoracic and lumbar regions, it is between 11 and 15 mm wide at the level of the intervertebral disc, while at the vertebral body, it is only 6–8 mm wide. This gives a cross-sectional area for the ligament of between 3 and 11 mm² in the lumbar region, considerably less than that of the anterior longitudinal ligament. It extends from the posterior surface of the first sacral segment to the posterior aspect of the body of the second cervical vertebra, where it becomes continuous with the tectorial membrane (p. 639).

The posterior longitudinal ligament is generally not considered to be as strong as the anterior ligament.

JOINTS BETWEEN VERTEBRAL ARCHES

The vertebral arches are united by synovial joints (zygapophyseal joints) between their articular processes, as well as by ligaments passing between the laminae, transverse and spinous processes. In the thoracic region, the joints lie anterior to the transverse process, while in the lumbar region, they lie posterior to them (Fig. 4.12). Anterior to the zygapophyseal joints in all regions are the intervertebral foramina: arthritic changes associated with these joints may give rise to the formation of bony projections (osteophytes) which may compress the spinal nerve within the foramen.

ZYGAPOPHYSEAL JOINTS

Articular Surfaces

Although these synovial joints are of the plane variety, the shape and orientation of the joint surfaces on the articular processes vary in the different regions of the vertebral column (Fig. 4.12, see also Fig. 5.8).

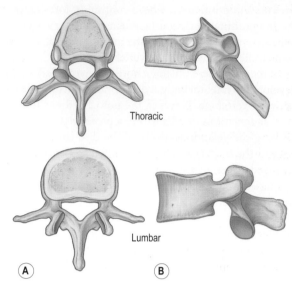

Fig. 4.12 Superior (A) and lateral (B) aspects of thoracic and lumbar vertebrae showing the orientation of the articular facets of the zygapophyseal joints.

In the thoracic region, the articular processes are thin, more or less triangular and project almost vertically. The articular facet on the superior processes faces mainly posteriorly but also slightly superolaterally so that it lies on the circumference of a circle whose centre is either just anterior to or in the anterior part of the vertebral body (Fig. 4.12). The inferior processes also have a circumferential arrangement so that their articular facets are directed anteriorly and slightly inferomedially: they do not project very far below the laminae.

The lumbar articular processes are strong and have a marked superior and inferior projection (Fig. 4.12): the articular facets are reciprocally curved in a horizontal plane, but virtually straight in a vertical plane. The facets on the superior processes are concave and face posteromedially, while those on the inferior processes are convex and face anterolaterally.

All articular surfaces are covered with hyaline cartilage. The shape and orientation of the articular processes play an important part in determining the type of movement possible within the thoracic and lumbar regions of the vertebral column. Those in the thoracic region favour lateral flexion/bending and rotation, while, in the lumbar region, they facilitate flexion, extension and lateral flexion/bending. An account of vertebral column movements is given on pages 517–522.

Joint Capsule and Synovial Membrane

Each joint is surrounded by a thin fibrous capsule attached to the margins of the articular surfaces. It is lax, particularly in the cervical region, to facilitate gliding movements between the two vertebrae. Synovial membrane lines the capsule and also attaches to the margins of the articular surfaces.

Accessory Ligaments

There are no ligaments or thickenings associated directly with the joint capsule; however, a number of accessory ligaments pass between the vertebral arches helping to stabilise the joints.

Ligamentum Flavum

Passing between the laminae of adjacent vertebrae from between C1 and C2 to between L4 and L5 is the ligamentum flavum (Fig. 4.13). Its yellowish appearance is due to the presence of a large amount of elastic tissue within it: it is the only true elastic ligament in the human body. At each intervertebral interval, there are two ligaments (right and left) each attached to the anterior aspect of the inferior border of the lamina above, passing posteroinferiorly to the posterior aspect of the superior border of the lamina below. The medial borders of the two ligaments meet at the root of the spinous process, elsewhere they are separated by a narrow cleft through which pass veins connecting the internal and external vertebral venous plexuses. Laterally, the ligaments extend as far as the joint capsules of the zygapophyseal joints, although they do not blend with them.

Studies in nonhuman primates have shown that the ligamentum flavum has a cross-sectional area greater than that of the anterior longitudinal ligament: there is no reason to suggest that the same is not true in humans. They assist the postvertebral muscles in maintaining the erect posture, as well as helping to return the trunk to the neutral position following flexion. Because of their elasticity, the ligamenta flava permit separation of the laminae during flexion. This same property also prevents them forming folds when the vertebral column returns to the erect position: such folds, if present, could become caught between the laminae or press upon the dura mater.

Supraspinous Ligament

Band of longitudinal fibres running superficial to and connecting the tips of the spinous processes (Fig. 4.13), it is continuous with the posterior edge of the interspinous ligament. The deeper shorter fibres connect adjacent spinous processes, while more superficial longer fibres extend over three or four spinous processes. In the cervical region, it merges with, and to a large extent becomes replaced by, the ligamentum nuchae (p. 633).

Interspinous Ligaments

Thin, membranous, relatively weak bands passing between and uniting adjacent vertebral spinous processes (Fig. 4.13), the interspinous ligaments are insignificant or absent at cervical levels, but longer and stronger at lumbar levels.

Intertransverse Ligaments

Generally insignificant bands connecting adjacent transverse processes, intertransverse ligaments tend to be absent at cervical levels, only becoming obvious in the lumbar region. In the upper part of the vertebral column, they are often replaced by intertransverse muscles.

Blood Supply and Innervation
Arterial Supply

The vertebral column receives its arterial supply segmentally from branches of vessels which lie adjacent to it. In the cervical region, these are from the vertebral and ascending cervical arteries; in the thoracic region, they are from the costocervical and posterior intercostal arteries; in the lumbar region from the lumbar and iliolumbar arteries; and in the pelvis from the lateral sacral arteries. All branches anastomose with and

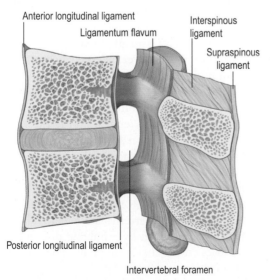

Anterior longitudinal ligament
Ligamentum flavum
Interspinous ligament
Supraspinous ligament
Posterior longitudinal ligament
Intervertebral foramen

Fig. 4.13 Sagittal section through the lumbar vertebral column showing the position and attachment of accessory ligaments associated with the zygapophyseal joints.

reinforce the anterior and posterior spinal arteries (p. 572) supplying the spinal cord.

As the branches from the segmental arteries pass around the middle of the vertebral body towards the intervertebral foramen, they supply it. Microradiographic studies have shown extensive horizontal and vertical anastomoses between the segmental vessels (Fig. 4.14A).

It is interesting to note that blood vessels surrounding the intervertebral disc during the early part of its development subsequently disappear, leaving an essentially avascular structure. Except perhaps for its most peripheral part, which receives a supply from adjacent blood vessels, mature discs are supported by diffusion through the spongy bone of the adjacent vertebral body surfaces.

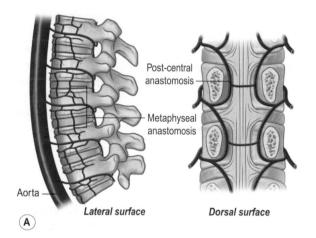

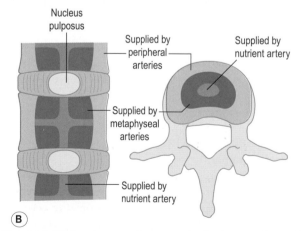

Fig. 4.14 (A) Anastomoses between the lumbar arteries and their branches; (B) zonal arrangement of the blood supply to the intervertebral disc. (Adapted from Ratcliffe, J.F., 1980. The arterial anatomy of the adult human lumbar vertebral body: a microarteriographic study. J. Anat. 131, 57–79.)

The blood supply to the vertebral body, as well as its possible disruption, is, therefore, extremely important.

The organisation of the arterial supply to the vertebral body appears to be zoned (Fig. 4.14B): the body immediately adjacent to the intervertebral disc is relatively avascular, with more central regions being more vascular. However, this central region can be subdivided into that supplied by the tortuous nutrient artery and that by metaphyseal arteries: the peripheral region of the vertebral body is supplied by short straight peripheral arteries. Diffusion of oxygen and nutrients for disc metabolism is also probably zoned because of the arrangement of the lamellae of the annulus fibrosus, with fluid trapped between lamellae channelled in a vertical plane: frequent movement of the lamellae probably speeds up diffusion. One consequence of ageing is the gradual narrowing of the lumen of arteries, resulting in a reduced, and eventually obliterated, blood flow. The arteries affected initially are those with a tortuous course, with the nutrient and metaphyseal arteries supplying the vertebral body probably being the first to suffer. With increasing age, peripheral arteries apparently become more numerous, so that the outer aspect of the vertebral body may get a relatively better blood supply than the central region. Disc degeneration and desiccation have been observed to appear at the centre of the disc earlier than at the periphery: the periphery may remain healthy and capable of repair long after disintegration and extrusion of the central part of the disc.

Although disc degeneration and low back pain due to disc hypoxia and starvation (as a secondary effect of reduced blood supply) is an attractive theory, it is, however, difficult to prove. Nevertheless, symptomatic discs differ from normal in their pH and lactic acid concentrations, suggesting that these biochemical changes are due to anoxic respiration of the disc.

Where the segmental arterial supply to the vertebral column is reduced (by the natural calibre of the vessels) or jeopardised (by compression of the vessels), it might be expected that the adjacent intervertebral discs would be liable to degenerative change at an earlier age than elsewhere. One such region is the lower lumbar where the fifth pair of lumbar arteries are small and may be subjected to compression by a bulging disc: the intervertebral discs on either side might be expected to have reduced nutrition and oxygenation. Studies have suggested that 95% of disc lesions involved one or both discs on either side of L5. Although the evidence is circumstantial, reduced blood supply to the vertebrae, and, therefore, to the disc, is strongly implicated in disc pathology.

Venous Drainage

The veins of the vertebral column form complex freely communicating plexuses extending the whole length of the column, both inside and out (Fig. 4.15). The plexuses are drained by a series of intervertebral veins which join the vertebral veins in the neck, posterior intercostal veins in the chest, lumbar veins in the lower back and lateral sacral veins in the pelvis.

The internal vertebral plexuses form a continuous network between the spinal dura and walls of the vertebral canal (Fig. 4.15B). Two anterior channels lie on either side of the posterior longitudinal ligament, anastomosing across the midline anterior to the ligament, receiving the basivertebral vein (Fig. 4.15B): they communicate superiorly with the basilar, occipital and sigmoid sinuses within the skull (p. 696). The posterior internal plexuses lie on the deep surfaces of the laminae and ligamenta flava: they anastomose across the midline, with some vessels emerging to join the posterior external plexus by passing between the free medial edges of the ligamenta flava. This latter connection may provide a venous pump mechanism as the vessels become squeezed during movements of the vertebral column. The main communication between the internal and external plexuses, however, is via the intervertebral veins passing through the intervertebral foramina.

The external plexuses are located along the anterior aspect of the vertebral column, as well as around the spinous, articular and transverse processes of the vertebrae.

Although the precise arrangement of the venous plexuses associated with the vertebral column may not be of interest *per se*, it must be remembered that they form a system of great blood-carrying capacity extending, with few if any valves, from the pelvis to inside the skull, communicating at all levels with the major venous systems of the abdomen, chest, neck and head. This complex venous network almost certainly plays a significant role in the transfer of metastatic cancer cells to widely separated regions of the body under the influence of differences in venous pressure. Secondary metastases associated with cancer of the breast and of the prostate invariably involve the vertebrae.

Innervation

The nerve supply of the intervertebral disc and the existence of nervous tissue within related structures (ligaments) is of considerable clinical importance. The sinuvertebral nerve is a recurrent nerve of the vertebral canal supplying the fibrous connective tissue associated with the spinal canal (posterior longitudinal ligament, periosteum), together with the venous sinuses and spinal dura: it may be considered equivalent to the recurrent meningeal branch of a cranial nerve. It has a dual origin from the spinal nerve and the sympathetic nervous system: the spinal part arises just distal to the dorsal root ganglion reentering the spinal canal to reach the midline, giving branches directly towards the discs above and below each level. It is also likely that some fibres innervate the medial aspect of the zygapophyseal joint capsule.

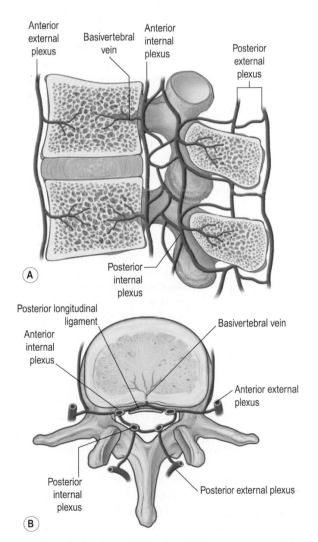

Fig. 4.15 Sagittal section (A) and superior view (B) of the venous drainage of the vertebral column.

Numerous fine nerve filaments, as well as encapsulated and nonencapsulated receptors, have been found in the anterior and posterior longitudinal ligaments and superficial layers of the annulus fibrosus. Innervation of the anterior longitudinal ligament and lateral aspect of the disc appears to be extensive and complex, particularly in the lumbar region, involving branches from the ventral ramus. The lateral aspect of the zygapophyseal joint capsule probably also receives an innervation from the dorsal ramus as it passes towards the postvertebral muscles.

With both C and A fibres involved in pain transmission, it is clear that structures exist in and around the intervertebral disc whose presence could explain the pain caused by mechanical compression of the anterior and posterior nerve fibres in the periphery of the annulus fibrosus.

Relations

Because the vertebral column extends from the base of the skull to the pelvis, it is associated with several distinct regions of the body: its relations change as various structures at first approach and then move away from it. It is not practical to consider in detail all of these relations; however, an attempt is made to illustrate the major relations in the thoracic and lumbar regions.

One major function of the vertebral column is to support and protect the spinal cord against physical trauma. Within the vertebral canal is the spinal cord and its meningeal coverings (p. 567), together with the internal vertebral venous plexus embedded in loose areolar tissue. The spinal cord ends at the level of the L1/L2 intervertebral disc, below which is the cauda equina (p. 571), still within the meningeal coverings as far as the level of S2.

In the thoracic region, the anterior relations of the vertebrae differ depending on the level at which the section is taken. In general, above the level of T8, thoracic contents only are seen (lungs, heart, great vessels and oesophagus: Fig. 4.16). Below this level and separated from the thoracic contents by the diaphragm, the liver and stomach become anterior relations (Fig. 4.17). Posterior and lateral to the vertebrae are the postvertebral muscles.

Anterior to the lumbar vertebrae lie the major vessels of the abdomen (aorta, inferior vena cava). Immediately lateral to the upper three lumbar vertebrae lie the kidneys, with various parts of the gastrointestinal tract

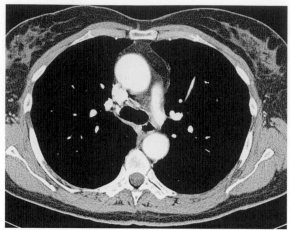

Fig. 4.16 Transverse section of the thorax above the level of T8. (Reproduced with permission from Standring, S., 2004. Gray's Anatomy, 39th ed. Elsevier, Churchill Livingstone, London.)

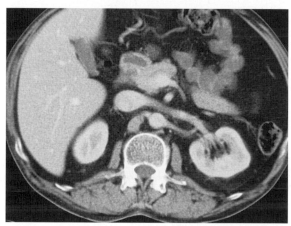

Fig. 4.17 Transverse section of the thorax below the level of T8. (Reproduced with permission from Standring, S., 2004. Gray's Anatomy, 39th ed. Elsevier, Churchill Livingstone, London.)

generally lying anteriorly (Fig. 4.18). The main posterior relation, situated between the transverse and spinous processes, as in other regions, is the postvertebral muscle mass; at lumbar levels, it is difficult to differentiate the individual components. Also in this region, the thick and strong thoracolumbar fascia can be readily seen (see Fig. 4.35C).

Stability

Despite its multisegmental nature, the vertebral column is a relatively stable structure. The ease with which the trunk can be held erect with a small amount of muscle

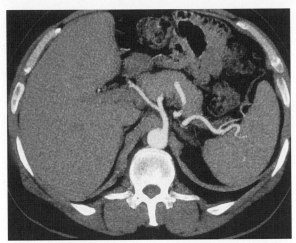

Fig. 4.18 Transverse section of the abdomen at the level of L1. (Reproduced with permission from Standring, S., 2004. Gray's Anatomy, 39th ed. Elsevier, Churchill Livingston, London.)

activity is in contrast to that required to hold the lower limbs in equilibrium against gravity. After a long illness, many individuals are able to sit up with relatively little effort long before they can stand, suggesting that the arrangement of the various elements of the vertebral column provide a high degree of inherent stability requiring little, if any, muscle activity to maintain the position of the trunk. It has been shown that a vertebral column devoid of all musculature does not collapse, but remains erect and can support 2 kg placed on its upper end without collapsing. How is this possible when the partial centres of gravity of the various links do not lie in the line of the centre of gravity? Furthermore, the centres of the articulations (except for a few) do not fall on this line. Clearly, rotational stresses between vertebrae must be neutralised, otherwise the column would lose its equilibrium and collapse.

What features contribute to this equilibrium and stability? Of considerable importance is the arrangement and nature of the joints between individual vertebrae, particularly those between the bodies. Being secondary cartilaginous joints, they do not permit a large amount of movement; together with the interaction of the components of the intervertebral disc with adjacent vertebrae they produce a unit (two vertebrae and intervening disc) which is self-stabilising. Whether loaded or at rest, the annulus fibrosus fibres are under tension because of the preloaded state of the disc due to its water-absorbing capacity: tension developed in these fibres tends to keep the vertebrae aligned. When a force is applied to

the upper vertebra causing it to move (as in extension), the nucleus pulposus moves anteriorly, increasing tension in the anterior part of the annulus, which tends to restore the upper vertebra to its original position (Fig. 4.19A). This mechanism works well with asymmetrically applied forces causing movement in extension, flexion or lateral flexion/bending. But what about axial rotation? During rotation, fibres in the annulus running counter to the movement are stretched, while those running in the opposite direction become relatively relaxed (Fig. 4.19A). Tension is maximum in the central annulus fibres compressing the nucleus pulposus, with its internal pressure rising in proportion to the extent of angular rotation. Compression of the nucleus pushes back against the annulus, with a tendency to put the relaxed fibres under tension, not only helping to limit movement but also restoring the upper vertebra to its original position. It appears that, irrespective of the direction of force applied to the intervertebral disc, it increases the internal pressure of the nucleus pulposus stretching the annulus fibrosus: this stretching tends to oppose the movement and restore the system to its initial state.

The unique hydrostatic properties of the intervertebral disc are the result of interaction between the annulus fibrosus and water-binding capacity of the proteoglycans in the nucleus pulposus, as well as from their interaction with the loading exerted by the longitudinal ligaments binding the vertebrae together. With the intake of water and subsequent increase in nuclear pressurisation, the disc increases in height. Not only does this height increase decrease displacement in all directions, it reduces ligament laxity by pushing adjacent vertebrae apart, putting the longitudinal ligaments under tension (Fig. 4.19B); however, if the vertebral column is deprived of ligaments, as well as muscles, it automatically collapses. As long as the ligaments and discs are intact, it preserves considerable resistance against deformation, being the result of elastic tension resistance in the ligaments and elastic compression resistance in the discs.

As can be seen from Fig. 4.19B, it is not only the longitudinal ligaments that interact with the disc to provide intrinsic stability, the ligamenta flava, interspinous and supraspinous ligaments are all equally as important. For the system to work efficiently and effectively, the vertebral arches must remain firmly attached to the vertebral bodies. It has been shown that if the entire column of arches is separated from the bodies, then the column of

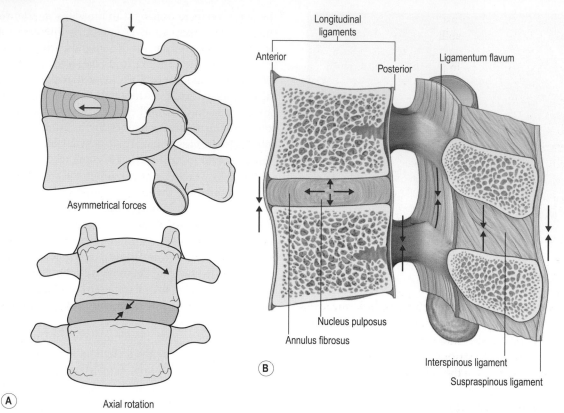

Fig. 4.19 (A) Reaction of the intervertebral disc to asymmetrically applied forces and axial rotation; (B) sagittal section showing the interaction of the intervertebral disc and vertebral ligaments providing an inherent stability of the vertebral column.

arches shrinks by 14%. As long as the arches are united with the bodies, they are spread apart, putting the ligaments under tension.

The inherent stability of the vertebral column has led to the development of a simple mechanical model (Fig. 4.20) in which adjacent vertebrae move with respect to each other guided by the zygapophyseal joints: the elastic properties of the disc and ligaments being replaced by springs. Each vertebra can then be considered to act as a first class lever, with the articular process acting as the fulcrum. Within such a model, the vertebral bodies and intervening disc are essentially the supporting structures and have a static role, while the articular and spinous processes, together with adjacent ligaments, have a dynamic role permitting, guiding and limiting movement.

The thoracic cage and its articulation posteriorly with the thoracic vertebrae confers some stability to the vertebral column in this region. The ribs themselves are forced into the thoracic cage under considerable stress

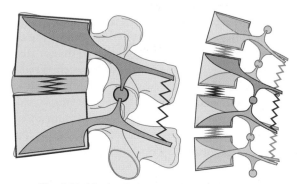

Fig. 4.20 Mechanical model of a vertebral unit.

(tearing or rupture of a costal cartilage through trauma results in the rib springing out slightly): in addition, the costal cartilages constantly change shape during respiration. In some respects, the thoracic vertebral bodies can be considered to be held between the heads of the ribs. This arrangement increases the elastic resistance of the thorax, some of which is used in respiration, but the greater part is exerted against the vertebral column contributing to its intrinsic stability.

That the vertebral column has some intrinsic stability is of practical and clinical importance: less muscle activity and, therefore, less energy expenditure are required to maintain an erect posture. However, as with all joints, ligaments are not sufficient to maintain stability: they need to be reinforced by muscles. Without the presence and intermittent activity of muscles, ligaments would gradually stretch and stability would be lost: the large postvertebral muscle mass plays an extremely important role in supporting ligaments and, therefore, to intrinsic stability. Just as importantly, these muscles are primarily responsible for stability during dynamic movements (extrinsic stability). However, in explosive dynamic movements, the postvertebral muscles by themselves may not be capable of providing the required stability.

With increased dynamic loading of the vertebral column, both intra-abdominal and intrathoracic pressures increase (Fig. 4.21). The increase in intra-abdominal pressure and its maintenance act as a pneumatic cushion, supporting the anterior aspect of the lumbar and lower thoracic regions of the vertebral column.

MOVEMENTS OF THE TRUNK

Movement between adjacent vertebrae occurs because the resilient intervertebral discs are slightly flexible, with the type of movement permitted in each region being largely determined by the shape and orientation of the articular processes. Where the discs are thick in relation to the vertebral bodies (lumbar region), the range of movement between adjacent vertebrae is increased. Even so, the amount of movement between successive vertebrae is slight, being limited by the arrangement of fibres within the annulus fibrosus of the intervertebral disc. Nevertheless, when added over the whole of the vertebral column, the total range of movement becomes considerable.

The basic movements of the vertebral column are flexion and extension about a transverse axis, lateral flexion/bending about an anteroposterior axis and rotation to the right or left about a vertical axis (Fig. 4.22). Of these, lateral flexion/bending and rotation are always associated movements, with neither being able to occur independently: in the lumbar region, there is always coupling of movement, so pure movement in any direction does not occur. Even though the coupled movements

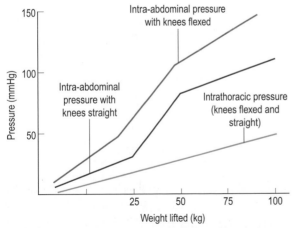

Fig. 4.21 Increases in intra-abdominal and intrathoracic pressure with increased dynamic loading of the vertebral column. (Adapted from Morris, J.M., Lucas, S.B., Breslar, B., 1961. Role of the trunk in stability of the spine. J. Bone Joint Surg. 43A, 327–351.)

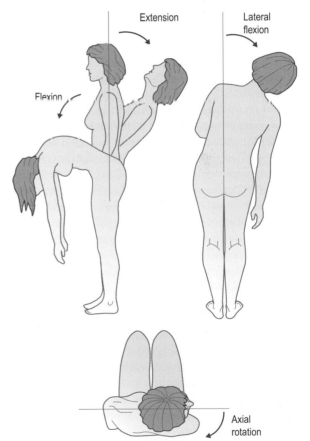

Fig. 4.22 Movement of the vertebral column as a whole.

are small, they are, nevertheless, important and probably serve to help maintain the inherent stability present within the vertebral column during movement. All movements are possible in each region, with the range being determined by disc thickness and articular process geometry. Flexion, extension and lateral flexion/bending all involve compression of the intervertebral discs at one edge and stretching at the other. During flexion, the anterior borders of vertebrae come together and the posterior borders separate: as full flexion is reached, the anterior part of the disc becomes compressed, tending to push the nucleus pulposus posteriorly. The posterior part of the disc, posterior longitudinal ligament and ligaments of the vertebral arches all become taut: the principal limiting factor to movement is tension in the postvertebral muscles. In extension, the posterior borders of the vertebrae become approximated and the anterior separate: the anterior longitudinal ligament becomes increasingly taut, while all posterior ligaments become relaxed. Extension is freer and has a wider range of movement than flexion: much of the apparent movement of flexion is due to flexion of the trunk at the hips, as well as movement of the head at the atlanto-occipital joints (p. 642).

The importance of the posterior ligaments and intervertebral discs in limiting movement of the vertebral column has been demonstrated by successive sectioning of these structures, and observing and measuring the subsequent movements between adjacent vertebrae. Progressive sectioning of the supra- and interspinous ligaments, ligamentum flavum, bilateral severing of the articular processes, sectioning the posterior longitudinal ligament and cutting the posterior and lateral parts of the annulus fibrosus results in a 100% increase in flexion–extension (from 8.4 to 17.3 degrees), a 70% increase in lateral flexion/bending (from 4.9 to 8.3 degrees) and a 650% increase in rotation (from 2.2 to 14.6 degrees) at the thoracolumbar junction. A similar pattern of changes would be expected elsewhere in the vertebral column, although they would be modified by the orientation of the articular processes, particularly regarding the percentage change in rotation.

An important structural component of the trunk is the thoracic cage, with the ribs, articulating with the thoracic vertebrae and sternum, providing protection to the underlying soft tissues. The anterior abdominal wall muscles, as well as being involved in producing trunk movements, also raise intra-abdominal pressure, aiding expiration and all straining activities (micturition, parturition, coughing, vomiting).

Although the intervertebral discs are thick in the lumbar region, and in theory would facilitate relatively large movements between adjacent vertebrae, the orientation of the articular processes (Fig. 4.12) tends to confer a certain degree of stability to this region, restricting rotation in particular. Of the lumbar vertebrae, the inferior facets of L5 face mainly anteriorly to articulate with the superior facets on the sacrum: movement between L5 and the sacrum is not the same as that between two typical lumbar vertebrae.

In the thoracic region, the intervertebral discs are relatively thin with respect to the vertebral bodies, which with the ribs and sternum limit movement. The orientation of the articular processes of the thoracic vertebrae, which lie on the arc of a circle with its centre close to the anterior part of the vertebral body, permits flexion, extension, lateral flexion/bending and rotation. The inferior processes of T12 resemble those in the lumbar region, with movements at the thoracolumbar junction being similar to those between adjacent lumbar vertebrae.

Flexion and Extension

Flexion occurs when the lumbar and thoracic regions bend forwards, with movement in the opposite direction being extension: these two movements are of considerable functional significance, particularly when they accompany flexion and extension of the thigh at the hip joint. Care must be taken when determining the range of movement of the trunk to exclude that of the hip.

Lumbar Region. Flexion is relatively free in the lumbar region, having a total range of 55 degrees, while extension has a range of 30 degrees (Fig. 4.23A). There is less movement at the thoracolumbar junction than between adjacent vertebrae and most movement at the lumbosacral junction. The total range of movement decreases with age, so that at 65 years it is between a half and a third that at age 10.

In flexion, the vertebrae tilt forward on each other so that the inferior articular processes of the upper vertebrae glide anterosuperiorly on the superior processes of the lower vertebrae (Fig. 4.23B). The spatial orientation of these joints allows the upper vertebrae to move slightly forwards over the lower vertebrae: this forward movement increases the superoinferior and decreases the anteroposterior diameter of the intervertebral foramen. Flexion from the erect position is controlled by the

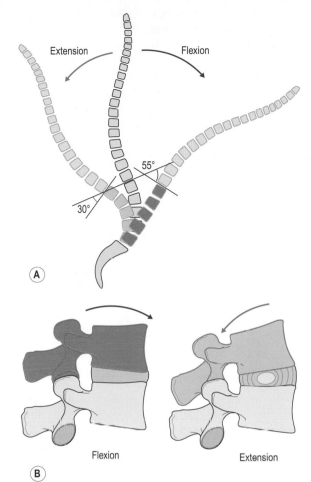

Fig. 4.23 (A) Range of flexion and extension of the lumbar region of the vertebral column; (B) movement between adjacent lumbar vertebrae.

postvertebral muscles on both sides, limited by tension in the posterior part of the intervertebral disc, posterior longitudinal ligament, ligamenta flava, interspinous and supraspinous ligaments. Flexion from the supine position is brought about by psoas major and the anterior abdominal muscles, especially rectus abdominis.

During extension, the inferior articular processes of the upper vertebra glide inferiorly against the hollowed superior processes of the lower vertebra, causing the upper vertebra to move slightly posteriorly on the lower vertebra (Fig. 4.23B). It is limited by the anterior longitudinal ligament, anterior part of the intervertebral disc, apposition of the lumbar spinous processes and close-packing of the facet joints. Extension from the erect

position is controlled by psoas major and the anterior abdominal muscles, while from the prone position, it is produced by the postvertebral muscles.

Thoracic region. The combined range of flexion and extension in the thoracic region is between 50 and 70 degrees, with extension being much more limited than flexion (Fig. 4.24A). Flexion is much freer in the lower half of the region as the lower ribs tend to be longer and more flexible because of their longer costal cartilages.

In flexion, the inferior articular processes of the vertebra above slide superiorly over the superior processes of the lower vertebra (Fig. 4.24B), with the interspace between the two vertebrae opening out posteriorly compressing the anterior part of the intervertebral disc. Flexion is limited by the presence of the thoracic cage and by tension developed in the supra- and interspinous ligaments, ligamenta flava, and posterior longitudinal ligament. From the erect position, flexion is controlled by the postvertebral muscles of both sides, while flexion from the supine position is brought about by the anterior abdominal muscles of both sides, especially rectus abdominis. During flexion, the angles between the various segments of the thorax and between the thorax and vertebral column increase (Fig. 4.24C).

Extension of the thoracic region approximates the vertebrae posteriorly (Fig. 4.24B); it is limited by impact of the articular and spinous processes of adjacent vertebrae, as well as tension in the anterior longitudinal ligament. The effect of extension on the thoracic cage flattens it by decreasing all angles between the various segments of the thoracic cage and the vertebral column (Fig. 4.24C). Extension from the erect position is controlled by the anterior abdominal wall muscles and from the prone position by the postvertebral muscles.

The total range of thoracolumbar flexion and extension may be as much as 135 degrees; however, the American Association of Orthopedic Surgeons (1994) give a value of 110 degrees, with flexion exceeding extension. Flexion in the thoracic region is approximately half that in the lumbar region (30 and 55 degrees, respectively) due to the presence of the ribs, while extension is two-thirds that in the lumbar region (20 and 30 degrees, respectively). Males tend to have a greater range of both flexion (Macrae and Wright, 1969) and extension (Moll and Wright, 1971) than females at all ages: both flexion and extension decrease with age (Fitzgerald et al., 1983), with the change in extension being greater than that in flexion (Sugahara et al., 1981).

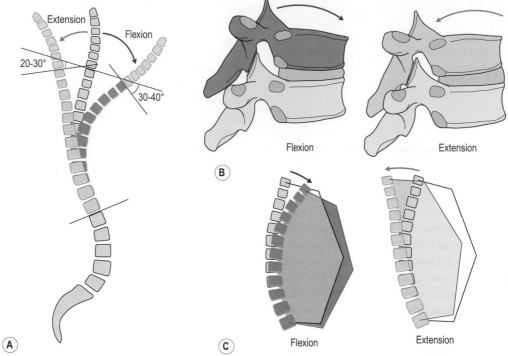

Fig. 4.24 (A) Range of flexion and extension of the thoracic region of the vertebral column; (B) movements between adjacent thoracic vertebrae; (C) effect of flexion/extension on the thoracic cage.

Lateral Flexion/Bending

Lateral flexion/bending occurs when the level of the shoulders becomes inclined with respect to that of the pelvis; it can occur on both left and right sides. In this movement, adjacent parts of the vertebral bodies on one side come closer together, while those on the opposite side separate.

Lumbar region. The range of lateral flexion/bending in the lumbar region, as with that of flexion and extension, varies between individuals and with age. In preteenage years, the range may be as large as 60 degrees on either side of the midline; however, by age 30, this has been halved. On average, the adult range of movement is between 20 and 30 degrees to each side (Fig. 4.25A). Throughout the total age range, lateral flexion/bending at the lumbosacral junction is minimal. Because of the small range of lateral flexion/bending in the lumbar region, there is very little associated vertebral rotation. Lateral flexion/bending is greatest in the erect position, being greatly diminished when the vertebral column is flexed and the lumbar curve lost.

In lateral flexion/bending, the articular processes of the flexed side become close-packed, while the superior process on the opposite side is withdrawn from the inferior (Fig. 4.25B). Because the articular surfaces also slope slightly, a narrow gap appears between the articular processes on the unflexed side. As a result, the intervertebral foramen on the unflexed side enlarges in all directions, while that on the flexed side narrows. Lateral flexion/bending initially requires active muscle contraction: it is not brought about by controlled relaxation (eccentric contraction) of the muscles of the opposite side. Lateral flexion/bending to the right requires contraction of muscles on the right side (anterior abdominal muscles, quadratus lumborum). However, once a certain degree of lateral flexion/bending has been reached (~10 degrees), then movement is controlled by the eccentric contraction of the muscles of the opposite side. Movement is limited by the intertransverse ligaments of the opposite side, as well as opposing muscle groups.

Thoracic region. In the thoracic region, the range of lateral flexion is 20–25 degrees to each side (Fig. 4.26A), being freer in the lower half of the region. During lateral

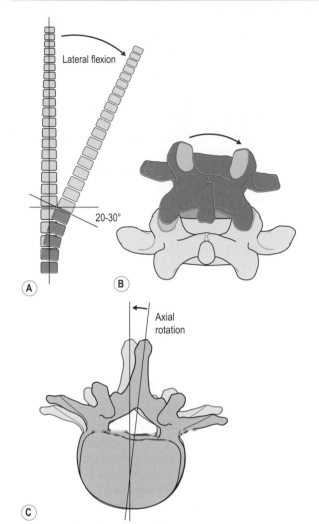

Fig. 4.25 (A) Range of lateral flexion in the lumbar region of the vertebral column; (B) movement between adjacent lumbar vertebrae; (C) axial rotation.

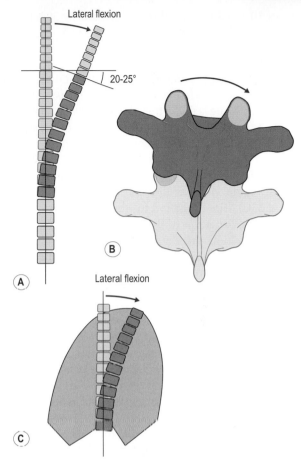

Fig. 4.26 (A) Range of lateral flexion of the thoracic region of the vertebral column; (B) movement of adjacent thoracic vertebrae; (C) effect of lateral flexion on the thoracic cage.

flexion/bending, the articular processes of two adjacent vertebrae slide relative to each other, with those on the contralateral side moving as during flexion, and those on the ipsilateral side as during extension (Fig. 4.26B). Lateral flexion/bending is limited by the impact of the articular processes on the side of the movement and tension developed in the ligamenta flava and intertransverse ligaments of the opposite side. In the thoracic region, lateral flexion/bending is associated with rotation of the vertebrae. In full lateral flexion/bending, the degree of rotation is approximately 20 degrees: for each degree of lateral flexion/bending, there is almost 1 degree of accompanying rotation, with rotation being such that the

spinous processes of the thoracic vertebrae point towards the concavity of the curve (they rotate contralaterally).

As with flexion and extension, lateral flexion/bending modifies the shape of the thoracic cage (Fig. 4.26C). On the contralateral side, the thorax is elevated, the intercostal spaces widen, the thoracic cage enlarges and the costochondral angle of the 10th rib tends to open out. On the ipsilateral side, the reverse occurs: the thoracic cage is lowered and shrinks, the intercostal spaces narrow and the costochondral angle decreases.

As in the lumbar region, lateral flexion/bending is brought about by the contraction of muscles on the same side.

The total range of lateral flexion is 55 degrees to each side with that in the thoracic and lumbar regions being similar (25 and 30 degrees, respectively). Between the ages of 30 and 80, lateral flexion decreases by 50% (Fitzgerald et al., 1983).

Rotation

This is produced by summation of individual vertebral movements which enable the trunk to be twisted to the right or left while keeping the shoulders level: rotation of the pelvis at the hip joint increases rotation of the shoulders. Again, care must be taken to fix the pelvis when assessing the degree of trunk rotation.

Lumbar region. Rotation is extremely limited in the lumbar region, being of the order of only a few degrees (Fig. 4.25C). The limitation to movement is due to the shape and orientation of the lumbar articular facets. In the erect position, there is a narrow gap between opposing articular processes: rotation occurs until all gaps on one side become obliterated. Narrowing and eventual obliteration of the gaps on one side produce widening of the gaps on the opposite side.

The rotation possible, however small, depends on the position of the lumbar column. When it is extended, no rotation at all is possible because of the close-packed position of the zygapophyseal joints; however, the range of possible rotation increases with increasing flexion.

Thoracic region. The orientation of the articular processes in the thoracic region promotes rotation: this may be a necessary adaptation due to the presence of the ribs. Were it not for the presence of the thoracic cage, the range of rotation of the thoracic column would be greater: even so, it is some 35 degrees in each direction (Fig. 4.27A). During rotation, the inferior processes of the upper vertebrae slide sideways outside the superior processes of the lower vertebrae, leading to rotation of one vertebral body with respect to the other about a common axis (Fig. 4.27B): a small degree of lateral flexion/bending accompanies the rotation. Movement of the vertebrae is accompanied by rotation and twisting of the intervertebral disc, which has a tendency to pull the adjacent vertebrae together. When the thoracic vertebral column is fully extended, both rotation and lateral flexion/bending are greatly reduced and may be lost completely.

Rotation is limited by tension in the supraspinous and interspinous ligaments and ligamenta flava: it is brought about largely by the abdominal oblique muscles (rotation of the trunk to the left is achieved by contraction of the right external oblique and left internal oblique).

Because of the articulation of the ribs with the vertebrae, any rotatory movement of the vertebrae induces a similar movement in the corresponding ribs; however, the movement is limited due to the articulation of the ribs anteriorly with the sternum. Instead, there is a distortion of the ribs as follows: an accentuation of the concavity of the rib on the side of rotation, with a flattening of the concavity on the opposite side (Fig. 4.27C). These changes are possible because of the elasticity of the rib and its costal cartilage: the movements of the ribs subject the sternum to shearing forces.

Rotation of the thoracolumbar part of the vertebral column is extremely important during walking. However, the rotation is not simple but rather complex, occurring in opposite directions in the upper and lower parts of the region. As one leg swings through, ready for the next heel-strike, the pelvis rotates about the hip joint of the supporting leg, carrying the trunk with it. In an attempt to keep the head facing forwards, the pectoral girdle rotates in the opposite direction. Studies have shown that the intervertebral disc between the seventh and eighth thoracic vertebrae is not subjected to any rotation (or at least very little), yet maximum rotation occurs (in opposite directions) in the discs immediately above and below it (Fig. 4.27D). The degree of rotation decreases towards the pelvic and pectoral girdles.

The total range of rotation to each side is 40 degrees, the majority of which (35 degrees) is associated with the thoracic region, being greatest in the mid-thoracic region (Fig. 4.27D). A 50% reduction in range has been observed between age 30 and 80 (Fitzgerald et al., 1983). The age-related changes reported for all movements are consistent with the age-related changes observed in intervertebral discs.

Accessory Movements

Rotation is really an accumulation of accessory movements occurring at each of the zygapophyseal joints, consisting of a rocking movement of the inferior articular process of the vertebra above within the hollow of the superior process of the lower vertebra. These same accessory movements can be demonstrated by applying pressure to one side of a lumbar spinous process when the individual is lying prone with the lumbar column slightly flexed.

Downward pressure applied to the mamillary processes (or spinous process) of lumbar vertebrae causes

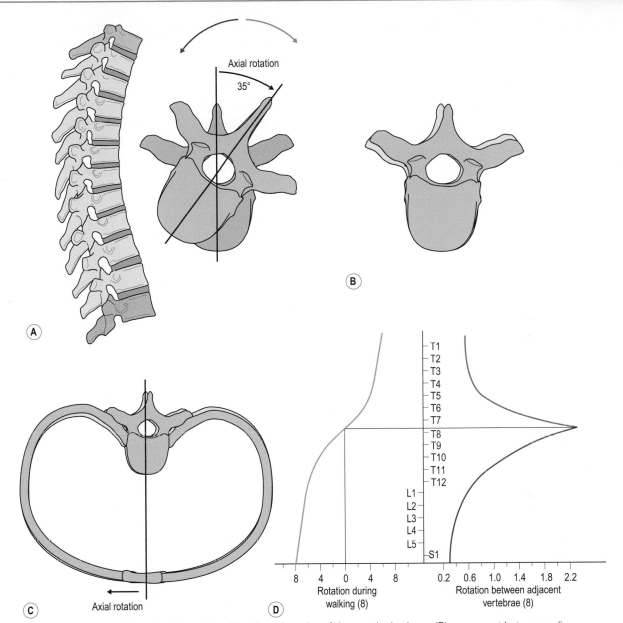

Fig. 4.27 (A) Range of axial rotation of the thoracic region of the vertebral column; (B) movement between adjacent thoracic vertebrae; (C) effect of rotation on the thoracic cage; (D) rotation in the thoracic region during walking.

a slight forward gliding of the body of the same vertebra with respect to the body above. At the same time, the superior articular processes move forward away from the inferior processes of the vertebra above, while the inferior processes are pushed into the superior processes of the vertebra below.

Accessory movements of the thoracic part of the vertebral column are difficult to demonstrate and usually only used therapeutically. Nevertheless, pressure on a spinous process will, because of its length and angulation, produce a slight rocking of the vertebral body and apposition of the articular surfaces of the zygapophyseal joints associated with its articular processes. A localised pressure applied to the posterior aspect of the base of the transverse process just below the zygapophyseal joint will slightly separate the joint by pushing the upper articular process forwards.

Application of Accessory Movements of the Trunk

A detailed knowledge of the accessory movements of the vertebral column, particularly in the lumbar region, is essential for those using manipulation and movement techniques. There is considerable misunderstanding of how the application of this knowledge can benefit the individual. Although manipulative and movement techniques are not discussed, certain facts are worth stating as they will be of help when consulting the manipulation and movement literature. Because many individuals suffer from back problems of one sort or another, comment will be restricted to the lumbar region. Rotation movements of the lumbar spine (rotation of the thorax on a fixed pelvis) open out the zygapophyseal joints on the side to which the thorax is rotating, with the extent of gapping and rotation increasing with flexion of the lumbar region: this is similar to that seen in the cervical region upon rotation. However, unlike the cervical region, where the orientation of the articular facets produces an increase in the size of the intervertebral foramen of the opposite side, in the lumbar region, the opposite side joints become compressed, preventing further movement.

If, as in most cases, when these accessory movements are being applied therapeutically, the trunk is fixed, and the lower limbs and pelvis are the mobile segments, then rotation of the pelvis to one side has the same effect on the joints as rotating the thorax to the opposite side. Flexing the lumbar region and applying traction to one leg produces a lateral flexion/bending of the lumbar region to the opposite side. This further increases separation of the zygapophyseal joints on the side of traction, stretching the joint capsule and adjacent part of the intervertebral disc, increasing the size of the intervertebral foramen and releasing trapped nerve roots.

The major muscles producing movements of the vertebral column are shown in Table 4.1: further details of each muscle can be found in the following sections.

BIOMECHANICS

Trabecular Systems

Within vertebrae are extensive and complex trabecular systems reflecting the stresses to which each vertebra is exposed. Within the vertebral body, three distinct zones of trabecular bone can be distinguished superoinferiorly

(Fig. 4.28A). The central zone essentially consists of vertically arranged large-diameter cylinders whose walls are formed by thin solid plates of lamellar bone, with circularly orientated trabeculae arranged around the basivertebral veins. The zones on either side directly beneath the end plate region are composed of regularly spaced longitudinal and transverse trabeculae. The anterior superior and inferior regions contain decreased trabecular bone and are regions of mechanical weakness: this helps to explain the wedge-shaped vertebral body seen in compression fractures (Fig. 4.28B).

There is one principal vertical and several secondary oblique and horizontal systems within each vertebral body: except for interruption by the intervertebral discs, the vertical system runs throughout the entire column of vertebral bodies from the odontoid process to the sacrum. The oblique accessory systems run in four tracts: a superior and inferior oblique system on each side. Each superior oblique system runs from the superior articular process of one side inferiorly through the pedicle to the inferior surface of the vertebral body on the opposite side (Fig. 4.28C). The inferior oblique system runs from the inferior articular process of one side superiorly via the pedicle to the superior surface of the vertebral body on the opposite side (Fig. 4.28C). The oblique systems do not reach the anterior margin of the vertebral body: this region consists of vertical compression trabeculae only (Fig. 4.28A). Posterior to the articular processes, the oblique systems are continuous with trabeculae within the spinous process (Fig. 4.28C).

Horizontal accessory systems begin in each transverse process, passing into the vertebral body where they intersect in the midline (Fig. 4.28D).

Mechanically, the vertical system sustains body weight and all the jars and shocks which reach the vertebral column perpendicularly: it is the principal trabecular system, resisting atrophy more than the other systems. In osteoporotic spines, the secondary systems atrophy first: their disappearance makes the vertical system stand out more sharply on radiographs. The spirally wound oblique systems resist torsion and, with the vertical system, share in the resistance to bending and shear. The horizontal systems are principally tension resistant, as are the minor accessory systems of the transverse and spinous processes: they resist muscular pull.

It is interesting to note that the compressive breaking strains of lumbar vertebrae tested at physiological strain rates are generally between 7 and 9 kN, with strength

TABLE 4.1 Muscles Associated With and Producing Movements of the Vertebral Column

Muscle	Attachments	Action	Innervation (root value)
Erector spinae: Iliocostalis (lumbar, thoracis and cervicis parts): lateral column	From a thick strong flat tendon along a U-shaped line around the attachment of multifidus: medial limb from T11 to L5 spinous processes and lateral limb from lateral and posterior sacral crest, sacrotuberous, sacrospinous and posterior sacroiliac ligaments. Lumborum attaches to lower six ribs; thoracis to upper six ribs and transverse process of C7; cervicis to posterior tubercles of transverse processes of C7–C4	All three columns of both sides extend vertebral column, as well as head on neck: also important in controlling flexion of trunk. One side produces combined lateral flexion/bending and rotation. When standing on one leg lower part on non-weight-bearing side prevents pelvis from dropping	Dorsal rami of adjacent spinal nerves
Longissimus (thoracis, cervicis, and capitis parts): intermediate column	Thoracis from transverse processes of lumbar vertebrae and adjacent thoracolumbar fascia to transverse processes of all 12 thoracic vertebrae and adjacent regions of lower 10 ribs; cervicis from transverse processes of T6–T1 to posterior tubercles of transverse processes of C6–C2; capitis from transverse processes of T5–T1 and articular processes of C7–C4 to posterior aspect of mastoid process		
Spinalis (thoracis, cervicis, capitis parts): most medial column	Thoracis from spinous processes of L2–T11 to those of T6–T1; cervicis and capitis are poorly developed often blending with adjacent muscles		
Interspinales (best developed in cervical and lumbar regions)	Between adjacent spinous processes	Extends lumbar and cervical spine: stabilises vertebral column during movement	Dorsal rami of adjacent spinal nerves
Semispinalis (thoracis, cervicis and capitis parts)	Thoracis from transverse processes of T10–T6 to spinous processes of T4–C6; cervicis from transverse processes of T6–T1 to spinous processes of C5–C2; capitis from transverse processes of T6–T1 and articular processes of C7–C4 to an impression between superior and inferior nuchal lines	Both sides extend thoracic and cervical parts of vertebral column. Individually each produces rotation of trunk and neck to opposite side	Dorsal rami of adjacent spinal nerves

Continued

TABLE 4.1   Muscles Associated With and Producing Movements of the Vertebral Column—cont'd

Muscle	Attachments	Action	Innervation (root value)
Multifidus	Posterior aspect of sacrum and fascia covering erector spinae, mamillary processes of lumbar vertebrae, transverse processes of all thoracic vertebrae and articular processes of C7–C4/3 to spinous processes of L5–C2	Extends, rotates and laterally flexes vertebral column at all levels: stabilises vertebral column	Dorsal rami of adjacent spinal nerves
Rotatores	Transverse process of one vertebra to lamina and spinous process of vertebra above, being best developed in thoracic region	Rotates adjacent vertebrae: stabilises vertebral column	Dorsal rami of adjacent spinal nerves
Quadratus lumborum	Iliac crest to medial half of lower border of 12th rib, attaching to lateral half of anterior surface of lumbar transverse processes	Together extend trunk; individually each laterally flexes vertebral column to same side	Subcostal and lumbar nerves (T12 and L1–L4)
Rectus abdominis	Symphysis pubis and pubic crest to xiphoid process and costal cartilages of fifth–seventh ribs: it is enclosed within rectus sheath	Both sides flex trunk or with thorax fixed lifts anterior part of pelvis reducing lumbar lordosis; individually it laterally flexes trunk	(T5/T6–T12)
External oblique	Lateral aspects of lower eight ribs and costal cartilages, fibres run inferomedially to anterior two-thirds of iliac crest and rectus sheath: has a free posterior border between 12th rib and iliac crest with lower free border forming inguinal ligament	Both sides flex trunk or with thorax fixed lifts anterior part of pelvis reducing lumbar lordosis; individually it laterally flexes and rotates trunk	(T7–T12)
Internal oblique	Lateral two-thirds of inguinal ligament, anterior two-thirds of iliac crest and thoracolumbar fascia, fibres fan out running superolaterally to lower four ribs posteriorly and rectus sheath anteriorly: lower part blends with lower part of transversus abdominis forming conjoint tendon, which attaches to pubic crest	Both sides flex trunk or with thorax fixed lifts anterior part of pelvis reducing lumbar lordosis; individually it laterally flexes and rotates trunk	(T7–T12 and L1)

TABLE 4.1 **Muscles Associated With and Producing Movements of the Vertebral Column—cont'd**

Muscle	Attachments	Action	Innervation (root value)
Transversus abdominis	Lateral one-third of inguinal ligament, anterior two-thirds of iliac crest and thoracolumbar fascia and lower six ribs the fibres run horizontally to rectus sheath: fibres arising from inguinal ligament blend with lower part of internal oblique forming conjoint tendon, which attaches to pubic crest	Helps to increase intra-abdominal pressure during expulsive acts; compresses the abdominal viscera	(T7–T12 and L1)

increasing at faster strain rates. However, at least half of the lumbar vertebrae tested in one study were found to have compressive strengths less than the calculated compressive forces.

Vertebral Unit

This is a useful concept when modelling the vertebral column: it consists of two adjacent vertebrae and the intervening intervertebral disc. In terms of functional components, the vertebral column can be considered to consist of an anterior supporting pillar comprising the vertebral bodies and intervertebral disc, and a posterior pillar comprising the articular processes joined by the vertebral arch. While the anterior pillar plays an essentially static role, the posterior pillar has a dynamic role in vertebral column mechanics.

A further differentiation of vertebral unit components can be distinguished as horizontal layers sandwiched together. The vertebrae form a passive segment while the intervertebral disc, posterior ligamentous structures and articular processes form an active unit: it is mobility of the active segment which underlies movements of the vertebral column.

The oblique trabecular systems described above functionally link the anterior and posterior pillars. With these systems as a basis, each vertebra can be compared to a first class lever with the articular processes acting as the fulcrum (Fig. 4.20), allowing the absorption of axial compression forces applied to the vertebral column by direct and passive absorption by the intervertebral disc, and by indirect and active absorption by the posterior ligaments and paravertebral muscles.

Intervertebral Disc Mechanisms

Ultrastructurally, the nucleus pulposus, annulus fibrosus and cartilage end plate appear as a close-packed system, postulated to act as a buffer against gravity and torsion by acting as a shock absorber of forces transmitted to the vertebral column. The ability to absorb shock is due to the construction of the disc, in which the soft fluidlike nucleus pulposus is encapsulated within the connective tissue lamellae of the annulus fibrosus. Vertical pressure on the vertebral column compresses the disc deforming the nucleus pulposus, causing it to expand radially against the surrounding annulus fibrosus: outward annulus fibrosus expansion is necessary for the disc to absorb shock.

Examining lateral, posterolateral and posterior disc bulging under compressive loading and applied movements has shown that the disc may bulge up to 2.7 mm beyond its unloaded state, with the largest bulges being associated with lateral flexion/bending: no clear relationship has been observed between intradiscal pressure and disc bulging. End plate bulging was found to be negligible (~0.1 mm) compared with disc bulging. When degenerated discs were tested, a greater degree of bulging was observed than nondegenerated discs, presumably because they are less efficient. The clinical manifestation of disc bulging, particularly in degenerating discs, may be entrapment of the nerve roots as they pass through the narrowed intervertebral foramen.

It has been suggested that the nucleus pulposus plays a major mechanical role in determining compressive deformation of the disc. However, studies have shown that the annulus fibrosus appears to be the primary

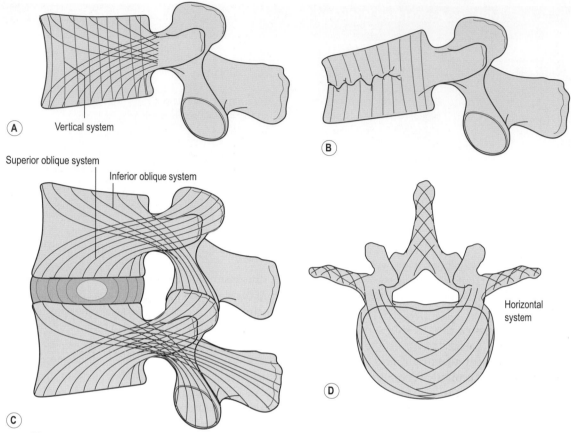

Fig. 4.28 Trabecular patterns within vertebrae: (A) in the body; (B) a compression fracture; (C) superior and inferior oblique systems; (D) horizontal system.

load-bearing structure, capable of performing this function in a near normal fashion even when part or all of the nucleus has been removed. Nevertheless, efficient functioning of the disc depends, to a large extent, on the elasticity of the nucleus, which is closely related to its water-binding capacity. Increased pressure within the nucleus (by the imbibition of water) increases disc height, prestressing the disc, reducing its laxity and increasing vertebral joint stiffness (Fig. 4.29).

Measurements of disc strength and pressure show that the tensile strength of the annulus fibrosus is between 15 and 50 kg/cm^2, while that of vertebral bodies varies between 8 and 10 kg/cm^2. In tension, failure is routinely observed at the disc end plate at forces of 850 N at cervical levels and 3000 N at lumbar levels: in compression vertebral bodies in the cervical and lumbar regions fail at 3000 and 5000 N, respectively. The tensile strength of the longitudinal ligaments is approximately 200 kg/cm^2 and

could provide considerable resistance to disc rupture. The ultimate torsional strength of the intervertebral disc in an intact vertebral column is approximately 40 kg/cm^2. It is, therefore, possible to appreciate why vertebral bodies may fracture without evidence of disc rupture.

Mechanically, the intervertebral disc may be regarded as a viscoelastic structure capable of maintaining very large loads without disintegrating (Fig. 4.30A): the end point is similar to that of steel. However, when the end point is exceeded, the disc retains some power of recovery after rest, retaining its properties of elasticity. The mechanical efficiency of the disc appears to improve with use, with the energy lost during recovery being decreased. This is significant in lifting heavy loads, providing a theoretical basis for the custom of taking the strain before a heavy load is lifted. Complete recovery of a disc after loading is modified by the duration of force application and the interaction of the various structural elements.

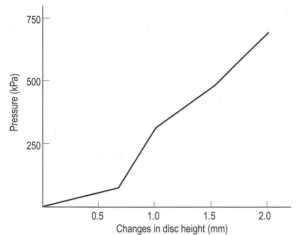

Fig. 4.29 Disc height changes with increasing nuclear pressurisation. (Adapted from Tencer, A.F., Ahmed, A.M., 1981. The role of secondary variables in the measurements of the mechanical properties of the lumbar intervertebral joint. J. Biomech. Eng. 103, 129–137.)

With static loading, disc deformation depends on the duration of loading, becoming stable after approximately 5 minutes. With loads up to 130 kg, most deformation occurs in the first 30 seconds following loading, with no absolute equilibrium being reached even after a few hours: the disc exhibits creep characteristics. The nucleus pulposus appears to act as an incompressible medium of short duration (~1 second): the nucleus and annulus interact to redistribute, equilibrate and adapt to the load. The creep characteristic is a mechanism by which the disc distributes the stress and occurs until it adapts or reaches a stable state with respect to a particular load: to some extent this is determined by the zygapophyseal articulations. However, when a dynamic load is applied, the intervertebral disc may begin to vibrate (this occurs in less than 1 second then dies out) (Fig. 4.30B): the disc acts as a shock absorber damping the oscillations.

The disc therefore has mechanical properties similar to many elastic and semielastic systems: it is important to be aware of these properties to understand the mechanisms of disc damage. For example, when loaded statically approaching its elastic limit, and then dynamically, the vibrations which occur may exceed the tensile limit of the annulus fibrosus or its attachment to bone, resulting in disc damage. The extent and site of disc failure appear to be related to the morphology of the nucleus pulposus: only when considerable weakness is already present does prolapse at a specific site occur.

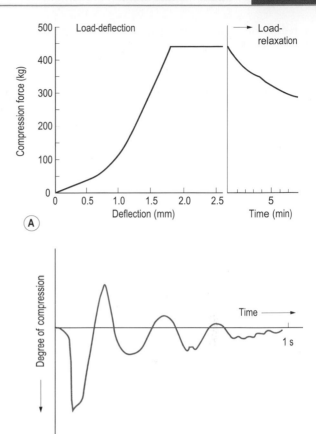

Fig. 4.30 Load–deflection and load–relaxation curves (A) and dynamic loading (B) of an intervertebral disc. (Adapted from (A) Markolf, K., Morris, J., 1974. The structural components of the intervertebral disc. J. Bone Joint Surg. 56A, 675–687; (B) Hirsch, C.S., 1995. The reaction of the intervertebral disc to compressive forces. J. Bone Joint Surg. 37A, 1188–1192.)

In vivo measurements of intradiscal pressures have shown that the force acting across the L5/S1 joint in an individual lifting loads is 30% less than that calculated theoretically: more impressively it is 50% less in the lower thoracic region. This difference between measured and theoretical findings is thought to be due to absorption of part of the load by the anterior abdominal muscles contracting in response to loading. Increases in disc pressure compared with quiet standing have been recorded when coughing (40%), stair climbing (40%) and walking slowly (15%). The significance of intradiscal pressure is important with respect to disc fluid transport and nutrition. Sustained flexion-loading of a lumbar segment results in fluid loss from the disc, with a reduction in its height. Sitting postures which entail flexion of the lumbar column cause more fluid to be expressed from the lumbar discs than erect postures: the effect is particularly marked in the nucleus pulposus. Fluid flow in flexed postures is sufficiently large to aid disc nutrition. The links between posture, fluid flow and disc nutrition may explain why societies that habitually adopt flexed or squatting postures have a low incidence of lumbar disc degeneration.

With ageing, the mechanical arrangement and biomechanical response of the intervertebral disc in relation to the zygapophyseal joints depart from that observed in earlier life. The disc space narrows and the surface contact area of the joints increases: the loss of disc space is attributed to thinning of the disc. However, it could equally be due to the disc sinking into the vertebral body, which itself weakens with age due to osteoporosis. Whatever the cause, the result is that the anterior and posterior joints of the vertebral column become less protected by the load-attenuating and load-distributing properties of the nucleus with respect to the annulus, decreasing the range of movement as well as the tolerance to impact. A commonly observed radiographic manifestation in disc/joint degeneration is the appearance of bony spurs, ridges or transverse bars along the superior, inferior and lateral margins of the vertebral bodies, intervertebral foramen and articular surfaces.

What is not certain is whether these changes are the result of purely mechanical factors causing a disturbance in equilibrium of the surrounding tissues, or whether it is the result of localised disruption of the periosteum altering the relationship of normal form and bony contour, or whether other factors are involved. There appears to be sufficient clinical and radiological evidence to suggest that the changes in the discs occur with changes in the posterior vertebral column at levels where stresses and strains are greatest (lower cervical and thoracolumbar areas), adversely affecting vertebral column kinematics. For example, with structural changes within the disc, over time there occurs an associated alteration in the zygapophyseal joints (or vice versa), affecting local biomechanics. The altered biomechanics of one component of the vertebral column may result in asymmetric motion between its components, in turn causing accelerated damage and degeneration that could eventually affect the entire vertebral region.

Changes in the relative position of the vertebral body also involve changes in the relative positions of the zygapophyseal joints. As nucleus turgor is lost and the disc space decreases, the joints become partially weight-bearing. Although there is convincing radiographic evidence of osteophyte formation, there is no experimental evidence confirming that osteophyte presence is indicative of degenerative disc disease.

With the intervertebral disc being indispensable for normal functioning of the vertebral column, it is not surprising that artificial discs are being developed to replace a degenerated disc. Although such discs have been developed, they, as yet, do not offer the same degree of efficiency as a replacement hip or knee joint does. There are, of course, fundamental differences in the design of joint prostheses and the design of an acceptable viscoelastic component. In addition, major problems are associated with removal of the degenerated disc and implantation of the prosthesis, not least of which is the proximity of the spinal cord posteriorly and the emergence of the nerve roots through the intervertebral foramen. Nevertheless, further development of such prostheses and their implantation offers tremendous benefits over plating and fixation of vertebral segments.

Pathology

The result of spinal fusion to counteract the effects of disc degeneration creates stress concentrations at either end of the fused segment: these increased stresses increase the chance of degeneration or instability in these regions. The greater the number of segments fused, the more the remaining segments must move to achieve the same overall range of movement.

Rotatory injuries of the vertebral column are associated with fracture of the articular facets, which tend to limit excessive rotation. At lower levels of the vertebral column, the common torsional injury is a fracture-dislocation at the thoracolumbar junction. Above this level, the thoracic column is relatively stiff due to the presence of the thoracic cage: the articular processes offer little resistance to rotation. Below this junction, the lumbar region gains increased resistance to deformation by the orientation of the articular processes. The T12/L1 area, being a transitional area, has neither the thoracic supplementary protective elements nor the lumbar protective bony geometry, thus torsional deformation and stress tend to be concentrated at the thoracolumbar junction.

The vertebral column possesses natural curvatures in the sagittal plane. Scoliosis is a lateral curvature of the column in a coronal plane: it is a three-dimensional deformity consisting of lateral flexion/bending and a rotational abnormality. The curves can be broadly subdivided into two types: nonstructural and structural. Nonstructural curves have no structural abnormality and can easily be reversed by changing posture or by traction: included in this group are postural curves eliminated on forward flexion with no fixed vertebral rotation, and compensatory curves devoid of vertebral rotation or structural changes. Compensatory curves develop above and below a single structural curve to maintain alignment of the body.

Structural curves on the other hand can be readily identified as they demonstrate rib and vertebral rotation to the convexity of the curve on forward flexion. Radiographs of the curve show vertebral rotation with the bodies rotated to the convexity and spinous processes to the concavity of the curvature (Fig. 4.31).

In theory, scoliotic curves can occur anywhere along the length of the vertebral column; however, in practice they are most commonly found in thoracic and lumbar regions. Involvement of the thoracic region is not surprising, considering there is little resistance to rotation in this region: involvement of the lumbar region is more difficult to account for, although the importance

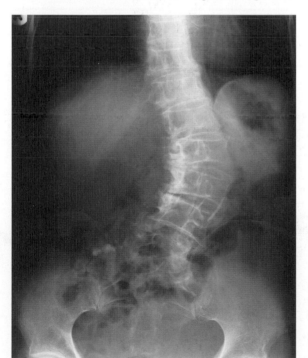

Fig. 4.31 Anteroposterior radiograph showing thoracolumbar scoliosis.

of lordosis in the development of scoliosis has been stressed by some authorities.

One way of classifying scoliotic curves is in terms of the age of the individual. This is particularly important in idiopathic scoliosis, which accounts for some 85% of all scolioses, where the side of the convexity of the curve is related to the age of onset. Infantile scoliosis (under age 4) is seen most commonly as a left thoracic curve, while right thoracic curves are most common in adolescent scoliosis (puberty to skeletal maturity): of these infantile scoliosis often regresses naturally. Juvenile scoliosis (age 4 to puberty) occurs with almost equal frequency to the right and left sides.

A further, and perhaps more important, classification of scoliosis is in terms of its aetiology and pathogenesis. Three classes of curves are considered:

1. Congenital: arising as a result of congenital vertebral anomalies which themselves can be classified.
2. Neuromuscular: due to an obvious neurological or muscular impairment. This type of curve was very common until recently, frequently developing following poliomyelitis.
3. Idiopathic: the aetiology is unclear, although many causes have been postulated. Within this class are four main groups: primary skeletal, neuromuscular, metabolic and hereditary.

Although the aetiology of many curves is understood, or at least postulated, the mechanisms by which the deformity develops are less certain.

The incidence of clinically evident scoliosis is 1–5 per 1000 of the population. However, screening programmes have suggested that as many as 15% of the population show some form of lateral curvature of the vertebral column. Presumably, many of these are nonstructural or never develop to any significance. Nevertheless, scoliosis is more common in the White population than the Black and is more prevalent in females than males (ratio of 5:1).

MUSCLES FLEXING THE TRUNK

Rectus abdominis
External oblique
Internal oblique
Psoas minor
Psoas major (p. 299)

Rectus Abdominis

Running vertically on the anterior aspect of the abdomen, rectus abdominis is enclosed within the rectus sheath (Fig. 4.32A). Arising from the anterior aspect of the symphysis pubis and pubic crest via two tendons, it passes superiorly, widening as it does so, to attach to the anterior surfaces of the xiphoid process and costal cartilages of the fifth, sixth and seventh ribs. Its slightly convex lateral border presents as a groove (linea semilunaris) on lean individuals: the two muscles are separated by the linea alba. Transverse tendinous intersections (usually three) are found in the anterior part of the muscle firmly attached to the rectus sheath: the lowest lies at the level of the umbilicus, the highest at the level of the xiphoid, and the third approximately midway between.

Each muscle is enclosed in a fibrous sheath formed by the aponeuroses of external and internal oblique and transversus abdominis (Fig. 4.32B): the two sheaths fuse along their medial borders in the region of the linea alba. Formation of the rectus sheath differs at different levels. Above the costal margin, it is only present anteriorly, being formed entirely by the aponeurosis of external oblique. Between the costal margin and midway between the umbilicus and symphysis pubis, it is formed anteriorly by the aponeuroses of external and internal oblique, and posteriorly by the aponeuroses of internal oblique and transversus abdominis (Fig. 4.32B(i)). Below this level the aponeuroses of all three muscles pass anterior to rectus abdominis so that the posterior wall of the sheath is deficient (Fig. 4.32B(ii)): the inferior limit of the posterior layer is marked by a crescentic border (arcuate line). Below the arcuate line, rectus abdominis lies directly on the transversalis fascia, separating it from extraperitoneal fat. Above the costal margin, the posterior layer is also deficient so that rectus abdominis lies directly on the thoracic wall.

When present, pyramidalis lies within the sheath: this small muscle, supplied by the subcostal nerve (T12), lies anterior to rectus abdominis, arising from the pubic crest and attaching to the linea alba. It tenses the linea alba, presumably to help provide a stable attachment from which the abdominal muscles can work, particularly when the trunk is flexed.

In the latter stages of pregnancy, the linea alba stretches increasing the distance between the two rectus abdominis muscles (divarication/diastasis recti). Separation of 5 cm or more can occur: postpartum it returns to normal providing undue strains are avoided.

Innervation.

From the lower six or seven thoracic nerves (T6/T7–T12). Skin over the muscle is supplied by nerves with root values (T4–L1).

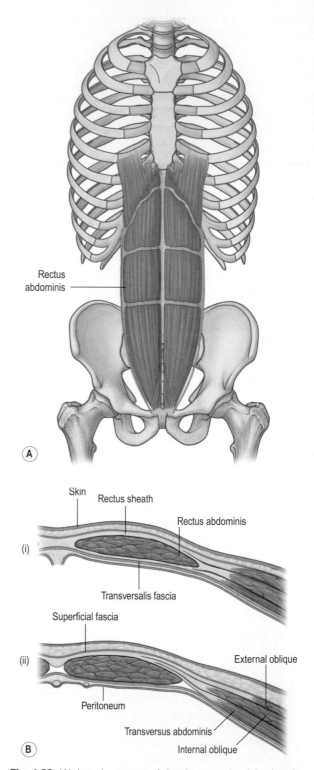

Rectus abdominis

(A)

Skin

Rectus sheath

Rectus abdominis

(i)

Transversalis fascia

Superficial fascia

(ii)

External oblique

Peritoneum

Transversus abdominis

Internal oblique

(B)

Fig. 4.32 (A) Anterior aspect of the thorax and pelvis showing the position and attachments of rectus abdominis; (B) formation of the rectus sheath.

Palpation

Rectus abdominis can be readily palpated as it runs vertically and centrally on the anterior abdominal wall when the trunk is flexed against resistance. In an athletic individual, it should also be possible to palpate the three transverse tendinous intersections, as well as the linea alba and semilunaris at the sides of each muscle.

External Oblique

Situated on the anterolateral aspect of the abdominal wall, the fibres of external oblique run inferomedially from the ribs towards the midline (Fig. 4.33): it is the most superficial of the three sheets of muscle forming the anterior abdominal wall. The upper attachment is by fleshy slips to the outer borders of the lower eight ribs and their costal cartilages, interdigitating with serratus anterior above and latissimus dorsi below. From here, the muscle fibres sweep inferomedially, with those from the lower two ribs passing almost vertically to attach to the anterior two-thirds of the lateral lip of the iliac crest, leaving a free posterior border of the muscle running between the 12th rib and iliac crest. The remaining fibres give rise to a large aponeurosis broader inferiorly than superiorly, with each aponeurosis passing across rectus abdominis, participating in the formation of the rectus sheath, towards the midline fusing with that of the opposite side at the linea alba. (The linea alba is a fibrous raphe running from the tip of the xiphoid process of the sternum to the symphysis pubis.)

The lower free border of the aponeurosis stretches between the pubic tubercle and anterior superior iliac spine forming the inguinal ligament, which folds back on itself so that it is convex inferiorly, caused by the pull of the fascia lata of the thigh attaching along its length. The medial part of the inguinal ligament is expanded along the pecten pubis, forming the lacunar ligament: a further extension of the lacunar ligament along the pecten is the pectineal ligament. In the anatomical position, the lacunar ligament lies almost horizontal. Above the pubic tubercle is a triangular cleft in the aponeurosis, the superficial inguinal ring (see Fig. 4.41): its base is at the pubic crest and the apex is directed superolaterally, with the sides bound by the medial and lateral crura.

Innervation

From the anterior primary rami of the lower six thoracic nerves (T7–T12). Skin over the muscle is supplied by the same nerve roots.

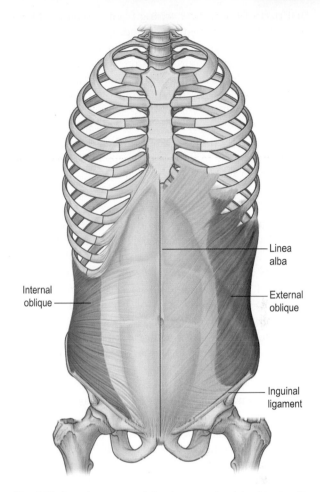

Fig. 4.33 Anterior aspect of the thorax and pelvis showing the position and attachment of the right internal oblique and left external oblique.

Internal Oblique

Lying deep to external oblique, internal oblique (Fig. 4.33) is the middle of the three sheets of abdominal muscles. Its muscle fibres arise from the lateral two-thirds of the inguinal ligament, anterior two-thirds of the intermediate line of the iliac crest and thoracolumbar fascia (see Fig. 4.35C). From this extensive attachment, the fibres fan outwards: the most posterior fibres pass almost vertically to attach to the inferior border of the lower four ribs; the more anterior and inferior fibres pass superomedially giving way to an aponeurosis along a line extending inferomedially from the 10th costal cartilage to the body of the pubis. The aponeurosis has a complex involvement in the formation of the rectus sheath (p. 531) before interlacing with that of the opposite side at the linea alba.

That part of the muscle arising from the inguinal ligament passes inferomedially, blending with the inferior part of transversus abdominis to form the conjoint tendon which attaches to the pubic crest and pecten pubis. A few fibres from the inferomedial part pass along the spermatic cord as the cremaster muscle (p. 541).

Innervation

By the lower six thoracic and first lumbar nerves (T7–T12 and L1).

Action

Flexion of the trunk is produced by concentric contraction of external oblique, internal oblique and rectus abdominis of both sides. If the thoracic cage is the fixed point, then these same muscles can lift the anterior part of the pelvis and change the pelvic tilt. This latter action has a significant effect in decreasing lumbar lordosis: it is advocated by some in the management of low back pain. The muscles are also involved in rotation and lateral flexion/bending of the trunk, as well as in general functional activities involving the abdomen which are discussed later (p. 546).

Palpation

The flat nature of the oblique muscles makes their palpation difficult in all but muscular individuals. Nevertheless, a flat hand placed over the lower lateral aspect of the ribs may allow the contraction of external oblique to be felt on resisted flexion. Internal oblique may be similarly palpated if the hand is placed over the lower abdomen just above the anterior part of the iliac crest.

Psoas Minor

A weak muscle, not always present; however, when present it arises from the lateral aspect of the bodies of T12 and L1 and intervening intervertebral disc. The fleshy belly soon gives way to a long tendon lying on psoas major and attaches to the iliopubic eminence and iliac fascia.

The muscle is supplied by the anterior primary ramus of L1 and acts as a weak flexor of the lumbar spine.

MUSCLES EXTENDING THE TRUNK

Erector spinae
Interspinales
Quadratus lumborum (p. 537)
Multifidus (p. 537)
Semispinalis (p. 538)

Erector Spinae

A large, complex, powerful mass of muscle consisting of several parts running the length of the vertebral column (Figs 4.34 and 4.35C).

In the lumbar region, erector spinae has a broad belly with a well-defined lateral border, but as it extends superiorly, it divides into three parallel columns, each of which is divided into three parts according to their relative positions (Fig. 4.34).

Erector spinae arises inferiorly from a strong, thick, flat tendon attached along a U-shaped line around the origin of multifidus. The medial limb arises from the spinous processes of T11–L5, spreading onto the supraspinous ligaments and associated median sacral crest. The lateral limb attaches to the lateral sacral crest, the sacrotuberous, sacrococcygeal and posterior sacroiliac ligaments, and posterior part of the iliac crest medial to internal oblique. Deep to the lateral limb, erector spinae has a fleshy attachment to the iliac tuberosity and medial lip of the iliac crest. From this extensive attachment, the muscle fibres pass superiorly deep to latissimus dorsi, splitting into three columns.

Iliocostalis

The most lateral of the three columns, iliocostalis is divided into lumbar, thoracic and cervical parts. Iliocostalis lumborum attaches by six slips into the inferior border of the lower six ribs near their angles. Medial to each slip arises iliocostalis thoracis which attaches near the angles of the upper six ribs and transverse process of C7. Finally, iliocostalis cervicis arises medial to the slips of thoracis to attach to the posterior tubercles of the transverse processes of C4–C7.

Longissimus

The intermediate column of erector spinae is the longest and thickest: it can be divided into thoracic, cervical and capitis parts. Longissimus thoracis runs from the transverse and accessory processes of lumbar vertebrae and adjacent thoracolumbar fascia to attach by two sets of slips to the transverse processes of all 12 thoracic vertebrae and adjacent regions of the lower 10 ribs. Longissimus cervicis runs from the transverse processes of T1–T6, medial to thoracis, to the posterior tubercles of the transverse processes of C2–C6. Longissimus capitis arises from the transverse processes of T1–T5, in common with longissimus cervicis, and articular processes of C4–C7 attaching to the posterior aspect of the mastoid process.

Spinalis

The medial relatively insignificant column of erector spinae is divided into thoracic, cervical and capitis parts. Spinalis thoracis, the most clearly demarcated part, runs from the spinous processes of T11–L2 to those of T1–T6. Spinalis cervicis and capitis are poorly developed, frequently blending with adjacent muscles.

Innervation

All parts of erector spinae are supplied by adjacent dorsal rami according to their position.

Action

When the three muscle columns of both sides act together, they extend the lumbar, thoracic and cervical regions, as well as the head on the neck, being the major extensor of the trunk: however, it is also important in controlling trunk flexion. When the three columns of one side act together, they produce combined lateral flexion/bending and rotation to the same side. When standing on one leg, the inferior part of erector spinae on the non-weight-bearing side works strongly to prevent the pelvis from dropping. During walking, erector spinae contracts alternately steadying the vertebral column on the pelvis.

Because the main mass of muscle is situated in the lumbar region, it (particularly longissimus thoracis) is responsible for maintaining the secondary lumbar curvature during sitting and standing.

Palpation

Each erector spinae can be felt and seen as a column of muscle on either side of the lumbar region, particularly during extension. Each muscle mass can also be felt contracting when alternately standing on one and then the other leg.

Interspinales

Short insignificant muscles of the back, the interspinales (Fig. 4.35B) extend between adjacent spinous processes. They are best developed in the cervical and lumbar regions where they consist of bundles of muscle fibres either side of the interspinous ligament: in the thoracic region they are poorly developed or absent.

Innervation

By the dorsal rami of adjacent spinal nerves.

Action

Interspinales can produce extension of the cervical and lumbar spine, but have a more significant role in stabilising the vertebral column during movement.

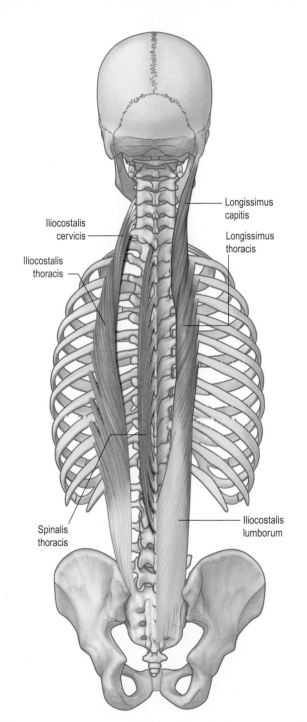

Iliocostalis cervicis

Iliocostalis thoracis

Spinalis thoracis

Longissimus capitis

Longissimus thoracis

Iliocostalis lumborum

Fig. 4.34 Posterior aspect of the skull, neck, thorax, vertebral column and pelvis showing the position and attachments of the constituent parts of the erector spinae muscle mass.

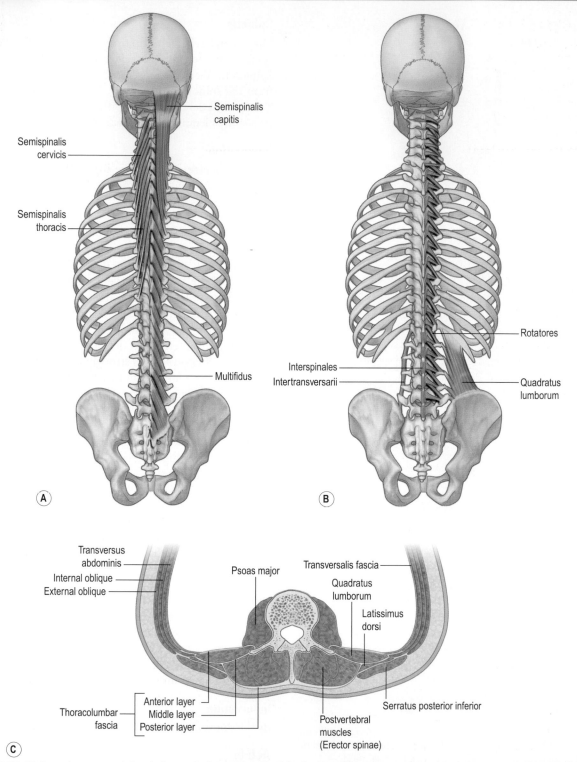

Fig. 4.35 (A) Posterior aspect of the skull, vertebral column and pelvis showing the position and attachments of the right multifidus and semispinalis capitis and left semispinalis thoracis and cervicis; (B) posterior aspect of the lower thoracic and lumbar vertebrae, lower ribs and pelvis showing the position and attachments of the right quadratus lumborum and the rotatores, and the left lumbar intertransversarii and interspinales; (C) transverse section through the upper lumbar spine showing the formation and arrangement of the thoracolumbar fascia.

MUSCLES LATERALLY FLEXING/BENDING THE TRUNK

Quadratus lumborum
Intertransversarii
External oblique (p. 533)
Internal oblique (p. 533)
Rectus abdominis (p. 531)
Erector spinae (p. 534)
Multifidus (p. 537)

Movement of the trunk to one side is called lateral flexion/bending: it is produced by muscles of the same side (rectus abdominis, external and internal oblique, quadratus lumborum and erector spinae).

Quadratus Lumborum

Large, flat, quadrilateral muscle of the posterior abdominal wall (Fig. 4.35B) running between the pelvis and 12th rib deep to erector spinae. It attaches inferiorly to the iliolumbar ligament and adjacent posterior part of the iliac crest. From here, fibres run superiorly and slightly medially to attach to the medial half of the inferior border of the 12th rib. During its course, the medial border of quadratus lumborum attaches to the lateral part of the anterior surface of the transverse processes of all lumbar vertebrae. The muscle is enclosed by the anterior and middle layers of the thoracolumbar fascia (Fig. 4.35C).

Innervation

By the subcostal nerve and the upper three or four lumbar nerves (T12 and L1–L3/L4).

Action

Contraction of quadratus lumborum produces lateral flexion/bending of the trunk to the same side. When standing on one leg, it acts strongly on the non-weight-bearing side to stop the pelvis dropping inferiorly. It also steadies the 12th rib during deep inspiration so that the attachment of the diaphragm is fixed. Acting together, both muscles help extend the lumbar vertebral column, giving it lateral stability.

Intertransversarii

Small slips of muscle (Fig. 4.35B) passing between adjacent transverse processes in the cervical and lumbar regions. In the cervical region, they are reasonably well developed, each muscle consisting of up to four slips between adjacent transverse processes from the atlas (C1) to T1. In the lumbar region, the intertransversarii exist as pairs of muscular slips, the lateral slip passing between adjacent transverse processes and medial slip between the accessory process of one vertebra to the mamillary process of the vertebra above: the lateral slips may extend as far as the transverse process of T10. In the cervical region, the intertransversarii slips lie both anterior and posterior to the emerging ventral ramus of the spinal nerve, while in the lumbar region they lie posterior to the ventral ramus.

Innervation

In the cervical region and lateral part in the lumbar region, the intertransversarii are supplied by the ventral rami of adjacent spinal nerves, while the medial lumbar slips are supplied by the dorsal rami of adjacent nerves.

Action

The intertransversarii on one side can produce lateral flexion/bending to the same side in the lumbar and cervical regions. However, their main function is as extensile ligaments stabilising adjacent vertebral segments during movements of the trunk.

MUSCLES ROTATING THE TRUNK

Multifidus
Rotatores
Semispinalis
Internal oblique (p. 533)
External oblique (p. 533)

Rotation of the trunk to the left is produced by the simultaneous contraction of the right external and left internal oblique. Conversely, rotation to the right is produced by the left external and right internal oblique. These movements may be accompanied by some flexion of the trunk.

Multifidus

It lies deep to semispinalis and erector spinae in the gutter between the spinous and transverse processes of the vertebrae at all levels. From inferior to superior, its lateral attachment is from the posterior aspect of the sacrum and fascia covering erector spinae, mamillary processes of the lumbar vertebrae, transverse processes of the thoracic vertebrae and articular processes of the lower four or five cervical vertebrae (Fig. 4.35A). From this extensive attachment, the muscle fibres are arranged in three layers as they pass superomedially to attach to the spines of all vertebrae from the L5 to C2. The deepest layer attaches to the vertebrae immediately above, the middle layer to the second or third vertebra above and the superficial layer to the third or fourth vertebra above.

Innervation

By the dorsal rami of adjacent spinal nerves.

Rotatores

Best developed in the thoracic region (Fig. 4.35B), the rotatores are represented by variable bundles in the lumbar and cervical regions. They lie adjacent to the transverse process of one vertebra passing superiorly to attach to the lamina of the vertebra above.

Innervation

By the dorsal rami of adjacent spinal nerves.

Action

Multifidus can produce rotation, as well as extension and lateral flexion/bending, of the vertebral column at all levels: rotatores only produce rotation in the thoracic region. Both muscles, however, probably have more functional importance in their role as extensible ligaments stabilising the vertebral column, adjusting their length to stabilise adjacent vertebrae irrespective of the position of the vertebral column.

Semispinalis

In three parts (Fig. 4.35A), semispinalis extends from the lower thoracic region to the base of the skull. Semispinalis thoracis arises from the transverse processes of the lower thoracic vertebrae (T6–T10) attaching to the spinous processes of the lower cervical and upper thoracic vertebrae (C6–T2). The larger semispinalis cervicis runs from the transverse processes of T1–T6 to the spinous processes of C2–C6. The largest part (semispinalis capitis) runs from the transverse processes of T1–T6 and articular processes of C4–C7 to attach to a medial impression between the superior and inferior nuchal lines on the base of the skull. The most medial part of semispinalis capitis may be separate from the remainder: if so, it is known as spinalis capitis.

Innervation

By the dorsal rami of adjacent spinal nerves.

Action

When both sides act together, semispinalis produces extension of the thoracic and cervical parts of the vertebral column. When only one side acts, it produces rotation of the trunk and neck to the opposite side.

CLINICAL EXAMINATION AND EVALUATION

Angular measurements of flexion and extension is difficult without using specialised goniometers: the easiest method for obtaining an estimate of the ranges of flexion and extension is with a tape measure.

Flexion

With the individual standing with the feet slightly apart and spine in neutral lateral flexion and rotation:
- Stabilise the pelvis to prevent tilting by placing one hand over the anterior aspect of the pelvis.
- Place the ends of the tape measure over the S1 and C7 spinous processes.

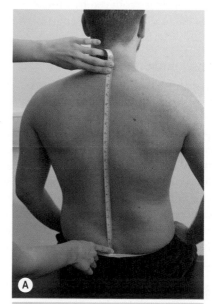

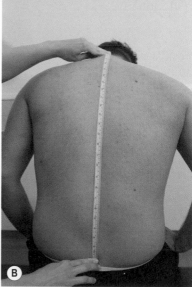

Fig. 4.36 Determination of the range of flexion of the thoraco-lumbar spine with the spine in neutral (A) and flexed (B).

- Take a reading when standing erect.
- Take a second reading in full flexion (Fig. 4.36).

The difference in readings is a measure of thoracolumbar flexion: a difference of 10 cm is considered normal. By having the ends of the tape over the spinous processes of T12 and C7, and S1 and T12, the contribution to the total movement made by the thoracic and lumbar regions can be determined.

An alternative method is the Modified Schober Technique in which the lumbosacral junction is marked, with a second mark made 10 cm above the first and a third mark 5 cm above the second. The tape is aligned between the top and bottom marks, and a reading taken with the individual erect and in full flexion; the range is the difference between the initial 15 cm and the length when flexed. This technique is essentially a measure of lumbar flexion.

Extension

With the individual in the same initial posture:
- Prevent pelvic tilting by placing one hand over the anterior aspect of the pelvis and the other over the posterior pelvis.
- Place the ends of the tape over the S1 and C7 spinous processes.
- Take a reading when standing erect.
- Take a second reading in full extension (Fig. 4.37).

The difference in readings between the erect position and full extension is an indication of thoracolumbar

extension. The measurements can be taken with the individual either prone or when lying on the side: it is easier to stabilise the pelvis with the individual lying prone.

Alternatively, the Modified Schober Technique can be used as for flexion, in which case the individual should place their hands on the buttocks and bend backwards as far as possible. The difference in readings between the initial 15 cm and that observed when bending backwards is an indication of lumbar extension.

Lateral Flexion/Bending

With the individual standing with the feet slightly apart and spine in neutral flexion/extension and rotation:
- Stabilise the pelvis to prevent lateral tilting by placing the hand over the opposite iliac crest to the direction of bending (Fig. 4.38).

Place the centre of the goniometer over the posterior aspect of the S1 spinous process, with the proximal arm aligned with the spinous process of C7 and the distal arm aligned perpendicular to the ground. During movement, the proximal arm is kept aligned with C7 and not the vertebral column as the lower thoracic and lumbar region becomes convex to the side of flexion/bending.

Rotation

With the individual seated comfortably erect on a stool with the feet on the floor and the spine in neutral flexion/extension and lateral flexion:

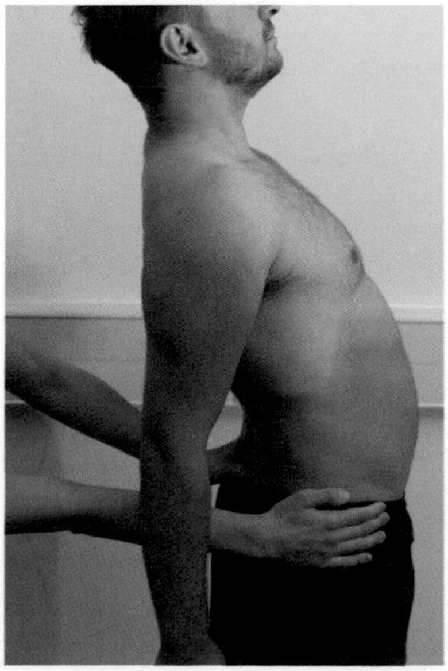

Fig. 4.37 Determination of the range of extension of the thoracolumbar spine.

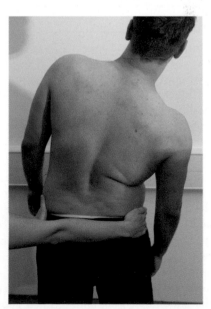

Fig. 4.38 Determination of the range of lateral flexion/bending of the thoracolumbar spine.

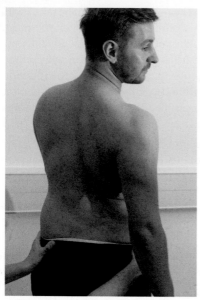

Fig. 4.39 Determination of the range of rotation of the thoracolumbar spine.

- Place the hands on both iliac crests to prevent pelvic rotation (Fig. 4.39).
  Place the centre of the goniometer over the centre of the vertex of the head with one arm parallel to a line passing between the acromion process and the other aligned parallel to a line passing through the iliac tubercles.

MUSCLES RAISING INTRA-ABDOMINAL PRESSURE

Transversus abdominis
Cremaster
External oblique (p. 533)
Internal oblique (p. 533)
Rectus abdominis (p. 531)

Transversus Abdominis

Deepest of the three sheets of abdominal muscles, transversus abdominis is named because of its transversely arranged fibres (Fig. 4.40). It arises from the lateral one-third of the inguinal ligament and anterior two-thirds of the medial lip of the iliac crest inferiorly, thoracolumbar fascia posteriorly and deep surface of the costal cartilages of the lower six ribs superiorly, where it interdigitates with the attachment of the diaphragm (see Fig. 4.51).

The fibres of transversus abdominis pass horizontally around the abdominal wall, ending in an aponeurotic

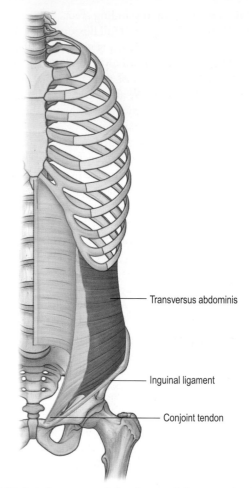

Fig. 4.40 Anterior aspect of the thorax, abdomen and pelvis showing the position and attachments of the left transversus abdominis.

sheet fusing with the posterior layer of the aponeurosis of internal oblique to reach the linea alba; it is therefore involved in forming the rectus sheath (p. 531).

Fibres arising from the inguinal ligament arch inferiorly to join those from internal oblique to form the conjoint tendon, which attaches to the pubic crest and pecten pubis behind the superficial inguinal ring.

The inferior free border of transversus abdominis between its attachment to the inguinal ligament and pecten pubis is concave inferiorly. Below this border, its fascial covering (transversalis fascia) comes into contact with both the internal and external oblique and with the inguinal ligament. In the lateral part of this fascia is a round opening (deep inguinal ring) (Fig. 4.41).

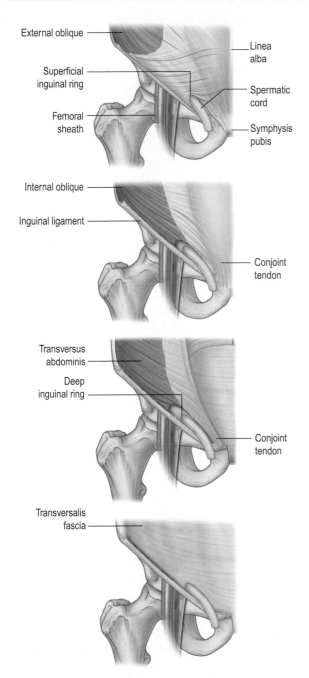

External oblique

Linea alba

Superficial inguinal ring

Spermatic cord

Femoral sheath

Symphysis pubis

Internal oblique

Inguinal ligament

Conjoint tendon

Transversus abdominis

Deep inguinal ring

Conjoint tendon

Transversalis fascia

Fig. 4.41 Lower anterior abdominal wall showing the muscles involved in forming the inguinal canal.

Innervation

By the lower six thoracic and first lumbar nerves (T7–T12 and L1).

Action

The actions of all eight muscles of the abdominal wall (four each side) can be related to the function of increasing intra-abdominal pressure: this is achieved by the sheet muscles pulling on the rectus sheath via their aponeuroses, flattening the abdomen and compressing the abdominal viscera. If the diaphragm maintains its tone and resists superior displacement, the increase in intra-abdominal pressure is important in producing the expulsive acts. Combined with appropriate sphincter relaxation, increased pressure on the bladder aids micturition; on the rectum it assists defecation; and on the stomach it helps in vomiting. In the final stages of childbirth, the compressive force produced helps to expel the foetus from the uterus.

When the diaphragm is relaxed, the increased intra-abdominal pressure presses the abdominal viscera against its inferior surface, pushing the diaphragm superiorly, increasing intrathoracic pressure so that, when the glottis is opened, air is forced from the lungs in a violent, explosive cough or sneeze. The coughing action is reinforced by the abdominal muscles acting on the lower ribs, pulling them inferiorly. Pain resulting from surgical incision of the abdominal wall frequently causes inhibition of these muscles, making coughing very difficult.

The combined action of the abdominal muscles, together with the diaphragm, also produces a muscular corset holding the abdominal viscera in place. This action can be increased during activities (lifting), in which a form of pneumatic cushion is formed anterior to the vulnerable lumbar spine. This action is frequently seen when people hold their breath, anchoring the diaphragm, prior to and when moving a heavy object.

Palpation

Combined contraction of all abdominal muscles can be felt if the hand is placed over the centre of the abdomen while the individual coughs. Increased tension within the anterior abdominal wall can also be appreciated during any of the expulsive acts described.

Cremaster

Loose arrangement of muscle fibres looping around the spermatic cord and testes, cremaster is continuous with the inferior edge of internal oblique and the adjacent part of the inguinal ligament attaching to the pubic tubercle: it is usually well developed in males, but sparse in females. It is supplied by the genital branch of the genitofemoral nerve (root value L1 and L2), although voluntary control over the muscle is not possible. A cremasteric reflex is present which raises the testes when the medial side of the thigh is stroked: the reflex is very active in infants, but much reduced by puberty.

Cremaster, together with dartos, helps in the mechanism of controlling the temperature of the testes. Relaxation of the muscles allows the testes to hang well down in the scrotum, reducing their temperature: contraction of the muscles draws the testes towards the superficial inguinal ring, raising their temperature. Precise regulation of the temperature of the testes is important for the proper formation of spermatozoa, which require a constant temperature approximately 3 degrees lower than core body temperature.

INGUINAL CANAL

An oblique passage through the anterior abdominal wall (Fig. 4.41), the inguinal canal is approximately 4 cm long: it transmits the spermatic cord in males and the round ligament of the uterus in females, as well as the ilioinguinal nerve in both sexes.

The inguinal canal begins at the deep inguinal ring (round opening in the transversalis fascia ~1.5 cm above the midpoint of the inguinal ligament) and ends at the superficial inguinal ring (deficit in the aponeurosis of external oblique above the pubic tubercle and medial end of the inguinal ligament). In the foetus and young children, the deep and superficial rings lie opposite each other facilitating, in males, passage of the testes and associated structures into the scrotum from the abdomen. With growth, the two rings separate so that, in adults, the inguinal canal runs inferomedially from the deep to superficial rings.

Throughout its course, the floor of the canal is formed by the inguinal ligament, with the lacunar ligament medially. The anterior wall is formed by the external oblique aponeurosis throughout, reinforced in its lateral third by muscular fibres of internal oblique. Posteriorly, the wall is formed throughout by the transversalis fascia, reinforced by the conjoint tendon in its medial third. The reinforcements of the anterior and posterior walls lie opposite the deep and superficial rings, respectively. The roof of the canal is formed by the arching fibres of internal oblique and transversus abdominis passing from anterior to posterior (conjoint tendon).

As the spermatic cord (or round ligament of the uterus) passes through the canal, it acquires coverings from some structures forming the canal. On entering the canal, the spermatic cord acquires a covering from the margins of the deep inguinal ring (internal spermatic fascia from the transversalis fascia); from the lower border of internal oblique a second covering is acquired (cremasteric fascia containing cremaster); and finally as the spermatic cord emerges from the canal a third covering is acquired from the margins of the superficial inguinal ring (external spermatic fascia from the external oblique aponeurosis).

The inguinal canal is a weak point in the anterior abdominal wall, although reinforcements opposite the deep and superficial inguinal rings provide some protection. Nevertheless, there is a tendency for contraction of the abdominal muscles to push mobile abdominal contents along the canal; however, contraction of these same muscles also narrows the canal, reducing the size of the inguinal rings. Internal oblique is in more or less continuous contraction when standing, so it will tend to have a protecting and supporting role as far as the inguinal canal is concerned. Some activities, such as heavy exertion with the trunk rotated, may cause the canal to open.

Because of this weakness, part of the mobile abdominal viscera may be squeezed through the superficial inguinal ring (hernia): for obvious reasons inguinal hernias tend to be twice as common in males as in females. One of two types of inguinal hernia may occur: indirect (oblique) or direct. An indirect hernia follows the course of the testis through the abdominal wall to appear at the superficial ring, being lateral to the inferior epigastric vessels at the deep inguinal ring. A direct hernia pushes through the posterior and sometimes anterior wall of the canal following no preformed path: it lies medial to the inferior epigastric vessels and may also appear lateral to the superficial ring.

Both forms of inguinal hernia can be distinguished from a femoral hernia, which emerges through the femoral canal, because its root lies above the inguinal ligament: in femoral herniae its root is below the inguinal ligament.

Herniae

An abdominal hernia is a protrusion of gut and covering peritoneum into a space where it is not normally found: it may be internal (nonpalpable) or external providing an obvious palpable protrusion. Hiatus hernia is the commonest form of internal hernia in which either the gastrointestinal junction and upper stomach passes through the oesophageal opening in the diaphragm to the posterior mediastinum, or part of the stomach passes through to lie adjacent to the oesophagus.

The commonest type of external hernia is inguinal hernia (75%) and then femoral hernia, both of which need to be distinguished from other lumps in the groin (enlarged superficial inguinal lymph nodes). Factors predisposing to external hernias include: sex, males are more commonly affected than females because of the differing contents of the inguinal canal; raised intra-abdominal pressure through obesity, coughing, straining or lifting; patent processus vaginalis; and abdominal muscle weakness.

Most inguinal hernias are indirect, occurring predominantly in males, in which a loop of small intestine follows the course of the spermatic cord through the abdominal wall so that a bulge appears above the inguinal ligament medial to the pubic tubercle. Once through the superficial ring, the hernia enters the scrotum (or rarely labium major in females). In direct inguinal hernias, the protruding gut pushes through the posterior wall of the inguinal canal, usually deep to or slightly lateral to the superficial ring.

Femoral hernia is twice as common in females as in males, particularly in women who have had children. Here, a loop of gut pushes through the femoral ring into the femoral sheath appearing below the inguinal ligament lateral to the pubic tubercle: the hernia is limited by the fascia lata except at the saphenous opening,

through which it may progress. With all external hernias, there is a danger of strangulation (twisting of the intestine and occlusion of its blood supply). Prompt surgical intervention is required to prevent gangrenous necrosis.

MUSCLES OF THE PELVIC FLOOR

Levator ani
Coccygeus

Levator Ani

The two levator ani muscles are broad but thin, forming a gutter-like floor across the inferior aspect of the pelvis: they separate the pelvic cavity from the perineum (Fig. 4.42). The two muscles unite in the midline, but for most of their extent are separated by the prostate in males and the urethra and vagina in females. Each muscle arises in a continuous manner from the medial deep surface of the pubic body anteriorly, obturator membrane and pelvic surface of the ischial spine laterally. The muscle fibres run posteriorly, inferiorly and medially towards the midline, attaching to the perineal body, sides of the anal canal and anococcygeal raphe between the anal canal and coccyx. Levator ani usually consists of least two distinct parts (iliococcygeus, pubococcygeus).

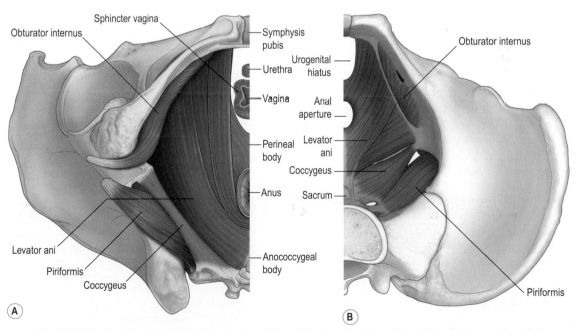

Fig. 4.42 Inferior (A) and superior (B) aspects of the pelvis showing the relationship of the muscles of the pelvic floor in females.

The pubococcygeal part arises anterior to the obturator canal. The most anterior fibres pass posteriorly around either the prostate (males) or vagina (females) to the perineal body: more posterior fibres pass to the prostate or vagina looping around the superior part of the anal canal pulling the anorectal junction towards the symphysis pubis. Some of these latter fibres fuse with the longitudinal muscle of the rectum and, via a series of fibroelastic slips, pass through the external anal sphincter to attach to the skin around the anus. The most posterior fibres of pubococcygeus attach to the anococcygeal body and sides of the coccyx.

Iliococcygeus arises from the fascia over obturator internus, attaching to the anococcygeal body and sides of the coccyx: on its deep surface it is partly overlapped by the posterior part of pubococcygeus.

Innervation

Levator ani has a dual nerve supply: from S3 and S4, and by a branch from the perineal branch of the pudendal nerve (root value S4), which enters the muscle on its perineal surface.

Action

Levator ani, with coccygeus, plays an important role in supporting the pelvic viscera, particularly in females: it is constantly active.

Contraction of both levator ani has a constricting effect on openings in the pelvic floor, either reflexly or voluntarily. For example, when intra-abdominal pressure is raised as in coughing, reflex contraction of levator ani closes the urethra and anus to prevent unwanted micturition or defecation. This action becomes voluntary when the muscles supplementing the appropriate sphincters contract to resist an inconvenient urge to micturate or defecate.

In females, the position of levator ani surrounding the vagina is important in supporting the uterus. Here, the muscle may become excessively stretched during childbirth or surgically traumatised by episiotomy. This stretching may adversely affect the action of levator ani on the anus and, more commonly the urethra, leading to stress incontinence, resulting in leakage of urine and possibly faeces whenever intra-abdominal pressure is raised. Active exercises are necessary to regain normal muscle tone: pelvic floor exercises are taught to restore normal function. Unfortunately, these exercises can be difficult to teach, and electrical stimulation may be necessary. It is possible to test and assess the power of contraction of levator ani by inserting the compressible bulb of a perineometer into the vagina. Failing this, the strength of contraction can be felt against a gloved finger placed in the vagina.

In males, the problems of stress incontinence are much less common, but are sometimes seen following prostatectomy. Pelvic floor exercises are again necessary to restore the tone of levator ani.

Coccygeus

Posterior to and in the same plane as levator ani (Fig. 4.42), coccygeus is a flat triangular sheet of muscle and fibrous tissue stretching from the spine of the ischium to the margin of the coccyx and lower two segments of the sacrum. The more fibrous gluteal surface forms the sacrospinous ligament.

Innervation

By the ventral rami of S4. Skin covering the inferior surface of the muscles is supplied by the anterior primary rami of S3 and S4.

Action

Forming the posterior part of the pelvic floor, coccygeus assists levator ani in its role in supporting the pelvic viscera and maintaining intra-abdominal pressure. It also pulls the coccyx anteriorly after it has been pushed posteriorly during defecation or parturition.

SECTION SUMMARY

Typical Lumbar Vertebra
- Large kidney-shaped body
- Short strong pedicles arising from superior half of body
- Horizontally projecting spinous process with thick posterior border
- Triangular vertebral canal
- Thin short transverse process
- Vertically projecting articular processes; superior transversely concave, facing medially; inferior transversely convex, facing laterally

Typical Thoracic Vertebra
- Heart-shaped bodies with demifacets for articulation with head of corresponding rib and rib below
- Short pedicles arising from superior half of body
- Small, almost circular vertebral canal
- Long inferiorly pointing spinous process
- Overlapping laminae between vertebrae
- Long, thick, rounded transverse processes with facet for articulation with tubercle of corresponding rib

SECTION SUMMARY—CONT'D

- Vertically projecting flat articular processes; superior facing posteriorly; inferior facing anteriorly

Joints Between Vertebral Bodies

Type	Secondary cartilaginous-symphysis
Articular surfaces	Adjacent vertebral bodies
Intervertebral disc	Consists of three integrated tissues: nucleus pulposus, annulus fibrosus and cartilage end plate
Ligaments	Anterior and posterior longitudinal

Joints Between Vertebral Arches (Zygapophyseal Joints)

Type	Plane synovial joint
Articular surfaces	Facets on superior and inferior articular processes
Capsule	Thin fibrous capsule surrounds joint attaching to articular margins
Ligaments	Ligamentum flavum; supraspinous, interspinous and intertransverse
Stability	Provided by interaction between intervertebral disc and associated ligaments; shape of facet joints
Movements	Lumbar region: 55 degree flexion and 30 degree extension 20-30 degree lateral flexion/bending to each side Minimal axial rotation Thoracic region: 50-70 degree combined flexion/extension 20-25 degree lateral flexion/bending to each side 35 degree axial rotation to each side

Movements of the Trunk

Movements of the trunk include those of the thoracic and lumbar spine. Many of the muscles are involved in producing several different movements which are given below.

Movement	Muscles (Root Value of Nerve Supply)
Flexion	Rectus abdominis (T6/7–T12) External oblique (T7–T12) Internal oblique (T7–T12 and L1) Psoas major (L1–L3 and L(4)) Psoas minor (L1)
Extension	Quadratus lumborum (T12 and L1–L4) Multifidus (segmental by dorsal rami) Semispinalis (segmental by dorsal rami) Erector spinae (segmental by dorsal rami)
Lateral flexion	Quadratus lumborum (T12 and L1–L4) Intertransversarii (cervical and lateral lumbar by ventral rami: medial lumbar by dorsal rami) External oblique (T7–T12) Internal oblique (T7–T12 and L1) Rectus abdominis (T6/7–T12) Multifidus (segmental by dorsal rami)
Rotation	Internal oblique (T7–T12 and L1) External oblique (T7–T12) Multifidus (segmental by dorsal rami) Rotatores (segmental by dorsal rami) Semispinalis (segmental by dorsal rami)

- In movements such as flexion and extension, the muscles on both sides of the trunk work. In lateral flexion/bending, muscles on one side work and, in rotation, it is a combination of some muscles from both sides.
- Many of the muscles (particularly the abdominals) work to raise intra-abdominal pressure for expulsive acts where the diaphragm is fixed, and also forced expiration where the diaphragm moves superiorly.

SELF-ASSESSMENT QUESTIONS

1. What is the innervation of erector spinae?
2. What feature(s) disstinguish(es) a thoracic vertebra?
3. Which structure is responsible for producing the curvatures of the vertebral column in adults?
4. In which direction do the superior articular processes in the thoracic region face?
5. In the lumbar region, how many layers of thoracolumbar fascia are there?
6. What are the components of the neural arch?
7. Which muscles are responsible for flexing the trunk?
8. What are the attachments of internal oblique?
9. What is the nerve supply to quadratus lumborum?
10. What are the attachments of multifidus?
11. Which muscles are enclosed by the thoracolumbar fascia?
12. What and where is the inguinal canal?
13. What is the action of the interspinales?
14. How much of the length of the vertebral column is contributed to by the intervertebral discs?
15. In the lumbar region, what is the average thickness of intervertebral discs?
16. What is the organisation of the intervertebral disc?
17. What are the attachments of the posterior longitudinal ligament?
18. What type of joint is the zygapophyseal joint?
19. What are the attachments of the ligamentum flavum?
20. What movements are possible in the lumbar region?
21. What is the most mobile segment of the trunk?
22. Which arteries supply the vertebral column?
23. What is the action of multifidus?
24. What are the named columns of erector spinae?
25. Are inguinal herniae more common in males or females?
26. Which abdominal oblique muscle does not have an attachment to the thoracolumbar fascia?
27. What are the three named parts of semispinalis?
28. Give three functions of the vertebral column.
29. How many free vertebrae are there?
30. What shape are the lumbar spinous processes?
31. What shape are the bodies of thoracic vertebrae?
32. Above the level of the umbilicus, how is the rectus sheath formed?
33. What is the nerve supply of the muscles of the pelvic floor?
34. What type of joint is between adjacent vertebral bodies?
35. Which part of the intervertebral disc is hydrophilic?
36. In the thoracic region, do the zygapophyseal joints lie anterior or posterior to the transverse processes?
37. What contributes to the inherent stability of the vertebral column?
38. A lateral curvature of the vertebral column is known as what?
39. Which region of the trunk permits the greatest range of flexion?
40. Which region of the trunk permits the greatest range of lateral flexion?

SIMPLE ACTIVITIES OF THE TRUNK

As in previous sections, this short description is included to show how different muscle groups cooperate in producing a desired movement. The sequence of movements involved, together with the joints involved and muscles are described.

A Sit-Up
Starting Position
The individual is lying on their back.

Sequence of Movements. The thoracolumbar spine is flexed by rectus abdominis and all four abdominal oblique muscles, each working concentrically. Once the trunk has been raised several centimetres from the ground, a position is reached where psoas major can work: pulling on the lumbar spine it increases flexion of the lumbar spine and hips. As this occurs, there is a tendency for psoas to lift the legs off the floor unless the feet are fixed. This is opposed by synergic activity in the hamstrings which holds the legs against the floor, but which unfortunately also tends to flex the knees. This latter action is opposed by the quadriceps which keeps the knees extended.

As the body returns to its lying position from sitting, involving extension of the hips and trunk, these same muscles now work eccentrically to control the downward movement which is produced by gravity. If the sit-up is performed with the hands behind the neck, and rotation of the trunk is also included (so that the right elbow moves to the left knee) then the left internal and right external oblique muscles will be working strongly to bring about the rotation.

Bending Down to Touch Toes and Straightening up Again

Starting Position

The individual starts in the anatomical position.

Sequence of Movements

The thoracolumbar spine and hip joints are both flexed. From the starting position, a brief concentric contraction of the trunk and hip flexors moves the trunk forwards, gravity then takes over, being the force producing the movement. Following this, flexion of the trunk is controlled by the eccentric contraction of erector spinae and quadratus lumborum, and that of the hip by eccentric contraction of gluteus maximus and the hamstrings.

Returning to the erect position, in which the trunk and hips are extended, is produced by concentric contraction of these same muscles.

Sideways Flexion/Bending

Starting Position

The individual starts by standing in full lateral flexion/bending to the left.

Sequence of Movements

The trunk is moved from full lateral flexion/bending to the erect position by concentric contraction of the following muscles on the right side of the body: external and internal oblique, rectus abdominis, quadratus lumborum and erector spinae. Once the trunk has moved past the vertical into right lateral flexion/bending, gravity continues the movement. Corresponding muscles on the left, working eccentrically, now take over to control the movement.

Increasing and Decreasing Lumbar Lordosis

Starting Position

The individual starts by standing with a deep lumbar lordosis.

Sequence of Movements

The lumbar spine is moved from its extended position to a more neutral position by rotation of the pelvis. The anterior part of the pelvis is raised by concentric contraction of rectus abdominis, while at the same time the posterior part is pulled inferiorly by the hamstrings and gluteus maximus, also working concentrically. The pelvis is returned to its neutral position by concentric contraction of erector

spinae and quadratus lumborum. If contraction of these muscles continues, then the lordosis may be increased as the posterior part of the pelvis becomes raised.

THORAX

LEARNING OUTCOMES

By the end of the section, you should be able to:
1. Identify, palpate and examine thoracic vertebrae, ribs and the sternum
2. Describe the joints of the thorax
3. Describe and explain movement of the thorax during inspiration and expiration
4. Describe the muscles associated with the thorax and give their attachments, action and innervation
5. Examine and assess movements of the thorax
6. Appreciate the influence of pathology and/or trauma on the function of the thorax

INTRODUCTION

The thorax is a bony and muscular structure (Fig. 4.43) surrounding, protecting and supporting the heart and lungs, amongst other structures. It is egg-shaped, with the narrower end superior towards the neck and the wider end inferior. However, the superior and inferior parts of the thoracic cage are cut off obliquely so that the superior opening (thoracic inlet) slopes anteroinferiorly at ~45 degrees, while the inferior opening (thoracic outlet) slopes posteroinferiorly.

The thoracic inlet is bounded by the anterior surface of the body of the first thoracic vertebra posteriorly, medial border of the first rib and its costal cartilage on each side, and the superior surface of the manubrium sterni anteriorly. Through this opening, the oesophagus and trachea pass, as well as the vessels and nerves which enter or leave the thorax: in the lateral part of the inlet is the apex of the lung, supported and covered by the suprapleural membrane. The thoracic outlet is much larger, bound by the anterior surface of the body of the 12th thoracic vertebra posteriorly, the 12th and anterior half of the 11th rib on either side, together with the 6th–10th costal cartilages and xiphisternal junction anteriorly. The diaphragm covers most of the outlet but has in it openings for the passage of the aorta, oesophagus and inferior vena cava: other smaller structures also pierce the diaphragm to pass between the thorax and abdomen.

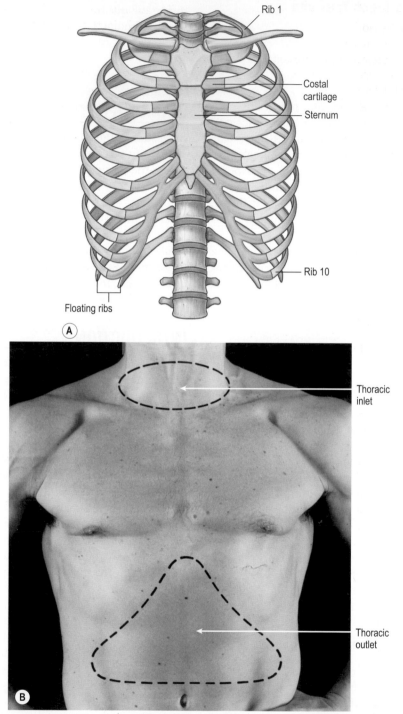

Rib 1

Costal
cartilage

Sternum

Rib 10

Floating ribs

(A)

(B)

Thoracic
inlet

Thoracic
outlet

Fig. 4.43 (A) Anterior aspect of the thoracic cage; (B) positions of the thoracic inlet and outlet superimposed on the anterior aspect of the chest and upper abdomen in a living subject.

The bony components of the thoracic cage are the 12 thoracic vertebrae posteriorly, 12 pairs of ribs laterally and sternum anteriorly. In general, the ribs pass from posterior to anterior, connecting the thoracic part of the vertebral column to the sternum: as the ribs pass forwards they also slope inferiorly so that the anterior end of the rib is at a lower level than its posterior part. The space between adjacent ribs (intercostal space) is filled by muscles, among which are found the intercostal vessels and nerves. The sixth intercostal space is probably the longest, with those above and below gradually decreasing in length: upper spaces are wider than lower ones, which also tend to be narrower posteriorly. The articulation of these bony parts is such that the thorax is flattened anteroposteriorly so that its transverse diameter is larger than its anteroposterior diameter. In children, the anteroposterior and transverse diameters are more or less equal because the ribs pass more horizontally around the thorax.

THORACIC VERTEBRAE

Details of the thoracic vertebrae can be found on page 501.

RIBS

Long flat bones which ossify from a cartilage model, part of which persists anteriorly as the costal cartilage of the rib. The costal cartilage of the first rib is very short and often ossified, particularly later in life, while the remainder gradually increase in length from superior to inferior, with the 10th costal cartilage being the longest. The costal cartilages of the upper seven ribs articulate directly with the sternum, while the 8th, 9th and 10th do so via the costal cartilage above. The 11th and 12th ribs merely have cartilage caps anteriorly and end within the abdominal wall musculature: they are often referred to as floating ribs. Each rib has a head, neck, angle and shaft. Some ribs (1st, 10th, 11th and 12th) exhibit certain features which distinguish them from the rest: the remainder are typical ribs.

Typical Rib

Each rib (Fig. 4.44) has an enlarged head at its posterior end, on which are two flattened articular facets with an intervening ridge. The facets articulate with the superior border of the body of its own vertebra and the inferior border of the body of the vertebra above.

The head is joined to the shaft by a short flattened neck, with superior and inferior borders, and anterior and posterior surfaces. The neck continues laterally as the shaft, marked at the junction on its posterior aspect by the tubercle of the rib, which has a small oval articular facet on its medial part: it is roughened laterally. The shaft is flattened having smooth medial and lateral surfaces, and rounded superior and sharp inferior borders. The inferior border forms the lateral margin of the subcostal groove, the medial margin being higher on the medial surface of the rib about a third of the way up. Approximately 3 cm lateral to the tubercle the shaft turns posteromedially, giving it a twisted appearance (angle of the rib). Only the second rib does not show twisting of the shaft, in addition to which its lateral surface faces superolaterally. The anterior end of the rib widens and ends as a roughened hollow being continuous with its costal cartilage.

First Rib

Short and sharply curved, the first rib is C-shaped (Fig. 4.45): the head has a single facet for articulation with the body of the first thoracic vertebra. Joining the head to the shaft is a relatively long narrow neck. The tubercle of the rib is large and situated on the lateral border; from here, the rib slopes anteroinferiorly. The shaft has superior and inferior surfaces, and medial and thickened lateral borders: it is not angled and remains broad throughout its length. Its inferior surface has a shallow subcostal groove running longitudinally, while the superior surface has two shallow transverse grooves on either side of the scalene tubercle projecting from the medial border. The anterior groove transmits the subclavian vein and the posterior groove the subclavian artery and first thoracic nerve: the two vessels are separated by scalenus anterior attaching to the scalene tubercle. Anteriorly, it articulates with the manubrium sterni by its costal cartilage.

10th Rib

Showing many of the features of a typical rib, being long with a definite angle: the 10th rib has, however, only one facet on the head for articulation with the body of the 10th thoracic vertebra.

11th Rib

Approximately half the length of the 10th rib, the 11th rib also possesses a single facet on its head

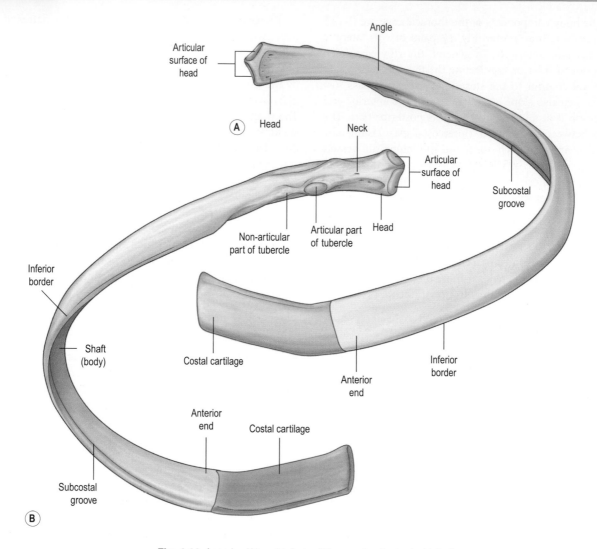

Fig. 4.44 Anterior (A) and inferior (B) aspects of a typical left rib.

for articulation with its corresponding vertebral body. It does not, however, have an articular facet on its tubercle for articulation with the transverse process.

12th Rib

Very short and dagger-like in appearance: the head of the 12th rib has one complete articular facet for articulation with the body of the 12th thoracic vertebra. There is no tubercle or articular surface for articulation with the transverse process, angle or subcostal groove: its anterior end is tapered in contrast to the widening of the other ribs.

Ossification

A primary ossification centre appears near the angle of the rib at 6 weeks *in utero*. In the second to sixth ribs, secondary centres appear in the head and each part of the tubercle: the 11th and 12th ribs only have a secondary centre in the head. All secondary centres appear at puberty, fusing with the remainder of the bone by the age of 25.

Costal Cartilages

The hyaline costal cartilages are continuous with their respective ribs, connecting them either directly (ribs 1–7) or indirectly (ribs 8–10) to the sternum. The perichondrium

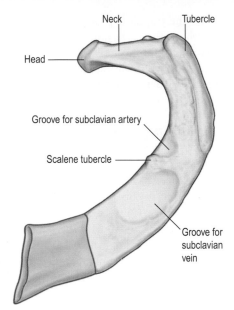

Fig. 4.45 Superior surface of the left first rib.

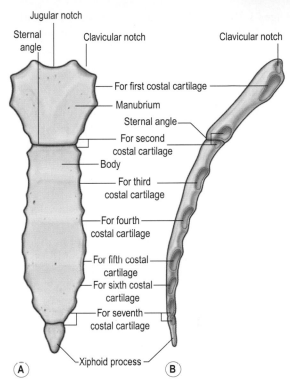

Fig. 4.46 Anterior (A) and lateral (B) aspects of the sternum.

of the cartilage is continuous with that of the rib: it is possible to rupture the cartilage within the perichondrium without obvious displacement of the cartilage.

STERNUM

Elongated flat bone (Fig. 4.46) situated in the midline of the anterior chest wall, the sternum extends from the root of the neck to the abdominal wall. It consists of three parts: the manubrium superiorly, the large body and the small irregular xiphoid process inferiorly. All three parts have anterior and posterior surfaces, and lateral, superior and inferior borders: adjacent parts articulate by secondary cartilaginous joints.

The manubrium is the widest part of the sternum, roughened on its anterior surface and smooth posteriorly. On its superior border is the jugular (suprasternal) notch, with smaller clavicular notches on either side for articulation with the clavicles. Below the clavicular notch on the lateral border is a roughened area for articulation with the first rib costal cartilage and, lower down, a demifacet for the second rib costal cartilage. The oval inferior surface is roughened for the attachment of the fibrocartilaginous disc of the manubriosternal joint.

The body is composed of four fused segments (sternebrae): again, it is roughened on its anterior surface and smooth posteriorly. It does not lie directly in line with the manubrium but rather forms an obtuse angle of 160 degrees which can be palpated and, as such, forms a useful landmark even in obese individuals. The superior surface receives the fibrocartilaginous disc, while the lateral borders show articular facets for the costal cartilages of the second to seventh ribs: the second and seventh facets are demifacets, while those between are full facets. Inferiorly, the body is continuous with the irregularly shaped xiphoid process at the secondary cartilaginous xiphisternal joint. The xiphoid process may be perforated or bifid; nevertheless, it is thinner than the body, being flush with its posterior surface.

The jugular notch is level with the inferior border of the body of the second thoracic vertebra, the sternal angle with the inferior border of the body of the fourth and xiphisternal junction with the ninth thoracic vertebra.

Ossification

Primary ossification centres appear in the manubrium during the fifth month *in utero*, and then in the four sternebrae in the sixth, seventh, eighth and ninth months *in utero* from superior to inferior. They fuse in sequence from inferior to superior in childhood, at puberty and at age 21; the manubrium does not usually fuse with the body until old age. Ossification of the xiphoid process can begin any time after age 3; however, it does not fuse with the body until middle age.

Palpation

With the individual seated, a deep hollow can be seen at the base of neck, the inferior margin is the jugular (suprasternal) notch, either side of which the medial ends of the clavicle can be palpated. Following the clavicle laterally, both its anterior and superior convex surfaces can be easily distinguished: further laterally, the concave anterior border can be traced to the lateral end of the bone. Beyond this, the anterior, lateral and posterior borders and superior surface of the acromion process can be palpated.

Approximately 2 cm below the suprasternal notch, a ridge of bone can be felt beyond which the sternum changes direction: this is the sternal angle at the level of the manubriosternal joint. On either side, the costal cartilage of the second rib can be palpated, with the space below the second rib and its costal cartilage being the second intercostal space.

At the inferior end of the sternum, the pointed xiphoid process can be identified with the costal cartilages of the 7th–10th ribs running laterally away from it. At the junction of the ninth costal cartilage is a marked angle on the anterior rim of the rib cage: this is level with the tip of the 12th rib and spinous process of the first lumbar vertebra posteriorly, and pylorus of the stomach internally. A transverse plane at this level is the transpyloric plane. The lateral border of rectus abdominis also crosses the costal margin at this level; at this junction on the right side, the fundus of the gall bladder may be palpated.

The upper two ribs are difficult to palpate: the first is almost completely covered by the clavicle anteriorly and thick muscle posteriorly. However, with deep pressure applied to the anteromedial part of the supraclavicular fossa, the superior surface of the first rib can be identified. It should be remembered that this manoeuvre may be painful because pressure is put on the structures running over the rib at this point.

The second rib is easily identifiable at the sternal angle but soon becomes lost in thick muscle as it passes posteriorly. The third to eighth ribs are easily identified throughout most of their length, except that posteriorly they are covered to a variable extent by the scapula. Posterolaterally, the angles of the ribs are quite clear, particularly if the scapula is protracted (p. 69), lateral to the paravertebral gutter. The anterior half of the 11th rib is quite clear, running anteriorly to the mid-axillary line, while the tip of the 12th rib can be palpated at the level of the transpyloric plane just beyond the bulk of the long back muscles.

JOINTS OF THE THORAX

Introduction

The bony components of the thorax articulate with one another in such a way to provide a rigid, yet slightly mobile thoracic cage (Fig. 4.47). Posteriorly, adjacent thoracic vertebrae articulate with one another by both secondary cartilaginous and synovial joints. Anteriorly, the various parts of the sternum are joined by secondary cartilaginous joints, while laterally, each rib is joined to its costal cartilage by a primary cartilaginous joint. However, it is the articulation of the rib with the vertebral column posteriorly and the costal cartilage with the sternum anteriorly, either directly or indirectly, which provides the mobility necessary during respiration. By the action of muscles, the ribs move to change both the anteroposterior and transverse diameters of the thorax. The precise nature of rib movement differs in different regions of the thorax, being determined by the shape of the articulating surfaces, as well as their anterior articulations.

The articulations within a rib (costochondral joint) and the sternum (manubriosternal and xiphisternal joints) are considered before the articulations of the rib with the vertebrae and sternum.

Costochondral Joints

Primary cartilaginous joint between the anterior roughened end of a rib and lateral end of the costal cartilage (Fig. 4.47A), it is surrounded by perichondrium continuous with that of the rib. Movement at these joints is confined to a slight bending of the cartilage at the junction with the rib: the cartilage, however, may undergo some twisting during the movement of the rib.

The costochondral joints can be stressed by applying continuous pressure to the anterior aspect of the chest wall, as in leaning against a table whilst sitting or against a fence when standing. Continued stress often results in the joint becoming extremely painful and possibly swollen (Tietze syndrome/chondritis). Depending on its location, the pain may be misdiagnosed as a cardiac problem, causing the individual further unnecessary stress.

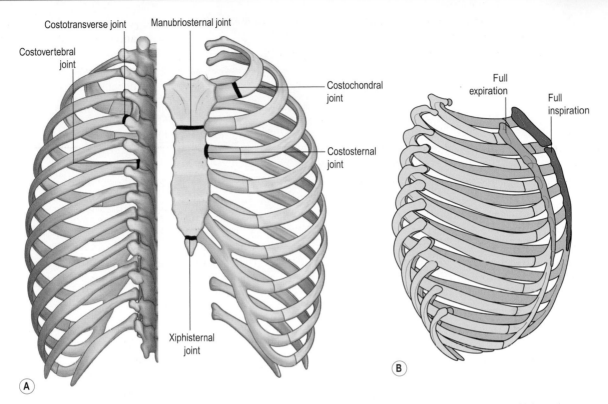

Fig. 4.47 (A) Posterior and anterior views of the thoracic cage showing the joints of the thorax; (B) lateral aspect of the thorax showing movements of the sternum during respiration.

Sternal Joints
Manubriosternal Joint

Secondary cartilaginous joint between the inferior surface of the manubrium and superior surface of the body of the sternum (Fig. 4.47A). The opposing surfaces of the two bones are covered with a thin layer of hyaline cartilage, between which is a fibrocartilaginous disc, often hollow at its centre. The joint is strengthened anteriorly and posteriorly by longitudinal fibrous bands and the adjacent sternocostal ligaments. Occasionally, the joint resembles a primary cartilaginous joint: in later life it may begin to ossify.

It permits a small amount of movement (~7 degrees): during inspiration, there is a decrease in the obtuse angle between the manubrium and body of the sternum. There is also a very slight shift of the body superiorly (Fig. 4.47B), which is noticeable when pressure is applied to the anterior aspect of the chest.

Xiphisternal Joint

The xiphoid process is an irregularly shaped piece of cartilage joined to the body of the sternum by a secondary cartilaginous joint, supported all around by a fibrous capsule. Late in life the xiphoid process and, with it, the xiphisternal joint ossify. While it remains cartilaginous, there is a certain amount of flexibility of the xiphoid process at the joint.

ARTICULATIONS OF THE RIBS AND THORACIC VERTEBRAE

Posteriorly, the typical ribs articulate with the sides of the bodies of two adjacent vertebrae (costovertebral joints) and with the transverse process of its corresponding vertebra (costotransverse joint): the 1st, 10th, 11th and 12th ribs articulate with only one vertebra.

COSTOVERTEBRAL JOINTS

Articular Surfaces

Between the convex articular facets on the head of the rib and a large concave demifacet on the superior border of the corresponding vertebra, and a smaller demifacet on the inferior border of the vertebra above (Fig. 4.48A and B). The crest on the head of the rib articulates with a slightly cupped depression on the posterolateral aspect of the intervening intervertebral disc. The joint surfaces are covered with hyaline cartilage.

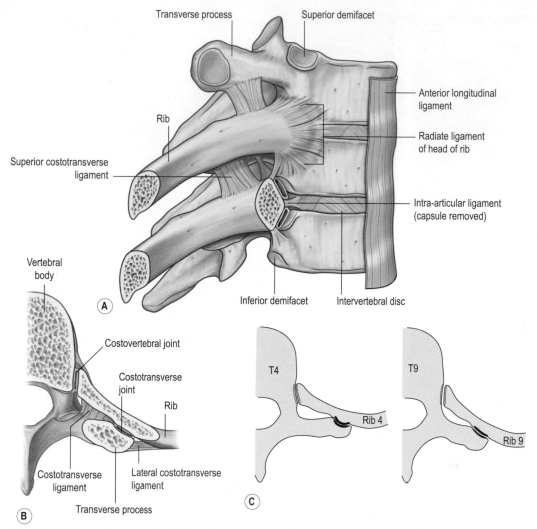

Fig. 4.48 (A) Lateral aspect of mid-thoracic vertebrae and their associated ribs showing the costovertebral joint and its associated ligaments; (B) horizontal section showing the costovertebral and costotransverse joints; (C) shape of the costotransverse joint surfaces at different vertebral levels.

Joint Capsule

A loose fibrous capsule surrounds the joint: anteriorly it is thickened forming the radiate ligament of the head of the rib (Fig. 4.48A), while posteriorly it blends with, and is reinforced by, the adjacent denticulation of the posterior longitudinal ligament. An intra-articular ligament completely divides the joint space, each part of which is lined by synovial membrane.

Ligaments
Intra-Articular Ligament

Short thick band passing from the crest of the head of the rib to the intervertebral disc: it divides the joint cavity into two parts (Fig. 4.48A).

Radiate Ligament of the Head of the Rib

Passing medially from the anterior aspect of the rib head deep to the lateral part of the anterior longitudinal ligament, its three bands of fibres radiate superiorly to the body of the vertebra above, horizontally to the anterior aspect of the intervertebral disc and inferiorly to the body of the vertebra below (Fig. 4.48A).

The 1st, 10th, 11th and 12th ribs articulate with their own vertebrae only. Consequently, there is a single joint cavity, no intra-articular ligament and a poorly developed radiate ligament.

COSTOTRANSVERSE JOINTS

Only present between the tubercles of the upper 10 ribs and transverse processes of their corresponding vertebrae (Fig. 4.48B).

Articular Surfaces

Between the articular facet on the anterior aspect of the transverse process, near its tip, and an oval facet on the posteromedial aspect of the tubercle of the rib: the shape of the joint surfaces changes from superior to inferior (Fig. 4.48C). In upper costotransverse joints the facet on the rib tubercle is convex and that on the transverse process is reciprocally concave; however, this arrangement differs inferiorly, with the facets on the rib and transverse process becoming flatter. This change in shape is one of the factors responsible for the different movements of the upper and lower ribs during respiration (p. 556).

Joint Capsule

A thin fibrous capsule completely surrounds the joint, strengthened posterolaterally by the lateral costotransverse ligament, which, although in contact with the capsule, does not fuse with it.

Ligaments

Lateral Costotransverse Ligament

Stout band passing between the tip of the transverse process, beyond the articular facet and roughened lateral part of the costal tubercle (Fig. 4.48B).

Costotransverse Ligament

Short fibres binding the rib to the transverse process, passing from the posterior aspect of the neck of the rib to the anterior aspect of the transverse process medial to the facet (Fig. 4.48B).

Superior Costotransverse Ligament

An anterior band of fibres passing from the rib superolaterally, and a posterior band passing superomedially (Fig. 4.48A). The bands attach to the inferior surface of the transverse process of the vertebra above, being separated by the external intercostal muscle. The fibres of the anterior band blend laterally with the internal intercostal membrane.

Movements

Movements at the costovertebral and costotransverse joints are dealt with together. Although each movement is small, because of the length of the rib, it is considerably magnified anteriorly. As the rib is raised or lowered, there is a twisting and gliding movement at the costovertebral joints, limited by the radiate and intra-articular ligaments.

At the same time there is movement at the costotransverse joint: in lower joints there is gliding and rotation of one plane surface against another; superiorly, because of the curved nature of the articular surfaces, the movement tends to be one of rotation only.

ARTICULATIONS OF THE COSTAL CARTILAGES AND STERNUM

Anteriorly, the costal cartilages articulate directly with the sternum by costosternal joints or with each other by interchondral joints: the 11th and 12th do not articulate with their corresponding transverse process posteriorly or with the preceding costal cartilage anteriorly.

Sternocostal Joints

Between the medial end of the costal cartilage of the first to seventh ribs and sternum (Fig. 4.49): that between the first costal cartilage and sternum is a primary cartilaginous joint (synchondrosis). The cartilage attaches to the socket on the superior part of the lateral border of the manubrium, preventing any appreciable movement, an important factor in respiration. The remaining joints are synovial, surrounded by a fibrous capsule supported anteriorly and posteriorly by the radiate ligaments. The joint cavity for the second rib is usually divided into two by an intra-articular ligament. With increasing age, however, these cavities, except for that of the second costal cartilage, become obliterated.

The anterior radiate ligament passes from the medial end of the costal cartilage over the joint to the anterior aspect of the sternum: the superior fibres pass superomedially, middle fibres horizontally and inferior fibres inferomedially (Fig. 4.49). The fibres interlace with those from the joints above and below and from the opposite side, forming a criss-cross feltwork covering the anterior aspect of the sternum: this feltwork fuses with tendinous fibres of pectoralis major. The posterior radiate ligament has a similar arrangement over the posterior aspect of the sternum.

The second sternocostal joint is similar to those above except that the anterior and posterior radiate ligaments attach superiorly to the manubrium, horizontally to the fibrocartilaginous pad between the manubrium and body and inferiorly to the body (Fig. 4.49). The intra-articular ligament of the joint restricts its movement.

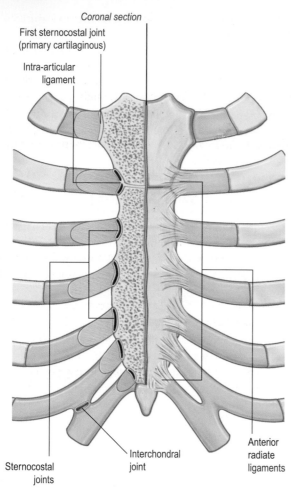

Coronal section

First sternocostal joint
(primary cartilaginous)

Intra-articular
ligament

Sternocostal
joints

Interchondral
joint

Anterior
radiate
ligaments

Fig. 4.49 Anterior aspect of the sternum and associated costal cartilages showing the sternocostal and interchondral joints.

These synovial joints allow the medial end of the cartilages to glide superiorly and inferiorly in the sockets on the lateral border of the sternum when the rib is raised and lowered during respiration.

Interchondral Joints

Between the tips of the costal cartilages of the 8th, 9th and 10th ribs and the inferior border of the cartilage above (Fig. 4.49): the 8th and 9th joints are synovial and the 10th is more like a fibrous joint. Small synovial joints are also formed between the adjacent margins of the fifth to ninth costal cartilages.

All the synovial joints are surrounded by fibrous capsules, and strengthened anteriorly and posteriorly by oblique ligaments: they allow a slight gliding movement adding to the general mobility of the region. The

interchondral joints can be strained under similar circumstances as the costochondral joints, leading to pain radiating from the area of the costal cartilage.

MOVEMENTS OF THE THORACIC CAGE

During respiration, the volume of the thorax changes by movement of the diaphragm, ribs and sternum: the vertical, transverse and anteroposterior diameters of the thorax increase and decrease during inspiration and expiration, respectively. Each rib and its costal cartilage can be considered as a lever which moves up and down, with the nature of the movement depending on several factors including its length and whether it articulates directly with the sternum or not. Ribs that articulate with the sternum gradually increase in length from superior to inferior, with their anterior ends lying at a lower level than the posterior ends (Fig. 4.50A). Although the eighth and ninth ribs are shorter, the nature of their attachment to the costal margin means that the transverse diameter of the thorax continues to increase as far as the ninth rib, after which it decreases.

The axis about which the rib moves runs posterolaterally along its neck through the costovertebral and costotransverse joints (Fig. 4.50B): it follows the inclination of the transverse processes of the vertebrae. However, the inclination of the transverse processes is less oblique in upper thoracic vertebrae, gradually increasing as the thoracic vertebral column is descended. Therefore, although the axis of movement relative to each rib remains unchanged, the resultant movement of the upper and lower ribs differs.

Movement of the upper ribs (second to fifth) about an axis along their necks raises their anterior ends, and with them, the body of the sternum. Because the first costal cartilage is firmly attached to the manubrium, as well as the first rib being much shorter, movement of its anterior end is slight, the longer second to fifth ribs lift the body of the sternum anterosuperiorly, resulting in bending of the manubriosternal joint (Fig. 4.47B). In this way, the anteroposterior diameter of the thorax increases (Fig. 4.50B). There is little lateral movement of these ribs except perhaps during the terminal part of a deep inspiration, because the axis of movement is less oblique than lower down. The movement has been likened to that of the handle of a pump when drawing water from a well, often being referred to as the *pump-handle* movement.

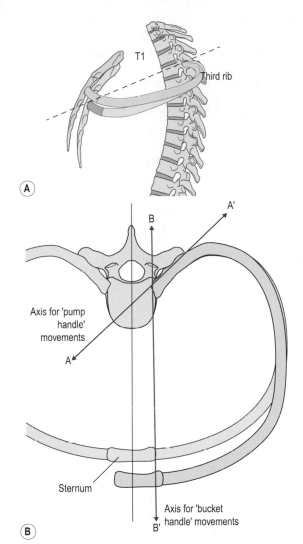

T1

Third rib

(A)

A'

B

Axis for 'pump handle' movements

A

Sternum

Axis for 'bucket handle' movements

B'

(B)

Fig. 4.50 (A) Relationship between the anterior and posterior ends of a rib; (B) horizontal section showing the axes about which the ribs move during respiration.

Movement of the 8th–10th ribs results in a superolateral movement of their anterior ends, resulting in a widening of the infrasternal angle and a consequent increase in the transverse diameter of the thorax (Fig. 4.50B). Because the shape of the costotransverse joints of these lower ribs is flat, there is both rotation and gliding of one bone against the other (Fig. 4.48C). Therefore it appears that the axis of movement of the ribs passes through the costovertebral and sternocostal or interchondral joints (Fig. 4.50B). The superolateral movement of the shaft of the rib has been likened to raising the handle from the

side of a bucket, often being referred to as the *bucket-handle* movement.

The intermediate sixth and seventh ribs show both pump-handle and bucket-handle types of movement. The 11th and 12th ribs are not attached anteriorly and thus have very little influence on changing the transverse diameter of the thorax. However, they do give attachment to some of the inferior fibres of the diaphragm and, with the aid of quadratus lumborum, provide a firm attachment for the diaphragm.

During expiration, the reverse movements of the ribs and sternum occur, with a decrease in both the anteroposterior and transverse thoracic diameters.

As well as these respiratory movements, the ribs also move passively, following changes in the thoracic part of the vertebral column. Flexion causes the ribs to move closer together, extension causes them to move further apart, lateral flexion/bending causes those on the concave side to come together and those on the convex side to separate, while rotation causes a slight relative horizontal displacement of one rib with respect to its neighbour.

MUSCLES PRODUCING INSPIRATION

Diaphragm
Intercostal muscles
Levatores costarum
Serratus posterior superior

In extreme respiratory distress, other muscles, whose primary actions are described elsewhere, may assist in increasing thoracic dimensions in an attempt to draw more air into the lungs. These muscles are often referred to as accessory muscles of respiration (serratus anterior, p. 74; sternomastoid, p. 644; the scalenes, p. 647; subclavius, p. 78; pectoralis minor, p. 75; and pectoralis major, p. 102). However, to use these muscles effectively, their attachment to the ribs and sternum must be free to move, with their other attachment being the fixed point.

Diaphragm

Musculotendinous sheet (Fig. 4.51) separating the thoracic and abdominal cavities, it consists of muscle fibres attached around the thoracic outlet, which converge to a central trefoil-shaped tendon. The lumbar part of the diaphragm arises in part from two crura which attach to the anterolateral aspects of the bodies of the lumbar vertebrae: the larger right crus from the bodies and

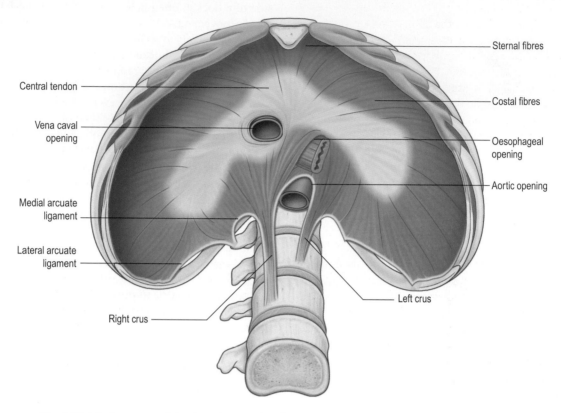

Fig. 4.51 Inferior aspect of the thoracic cage showing the position and attachments of the diaphragm.

intervening discs of L1–L3 and smaller left crus from the bodies and disc of L1 and L2. The aorta enters the abdomen behind the two crura as they cross one another anterior to the body of T12: at this point the crura are connected by a tendinous band (median arcuate ligament). Fibres of the right crus generally pass towards the left, separating to surround the oesophagus before attaching to the central tendon: fibres of the left crus may also pass behind the oesophageal opening, separating it from the aortic opening. From near the oesophageal opening, the suspensory ligament of the duodenum arises from the right crus to attach to the terminal part of the duodenum.

The remainder of the lumbar part of the diaphragm arises from the medial and lateral arcuate ligaments immediately lateral to the crura. The medial arcuate ligament is a thickening of the fascia covering psoas major: it runs from the side of the body of L2 to the transverse process of L1. The lateral arcuate ligament is a thickening of the anterior layer of the thoracolumbar fascia covering

quadratus lumborum: it passes from the transverse process of L1 to the tip of the 12th rib. Lateral to the arcuate ligaments, the costal part of the diaphragm arises from the deep surface of the lower six ribs and their costal cartilages, interdigitating with transversus abdominis, to attach to the anterolateral part of the central tendon.

The most anterior (sternal) part of the diaphragm arises by two slips from the posterior surface of the xiphoid process of the sternum.

All muscle fibres arch superomedially to their attachment to the central tendon situated towards the anterior part of the muscle: the short anterior fibres and longer posterior fibres give the appearance of an inverted letter J when viewed from the side. When viewed anteriorly, two small domes (cupolae) on either side of the central tendon can be seen, that on the right being at a slightly higher level than the left: the central part lies opposite the xiphisternal joint.

The superior surface of the diaphragm is covered with parietal pleura lining the thoracic cavity. A potential space (costodiaphragmatic recess) separates the parietal and visceral pleurae, the latter covering the lungs. The fibrous pericardium enclosing the heart is firmly attached to the central tendon. The inferior surface of the diaphragm is lined by the parietal layer of peritoneum: this surface is related on the right to the right lobe of the liver and right kidney, and on the left to the left lobe of the liver, fundus of the stomach and left kidney.

Several structures pass between the thorax and abdomen by either passing through or posterior to the diaphragm. The major tubular structures (inferior vena cava, oesophagus and aorta) do so by named openings and may be accompanied by nerves and/or other vessels. The caval opening in the central tendon lies to the right of the midline and transmits the inferior vena cava and right phrenic nerve: the wall of the vena cava is firmly adherent to its margin so that it is constantly held open. It is level with the lower border of T8.

The oesophageal opening, at the level of T10, is to the left of the midline and surrounded by fibres of the right and left crura. As well as the oesophagus, the trunks of the vagus nerves (now the gastric nerves) and the oesophageal branches of the left gastric vessels pass through the opening. The left phrenic nerve pierces the muscular part of the diaphragm near the oesophageal opening anterior to the left part of the central tendon.

The aortic opening lies posterior to the diaphragm, anterior to T12, as the two crura cross each other: it enables the aorta and thoracic duct to pass into and out of the abdomen, respectively. The azygos vein is partly covered by the right crus, while the greater and lesser splanchnic nerves pierce the crura to enter the abdomen and pass towards the coeliac ganglion.

Posterior to the medial and lateral arcuate ligaments, the sympathetic trunk and subcostal nerve pass, respectively. Anteriorly between the sternal and costal attachments of the diaphragm, the superior epigastric artery enters the rectus sheath to supply the upper part of rectus abdominis.

Innervation

The diaphragm is supplied with motor and sensory innervation by the left and right phrenic nerves (root value C3, C4 and C5). Additional sensory fibres to the peripheral part of the diaphragm are supplied by the lower six intercostal (thoracic) nerves.

Action

The diaphragm is the major muscle of inspiration: its downward movement, elevation of the ribs and anterior movement of the sternum all increase thoracic dimensions, causing air to be drawn into the lungs. From its resting position, sequential contraction of the diaphragm can be described as follows.

Contraction of the peripheral muscular portion against the fixed ribs flattens the two cupolae, pulling the central tendon inferiorly from the level of T8/T9: further descent is arrested by compression of the abdominal viscera, which is prevented from bulging outwards by tone in the abdominal muscles and, to a lesser extent, tension on the pericardium. At this point, the central tendon becomes the fixed point, with further contraction of the muscle fibres causing movement of the ribs and sternum. The lower ribs are lifted anterosuperiorly, increasing the lateral thoracic diameter, and the upper ribs raised carrying the body of the sternum anteriorly, increasing the anteroposterior diameter. These rib movements (*bucket-handle* and *pump-handle*, respectively) (p. 565) occur at the costovertebral, costotransverse, sternocostal and interchondral joints. In shallow respiration, descent of the diaphragm can be as little as 1.5 cm, while in deep inspiration it can be as much as 10 cm. This descent, together with movement of the ribs and sternum, produces a very efficient mechanism for drawing air into the lungs. From the position of full inspiration, the diaphragm relaxes to control the rate of expiration produced by the elastic recoil of the lungs.

The diaphragm also plays an important role in increasing intra-abdominal pressure, where it resists superior movement of the abdominal contents when the abdominal muscles contract to produce the expulsive acts (defecation, vomiting, micturition and parturition). This action is also important in supporting the lumbar spine during lifting activities by creating a pneumatic cushion to support it. It is likely that compression of the oesophagus by fibres of the right crus prevents regurgitation of food from the stomach.

Changes in pressure in the thoracic and abdominal cavities caused by movement of the diaphragm assist venous and lymphatic drainage from the abdomen to the thorax.

Palpation

The diaphragm is too deep to be directly palpable, but the effects of its contraction can be seen and felt. With the individual sitting and relaxed, the examiner's flat hand should be placed over the subcostal angle. After full expiration as a breath is taken, the abdominal wall can be felt pushing outwards. If the hands are now placed along the lower ribs, these will be felt rising superiorly and outwards at the same time as the sternum moves anteriorly.

Frequently, accessory muscles of respiration are used during breathing. In many instances, this leads to apical breathing, in which only the superior parts of the lungs are used. Instruction in the correct method of diaphragmatic breathing greatly increases the efficiency of breathing and is essential in activities which require breathing control (singing).

Intercostal Muscles

Group of muscles passing between adjacent ribs arranged in three layers (Fig. 4.52): the region between the ribs in which the muscles are situated is the intercostal space.

The most superficial muscle layer is the external intercostal, with fibres passing obliquely inferomedially from the inferior border of the rib above to the superior border of the rib below. It extends from the tubercles of the ribs posteriorly, becoming thinner anteriorly, until it is replaced by and becomes continuous with the external intercostal membrane in the region of the costochondral junction. In the lower part of the thorax, the fibres of the external intercostals blend with those of external oblique.

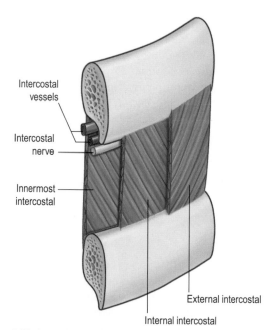

Intercostal vessels

Intercostal nerve

Innermost intercostal

External intercostal

Internal intercostal

Fig. 4.52 Lateral aspect of the thorax showing the intercostal muscles and the position and relationship of the neurovascular bundle within an intercostal space.

The middle muscle layer is the internal intercostal, with fibres passing from the inferior border of the costal cartilage and costal groove of the rib above to the superior border of the rib below. It extends from the side of the sternum to the angle of the rib, where it is replaced by the internal intercostal membrane: it is thicker anteriorly than posteriorly. The muscle fibres pass obliquely inferolaterally from the costal groove on the rib above to the superior border of the rib below at 90 degrees to those of external intercostal.

The deepest muscle layer is the innermost intercostal, which, although not complete, runs between the deepest surfaces of adjacent ribs: it is poorly developed in the upper intercostal spaces. The muscle fibres run in a similar direction to those of internal intercostal, but are separated from them by the intercostal nerve and vessels running in the neurovascular plane between the deep and intermediate muscle layers.

Innervation

By the intercostal (thoracic) nerves. Skin over each intercostal space is supplied by cutaneous branches of the same nerves.

Action

It is generally accepted that some external intercostals are active during inspiration, causing elevation of the rib below towards the rib above. The precise role of the internal and innermost intercostals has not been fully established; however, it seems likely that their contraction resists the blowing in and out of the intercostal spaces during respiration, producing a more rigid cavity upon which the diaphragm can act. Marked caving in and bulging out of the intercostal spaces occurs when the intercostal muscles are paralysed (quadriplegia). Action in the intercostals has been recorded during many movements involving the trunk: again, it appears that their role is one of stabilisation of the chest wall.

Levatores Costarum

Small, strong, triangular muscles found between C7 and T11 (Fig. 4.53A). Each of the 12 muscles of each side runs from the tip of the transverse process of the vertebra above to the superior border of the rib below near its tubercle: the fibres fan out as they pass inferolaterally.

Innervation

By adjacent thoracic nerves.

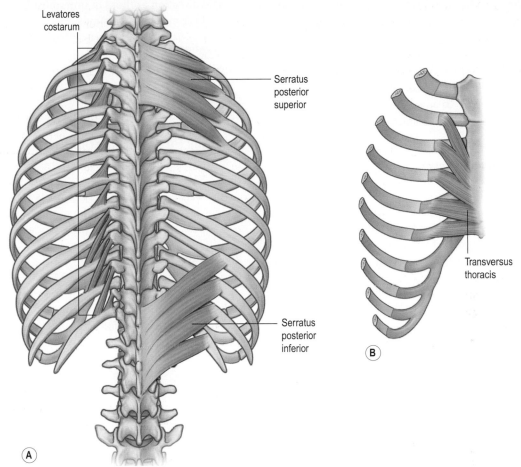

Fig. 4.53 (A) Posterior aspect of the vertebral column and thorax showing the position and attachments of the left levatores costarum and right serratus posterior superior and inferior; (B) deep aspect of the sternum and left side of the thoracic cage showing the position and attachments of transversus thoracis.

Action

These small muscles elevate the ribs during inspiration; however, their position enables them to also produce a slight degree of rotation and lateral flexion/bending of the trunk.

Serratus Posterior Superior

Thin flat muscle (Fig. 4.53A) lying deep to the rhomboids. It arises from the inferior part of the ligamentum nuchae and spinous processes of C7–T3, the fibres pass inferolaterally to attach lateral to the angles of the second to fifth ribs.

Innervation

By thoracic nerves (T2–T6).

Action

Their attachment to the ribs causes them to be elevated, thus assisting inspiration.

MUSCLES PRODUCING EXPIRATION

Transversus thoracis
Subcostals
Serratus posterior inferior
External oblique (p. 533)
Internal oblique (p. 533)
Transversus abdominis (p. 540)
Latissimus dorsi (p. 103)

The role of the abdominal muscles in forced expiration is considered on page 540.

Transversus Thoracis

Found on the deep aspect of the anterior thoracic wall (Fig. 4.53B), transversus thoracis arises from the posterior surface of the xiphoid process, lower half of the body of the sternum and fourth to seventh costal cartilages. The inferior fibres pass horizontally and superior ones superolaterally to attach to the deep surface of the second to sixth costal cartilages.

Innervation

By adjacent thoracic nerves.

Action

Transversus thoracis pulls the costal cartilages articulating with the sternum inferiorly and so contributes to expiration.

Subcostals

Irregular slips of muscle extending across one or two intercostal spaces attaching to the deep surface of the rib near the angle, the subcostals are best developed in the lower thoracic region, where their fibres run in the same general direction as those of innermost intercostal, with which they may be continuous.

Innervation

By adjacent thoracic nerves.

Action

The subcostals depress the ribs and so aid expiration.

Serratus Posterior Inferior

Lying deep to latissimus dorsi, serratus posterior inferior (Fig. 4.53A) arises from the spinous processes of T11–L2 and associated supraspinous ligaments via the thoracolumbar fascia (Fig. 4.35C). The muscle fibres run horizontally to attach to the lower four ribs at their angles.

Innervation

By adjacent thoracic nerves (T9–T11).

Action

Serratus posterior inferior helps pull the lower four ribs inferoposteriorly and as such may assist expiration.

SECTION SUMMARY

Typical Thoracic Vertebra
- Heart-shaped bodies with demifacets for articulation with head of corresponding rib and rib below
- Short pedicles arising from superior half of body
- Small, almost circular vertebral canal
- Long downward-pointing spinous process
- Overlapping laminae between vertebrae
- Long, thick, rounded transverse processes with facet for articulation with tubercle of corresponding rib
- Vertically projecting flat articular processes; superior facing posteriorly; inferior facing anteriorly

Ribs and Sternum
Typical rib
- Large head with two facets for articulation with body of own vertebra and that above
- Short flattened neck
- Prominent tubercle for articulation with transverse process of corresponding vertebra
- Long slender shaft with subcostal groove
- Articulates anteriorly with its corresponding costal cartilage

First Rib
- Short and sharply curved with superior and inferior surfaces: superior surface has two grooves separated by scalene tubercle

Sternum
- Elongated flat bone consisting of three parts: manubrium, body, xiphoid process
- Xiphoid process remains cartilaginous until middle age

Joints of the Thorax

Costochondral joints

Type	Primary cartilaginous
Articular surfaces	Anterior end of rib and costal cartilage

Manubriosternal joint

Type	Secondary cartilaginous
Articular surfaces	Inferior surface of manubrium and superior surface of body of sternum
Movements	Small amount of movement associated with inspiration, body carried anterosuperiorly

Xiphisternal joint

Type	Secondary cartilaginous
Articular surfaces	Xiphoid process and inferior of body of sternum; supported by fibrous capsule

SECTION SUMMARY—CONT'D

Costovertebral joints

Type	Synovial plane joint
Articular surfaces	Facet(s) on head of rib with facet(s) on vertebral bodies; crest of rib head with posterolateral depression on intervertebral disc
Capsule	Loose fibrous capsule surrounds joint; intra-articular ligament divides joint into two compartments
Ligaments	Radiate ligament formed by anterior thickening of capsule; posterior longitudinal ligament blends with capsule; intra-articular

Costotransverse joints

Type	Synovial plane joint
Articular surfaces	Facet on transverse process of vertebra with facet on tubercle of rib
Capsule	Thin fibrous capsule completely surrounds joint
Ligaments	Lateral costotransverse; costotransverse; superior costotransverse

First sternocostal joint

Type	Primary cartilaginous
Articular surfaces	Anterior end of first costal cartilage with lateral aspect of manubrium

Second to seventh sternocostal joints

Type	Synovial plane joints
Articular surfaces	Anterior end of costal cartilages with facets on side of manubrium (second), body (second to seventh) and xiphoid process (seventh) of sternum
Capsule	Fibrous capsule surrounds joint
Ligaments	Anterior and posterior radiate

Interchondral joints

Type	Synovial plane joints
Articular surfaces	Tips of 8th, 9th and 10th costal cartilages with cartilage above
Capsule	Fibrous capsule surrounds joint, strengthened anteriorly and posteriorly by oblique ligaments

Movements of Respiration

Respiration is produced by movements of the diaphragm and ribs. These movements are produced by the following muscles:

- Expiration is normally passive, produced by the elastic recoil of the lungs.
- In addition to the muscles listed below, other muscles (pectoralis major and pectoralis minor) attaching to the ribs can assist inspiration when more effort is required to draw air into the lungs.
- Raising the anterior end of the upper ribs and lateral part of the lower ribs is produced by: twisting and gliding at the costovertebral joints, simultaneous gliding and rotation at the costotransverse joint and gliding at the interchondral joint.
- Upper ribs movement increases the anteroposterior diameter of the thorax.
- Lower ribs movement increases the transverse diameter of the thorax.

Movement	Muscles (root value of nerve supply)
Inspiration	Diaphragm (C3, C4 and C5)
	Intercostals (segmental)
	Levatores costarum (segmental by dorsal rami)
	Serratus posterior superior (T2–T6)
Expiration	Transversus thoracis (segmental)
	Subcostals (segmental)
	Serratus posterior inferior (T9, T10 and T11)
	External oblique (T7–T12)
	Internal oblique (T7–T12 and L1)
	Transversus abdominis (T7–T12 and L1)
	Latissimus dorsi (C6, C7 and C8)

❓ SELF-ASSESSMENT QUESTIONS

41. How many ribs articulate with the second thoracic vertebrae?
42. What attaches to the scalene tubercle on the first rib?
43. What type of joint is the first sternocostal joint?
44. How many ribs articulate directly with the sternum?
45. What is the nerve supply to the diaphragm?
46. What is the action of serratus posterior superior?
47. What is the nerve supply to serratus posterior inferior?
48. What passes through the central tendon of the diaphragm?
49. What are the named parts of the sternum?
50. What type of joint is the manubriosternal joint?
51. With which vertebrae does the seventh rib articulate?
52. With which rib does the transverse process of T5 articulate?
53. The axis for the so-called pump-handle movements passes through which joints?
54. The anterior radiate ligaments are associated with which joints?
55. Which are the floating ribs?
56. What runs in the subcostal groove of a rib?
57. Between which muscles is the intercostal plane?
58. What are the peripheral attachments of the diaphragm?

8. Describe the formation of the cervical, brachial, lumbar, lumbosacral and sacral plexuses from the ventral rami of spinal nerves
9. Describe the autonomic nervous system (ANS) and its two component parts
10. Describe the outflow of the sympathetic and parasympathetic parts of the autonomous nervous system
11. Describe the arrangement of preganglionic and postganglionic fibres in both the sympathetic and parasympathetic nervous systems
12. Describe the formation of the splanchnic nerves
13. Describe the effects of the sympathetic and parasympathetic nervous system on the body

SPINAL CORD AND AUTONOMIC NERVOUS SYSTEM

LEARNING OUTCOMES

By the end of the section, you should be able to:
1. Describe the organisation of the white and grey matter in the spinal cord
2. Describe the surface features of the spinal cord
3. Describe the formation and branches of spinal nerves
4. Describe the organisation of the meningeal coverings of the spinal cord
5. Appreciate that the spinal cord terminates at the level of L1/L2 and that the dural sac extends to the level of S2
6. Appreciate that the cauda equina is a collection of elongated L2–Co1 nerve roots
7. Describe the blood supply to the spinal cord

INTRODUCTION

The central nervous system (CNS) is formed by the aggregation of bundles of axons and clusters of nerve cell bodies: its internal appearance and external form reflect the manner in which these components are arranged (a more detailed account can be found on page 682).

The central part of the spinal cord is formed by nerve fibres and nerve cell bodies, appearing grey in transverse sections. The outer part of the spinal cord consists mainly of myelinated axons, giving it a white appearance in transverse sections. As cell bodies are not myelinated, ganglia and nuclei form grey matter and myelinated axons form white matter. Thus areas in the CNS formed mainly by axons are referred to as white matter, while areas formed mainly by cell bodies appear grey and are referred to as grey matter (Figs 4.54 and 5.42).

Collections of cell bodies forming a prominent, usually rounded swelling are referred to as ganglia, while

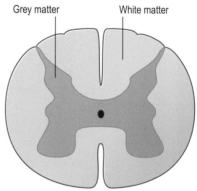

Grey matter   White matter

Fig. 4.54 Organisation of grey and white matter as seen in a transverse section of the spinal cord.

clusters of axons forming recognisable bundles within the CNS are referred to as fasciculi. A bundle of axons forming a raised bump or convex contour on the surface of the spinal cord is a funiculus. These terms refer to the topographic appearance of collections of axons or cell bodies without regard to their function. However, other terms have functional implications: a group of axons with a similar function is a tract, while a group of cell bodies with a similar function is a nucleus.

Development

The CNS develops from a single tubular structure (neural tube) formed along the dorsal surface of the embryo from the site of the future head to the tail (Fig. 4.55): it has two ends (head and tail). Because the tube bends in the sagittal plane during development of the brain, the terms anterior, posterior, superior and inferior cannot be applied to the nervous system without confusion: different terms of reference are, therefore, used with respect to the CNS.

The tail is the caudal end, and the head, irrespective of the direction it points with respect to the rest of the body, is the rostral end (Fig. 4.55). The surface of the neural tube facing the belly of the embryo is its ventral surface, irrespective of whether the tube is straight or curved in the sagittal plane; the opposite surface is the dorsal surface. These directional terms are equally applicable in descriptions of the adult CNS.

The neural tube maintains a narrow cavity along its length; however, the thickness of its walls increases as the constituent cells multiply and grow. Most of the caudal part simply grows in length and diameter: its walls get thicker, but its cavity remains narrow. This part forms the future spinal cord, with its cavity becoming the central canal (Fig. 4.55).

Details of the development of the brain can be found on page 683.

Glial Cells

Nerve cells are not the only constituents of the CNS: interspersed between them are several types of cells collectively referred to as glial cells (glia: Latin, meaning glue) whose function, in general, is to hold the neurons of the CNS together. As a whole, glial cells outnumber nerve cells and constitute almost half the total volume of the CNS. Details of glial cells can be found on page 682.

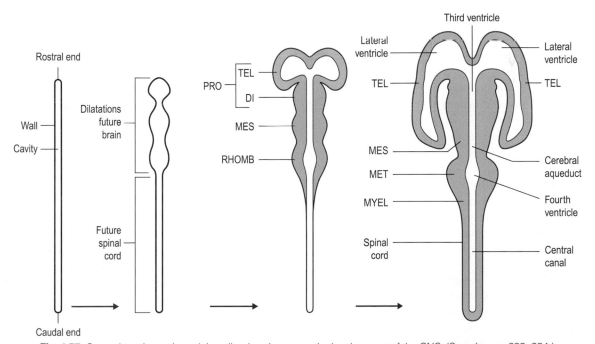

Fig. 4.55 Coronal sections, viewed dorsally, showing stages in development of the CNS. (See also pp. 683–684.)

SPINAL CORD

Essentially the spinal cord is a long thick cable formed by thousands of longitudinally running axons surrounding a central core of grey matter: it is approximately 45 cm long and occupies the vertebral canal at cervical, thoracic and upper lumbar levels.

The external surface has only a few named features (Fig. 4.56). Running along the midline on the ventral surface is a pronounced depression (anterior median fissure) dividing the ventral part of the spinal cord into left and right halves. Dorsally, the spinal cord is marked by several less pronounced longitudinal depressions, one of which lies in the midline (posterior median sulcus), separating the left and right halves of the spinal cord: posterior lateral sulci run along the entire length of the spinal cord on its posterolateral aspects. A further sulcus (posterior intermediate sulcus) on each side of the rostral half of the spinal cord runs longitudinally between the posterior median and posterior lateral sulci.

Between the three sulci on each side of the rostral half of the spinal cord are two slightly rounded prominences extending longitudinally. The medial prominence (fasciculus gracilis) lies between the posterior median and posterior intermediate sulci, and the lateral prominence (fasciculus cuneatus) lies between the posterior intermediate and posterior lateral sulci. These fasciculi are formed by bundles of sensory axons destined to synapse in the nucleus gracilis and nucleus cuneatus, respectively. Only the fasciculus gracilis is present in the caudal half of the spinal cord: this region lacks a posterior intermediate sulcus.

The width of the spinal cord is not uniform along its length: it is expanded a short distance below its rostral end, as well as near its caudal end (Fig. 4.56). These expansions occur at levels concerned with innervation of the upper and lower limbs (cervical and lumbar enlargements, respectively), being formed by larger numbers of cell bodies and axons associated with limb functions. The caudal end of the spinal cord tapers to a pointed tip (conus medullaris).

Internal Structure

The central core of the spinal cord consists of grey matter which has a characteristic butterfly appearance in transverse section (Fig. 4.57). The area surrounding the central canal is the central grey matter: projecting dorsolaterally and ventrally from this central area are

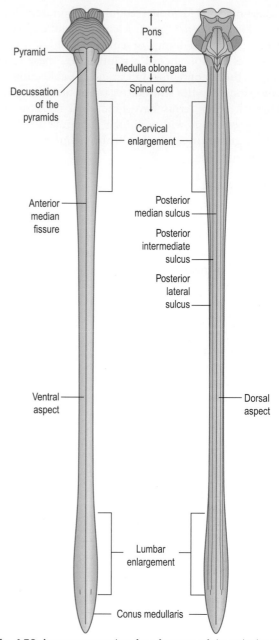

Fig. 4.56 Appearance and surface features of the spinal cord.

extensions of grey matter, the dorsal (posterior) and ventral (anterior) horns (Fig. 4.57B).

The ventral horns are formed by the cell bodies of neurons innervating voluntary muscles: the axons leave the spinal cord through the ventral roots. The dorsal horns consist of cells concerned with processing sensory information entering the spinal cord through the dorsal

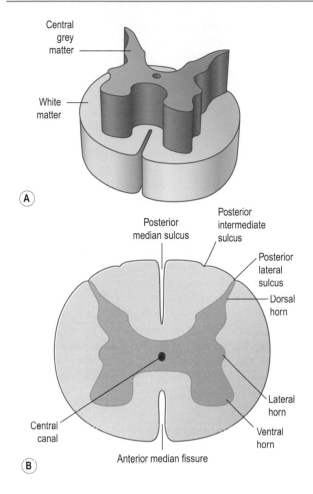

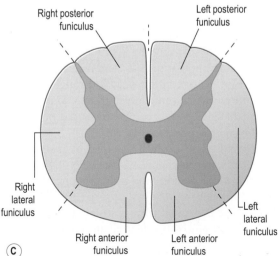

Fig. 4.57 (A) Internal organisation of the spinal cord and its appearance in transverse section; (B) organisation between T1 and L2; (C) location of funiculi.

roots. In general, sensory fibres entering the spinal cord synapse on neurons in the dorsal horn, with their axons forming tracts running rostral or caudal in the spinal cord.

Between the T1 and L2 segments of the spinal cord, there is an additional small horn of grey matter (lateral horn) projecting laterally in the angle between the dorsal and ventral horns (Fig. 4.57B): it contains cell bodies of neurons whose axons are part of the autonomic nervous system (ANS) (p. 575).

The peripheral part of the spinal cord consists of white matter formed by axons arranged in tracts conveying information to or from the brainstem, or between different segments of the spinal cord. The white matter is divided into sectors by imaginary radial lines through the dorsal and ventral horns (Fig. 4.57C), giving three regions of white matter in each half of the spinal cord. Between the ventral and dorsal horns laterally is the lateral funiculus, formed by descending tracts conveying motor information and ascending tracts concerned with pain, temperature, touch and pressure sensation. The white matter between the dorsal horn and midline dorsally is the posterior funiculus, consisting largely of ascending tracts conveying information on pressure, touch and position sense. Finally, the region between the ventral horn and midline anteriorly is the anterior funiculus, formed by a mixture of descending motor and ascending sensory tracts.

The white matter embracing the anterolateral aspect of the ventral horn is occasionally referred to as the anterolateral funiculus, because axons in this region overlap both anterior and lateral funiculi: they constitute the largest single collection of ascending sensory fibres conveying sensations of pressure, touch, pain and temperature.

Meninges

Although glial cells hold the neurons of the CNS together and provide protection against metabolic insults, the CNS is nonetheless a soft cellular mass. It is, therefore, vulnerable to external mechanical insult which might arise were it freely mobile within the vertebral canal or skull. To protect against such insult, the CNS is surrounded by three membranes (meninges) and bathed in cerebrospinal fluid (CSF).

Meninges of the Spinal Cord

The outermost meningeal covering is a tough fibrous layer (dura mater): in the vertebral canal it forms a long sac (dural sac) housing the spinal cord (Fig. 4.58).

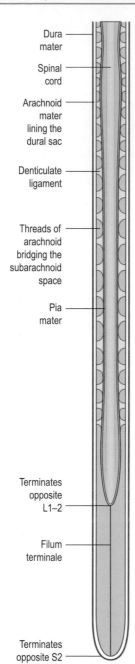

Dura mater

Spinal cord

Arachnoid mater lining the dural sac

Denticulate ligament

Threads of arachnoid bridging the subarachnoid space

Pia mater

Terminates opposite L1–2

Filum terminale

Terminates opposite S2

Fig. 4.58 Meningeal coverings of the spinal cord showing the threads of arachnoid mater bridging the subarachnoid space and the denticulate ligaments holding the spinal cord in place.

Rostrally, the dural sac attaches to the margins of the foramen magnum, but within the vertebral canal it is relatively mobile, attached to the vertebral canal by modest fibrous ligaments only: the dural sac is much longer than the spinal cord, reaching as far as S2.

The deepest meningeal covering is a thin transparent membrane (pia mater), intimately investing the entire surface of the spinal cord like a fine skin (Fig. 4.58). From the caudal end of the spinal cord, it continues as a thread of tissue (filum terminale) devoid of neural elements: it pierces the tip of the sac to attach to the coccyx (Fig. 4.58).

The middle meningeal covering is a shiny membrane (arachnoid mater) lining the internal surface of the dura mater (Fig. 4.58). A substantial space (subarachnoid space) persists between the pia mater covering the spinal cord and the arachnoid and dura mater. The subarachnoid space is permeated by a network of threads connecting the arachnoid and dura mater to the pia mater.

Spanning the subarachnoid space is a series of ligaments formed by the pia mater (denticulate ligaments): these triangular tooth-like extensions have their bases attached at regular intervals along the lateral aspect of the spinal cord and their apices to the dural sac (Fig. 4.58). Between the foramen magnum and tip of the spinal cord, 21 pairs of ligaments project to the dural sac, anchoring the spinal cord and protecting it from injury due to violent contact with the walls of the vertebral canal during movement of the trunk.

Cerebrospinal Fluid

Running between the threads of arachnoid mater and filling the subarachnoid space is cerebrospinal fluid (CSF): it is secreted by strings of capillaries projecting into the lateral, third and fourth ventricles of the brain. Filling the cavities of the CNS, it emerges through apertures in the roof of the fourth ventricle to fill the subarachnoid space surrounding the brain and spinal cord.

CSF is continuously secreted and reabsorbed into the bloodstream. Reabsorption occurs through extensions of arachnoid mater (arachnoid granulations) piercing the dura mater of the falx cerebri and projecting into the superior sagittal sinus (see Fig. 5.57B).

Chemically, CSF protects the CNS by maintaining a constant pH environment: mechanically it endows the CNS with a cushioning fluid environment. Within the skull, the brain is buoyant in a pool of CSF, while within the dural sac the spinal cord is suspended in a pool of CSF, held centrally by the denticulate ligaments.

Spinal Nerves

Short nerves within the intervertebral foramina of the vertebral column (Fig. 4.59A). Outside the vertebral

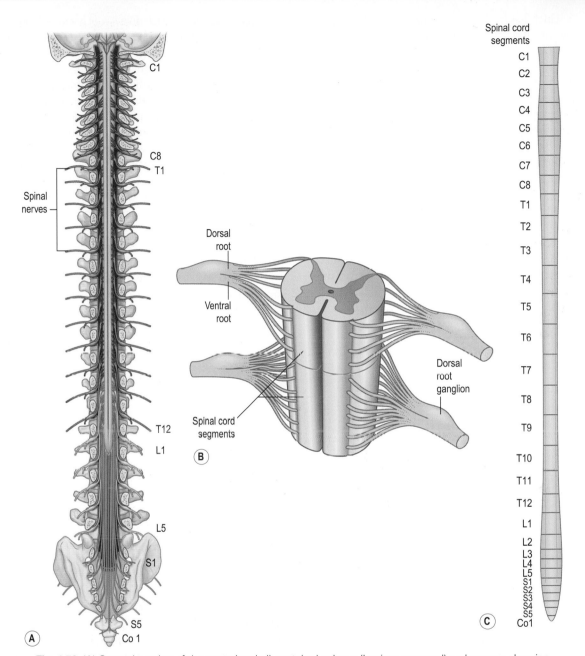

Fig. 4.59 (A) Coronal section of the posterior skull, vertebral column (laminae removed) and sacrum showing the spinal cord in the vertebral canal and spinal nerves in the intervertebral foramina; (B) two segments of the spinal cord showing the formation of spinal nerves and position of the dorsal root ganglion; (C) segmental arrangement of the spinal cord.

column, they are part of the peripheral nervous system, but within the vertebral canal, each spinal nerve is connected to the spinal cord by ventral and dorsal nerve roots (Fig. 4.59B), components of the CNS.

There are 31 pairs of spinal nerves, each named according to the vertebra they are related to. There are eight pairs of cervical spinal nerves (C1–C8), each lying above the cervical vertebra with the same segmental number, except for C8 which lies below C7. The remaining spinal nerves take the number of the vertebra lying above them: the nerve below T6 is the T6 spinal nerve, and that below L2 is the L2 spinal nerve. In total there are 8 cervical (C1–C8), 12 thoracic (T1–T12), 5 lumbar (L1–L5), 5 sacral (S1–S5) and a pair of coccygeal (Co1) spinal nerves.

The ventral roots of all spinal nerves attach in series on each side along the ventrolateral aspect of the spinal cord (Fig. 4.57B): in a similar way, the dorsal roots attach to the posterolateral aspect of the spinal cord along the posterior lateral sulcus. As each dorsal root approaches the spinal cord, it divides into a series of small branches (rootlets) forming the junction with the spinal cord. Correspondingly, each ventral root is formed by a series of rootlets emerging from the spinal cord to form the ventral root proper.

The dorsal roots convey only sensory fibres from the spinal nerves to the spinal cord: the ventral roots convey motor fibres from the spinal cord to the spinal nerves, but also contain some sensory fibres. Near its junction with the ventral root and spinal nerve, each dorsal root has a swelling (dorsal root ganglion) formed by the cell bodies of all sensory fibres running in the related spinal nerve (Fig. 4.59B).

Each spinal nerve attaches by its roots to a discrete section of the spinal cord (spinal cord segment): the limits of each segment are demarcated by an imaginary transverse plane drawn through the spinal cord midway between the sites of attachment of the most rostral rootlets of one spinal nerve and most caudal rootlets of the nerve above or below. Each spinal cord segment is named after the spinal nerve attached to it (Fig. 4.59C): the spinal cord, therefore, consists of 8 cervical, 12 thoracic, 5 lumbar, 5 sacral segments and 1 coccygeal segment.

Nerve Root Sheaths

To reach the peripheral nervous system, spinal nerve roots must penetrate the meninges. On leaving the spinal cord, the proximal ends of spinal nerve roots are invested by the pia mater (Fig. 4.60): this is one

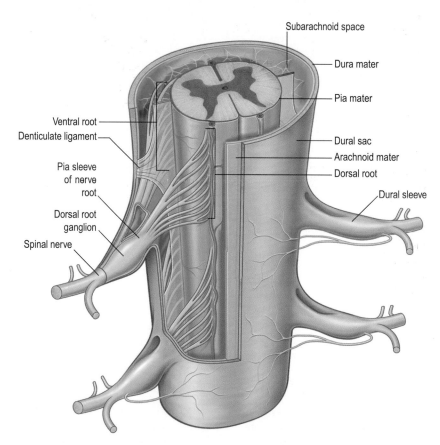

Fig. 4.60 Organisation of the meninges surrounding the spinal cord and spinal nerve roots, also showing the relationship between the meningeal sheaths and spinal nerves.

morphological reason for classifying the spinal nerves as part of the CNS. The pia mater spreads like a tubular extension over the surface of each spinal nerve from its attachment to the spinal cord as far as where it leaves the vertebral canal. As the spinal nerve roots leave the dural sac, they take a funnel-shaped extension of dura and arachnoid mater with them (dural sleeves) extending as far as the spinal nerve (Fig. 4.60): throughout their entire length the spinal nerve roots are bathed in CSF.

Cauda Equina

In early development of the CNS, the spinal cord is the same length as the vertebral column, with each spinal nerve running transversely from the spinal cord to its corresponding intervertebral foramen (Fig. 4.61). As the foetus develops, differential growth of the vertebral column and spinal cord results in the vertebral column becoming substantially longer than the spinal cord. The dural sac grows to accommodate this difference: in adults it terminates at the level of S2, with the spinal cord ending opposite the L1/L2 intervertebral disc.

In spite of this differential growth, the spinal nerves retain their original relationship with their respective intervertebral foramina: the spinal nerve roots also remain attached to their respective spinal cord segments. The difference in length between the spinal cord and vertebral column is accommodated by elongation of the more caudal nerve roots becoming increasingly oblique within the dural sac (Fig. 4.61).

Cervical spinal cord segments remain related to their vertebrae, with the cervical nerve roots more or less retaining their original transverse course. Upper thoracic spinal cord segments are displaced from their respective intervertebral foramina by approximately one segmental level, with progressively lower spinal cord segments being displaced by an increasing margin, until the S5 segment lies 10 vertebral segments short of the S5 intervertebral foramen. Thoracic, lumbar, sacral and coccygeal nerve roots are, therefore, progressively longer.

Below the caudal tip of the spinal cord, the L2–Co1 nerve roots form a leash of nerves hanging freely in the dural sac (cauda equina) (Fig. 4.61), with each root ensheathed in its own sleeve of pia mater and bathed in CSF. As each set of dorsal and ventral nerve roots descends to its respective intervertebral foramen, it passes to the lateral side of the dural sac, penetrating it just above the appropriate intervertebral foramen.

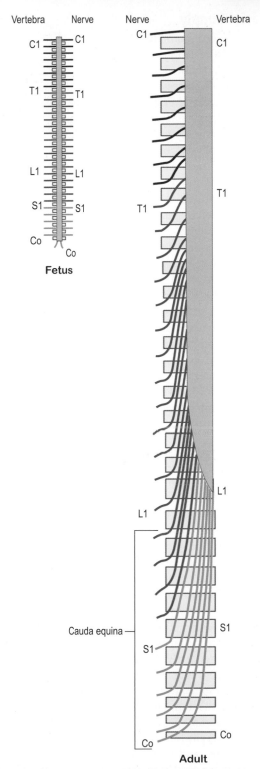

Fig. 4.61 Relationship between the intervertebral foramina, spinal nerves and spinal cord in the foetus and adult.

Arterial Supply

This is derived from the internal carotid and vertebral arteries. The vertebral arteries pierce the dural sac, entering the subarachnoid space just above the first cervical vertebra: each passes anterosuperiorly through the foramen magnum, joining in the midline anterior to the medulla oblongata, to form the basilar artery, which runs superiorly anterior to the pons (see Figs 5.59 and 5.60). Branches of the vertebral and basilar arteries pass laterally, supplying the medulla oblongata, pons and cerebellum.

Each vertebral artery gives an anterior spinal artery, which descends obliquely anterior to the medulla oblongata towards the spinal cord (see Fig. 5.59). The anterior spinal arteries form a single anterior spinal artery descending along the anterior median sulcus: most of the blood supply to the spinal cord is derived from this single vessel (Fig. 4.62). Smaller branches (posterior spinal arteries) of the vertebral artery descend along the posterolateral aspect of the spinal cord supplying only the posterolateral corners (Fig. 4.62). At variable distances along the spinal cord, the anterior and posterior spinal arteries are reinforced by vessels passing along the spinal nerve roots. In the cervical region, these are from the vertebral artery, at thoracic levels from posterior intercostal arteries, and at lumbar levels from lumbar arteries (Fig. 4.62).

SOMATIC NERVOUS SYSTEM

Formed by peripheral branches of cranial and spinal nerves the somatic nervous system conveys motor axons to the muscles of the body and sensory fibres to the CNS.

Each spinal nerve contains sensory and motor axons connected to the spinal cord by dorsal and ventral nerve roots, respectively: because the ventral and dorsal roots lie within the vertebral canal and dural sac they are classified as being part of the CNS. The peripheral nervous system is formed by the branches of the spinal nerves outside the vertebral column.

Immediately beyond the intervertebral foramen, each spinal nerve divides into two branches (dorsal and ventral rami) (Fig. 4.63). With the exception of the first two cervical spinal nerves, the ventral ramus of each spinal nerve is substantially larger than the dorsal ramus.

All dorsal rami pass posteriorly into the tissues of the trunk, principally innervating the postvertebral muscles, and ligaments and joints of the vertebral arches. Most also give cutaneous branches to skin over the posterior aspect of the head, neck, trunk and pelvic girdle. The dorsal rami of C1, L4 and L5 lack cutaneous branches, while those of C4–C6 are inconstant. That is not to say that these dorsal rami are entirely motor, although lacking cutaneous branches they do convey sensory fibres from the muscles, joints and ligaments they innervate.

The ventral rami supply the sides and anterior aspects of the body wall, limbs and perineum. In the thoracic region, they have a simple arrangement: except for the first, each thoracic ventral ramus forms a typical intercostal nerve, passing laterally from the intervertebral foramen inferior to the rib of the same segment (Fig. 4.64). The first thoracic ventral ramus gives a small branch constituting the first intercostal nerve: the main part passes over the first rib contributing to the formation of the brachial plexus (p. 225). Peripherally, each intercostal nerve innervates muscles in its intercostal space and the overlying skin. The lower six intercostal nerves extend into the anterior abdominal wall to segmentally innervate muscles of the anterior abdominal wall and overlying skin.

At cervical, lumbar and sacral levels, the simple segmental pattern of thoracic levels is modified as the ventral rami form plexuses: a plexus is a network of interconnections between several adjacent ventral rami allowing them to exchange nerve fibres before forming discrete peripheral nerves. The cervical, lumbar and sacral ventral rami form five named plexuses on either side of the vertebral column (Fig. 4.65):

1. The cervical plexus is formed by the C1–C4 ventral rami: the peripheral nerves are distributed to the prevertebral muscles, levator scapulae, sternomastoid, trapezius, diaphragm and skin of the anterior and lateral aspects of the neck from the shoulder to the mandible and external ear (p. 650).
2. The brachial plexus is formed by the C5–T1 ventral rami: nerves derived from this plexus innervate the musculature and joints of the pectoral girdle and upper limb, and skin of the upper limb (p. 225).
3. The lumbar plexus is formed by the L1–L4 ventral rami, with a contribution from the T12 ventral ramus: the smaller nerves innervate muscles of the lower anterolateral abdominal wall and skin of the groin, lateral thigh and anterior parts of the external genitalia. The femoral and obturator nerves are the largest arising from the lumbar plexus: they innervate muscles and skin in the lower limb (p. 466).

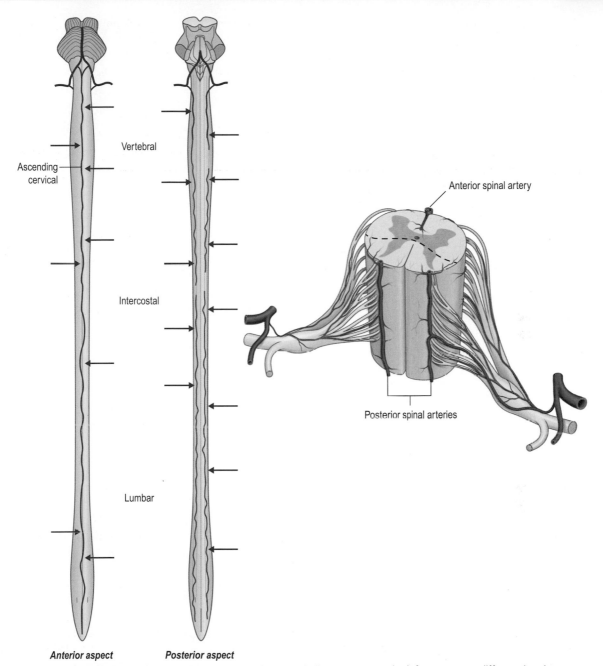

Anterior aspect   **Posterior aspect**

Fig. 4.62 Arterial supply of the spinal cord: arrows indicate segmental reinforcement at different levels.

4. The lumbosacral plexus is formed by the L4–S3 ventral rami; branches innervate muscles and skin of the lower limb (p. 470).
5. The sacral plexus is formed by the S3–S5 ventral rami and gives rise to nerves innervating the pelvic floor and perineum (p. 476).

Knowledge of the distribution of major peripheral nerves is necessary in clinical practice for the diagnosis and assessment of peripheral nerve injuries and other neurological disorders. The course and distribution of the various peripheral nerves are described in more detail in the relevant sections dealing with the regions

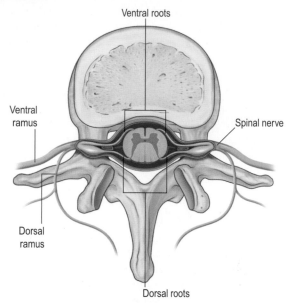

Fig. 4.63 Dorsal and ventral rami of a typical spinal nerve.

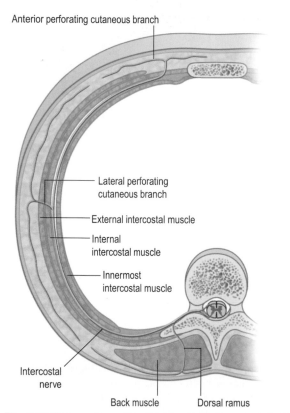

Fig. 4.64 Transverse section showing the course and distribution of a typical intercostal nerve.

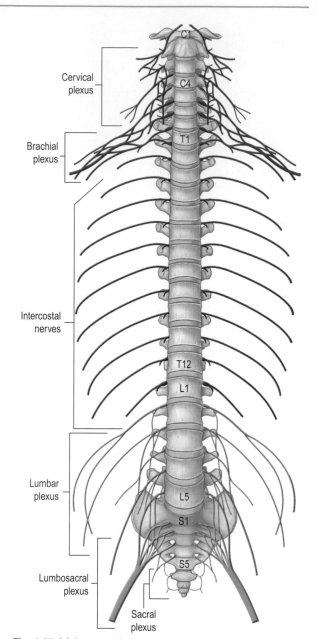

Fig. 4.65 Major somatic nerve plexuses arising from the spinal cord.

of the body in which they are found. Their cutaneous distribution follows and complements the segmental dermatome arrangement.

Muscles of the pelvic and pectoral (shoulder) girdles are not grouped into compartments and are not covered by such rules. These muscles usually receive a unique nerve supply or a single nerve may innervate two or three muscles. These relationships are described in the sections dealing with the muscles of the pelvic and pectoral (shoulder) regions.

AUTONOMIC NERVOUS SYSTEM

The autonomic nervous system (ANS) consists of nerves innervating the viscera of the body, its blood vessels, salivary, lacrimal and sweat glands and muscles (arrectores pilorum) associated with hairs. On topographical, anatomical and physiological grounds, the ANS is divided into two discrete parts (sympathetic and parasympathetic nervous systems).

Topographically, the two systems differ with respect to where they are connected to the CNS. Parasympathetic nerves emerge from the CNS in cranial nerves III, VII, IX and X and the S2–S4 spinal nerves: axons of the sympathetic nervous system emerge from the spinal cord in the T1–L2 spinal nerves. Parasympathetic nerves are, therefore, described as having a craniosacral outflow and sympathetic nerves as having a thoracolumbar outflow.

Anatomically, both systems are similar at the microscopic level as any target organ is connected to the CNS by two neurons in series (Fig. 4.66). The axon of the first nerve emerges from the CNS and synapses with the second neuron, with the collections of cell bodies of the second neurons forming swellings (ganglia). Axons conveying information from the CNS to such ganglia are preganglionic axons, those forming the ganglia whose axons lead from them to the peripheral target organ are postganglionic axons.

Anatomically the difference between the sympathetic and parasympathetic nervous systems is that parasympathetic ganglia lie close to the target organ, while sympathetic ganglia lie some distance away. As a result, postganglionic parasympathetic fibres tend to be short, and postganglionic sympathetic fibres considerably longer.

Pharmacologically, the parasympathetic and sympathetic nervous systems differ in that parasympathetic postganglionic neurons have acetylcholine as their neurotransmitter and sympathetic postganglionic neurons have noradrenaline. However, preganglionic neurons in both systems have acetylcholine as their neurotransmitter (Fig. 4.66).

Physiologically, the ANS exerts a variety of effects on different types of tissues; however, in general, these are all as a result of contraction or relaxation of smooth muscle or myoepithelial cells in exocrine glands. Generally, acetylcholine secreted by parasympathetic neurons excites smooth muscle causing it to contract. Noradrenaline can either excite or inhibit smooth muscle depending on the molecular receptors found on the smooth muscle membrane: α-receptors cause smooth muscle to contract, β-receptors cause it to relax. Different tissues are endowed with either α- or β-receptors: some contain both types of receptors in different regions or even in the same region. These variations give rise to the diversity of effects of the sympathetic nervous system.

The sympathetic nervous system stimulates the sinoatrial node of the heart, increasing heart rate: it also stimulates cardiac muscle directly, increasing the power of cardiac contraction. In the peripheral vascular system, the effects of the sympathetic nervous system are variable. Acting on α-receptors, sympathetic nerves cause smooth muscle in arterioles to contract causing vasoconstriction: acting on β-receptors, they cause

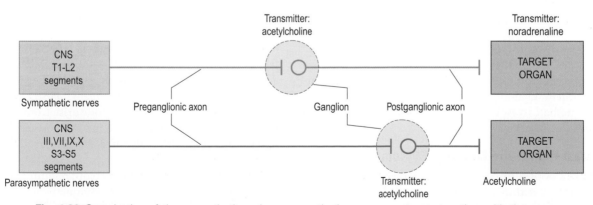

Fig. 4.66 Organisation of the sympathetic and parasympathetic nervous systems, together with the neurotransmitter at each site of synapse.

vasodilation. In the digestive tract, the sympathetic nervous system relaxes smooth muscle of the tract, but stimulates its sphincters to contract. In the respiratory tract, it relaxes smooth muscle of the bronchi. It also causes the bladder sphincter to contract and mediates ejaculation in males, causing contraction of the smooth muscle in the vas deferens, seminal vesicle and prostate gland. In the eye, it causes dilation of the pupil, while in skin it causes erection of the hairs and sweating.

These diverse effects may be summarised by an aphorism: the effects of the sympathetic nervous system are those that would be evident in the functions of Fright, Flight, Fight and Fill. The reaction of fright is manifest by pupillary dilation, hair standing on end, sweating and increased heart rate; flight (running away) and fight involve increased heart rate, increased circulation (vasodilation) to muscular blood vessels and diversion (vasoconstriction) of blood away from the digestive tract. All of these actions are mediated by the sympathetic nervous system. The function of fill refers to the relaxation of bronchial smooth muscle, increasing air entry and allowing air to be drawn into the lungs. The combination of relaxation of smooth muscle of the digestive tract and contraction of its sphincters results in filling of its lumen.

In a sense, the parasympathetic nervous system exerts opposite effects. It slows the sinoatrial node reducing heart rate. In the eye, it causes pupillary constriction and accommodation of the lens. It causes contraction of bronchial musculature and contracts smooth muscle of the digestive and urinary tracts while relaxing their sphincters. Its action on hollow organs is designed to empty them. This emptying effect is further evident in salivary and lacrimal glands where the parasympathetic nervous system causes secretion of their respective fluids. Its effect on glands is also evident in the respiratory and digestive tracts, where it causes secretion of mucus and acid. The parasympathetic nervous system also has effects on blood vessels, causing vasodilation in the genital system, enabling erection of the penis or clitoris; it also mediates vasodilation of the internal and external carotid circulations.

Parasympathetic Nervous System

The cell bodies of preganglionic parasympathetic neurons are located in special nuclei in the brainstem associated with the nuclei of cranial nerves III (oculomotor), VII (facial), IX (glossopharyngeal) and X (vagus). Axons

of these neurons emerge from the brainstem in these cranial nerves travelling with their sensory and somatic motor fibres (p. 572).

Located near the back of the orbit close to the optic nerve, the ciliary ganglion is formed by postganglionic parasympathetic neurons innervating the sphincter pupillae and ciliary muscle of the eye (Fig. 4.67A). The preganglionic neurons from the oculomotor nerve synapse with postganglionic neurons in the ciliary ganglion. Stimulation of the postganglionic neurons causes the sphincter pupillae and ciliary muscle to contract, narrowing the pupil and increasing the refractive (focusing) power of the lens, respectively.

Located in the pterygopalatine fossa associated with the maxillary nerve is the pterygopalatine ganglion, formed by postganglionic parasympathetic neurons innervating the mucous glands of the nose and lacrimal gland (Fig. 4.67A). The ganglion receives preganglionic neurons from the facial (VII) nerve: when stimulated the postganglionic fibres cause lacrimation, as well as nasal and palatine secretion.

The submandibular and sublingual salivary glands are innervated by postganglionic parasympathetic nerves which form a ganglion located in the submandibular region (submandibular ganglion) (Fig. 4.67A): the preganglionic neurons are from the facial nerve via the chorda tympani.

The parotid gland is innervated by postganglionic parasympathetic neurons whose cell bodies form the otic ganglion associated with the mandibular division of the trigeminal nerve just below the foramen ovale. It receives preganglionic neurons predominantly from the glossopharyngeal nerve, with a small contribution from the facial nerve (Fig. 4.67A).

The parasympathetic distribution of the vagus nerve includes the heart, larynx, trachea and bronchi, pharynx, oesophagus, stomach, small intestine, large intestine as far as the splenic flexure, as well as the liver, biliary tract and pancreas (Fig. 4.67A): both vagus nerves convey preganglionic axons to these organs. Postganglionic fibres innervating the sinoatrial node arise from ganglia lying on the surface of the heart, but the postganglionic fibres of the respiratory, digestive and urinary tracts lie embedded in the tract walls.

The descending and sigmoid colon, rectum and pelvic viscera are innervated by parasympathetic neurons arising from the S2–S4 spinal nerves. Their cell bodies are in the S2–S4 segments of the spinal cord: the axons

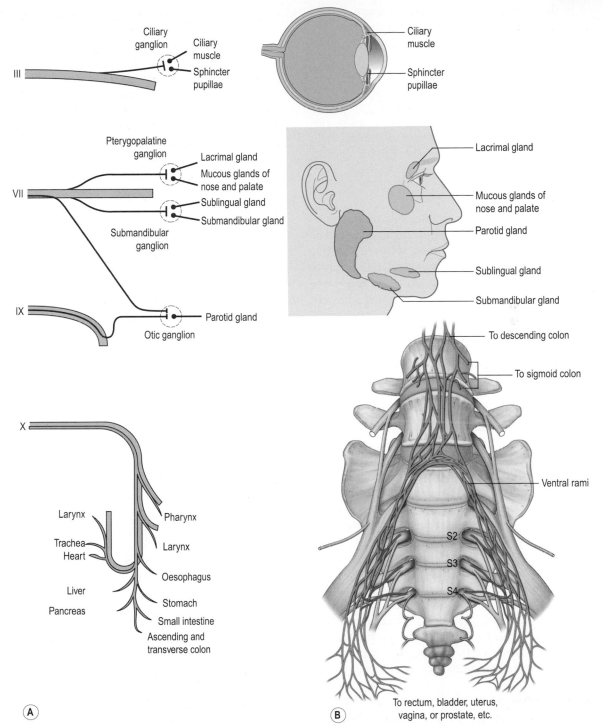

Fig. 4.67 (A) Distribution of the parasympathetic fibres in the III (oculomotor), VII (facial), IX (glossopharyngeal) and X (vagus) cranial nerves; (B) the pelvic splanchnic nerves.

travel in the ventral roots of the S2–S4 spinal nerves. As they emerge from the anterior sacral foramina, the parasympathetic axons (pelvic splanchnic nerves) pass directly to their target viscera (Fig. 4.67B).

Fibres destined for the pelvic viscera pass directly into them, synapsing on postganglionic parasympathetic neurons located within their walls. Those destined for the descending and sigmoid colon pass superiorly out of the pelvis, across the left posterior abdominal wall, reaching the descending colon or entering the sigmoid mesocolon to reach the sigmoid colon.

Sympathetic Nervous System

Running longitudinally along either side of the vertebral column from C1 to the coccyx, crossing the tips of cervical transverse processes, heads of the ribs at thoracic levels and anterolateral aspects of the vertebral bodies at lumbar and sacral levels, are two sets of nerve fibres (sympathetic trunks/chains) (Fig. 4.68). They are formed by preganglionic and postganglionic neurons of the sympathetic nervous system; sites along the trunks where preganglionic and postganglionic neurons synapse are marked by swellings (sympathetic ganglia).

Embryologically, a sympathetic ganglion is formed opposite each spinal nerve, but later in development, some ganglia divide and reform in a variable pattern giving fewer ganglia: eventually 11 thoracic, between 1 and 6 (usually 4) lumbar and 4 sacral ganglia, are formed. Anterior to the coccyx, the sympathetic trunks join, forming a single common ganglion (ganglion impar). At cervical levels, two main ganglia are formed: a large one at the level of C1–C3 (superior cervical ganglion) and one at the cervicothoracic level (cervicothoracic (stellate) ganglion). A third ganglion (middle cervical ganglion) is frequently, but not constantly, formed at the level of C6.

Cell bodies of preganglionic sympathetic neurons are located in the lateral horns of the grey matter in the T1–L2 segments of the spinal cord: their axons leave the spinal cord in the ventral roots of the spinal nerves at these same levels (Fig. 4.69). Preganglionic sympathetic neurons are not found in spinal nerves or nerve roots at other levels.

After traversing the spinal nerve, preganglionic sympathetic neurons enter the ventral ramus of the spinal nerve: just beyond the intervertebral foramen they leave the ventral ramus, forming a branch entering the sympathetic trunk conveying preganglionic neurons from

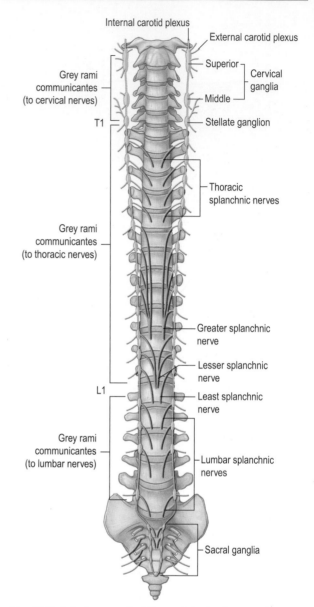

Fig. 4.68 Anterior aspect of the vertebral column and sacrum showing the position of the sympathetic trunks/chains and their branches.

the ventral ramus to the sympathetic trunk (Fig. 4.69). Because it is a branch, it is a ramus, and because it communicates with the sympathetic trunk, it is a ramus communicans, and because preganglionic neurons are myelinated (in fresh specimens), they have a whitish appearance and are referred to as a white ramus communicans (plural: rami communicantes).

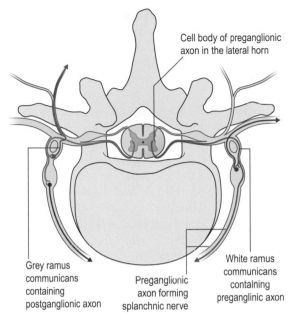

Fig. **4.69** Arrangement of the white and grey rami communicantes and course of the pre- and postganglionic sympathetic axons seen in transverse section.

Upon entering the sympathetic trunk, preganglionic sympathetic neurons terminate, or pass superiorly or inferiorly within it. Preganglionic neurons from white rami communicantes from upper thoracic ventral rami tend to pass superiorly to reach cervical levels before terminating. Those from lower thoracic and lumbar white rami communicantes tend to pass inferiorly to lower lumbar and sacral levels before terminating. Those from mid-thoracic white rami communicantes pass superiorly or inferiorly for short distances or terminate at their level of entry.

When they terminate, preganglionic sympathetic neurons do so by synapsing with cell bodies of postganglionic sympathetic neurons located in sympathetic ganglia. Axons of postganglionic sympathetic neurons then leave the sympathetic trunk or pass superiorly or inferiorly before leaving.

Postganglionic sympathetic neurons leave the sympathetic trunk in one of three ways. Most do so by joining a ventral ramus; others leave following arteries or form distinct branches passing directly to certain viscera or plexuses (Fig. 4.70).

Postganglionic neurons joining a ventral ramus do so by forming a small branch passing from the sympathetic trunk to the ventral ramus (Fig. 4.69). Because these branches are unmyelinated postganglionic sympathetic

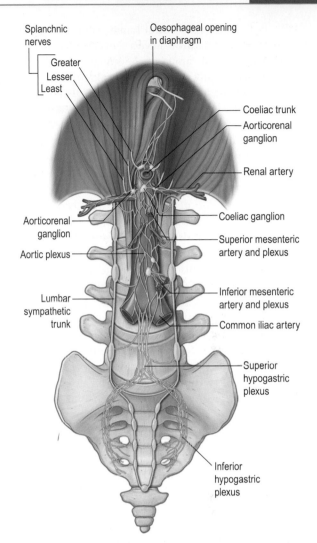

Fig. **4.70** Anterior aspect of the lumbar spine and sacrum showing the sympathetic nerves, ganglia and plexuses in the abdomen and pelvis.

neurons, they appear greyish and are referred to as a grey ramus communicans. Grey rami communicantes leave the sympathetic trunk at all levels so that every ventral ramus receives a grey ramus communicans: this is distinct from the pattern of white rami communicantes, which are found only at the T1–L2 levels. Although every ventral ramus is connected to the sympathetic trunk by a grey ramus communicans, those at T1–L2 levels have both grey and white rami communicantes. White and grey rami cannot be distinguished by the naked eye: generally, grey rami join the ventral rami slightly proximal to the origin of the white rami.

Once they join the ventral ramus, some postganglionic sympathetic neurons have a short recurrent course entering the dorsal ramus of the spinal nerve, but the majority pass distally within the ventral ramus. Postganglionic neurons use the course of the dorsal and ventral rami of the spinal nerves to reach their destinations, principally blood vessels in the tissues supplied by the ventral and dorsal rami. Some postganglionic sympathetic neurons follow the course of cutaneous branches of somatic nerves to reach sweat glands in the skin and arrectores pilorum muscles.

Because skin and deep tissues of the head are supplied by cranial nerves and not by spinal nerves, blood vessels and sweat glands of the head cannot receive their sympathetic nerve supply via grey rami communicantes: a different strategy is used to innervate them.

Running rostrally in the neck, the common, internal and external carotid arteries pass close to the cervical portion of the sympathetic trunk. Postganglionic sympathetic neurons destined to supply structures in the head leave the sympathetic trunk to join these arteries either forming distinct nerves running parallel to the artery (internal carotid nerves) or plexuses weaving around the artery: the plexuses are named according to the associated artery (internal and external carotid plexuses).

The nerves and plexuses follow their respective arteries, giving branches that follow branches of the artery. Generally, any structure in the head derives its sympathetic innervation from the sympathetic plexus on the nearest available main artery.

A modification to this rule relates to sympathetic innervation of the eye. Internal carotid nerves accompany the internal carotid artery through the carotid canal and foramen lacerum (p. 660) as far as the cavernous sinus (p. 696). Here, some sympathetic nerves leave the internal carotid artery and pass independently through the superior orbital fissure to reach the ciliary ganglion. Others leave the internal carotid artery to join the ophthalmic division of the trigeminal nerve, entering its nasociliary branch. Sympathetic nerves reach the eye either through the short ciliary branches of the ciliary ganglion or along the long ciliary branches of the nasociliary nerve: within the eye they are distributed to dilator pupillae and blood vessels.

Sympathetic nerves to thoracic, abdominal and pelvic viscera pass directly from the sympathetic trunk as splanchnic nerves: those to the heart and lungs are formed by postganglionic sympathetic axons arising from the upper four thoracic sympathetic ganglia (Fig. 4.68) forming plexuses around the bronchi and coronary arteries to reach their respective destinations.

The abdominal viscera are innervated by the greater, lesser and least splanchnic nerves with variable origins from the lower seven or eight thoracic spinal cord segments (Fig. 4.68). All three nerves enter the abdominal cavity by piercing the ipsilateral crus of the diaphragm and form dense plexuses around the coeliac and renal arteries and the abdominal aorta (Fig. 4.70).

The greater, lesser and least splanchnic nerves are formed by preganglionic sympathetic axons passing through the sympathetic trunk without synapsing. Instead, they synapse with postganglionic neurons whose cell bodies form large ganglia surrounding the coeliac and renal arteries (coeliac and aorticorenal ganglia). The axons of these postganglionic neurons reach their target organs by forming plexuses surrounding and following the arteries to abdominal viscera: abdominal organs receive their sympathetic innervation along the artery supplying it.

One modification to this pattern relates to the adrenal gland. Embryologically, the medulla of the adrenal gland has the same origin as the sympathetic nervous system: its cells are equivalent to postganglionic sympathetic neurons. The adrenal gland, therefore, is innervated directly by preganglionic neurons from the coeliac plexus and not by postganglionic neurons.

Pelvic viscera receive their sympathetic innervation from postganglionic neurons descending from the coeliac plexus along the aorta via the abdominal aortic plexus, which is supplemented by postganglionic neurons from lumbar splanchnic nerves arising from the lumbar sympathetic ganglia. At the level of L4 the aorta terminates, but its sympathetic plexus continues on to the anterior surface of L5 and the promontory of the sacrum (superior hypogastric plexus) (Fig. 4.70). Leashes of nerves derived from this plexus descend either side of the sacrum with the internal iliac arteries, joining the pelvic splanchnic nerves, forming the inferior hypogastric plexuses. From these latter plexuses, postganglionic sympathetic neurons enter the bladder, rectum and other pelvic viscera.

SECTION SUMMARY

Spinal Cord
- Continuation of the medulla oblongata of the brain to the conus medullaris at the level of L1/L2
- Long tubular structure lying within the vertebral canal
- Has cervical and lumbar enlargements
- Central H-shaped core of grey matter (cell bodies) presenting ventral (anterior) and dorsal (posterior) horns
- White matter (axons) surrounds grey

Meninges
- Three coverings: outer fibrous dura mater; middle arachnoid mater; inner pia mater
- Arachnoid and pia mater separated by subarachnoid space containing CSF
- Dural sac ends at S2 where pia mater continues as filum terminale to attach to coccyx

Arterial Supply
- From single anterior and paired posterior spinal arteries supplemented by adjacent arteries

Spinal Nerves
- 31 pairs, each pair associated with a spinal cord segment; 8 cervical (C), 12 thoracic (T), 5 lumbar (L), 5 sacral (S) and 1 coccygeal (Co)
- Formed within the vertebral canal by ventral (motor) and dorsal (sensory) roots from the spinal cord

Autonomic Nervous System
Function and organisation
- Innervates viscera, blood vessels and glands
- Preganglionic fibres pass from the CNS to synapse in a ganglion
- Postganglionic fibres pass to target organ/structure
- Has sympathetic and parasympathetic parts

Parasympathetic nervous system
- Craniosacral outflow with preganglionic fibres in cranial nerves III, VII, IX and X and S2, S3 and S4 (craniosacral outflow)
- III fibres innervate ciliary muscles and sphincter pupillae (iris) of eye
- VII fibres innervate nasal, lacrimal, submandibular and sublingual salivary glands
- IX fibres innervate parotid salivary gland
- X fibres are distributed to heart, lungs, trachea, bronchi, oesophagus, small intestine, large intestine, liver and pancreas
- S2, S3 and S4 (pelvic splanchnic nerves) are distributed to the descending and sigmoid colon, rectum and pelvic viscera

Sympathetic nervous system
- Preganglionic fibres emerge from spinal cord between T1 and L2 (thoracolumbar outflow)
- Enter sympathetic trunk/chain where they synapse with cell bodies of postganglionic fibres
- Sympathetic chain extends whole length of and is parallel to vertebral column
- Postganglionic fibres distributed to all regions and structures within body
- Some fibres (T5–T12) form splanchnic nerves which pass into abdomen

SELF-ASSESSMENT QUESTIONS

59. How many pairs of spinal nerves are there?
60. What name is given to a collection of cell bodies forming a swelling?
61. From which part of the spinal cord do motor fibres emerge?
62. At which level does the spinal cord terminate?
63. Between which meningeal layers is cerebrospinal fluid (CSF) found?
64. Which three arteries supply the spinal cord?
65. What type of nerve fibres are found in the dorsal root?
66. At which vertebral level does the dural sac end?
67. In the sympathetic nervous system what is the neurotransmitter at the synapse between pre- and postganglionic fibres?
68. Which cranial nerves contain parasympathetic fibres?
69. Between which vertebral levels is sympathetic outflow?
70. From which part of the spinal cord do sympathetic fibres emerge?
71. Apart from cranial nerves, which other nerves contain parasympathetic nerve fibres arising from the spinal cord?
72. What type of fibres does a white ramus communicans contain?

BODY SYSTEMS

LEARNING OUTCOMES

By the end of the section, you should be able to:

1. Describe and locate the surface markings of the heart and heart valves
2. Describe the arterial supply, venous drainage and conducting system of the heart
3. Describe the four chambers of the heart and the pattern of blood flow through them in the foetus and adult
4. Describe and understand the function of the foramen ovale and ductus arteriosus
5. Describe and locate the surface markings of the right and left lungs, their lobes, fissures and bronchopulmonary segments
6. Describe and understand the function of the parietal and visceral pleurae
7. Describe the components of the digestive system
8. Describe and locate the nine regions and four quadrants of the abdomen and the contents of each
9. Describe the components of the urinary system
10. Describe the components of the male and female genital systems
11. Appreciate the changing position of the uterus during pregnancy
12. Describe the components and functions of the endocrine system

CARDIOVASCULAR SYSTEM

Introduction

The cardiovascular system comprises the heart and blood vessels (arteries, veins) conveying blood to and from various body organs and tissues. Although appearing as a single organ, the heart is functionally a double muscular pump: the two parts being linked via the pulmonary circulation. The right pump receives deoxygenated blood via the superior and inferior venae cavae and coronary sinus and conveys it to the lungs, while the left pump delivers oxygenated blood to the aorta for distribution to the body.

Development

The cardiovascular system begins to develop during the third week *in utero* with all component parts (heart, blood vessels, blood cells) derived from the mesodermal germ layer. It is the first system to function in the embryo with blood beginning to flow and the first heart

beats occurring by the end of the third week. The area giving rise to the heart is initially anterior to the prochordal and neural plates; however, with rapid growth of the CNS and closure of the neural tube, the developing heart and pericardial cavity come to lie anterior to the future foregut (Fig. 4.71A). It is at this time that the single heart tube is formed, then elongates, developing alternate constrictions and expansions which give rise to the future parts of the heart.

Identifiable parts of the heart tube are the horns of the sinus venosus, pulmonary atrium, atrioventricular canal, pulmonary ventricle, bulbus cordis and truncus arteriosus, the latter being continuous with the aortic sac giving rise to the aortic arches (Fig. 4.72A). Between the fourth and seventh weeks *in utero*, the heart tube undergoes considerable change, with all except the sinus venosus becoming divided by septa, giving rise to the human four-chambered heart.

The right horn of the sinus venosus is incorporated into the right atrium forming the smooth-walled part: the left horn forms the coronary sinus. The pulmonary atrium contributes the rough-walled parts to both adult atria: the smooth wall in the left is from incorporation of the pulmonary veins. The pulmonary ventricle forms the adult left ventricle, while the adult right ventricle arises from the proximal part of the bulbus cordis: the middle part gives the outflow tracts of both ventricles and the distal part the roots of the aorta and pulmonary trunk.

The pulmonary atrium is divided by two septa. The septum primum grows from the dorsal wall of the atrium towards the endocardial cushions: just prior to fusion perforations appear in its upper part maintaining communication between right and left sides (Fig. 4.71C). At the same time, the incomplete septum secundum grows to the right of the septum primum from the ventral wall of the atrium forming the foramen ovale (Fig. 4.71C). Prior to birth, the septa remain separate allowing blood from the inferior vena cava to pass freely from the right to left atrium: after birth the septa fuse forming a complete partition between the two atria.

Endocardial cushions gradually project into the atrioventricular canal: fusion of their intermediate parts gives rise to the right (tricuspid) and left (mitral) atrioventricular openings (Fig. 4.71C).

A spiral septum develops, splitting the bulbus cordis and truncus arteriosus longitudinally, separating the aorta from the pulmonary trunk and becoming

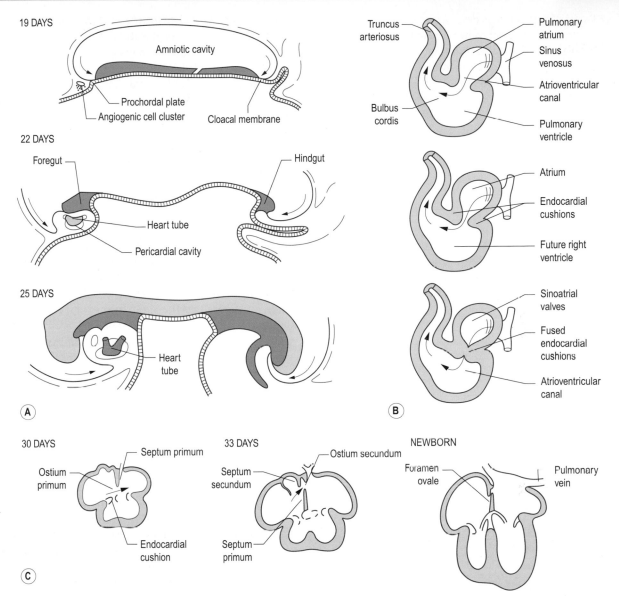

Fig. 4.71 (A) Sagittal sections through the embryo at various stages of development showing formation and migration of the heart tube; (B) heart at 4–5 weeks *in utero* showing formation of the atrioventricular canal; (C) formation of the interatrial septum.

continuous with the developing muscular interventricular septum. This division brings the aorta into communication with the left ventricle and pulmonary trunk with the right ventricle.

Heart malformations are relatively common, the majority being due to multiple factors, both genetic and environmental. Although some congenital cardiac malformations cause very little disability, others are incompatible with extrauterine life; however, many can be surgically corrected. Abnormalities may involve the interventricular system, truncus arteriosus and bulbus cordis, and formation of the valves. The heart may be normal, but its position may be on the right rather than the left (dextrocardia) and may be associated with a complete or partial transposition of the abdominal viscera (situs inversus).

A pair of aortic arches develop associated with each of the six pairs of branchial arches. The important derivatives from these arches are: the common carotid and first part of the internal carotid arteries from the third aortic arch; the aortic arch from the fourth left and proximal part of the right subclavian artery from the fourth right aortic arch; the proximal parts of the right pulmonary artery from the right sixth and similarly on the left, as well as the ductus arteriosus (shunt from the left pulmonary artery to the aorta) from the left sixth aortic arch (Fig. 4.72A).

Foetal Circulation

In the foetus, blood returns from the placenta in the umbilical vein, bypassing the liver via the ductus venosus, flowing directly into the inferior vena cava, mixing with deoxygenated blood returning from the lower limbs, abdomen and pelvis (Fig. 4.72B). From the right atrium, blood is directed towards the foramen ovale with most entering the left atrium, then to the aorta supplying the head, neck and upper limbs. Blood entering the right atrium via the superior vena cava passes to the right ventricle and pulmonary trunk. The high resistance to blood flow in the pulmonary vessels results in blood passing to the descending aorta via the ductus arteriosus. From the descending aorta, blood flows towards the placenta via the two umbilical arteries to be reoxygenated, beginning the cycle once again.

Changes After Birth

At birth, important circulatory changes occur associated with the cessation of blood flow through the placenta and functioning of the infant's lungs. The foramen ovale closes with the first good breath as the septum primum is pushed against the septum secundum (fusion occurs by the end of the first year). The ductus arteriosus closes with complete anatomical closure by age 3 months: the obliterated ductus arteriosus forms the ligamentum arteriosum (Fig. 4.72C). The umbilical vein and ductus venosus become obliterated after birth, forming the ligamentum teres in the free edge of the falciform ligament and the ligamentum venosum, respectively. The distal parts of the umbilical arteries close becoming the medial umbilical ligaments.

HEART

Surface Markings

Although the heart changes its position with respiration and posture, its position within the thorax is as follows:

a third lies to the right of the midline with the right border extending from the right third to sixth costal cartilage, approximately 1 cm to the right of the sternal border; the left border slopes from the left second intercostal space, 1 cm to the left of the sternal border to the apex of the heart in the left fifth intercostal space 9 cm from the midline (the apex can usually be palpated in the living); the inferior border sits on the central tendon of the diaphragm indicated by a shallow concavity joining the two inferior points of the right and left borders; joining the superior points of the right and left borders gives the remaining surface marking (Fig. 4.73A).

The heart itself is pyramidal having three surfaces: sternocostal (anterior), diaphragmatic (inferior) and a base (posterior). The sternocostal surface is formed mainly by the right atrium and right ventricle, separated by the atrioventricular groove. The right border of this surface is formed by the right atrium, and the left border by the left ventricle and part of the left atrium. The ventricles are separated by the anterior interventricular groove. The diaphragmatic surface is formed by the right and left ventricles, separated by the posterior interventricular groove and part of the right atrium. The base is formed by the left atrium and a small contribution from the right atrium.

Pericardium

The heart lies within the middle mediastinum (Fig. 4.73B), surrounded by a double fold of serous membrane (serous pericardium), contained within a dense connective tissue sac (fibrous pericardium) and attached to the central tendon of the diaphragm (Fig. 4.73B). The outer (parietal) layer of the serous pericardium attaches to the deep surface of the fibrous pericardium, with the deep (visceral) layer being adherent to the heart wall. The two layers are continuous at the roots of the great vessels (Fig. 4.73C) forming a closed pericardial space, which may become filled with blood or other fluid (cardiac tamponade) and interfere with normal functioning of the heart.

Structure

The greater part of the heart wall is cardiac muscle (myocardium), the serous pericardium with a thin subserous layer of connective tissue is the epicardium: the heart chambers are lined by endocardium. Within the heart wall, a connective tissue skeleton of four firmly

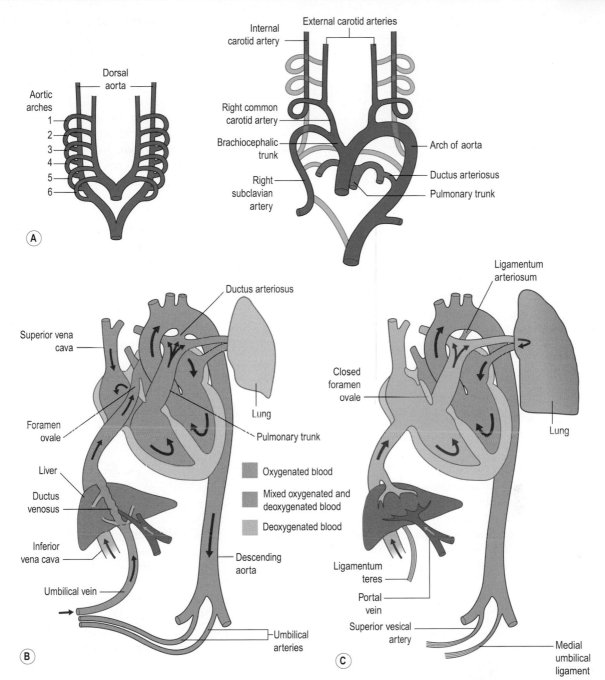

Fig. 4.72 (A) The six pairs of aortic arches and their derivatives: (B) the pattern of blood flow through the heart before (B) and after (C) birth.

connected rings of fibrous tissue provides a relatively rigid attachment for the valves and myocardium (Fig. 4.73D). The myocardium consists of two separate systems of spiralling and looping bundles of fibres, one associated with the atria and the other with the ventricles. Nowhere are the two systems continuous with each other, hence the need for a specialised atrioventricular conducting system.

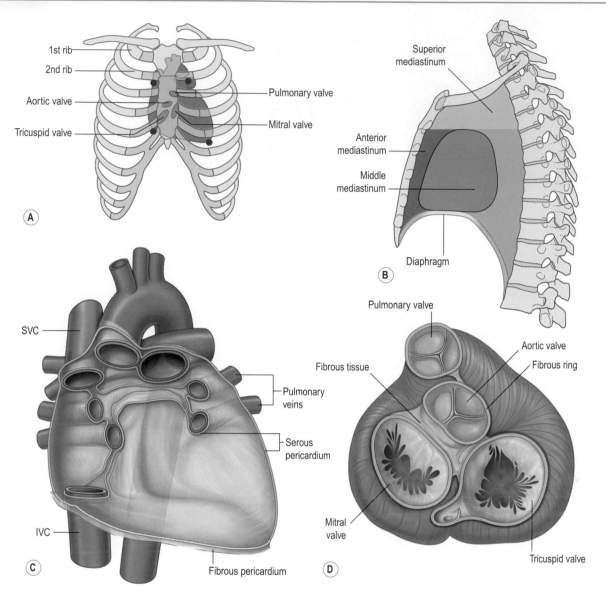

Fig. 4.73 (A) Anterior aspect of the thorax showing the position and surface markings of the heart and heart valves, with the best sites (*blue dots*) for listening to each valve sound; (B) sagittal section of the thorax showing the mediastinum and its divisions; (C) posterior aspect of the heart showing the reflection of the serous and fibrous pericardium; (D) fibrous framework of the heart supporting the heart valves.

Chambers of the Heart

The heart has four chambers: right and left atria, and right and left ventricles. The right atrium receives deoxygenated blood from the systemic circulation via the superior and inferior venae cavae and coronary sinus opening into the smooth posterior part, derived from the sinus venosus (p. 582). The rough anterior part, derived from the pulmonary atrium (p. 582), is separated from the posterior part by the crista terminalis (Fig. 4.74A): the thickenings are the musculi pectinati. The superior end of the crista terminalis surrounds the sinoatrial node. On the interatrial septum, a shallow oval depression (fossa ovalis) indicates the site of the foetal foramen ovale, which enables blood to enter

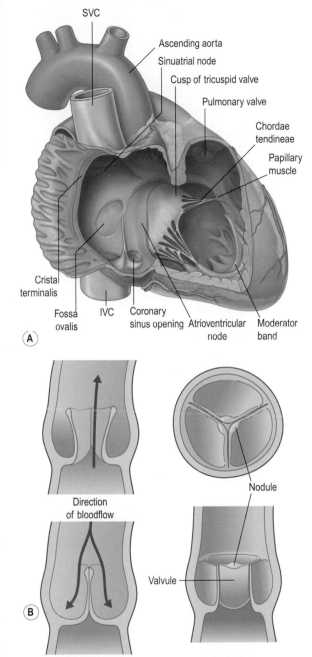

SVC

Ascending aorta

Sinuatrial node

Cusp of tricuspid valve

Pulmonary valve

Chordae tendineae

Papillary muscle

Crista terminalis

Fossa ovalis

IVC

Coronary sinus opening

Atrioventricular node

Moderator band

(A)

Direction of bloodflow

Nodule

Valvule

(B)

Fig. 4.74 (A) Right atrium and ventricle opened showing internal features of each chamber; (B) structure of the semilunar (pulmonary and aortic valves), with opening and closing of the valves being dependent on the direction of blood flow.

the left atrium bypassing the pulmonary circulation (p. 582). From the right atrium, blood enters the right ventricle via the right atrioventricular (tricuspid) valve.

The right ventricle is separated from the left by the interventricular septum. Its internal surface shows irregular muscle projections (trabeculae carnae), some of which attach to the ventricular wall along their whole length, while others are free at one end. The latter pass into the ventricular cavity becoming attached to the chordae tendineae of the cusps of the tricuspid valve by the papillary muscles (Fig. 4.74A). The moderator band lies partly free in the ventricle carrying the right branch of the atrioventricular bundle of the conducting system. The pulmonary opening leading to the pulmonary trunk is guarded by the pulmonary valve. During ventricular systole (contraction), the papillary muscles contract, pulling on the chordae tendineae, preventing the cusps of the tricuspid valve inverting and allowing blood to flow back into the right atrium.

The left atrium has two pulmonary veins opening into it on each side bringing freshly oxygenated blood from the lungs. Most of the lining is smooth due to incorporation of the terminal parts of the pulmonary veins: only the auricle develops from the pulmonary atrium of the foetus. Blood passes into the left ventricle via the left atrioventricular (mitral) valve.

The left ventricle has the thickest walls of all four chambers due to the extremely high pressures it has to generate to force blood into the systemic circulation. The wall also possesses trabeculae carnae: three papillary muscles attach to the free margins of the cusps of the mitral valve. The opening leading to the aorta is guarded by the aortic valve: above each semilunar valvule is an aortic sinus, the right and left of which give rise to the right and left coronary arteries, respectively.

The pulmonary and aortic valves each consist of three semilunar valvules attached to the vessel wall: the free border projects into the vessel lumen. In the middle of the free border, a thickened nodule assists in approximating the central areas of the edges of the valvule (Fig. 4.74B). Concavities formed by the valvules face away from the direction of blood flow so that, during ventricular systole, they lie against the vessel wall. In diastole when interventricular pressure falls, there is a tendency for blood to return to the ventricle: the valvules fill approximating their free borders preventing further blood flow (Fig. 4.74B). The surface markings of the tricuspid, mitral, pulmonary and aortic valves are shown in Fig. 4.73A, which also shows the most appropriate site for listening to each valve with a stethoscope.

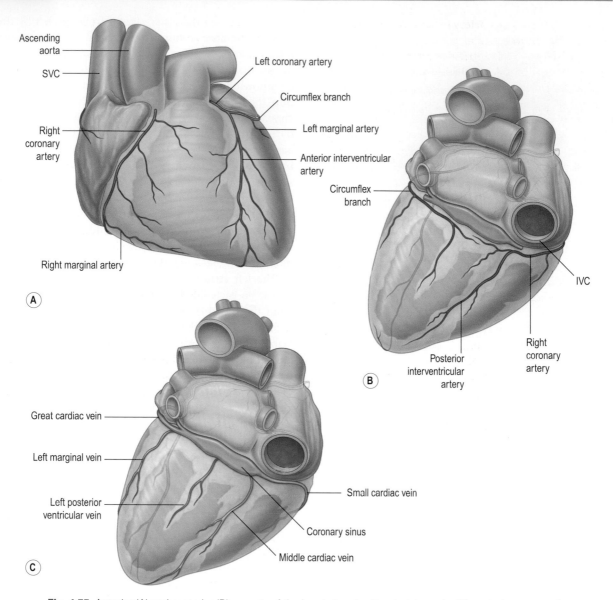

Fig. 4.75 Anterior (A) and posterior (B) aspects of the heart showing its arterial supply; (C) posterior aspect of the heart showing its venous drainage. *IVC*, Inferior vena cava; *SVC*, superior vena cava.

Blood Supply

The arterial supply to the heart is provided by the right and left coronary arteries, branches of the ascending aorta just above its origin from the left ventricle (Fig. 4.75A). The right coronary artery arises from the right aortic sinus, passing anteriorly between the pulmonary trunk and right auricle, to enter the atrioventricular groove between the right atrium and ventricle (Fig. 4.75A). It continues in the groove around the inferior

margin of the heart, giving the right marginal artery towards the posterior interventricular groove, where it anastomoses with the circumflex branch of the left coronary artery, giving the posterior interventricular artery, which runs in the posterior interventricular groove (Fig. 4.75B). The right coronary artery gives branches supplying both atria and ventricles, as well as providing the major blood supply to the conducting system. The sinoatrial node is supplied by a sinoatrial branch from the right coronary artery in 60%–70% of individuals, with the atrioventricular node artery given off close to the posterior interventricular artery, supplying the atrioventricular bundle and its branches.

The left coronary artery arises from the left aortic sinus passing anteriorly between the pulmonary trunk and left auricle towards the atrioventricular groove. Here, it divides into a circumflex branch continuing around the atrioventricular groove, giving the left marginal artery, towards the posterior of the heart anastomosing with the right coronary artery, and the anterior interventricular artery, passing in the anterior interventricular groove towards the apex of the heart, supplying both ventricles and the interventricular septum (Fig. 4.75A).

The coronary arteries and their larger branches are functional end-arteries, with the anastomoses between them not being sufficient to provide an alternative blood supply should the main artery become blocked: sudden blockage of a coronary artery or one of the large branches is almost invariably fatal. Blockage of smaller vessels leads to necrosis of the heart tissue supplied by that vessel (heart attack). Narrowing of the lumen of the coronary arteries or major branches results in a reduction in blood supply to the muscle (ischaemia) with the individual complaining of pain behind the sternum: pain often radiates down the left arm (angina pectoris).

The greater part of the venous drainage is by a system of veins draining into the coronary sinus lying in the posterior part of the atrioventricular groove and emptying into the right atrium (Fig. 4.75C): the larger veins follow the arteries. The great cardiac vein lies in the anterior interventricular groove beginning at the apex of the heart, and receives the left posterior ventricular vein and left marginal vein, forming the coronary sinus. Close to its termination, the coronary sinus is joined by the small and middle cardiac veins (Fig. 4.75C). In addition, two or three anterior cardiac veins from the surface of the right ventricle drain directly into the right atrium, and a number of very small veins drain directly into the atria from the myocardium (venae cordae minimae).

Conducting System

The conducting system consists of specialised cardiac muscle fibres arranged as groups of cells (nodes) or bundles of fibres responsible for the rhythmic initiation and propagation of the impulse associated with the heart beat and coordinated contraction of the atria and ventricles. Contraction is initiated at the sinoatrial node in the right atrium: the impulse spreads through the two atria to the atrioventricular node (Fig. 4.76A) in the interatrial septum close to the opening of the coronary sinus. The atrioventricular node passes the impulse to the atrioventricular bundle in the interventricular septum: within the septum, the bundle divides into right and left bundle branches. The right bundle branch runs towards the apex of the heart and enters the moderator (septomarginal) band, supplying the papillary muscles, and then divides into fine (Purkinje) fibres supplying the remainder of the right ventricle. The left bundle branch divides into two or more strands as it passes towards the apex of the heart. If the atrioventricular bundle is interrupted (lack of blood supply) total heart block results, with the ventricles beating slowly and rhythmically at their own rate independent of the atria, which continue to contract at a rate determined by the sinoatrial node.

The nerve supply is from both sympathetic and parasympathetic parts of the ANS reaching the sinoatrial node via cardiac plexuses of nerves associated with the arch of the aorta and bifurcation of the trachea. The cell bodies of sympathetic fibres are in the first four or five thoracic spinal cord segments, reaching the heart by the superior and middle cervical sympathetic ganglia: parasympathetic fibres come from the vagus. Increased sympathetic stimulation increases heart rate, while increased parasympathetic stimulation slows heart rate.

Great Vessels

The great vessels (Fig. 4.76B) connect the heart to the pulmonary and systemic circulations. The superior vena cava carries blood from the thorax, upper limbs, head and neck, and the inferior vena cava from the abdomen, pelvis and lower limbs. The superior vena cava is formed by the union of the left and right brachiocephalic veins behind the first costal cartilage. The inferior vena cava passes through the central tendon of the diaphragm, almost immediately entering the right atrium.

The pulmonary trunk divides into right and left pulmonary arteries just inferior to the sternal angle and pass towards the lung root. Close to the bifurcation, the left pulmonary artery is joined to the inferior aspect of the aortic arch by the ligamentum arteriosum (remnant of the foetal ductus arteriosus) (p. 584).

The aorta leaves the left ventricle passing posterosuperiorly to the right as far as the level of the sternal angle (ascending aorta), curving over the anterior aspect of the vertebral column at T4 (aortic arch) to pass inferiorly

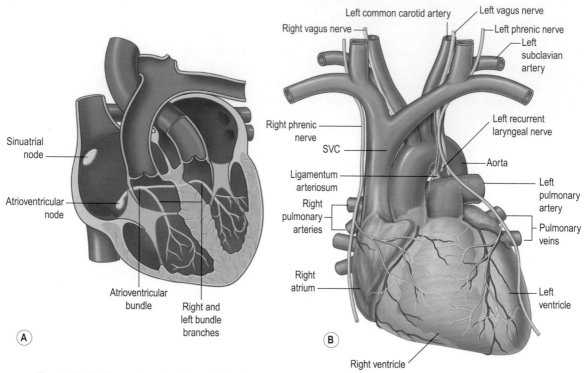

Fig. 4.76 (A) Coronal section through the heart showing the conducting system; (B) anterior aspect of the heart, great vessels and related nerves. *SVC*, Superior vena cava.

through the thorax anterior to the vertebral column (descending aorta). The aorta passes posterior to the diaphragm at the level of T12 to enter the abdomen.

RESPIRATORY SYSTEM

Introduction

The respiratory system is concerned with the exchange of gases (oxygen and carbon dioxide) between air in the lungs and blood in the capillaries of the pulmonary circulation: this is referred to as external respiration. (Internal respiration occurs between blood in the systemic capillaries and cells and tissues of body organs.) In inspiration, muscle action increases the diameters of the thorax, with pressures in the pleural cavity and lung spaces becoming less than that of the atmosphere: the lungs expand and air rushes in. Expiration, unless forced, is relatively passive due to recoil of the lungs, muscular relaxation and atmospheric pressure acting on the chest wall. The maximum amount of air that can be exhaled (vital capacity) following the deepest inspiration is 3000/3500 mL (females/males): the amount of air breathed in and out (tidal volume) during quiet respiration is 500 mL. The total lung surface area available for respiratory exchange is approximately 70 m².

Rigid or semirigid walls in the nasal cavity, pharynx, larynx, trachea and larger bronchi keep the upper airways open at all times. The soft, flexible, elastic lungs respond passively to changes in thoracic diameter, having more room for expansion laterally, inferiorly and anteriorly, where chest enlargement is not limited, than in apical, upper anterior and posterior mediastinal regions. Respiration predominantly occurs in the peripheral (superficial) lung zone, most immediately expanded by thoracic enlargement, being some 5 mm deep in quiet respiration and up to 30 mm in forced respiration.

Development

During the fourth week of development, the respiratory system (larynx, trachea, bronchi and lungs) appears as an outgrowth from the anterior wall of the primitive pharynx (Fig. 4.77A): the epithelium and glands are of endodermal origin, while the connective tissue and

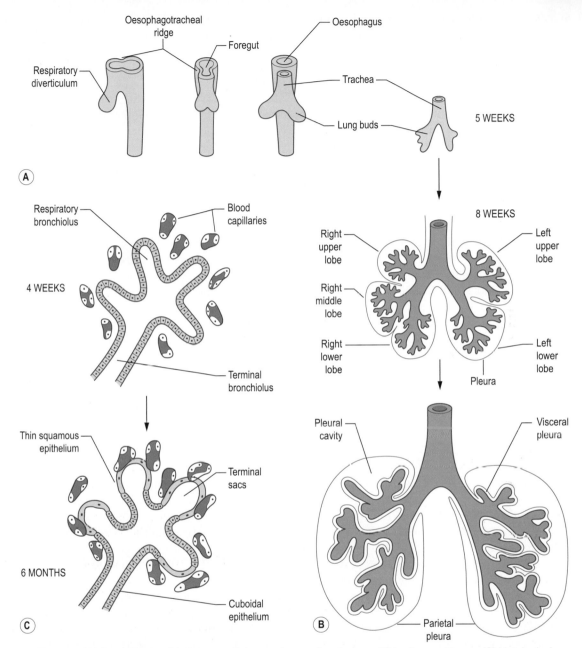

Fig. 4.77 (A) Stages in the development of the respiratory diverticulum; (B) trachea and lungs; (C) histological and functional development of the lungs.

muscular components are derived from splanchnic mesoderm surrounding the developing foregut. With expansion of the distal end of the respiratory diverticulum to form the lung buds, a septum forms dividing the foregut into the oesophagus and trachea, and the lung buds (Fig. 4.77A).

The developing lung buds expand growing into the primitive pleural cavities, which become separated from the pericardial and peritoneal cavities. The parietal and visceral pleura develop from mesoderm lining the body wall and covering the outside of the lungs, respectively: they are continuous at the lung root. During the fifth week *in utero*, the right lung bud divides into three main bronchi and the left lung bud into two, foreshadowing the adult pattern (Fig. 4.77B). Secondary bronchi undergo progressive branching, giving rise to 10 segmental bronchi in each lung, representing the future bronchopulmonary segments, each surrounded by mesenchymal tissue.

The main bronchi continue to divide repeatedly until the end of the sixth month *in utero* when there have been approximately 17 divisions (Fig. 4.77B): an additional six divisions occur postnatally. Until the seventh month bronchioles continue to divide into smaller and smaller canals as the vascular supply to the lungs increases. However, respiration is not possible until cells of the respiratory bronchioles become flat and thin (Fig. 4.77C). By the seventh month, an adequate gas exchange is possible so that premature infants are capable of surviving. There is considerable growth of the lungs, both of respiratory bronchioles and alveoli, after birth.

In addition to alveolar epithelial cells surrounding the capillaries, other cells produce surfactant, lowering surface tension at the air–blood barrier. Prior to birth, the lungs are filled with fluid, but with the beginning of respiration, most fluid is rapidly resorbed by the blood and lymphatic capillaries: a small amount is expelled during parturition. However, the surfactant remains in the lungs as a thin lining on the alveolar cell membrane.

UPPER RESPIRATORY TRACT

The upper respiratory tract (Fig. 4.78A) is lined by pseudostratified, ciliated, columnar respiratory epithelium, beneath which lies lymphoid tissue, further mucous and serous glands and a rich vascular plexus, hence the cleansing, warming and moistening of the inspired air that occur. In forced respiration or respiratory distress, the oral cavity also becomes part of the upper respiratory tract, but the function of the respiratory epithelium is lost.

Nasal Cavity

This communicates anteriorly with the external environment, by the nostrils (nares) of the largely cartilaginous external nose, and posteriorly with the nasopharynx, via the choanae, as well as with paranasal sinuses, which, although they have no respiratory function, are important in vocalisation. The nasal septum divides the cavity into two parts, each having a roof, floor, lateral and medial walls, with the latter being the nasal septum. Each irregular lateral wall has inferomedial projections

(superior, middle and inferior conchae) (Fig. 4.78B) causing turbulence of the inspired air: its thick lining may swell due to infection, blocking the nasal cavity.

Pharynx

Fibromuscular tube extending from the base of the skull to the cricoid cartilage at the level of C6, lying posterior to and communicating with the nasal cavity (nasopharynx), oral cavity (oropharynx) and larynx (laryngopharynx) (Fig. 4.78C). Its inner epithelial lining (respiratory in the nasopharynx, stratified squamous in the oropharynx and laryngopharynx) is separated from an incomplete muscular layer (constrictor muscles) by the pharyngobasilar fascia: it is surrounded by the buccopharyngeal membrane. The nasopharynx is part of the respiratory system, the oropharynx is part of both the respiratory and digestive systems, and the laryngopharynx is part of the digestive system. During swallowing, respiration is temporarily suspended as the nasopharynx is closed by raising the soft palate and partly closing the laryngeal inlet by the epiglottis as the bolus of food passes towards the oesophagus.

Larynx

The framework of cartilages forming the larynx is maintained by membranes and muscles (Fig. 4.79A), with the muscles primarily acting as sphincters to protect the lower respiratory tract or increase intrathoracic pressure, as well as move the vocal ligaments during respiration and phonation. The larynx narrows at the vestibular folds, widens between the vestibular and vocal folds and narrows again at the vocal folds (rima glottidis). Below the vocal folds, the larynx again widens, becoming continuous with the trachea (Fig. 4.79B).

Trachea and Principal Bronchi

The trachea extends from the cricoid cartilage to its bifurcation into right and left main bronchi (Fig. 4.79C) at the level of T4/T5: in full inspiration the bifurcation (carina) extends as low as T6. The fibromembranous trachea and principal bronchi are reinforced by incomplete cartilage rings, completed posteriorly by smooth muscle (trachealis). The right bronchus is shorter, straighter, larger and a more direct continuation of the trachea than the longer narrower left bronchus: inhaled foreign bodies tend to pass into the right lung. The principal bronchi divide into secondary bronchi, one for each lobe of the lung, which in turn divide into tertiary bronchi, one for each bronchopulmonary segment.

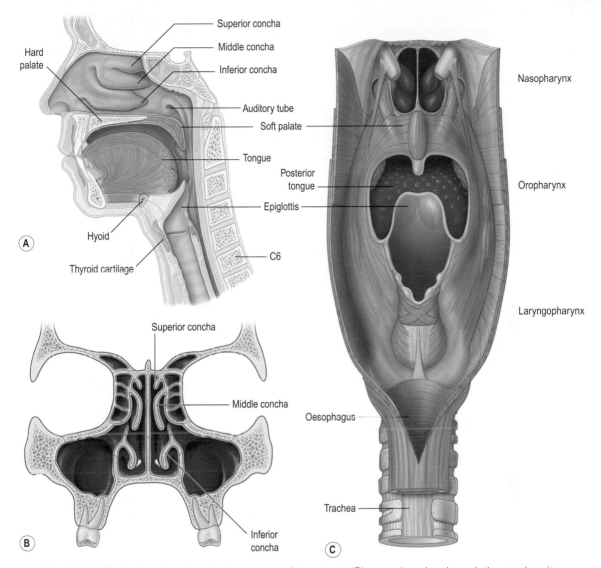

Fig. 4.78 (A) Sagittal section through the upper respiratory tract; (B) coronal section through the nasal cavity showing the conchae; (C) the pharynx opened and viewed posteriorly showing the nasopharynx, oropharynx and laryngopharynx.

LUNGS AND PLEURA

Lungs

Occupying most of the space in the thoracic cavity, each lung lies free within its pleural cavity attached only by its root to the mediastinum. Conforming to the outline of the thoracic cage, each lung has an apex, base, costal and mediastinal surfaces, and anterior, inferior and posterior borders (Fig. 4.80). The anterior border is sharp, with that of the left lung having a shallow (cardiac) notch below which is the lingula: the posterior border is rounded lying in the paravertebral gutter. The shorter, wider and heavier right lung is divided into three lobes (superior, middle and inferior) by two fissures (oblique and horizontal): the smaller left lung has only two lobes (superior (including lingula) and inferior) separated by the oblique fissure (Fig. 4.80).

Due to the obliquity of the thoracic inlet the rounded apex of the lung projects into the neck: the concave

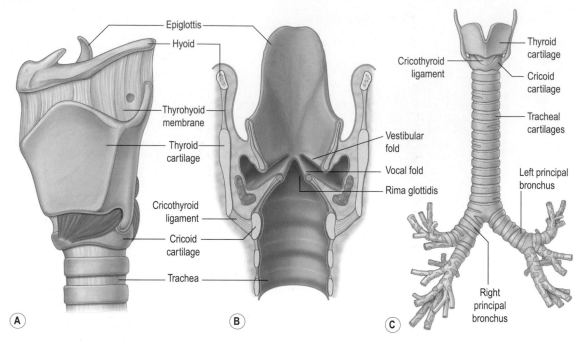

Fig. 4.79 (A) Components of the larynx; (B) coronal section through the larynx viewed posteriorly showing the position of the vestibular and vocal folds (cords); (C) anterior aspect of the trachea and principal bronchi.

base is separated from the liver (on the right) and liver, spleen and stomach (on the left) by the diaphragm. The medial surface of the right lung is related to the right atrium, oesophagus, azygos vein, trachea, superior vena cava and subclavian artery, with that of the left lung being related to the left ventricle, oesophagus, arch and descending aorta, subclavian and common carotid arteries (Fig. 4.80).

The lung root is the only part not covered with pleura, being the entry and exit site for structures entering and leaving the lung (Fig. 4.80): bronchus (posterior), pulmonary artery (anterosuperior) and pulmonary veins (anteroinferior). Also present are bronchial vessels (lying close to the bronchi) and lymph nodes. An inferior extension of pleura surrounding the lung root forms the pulmonary ligament. Passing anterior to the lung root is the phrenic nerve and anterior pulmonary plexus, and posterior is the vagus and posterior pulmonary plexus.

Pleura

Each lung is surrounded by a pleural sac having two serous membranous layers (visceral and parietal pleura) continuous with each other at the lung root/hilum

(Fig. 4.81). The visceral pleura is firmly adherent to the lung tissue and extends deep into the fissures, while the parietal pleura lines the thoracic wall (costal pleura), covers the superior surface of the diaphragm (diaphragmatic pleura) and mediastinum (mediastinal pleura). At the thoracic inlet, the parietal pleura arches over the apex of the lung (cervical pleura) reinforced superiorly by dense connective tissue (suprapleural membrane).

The potential space (pleural cavity) between the visceral and parietal pleurae contains a thin film of fluid (surfactant) to reduce friction during movement. Pleural inflammation elicits pain and may give rise to audible and palpable friction (crepitus). Excess fluid within the pleural cavity (hydrothorax) produces a dullness on percussion and reduction in breath sounds, while air (pneumothorax) produces a resonance and absence of breath sounds.

The parietal pleura is supplied with blood from the intercostal and internal thoracic arteries, with venous drainage being to corresponding veins, lymphatics pass to nodes on the deep aspect of the chest wall and innervation is by intercostal (mediastinal pleura) and phrenic (diaphragmatic pleura) nerves. Pain may be referred to the thoracic and/or abdominal walls or neck

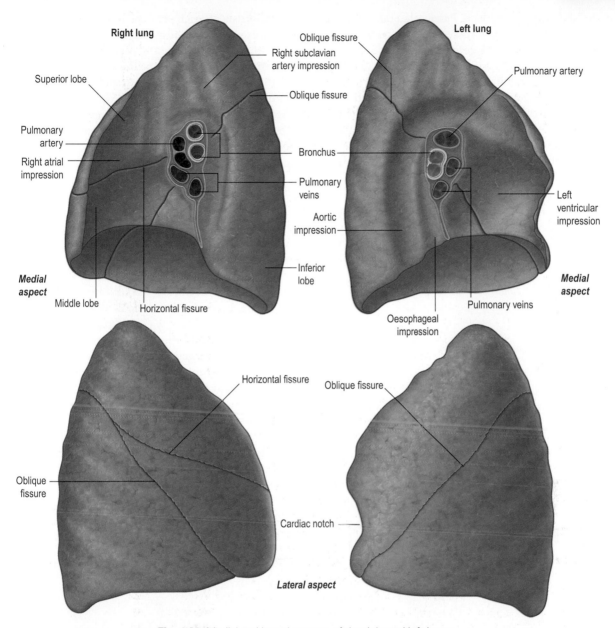

Fig. 4.80 Medial and lateral aspects of the right and left lungs.

and shoulder (mediastinal pleura). The visceral pleura is supplied by bronchial arteries, with its venous and lymphatic drainage being similar to that of the lung: innervation is from the ANS and is not sensitive to pain.

Surface Markings

The surface markings of the lungs and pleura are important in any physical examination of the chest (Fig.

4.82). On both sides, the parietal pleura and lung surface markings run from the apex 3 cm above the medial one-third of the clavicle, passing deep to the sternoclavicular joint to the sternal angle close to the midline. On the right, both parietal pleura and lung surface markings run to the sixth costal cartilage then diverge, while on the left the pleura and lung surface markings deviate to the left 3 cm at the fourth costal cartilage before passing to the sixth costal cartilage. Passing laterally, the inferior border of each lung crosses the mid-clavicular line at the sixth costal cartilage and parietal pleura at the eighth rib. In the mid-axillary line, the lungs lie at the eighth rib and parietal pleura at the 10th: posteriorly, the lungs cross the 10th rib and parietal pleura at the 12th rib, both 5 cm from the midline. Posteriorly, the inferior border of parietal pleura on each side dips below the costal margin. The posterior borders of both lung and parietal pleura pass superiorly towards the apex of the lung.

As the lungs do not extend as far inferiorly as the parietal pleura, a potential space (costodiaphragmatic recess) exists on each side: the lung does not enter this recess except in deep respiration.

With the arm abducted 90 degrees, the oblique fissure corresponds to a line running from the spinous process of T3 (level with the spine of the scapula) along the medial border of the scapula as far as the mid-axillary line and then anteriorly along the sixth rib and costal cartilage. The horizontal fissure of the right lung runs laterally along the inferior margin of the fourth costal cartilage and rib, meeting the oblique fissure in the mid-axillary line.

Bronchopulmonary Segments

Each bronchopulmonary segment is functionally independent and can be defined radiographically and often removed surgically. Their location and relation to the relevant tertiary bronchus are important when drainage of a particular lung segment is required. Within a bronchopulmonary segment, tertiary bronchi repeatedly subdivide, becoming bronchioles when cartilage is no longer present in their walls. Bronchioles further subdivide, eventually becoming distributed as alveoli where respiratory exchange occurs.

In the right lung, the superior lobe bronchus arises from the main bronchus 2.5 cm from the carina, and soon divides into tertiary segmental bronchi (apical, posterior and anterior) passing to similarly named bronchopulmonary segments in the superior lobe (Fig. 4.83). Five centimetres from the carina, the main bronchus divides into middle and inferior lobe bronchi, passing

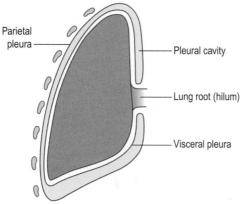

Fig. 4.81 Parietal and visceral pleura covering the lungs, also showing formation of the pleural cavity.

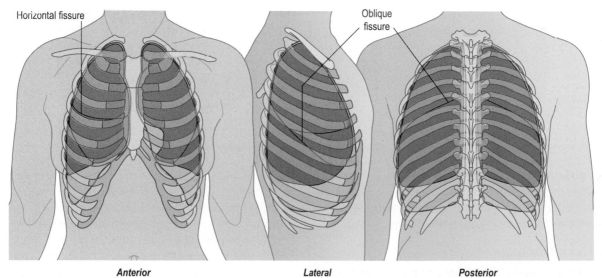

Anterior   *Lateral*   *Posterior*

Fig. 4.82 Surface markings of the lungs (and visceral pleura) and fissures (—): parietal pleura (*shaded*).

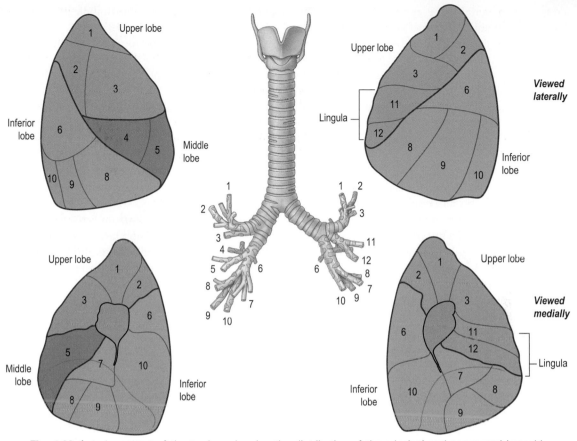

Fig. 4.83 Anterior aspect of the trachea showing the distribution of the principal and segmental bronchi. Bronchopulmonary segments: (1) apical, (2) posterior, (3) anterior, (4) lateral, (5) medial, (6) apical basal, (7) medial basal, (8) anterior basal, (9) lateral basal, (10) posterior basal, (11) superior and (12) inferior.

to the middle and inferior lobes of the lung, respectively. The middle lobe bronchus divides into lateral and medial segmental bronchi, supplying corresponding bronchopulmonary segments in the middle lobe: the inferior lobe bronchus gives the apical basal segmental bronchus opposite the origin of the middle lobe bronchus, and then divides into the medial basal, anterior basal, lateral basal and posterior basal segmental bronchi (Fig. 4.83).

In the left lung, the superior lobe bronchus arises 4–5 cm from the carina then divides into superior and inferior (lingular) parts supplying the superior lobe and lingula, respectively (Fig. 4.83). The superior division gives three segmental bronchi (apical, posterior and anterior) passing to similarly named bronchopulmonary segments. The lingular division gives superior and inferior segmental bronchi. (The lingula of the left lung is comparable to the middle lobe of the right lung.) The inferior

lobe bronchus continues for another 1.5 cm before giving rise to the apical basal segmental bronchus, and then divides into the medial basal, anterior basal, lateral basal and posterior basal segmental bronchi (Fig. 4.83).

It should be noted that variations in the pattern of branching of tertiary bronchi have been observed, giving rise to fewer bronchopulmonary segments in either lung than described above.

DIGESTIVE SYSTEM

Introduction

The digestive tract is essentially a long tube extending from the oral cavity to the anus: it comprises the mouth, pharynx, oesophagus, stomach, small and large intestines, rectum and anal canal. Ingested food is broken down, some of which is absorbed through the wall of the digestive tract, with indigestible material being excreted. It has a moist epithelial lining containing numerous glands secreting either mucous or digestive enzymes: some enzymes are produced by associated organs (salivary glands, liver and pancreas). In specific regions, the epithelium has a specialised surface for absorption of simple chemical compounds. Relatively thick internal circular and external longitudinal muscle layers surround the epithelium keeping the mixed food and enzymes moving along the tract (peristalsis).

Development

The primitive gut (foregut, midgut and hindgut) forms during the fourth week *in utero* resulting from lateral folding of the embryo and incorporation of the dorsal part of the yolk sac (see Fig. 1.5): the rest of the yolk sac and allantois remain outside the embryo. Endoderm of the primitive gut gives rise to the epithelial lining of most of the digestive tract and its derivatives (biliary system, parenchyma of the liver and pancreas), except at the cranial and caudal extremities where it is derived from ectoderm of the stomodeum and proctodeum, respectively. The splanchnic mesoderm surrounding the primitive gut gives rise to the muscular and connective tissue (peritoneal) components.

The foregut gives rise to the oesophagus, trachea and lung buds (Fig. 4.77A), stomach, proximal duodenum, liver and biliary system, and pancreas; the midgut forms the primary intestinal loop giving rise to the distal duodenum, jejunum, ileum, caecum, vermiform appendix, ascending and proximal transverse colon; the hindgut forms the distal transverse, descending and sigmoid colon, rectum and proximal part of the anal canal: the distal part of the anal canal is derived from the proctodeum.

The stomach appears as a dilation beyond the oesophagus in the fourth week of development. Due to differential growth, it rotates 90-degree clockwise about its long axis acquiring greater and lesser curvatures: the dorsal mesentery is carried to the left forming the omental bursa and lesser sac behind the stomach (Fig. 4.84A).

The liver, gall bladder and biliary system appear as an outgrowth (liver bud) from the proximal duodenum during the fourth week (Fig. 4.84B), dividing into two parts, enlarging and growing between layers of the ventral mesentery. The liver grows rapidly, filling most of the abdominal cavity by the ninth week: part of the liver (bare area) outgrows the ventral mesentery, coming to lie in direct contact with the diaphragm (Fig. 4.84B).

Elongation of the midgut forms the primary intestinal loop, which, because of rapid growth of the liver

and kidneys, projects into the umbilical cord during the sixth to tenth weeks (Fig. 4.84B).

The endoderm of the hindgut, as well as giving rise to the remainder of the digestive tract, also forms the internal lining of the bladder and urethra. The terminal part of the hindgut is an endoderm-lined cavity (cloaca) in direct contact with the surface ectoderm at the cloacal membrane. The urorectal septum divides the cloaca into anterior (urogenital) and posterior (anorectal) parts, with the cloacal membrane dividing into urogenital (anterior) and anal (posterior) membranes (Fig. 4.84C). The anal membrane becomes surrounded by mesenchymal swellings so that, at 8 weeks, it is at the deepest part of the proctodeum (anal pit). During the ninth week, the anal membrane ruptures allowing communication between the rectum and the outside (Fig. 4.84C). The proximal part of the anal canal is derived from endoderm of the hindgut and distal part from ectoderm.

Oral Cavity

Divided into the vestibule between the lips and cheeks externally and gums and teeth internally, it receives secretions of the parotid salivary gland, and the oral cavity proper (mouth) internal to the teeth (Fig. 4.85A). The hard and soft palates form the roof of the mouth, and mylohyoid the floor: it contains the tongue and receives secretions from the submandibular and sublingual salivary glands. The mouth is continuous posteriorly with the oropharynx via the oropharyngeal isthmus.

The highly mobile upper and lower lips help keep saliva and food within the mouth, as well as changing their shape to produce different sounds in speech (phonation). The cheek has buccinator as the principal muscle acting to prevent food from accumulating in the vestibule. The lining of the cheek is continuous with that covering the gums (gingivae) and, in turn, is continuous with the periosteum lining the alveolar sockets.

Teeth

Each tooth has a crown above and root below the gum margin (Fig. 4.85B), with the greater part formed by dentine covered by enamel over the crown and cementum over the root: within the dentine is the pulp cavity containing vessels and nerves. Each tooth is anchored to the surrounding alveolar bone by the periodontal membrane/ligament (Fig. 4.85B). The teeth of the maxilla are innervated by anterior, middle and posterior superior

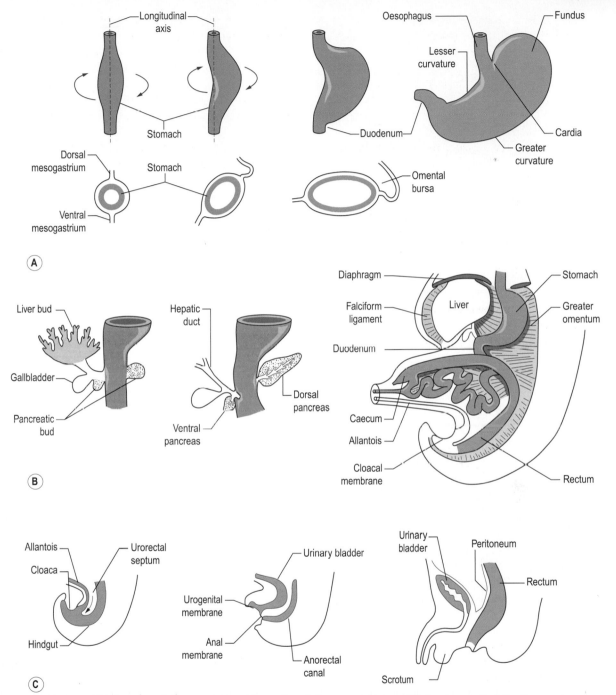

Fig. 4.84 (A) Rotation of the stomach and formation of the omental bursa; (B) development of the liver and pancreas, together with herniation of the midgut; (C) development of the urinary bladder and anorectal canal.

alveolar nerves from the maxillary division of the trigeminal nerve, and those of the mandible by the inferior alveolar nerve from the mandibular division of the trigeminal nerve. Superior and inferior alveolar arteries from the maxillary artery accompany the nerves.

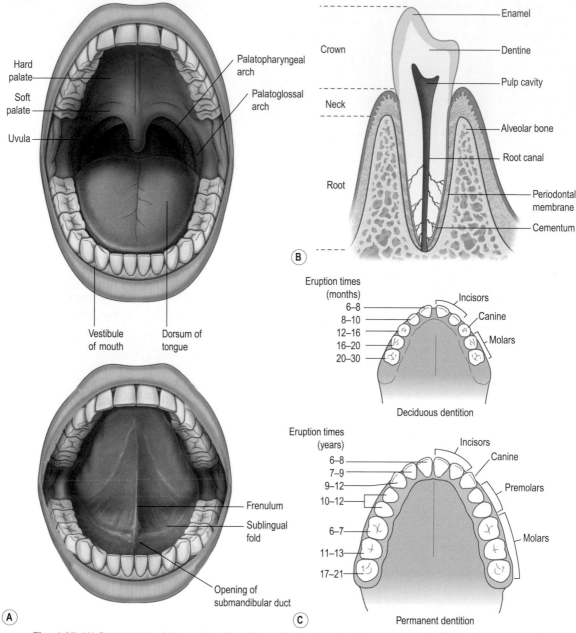

Fig. 4.85 (A) Boundaries of the oral cavity; (B) longitudinal section through a tooth; (C) the deciduous and permanent dentition, together with average eruption times for each tooth.

There are two sets of teeth (deciduous and permanent) whose components (incisor, canine, premolar and molar) erupt at specific times (Fig. 4.85C). The deciduous dentition begins to appear by 6 months and is completed by eruption of the second molar at 2 years. From age 6, the deciduous dentition is gradually replaced by the permanent dentition, which is usually complete by age 20:

the third molar may remain unerupted. As permanent teeth are lost, the surrounding alveolar bone gradually resorbs, reducing the depth of the mandible (p. 665).

Tongue

The mobile muscular tongue is divided into anterior two-thirds (within the mouth) and posterior one-third (in the oropharynx) by the sulcus terminalis with the foramen caecum (origin of the thyroglossal duct which gave rise to the thyroid) at the apex (Fig. 4.86A): the upper surface of the tongue is the dorsum. The extrinsic muscles (genioglossus, hyoglossus, styloglossus and palatoglossus) attach the tongue to the skull and mandible, and are responsible for changing its position: the intrinsic muscles have no bony attachment and change its shape. All except palatoglossus are supplied by the hypoglossal nerve.

The roughness of the anterior part is due to filiform (white conical) and fungiform (red globular) papillae under the mucous membrane. Anterior to the sulcus terminalis are 8–12 circumvallate papillae, the walls of which contain numerous taste buds. The nodular appearance of the posterior part is due to the underlying lingual tonsil. The mucous membrane is richly innervated: the anterior two-thirds by the lingual nerve of the mandibular division of the trigeminal nerve (general sensation) and chorda tympani of the facial nerve (taste); and the posterior one-third, including the circumvallate papillae, by the glossopharyngeal nerve for both general sensation and taste.

Palate

The palate is divided into the larger anterior hard palate, formed by the maxilla and palatine bones, which gives attachment posteriorly to the soft mobile (muscular) palate (Fig. 4.85A). During swallowing and phonation, the soft palate tenses and elevates, closing off the nasopharynx.

Pharynx and Oesophagus

Extending from the base of the skull to the level of the cricoid cartilage at C6, the pharynx consists of three overlapping, circularly arranged muscles (superior, middle and inferior constrictor) and three longitudinal muscles (stylopharyngeus, palatopharyngeus and salpingopharyngeus). It communicates with the nasal cavity, mouth and larynx anteriorly: only the oropharynx and laryngopharynx are involved in the passage of the bolus of food from the mouth to the oesophagus.

The oesophagus begins at the level of the cricoid cartilage (C6), descending through the thorax posterior to the trachea and left atrium, passing through the diaphragm at the level of T10 to the left of the midline, entering the cardiac region of the stomach (Fig. 4.86B). The oesophagus is constricted at its origin, at the level of T4/T5 where the arch of the aorta and left bronchus cross anteriorly, and where it pierces the diaphragm: these are the commonest sites of stricture and cancer.

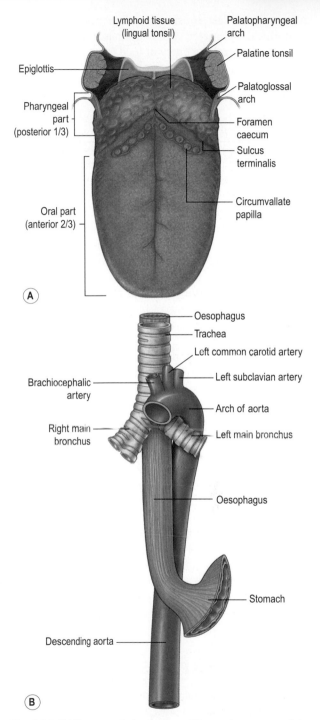

Fig. 4.86 (A) Dorsum of the tongue; (B) anterior aspect of the oesophagus showing its relations in the thorax.

Although the last constriction does not constitute an anatomical sphincter, it is an important functional sphincter controlling entry of food into the stomach, as well as preventing reflux of stomach contents.

Chewing and Swallowing

Chewing is the process of breaking food into smaller parts, during which time digestion begins by the action of salivary enzymes. Chewing is achieved by alternate protraction and retraction of the mandible on each side coupled with elevation on the side of protraction (p. 602). The tongue and buccinator keep food between the teeth, preventing it from accumulating in the mouth or vestibule, respectively: the resulting mass is then formed into a bolus in preparation for swallowing.

In the voluntary stage of swallowing, the bolus is pushed posteriorly, between the tongue and hard palate, towards the oropharynx: the floor of the mouth is raised by contraction of mylohyoid, which also elevates the hyoid. At the same time, the soft palate tenses and is elevated, preventing food from entering the nasopharynx and nasal cavity. When the bolus has passed the palatoglossal folds/arches, they are brought together, closing the oropharyngeal isthmus preventing food returning to the mouth: contraction of the palatoglossal muscles helps push the bolus into the oropharynx.

Once the bolus makes contact with the pharyngeal wall, the swallowing reflex is initiated. Respiration is temporarily suspended by closure of the nasopharynx above and laryngeal inlet below as the bolus is propelled towards the oesophagus by serial contractions (peristalsis) of the constrictor muscles. Simultaneous contraction of the longitudinal pharyngeal muscles pulls the laryngeal walls superomedially, elevating the larynx and pharynx to receive the bolus: in this way, the bolus is forced into the oesophagus.

When swallowing fluids, the tongue forms a longitudinal midline furrow along which fluid flows, passing either side of the epiglottis into the piriform fossae, entering the oesophagus.

ABDOMEN AND PELVIS

The greater part of the remainder of the digestive tract lies within the abdomen and pelvis.

Stomach

Lying free within the abdominal cavity, the stomach is anchored only at its proximal and distal ends. It is divided into the fundus above the oesophageal opening, body below the fundus and pylorus separated from the body by the angular notch (incisura angularis) (Fig. 4.87A): the pyloric antrum lies next to the body, with the thickened pyloric sphincter controlling the passage of gastric contents into the duodenum. The muscular wall of the stomach contains an internal oblique layer in addition to the longitudinal and circular layers: its interior is thrown into a series of longitudinal folds (rugae).

The stomach produces 2500 mL of secretions per day: it has a rich blood supply from the coeliac trunk (artery of the foregut) with blood draining into the portal vein and then to the liver.

Small Intestine

The C-shaped duodenum (first part of small intestine) (Fig. 4.87B) lies directly on the posterior abdominal wall and overlies the vertebral column: it has a thick muscular wall with the interior thrown into irregular circular folds. The duodenum receives secretions from both the pancreas (pancreatic juice for digestion of proteins, fats and carbohydrates) and the liver (bile for digestion of fats) via the gall bladder: the two ducts have a common site of entry (major duodenal papilla).

The jejunum and ileum (remainder of the small intestine) are relatively mobile, filling any available space in the abdominopelvic cavity, being the most common parts of the digestive tract found within hernias (p. 542). The jejunum and ileum are fixed to the posterior abdominal wall at the duodenojejunal and ileocaecal junctions, respectively. The blood supply to the small intestine, beyond the first part of the duodenum, as far as the transverse colon of the large intestine, is by branches from the superior mesenteric artery (artery of the midgut).

Large Intestine

The caecum (first part of the large intestine) is a blind-ending pouch below the ileocaecal junction and has the appendix attached to its medial aspect (Fig. 4.87C). The extremely mobile appendix is of variable length (3–20 cm) and may be found lying behind the caecum or over the pelvic brim.

The ascending colon lies directly on muscles of the posterior abdominal wall on the right side from the caecum to just inferior to the liver: it bends sharply becoming the transverse colon. The transverse colon is suspended from the posterior abdominal wall inferior

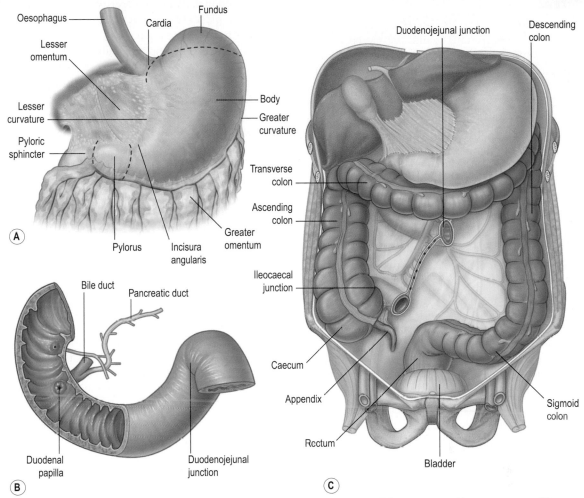

Fig. 4.87 (A) Anterior aspect of the stomach showing the attachments of the greater and lesser omenta; (B) duodenum and its relation to the bile and pancreatic ducts; (C) large intestine within the abdomen.

and posterior to the stomach: on reaching the spleen it bends sharply inferiorly becoming the descending colon. The descending colon also lies directly on the posterior abdominal wall, descending as far as the pelvic brim (Fig. 4.87C).

The sigmoid colon joins the descending colon to the rectum, which begins at the level of the third sacral vertebra and follows the curve of the distal sacrum and coccyx to the pelvic floor, where it is supported by levator ani. The rectum pierces the pelvic floor, becoming the anal canal at the anorectal junction: the anal canal extends posteroinferiorly ending at the anus.

From partway along the transverse colon to halfway along the anal canal, the blood supply to the digestive tract is from branches of the inferior mesenteric artery (artery of the hindgut): the distal half of the anal canal is supplied by branches from the internal iliac artery.

Venous drainage of the digestive tract below the diaphragm to halfway along the anal canal is via the portal vein and then to the liver. The transition in the anal canal between systemic and portal drainage is the site of a portosystemic anastomosis: a similar arrangement exists in the distal third of the oesophagus. In cases of portal hypertension, venous vessels at the sites of these anastomoses may distend (varices) and rupture causing bleeding: in the anal canal the varices are known as haemorrhoids.

Pancreas

Both an endocrine (insulin secretion) and exocrine (pancreatic juice secretion) gland, the pancreas has a rich blood supply as well as a substantial duct system. Lying obliquely across the posterior abdominal wall at the level of L1, it is divided into head, neck, body and tail (Fig. 4.88A). The expanded head lies within the C-shaped duodenum, with the body extending to the left as far as the hilum of the left kidney and the tail ending at the hilum of the spleen.

Liver and Biliary Tract

A large solid organ about 2.5% of adult body weight (5% at birth) lying under cover of the costal margin, the liver is directly related to the inferior surface of the diaphragm. It has main right and left lobes and smaller caudate and quadrate lobes (Fig. 4.88B), both being functionally part of the left lobe. The liver receives a large blood supply (30% from the hepatic artery and 70% from the portal vein) and produces bile: venous drainage is by hepatic veins into the inferior vena cava. The porta hepatis is where the bile ducts leave and hepatic artery and portal vein enter the liver.

Right and left hepatic bile ducts form the common hepatic duct just below the liver. The cystic duct from the gall bladder joins the common hepatic duct forming the common bile duct (Fig. 4.88C) emptying into the duodenum with the pancreatic duct. The liver produces 1500 mL of bile each day: it is stored and concentrated (by a factor of 10) in the gall bladder, an accessory organ of the biliary tract, and periodically released.

Spleen

Although not part of the digestive system, the spleen is closely related to the stomach and pancreas, as well as the left kidney, and transverse and descending colon. It is part of the reticuloendothelial system concerned with haematopoiesis in the foetus, as well as with reutilisation of iron from haemoglobin of destroyed red blood cells.

The spleen lies under cover of the thoracic cage on the left side of the body between the 9th and 11th ribs. Rupture of the spleen following a violent blow to the lower left ribs may produce massive intraperitoneal haemorrhage, which if left untreated or undiagnosed, may be fatal.

ABDOMINAL REGIONS

For descriptive purposes, the abdomen can be divided into nine regions projected onto the anterior abdominal wall by the intersection of horizontal transpyloric and transtubercular planes and vertical right and left midclavicular planes (Fig. 4.89A). The transpyloric plane lies midway between the jugular notch (sternum) and superior border of the symphysis pubis: the transtubercular plane passes through the iliac tubercles (p. 259). Alternatively, the abdomen can be divided into quadrants centred on the umbilicus (Fig. 4.89B). Even though the position of the umbilicus is variable, the quadrants are extensively used in clinical practice.

Palpation

In adults, virtually no normal abdominal viscus is palpable. The anteroinferior edge of the liver may be palpated in infants below the right costal margin extending from the right hypochondrium. As the liver moves with the diaphragm during respiration, it may become palpable below the right costal margin on full inspiration in adults. The gall bladder is not normally palpable; however, the fundus lies at the intersection of the right costal margin and linea semilunaris. In infants the spleen can be palpated in the left hypochondrium as it moves with respiration: in adults it cannot be felt until about three times its normal size. The digestive tract is not normally palpable; however, an enlarged caecum or sigmoid colon may be felt in the right or left iliac fossae, respectively. In thin individuals, pulsation of the abdominal aorta is transmitted to the anterior abdominal wall and can be easily seen. Movements of the digestive tract are rarely visible: if seen, such movements are abnormal.

UROGENITAL SYSTEM

Introduction

The urinary part of the urogenital system is concerned with the formation, concentration, storage and excretion of urine. It lies partly in the abdomen (kidneys and ureters) and partly in the pelvis (bladder), with the remainder passing through the perineum (urethra).

URINARY SYSTEM

Introduction

On the basis of function, the urogenital system can be considered as two different components: the urinary system and the genital system. However, they are embryologically and anatomically intimately related, developing from a common mesodermal ridge (intermediate mesoderm) along the entire length of the posterior body wall, with the excretory ducts of both systems initially entering a common cavity (cloaca).

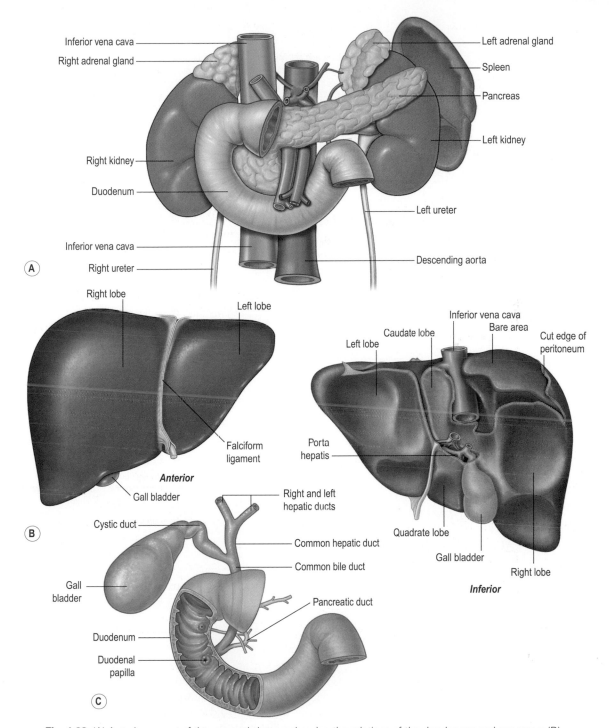

Fig. 4.88 (A) Anterior aspect of the upper abdomen showing the relations of the duodenum and pancreas; (B) anterior and inferior aspects of the liver; (C) biliary system.

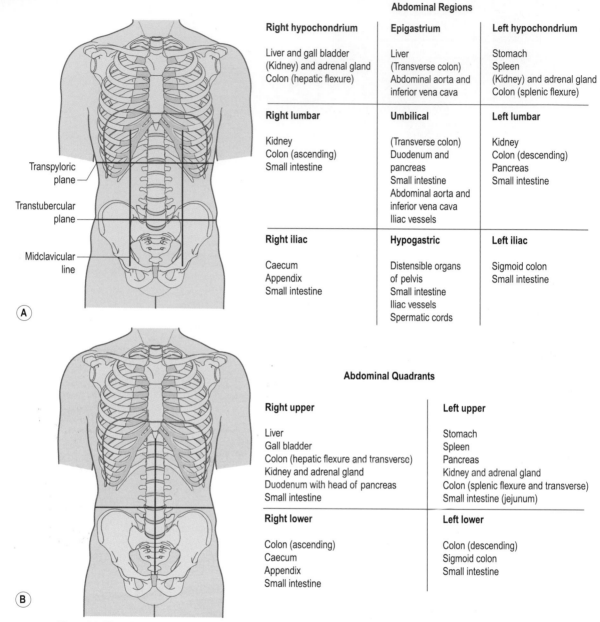

Transpyloric plane

Transtubercular plane

Midclavicular line

Abdominal Regions

Right hypochondrium	Epigastrium	Left hypochondrium
Liver and gall bladder (Kidney) and adrenal gland Colon (hepatic flexure)	Liver (Transverse colon) Abdominal aorta and inferior vena cava	Stomach Spleen (Kidney) and adrenal gland Colon (splenic flexure)
Right lumbar	**Umbilical**	**Left lumbar**
Kidney Colon (ascending) Small intestine	(Transverse colon) Duodenum and pancreas Small intestine Abdominal aorta and inferior vena cava Iliac vessels	Kidney Colon (descending) Pancreas Small intestine
Right iliac	**Hypogastric**	**Left iliac**
Caecum Appendix Small intestine	Distensible organs of pelvis Small intestine Iliac vessels Spermatic cords	Sigmoid colon Small intestine

Abdominal Quadrants

Right upper	Left upper
Liver Gall bladder Colon (hepatic flexure and transverse) Kidney and adrenal gland Duodenum with head of pancreas Small intestine	Stomach Spleen Pancreas Kidney and adrenal gland Colon (splenic flexure and transverse) Small intestine (jejunum)
Right lower	**Left lower**
Colon (ascending) Caecum Appendix Small intestine	Colon (descending) Sigmoid colon Small intestine

Fig. 4.89 The nine abdominal regions (A) and four quadrants (B), together with the viscera found in each.

Development

During development, three different kidney systems are formed (pronephros, mesonephros and metanephros), with the metanephros forming the permanent kidney. The pronephros appears during the fourth week *in utero* as a few cell clusters in the cervical region which soon degenerate (Fig. 4.90A). However, most of their ducts are used by the developing mesonephros, appearing later in the fourth week caudal to the pronephros, forming large ovoid structures either side of the midline (Fig. 4.90A). At the end of the ninth week, all that remains of the mesonephros are a few caudal tubules in both sexes and the mesonephric duct in males.

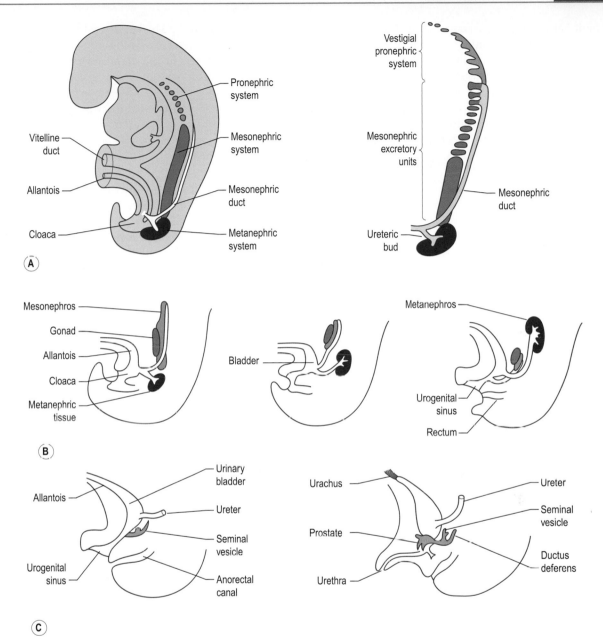

Fig. 4.90 (A) Sagittal section of the embryo showing the pronephric, mesonephric and metanephric systems and their contributions to the adult urinary system; (B) ascent of the kidney; (C) development of the urogenital sinus into the urinary bladder.

The metanephros begins to develop in the fifth week, becoming functional 6 weeks later. The permanent kidneys develop from two sources: the metanephric diverticulum (ureteric bud) giving rise to the ureter, renal pelvis, calyces and collecting tubules, and metanephric mesoderm giving rise to the nephrons (excretory units) of the kidney (Fig. 4.90B). No new nephrons are formed after birth.

The kidneys migrate from the pelvis into the abdomen, attaining their adult position by the ninth week (Fig. 4.90B), eventually coming to lie close to the vertebral column at the level of L1. They become fully functional during the second half of pregnancy, with urine passing into the amniotic cavity forming the major part of amniotic fluid. However, because the placenta eliminates metabolic waste products from the foetal blood, the kidneys do not need to be functional prior to birth.

The epithelium of the bladder arises from the urogenital sinus: the other layers develop from adjacent splanchnic mesoderm. The distal parts of the mesonephric ducts become incorporated into the bladder: their proximal parts degenerate in females but persist in males, forming the epididymis, vas deferens and ejaculatory duct when the mesonephros degenerates. In males, the pelvic part of the urogenital sinus forms the prostatic and membranous parts of the urethra (Fig. 4.90C). The epithelium of both the male and female urethra is of endodermal origin, with the surrounding connective tissue and smooth muscle being derived from adjacent splanchnic mesoderm. In males at the end of the 12th week, the epithelium of the prostatic urethra proliferates, penetrating the surrounding mesenchyme to form the prostate gland: in females, the proximal part of the urethra gives rise to the urethral and paraurethral glands.

Kidneys and Ureters

The kidneys lie on the posterior abdominal wall in the paravertebral gutters opposite L1–L3, with the left slightly higher than the right: their exact position varies with respiration and body posture. Their anterior relations are (Figs 4.88A and 4.91A): medial aspect of the proximal poles to the adrenal (suprarenal) glands; the hilar region of the left kidney to the pancreas and that of the right kidney to the duodenum; part of the distal pole of each kidney to the flexures of the large intestine, the remainder to small intestine; the liver overlies the right kidney and the stomach and spleen the left. Posteriorly, each kidney lies on psoas, quadratus lumborum and transversus abdominis (from medial to lateral), with the diaphragm superiorly (Fig. 4.91A). Except in thin individuals, the kidneys are not palpable.

Each kidney is covered by a fibrous capsule surrounded by perirenal fat, which in turn is enclosed by anterior and posterior layers of the perirenal fascia. The layers fuse superiorly but remain separate inferiorly: in wasting diseases the fat disappears and the kidneys move inferiorly. The kidney has outer convex and inner concave borders: the hilum, where structures enter and leave, is on the concave border. At the hilus, the renal

vein is anterior to the renal artery, which is anterior to the pelvis of the ureter (Fig. 4.91B).

When sectioned in the coronal plane, the internal structure of the kidney can be clearly seen (Fig. 4.91C). The cortex lies deep to the capsule extending inwards (renal columns) between medullary pyramids: the apex of each pyramid leads to minor calyces draining into major calyces then to the pelvis and ureter.

The functional unit of the kidney is the nephron (more than 1 million per kidney) comprising the glomerulus (filtration of blood plasma), proximal convoluted tubule, loop of Henle (straight tubule), distal convoluted tubule (together with the proximal tubule resorbs water and dissolved materials back into the circulation) and collecting ducts. Both cortex and outer medulla contain glomeruli: some convoluted tubules are found in the cortex, but the majority are in the medulla, together with the loops of Henle and collecting ducts.

The ureter (continuation of renal pelvis) passes inferiorly over psoas and the pelvic brim anterior to the bifurcation of the common iliac artery, entering the bladder obliquely at the proximal lateral angle of the trigone (Fig. 4.92A and B). Close to the bladder, it is crossed by the vas deferens (males), while in females, it lies below the broad ligament (see Fig. 4.94) lateral to the cervix where it can be palpated. Along its length, the ureter has three constrictions (at the junction with the renal pelvis, as it crosses the pelvic brim, where it enters the bladder): renal stones may become impacted at these sites causing intense pain.

Bladder

A hollow muscular organ, the bladder varies in shape and size depending on the amount of urine contained: when empty it lies in the pelvis, but as it fills (up to 500 mL) it enlarges superiorly into the abdominal cavity. It has outer longitudinal, middle circular and inner longitudinal muscle layers (detrusor muscle). The mucous membrane lining (transitional epithelium) is thrown into folds due to its loose attachment to the underlying tissue, except at the trigone (triangular area between the openings of the ureters and urethra) where it is firmly attached and appears smooth (Fig. 4.92B).

When empty, the bladder has four pyramidal sides: the base (posterior), superior and inferolateral surfaces, which meet at the apex (Fig. 4.92A). Anteriorly, the apex lies posterior to the symphysis pubis; the superior surface has coils of small intestine resting on it; the

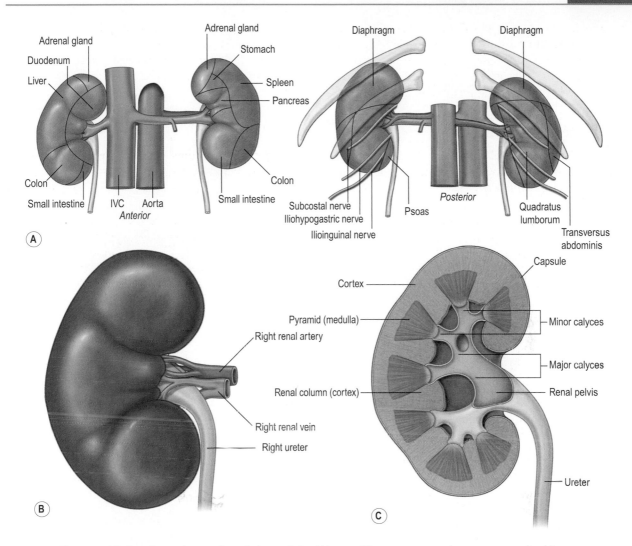

Fig. 4.91 (A) Anterior and posterior relations of the kidneys; (B) arrangement of structures at the hilum, anterior aspect; (C) coronal section through the kidney showing the internal organisation of the kidney. *IVC,* Inferior vena cava.

inferolateral surfaces rest on levator ani (pelvic floor) and against obturator internus; posteriorly, the base is related to the uterus (females) or seminal vesicles and vas deferens (males), further posteriorly is the rectum (Fig. 4.92C). The bladder is relatively immobile where the urethra leaves (neck) being fixed by ligaments in both sexes: it is also firmly adherent to the prostate in males.

In infants, the bladder is an abdominal organ and readily palpable in the hypogastrium when full. A completely full bladder in adults is theoretically palpable above the pubis; however, rectus abdominis makes this difficult.

Urethra

The urethra is much longer in males than females (20 cm compared with 4 cm). In males, it passes from the neck of the bladder through the prostate (prostatic urethra), pelvic floor and perineal membrane (membranous urethra) and penis (penile/spongy urethra), ending at the external urethral opening at the tip of the glans penis (Fig. 4.92C): the prostatic urethra has the ejaculatory and prostatic ducts opening into it.

In females the urethra runs from the neck of the bladder through the pelvic floor and perineal membrane, opening into the vestibule (between the labia

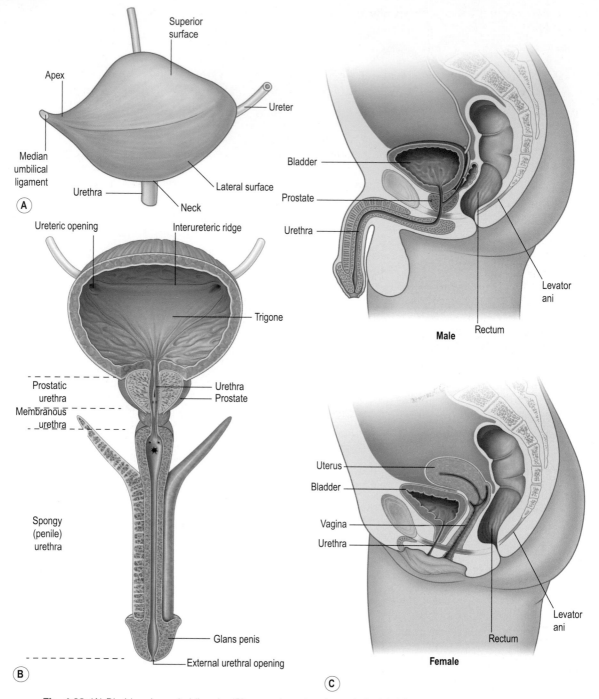

Fig. 4.92 (A) Bladder viewed obliquely; (B) coronal section through the bladder, prostate and penis; (C) coronal sections through the abdomen and pelvis in males and females.

minor) just anterior to the vagina, firmly attached to its anterior wall.

Micturition

When the bladder contains more than 300–400 mL of urine, the desire to micturate increases: although some individuals can hold 600 mL, there comes a point when emptying becomes involuntary. The voluntary act of micturition initially involves contraction of the abdominal muscles and diaphragm, raising intra-abdominal pressure, followed by contraction of detrusor and relaxation of the sphincter mechanisms in the proximal part of the urethra in males and along most of the urethra in females. Towards the end of micturition, the abdominal muscles contract again then relax; detrusor relaxes and the sphincters contract.

During micturition, the neck of the bladder becomes funnel-shaped due to relaxation of the pelvic floor. If these muscles are torn during childbirth, the ability to lift the neck of the bladder becomes impaired, with the sphincter mechanism unable to prevent urine being expelled when intra-abdominal pressure increases (stress incontinence). In males, hypertrophy of the middle lobe of the prostate may act as a valve at the internal urethral opening, forming a recess in which urine collects and remains after micturition: in some cases, the amount of urine retained may be sufficient that the individual has a constant urge to micturate yet is only able to void a relatively small amount.

GENITAL SYSTEM

Development

The early genital systems of both sexes are similar: it is only later, under the influence of the testis-determining factor gene on the Y chromosome, that a series of events occurs determining the fate of the rudimentary sexual organs.

The gonads appear as a pair of longitudinal (genital) ridges formed by mesodermal epithelium and underlying mesenchyme, from which primary sex cords develop and, after the sixth week *in utero*, primordial germ cells. Up to the seventh week, the gonads of both sexes are identical (indifferent gonads). In males, the primary sex cords form the testes and become connected to the epididymis. In females, the primary sex cords degenerate; however, secondary sex cords extend from the surface epithelium of the developing ovary into the underlying mesenchyme incorporating the primary germ cells. As the ovary separates from the regressing mesonephros, it becomes suspended by its own ligament (mesovarium).

Both males and females initially have two pairs of genital ducts: mesonephric and paramesonephric ducts. The fate of the mesonephric duct in males has already been discussed (p. 606): the paramesonephric ducts degenerate. In females, the paramesonephric ducts form the main genital duct with three recognisable parts: the first two parts form the uterine (fallopian) tubes, with the fused parts becoming the body and cervix of the uterus (Fig. 4.93A). The surrounding mesenchyme forms the myometrium of the uterus and its peritoneal covering (perimetrium).

The fibromuscular wall of the vagina develops from mesenchyme with the epithelial lining being derived from the urogenital sinus. Until late in foetal life, the lumen of the vagina is separated from the cavity of the urogenital sinus by a membrane (hymen) (Fig. 4.93A), which usually ruptures during the perinatal period.

Descent of the Gonads

As the mesonephros degenerates, the gubernaculum descends from the inferior pole of each gonad, passing obliquely from the anterior abdominal wall at the site of the future inguinal canal, attaching to the labioscrotal swelling. The processus vaginalis (evagination of peritoneum) develops anterior to the gubernaculum, passing through the abdominal wall along the same path, pushing before it layers of the abdominal wall. In males, these layers become the coverings of the spermatic cord (p. 542).

In males, by week 28, the testes have descended from the posterior abdominal wall to the deep inguinal ring, the internal opening of the inguinal canal (p. 542). Their passage through the inguinal canal usually takes 2 or 3 days, passing outside the peritoneum and processus vaginalis (Fig. 4.93B). By week 32, the testes have entered the scrotum, after which the inguinal canal contracts and closes around the spermatic cord (Fig. 4.93C).

In females, the ovaries descend from the posterior abdominal wall to just below the pelvic brim. The proximal gubernaculum attaching to the uterus inferior to the fallopian tubes becomes the round ligament of the ovary, and the distal part the round ligament of the uterus, passing through the inguinal canal terminating in the labia major.

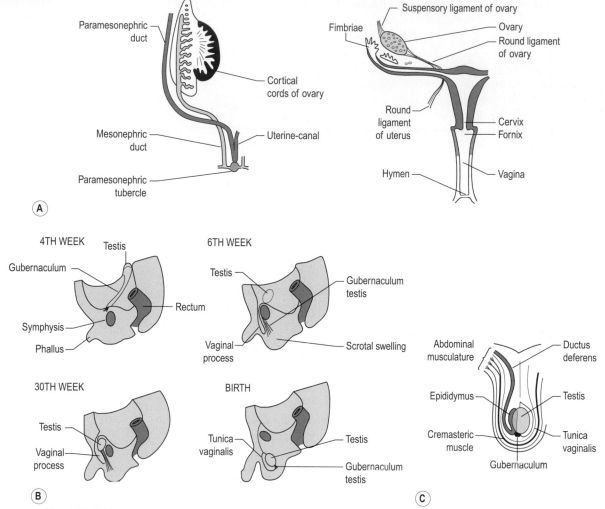

Fig. 4.93 (A) Female genital ducts at 8 weeks together with their contribution to the female genital system; (B) descent of the testes; (C) adult relationship of the testes and their coverings.

FEMALE REPRODUCTIVE SYSTEM

Introduction

The greater part of the female reproductive system (ovaries, uterine tubes, uterus and proximal part of the vagina) lies in the pelvis, with only a small part lying in the perineum (distal part of the vagina). The ovaries are the female gonads analogous to the testes in males; the uterine tubes convey the ovum (egg) to the uterus where, following fertilisation, the zygote becomes implanted: development into the embryo and foetus takes place in the uterus. The vagina connects the uterus to the exterior, enabling the introduction of sperm, as well as acting as the birth canal.

The peritoneal lining of the pelvic cavity extends laterally as a horizontal fold over the uterus and uterine tubes, dividing the cavity into anteroinferior and posterosuperior compartments containing the bladder and rectum, respectively (Fig. 4.92C): anterior and posterior layers of the fold on either side of the uterus form the broad ligaments.

Ovaries and Uterine Tubes

Each ovary (3 cm long, 2 cm wide and 1 cm thick) lies in the posterior layer of the broad ligament related to the opening (infundibulum) of the uterine tube (Fig. 4.94A). The distal pole is connected to the uterus by the

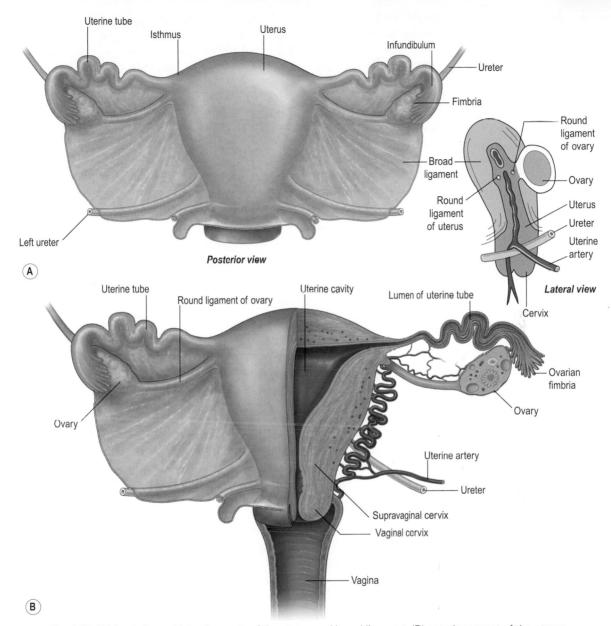

Fig. 4.94 (A) Posterior and lateral aspects of the uterus and broad ligament; (B) anterior aspect of the uterus with the right side seen in coronal section.

round ligament of the ovary, being continuous with the round ligament of the uterus passing through the inguinal canal to the labia major. At approximately monthly intervals, a single ovum (Graafian follicle) is shed by one ovary and enters the peritoneal cavity where it is immediately engulfed by the infundibulum and conveyed to the uterus, which takes 4 days.

The ovary develops on the posterior abdominal wall, lying in the iliac fossa until age 6, after which it moves into the pelvis. During pregnancy, the ovary is pulled superiorly by the enlarging uterus, returning to the pelvis after childbirth, with its position being more variable than prior to childbirth and no longer vertical. The surface of the ovary is smooth in the child, becoming more irregular due to successive ovulations resulting in the formation of areas of fibrous tissue: after the menopause it becomes smaller.

The uterine tubes extend laterally from the junction of the fundus and body of the uterus: its lumen communicates with that of the uterus (Fig. 4.94B). The narrowest part (isthmus) is where it joins the uterus, widening (ampulla) as it passes laterally, ending as the funnel-shaped infundibulum fringed with fimbriae, one of which (ovarian fimbria) attaches to the superior pole of the ovary.

Fertilisation takes place in the uterine tube, with the fertilised ovum moved by contraction of the smooth muscular wall of the uterine tube, as well as by the action of cilia, towards the uterus. Delay in its passage may result in the dividing ovum becoming lodged in the uterine tube (tubal pregnancy): rupture of the tube with severe haemorrhage usually follows within 4–6 weeks, occasionally being fatal.

Hormonal changes during the menstrual cycle produce changes in the vascularity of the lining of the uterine tubes.

Uterus

Thick-walled muscular organ lying in the pelvic cavity, the uterus can be divided into three parts: fundus above the opening of the uterine tubes, body narrowing inferiorly and neck (cervix) projecting into the vagina. The cavity of the uterus (triangular mediolaterally but a slit anteroposteriorly) is continuous with the cervical canal through the isthmus: the canal opens into the vagina through the external os (Fig. 4.95A).

Mucous membrane lining the uterus (endometrium) undergoes extensive changes during the menstrual cycle in response to circulating levels of ovarian hormones: the lining is shed each month if fertilisation of the ovum does not occur. If fertilisation occurs, the ovum becomes embedded in the uterine wall through which it acquires its nutrients for growth into a full-term foetus.

Apart from the vaginal part of the cervix, the uterus is relatively free and mobile. In the majority of women, the body overlies the superior surface of the empty bladder (normal anteverted position) (Fig. 4.95B): the uterus is also bent forward along its own axis (anteflexed) (Fig. 4.95B). The uterus can also slope backwards (retroverted) and/or be bent backwards along its own axis (retroflexed).

Lying superior to the bladder, the uterus is separated from it by the uterovesical pouch, posteriorly it is separated from the middle third of the rectum by the rectouterine pouch. Inferiorly, the cervix is supported by the muscular pelvic diaphragm (levator ani) and condensations of pelvic fascia which form three ligaments (transverse cervical, pubocervical and sacrocervical). The fibromuscular perineal body, to which part of levator ani attaches, is important in maintaining the pelvic floor: if it becomes damaged during childbirth, prolapse of pelvic viscera may occur, particularly the uterus, but in severe cases also the bladder (p. 608).

Pregnancy

During pregnancy, the foetus and uterus enlarge, occupying more and more of the abdominal cavity (Fig. 4.95C); from being a pelvic organ, the uterus enlarges superiorly reaching the symphysis pubis by 12 weeks, the umbilicus by 24 weeks and xiphisternum by 36 weeks. In the last 4 weeks, the foetal head may descend into the pelvis (engagement of the head), and the fundus may also descend to some extent. Within 6 weeks of the end of labour, the uterus returns to almost its former size (7.5 cm long, 5 cm broad and 2.5 cm thick).

Vagina

Terminal part of the female reproductive tract continuous with the uterine cavity at the external os: it opens into the vestibule between the labia minor, lying parallel with the pelvic inlet. The anterior and posterior walls are usually opposed, becoming widely distended and elongated during parturition. The space between the cervix and vagina (fornix) is divided into anterior, posterior and lateral parts: the posterior wall of the vagina is longer than the anterior, so the posterior fornix is deeper than the anterior.

Anteriorly, the vagina is related to the base of the bladder and urethra, which is bound to it, posteriorly is the rectouterine pouch and ampulla of the rectum, and inferiorly, the perineal body. Laterally, the proximal part of the vagina is related to the broad ligament containing the ureter and uterine artery. Levator ani surrounds the vagina.

The mucous membrane lining the vagina is firmly attached to the underlying muscular coat, being thick and corrugated by transverse elevations (vaginal rugae): longitudinal ridges form the anterior and posterior rugal columns in the corresponding walls. The musculature is arranged longitudinally, having a thin layer of erectile tissue between the mucosal and muscular coats.

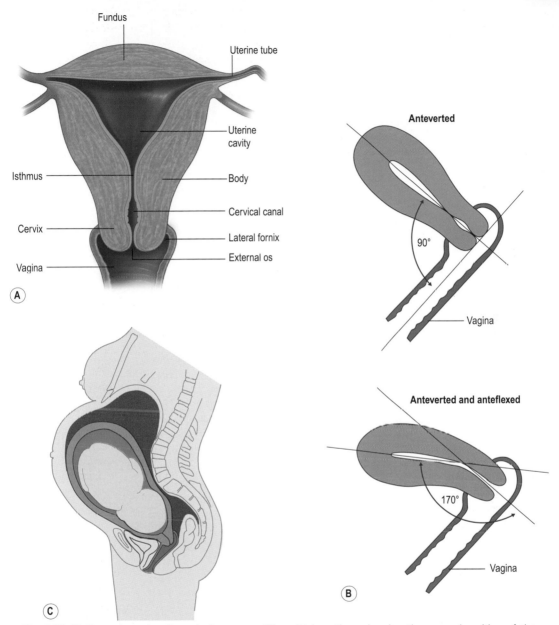

Fig. 4.95 (A) Coronal section through the uterus; (B) sagittal sections showing the *normal* position of the uterus; (C) sagittal section showing the enlarged uterus occupying most of the abdominal and pelvic cavities near full term.

ENDOCRINE SYSTEM

Introduction

A major communication system of ductless glands (Fig. 4.96) collectively forming the endocrine system, which, with the nervous system, regulates and coordinates body functions. The system comprises the pituitary (hypophysis), thyroid, parathyroid, adrenal (suprarenal) glands, pancreas (islets of Langerhans) and gonads; other regions (hypothalamus, kidneys, digestive tract, thymus and pineal gland) also have endocrine functions. Disorders of the endocrine glands are numerous and may result in disturbances of growth and development, metabolism and reproduction.

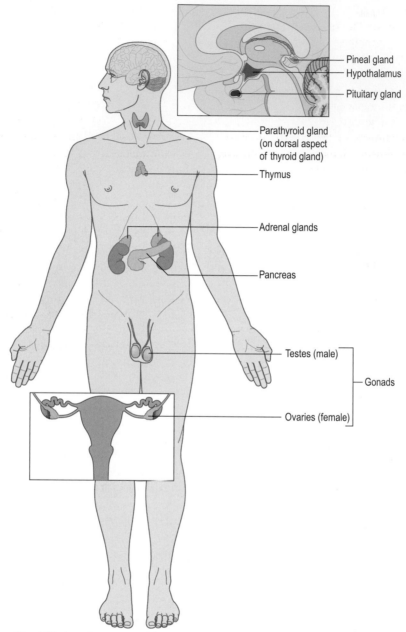

Fig. 4.96 Anterior aspect of the body showing the position of endocrine glands.

Glands
Pituitary

Small gland (1 cm diameter) in two parts situated within the skull: the anterior lobe (adenohypophysis) develops from ectoderm of the oral cavity and posterior lobe (neurohypophysis) from the brain: it is connected to the hypophysis by the infundibulum. It acts mainly by controlling the activity of all other endocrine glands.

Thyroid

Largest of the endocrine glands, the thyroid consists of two lobes joined across the midline by an isthmus: it lies in the neck with the lobes covering the lower part of the larynx and upper part of the trachea, with the isthmus overlying the second to fourth tracheal rings. It secretes the hormones thyroxine and tri-iodothyronine, which are important in controlling the rate of oxidation (metabolic rate) in the body, and calcitonin (from C-cells), lowering both calcium and phosphate levels in the plasma. Unlike other endocrine glands, the thyroid maintains a large store of hormones.

Because of its attachment to the larynx, it moves superiorly during swallowing. Its size varies with age, sex and general nutritional status, increasing slightly in women during menstruation and pregnancy. Pathological enlargement produces a goitre.

Parathyroid

Four small glands (3 mm wide, 1 mm deep and 6 mm long) lying on or embedded in the posterior aspect of the lobes of the thyroid. Each gland consists of chief cells producing parathyroid hormone (parathormone), maintaining the normal relation between blood and skeletal calcium levels, and oxyphil cells, whose function is unknown. Removal of the parathyroids is followed by increased neuromuscular excitability and muscle spasms, eventually leading to death within a few days.

Adrenal

Each adrenal gland lies on the superior pole of its respective kidney: the right is triangular and left crescentic. Each gland consists of an outer cortex and inner medulla, which function as separate endocrine glands: the medulla develops from the same cells giving rise to the sympathetic nervous system. The cortex consists of three zones producing specific steroid hormones: the outer zone produces mineralocorticoids (e.g., aldosterone), the intermediate and inner zones produce glucocorticoids (e.g., cortisol) and sex hormones (e.g., androgens). The cortex is essential to life, with interference in its function causing disruption of fluid and electrolyte balance: it is also concerned with carbohydrate metabolism and is important in normal bodily reactions to stress.

The cells of the medulla secrete a specific catecholamine (adrenaline or noradrenaline). Adrenaline is released in response to stress, increasing heart rate, raising blood pressure and causing the release of sugar into the bloodstream from the liver: it may also be a neurotransmitter in the brain associated with many functions, including cardiovascular and respiratory responses. Noradrenaline has widespread actions including cardiac stimulation, blood vessel constriction

and relaxation of the bronchioles and of the digestive tract. Within the brain, it is involved in regulating body temperature, food and water intake, as well as cardiovascular and respiratory control.

Islets of Langerhans

Scattered throughout the pancreas they produce glucagon (secreted by A-cells) and insulin (secreted by B-cells). Glucagon is secreted in response to low blood glucose concentrations acting to raise blood glucose levels by stimulating conversion of liver glycogen into glucose. It also stimulates secretion of insulin, pancreatic somatostatin (inhibits insulin and glucagon release) and growth hormone. Insulin is released in response to increasing blood glucose levels (after a meal), acting to lower the level by accelerating glucose uptake by most tissues (except the brain), promoting its conversion into glycogen and fat.

Gonads

Steroid hormones are produced and secreted mainly by the gonads (testes in males and ovaries in females) and are necessary for sexual development and the control of reproductive function. The most important are certain androgens (testosterone and dihydrotestosterone), found predominantly in males, and progesterones (progesterone) and certain oestrogens (oestradiol, oestrone and oestriol), found predominantly in females. They probably act on the brain influencing sexual and other behaviour.

Androgens are necessary for the development of male genitalia in the foetus: during puberty, they promote development of secondary sexual characteristics (growth of the penis and testes; appearance of pubic, facial and body hair; increase in muscle strength; deepening of the voice). In adults, they are required for producing sperm and maintaining libido.

Oestrogens are responsible for the development of female secondary sexual characteristics, as well as promoting sexual readiness and preparing the uterus for implantation of the embryo. Progesterone is required for maintaining pregnancy and preparing the uterus for implantation: it also inhibits ovulation during pregnancy and prepares the breasts for lactation.

Hypothalamus

Part of the brain having an important role in regulating the internal environment (food intake, water balance, body temperature), as well as controlling the release of hormones from the pituitary. Through the limbic system it is also involved in controlling emotions.

Thymus

Lymphoid gland of variable size and shape located in the thorax, the thymus is present at birth, continuing to grow until puberty after which it usually regresses. Its presence is essential in newborns for the development of lymphoid tissue and immunological competence. In adults, it is concerned with lymphocyte production, most of which are destroyed by the gland itself with only a few released into the circulation.

Pineal

Small gland within the brain above the third ventricle separated by the blood–brain barrier, the pineal synthesises melatonin from serotonin. The secretion of melatonin and its concentration within blood both fluctuate, being highest during darkness. It may be associated with synchronisation of circadian rhythms (sleep and waking, the daily rise and fall of cortisol production).

SECTION SUMMARY

Cardiovascular System

Heart

Muscular double pump with the right side receiving and pumping deoxygenated blood to the lungs, and the left side receiving oxygenated blood from the lungs and pumping it to all tissues in the body.

Structure
- Four chambers, two atria (right and left) and two ventricles (right and left)
- Contained within a dense sac of connective tissue (fibrous pericardium) lined with serous pericardium

Right side
- Right atrium receives venous blood from the superior and inferior venae cavae and coronary sinus
- Tricuspid valve connects the right atrium and ventricle
- Right ventricle pumps blood to the lungs via the pulmonary trunk guarded by a semilunar valve

Left side
- Left atrium receives oxygenated blood from the lungs by pulmonary veins
- Mitral (bicuspid) valve connects the left atrium and ventricle
- Left ventricle has thickest walls; pumps blood into the aorta via the aortic valve

Conducting system
- Sinoatrial node initiates contraction, which spreads through the atria to the atrioventricular node, then via the atrioventricular bundles to the ventricles
- Sympathetic and parasympathetic stimulation increase and decrease heart rate, respectively

Blood supply
- Arterial supply from right and left coronary arteries from ascending aorta
- Venous drainage from system of veins draining into coronary sinus and then to right atrium

Respiratory System

Concerned with the exchange of oxygen and carbon dioxide between air in the lungs and blood in the pulmonary circulation (external respiration) and between the blood and cells and tissues (internal respiration).

Upper respiratory tract
- Comprises: nasal cavity, pharynx, larynx, trachea and main bronchi
- Trachea bifurcates into right and left principal bronchi
- Principal bronchi divide into secondary bronchi (one for each lobe), which divide into tertiary bronchi (one for each bronchopulmonary segment)

Lungs
- Right lung has three lobes (superior, middle and inferior) separated by two fissures (oblique and horizontal)
- Left lung has two lobes (superior and inferior) separated by the oblique fissure
- Bronchus and pulmonary artery enter and pulmonary veins leave at hilum
- Lungs surrounded by visceral pleura, being separated from parietal pleura, which lines thoracic cavity, by pleural cavity

Digestive System

Long tube extending from the oral cavity to the anus: it comprises the mouth, pharynx, oesophagus, stomach, liver, pancreas, small and large intestines, rectum and anal canal. Ingested food is broken down, some absorbed through the wall of the digestive tract and undigested material excreted.

Oral cavity
- Contains the teeth, tongue: receives secretions from salivary glands

Pharynx
- Fibromuscular tube communicates with the nasal and oral cavities, and larynx; continues as the oesophagus

SECTION SUMMARY—CONT'D

Stomach
- Lies free within abdominal cavity: has fundus, body and pylorus
- Pyloric sphincter controls the release of contents into duodenum

Small intestine
- Connects stomach and large intestine
- Has three parts: duodenum, jejunum and ileum
- Duodenum receives secretions from liver and pancreas

Large intestine
- Has six parts: ascending, transverse, descending and sigmoid colon, rectum and anal canal terminating at anus

Pancreas
- Endocrine and exocrine gland lying behind stomach
- Endocrine secretions enter bloodstream directly; exocrine secretions enter duodenum

Liver
- Large organ lying inferior to the diaphragm (mainly right side); divided into right, left, caudate and quadrate lobes
- Receives blood from digestive tract
- Produces bile, which is secreted into duodenum or stored and concentrated in gall bladder

Urinary System
Concerned with the formation, concentration, storage and excretion of urine: it comprises the kidneys, ureters, bladder and urethra.

Kidneys
- Lie on the posterior abdominal wall, covered by fibrous capsule and surrounded by fat
- Have cortex and medulla
- Functional unit is the nephron
- Renal artery enters and renal vein and ureter leave at hilum
- Ureter runs from hilum to bladder

Bladder
- Hollow muscular organ resting on levator ani posterior to the symphysis pubis
- Receives ureter from each kidney; drained by the urethra

- In males, the urethra passes through prostate gland, perineal membrane and penis
- In females, the urethra pierces the pelvic floor and perineal membrane, opening into the vestibule between the labia minor anterior to vagina

Genital System
Male reproductive system
- Comprises the testes, epididymis, vas/ductus deferens, seminal vesicles and urethra.

Female reproductive system
- Each ovary lies in the posterior layer of the broad ligament close to the opening (infundibulum) of the uterine (Fallopian) tubes.
- Ovary connected to the uterus by the round ligament of the ovary, which is continuous with the round ligament of the uterus.
- Uterine tubes extend laterally from sides of the uterus being narrow (isthmus) where they join.

Uterus
- Thick-walled muscular organ lying in pelvic cavity.
- Has fundus above opening of uterine tubes, body narrowing inferiorly to the cervix which projects into the vagina.
- Cervix is supported by levator ani and transverse cervical, pubocervical and sacrocervical ligaments (condensations of pelvic fascia).
- Is usually anteverted and anteflexed so that body lies superior to bladder.
- Separated from bladder and rectum by uterovesical and rectouterine pouches, respectively.

Vagina
- Proximal part surrounds cervix, distal part opens into vestibule between labia minor.
- Space between vagina and cervix is fornix (anterior, lateral and posterior).

Endocrine System
A collection of individual ductless glands communicating with the nervous system to regulate and coordinate body functions. It comprises the pituitary (hypophysis), thyroid gland, parathyroid glands, adrenal (suprarenal) glands, pancreas (islets of Langerhans) and gonads; other regions (hypothalamus, kidneys, digestive tract, thymus and pineal gland) also have endocrine functions.

❓ SELF-ASSESSMENT QUESTIONS

73. Which two structures are connected by the ductus arteriosus?
74. In which part of the heart is the foramen ovale?
75. What type of valve is the aortic valve?
76. From which part of the aorta do the coronary arteries arise?
77. Into which chamber of the heart does the coronary sinus drain?
78. Where on the chest wall would you listen for the apex beat?
79. Which side of the heart sends blood to the lungs?
80. Which vessel arises from the left ventricle?
81. How many lobes does the right lung have?
82. What is the surface marking of the oblique fissure of the left lung?
83. Which part of each lung is not covered by visceral pleura?
84. Anteriorly, how far superiorly does the parietal pleura extend?
85. In which abdominal quadrant is the liver?
86. Name the three parts of the small intestine.
87. What is the function of the gall bladder?
88. How many sets of teeth does an individual have?
89. What is the functional unit of the kidney?
90. What is the normal position of the uterus?
91. At approximately which level is the uterus at 36 weeks pregnancy?
92. What is the function of the endocrine system?

SELF-ASSESSMENT MULTIPLE CHOICE QUESTIONS

1. Which of the flowing muscles does NOT have an attachment to the thoracic cage?
   a. Trapezius
   b. Pectoralis minor
   c. Subclavius
   d. External oblique
   e. Pectoralis major
2. Which of the following is NOT a feature of thoracic vertebrae?
   a. Body
   b. Flat articular processes
   c. Spinous process
   d. Foramen transversarium
   e. Laminae
3. Which of the following is a feature of a typical rib?
   a. Has a groove for the subclavian artery.
   b. Articulates with the bodies of two adjacent vertebrae.
   c. Has a sharp superior border.
   d. Articulates directly with the sternum.
   e. Has a mamillary process.
4. At which vertebral level does the spinal cord terminate?
   a. L1
   b. L1/L2
   c. L2
   d. L2/L3
   e. L3
5. At which vertebral level does the dural sac terminate?
   a. S1
   b. S1/S2
   c. S2
   d. S2/S3
   e. S3
6. Concerning the anterolateral abdominal wall, which of the following statements is NOT correct?
   a. The fibres of internal oblique pass anterosuperiorly.
   b. Rectus abdominis is completely enclosed within the rectus sheath.
   c. Transversus abdominis is the deepest muscle layer.
   d. The lower free border of external oblique forms the inguinal ligament.
   e. The deep inguinal ring is a deficiency in the transversalis fascia.
7. Which of the following muscles does NOT have an attachment to the vertebral column?
   a. Rhomboid major
   b. Latissimus dorsi
   c. Transversus abdominis
   d. Internal oblique
   e. External oblique

8. Which vertebra lies level with the highest part of the iliac crest?
   a. L1
   b. L2
   c. L3
   d. L4
   e. L5
9. Which of the following pairs of ribs do NOT articulate directly with the sternum?
   a. First
   b. Third
   c. Fifth
   d. Seventh
   e. Ninth
10. Concerning the postvertebral muscles, which of the following statements is NOT correct?
    a. Iliocostalis is the most lateral column of the erector spinae muscle mass.
    b. Longissimus consists of thoracic, cervical and capitis components.
    c. Spinalis is the most well-defined column of the erector spinae muscle mass.
    d. Semispinalis consists of thoracic, cervical and capitis components.
    e. The interspinales are short insignificant muscles.
11. Concerning movements of the trunk, which of the following statements is correct?
    a. In the thoracic region the range of flexion is greater than that of extension.
    b. In the lumbar region the range of flexion is less than that of extension.
    c. There is no axial rotation associated with the thoracic region.
    d. Lateral flexion/bending in the lumbar region is greater to the right than to the left.
    e. Lateral flexion/bending is greater in the thoracic region than in the lumbar region.
12. Which of the following ligaments is NOT present throughout the length of the vertebral column?
    a. Anterior longitudinal ligament
    b. Ligamentum flavum
    c. Iliolumbar ligament
    d. Posterior longitudinal ligament.
    e. Interspinous ligament
13. Which of the following is NOT a function of the vertebral column?
    a. Provides attachment for many muscles which move the vertebral column.
    b. Surrounds and protects the spinal cord.
    c. Acts as a shock absorber.
    d. Gives attachment to muscles of the pectoral and pelvic girdles.
    e. Is unable to transmit forces from one part of the body to another.
14. In the adult vertebral column how many free vertebrae are there?
    a. 12
    b. 19
    c. 24
    d. 30
    e. 33
15. Concerning the thoracolumbar fascia, which of the following statements is NOT correct?
    a. It consists of two layers.
    b. It gives attachment to internal oblique.
    c. The anterior layer lies anterior to quadratus lumborum.
    d. The posterior layer is superficial to erector spinae.
    e. In the lumbar region it is important in filling the gap between the 12th rib and iliac crest.
16. What is the order of structures, from superior to inferior, in the subcostal groove?
    a. Artery, vein and nerve
    b. Artery, nerve and vein
    c. Vein, artery and nerve
    d. Vein, nerve and artery
    e. Nerve, artery and vein
17. What type of joint is the first costosternal joint?
    a. Primary cartilaginous
    b. Secondary cartilaginous
    c. Fibrous
    d. Syndesmosis
    e. Synovial
18. Which of the following joints does NOT contain a complete or partial intra-articular disc?
    a. Intervertebral
    b. Temporomandibular
    c. Sternoclavicular
    d. Acromioclavicular
    e. Manubriosternal
19. Concerning rectus abdominis, which of the following statements is NOT correct?
    a. It is wider superiorly.
    b. It has three tendinous intersections associated with its anterior surface.

c. It has an attachment to the anterior aspect of the pubis.

d. Above the costal margin it is completely enclosed by the rectus sheath.

e. It is innervated by the lower six or seven intercostal nerves.

20. Which of the following muscles does NOT have an attachment to the first rib?
   a. Scalenus anterior
   b. Scalenus medius
   c. Scalenus posterior
   d. External intercostal
   e. Internal intercostal

21. Which of the following joints is NOT associated with the vertebral column?
   a. Zygapophyseal
   b. Symphysis pubis
   c. Costovertebral
   d. Costotransverse
   e. Median atlantoaxial

22. Concerning the diaphragm, which of the following statements is NOT correct?
   a. It is innervated by nerves with a root value of C3, C4 and C5.
   b. It is attached to the upper three lumbar vertebrae.
   c. The aorta passes posterior to it at the level of T12.
   d. The oesophagus passes through the central tendon.
   e. It separates the thorax and abdomen.

23. Which of the following muscles is NOT involved during expiration?
   a. Serratus posterior inferior
   b. Levator costarum
   c. External oblique
   d. Latissimus dorsi
   e. Subcostals

24. How many pairs of spinal nerves are there?
   a. 27
   b. 29
   c. 31
   d. 33
   e. 35

25. Concerning spinal nerves, which of the following statements is NOT correct?
   a. They contain both motor and sensory fibres.

b. They emerge from the vertebral canal through the intervertebral foramina.

c. Each spinal nerve is attached to a specific segment of the spinal cord.

d. Each spinal nerve is formed by the union of ventral and dorsal roots.

e. Each spinal nerve is completely surrounded by the meninges.

26. Concerning the spinal cord, which of the following statements is NOT correct?
   a. Sympathetic outflow is between the levels of T1 and S2.
   b. It has a central canal.
   c. A lateral horn is present only in the grey matter in the thoracic region.
   d. The ventral horn contains the cell bodies of motor fibres.
   e. The dorsal horn contains cells concerned with sensory processing.

27. Concerning the meninges, which of the following statements is NOT correct?
   a. The tough outer layer is the dura mater.
   b. The filum terminale is an extension of the arachnoid mater.
   c. The subarachnoid space contains cerebrospinal fluid (CSF).
   d. The denticulate ligaments are lateral extensions of the pia mater.
   e. The pia mater invests the entire spinal cord.

28. Concerning the somatic nervous system, which of the following statements is NOT correct?
   a. The brachial plexus is formed by the ventral rami of C5–T2.
   b. The dorsal rami of spinal nerves innervate postvertebral muscles.
   c. The lumbar plexus is formed by the ventral rami of L1–L4.
   d. The ventral rami of thoracic nerves are the intercostal nerves.
   e. The sacral plexus gives rise to nerves innervating the pelvic floor and perineum.

29. Concerning the autonomic nervous system (ANS), which of the following statements is NOT correct?
   a. The S2–S4 spinal nerves contain preganglionic parasympathetic fibres.
   b. Preganglionic parasympathetic fibres tend to synapse close to the target organ.

c. Sympathetic nervous stimulation decreases heart rate.

d. Parasympathetic nervous stimulation results in secretion from salivary glands.

e. The sympathetic trunk gives rise to the greater, lesser, and least splanchnic nerves.

30. Concerning the heart, which of the following statements is correct?

a. The right border is formed by the right ventricle.

b. The entrance to the aorta is guarded by the tricuspid valve.

c. The pulmonary trunk arises from the left ventricle.

d. It lies in the middle mediastinum.

e. Semilunar valves are connected to the myocardium by papillary muscles.

31. Concerning the heart, which of the following statements is NOT correct?

a. The coronary sinus drains into the left atrium.

b. The fossa ovalis is associated with the interatrial septum.

c. The anterior interventricular artery is a branch of the left coronary artery.

d. Arteries supplying the myocardium are functionally end-arteries.

e. The great cardiac vein drains the anterior aspect of the heart.

32. Concerning the heart, which of the following statements is NOT correct?

a. The conducting system consists of specialised cardiac muscles fibres.

b. The great vessels connect the heart to the systemic and pulmonary circulations.

c. The sinoatrial node lies in the right atrium.

d. In the foetal heart blood flows from the right atrium to the left atrium.

e. The left atrium receives blood from the superior and inferior venae cavae.

33. Concerning the respiratory system, which of the following statements is NOT correct?

a. In adults tidal volume is 500 mL.

b. The left lung has three lobes.

c. The surface marking of the oblique fissure is along the inferior border of the fourth rib.

d. The apex of each lung projects into the neck.

e. The right principle bronchus is shorter than the left.

34. Concerning the respiratory system, which of the following statements is NOT correct?

a. The right lung has a middle lobe.

b. Parietal pleura is firmly adherent to lung tissue.

c. The pleural space contains a thin film of fluid reducing friction during movement.

d. The bronchus is the most posterior structure at the lung root.

e. The phrenic nerve passes anterior to the lung root.

35. Concerning the digestive system, which of the following statements is NOT correct?

a. The oral cavity contains the tongue.

b. The stomach lies in the left hypochondrium.

c. The pancreas is an exocrine and endocrine gland.

d. The jejunum of the small intestine opens into the ascending colon.

e. Normally the liver cannot be palpated.

36. Concerning the stomach, which of the following statements is NOT correct?

a. It has the greater omentum hanging from its greater curvature.

b. The lesser omentum connects it to the liver.

c. The pyloric sphincter controls the passage of gastric contents into the ileum.

d. It has three muscle layers.

e. It is supplied with blood from the coeliac trunk.

37. Concerning the urinary system, which of the following statements is NOT correct?

a. Each kidney lies on the posterior abdominal wall.

b. Each ureter has three constrictions along its length.

c. In males the bladder lies directly on the prostate gland.

d. The urethra is longer in males than females.

e. The base of the bladder rests on levator ani.

38. Concerning the female reproductive system, which of the following statements is NOT correct?

a. In the majority of females the uterus is anteverted and anteflexed.

b. The ovaries lie within the broad ligament.

c. The round ligament of the ovary passes through the inguinal canal into the labia major.

d. The endometrium undergoes extensive changes during the menstrual cycle.

e. The uterus is separated from the bladder by the uterovesical pouch.

39. Which of the following is NOT part of the endocrine system?
   a. Subthalamus
   b. Gonads
   c. Pituitary gland
   d. Thymus
   e. Thyroid gland

40. Which of the following statements is NOT correct?
   a. The total range of flexion/extension of the vertebral column is in excess of 200º.
   b. The costovertebral joints are associated with the bodies of thoracic vertebrae.
   c. The investing layer of superficial fascia encloses all muscles in the neck.
   d. The roots of the brachial plexus pass between scalenus anterior and scalenus medius.
   e. The phrenic nerve is enclosed within the carotid sheath.

REFERENCES

American Association of Orthopaedic Surgeons. (1994) Joint Motion: Methods of Measuring and Recording (edited by WB Greene and JD Heckman). American Association of Orthopaedic Surgeons. Illinois.

Fitzgerald, G.K., Wynveen, K.J., Rheault, W., et al., 1983. Objective assessment with establishment of normal values for lumbar spine range of motion. Phys. Ther. 63, 1776–1781.

Macrae, I.F., Wright, V., 1969. Measurement of back movement. Ann. Rheum. Dis. 28, 584–589.

Moll, J.M., Wright, V., 1971. Normal range of spinal mobility: an objective clinical study. Ann. Rheum. Dis. 30, 381–386.

Sugahara, M., Nakamura, M., Sugahara, K., et al., 1981. Epidemiological study on the change of mobility of the thoracolumbar spine and body height with age as indices for senility. J. Hum. Ergol. 10, 49–60.

Neck and Head

OUTLINE

KEY CONCEPTS

- The neck comprises the cervical region of the vertebral column.
- The first (C1) and second (C2) cervical vertebrae are specialised, permitting specific movements between the neck and base of the skull.
- The cervical vertebrae articulate with each other between the bodies by secondary cartilaginous (and synovial joints) and between the vertebral arches by synovial joints.
- Summation of small movements between cervical vertebrae gives the neck a wide range of movement in flexion/extension, lateral flexion/bending and rotation.
- The intervertebral disc and ligaments in the neck, and the uncovertebral joints, give the neck a high degree of stability despite its wide range of movement.
- The skull consists of the cranium and facial skeleton.
- The cranium houses and protects the brain: the orbits house and protect the eyes.

- Located within the petrous temporal bone, the middle and inner ear are protected from trauma.
- Bones of the skull are united by sutures.
- The mandible articulates with the skull via the temporomandibular joints, which have complete intra-articular discs.
- The muscles of facial expression are innervated by the facial nerve, and the muscles of mastication are innervated by the mandibular division of the trigeminal nerve.
- The skin of the face is innervated by the three divisions of the trigeminal nerve: each division is clearly demarcated.
- The brain and spinal cord constitute the central nervous system (CNS).
- The brain consists of two cerebral hemispheres divided into lobes by fissures, as well as the cerebellum, pons and brainstem.
- There are 12 pairs of cranial nerves.
- The ear is responsible for hearing and balance.
- The eye is responsible for vision.

OVERVIEW

This part considers the anatomy and function of the neck and head. It is organised into six major sections: neck, skull, mandible and hyoid, brain, ear and eye.

In the neck section the cervical vertebrae, their associated ligaments and muscles, as well as the joints between the upper cervical vertebrae and base of the skull are considered: palpation of bony and muscular structures is also included. In the skull section, the organisation of the bones of the cranium and face is considered, including their palpation, followed by the muscles of the face and scalp and their function. In the mandible and hyoid section, the individual bones are considered together with the temporomandibular joint, its palpation, movements possible and the muscles producing each movement. For each muscle mentioned, its attachments, innervation, action and palpation are given. The clinical examination and evaluation of movement of the mandible at the temporomandibular joint are given. In the brain, ear and eye sections, the appropriate anatomy and function are given.

At the end of each section, there is a summary of the bones, joints and muscles (including nerve supply) involved, as well as the clinical examination and evaluation of each movement (including maximum range and end feel). There is also a selection of self-assessment questions at the end of each section, with a selection of self-assessment multiple choice questions at the end of the chapter.

INTRODUCTION

Concomitant with changes in the vertebral column and trunk, the relation and form of the skull and its associated musculature have also changed dramatically. In quadrupeds, the head is supported by the postvertebral (nuchal) muscles and ligaments (which are under tension), producing compression of the cervical vertebrae. As the erect posture evolved, the strength required in the postvertebral muscles was reduced because more of the weight of the head was carried directly by the vertebrae. This was accompanied by a reduction in the size of the muzzle and an enlargement of the brain (Fig. 5.1A), causing the centre of gravity of the head to move more nearly over the point of support (occipital condyles). It would be undesirable to have the head perfectly balanced on the occipital condyles, because humans possess no powerful prevertebral muscles to support the skull anteriorly.

Consequently, the centre of gravity projection falls just anterior to the occipital condyles, being balanced by the postvertebral muscles (Fig. 5.1B). That the postvertebral muscles have been reduced in importance is evident from the relatively small area of their attachment to the skull in humans compared with other primates (Fig. 5.1C).

In the cervical region, the medial end of the costal element fuses with the side of the vertebral body: the presence of the vertebral vessels anterior to the true transverse process prevents complete fusion of the costal element with the transverse process. Instead, a costotransverse lamella (bar) joins the two parts laterally, leading to the formation of the foramen transversarium: consequently, the anterior tubercle of the transverse process is the lateral end of the costal element, while the posterior tubercle represents the lateral end of the transverse process (see Fig. 4.3). The first and second cervical vertebrae have no anterior tubercles. See also page 500 for the fate of the costal elements in other regions.

Details of curvatures of the vertebral column, and their development, can be found on page 496.

NECK

LEARNING OUTCOMES

By the end of this section, you should be able to:
1. Describe and explain the movements possible, and their restraints, in the cervical region of the vertebral column, including those between C2 and C1, and between C1 and base of the skull
2. Locate, palpate and examine the muscles associated with the neck and give their attachments, action and innervation
3. Examine and assess movements of the neck, neck and head, and head on the neck
4. Appreciate the influence of pathology and/or trauma on the function of the neck

CERVICAL VERTEBRAE

The characteristic feature of all cervical vertebrae is the presence of a foramen transversarium in each transverse process (Fig. 5.2): the vertebrae tend to be small as they do not carry much weight. The third, fourth, fifth and sixth cervical vertebrae are sufficiently similar to be considered together: the body is relatively small, appearing kidney-shaped when viewed superiorly. Its superior

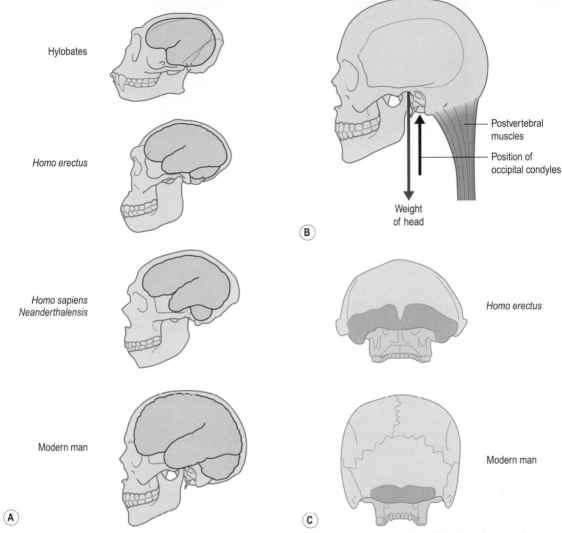

Fig. 5.1 (A) Reduction in muzzle size and increase in brain size from lower primates (Hylobates) to modern humans; (B) centre of gravity of the head in relation to the occipital condyles; (C) reduction in attachment area of the postvertebral muscles in modern humans.

surface projects superiorly at the sides, with its inferior surface being correspondingly bevelled. The anterior surface is marked by the attachment of the anterior longitudinal ligament: laterally, the body is hollowed, while posteriorly it is flat.

The short pedicles pass posterolaterally, which is why the vertebral canal in the cervical region is triangular and larger than elsewhere. The long narrow laminae pass posteromedially joining together to form the spinous process, which is short and bifid projecting posteriorly from the centre of the vertebral arch.

The stout composite transverse processes project from the lateral side of the body and pedicle, each ending in prominent anterior and posterior tubercles united by the costotransverse lamella. Within each process is a foramen transversarium bound posteriorly by the pedicle and anterolaterally by the various parts of the transverse process: it transmits the vertebral artery (except the seventh) and vein.

The large superior and inferior articular processes project from the articular mass located at the junction of the pedicle and lamina on each side: each process bears

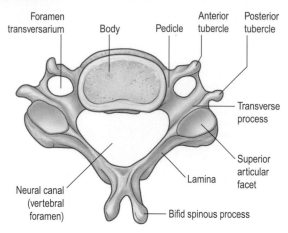

Fig. 5.2 Superior aspect of a typical cervical vertebra.

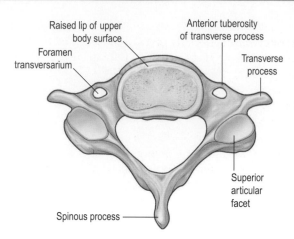

Fig. 5.3 Superior aspect of the seventh cervical vertebra.

an articular facet. The slightly convex superior facet faces superoposteriorly and the reciprocally concave inferior facet faces inferoanteriorly: they become more vertical in the lower part of the cervical spine.

Seventh Cervical Vertebra

The seventh vertebra (vertebra prominens) is noted for the length of its nonbifid spinous process (Fig. 5.3): it is larger than the preceding cervical vertebra having similarities to thoracic vertebrae. The body is larger, the pedicles directed more posteriorly than laterally, the inferior articular facets face more anteriorly than inferiorly, and the vertebral canal is generally smaller than that of other cervical vertebrae.

The transverse processes have a small foramen transversarium transmitting only the vertebral vein. Occasionally, the anterior costal element of the transverse process is longer than the posterior part, giving the appearance of a rudimentary rib extending anteriorly towards the first rib as either a fibrous or bony strip. This can lead to pressure on the eighth cervical nerve root as it passes over the first rib to take part in the brachial plexus.

Second Cervical Vertebra (Axis)

Strongest cervical vertebrae with many features of a typical cervical vertebra (Fig. 5.4); however, it has the separated body of the atlas fused with the superior surface of its body giving a superior tooth-like projection (odontoid process/dens). The dens is slightly pointed at its apex where the apical ligament attaches it to the anterior margin of the foramen magnum. From the sloping sides of the apex, alar ligaments pass to tubercles on the

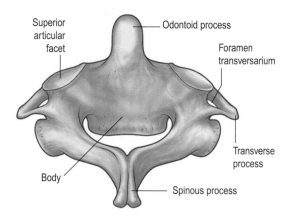

Fig. 5.4 Posterosuperior aspect of the axis (C2).

medial side of the occipital condyles. Its anterior surface has a small smooth facet, concave from superior to inferior and convex transversely, for articulation with the facet on the posterior aspect of the anterior arch of the atlas. Posteriorly, is a smooth constricted horizontal surface where the transverse ligament crosses; superior to the constriction is a slightly expanded area (head).

Large superior articular facets lie at the junction of the body and pedicle transmitting the weight of the head to the body of the axis, leaving the dens free to rotate with respect to the atlas. The articular facets are slightly convex superolaterally, resembling a segment of a dome, allowing anterior gliding of one lateral mass and posterior gliding of the other when the atlas rotates on the axis. The slightly concave inferior facets, situated just posterior to the transverse processes at the junction of the pedicles and laminae on either side, face inferoanteriorly.

The transverse processes are small and rounded, projecting laterally from the sides of the vertebral body. As there is no anterior tubercle, the foramen transversarium is closed anteriorly by the costotransverse lamella.

Thick and strong laminae pass posteromedially joining together to form the strong stout (usually bifid) spinous process. The spinous process projects almost 1 cm further posteriorly than the posterior tubercle of C1 covering the thinner spinous process of C3.

The inferior surface of the axis is similar to that of a typical cervical vertebra (Fig. 5.2).

First Cervical Vertebra (Atlas)

Ring of bone bearing little resemblance to a cervical or any other vertebra (Fig. 5.5). It has no body or spine, consisting only of slender anterior and posterior arches joined on each side by a lateral mass bearing superior and inferior articular facets and a transverse process laterally. The concave superior facets articulate with the condylar processes of the occipital bone, while the concave inferior facets articulate with the axis. The inferior articular facets are segments of a sphere facilitating rotation between the atlas and axis. Each lateral mass is marked medially by a small tubercle giving attachment to the transverse ligament of the atlas.

Passing between the lateral masses anteriorly is a short flattened anterior arch having in the middle of its anterior surface the anterior tubercle and posteriorly a facet for articulation with the dens of the axis. The posterior arch, representing the pedicles and laminae of typical vertebrae, is a long curved bar joining the lateral masses and roots of the transverse processes: posteriorly, the posterior tubercle represents the spinous process. On the superior surface of the posterior arch, running medially from the posterior aspect of each lateral mass, is a shallow groove for the vertebral artery before it enters the foramen magnum: the groove may be converted into a foramen by cartilaginous or bony tissue.

The strong transverse processes are large and wide: they may be bifid even though they represent only the posterior tubercle of a typical cervical vertebra. The foramen transversarium, lying close to the lateral mass, transmits the vertebral vessels as well as sympathetic nerves.

Ossification

The ossification of typical cervical vertebrae is similar to that of other vertebrae: details can be found on page 502.

The upper two cervical vertebrae cannot be considered typical in their pattern of ossification and are considered

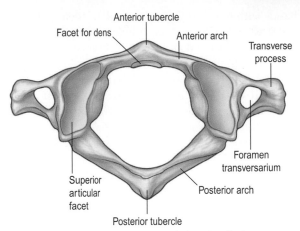

Fig. 5.5 Superior aspect of the atlas (C1).

here. In the atlas, a primary centre appears during the second month *in utero* for each half of the vertebral arch and associated lateral mass, with the two halves usually uniting during the third or fourth year: occasionally, a secondary centre appears in the intervening cartilage. At birth, the anterior arch is cartilaginous, but an ossification centre appears by the end of the second year to fuse with the lateral masses, including the anterior part of the superior articular surface, during the seventh year. An epiphysis for each transverse process appears and unites with the rest of the bone during puberty.

In the axis, primary centres for each vertebral arch appear during the second month *in utero*, one for the inferior part of the body and two more side by side for the dens and superior part of the body during the fifth month. Those for the dens fuse together 2 months later so that, at birth, the axis consists of four parts, which unite between the third and sixth year. Secondary centres appear in the tip of the dens between 2 and 6 years fusing with the dens by age 12, and for the inferior surface of the body during puberty, fusing between ages 18 and 25. Occasional additional ossification centres may be present.

Bifid cervical spinous processes each have a secondary ossification centre, in addition to which the sixth and seventh cervical vertebrae may have separate primary ossification centres for their costal elements. When present, these usually fuse with the rest of the bone during the fifth year; however, there may be a tendency for that of the seventh to remain separate as a cervical rib.

Palpation

The cervical region is most easily examined with the individual prone and the forehead supported on the hands with the chin slightly tucked in: even so, the central area (C3–C5) may be difficult to distinguish. The spines of the second and seventh cervical vertebrae are, however, unmistakable landmarks.

First, find the external occipital protuberance on the occipital bone (p. 659): this should be almost directly below the most prominent part of the posterior aspect of the skull. Approximately 2 cm below this, the large prominence of the spine of C2 will be encountered: because C1 has no spinous process just a relatively small tubercle, there is a deep hollow between the two landmarks. Moving inferiorly approximately 10 cm, the long spinous process of C7 (vertebra prominens) is the next large prominence encountered. Usually two prominences can be felt in this region as the spinous process of T1 is just below that of C7: occasionally, the spinous process of C6 can also be felt. If there is any doubt in the differential identification of C7, the individual should be asked to raise their forehead from the hands, in which case the C7 and T1 spines remain under the fingers, while that of C6 moves forwards and may not be palpable. If the cervical spine is flexed, the spinous processes may be a little easier to identify, but this depends, to some extent, on the tautness of the ligamentum nuchae.

Deep palpation lateral to the muscle mass either side of the spinous processes reveals another line of bony projections running up the side of the vertebrae: these are the tips of the transverse processes. They appear blunted because the fingers are feeling both the anterior and posterior tubercles at the same time (Fig. 5.2). Near the upper part of the neck, a series of cordlike structures can be felt running inferolaterally from the tubercles: these are the scalene muscles. The large transverse process of C1 can easily be felt below the mastoid process of the skull (p. 659). At the lower end of the cervical region, the tubercles become more pronounced with the seventh nearly always projecting further laterally than the rest: it may also be tender to the touch. In some individuals, the costal element of C7 may be longer than normal and slightly mobile, giving the appearance of a rudimentary rib (cervical rib). Occasionally, this may lead to pressure on the eighth cervical nerve root leading to neurological signs and symptoms in the area of its distribution.

JOINTS BETWEEN VERTEBRAL BODIES

Details of the joints between vertebral bodies, including the anterior and posterior longitudinal ligaments, can be found on page 504.

Intervertebral Discs

Intervertebral discs in the neck have the same organisation as those in the trunk (thoracic and lumbar regions), except that they do not extend across the full width of the vertebral body as the margins of the adjacent bodies articulate via uncovertebral joints. In the cervical region the nucleus pulposus is more centrally placed, similar to that in thoracic discs (Fig. 5.6).

Details of the intervertebral disc can be found on page 504.

UNCOVERTEBRAL JOINTS

In the cervical region, the intervertebral discs do not extend the full width of the vertebral bodies: small synovial joints (uncovertebral joints) are situated between the lateral parts of adjacent vertebral bodies (Fig. 5.7). The lateral edges of inferior vertebrae are lipped and fit the bevelled edges of the vertebra above: the cartilage-covered superior and inferior articular surfaces face inferolaterally and superomedially, respectively. Each joint is surrounded by a capsule continuous medially with the intervertebral disc.

Movement at these joints is intimately associated with movement of the cervical spine as a whole and, to some extent, help to control these movements and stabilise the neck.

The uncovertebral joints lie anterior to the intervertebral foramen. They can, and do, undergo arthritic changes, which can affect the relevant spinal nerves as well as restrict movement between adjacent vertebrae.

JOINTS BETWEEN VERTEBRAL ARCHES
Articular Surfaces

The articular processes form prominent lateral projections arising from the junction of the pedicles and

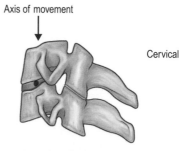

Fig. 5.6 Relative position of the nucleus pulposus in the intervertebral disc in the cervical region and its relation to the axis about which movements occur (cervical vertebra only).

laminae: they carry flat oval articular facets lying in an oblique plane. The superior facets face posterosuperiorly and slightly medially, while the inferior facets face inferoanteriorly and slightly laterally (Fig. 5.8): the obliquity of the plane of the joints increases slightly from superior to inferior. The joints are arranged to permit movement in all directions (flexion, extension, lateral flexion/bending and rotation). In the cervical region, the zygapophyseal joints are posterior to the transverse processes, forming a weight-bearing pillar of bone (Fig. 5.8).

Joint Capsule and Synovial Membrane

Each joint is surrounded by a thin lax fibrous capsule attached to the margins of the articular surfaces, facilitating gliding movements between the two vertebrae. Synovial membrane lines the capsule and also attaches to the margins of the articular surfaces.

Accessory Ligaments

Although there are no ligaments or thickenings directly associated with the joint capsule, a number of accessory ligaments help to stabilise the vertebral arches.

Ligamentum Nuchae

Triangular, midline, fibroelastic septum extending superiorly from the spinous process of the seventh cervical vertebra to attach to the external occipital protuberance and crest (p. 659). The deep part of the ligament attaches to the posterior tubercle of the atlas and spinous processes of all cervical vertebrae (Fig. 5.9). In humans, the ligamentum nuchae is a rudiment of the well-developed elastic ligament seen in quadrupeds, which assists in holding the head erect. Its principal role in humans is, perhaps, in providing muscle attachments without limiting extension of the neck, as would occur with long cervical spinous processes.

Details of the ligamentum flavum, supraspinous, interspinous and intertransverse ligaments can be found on page 511.

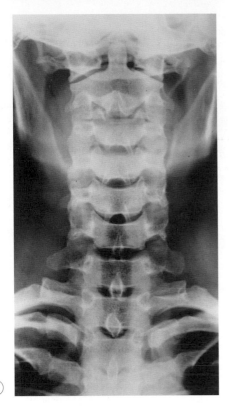

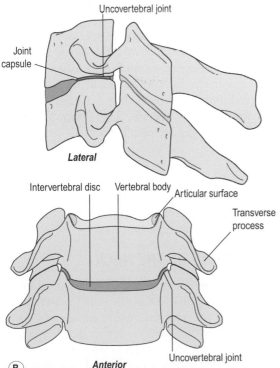

Fig. 5.7 (A) Anteroposterior radiograph of the cervical spine; (B) uncovertebral joints.

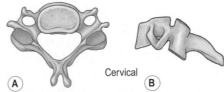

Fig. 5.8 Superior (A) and lateral (B) aspects of a typical cervical vertebra showing the orientation of the articular facets of the zygapophyseal joints.

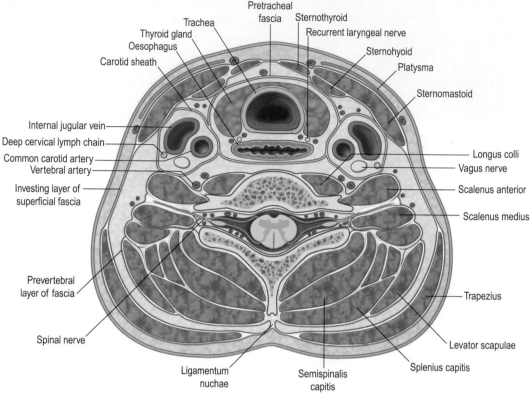

Fig. 5.9 Transverse section of the neck at the level of C6.

Relations

The neck is one of the most complex areas within the body: several named regions can be identified with respect to areas bound by specific muscles, some of which contain important structures (carotid arteries): the regions described often have no functional basis. Well-defined fascial sheets and membranes enclose the principal muscle masses, viscera, main nerves and blood vessels. These fasciae have continuities and bony attachments forming fascial planes and compartments in which deeper structures of the neck are confined. The cervical vertebrae are located towards the posterior part of the neck. Posteriorly are the postvertebral muscles, enclosed within the superficial layer of cervical fascia. Anterolaterally is the carotid sheath, enclosing the common carotid artery, internal jugular vein and 10th cranial nerve (vagus), with the cervical sympathetic trunk posteromedial and deep cervical lymph chain posterolateral to it. The anterior part of the neck essentially comprises two compartments: a superficial muscular compartment and a deeper visceral compartment

enclosing the pharynx, oesophagus, larynx, trachea, thyroid and parathyroid glands. The relationship of the various structures one to another and to the cervical vertebrae at the level of C6 is shown in Fig. 5.9. There are minor variations concerning the precise arrangement of these structures both superior and inferior to this level; nevertheless, the general plan is similar.

Stability

Similar features contribute to the stability of the neck as to the trunk, with the addition of the uncovertebral joints. Details of these features and how they interact can be found on page 514.

MOVEMENTS OF THE NECK

Taken as a whole, the neck consists of two anatomically and functionally distinct regions: the lower cervical region, extending from the inferior surface of C2 to the superior surface of T1 and the suboccipital region, consisting of the first and second cervical vertebrae, their articulation, and that between C1 and base of the skull.

Although each region is distinct functionally, they are complementary allowing flexion and extension, lateral flexion/bending and rotation of the neck, the neck and head, and the head on the neck.

MOVEMENTS IN THE LOWER CERVICAL REGION

The intervertebral discs in the lower cervical region are relatively thick (Fig. 5.6), together with the shape and orientation of the articular facets (Fig. 5.8), which means that flexion and extension, lateral flexion/bending and rotation are all extensive movements. As in the thoracic region, lateral flexion/bending and rotation occur as linked movements. Movements in the suboccipital region are considered on page 642.

Flexion and Extension

The total range of flexion and extension in the lower cervical region is approximately 110 degrees (Figs 5.10A and 5.17A), with that in the suboccipital segment being 20–25 degrees, giving a total range of cervical movement of 135 degrees (American Association of Orthopaedic Surgeons, 1994): the least movement is between the seventh cervical and first thoracic vertebrae. In both sexes up to age 20, the range of flexion is 64 degrees and extension 85 degrees (Youdas et al., 1992). The loss of motion is, on average, 3 degrees in both sexes with each 10-year increase in age for flexion and 5 degrees for extension; however, over age 30, females tend to have greater ranges of movement than males.

During flexion, the upper vertebral body tilts and slides anteriorly on the lower, compressing the intervertebral space anteriorly (Fig. 5.10B). Tilting of the upper vertebra is facilitated by the anterior ledge on the superior surface of the lower vertebra, allowing the inferiorly directed projection on the inferior surface of the upper vertebra to move past it. Flexion between two vertebrae does not occur about the centre of curvature of the facets on the articular processes: the inferior facet of the upper vertebra moves anterosuperiorly, widening the joint space posteriorly. Flexion is not limited by bony impact, but by tension developed in the posterior longitudinal ligament, zygapophyseal joint capsule, ligamenta flava, ligamentum nuchae and postvertebral muscles. From the erect position, flexion is controlled by the posterior neck muscles (trapezius, splenius capitis, longissimus capitis and semispinalis capitis) of both sides working against the weight of the

head and neck. In the supine position, the anterior muscles (sternomastoid, longus capitis, longus colli and scalene muscles) of both sides flex the lower cervical column.

In extension, the upper vertebra tilts and slides posteriorly over the lower (Fig. 5.10B). Because movement does not occur about the centre of curvature of the facets, the superior articular facet moves posteroinferiorly causing the anterior part of the joint space to widen and the intervertebral foramen to narrow. Extension is limited by tension developed in the anterior longitudinal ligament and by impact of the superior articular process of the lower vertebra on the transverse process of the upper vertebrae, as well as impact of the posterior arches through the ligaments. Extension from the erect position is controlled by the anterior neck muscles as described, while in the prone position, the posterior muscles produce extension.

Movements of the vertebral bodies during flexion and extension are, to some extent, guided by the uncovertebral joints, otherwise they would probably not be as pure as they are.

As there is no bony limitation to flexion, the cervical column is predisposed to a particular form of dislocation. During car accidents the neck is strongly extended and then flexed producing a whiplash injury, causing stretching or occasionally tearing of the ligamentous structures limiting flexion. In extreme cases, there may be anterior dislocation of the zygapophyseal joints in which the inferior articular facets of the upper vertebra become hooked over the anterosuperior margin of the superior facet of the lower vertebra (Fig. 5.10C). The dislocation is extremely difficult to reduce as it endangers the medulla oblongata and cervical spinal cord with the risk of paraplegia, quadriplegia or death.

Lateral Flexion/Bending

The total range of movement is 45 degrees on each side, with 40 degrees occurring in the lower cervical region (Figs 5.11A and 5.17B). After age 40, lateral flexion/bending gradually decreases so that, by age 90, it is 24 degrees (Youdas et al., 1992). Because of the orientation and shape of the articular facets, it not possible to get pure lateral flexion or pure rotation. When flexed to one side, the inferior articular process on that side glides posteroinferiorly on the superior process of the vertebra below: on the other side each articular process moves anterosuperiorly over the superior process of the vertebra below. Flexion to one side is accompanied by slight rotation to the same side (Fig. 5.11B). If the whole of the

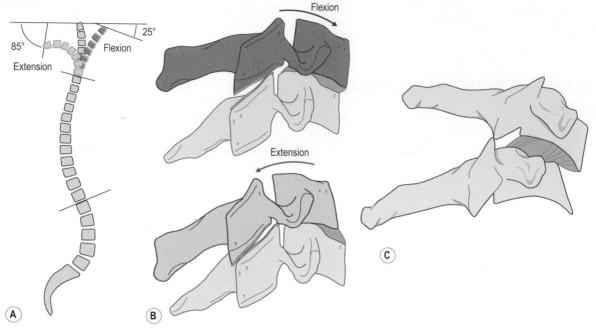

Fig. 5.10 (A) Range of flexion and extension of the lower cervical region; (B) movements between adjacent cervical vertebrae; (C) anterior dislocation of the zygapophyseal joints as in severe whiplash injury.

lower cervical region is considered, rather than movement between adjacent vertebrae, there is a slight extension accompanying lateral rotation of the cervical column.

During lateral flexion/bending, the joint spaces of the contralateral uncovertebral joints widen (Fig. 5.11C). The movement is quite complex because it involves not only lateral flexion/bending of one vertebra with respect to another but also rotation and slight extension.

As in the thoracic and lumbar regions, lateral flexion/bending of the neck requires muscle contraction on the side of flexion. The movement is arrested in part by apposition of the articular facets and in part by stretching of the contralateral zygapophyseal joint capsule and compression of the intervertebral disc.

Rotation

In the lower cervical region this amounts to 50 degrees in each direction (Fig. 5.12): the total range of rotation is 70 degrees to each side (Youdas et al., 1992), with the majority of rotation in the suboccipital region occurring at the atlantoaxial joint (C1 and the head move as a single unit) (p. 642). Rotation cannot occur without some associated lateral flexion to the same side. After age 30, rotation gradually decreases to 50 degrees at age 90 (Youdas et al., 1992), with females having a greater range in later years than males.

In rotation, the inferior facets on the opposite side of the vertebra above move against the superior facets of the lower vertebra producing a camber effect, resulting in an increase in size of the intervertebral foramen on that side. On the side to which rotation occurs, the articular facets separate slightly, reducing the size of the intervertebral foramen. The movement is limited by a grinding contact of the opposite side facets, tension within both joint capsules and torsion of the intervertebral disc. Rotation is produced by posterior muscles which pass superomedially posterior to the axis of rotation (semispinalis cervicis) and anterior muscles passing superolaterally anterior to the axis of rotation (sternomastoid): this combination produces rotation to the opposite side.

One practical consequence of rotation is that it can relieve pressure on the nerve root of the side opposite to the direction of rotation by increasing the size of the intervertebral foramen. At the same time, pressure is relieved on the same side facet joints; however, it decreases the size of the intervertebral foramen. Practical use is made of these movements in the application of traction, in which flexion is combined with rotation to relieve pressure on a nerve root: these movements are also utilised in mobilisation and manipulation techniques.

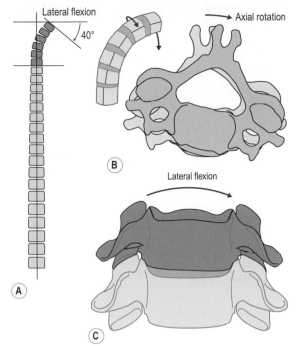

Fig. 5.11 (A) Range of lateral flexion/bending of the lower cervical region; (B) linked lateral flexion/bending and rotation; (C) movement between adjacent cervical vertebrae during lateral flexion/bending.

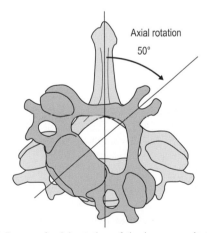

Fig. 5.12 Range of axial rotation of the lower cervical region of the vertebral column.

Circumduction

Circumduction is a combination of flexion, extension, lateral flexion/bending and rotation involving all joints in the cervical region: the limiting factors are those which limit the individual movements. Circumduction is a popular movement in fitness clubs in which *clicking* sounds may be sought by untrained practitioners. Combined movements as in circumduction, particularly when performed towards the extremes of the range of movement, bring into play certain locking mechanisms in some joints. The clicking sounds heard are often due to forcing a joint beyond one of these locking positions: this commonly leads to severe neck pain, often referred to the arm and upper chest, which usually appears within a day or two of performing the activity. Manipulators often make use of these locking mechanisms practically; however, they must be treated with great care and caution.

Muscles producing movements of the lower cervical region are shown in Table 5.1. Further details of each muscle are given in following sections.

SUBOCCIPITAL REGION

The joints between the atlas (C1) and axis (C2) are of two types: bilateral plane synovial joints between the surfaces of the articular processes and a median synovial pivot joint between the dens and anterior arch and transverse ligament of the atlas. The median joint is supported by a number of accessory ligaments.

LATERAL ATLANTOAXIAL JOINTS

Articular Surfaces

Between the articular facets on the superior articular processes of the axis (C2) and those on the inferior lateral masses of the atlas (C1) (Fig. 5.13). The articular surface on the axis is oval with its long axis running anterosuperomedial to posteroinferolateral, so that it is inclined obliquely inferolaterally (Fig. 5.13). The articular surface is slightly convex about both axes, with the convexity being greater about its short axis. The atlantal articular surface is also oval with corresponding long and short axes; however, it is much flatter showing only a slight concavity if any: occasionally, the surface may show a slight convexity. Both articular surfaces are covered with hyaline cartilage.

Joint Capsule and Synovial Membrane

Each joint is enclosed in a loose fibrous capsule lined by synovial membrane, which attaches to the margins of the articular surfaces.

Ligaments
Accessory Atlantoaxial Ligament

This passes obliquely inferomedially from the posterior aspect of the lateral mass of the atlas to the posterior aspect of the body of the axis. In its course, it runs in direct contact with the posterior part of the joint capsule.

TABLE 5.1   Muscles Producing Movements of the Lower Cervical Region of the Neck

Muscle	Attachments	Action	Innervation (root value)
Sternomastoid	Superior part of manubrium (sternal head) and superior surface of medial one-third of clavicle (clavicular head) to lateral half of superior nuchal line (sternal head) and lateral surface of mastoid process (clavicular head)	Individually each laterally flexes and rotates head to same side (bringing the ear to shoulder); together sternal fibres flex head and neck, and clavicular fibres extend head on neck	Spinal part of accessory nerve (XI), with proprioceptive fibres from C2 and C3
Longus colli	Anterior tubercles of C3–C5 to anterior tubercle of C1 (upper part); front of bodies of C1–C3 to front of bodies of C2–C4 (middle part); front of bodies of T1–T3 to anterior tubercles of C5 and C6 (lower part)	Flexes neck; individually each lower part may aid lateral flexion/bending to same side and rotation to opposite side	C3–C6
Scalenus anterior	Anterior tubercles of C6–C3 to scalene tubercle on first rib	Individually each laterally flexes neck to same side; together they flex neck	C4–C6
Scalenus medius	Transverse processes of C1 and C2, posterior tubercles of C3–C7 to superior surface of first rib posterior to subclavian groove	Individually each laterally flexes neck to same side; together they flex neck	C3–C8
Scalenus posterior	Posterior tubercles of C4–C6 to lateral surface of second rib	Individually each laterally flexes neck to same side; together they flex neck	C6–C8
Levator scapulae	Transverse processes of C1–C3/C4 to medial border of scapula superior to root of spine	Elevates and retracts pectoral girdle; also resists inferior movement when carrying a load; with trapezius both sides extend head and neck	Dorsal scapular nerve (C5) and directly from C3 and C4
Splenius cervicis	Spinous processes C3–C6 to posterior tubercles and transverse processes C1–C3/C4	Individually each laterally flexes and rotates neck to same side; together they extend neck	Posterior primary rami C5–C7
Semispinalis cervicis	Transverse processes of T6–T1 to spinous processes of C5–C2	Both sides produce extension of neck; individually each rotates trunk and neck to opposite side	Posterior primary rami of adjacent spinal nerves
Multifidus	Posterior aspect of sacrum and fascia covering erector spinae, mamillary processes of lumbar vertebrae, transverse processes of all thoracic vertebrae and articular processes of C7–C4/3 to spinous processes of L5–C2	Extends, rotates and laterally flexes/bends neck: stabilises neck	Posterior primary rami of adjacent spinal nerves

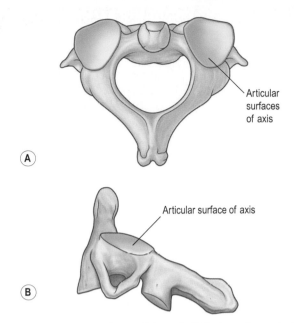

Fig. 5.13 Articular surfaces of the axis (C1) viewed superiorly (A) and laterally (B).

Relations

A membranous expansion from each side of the anterior longitudinal ligament near its attachment to the anterior tubercle of the atlas passes to the anterior aspect of the body of the axis. Posteriorly, bridging the gap between the arch of the atlas and that of the axis is a membrane lying in series with the ligamentum flavum, attaching to the vertebral arches of lower levels. The second cervical nerve pierces this membrane as it passes posterior to the lateral atlantoaxial joint, suggesting that these joints are of different morphological origin than those between the articular processes of lower vertebrae. Because these joints have a similar relationship to the nerve as the uncovertebral joints, they may be considered homologous to them, although they are much more specialised.

MEDIAN ATLANTOAXIAL JOINTS

Articular Surfaces

Between a more or less rectangular facet on the anterior aspect of the dens, convex vertically and transversely, and a reciprocally curved oval facet on the deep aspect of the arch of the atlas (Fig. 5.14A): both surfaces are covered with hyaline cartilage.

On the posterior surface of the dens is a further hyaline cartilage-covered surface, concave superoinferiorly and convex transversely, which articulates with the anterior fibrocartilaginous surface of the transverse ligament of the atlas (Fig. 5.14A).

Joint Capsule and Synovial Membrane

Each median joint is enclosed by a thin fibrous capsule lined by synovial membrane: the joint cavity formed between the dens and transverse ligament is the larger.

Ligaments
Transverse Ligament of the Atlas

Thick strong band passing posterior to the dens attaching to a small tubercle on the medial side of each lateral mass of the atlas (Fig. 5.14B and C). From the middle of the ligament, a small band of longitudinal fibres passes superiorly to attach to the anterior edge of the foramen magnum: a further band of fibres passes inferiorly to attach to the posterior aspect of the body of the axis. The two longitudinal bands, together with the transverse ligament, constitute the cruciform ligament of the atlas (Fig. 5.14C).

Accessory Ligaments/Membranes

A number of accessory ligaments are associated with the median atlantoaxial joints uniting the axis with the occipital bone: they serve to increase the stability of the suboccipital region.

Tectorial Membrane

Broad sheet continuous with the posterior longitudinal ligament: it extends from the posterior aspect of the body of the axis to the occipital bone within the anterior margin of the foramen magnum as far laterally as the hypoglossal canals (Fig. 5.14B). It covers the posterior aspect of the dens, cruciform and alar ligaments: occasionally a small synovial bursa exists between the membrane and median part of the transverse ligament of the atlas. The lateral parts of the membrane blend with and overlie the accessory atlantoaxial ligament.

As the membrane approaches the foramen magnum, it becomes closely applied to and eventually blends with the spinal dura mater.

Alar Ligaments

These pass obliquely superolaterally from each side of the apex of the dens to the medial side of the respective occipital condyle: each ligament is a short, strong and rounded band (Fig. 5.14C).

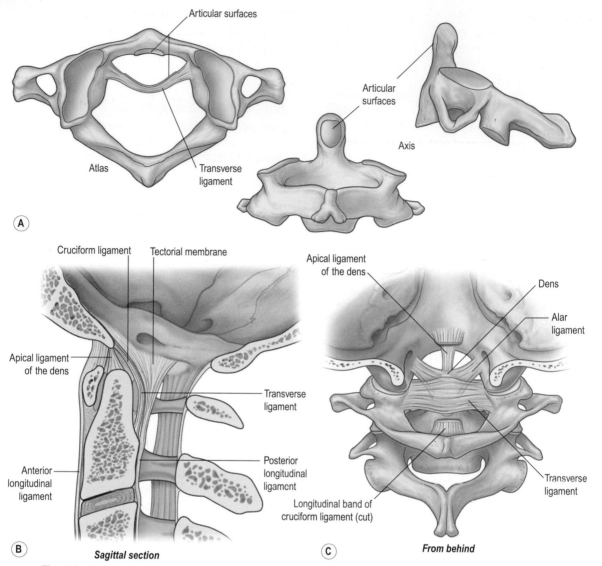

Fig. 5.14 (A) Articular surfaces of the median atlantoaxial joint; (B) sagittal section through the suboccipital region; (C) posterior view showing the position and attachments of the associated ligaments.

Apical Ligament of the Dens

Slender band lying immediately anterior to the upper longitudinal band of the cruciform ligament (Fig. 5.14B and C): it passes from the apex of the dens to the anterior edge of the foramen magnum between the diverging alar ligaments.

Ligamentum Nuchae

Details can be found on page 633.

Ligamentum Flavum

Details can be found on page 511.

ATLANTO-OCCIPITAL JOINT

Each synovial atlanto-occipital articulation is between the occipital condyle and the facet on the superior surface of the lateral mass of the atlas (Fig. 5.15A). The two joints are symmetrical and can be considered a single ellipsoid joint because, functionally, they act together: their movements are mechanically linked.

Articular Surfaces

The oval articular facets on the atlas are concave about both their long and short axes: occasionally, they may be narrowed in their middle part or even divided into two separate facets. The long axis of the oval runs obliquely from posterolateral to anteromedial, with that of each side converging to meet in the midline anterior to the anterior arch of the atlas.

The articular surfaces of the occipital condyles are reciprocally curved to those on the atlas, being elongated and convex, and converge anteriorly (Fig. 5.15A): both articular surfaces are covered with hyaline cartilage.

Joint Capsule and Synovial Membrane

Each joint is enclosed by a thin, loose, fibrous capsule attaching to the margins of the articular surfaces and lined with synovial membrane.

Ligaments and Membranes

To a large extent, the ligaments and membranes passing between the axis and occipital bone confer some stability on the atlanto-occipital joints; however, two membranes connect the arches of the atlas with the occipital bone.

Anterior Atlanto-Occipital Membrane

Between the anterior arch of the atlas to just anterior to the anterior margin of the foramen magnum on the base of the skull (Fig. 5.15B). It consists of densely woven fibres thickened in its central portion by a superior prolongation of fibres from the anterior longitudinal ligament: its lateral margins blend with the anteromedial part of the joint capsule.

Posterior Atlanto-Occipital Membrane

Attached superiorly to the posterior margin of the foramen magnum and inferiorly to the superior border of the posterior arch of the atlas (Fig. 5.15B), it reaches and blends with the posteromedial aspect of the joint capsule. In the lateral part of its attachment to the atlas, the membrane arches over the vertebral artery and first cervical nerve as they cross this part of the posterior arch. This arched part of the membrane is thickened and may become ossified. (It should be noted that the first cervical nerve passes posterior to the atlanto-occipital joint.)

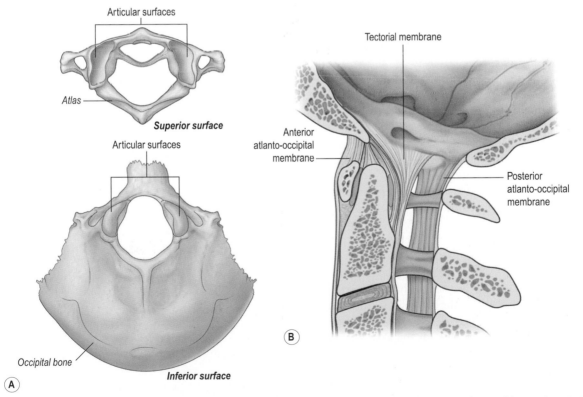

Fig. 5.15 (A) Articular surfaces of the atlanto-occipital joint; (B) sagittal section showing the position and attachments of associated ligaments.

Ligamentum Nuchae
Details can be found on page 633.

MOVEMENTS IN THE SUBOCCIPITAL REGION

The rather complex suboccipital region permits flexion and extension, lateral flexion/bending and rotation, but because of the nature of the articulations between the bones involved, it is best to consider movements between the first and second cervical vertebrae, and between the first cervical vertebra and base of the skull separately.

ATLANTOAXIAL (C1/C2) MOVEMENTS

Movements at the atlantoaxial joints are extremely complex because all joints (median and lateral) move together. The principal movement is rotation; however, a limited amount of flexion and extension may be possible.

Rotation

During rotation, the head and C1 move as a single unit with the range of movement being approximately 15 degrees to each side. As the anterior arch of the atlas and transverse ligament pivot around the stationary dens, the lateral masses of the atlas glide over the articular surfaces of the axis, one anteriorly and the other posteriorly. Because of the oblique orientation of the lateral joint surfaces, together with the slight convexity of the facets on the axis, rotation is accompanied by a slight vertical descent (~1 mm) of the head: this slackens the alar ligaments, delaying their action in limiting rotation. Rotation can be further increased by tilting the head posteriorly and to the opposite side.

Rotation is achieved by the suboccipital muscles, sternomastoid and trapezius.

Flexion and Extension

Some flexion and extension are possible at the atlanto-axial joints (Fig. 5.16): the axis about which movement occurs passes more or less through the centre of the dens. Due to the shape of the articular facets of the lateral joints, the lateral mass of the atlas rolls and slides on the superior articular facet of the axis. This is only permitted because of the nonrigid transverse ligament giving some flexibility to the median atlantoaxial joints. During flexion, the transverse ligament bends inferiorly, while during extension it bends superiorly.

Accessory Movements

There are few accessory movements possible at these joints. Anterior and posterior displacement is prevented by the odontoid process held between the anterior arch of the atlas anteriorly and transverse ligament posteriorly. Lateral flexion/bending is prevented by the odontoid process abutting against the medial side of the lateral mass of the atlas. Indeed, all movements between the two bones are positively discouraged.

ATLANTO-OCCIPITAL MOVEMENTS

Movement at the atlanto-occipital joints occurs primarily in two directions: flexion and extension, and lateral flexion/bending. There is, however, slight slipping between the skull and atlas constituting a form of rotation.

Flexion and Extension

The total range of flexion and extension is approximately 20 degrees (Fig. 5.17A) achieved by the occipital condyles

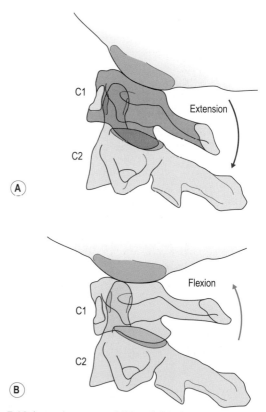

Fig. 5.16 Lateral aspects of C1 and C2 showing extension (A) and flexion (B) at the atlanto-occipital joint.

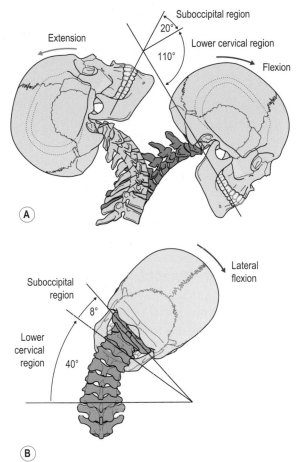

In extension, the occipital condyles slide anteriorly on the lateral masses of the atlas (Fig. 5.18B), bringing the occipital bone close to the posterior arch of the atlas: it tends to cause slight extension at the atlantoaxial joints so that the posterior arches of the atlas and axis become approximated. Extension is limited by the impact of the occipital bone and posterior arches of the atlas and axis. In forced extension, the posterior arch of the atlas, caught between the other two, may be fractured. Extension is produced in the erect position by the controlled action of the anterior muscles of both sides and from the prone position by the action of the postvertebral muscles.

Lateral Flexion/Bending

In the suboccipital region, lateral flexion/bending is limited to no more than 8 degrees to either side (Fig. 5.17B), consisting of movement of the skull against the atlas (5 degrees) and axis against C3 (3 degrees). The atlanto-occipital movement consists of slipping of the occipital condyles so that on the side of flexion, it moves towards the midline and on the opposite side away from the midline: it is limited by tension in the joint capsule and contralateral alar ligament.

Rotation

The small degree of rotation possible at the atlanto-occipital joints is secondary to the rotation of the atlas around the dens. With respect to the lateral masses of the atlas, one occipital condyle moves anteriorly while the other moves posteriorly. Rotation to one side is associated with a slight lateral flexion to the opposite side.

Accessory Movements

The lateral mass of the atlas can be slid anteriorly with respect to the occipital bone by applying pressure to the posterior arch when the muscles are relaxed. A forward and backward gliding of the head on the atlas can also be achieved, usually when using traction. The head can also be moved sideways, producing a sideways gliding of one articular surface against the other. Finally, distraction of the joints can be produced by applying traction to the head: in distraction, a rotatory movement can also be produced.

Loss of rotation to one side at the atlanto-occipital joint may lead to compensatory rotation of the rest of the cervical spine to the opposite side, often causing pain and discomfort. Restoration of the range can be achieved by fixing the spinous process of the axis and rotating the atlas and head: the movement can be forced

Fig. 5.17 Total range of (A) flexion and extension and (B) lateral flexion/bending in the lower cervical and suboccipital regions of the vertebral column.

sliding on the lateral masses of the atlas. During flexion, the condyles move posteriorly on the lateral masses: at the same time, the occipital bone moves away from the posterior arch of the atlas (Fig. 5.18A) causing slight flexion at the atlanto-occipital joints as the posterior arches of the atlas and axis become separated. Flexion is limited by tension developed in the joint capsules, posterior atlanto-occipital membrane, ligamentum nuchae and posterior suboccipital muscles. Flexion of the head from the erect position is controlled by the postvertebral neck muscles of both sides (trapezius, splenius capitis, longissimus capitis, semispinalis capitis and most short suboccipital muscles) acting against the weight of the head. From the supine position, the head is flexed by the anterior muscles of both sides (sternomastoid, longus capitis and short muscles between the atlas and occiput).

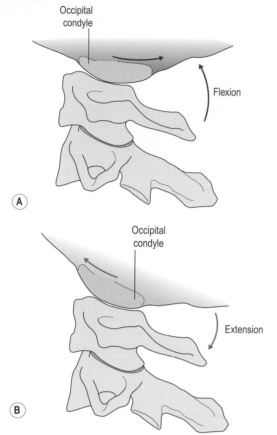

Fig. 5.18 Lateral aspect of C1 and base of the skull showing flexion (A) and extension (B) at the atlanto-occipital joint.

a little beyond the normal. However, this manoeuvre should only be performed by a qualified practitioner.

MUSCLES FLEXING THE NECK

Longus colli
Sternomastoid
Scalenus anterior (p. 647)

Longus Colli

Has three parts which lie on the anterior and lateral aspects of the upper thoracic and cervical vertebral bodies (Fig. 5.19A). The lowest part runs obliquely superiorly from the anterior aspect of the bodies of the first, second and third cervical vertebrae to the anterior tubercles of the transverse processes of the fifth and sixth cervical vertebrae. The middle part runs vertically from the anterior aspect of the bodies of the upper three thoracic and lower three cervical vertebrae to attach to

the anterior aspect of the bodies of the second, third and fourth cervical vertebrae. The upper part arises from the anterior tubercles of the transverse processes of the third, fourth and fifth cervical vertebrae to attach to the anterior tubercle of the atlas (Fig. 5.19A).

Innervation

By the ventral rami of C3, C4, C5 and C6.

Action

The main action of longus colli, acting either singly or together, is to flex the neck. When working singly, it is possible that the lower part aids lateral flexion/bending to the same side and rotation to the opposite side, but the central position of both attachments makes this questionable.

Sternomastoid (Sternocleidomastoid)

Long strap-like muscle arising from two heads running obliquely around the lateral aspect of the neck close to the midline anteriorly (Fig. 5.19B). The sternal head arises via a narrow rounded tendon from the superior aspect of the anterior surface of the manubrium sterni, while the broad clavicular head arises by a flattened muscular attachment to the superior surface of the medial one-third of the clavicle. The fibres from the two heads are initially separated by a small gap, with the clavicular head passing deep to the sternal head, but unite forming a relatively thick muscle belly. Superiorly, sternomastoid attaches by a short, strong, flat tendon into the lateral surface of the mastoid process of the temporal bone, and by a thin aponeurosis to the lateral one-third of the superior nuchal line of the occipital bone.

Innervation

The motor supply is by the spinal part of the accessory (11th cranial) nerve: it receives sensory fibres from the ventral rami of C2 and C3. Skin over the muscle is supplied by roots C2 and C3.

The spinal part of the accessory nerve enters the deep surface of the superior one-third of sternomastoid, exiting about halfway down its lateral border: the sensory fibres may join the accessory nerve.

Action

Contraction of sternomastoid tilts the head to the same side, producing lateral flexion/bending of the neck: at the same time the head rotates to the opposite side. The anterior fibres are said to flex the head on the neck, while the

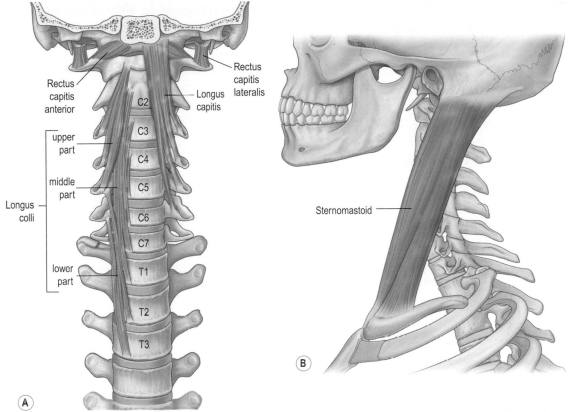

Fig. 5.19 (A) Anterior aspect of the cervical spine and skull showing the position and attachments of the right rectus capitis anterior and longus colli, and left rectus capitis lateralis and longus capitis; (B) lateral aspect of the cervical spine, skull, mandible and upper thorax showing the position and attachments of the left sternomastoid.

posterior fibres (those attaching to the superior nuchal line) may extend the head at the atlanto-occipital joint.

When both sides contract, they produce flexion of the neck by pulling the head forwards. If the head and neck are fixed, it is possible for both muscles to raise the clavicle, manubrium sterni and ribs, acting as accessory muscles of respiration (p. 557).

Palpation

Sternomastoid can be easily palpated if the individual is asked to laterally flex/bend the neck to the same side and then rotate the head to the opposite side against resistance. Both sternal and clavicular heads can be gripped between the fingers, with the gap between them easily identifiable. The round muscle belly is palpable throughout its length, as is the flat tendon attaching to the mastoid process.

Application

Spasm or contracture of sternomastoid on one side produces the characteristic deformity of lateral flexion/

bending of the neck to the same side with rotation of the head to the opposite side. This position is often seen in individuals with acute neck pain or in infants with torticollis (wry neck). Frequently, these conditions require that the muscle is stretched into its longest position by extending and laterally flexing/bending the neck, coupled with rotation of the head in the appropriate direction.

MUSCLES FLEXING THE NECK AND HEAD

Longus capitis
Sternomastoid (p. 644)

Longus Capitis

Long narrow muscle (Fig. 5.19A) running from the anterior tubercles of the transverse processes of the third, fourth, fifth and sixth cervical vertebrae, passing superomedially to attach to the basilar part of the occipital bone lateral to the pharyngeal tubercle.

Innervation

By the ventral rami of C1, C2, C3 and occasionally C4.

Action

Longus capitis flexes the upper cervical spine, as well as flexing the head on the neck. However, such a movement is usually achieved by relaxation of the extensors so that active flexion is only needed against resistance.

MUSCLES FLEXING THE HEAD ON THE NECK

Rectus capitis anterior

Rectus Capitis Anterior

Short strap muscle deep to longus capitis (Fig. 5.19A), rectus capitis anterior passes from the anterior surface of the lateral mass of the atlas superomedially to the basilar part of the occipital bone between longus capitis and the occipital condyle.

Innervation

By the ventral rami of C1 and C2.

Action

Rectus capitis anterior flexes the head on the neck; however, its main function is probably to stabilise the atlanto-occipital joint during movement.

MUSCLES EXTENDING THE NECK

Levator scapulae (p. 76)
Splenius cervicis (p. 648)

MUSCLES EXTENDING THE NECK AND HEAD

Trapezius (p. 73)
Splenius capitis (p. 648)
Erector spinae (p. 534)

MUSCLES EXTENDING THE HEAD ON THE NECK

Rectus capitis posterior major
Rectus capitis posterior minor
Superior oblique

Rectus Capitis Posterior Major

Small muscle (Fig. 5.20A) arising from the spinous process of the axis passing to attach to the lateral part of the inferior nuchal line of the occipital bone deep to superior oblique and semispinalis capitis.

Innervation

By the dorsal ramus of C1.

Action

Rectus capitis posterior major extends the head on the neck. Working singly, it may produce some rotation of the head to the same side; however, stabilisation of the atlanto-occipital joint during movement is probably its main role.

Rectus Capitis Posterior Minor

Small muscle (Fig. 5.20A) arising from the posterior tubercle of the atlas to attach to the medial part of the inferior nuchal line of the occipital bone medial and deep to rectus capitis posterior major.

Innervation

By the dorsal ramus of C1.

Action

Rectus capitis posterior minor extends the head on the neck and, like rectus capitis posterior major, stabilises the atlanto-occipital joint during movement.

Superior Oblique

Arising from the superior surface of the transverse process of the atlas, superior oblique (Fig. 5.20A) attaches between the superior and inferior nuchal lines of the occipital bone lateral to semispinalis capitis.

Innervation

By the dorsal ramus of C1.

Action

Superior oblique extends the head on the neck, as well as having an important stabilising role during movement.

MUSCLES LATERALLY FLEXING/BENDING THE NECK

Scalenus anterior
Scalenus medius
Scalenus posterior
Splenius cervicis
Levator scapulae (p. 76)
Sternomastoid (p. 644)

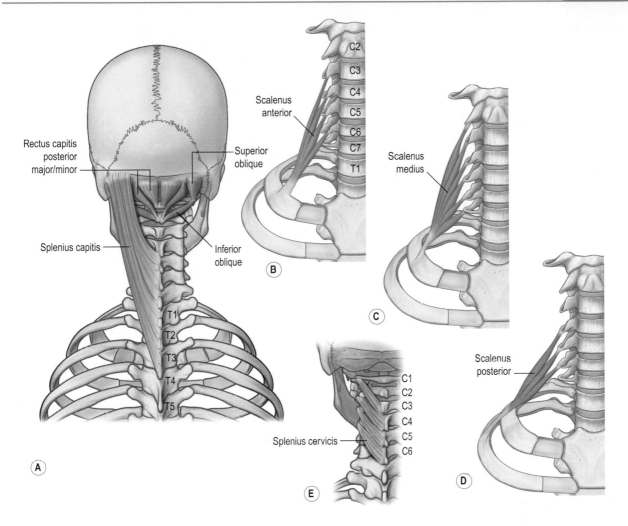

Fig. 5.20 (A) Posterior aspect of the skull, cervical and upper thoracic spine showing the position and attachments of the left splenius capitis, rectus capitis posterior minor and major, and right superior and inferior oblique. Anterior aspect of the cervical spine and superior aspect of the first rib showing the position and attachments of the right scalenus anterior (B), scalenus medius (C) and scalenus posterior (D); (E) posterior aspect of the cervical spine showing the position and attachments of the left splenius cervicis.

Scalenus Anterior

The most anterior (Fig. 5.20B), scalenus anterior lies deep to sternomastoid and anterior to scalenus medius. It arises from the anterior tubercles of the transverse processes of the third to sixth cervical vertebrae. The muscle fibres run almost vertically inferiorly deep to the prevertebral fascia, forming a narrow tendon attaching to the prominent scalene tubercle on the medial border of the first rib (Fig. 5.20).

Innervation

By the ventral rami of C4, C5 and C6.

Action

Each scalenus anterior laterally flexes/bends the neck to the same side with a limited amount of rotation to the opposite side. When both muscles contract, they flex the neck: if their superior attachments are fixed they act to steady the first rib during respiration and may assist in its elevation.

Scalenus Medius

The middle and largest of the scalene muscles (Fig. 5.20C), scalenus medius arises from the transverse processes of the first and second cervical vertebrae and the posterior tubercles of the third to seventh cervical vertebrae. The muscle fibres run inferolaterally to attach to a rough impression on the superior surface of the first rib posterior to the groove for the subclavian artery.

Innervation

By the ventral rami of C3–C8 inclusive.

Action

Working individually, scalenus medius produces strong lateral flexion/bending of the neck to the same side. If its superior attachment is fixed, it is very effective in steadying or elevating the first rib during respiration.

Scalenus Posterior

Smallest and most posterior scalene muscle (Fig. 5.20D), scalenus posterior arises from the posterior tubercles of the transverse processes of the fourth, fifth and sixth cervical vertebrae. Its fibres run inferolaterally to attach to the lateral surface of the second rib posterior to the attachment of serratus anterior.

Innervation

By the ventral rami of C6, C7 and C8.

Action

Scalenus posterior laterally flexes/bends the neck to the same side and may assist in steadying the second rib during respiration.

Splenius Cervicis

Arising from the spinous processes of the third to sixth cervical vertebrae from where its fibres run superolaterally to attach to the posterior tubercles of the transverse processes of the upper three or four cervical vertebrae anterior to levator scapulae (Fig. 5.20E).

Innervation

By the dorsal rami of C5, C6 and C7.

Action

Acting on its own, splenius cervicis laterally flexes/bends and slightly rotates the neck to the same side; together both muscles extend the neck.

MUSCLES LATERALLY FLEXING/BENDING THE NECK AND HEAD

Sternomastoid (p. 644)

Splenius capitis
Trapezius (p. 73)
Erector spinae (p. 534)

Splenius Capitis

Lying deep to the rhomboids, trapezius and sternomastoid, splenius capitis (Fig. 5.20A) arises from the lower half of the ligamentum nuchae and spinous processes of the seventh cervical to fourth thoracic vertebrae. It runs superolaterally to attach to the posterior aspect of the mastoid process of the temporal bone and lateral one-third of the superior nuchal line deep to sternomastoid.

Innervation

By the dorsal rami of C3, C4 and C5.

Action

Acting individually, splenius capitis extends the head and neck: this is usually accompanied by lateral flexion/bending of the neck and rotation of the face to the same side. Only when both muscles act together is pure extension of the neck and head achieved.

MUSCLES LATERALLY FLEXING/BENDING THE HEAD ON THE NECK

Rectus Capitis Lateralis

Short strap-like muscle that passes superiorly from the superior surface of the transverse process of the atlas to the jugular process of the occipital bone.

Innervation

By the ventral rami of C1 and C2.

Action

Rectus capitis lateralis produces lateral flexion/bending of the head to the same side. Its main action, however, appears to be stabilising the atlanto-occipital joint during movement.

MUSCLES ROTATING THE NECK

Semispinalis cervicis (p. 538)
Multifidus (p. 537)
Scalenus anterior (p. 647)
Splenius cervicis (p. 648)

MUSCLES ROTATING THE NECK AND HEAD

Sternomastoid (p. 644)
Splenius capitis (p. 648)

MUSCLES ROTATING THE HEAD ON THE NECK

Inferior oblique
Rectus capitis posterior major (p. 646)

Inferior Oblique

Largest (Fig. 5.20A) of the suboccipital muscles, inferior oblique arises from the spinous process of the axis and runs superolaterally to the posterior aspect of the transverse process of the atlas.

Innervation

By the dorsal ramus of C1.

Action

Inferior oblique turns the face to the same side: due to the lever arm afforded by the atlas, this is quite a strong movement. The muscle also acts as an extensile ligament stabilising the atlantoaxial joint during movement.

Palpation

Many of the muscles in the neck are extremely small and impossible to palpate. Nevertheless, their actions, individually or in groups, are important for the alignment and correct posture of the head and neck. Although many smaller muscles can be shown to have specific actions, their main role appears to be one of balancing the head on the neck.

Accessory Movements of the Neck as a Whole

These are present in the cervical joints; however, they are not easy to demonstrate: they fall into two groups (general and local).

1. Traction of the cervical spine is the most obvious general movement affecting the neck as a whole, producing distraction of the discs and facet joints throughout the region causing the nerve roots to be drawn back through the intervertebral foramina. With careful positioning, traction can be limited to specific areas; however, skill in location and handling is essential. In the neutral position, elongation of the neck by several millimetres can be achieved depending on the preparation of the individual. Such elongation reduces pressure on the intervertebral disc by 70% (from 30 to 10 kg/cm^2), as well as distraction of the facet joints.

2. Traction stretches all structures crossing the joints (capsules, ligamentum nuchae, anterior and posterior longitudinal ligaments, muscles). Because of ligaments passing between C2 and the base of the skull, traction has a negligible effect on the joints between the base of the skull and C1, and between C1 and C2. If traction at these joints is achieved, it may have undesirable effects, so care and caution must be exercised.

3. Side-to-side movement can be produced by keeping the head erect and moving it to the left or right: fixing the lower part of the cervical column and applying some traction increases this movement. It involves a sideways sliding of the vertebral bodies on each other, with an inferior gliding of the zygapophyseal facets and uncovertebral joints of one side and a superior gliding on the other.

4. Local accessory movements can be performed by applying precise pressure to the spinous processes, transverse processes or articular pillars of the vertebrae. Detailed information on the practical application of these procedures is best obtained by consulting the mobilisation and manipulation literature.

CLINICAL EXAMINATION AND EVALUATION

Flexion

With the individual seated:

- Support the pectoral girdle against a chair back to prevent thoracic and/or lumbar flexion/extension.
- Place the head in neutral flexion/extension, lateral flexion/bending and rotation.
- Apply pressure to the back of the head to maintain flexion, while gently pulling the chin towards the chest (Fig. 5.21A).

The centre of the goniometer is placed over the external auditory meatus with one arm vertical (a small plumb line attached to the proximal arm helps to achieve this) and the other aligned with the base of the nose; if a tongue depressor is held between the teeth, the distal arm can be aligned parallel with the tongue depressor: the mouth should remain closed. Care must be taken to prevent thoracic and/or lumbar flexion.

Extension

From the same starting position and goniometer alignment for flexion, the head is tilted backwards by applying pressure to the chin: rotation and lateral flexion/bending of the neck are prevented by holding the chin (Fig. 5.21B). Thoracic and lumbar extension are prevented by the presence of the chair back.

Lateral Flexion/Bending

With the individual seated:
- Support the thoracic and lumbar spine with a chair back.
- Place the head in neutral flexion/extension, rotation and lateral flexion/bending.
- Place one hand on the opposite shoulder to prevent lateral flexion/bending of the thoracic and lumbar spine.
- Laterally flex/bend the cervical spine by pulling the head laterally (Fig. 5.22A).

The centre of the goniometer is placed over the C7 spinous process with one arm aligned with the spinous processes of thoracic vertebrae and the other aligned with the external occipital protuberance. Alternatively, an estimate of lateral flexion can be achieved by measuring the distance between the mastoid process and acromion using a tape measure.

Rotation

With the individual seated:
- Support the thoracic and lumbar spine.
- Place the head in neutral flexion/extension, lateral flexion/bending and rotation.
- Place one hand on the opposite shoulder to prevent rotation of the thoracic and lumbar spine.
- Rotate the neck while preventing cervical flexion/extension and lateral flexion/bending (Fig. 5.22B).

The centre of the goniometer is placed over the centre of the vertex of the head with one arm aligned parallel to a line passing between the acromion processes and the other aligned with the tip of the nose. Alternatively, an estimate of rotation can be achieved by measuring the distance between the chin and acromion process using a tape measure.

CERVICAL PLEXUS

The cervical plexus (Fig. 5.23) is formed from the ventral rami of the upper four cervical nerves and consists of a series of loops between adjacent nerves. The first cervical nerve emerges between rectus capitis anterior and rectus capitis lateralis descending anterior to the transverse process of the atlas to join the ascending branch of the second cervical nerve. As it does so, it sends a large

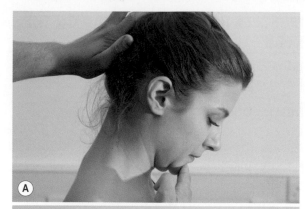

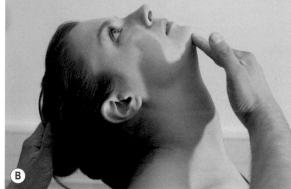

Fig. 5.21 Evaluation of the range of flexion (A) and extension (B) of the neck.

branch to join the hypoglossal nerve. The second, third and fourth nerves divide into upper and lower parts with adjacent parts joining together; the lower part of the fourth cervical nerve may participate in the brachial plexus. The loop communications of the plexus lie close to the vertebral column, anterior to levator scapulae and scalenus medius posterior to the prevertebral muscles. The branches arising from the loops lie posteromedial to the internal jugular vein deep to sternomastoid. The branches given off can be grouped into superficial and deep: the former supply skin of the lower part of the skull and neck, while the latter separate into medial and lateral divisions which supply muscles or communicate with other nerves.

Superficial Branches

Four cutaneous nerves appear in the posterior triangle of the neck superior to the midpoint of the posterior border of sternomastoid, before piercing the deep fascia to supply skin of the head and neck (Fig. 5.24).

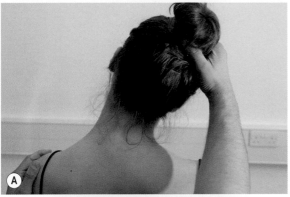

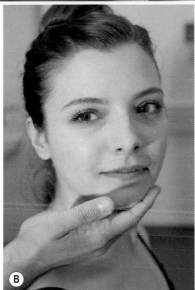

Fig. 5.22 Evaluation of the range of lateral flexion/bending (A) and rotation (B) of the neck.

Lesser Occipital Nerve

Hooking below the accessory nerve to emerge above the other three, the lesser occipital nerve (C2 and C3) ascends along the posterior border of sternomastoid, piercing the deep fascia at the apex of the posterior triangle. It then divides to supply skin and fascia on the superolateral part of the neck, cranial surface of the auricle and mastoid process, and adjacent part of the scalp (Fig. 5.24): occasionally, it is double.

Greater Auricular Nerve

Largest cutaneous branch, the greater auricular nerve (C2 and C3: sometimes just C3), emerges inferior to the lesser occipital nerve, passing anterosuperiorly over the superficial surface of sternomastoid deep to platysma towards the lower part of the auricle. During its course, it divides into a number of branches: anterior branches pass through the parotid gland and over the angle of the mandible to supply skin and fascia over the posteroinferior surface of the face (Fig. 5.24). Within the parotid, the branches communicate with the facial nerve. Intermediate branches supply both surfaces of the lower part of the auricle, while posterior branches supply an area of skin and fascia over the mastoid process: the posterior branches communicate with the lesser occipital nerve and posterior auricular branch of the facial nerve.

Transverse Cutaneous Nerve of Neck

Passing horizontally forwards around the posterior border of sternomastoid deep to platysma and the external jugular vein is the transverse cutaneous nerve of the neck (C2 and C3). It crosses sternomastoid, then divides into upper and lower branches supplying skin and fascia over the anterior triangle of the neck from the mandible to just superior to the clavicle near the midline (Fig. 5.24).

Supraclavicular nerves

These appear as a single large nerve (C3 and C4) at the posterior border of sternomastoid just inferior to its midpoint, to pass inferiorly through the lower part of the posterior triangle. The main trunk then divides into lateral, intermediate and medial supraclavicular nerves, which pierce the deep fascia superior to the clavicle to supply skin and fascia over the lower part of the side of the neck and anterior chest wall as far as the sternal angle (Fig. 5.24). The lateral nerve also supplies the acromioclavicular joint, while the medial supplies the sternoclavicular joint. Branches from the intermediate and lateral nerves may groove or pierce the clavicle.

Deep Branches

The muscular branches arise with other branches deep to sternomastoid: they can be divided into lateral and medial branches depending on whether they pass into the posterior or anterior triangles of the neck, respectively.

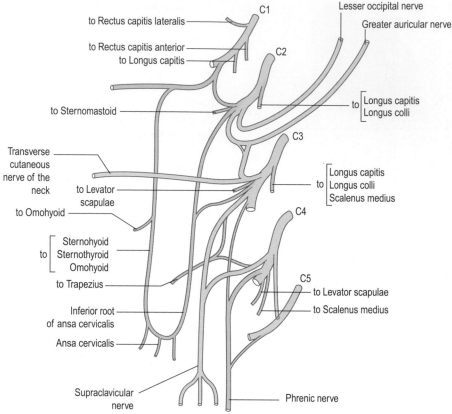

Fig. 5.23 Superficial (*blue*) and deep (*yellow*) branches of the cervical plexus.

Lateral Branches

A sensory branch from the second cervical nerve enters the deep surface of sternomastoid, while a sensory branch from the third and fourth cervical nerves crosses the posterior triangle to enter the deep surface of trapezius. Separate fibres from C3 and C4 innervate levator scapulae, and scalenus medius and posterior (Fig. 5.23).

Medial Branches

These innervate rectus capitis lateralis and anterior (C1 and C2), longus capitis (C1–C4) and longus colli (C2–C4) (Fig. 5.23). From the first cervical nerve, a branch joins the hypoglossal nerve: a smaller sensory branch (meningeal branch) passes superiorly with the hypoglossal nerve to supply the skull and dura mater of the posterior cranial fossa. The remaining fibres pass with the hypoglossal nerve and are given off in one of

three branches, none of which contain hypoglossal fibres. These are the superior root of the ansa cervicalis descending anterior to the internal and common carotid arteries to join the inferior root, formed by branches from C2 and C3 passing over the anterior surface of the internal jugular vein, to form the ansa cervicalis (Fig. 5.23) superficial to the carotid sheath: branches from the ansa cervicalis innervate sternohyoid, sternothyroid and omohyoid. The other two branches arising from the hypoglossal nerve containing C1 fibres are the nerves to thyrohyoid and to geniohyoid.

Communicating Branches

The cervical plexus sends fibres to the vagus, accessory and hypoglossal nerves, and receives grey rami communicantes from the superior cervical ganglion of the sympathetic trunk.

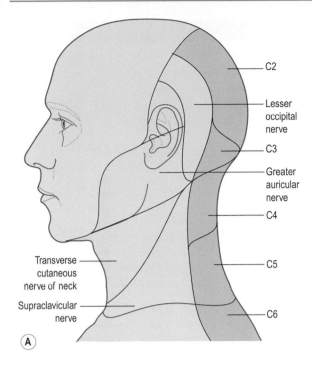

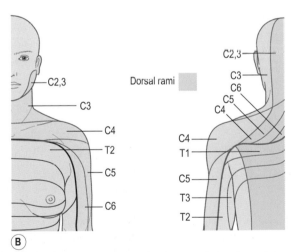

Fig. 5.24 (A) Cutaneous distribution of branches from the cervical plexus; (B) the C2–T2 dermatomes.

Phrenic Nerve

Arising from C3, C4 and C5, although its principal root is C4 (Fig. 5.23), is the phrenic nerve. Branches from C3 reach it directly or by the nerve to sternohyoid, while the C5 fibres reach it directly or via the accessory phrenic nerve from the nerve to subclavius. The phrenic nerve innervates the diaphragm, being its only motor supply: it passes through both the neck and thorax to reach the diaphragm.

In the neck, each phrenic nerve passes inferiorly from lateral to medial anterior to scalenus anterior posterior to sternomastoid, omohyoid, the internal jugular vein and suprascapular vessels: it is anterior to the cervical fascia. At the base of the neck, each phrenic nerve enters the thorax posterior to the subclavian vein and anterior to the subclavian artery.

In the thorax, the left and right phrenic nerves are separated from the pleural cavity by the mediastinal pleura.

Left Phrenic Nerve

Passing anterior to the internal thoracic artery, medial to the apex of the left lung and pleura, and between the left common carotid and subclavian arteries, the left phrenic nerve crosses the aortic arch anterior to the vagus nerve. It then passes anterior to the left lung root with the left ventricle and pericardium medially and visceral pleura laterally: it pierces the muscular part of the diaphragm lateral to the oesophageal opening, supplying its inferior surface mainly on the left.

Right Phrenic Nerve

Shorter and more vertical, the right phrenic nerve enters the thorax lateral to the right brachiocephalic vein and superior vena cava: it is not in contact with the vagus nerve. It then passes between the pleura and pericardium as it descends across the right atrium, reaching the inferior vena cava after passing anterior to the right lung root. It passes through the central tendon of the diaphragm through or adjacent to the inferior vena caval opening, supplying its inferior surface mainly on the right side.

In addition to providing the only motor supply to the diaphragm, the phrenic nerves are sensory to its central part as well as to the mediastinal and diaphragmatic pleura, fibrous pericardium, diaphragmatic peritoneum and probably also to the liver, gall bladder and inferior vena cava. The phrenic nerves receive fibres from the sympathetic trunk in the neck and coeliac plexus in the abdomen.

SECTION SUMMARY

Typical Cervical Vertebra

- Small kidney-shaped body with synovial uncovertebral joints at lateral margins of superior and inferior surfaces
- Short pedicles projecting almost laterally from body
- Long narrow laminae
- Large triangular vertebral canal
- Short bifid spinous process
- Composite transverse processes projecting from side of body ending in anterior and posterior tubercles: each process contains a foramen transversarium
- Large superior and inferior articular processes: superior face superoposteriorly, inferior anteroinferiorly

Atlas (C1)

- Lacks a body; consists of anterior and posterior arches
- Anterior arch articulates with odontoid process/dens of axis
- Superior articular facets articulate with occipital condyles of skull

Axis (C2)

- Strongest cervical vertebra
- Odontoid process/dens projects superiorly from body; articulates with atlas

Joints between vertebral arches (zygapophyseal joints)

Type	Plane synovial joint
Articular surfaces	Facets on superior and inferior articular processes
Capsule	Thin fibrous capsule surrounds joint attaching to articular margins
Ligaments	Ligamentum flavum; supra-spinous, interspinous and intertransverse; ligamentum nuchae
Stability	Provided by interaction between intervertebral disc and associated ligaments; shape of facet joints
Movements	Lower cervical region: 25 degree flexion and 110 degree extension, 40 degree lateral flexion/bending to each side and 50 degree axial rotation to each side

Atlantoaxial and atlanto-occipital articulations

Lateral atlantoaxial joint

Type	Plane synovial joint
Articular surfaces	Superior facet of axis (C2) with inferior facet of atlas (C1)
Capsule	Loose fibrous capsule enclosing joint attaching to articular margins
Ligaments	Accessory atlantoaxial ligament

Median atlantoaxial joint

Type	Synovial pivot joint
Articular surfaces	Anterior facet on dens of axis with facet on posterior aspect of arch of atlas; posterior facet on dens with anterior surface of transverse ligament of atlas
Capsule	Thin fibrous capsule encloses each joint
Ligaments	Transverse ligament of atlas, tectorial membrane, alar, apical ligament of the dens, ligamentum nuchae and ligamentum flavum
Movements	15 degree axial rotation of atlas (C1) and head around axis (C2): small amount of flexion and extension

Atlanto-occipital joint

Type	Synovial ellipsoid joint
Articular surfaces	Occipital condyle with facet on superior surface of atlas
Capsule	Thin loose capsule attaching to articular margins
Ligaments	Anterior and posterior atlanto-occipital membranes and ligamentum nuchae
Stability	From muscles crossing joints and associated ligaments
Movements	20 degree combined flexion/extension, 8 degree lateral flexion/bending to each side and small amount of rotation

SECTION SUMMARY—CONT'D

Movements of neck and head

Movements are described as of the neck, of the neck and head at joints of the lower cervical spine, and of the head on the neck at the atlanto-occipital joint. Frequently, the same muscles move both of these regions. Movements are produced by the following muscles:

Movement	Muscles
Flexion	Longus colli (C3, C4, C5 and C6)
	Sternomastoid (CN XI)
	Scalenus anterior (C4, C5 and C6)
	Longus capitis (C1, C2, C3 and C(4))
	Rectus capitis anterior (head only) (C1 and C2)
Lateral flexion	Scalenus anterior (C4, C5 and C6)
	Scalenus medius (C3–C8)
	Scalenus posterior (C6 and C7)
	Levator scapulae (C3, C4 and C5)
	Sternomastoid (CN XI)
	Splenius capitis (C3, C4 and C5 by posterior primary rami)
	Trapezius (CN XI)
	Erector spinae (segmental by posterior primary rami)
	Rectus capitis lateralis (head only) (C1 and C2)

Movement	Muscles
Extension	Levator scapulae (C3, C4 and C5)
	Splenius cervicis (C5, C6 and C7)
	Trapezius (CN XI)
	Splenius capitis (C3, C4 and C5 by posterior primary rami)
	Erector spinae (segmental by posterior primary rami)
	Rectus capitis posterior major (head only) (C1 posterior primary ramus)
	Rectus capitis posterior minor (head only) (C1 posterior primary ramus)
	Superior oblique (head only) (C1 posterior primary ramus)
Rotation	Semispinalis cervicis (segmental by posterior primary rami)
	Multifidus (segmental by posterior primary rami)
	Scalenus anterior (C4, C5 and C6)
	Splenius cervicis (C5, C6 and C7)
	Splenius capitis (C3, C4 and C5 by posterior primary rami)
	Sternomastoid (CN XI)
	Inferior oblique (head only) (C1 by posterior primary ramus)
	Rectus capitis posterior major (head only) (C1 by posterior primary ramus)

? SELF-ASSESSMENT QUESTIONS

1. What movement is possible between C1 and the base of the skull?
2. Which structures pass through the intervertebral foramina of the upper six cervical vertebrae?
3. How many cervical vertebrae are there in adults?
4. Which cervical vertebrae do not have a bifid spine?
5. How many joints are there between C1 and C2?
6. What and where are the uncovertebral joints?
7. How many parts does longus colli have and what are their attachments?
8. What is the action of scalenus anterior?
9. What is the nerve supply of rectus capitis lateralis?
10. What is the ligamentum nuchae?
11. What are the articular surfaces of the atlanto-occipital joint?
12. What type of joint is the median atlantoaxial joint?
13. Name the four cutaneous branches of the cervical plexus.
14. What holds the dens of C2 against the anterior arch of C1?
15. What is the possible consequence of arthritic changes in the uncovertebral joints?
16. In the neck, which layer of fascia splits to enclose trapezius and sternomastoid?
17. With what is the posterior longitudinal ligament continuous superiorly?
18. Which ligaments are associated with the atlanto-occipital joint?
19. What is the action of superior oblique?
20. What is the nerve supply to sternomastoid?

SKULL AND FACE

LEARNING OUTCOMES

By the end of the section, you should be able to:
1. Name and identify the bones, joints and muscles of the skull and face
2. Describe the role of the muscles of facial expression
3. Appreciate the influence of pathology and/or trauma on the skull and face

INTRODUCTION

An awesome-looking structure commonly used to portray death and instil terror, the skull is a complex arrangement of individual bones which form the skeleton of the head and face. It consists of two main elements: the large, hollow cranial cavity (the walls of which enclose the brain) and the bones of the face anteroinferiorly, which complete the walls of the orbits and nasal cavity, as well as forming the roof of the mouth. The mandible, a separate bone, completes the bony framework of the face (p. 665).

The discovery of many fossilised vertebrate remains, particularly skull fragments and teeth, has led to a detailed study of the skull, revealing a fascinating history of evolutionary development of the human skeleton. The size and shape of the cranial, orbital and nasal cavities, jaws and teeth have all provided a detailed catalogue of the probable evolutionary history of vertebrates. Estimates of relative brain size from the size and shape of the cranial cavity reveal information regarding possible intelligence. The size and shape of the jaws and teeth give clues to the type of food eaten, as well as indirectly providing information regarding changes in body posture in relation to adaptations to the gathering and the provision of food (running and hunting). The size and direction of the orbits, together with changes in the upper cervical spine, indicate the increasing importance of the power and range of vision. This, together with the erect bipedal posture adopted during the same period, gives an insight into the defence, protection and manipulation of tools necessary for survival.

SKULL

The cranial cavity of the human skull is relatively large and projects anteriorly over the facial skeleton (Fig. 5.25). Its walls are composed of plates of bone, arranged as two layers of compact bone, enclosing a central layer of cancellous bone (diploe). Bones of the skull vault ossify in membrane (intramembranous ossification) (p. 37) and are joined edge to edge by fibrous interlocking joints (sutures) (p. 40).

The superior aspect and most of the sides of the skull are formed by the two large parietal bones, which articulate along their medial borders at the sagittal suture (Fig. 5.25A). Anteriorly, the skull is formed by the frontal bone, which joins the two parietal bones at the coronal suture: the region where the coronal and sagittal sutures meet is the bregma. At birth, the region of the bregma is not ossified, appearing as an easily felt diamond-shaped area of connective tissue (anterior fontanelle): it gradually decreases in size and closes about 18 months after birth.

The frontal bone forms the forehead and separates the orbital cavities from the anterior cranial fossa: it forms the roof of each orbital cavity and floor of the anterior cranial fossa.

The remaining part of each side of the skull is formed by the squamous part of the temporal bone and part of the greater wing of the sphenoid. The region where the frontal, parietal, temporal and sphenoid bones almost meet is the pterion: it has a small, sphenoidal fontanelle which closes within 3 months of birth. Passing medially and slightly anteriorly from the squamous part of the temporal bone is the petrosal part of the temporal bone, which forms most of the floor of the middle cranial fossa: it contains and protects the organs of hearing and balance.

The most posterior section of the cranial cavity is formed by the occipital bone, which meets the posterior border of each parietal bone at the lambdoid suture: the meeting point of the lambdoid and sagittal sutures is the lambda. Again, at birth this region is not ossified and appears as a triangular area of connective tissue (posterior fontanelle): it rapidly decreases in size and closes between the third and sixth month after birth. The occipital bone curves anteriorly to surround the foramen magnum, projecting anteriorly as the basilar part of the occipital bone to join the body of the sphenoid.

The outer aspect of the top of the skull needs little description, as the parietal bones and the relevant parts of the frontal and occipital bones show few bony landmarks, except for the sutures where they join. It is, however, worth noting that the skull is widest posteriorly: its roundness means that the effects of a blow to the head can be distributed and minimised. On the deep aspect of the skull, in the region of the sagittal suture, is a faint groove formed by the superior sagittal sinus as it passes posteriorly between the two layers of the dura mater as

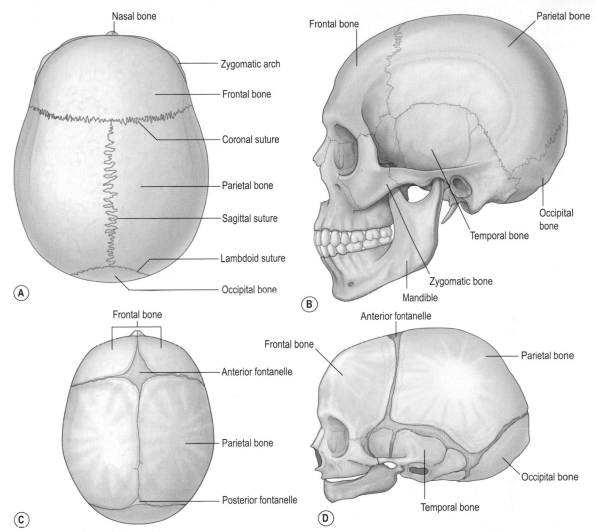

Fig. 5.25 Superior (A and C) and lateral (B and D) views of adult (A and B) and foetal (C and D) skulls.

far as the internal occipital protuberance. On either side of this groove, deeply pitted areas can usually be seen formed by the underlying arachnoid granulations, which are involved in regulating the flow of cerebrospinal fluid (CSF) into the systemic circulation. The base of the skull shows many features and openings which allow blood vessels and nerves to enter and leave the cranial cavity.

Growth of the Skull

At birth, the cranial cavity is relatively large, but the face is small (Fig. 5.25D), approximately an eighth of the whole skull compared with a third in adults. The teeth are not fully formed, and the paranasal sinuses are rudimentary, consequently both the jaws (maxillae,

mandible) and nasal cavities are small. The individual bones are joined by cartilage, ossification progressing with age. There is no mastoid process, so the styloid process and stylomastoid foramen are closer to the side of the head. Undue pressure applied during a forceps delivery in the region of the developing mastoid may, therefore, damage the facial nerve. The maxilla is shallow because it has no sinus, consisting mainly of alveolar processes and developing teeth. The nasal bones are flat, so that the infant has no bridge to the nose, which, together with the absence of superciliary arches, gives the forehead its prominent appearance. The orbits are relatively large and have the nasal cavity lying almost completely between them.

After birth, the skull grows rapidly until the seventh year, with the greatest increase in the size of the cranial cavity occurring during the first year. During the second year, the styloid process and stylomastoid foramen come to lie deeper as the mastoid process begins to grow. By the seventh year, the orbits are almost adult-sized: the petrous part of the temporal bone, body of the sphenoid and foramen magnum have, however, reached full-size. The jaws have enlarged in preparation for eruption of the permanent teeth. Growth of the skull after age 7 is slower than before, except during puberty when a rapid growth in all directions occurs, particularly in the frontal and facial regions, accompanying the increasing size of the paranasal sinuses.

From the early 20s to middle age, there is gradual fusion of the various sutures between the individual bones of the skull, beginning with the sagittal suture.

Viewed Anteriorly

When viewed from the front (Fig. 5.26), the upper third of the skull (forehead) consists of the cranial cavity formed by the frontal bone: parts of the parietal, sphenoid and temporal bones can also be seen in this region. Below the forehead are the two large orbital cavities, whose margins are formed by the frontal bone superiorly, the zygomatic bone inferolaterally and maxilla inferomedially. The walls of the orbital cavity are formed by: the maxilla inferiorly; zygomatic bone and greater wing of the sphenoid laterally; frontal bone and lesser wing of the sphenoid superiorly; and ethmoid and lacrimal bones medially. Deep within the cavity can be seen the superior and inferior orbital fissures and optic canal. Along the medial part of the superior margin is the supraorbital notch, transmitting the corresponding vessels and nerves. Towards the

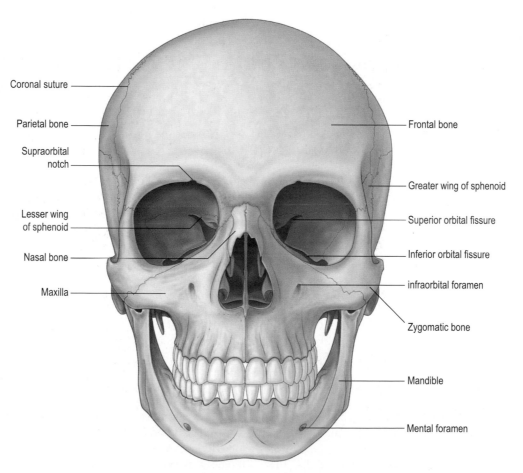

Fig. 5.26 Anterior aspect of an adult skull showing the bones involved and their features.

anterior part of the medial wall is the opening for the nasolacrimal duct, which conveys secretions from the eye (tears) to the nose for eventual swallowing. Below the inferior orbital margin on the anterior aspect of the face is the large infraorbital foramen, through which pass the infraorbital nerve and vessels onto the face.

Inferior and medial to the orbits is the pear-shaped nasal aperture, bound almost entirely by the maxillae, with only the superior part bound by the two nasal bones. Within the nasal cavity, a more-or-less midline septum can be seen formed by the vomer and perpendicular plate of the ethmoid. Projecting medially into the cavity from the lateral walls are the inferior and middle conchae: the superior conchae lie deep to the nasal bones. The inferior alveolar margin of the maxilla, supporting the teeth, forms an almost horizontal convex arch, which fits snugly with the corresponding arch of the mandible.

Viewed Laterally

The temporal bone is central to the lateral aspect of the skull (Fig. 5.25B). Superiorly, it joins the parietal bone posteriorly and greater wing of the sphenoid anteriorly; posteroinferiorly, it joins the occipital bone. It is marked just posterior and inferior to its centre by the external acoustic meatus, above which is a bony ramus passing anteriorly to meet a similar posteriorly projecting process from the zygomatic bone, forming the zygomatic arch. Just inferior to the posterior part of this arch is the mandibular fossa. The styloid process projects inferiorly from deep to the external acoustic meatus.

Viewed Inferiorly

The skeleton of the face attaches to the inferior surface of the anterior half of the cranial cavity. Consequently, a view from below reveals the mandible, maxilla and palatine bones: with the mandible removed, the maxilla and palatine bones can be seen (Fig. 5.27A).

The anterior and lateral margins of the maxilla are marked by sockets for the teeth, somewhat smaller anteriorly, increasing in size as they pass posteriorly around the alveolar margin. The area between these bony margins is formed by the palatine part of the maxilla anteriorly and horizontal plate of the palatine bone posteriorly. Projecting posteriorly in the midline from the posterior border of the palatine bones is the nasal spine, and laterally are the inferiorly directed medial and lateral pterygoid plates of the sphenoid: the medial pterygoid plate has the hook-like pterygoid hamulus. At the lateral edges of the palatine

bones are the greater and lesser palatine foramina transmitting the corresponding vessels and nerves. At the anterior part of the hard palate is the incisive canal, through which pass terminal branches of the greater palatine and sphenopalatine vessels, together with the nasopalatine nerves.

The central section of the base of the skull is formed mainly by the sphenoid, with its many bony processes and foramina. Laterally lies the temporal bone marked by the mandibular fossa, which receives the condyle of the mandible; posterolaterally lies the external acoustic meatus; and posteromedially the styloid process of the temporal bone, a long and slender projection passing inferiorly as well as anteromedially (Fig. 5.27A). Anteromedial to the styloid process is the carotid canal and posteriorly the jugular foramen.

Anterior to the carotid canal is the foramen spinosum, separated from it by the spine of the sphenoid. Posterior to the external acoustic meatus is the large mastoid process of the temporal bone, with the stylomastoid foramen lying medially between it and the styloid process. It is here that the facial nerve (cranial nerve VII) emerges from the skull. Centrally, the large foramen magnum is unmistakable with the occipital condyles on its anterolateral borders. The hypoglossal (anterior condylar) canal lies anterior to the condyle: posterior is the posterior condylar canal. Posterior to the foramen magnum, joined to it by the external occipital crest, is the external occipital protuberance. Passing laterally towards the mastoid process is the superior nuchal line; between this line and the foramen magnum are less distinct lines (inferior nuchal lines), which also curve laterally. The area between the two nuchal lines and foramen magnum gives attachment to the postvertebral muscles.

Palpation

Virtually the whole of the outer surface of the cranium is palpable, being either subcutaneous or lying just below a thin sheet of muscle. The superior aspect of the skull (parietal and frontal bones) can be taken between the examiner's hands as in giving a blessing. On the superior part of the occipital bone, the external occipital protuberance can be readily felt by the fingertips. On the temporal bone, to the side of the skull, the external acoustic meatus is visible, and posteriorly the pinna of the ear: the mastoid process can be identified, becoming pointed at the level of and posterior to the lobe of the ear. From just above the external acoustic meatus, the posterior part of the zygomatic arch can be identified running

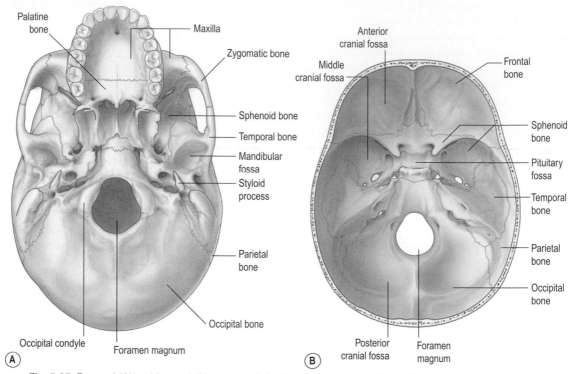

Fig. 5.27 External (A) and internal (B) aspects of the base of an adult skull showing the bones involved and their features.

anteriorly to join the zygomatic bone, which presents as the point of the cheek and is easily palpable.

Anterosuperior to the cheek, the margins of the orbit can be palpated, being particularly marked deep to the eyebrow.

Floor of the Cranial Cavity

The floor of the cranial cavity is formed by the base of the skull, with both the right and left sides having similar features (Fig. 5.27B). The two halves are separated in the sagittal plane by the crista galli anteriorly, body of the sphenoid centrally and foramen magnum and internal occipital protuberance posteriorly. The floor is further divided into anterior, middle and posterior cranial fossae by prominent ridges of bone: each fossa lies at a different level, with the anterior being the highest and posterior the lowest.

Anterior Cranial Fossa

This lies superior and anterior to the middle cranial fossa (Fig. 5.27B), separated from it by the posterior concave edge of the lesser wings of the sphenoid: it contains the inferior part of the frontal lobes of the brain. The walls and most of the floor are formed by the frontal bone, with the posterior part of the floor formed by the lesser wings of

the sphenoid. Between the two sides is a sagittally directed elongated hollow, in the centre of which is the crista galli. On either side of the crista galli is the perforated cribriform plate: it is through this plate that the olfactory nerves (cranial nerve I) from the superior part of the nasal cavity pass to the olfactory bulb, which sits on the cribriform plate.

Middle Cranial Fossa

Lying posterior and inferior to the anterior cranial fossa (Fig. 5.27B), the middle cranial fossa is formed by the temporal and sphenoid bones: it has a median and two lateral parts. The lateral parts contain the temporal lobes of the brain, with the raised median part being formed by the body of the sphenoid. Passing laterally from the body of the sphenoid are the greater wings of the sphenoid, which, with the squamous part of the temporal bone, turn superiorly to form the lateral wall of the skull in the temporal region. The floor of the middle cranial fossa is formed by part of the greater wings of the sphenoid anteriorly and the gently sloping superior surface of the petrous part of the temporal bone posteriorly. Anteriorly, each greater wing of the sphenoid turns superiorly, forming the anterior wall of the fossa. The superior part of this wall is overlapped by the posterior edge of the anterior cranial fossa (lesser wing of the sphenoid).

The body of the sphenoid has a smooth, hollowed depression superiorly (pituitary/hypophyseal fossa), which houses the pituitary gland. Small, hornlike (clinoid) processes project on either side from the anterior and posterior parts of the hollow, giving attachment anteriorly to a horizontal fold of dura mater (tentorium cerebelli) which passes between the cerebral and cerebellar hemispheres. The cavernous sinuses (p. 696), part of the intracranial venous sinus system, are formed between the two layers of the dura mater on either side of the body of the sphenoid. Within the walls, or through the sinuses, pass many of the nerves destined for the orbit, as well as the internal carotid artery: the internal carotid artery emerges from the sinus anterolateral to the anterior clinoid process. Anterior to this region, between the roots of the lesser wings of the sphenoid, is the optic canal running anterolaterally, conveying the optic nerve and ophthalmic artery to the orbit. Passing transversely between the two optic canals is a groove (sulcus chiasmatis); it does not lodge the optic chiasma. Between the greater and lesser wings of the sphenoid is a gap which narrows as it passes laterally (superior orbital fissure): it opens directly into the posterior part of the orbit. It transmits many structures to and from the orbit: third (III), fourth (IV), ophthalmic division of the fifth (V_1), and sixth (VI) cranial nerves, and the ophthalmic veins. Inferior to the superior orbital fissure in the anterior wall, close to the body of the sphenoid, is the rounded foramen rotundum, through which passes the maxillary division of the fifth (V_2) cranial nerve to enter the pterygopalatine fossa.

In the floor of the middle cranial fossa, between the greater wing of the sphenoid and petrous temporal bone, is the foramen lacerum. In life, its edges are connected by fibrous tissue, which supports the internal carotid artery as it passes medially from the carotid canal to the side of the body of the sphenoid. Lateral to the foramen lacerum are two openings in the greater wing of the sphenoid. The larger medial one (foramen ovale) transmits the mandibular division of the fifth (V_3) cranial nerve, as well as the lesser petrosal nerve and small blood vessels, while the more lateral opening (foramen spinosum) transmits the middle meningeal artery supplying the meninges of the brain.

Posterior Cranial Fossa

Largest and deepest of all three fossae (Fig. 5.27B), the posterior cranial fossa houses the cerebellum. The temporal bone is a hard ridge passing posterolaterally from the body of the sphenoid: along its superior border is a longitudinal groove for the superior petrosal sinus.

The floor and most of the posterior wall of the fossa are formed by the concave surface of the occipital bone, with a small part of the posterior wall being formed by the parietal bones. The anterolateral wall is formed by the posterior surface of the petrous part of the temporal bone, with the body of the sphenoid and basilar part of the occipital bone forming the anterior wall.

Its most obvious feature is the large oval foramen magnum, which is slightly narrower transversely than from anterior to posterior. It transmits the spinal cord at the junction of the spinal cord and brainstem, as well as a number of blood vessels and the spinal part of the accessory nerve (cranial nerve XI). Passing superiorly from the posterior margin of the foramen magnum is the internal occipital crest, ending at the internal occipital protuberance. Running inferiorly towards the protuberance is the continuation of the groove of the superior sagittal sinus. On approaching the protuberance, the groove passes to the right running transversely around the posterolateral wall of the fossa as the groove for the transverse sinus. On reaching the petrous part of the temporal bone, the groove turns inferiorly, continuing as an S-shaped groove towards the jugular foramen for the sigmoid sinus. A similar arrangement of transverse and sigmoid grooves is also present on the left-hand side of the fossa. The sigmoid sinus passes through the jugular foramen to become the internal jugular vein. As it does so, it is joined by the inferior petrosal sinus, which runs in the groove between the petrous temporal and basioccipital bones towards the jugular foramen. As well as these two venous channels, the jugular foramen also transmits the glossopharyngeal (IX), vagus (X) and accessory (XI) cranial nerves.

Anterior to the jugular foramen is the carotid canal, which transmits the internal carotid artery and its associated plexus of sympathetic nerves. In the posterior surface of the petrous part of the temporal bone is the opening of the internal auditory meatus; both the facial (VII) and vestibulocochlear (VIII) cranial nerves enter the canal.

Running anterosuperiorly from the anterior margin of the foramen magnum is the clivus, which has the basilar artery separating it from the brainstem. On the lateral part of the clivus, medial to the groove for the inferior petrosal sinus, runs the abducens (VI) cranial nerve before piercing the dura to run in the sinus. Above the lateral margin of the foramen magnum is the hypoglossal canal, which runs anterolaterally and transmits the hypoglossal (XII) cranial nerve.

FACE

MANDIBLE

Details of the mandible can be found on page 665.

MUSCLES CHANGING THE SHAPE OF THE FACE

The muscles which change the shape of the face are commonly known as the muscles of facial expression (Fig. 5.28). Although contraction of individual or groups of muscles enables human beings to smile, frown, look happy or sad and generally convey many emotions, it has to be remembered that their primary action is to dilate (open) or constrict (close) the eyes, nose and mouth. In addition, buccinator plays an important role in mastication (p. 680), while others are involved in forming and shaping the sounds produced by the larynx into recognisable words.

To perform these many complex actions, it is not surprising that the majority of muscles have only one attachment to bone, the other being to the superficial fascia and skin. Consequently, when the facial muscles contract, their secondary action has a profound effect on facial expression, through which an individual can convey their emotions to the world at large, as well as recognise the feelings of others.

All the muscles of facial expression are derived from the second pharyngeal arch and are consequently supplied by branches of the facial (seventh cranial) nerve. Damage to branches of the facial nerve results in the loss of tone in the muscles supplied by that branch, with a consequent sagging of that part of the face. The skin of the face is supplied by the ophthalmic, maxillary and mandibular branches of the trigeminal (fifth cranial) nerve.

The muscles are best considered in groups in relation to whether they act upon the eyes, nose or mouth: muscles which do not adhere to this plan are considered individually.

MUSCLES OF THE FOREHEAD AND EYEBROWS

Occipitofrontalis
Corrugator supercilii
Procerus

Occipitofrontalis

Raising the eyebrows, as in an expression of surprise, is produced by occipitofrontalis (Fig. 5.28), a two-part muscle united by the strong aponeurosis of the scalp. The posterior belly arises from the lateral part of the superior nuchal line and mastoid part of the temporal bone from where it passes

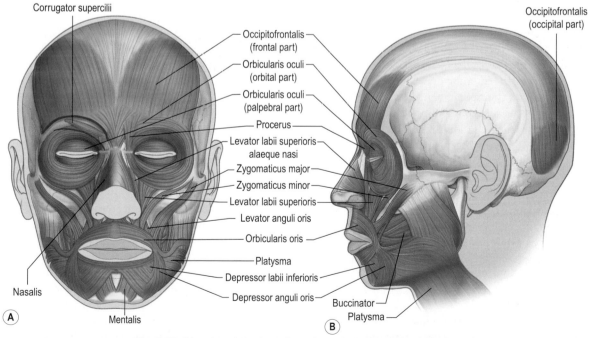

Fig. 5.28 Muscles of the face viewed anteriorly (A) and laterally (B).

to attach to the aponeurosis. The larger anterior belly runs from the aponeurosis to the superficial fascia of the forehead and eyebrow, interlacing with orbicularis oculi.

Action

Contraction of the posterior or anterior bellies of occipitofrontalis pulls the scalp posteriorly or anteriorly, respectively. Acting from the aponeurosis, the anterior bellies raise the eyebrows either together in surprise or individually as in a quizzical expression: this action produces the deep transverse lines on the forehead.

Corrugator Supercilii

Small muscle (Fig. 5.28) arising from the medial end of the superciliary arch (eyebrow), blending with orbicularis oculi: its fibres run superolaterally to attach to the skin of the eyebrows. On contraction, they pull the eyebrows together inferomedially as in a frown, so producing the deep vertical wrinkles between the eyebrows.

Procerus

Small muscles continuous with each other across the midline: they run from the inferior part of the nasal bone to the skin over the inferior part of the forehead, intermingling with the anterior belly of occipitofrontalis (Fig. 5.28). On contraction, they pull down the medial part of the eyebrow producing transverse wrinkles at the root of the nose.

MUSCLES AROUND THE EYE

Orbicularis Oculi

One of the most complex muscles of the face and by far the most important around the eye (Fig. 5.28), orbicularis oculi consists of three parts (orbital, palpebral and lacrimal). The orbital part surrounds the orbit, spreading onto the forehead, temple and cheek, having an attachment to the medial margin of the orbit and medial palpebral ligament: the fibres attaching above the medial palpebral ligament run elliptically around the orbit to attach again below it. The palpebral part of the muscle is much thinner and lies within the eyelids: these fibres arise from the medial palpebral ligament and run laterally within the eyelids to unite at the lateral palpebral raphe. The lacrimal part arises from fascia posterior to the lacrimal sac and crest of the lacrimal bone, passing laterally to attach to the tarsal plates of each eyelid.

Action

Orbicularis oculi plays an important role in protecting the eye by washing the eyeball with tears and firmly closing the eye to protect it against insult and injury. The orbital part of the muscle, which can act independently or with the other parts, draws the skin of the forehead and cheek towards the medial angle of the orbit, so that the eye is screwed up tightly as when a bright light is shone into the eyes or when dust blows towards them. This action produces the characteristic crow's feet at the lateral corner of the eye. The palpebral part of the muscle exerts much finer control over the individual eyelids: by reflex or voluntary contraction, it pulls the upper eyelid inferiorly and lower eyelid superiorly closing the eye. By pulling the eyelids medially during regular blinking, tears produced by the lacrimal gland are wiped over the surface of the eyeball to keep it moist, as well as washing particles towards the lacrimal puncta. The small movements of the eyelids are very important in nonverbal communication between humans. The lacrimal part of the muscle dilates the lacrimal sac.

Application

When orbicularis oculi is paralysed, there is an inability to close the eye resulting in the eyeball becoming red and inflamed.

MUSCLES AROUND THE NOSE

Nasalis
Levator labii superioris alaeque nasi
Depressor septi
Small muscles around the nose (Fig. 5.28) acting to dilate or constrict the nasal apertures. Although these actions are rudimentary in humans, they are of obvious importance in some animals (camels). The dilators are nasalis and levator labii superioris alaeque nasi, which also acts on the upper lip, and the constrictor is depressor septi.

MUSCLES AROUND THE MOUTH

Orbicularis oris
Buccinator
Levator labii superioris alaeque nasi
Levator labii superioris
Zygomaticus major and minor
Levator anguli oris
Depressor anguli oris and depressor labii inferioris
Risorius and mentalis

Orbicularis Oris

Surrounding the mouth (Fig. 5.28), orbicularis oris is a composite sphincter muscle with deep and superficial parts. Vertically, it extends from the nasal septum to midway between the chin and lower lip: the deep fibres are continuous with buccinator, while the superficial fibres are all derived from other muscles. The deep fibres attach to both the maxilla and mandible near the lateral incisor. Between the deep and superficial layers, the intrinsic fibres of orbicularis oris run elliptically around the mouth, having no bony attachment. Some superficial fibres decussate like those of buccinator.

Action

Orbicularis oris produces puckering of the lips as in kissing or whistling. It has an important role in (1) speech by changing the shape of the mouth and lips to help form recognisable sounds and (2) mastication as its contraction against the teeth helps keep food between the teeth during chewing. Contractions of the various muscles which blend with orbicularis oris change its shape.

Buccinator

Continuous with the deep part of orbicularis oris, buccinator forms the substance of the cheek (Fig. 5.28). It arises from both the maxilla and mandible opposite the molar teeth and from the pterygomandibular raphe between the pterygoid hamulus and posterior end of the mylohyoid line. The fibres run anteriorly to blend with those of orbicularis oris: the medial fibres decussate posterolateral to the angle of the mouth so that the lower fibres run to the upper lip and the upper fibres to the lower lip. The interlacing of the deep fibres of buccinator with some of the superficial fibres of orbicularis oris forms an easily felt nodule at the angle of the mouth (modiolus).

Action

Buccinator presses the cheek against the teeth or resists outward pressure against the cheek. The former action is important in mastication as it prevents the accumulation of food in the vestibule of the mouth (a common problem when buccinator is paralysed). When blowing up a balloon, buccinator can be felt resisting the outward pressure of air against the cheek. When the lips are protruded by orbicularis oris, buccinator causes the cheek to cave in, thereby producing a sucking action. It can also be used to pull orbicularis oris posteriorly against the teeth or to retract the angle of the mouth to expose the premolar and molar teeth.

Palpation

If a finger is placed between the cheek and teeth, buccinator can be felt contracting as the finger is pressed against the teeth.

Levator Labii Superioris Alaeque Nasi

Arising from the maxilla it attaches to the ala of the nose and skin and muscles of the upper lip (Fig. 5.28).

Levator Labii Superioris

Arising from the maxilla above the infraorbital foramen it attaches to the upper lip towards its lateral end (Fig. 5.28).

Zygomaticus Major and Minor

Both muscles arise from the zygomatic bone and attach to the upper lip near its angle (Fig. 5.28).

Levator Anguli Oris

Arising from the maxilla below the infraorbital foramen (Fig. 5.28), it attaches to the skin and muscle at the angle of the mouth: some fibres may pass to the lower lip.

Action

When contracting on both sides, all of the above muscles raise the upper lip as in smiling: contraction of one side produces a sneer. The tone of the muscles is important in maintaining the normal horizontal position of the mouth. When paralysed, there is gradual drooping of the angle of the mouth on the affected side leading to leakage of saliva and a constant dribble from the corner of the mouth. Zygomaticus major, assisted by levator anguli oris, raises and pulls the angle of the mouth laterally, as in laughing.

The following facial muscles have their effect on the lower lip.

Depressors Anguli Oris and Labii Inferioris

Depressor anguli oris arises from the anterior aspect of the mandible inferior to the mental foramen and blends with muscles of the lower lip at the angle of the mouth (Fig. 5.28), as well as attaching to the skin; some fibres may pass into the upper lip. It is continuous with platysma and overlaps depressor labii inferioris, which also arises from the mandible inferior to the mental foramen: its fibres attach to the skin and muscle of the lower lip, with fibres from each side blending together (Fig. 5.28).

Risorius and Mentalis

These two muscles, although considered as part of the lower lip musculature, usually only have connections to the skin of the lower lip. Risorius arises from the fascial covering of the parotid gland attaching to the skin at the angle of the mouth: mentalis arises from the mandible inferior to the incisors and passes to the skin of the chin (Fig. 5.28).

Platysma (Fig. 5.28), with which risorius may be completely fused, is considered on page 677.

Action

Depressor anguli oris and depressor labii inferioris pull the mouth inferolaterally giving an expression of sadness: by itself, depressor labii inferioris curls the lower lip inferiorly. Mentalis on the other hand pulls the skin of the chin superiorly, causing protrusion of the lower lip as in pouting: risorius merely pulls the angle of the mouth laterally.

Application

If the muscles on one side of the face are paralysed, as in Bell palsy, the typical problems encountered are an inability to close the eye, a tendency for food to accumulate in the vestibule of the mouth (between the cheek, lips and teeth of the paralysed side), the corner of the mouth droops downwards on the affected side, and, on smiling, the mouth is pulled towards the sound side by the unopposed action of the intact muscles.

SECTION SUMMARY

Skull
- The skeleton of the head and face consists of a large, hollow, cranial cavity (housing the brain) and bones of the face anteroinferiorly
- The cranial cavity is formed by the parietal, frontal, temporal, sphenoid and occipital bones
- The facial skeleton is formed by the frontal and zygomatic bones and maxillae, with the mandible inferiorly
- The floor of the cranial cavity is divided into anterior, middle and posterior cranial fossae

Muscles of the Face
These principally act to open or close the orbit, nose and mouth; however, because they attach to the skin, they are also intimately involved in changing facial expressions. All muscles are innervated by the facial (seventh) cranial nerve.

Muscles of the Forehead and Eyebrows
Occipitofrontalis, corrugator supercilii and procerus

Muscles Around the Eye
Orbicularis oculi

Muscles Around the Nose
Nasalis, levator labii superioris alaeque nasi and depressor septi

Muscles Around the Mouth
Orbicularis oris, buccinators, levator labii superioris alaeque nasi, levator labii superioris, zygomaticus major, zygomaticus minor, levator anguli oris, depressor anguli oris, depressor labii inferioris, risorius and mentalis

❓ SELF-ASSESSMENT QUESTIONS

21. Which of the following bones does not contribute to the skull vault?
    a. Parietal
    b. Occipital
    c. Maxilla
    d. Frontal
    e. Temporal
22. At what age does the anterior fontanelle close?
23. Between which bones is the posterior fontanelle?
24. Of which bone is the styloid process a part?
25. Which is the largest opening on the inferior aspect of the skull?
26. Which muscle presses the cheek against the teeth?
27. Which cerebral lobe is located within the anterior cranial fossa?
28. Which bones form the middle cranial fossa?
29. What is the innervation of the muscles of facial expression?
30. Which muscle is responsible for closing the eye?

MANDIBLE AND HYOID

LEARNING OUTCOMES

By the end of the section, you should be able to:
1. Identify, palpate and examine the mandible and hyoid
2. Locate, palpate (where possible) and examine the muscles of mastication and describe their attachments, action and innervation
3. Describe the movements possible and their restraints at the temporomandibular joint
4. Describe the role of the muscles of mastication
5. Examine and assess movements of the mandible
6. Appreciate the influence of pathology and/or trauma on the temporomandibular joint

MANDIBLE

The mandible (lower jaw) completes the skull: it consists of a horizontal convex body, with two rami projecting superiorly from the posterior ends of the body (Fig. 5.29). The rami and body present lateral and medial surfaces, with the body having superior and inferior borders and the rami anterior and posterior borders. The lateral surface of the body is slightly concave from superior to inferior and markedly convex from side to side: a vertical midline may be evident where the two halves have fused. Towards the anterior aspect of the body on each

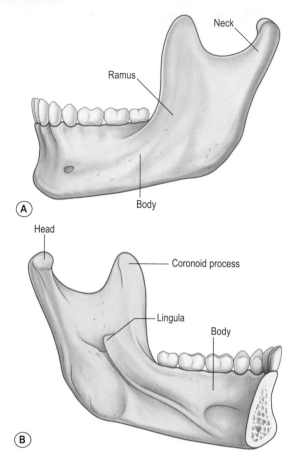

Fig. 5.29 Lateral (A) and medial (B) aspects of the ramus and body of the mandible.

side is the mental foramen transmitting the mental nerve and vessels. The medial surface of the body is divided by a slightly raised ridge (mylohyoid line) into superior and inferior areas. Posterior to the anterior aspect of the mandible, above the mylohyoid line, is the sublingual fossa which lodges the sublingual salivary gland: below the mylohyoid line, in the middle third of the body, is the submandibular fossa for the submandibular gland. On the medial surface of the anterior midline region are two pairs of bony projections (genial/mental spines): the superior pair lie above the mylohyoid line and give rise to part of the tongue (genioglossus), while the inferior pair lie below the line and give attachment to geniohyoid. The superior border of the body consists of a series of sockets for the teeth: the bone behind the third molar is thickened as it joins the anterior border of the ramus. The inferior border of the body is thick and rounded but has two fossae (digastric fossae) anteriorly, one on each side of the midline for

attachment of the anterior belly of digastric. Posteriorly, the body meets the inferior posterior part of the ramus at the angle, which tends to be everted in males and inverted in females. Just anterior to the angle, the inferior border is notched where the facial artery crosses it to enter the face.

Each ramus is continuous with the body but is flatter: the medial surface is marked by the mandibular foramen, which is partially covered by a small bony process (lingula), to which is attached the sphenomandibular ligament. The inferior alveolar nerve and vessels enter the mandible at the mandibular foramen, giving mylohyoid branches before they do so. The latter pass anteroinferiorly running in the mylohyoid groove, also seen on the medial surface of the ramus. The area behind the mylohyoid groove towards the angle of the mandible is roughened for attachment of medial pterygoid. The lateral surface of the ramus is roughened for the attachment of masseter. The posterior border is thick and rounded, particularly at its inferior end, and may show a shallow fossa for part of the parotid gland. The anterior border is also thick inferiorly but becomes a thin pointed projection superiorly (coronoid process). The superior border between the coronoid process anteriorly and condylar process (head) posteriorly is concave. The head, which articulates with the mandibular fossa of the temporal bone, is much broader transversely than anteroposteriorly: it is marked at its lateral and medial ends by prominent tubercles.

Palpation

The entire length and depth of the mandible are palpable with the angle posteriorly being prominent, particularly in males, even though the posterior border and lateral surface of the ramus is mainly covered by muscle and part of the parotid gland. The lateral tubercle on the condyle can be palpated anterior to the tragus of the ear inferior to the posterior part of the zygomatic arch. Identification is easier with the individual opening and closing the mouth, when the condyle can be felt gliding anteriorly on the articular surface of the temporal bone.

Development

At birth, the two halves of the mandible are separate, with the body being a shell of alveolar bone enclosing the developing teeth. The ramus is short, with the angle it makes with the body being obtuse (~175 degrees), so that the condyle lies nearly in line with the body (Fig. 5.30A). During the first year, the two halves begin to fuse at the symphysis menti, with union being complete by the end of the second year. The ramus gradually enlarges

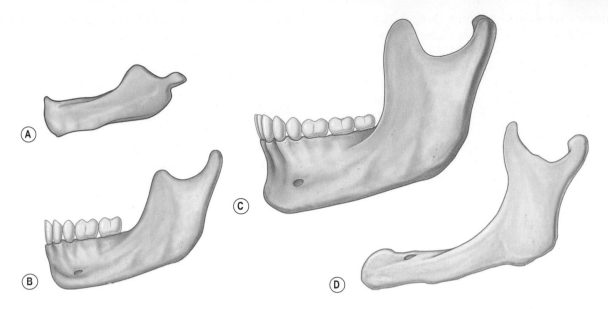

Fig. 5.30 Lateral aspect of the mandible: (A) at birth, (B) at age 4, (C) in adults and (D) in old age.

with a corresponding decrease in the angle between the body and ramus, so that by about age 4, it has decreased to 140 degrees (Fig. 5.30B). Progressive changes within the mandible continue so that, in adults, the angle has decreased to 110 degrees or less (Fig. 5.30C). With the loss of teeth in old age, the alveolar sockets are absorbed, and the angle between the body and ramus now increases to 140 degrees due to bony remodelling (Fig. 5.30D). The condyle becomes directed posteriorly widening the mandibular notch.

The mandible grows in width between its angles, as well as in length, height and thickness. The condylar process grows not only superiorly but also posteriorly and laterally, contributing to its increase in total length, height and width. Modelling maintains the shape of the condyle and the curves of the anterior margin of the ramus and coronoid process.

In adults, the long axis of the condyle is directed posteromedially, forming an angle of approximately 30 degrees with the frontal plane (Fig. 5.31): the angle is not always consistent from side to side. If prolonged, the two axes meet in the median plane at the anterior margin of the foramen magnum.

TEMPOROMANDIBULAR JOINT

Indirect articulation between the mandible (lower jaw) and skull: it is one of the few joints containing a complete

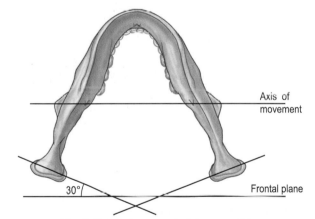

Fig. 5.31 Inferior aspect of the mandible.

intra-articular disc dividing the joint space into superior and inferior compartments. The disc facilitates the movements which are possible at the joint so that the combined gliding and hinge actions produce rotation of the mandible about a transverse axis between the lingulae. The position of the axis means that, during mandibular movements, structures entering the mandibular foramen (inferior alveolar neurovascular bundle) are not put under tension.

The articular surfaces of the two components of the joint are highly incongruent: the intra-articular disc improves congruence between them. It is probably a functional advantage to have highly incongruent joint surfaces at the temporomandibular joint because of the growth changes associated with the mandible and, therefore, the changing demands made upon the joint.

The temporomandibular joint, together with its associated ligaments and muscles, as well as the occluding surfaces of the teeth, limits the forcible opposition of the jaws during biting. However, this is only one aspect of normal function which includes mastication, suckling, swallowing, yawning and speaking, although this latter activity involves little force at the joint.

Articular Surfaces

Each temporomandibular joint is a synovial condyloid joint between the mandibular fossa of the temporal bone on the base of the skull and the corresponding condyle of the mandible: between each pair of joint surfaces is a complete intra-articular disc. The bony articular surfaces are covered by fibrocartilage, with the superficial part having a large fibrous element and only the deeper parts containing cartilage.

Mandibular Fossa

The temporal articular surface extends from the squamotympanic fissure to the anterior margin of the articular eminence: it is concavoconvex from posterior to anterior (Fig 5.32). It is oval, wider mediolaterally than anteroposteriorly (~23 and ~19 mm, respectively): at birth, this surface is more-or-less plane, with the lateral part higher than the medial. Changes during childhood result in the sinuous surface shape seen in sagittal section: mediolaterally, the surface becomes more horizontal. In adults, the fossa consists of a continuous plate of

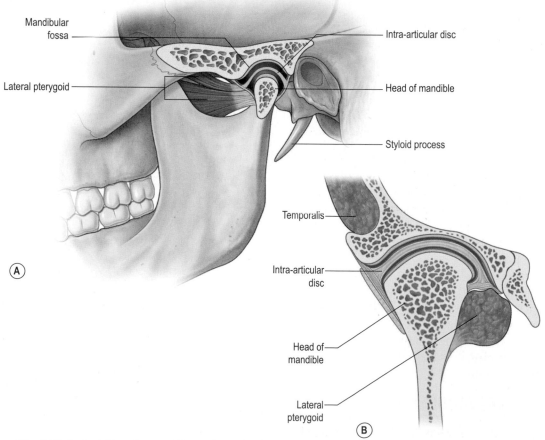

Fig. 5.32 Sagittal (A) and coronal (B) sections of the temporomandibular joint showing the intra-articular disc between the articular surfaces, as well as the relationship of lateral pterygoid.

compact bone with no underlying spongy bone. Remodelling of the bony plate occurs throughout life and may lead to deviations from the usual joint shape.

Condyle of the Mandible

The spindle-shaped condyle lies at right angles to the ramus of the mandible, with its long axis passing posteromedially: it is slightly smaller than the mandibular fossa (~20 mm mediolaterally and ~10 mm anteroposteriorly). The articular surface of the condyle is curved and displaced slightly posteriorly with respect to the highest point of the condyle (Fig. 5.32): mediolaterally, there is a great degree of symmetry.

Intra-Articular Disc

Separating the incongruent bony articular surfaces, the intra-articular disc moulds itself to them during movements at the joint (Fig. 5.32). The disc is thought to be derived from the tendon of lateral pterygoid, which in the embryo passes posteriorly between the head of the mandible and temporal bone to attach to the malleus: the tendon compressed between the two bones is said to form the disc. In adults, when viewed from above, it is an avascular oval plate of fibrous tissue. At birth, it is relatively flat, but with development of the bony constituents of the joint, the disc becomes shaped like a jockey's cap so that its superior surface is concavoconvex to fit the mandibular fossa and articular eminence, while the inferior surface is concave over the condyle.

The central region of the disc, although the most dense, is the thinnest (1.1 mm): anteriorly and posteriorly its thickness varies up to 2.0 and 2.8 mm, respectively. Very rarely, the disc is perforated in its central region. Although essentially avascular, the periphery of the disc, which is attached to the deep aspect of the joint capsule, is highly vascular and innervated. Anteriorly, the disc attaches near the condyle and receives, together with the adjoining capsule, the attachment of the upper fibres of lateral pterygoid. Posteriorly, it attaches nearer to the temporal bone than the mandible and is, therefore, not as freely mobile as elsewhere. This region is less dense than other parts, with the fibres having a crinkled arrangement enabling a small degree of elongation and recoil.

At birth, the central region consists of relatively soft collagenous tissue, which becomes coarser with age and use. The functional wear that occurs is thought to be a major factor in the conversion of the region into a disc of fibrocartilage.

Surface Marking and Palpation

The line of the temporomandibular joint can be easily identified by placing the tip of the finger immediately anterior to the tragus of the ear. As the individual opens their mouth, the mandibular condyle moves anteriorly and a large depression can then be felt: this is the joint cavity.

Joint Capsule and Synovial Membrane

The strong fibrous joint capsule is thin and loose, surrounding the articular surfaces and enclosing the intra-articular disc. It attaches superiorly to the margins of the mandibular fossa as far anteriorly as the transverse prominence of the articular eminence: inferiorly, the capsule attaches to the neck of the mandible (Fig. 5.33). The intra-articular disc is attached to the deep aspect of the capsule (Fig. 5.32). Above this attachment, the capsule is loose permitting free movement of the disc with respect to the mandibular fossa: inferiorly, the capsule is much more taut with the fibres of the medial and lateral parts being short so that the disc appears to be attached directly to the medial and lateral ends of the condyle. Part of the tendon of lateral pterygoid attaches to the anterior aspect of the joint capsule and, therefore, indirectly to the intra-articular disc.

The capsular attachments allow rotatory movements to occur between the condyle and inferior surface of the disc, as well as enabling the disc and condyle to move anteriorly and posteriorly as a single unit against the mandibular fossa.

Two synovial membranes are associated with the joint, one for each compartment (superior and inferior to the disc): each membrane lines all nonarticular surfaces and fuses with the periphery of the disc.

Ligaments

Three ligaments are associated with the joint: the lateral ligament blends with the capsule, while the sphenomandibular and stylomandibular ligaments are accessory to the joint. The accessory ligaments play an important role in guiding movement of the mandible against the base of the skull during muscle contraction: the pterygomandibular raphe also acts to guide movement of the mandible.

Lateral Ligament

A broad attachment to the inferior border and tubercle of the zygomatic bone, from where fibres pass posteroinferiorly blending with the joint capsule to attach to the lateral and posterior parts of the neck of the mandible (Fig. 5.33A): it reinforces the lateral aspect of the joint capsule.

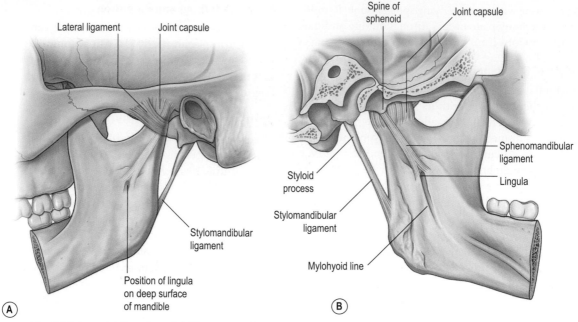

Fig. 5.33 Lateral (A) and medial (B) aspects of the temporomandibular joint showing ligaments associated with the joint.

Sphenomandibular Ligament

Strong, thin, flat band lying on the medial side of the joint, passing anteroinferiorly from the spine of the sphenoid to the lingula and adjacent area on the medial surface of the ramus of the mandible (Fig. 5.33B). The sphenomandibular ligament develops from the sheath of that part of the cartilage of the first pharyngeal arch (Meckel's cartilage) lying between the base of the skull and mandibular foramen.

Stylomandibular Ligament

Thickening of the deep cervical fascia extending from near the apex of the styloid process to the inferior part of the posterior border of the ramus of the mandible close to the angle (Fig. 5.33). It separates the parotid (posterior) and submandibular (anterior) salivary glands.

Blood Supply, Lymphatic Drainage and Innervation

The arterial supply to the temporomandibular joint is from branches of the middle meningeal and anterior tympanic branches of the maxillary artery, as well as the superficial temporal and ascending pharyngeal arteries. The superficial temporal and maxillary arteries are the terminal branches of the external carotid artery, while the ascending pharyngeal arises from the external

carotid lower down in the neck. Venous drainage is to the retromandibular vein and then to the jugular system within the neck. Lymphatic drainage of the joint is to the deep parotid lymph nodes.

The nerve supply to the joint is by twigs from the auriculotemporal and masseteric branches of the mandibular division of the trigeminal (fifth cranial) nerve.

Relations

The joint is relatively superficial, covered by skin and subcutaneous tissue only. The condyle can be palpated immediately below the middle third of the zygomatic arch. Crossing the zygomatic arch posteriorly, but anterior to the external auditory meatus, are the superficial temporal vessels (Fig. 5.34): pressure applied in this region reveals the pulse.

Anteriorly is the tendon of lateral pterygoid passing from its anterior and deep attachments to attach partly to the anterior joint capsule and partly to the neck of the mandible. Also anteriorly is the tendon of temporalis (Fig. 5.34), lying superficial to lateral pterygoid, as it passes deep to the zygomatic arch from the temporal fossa to attach to the anterior and medial aspects of the coronoid process.

The root of the styloid process is posteromedial to the mandibular fossa, which has the carotid sheath and its contents medial to it.

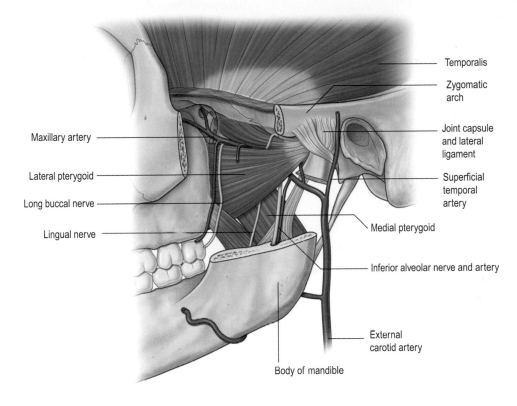

Temporalis

Zygomatic arch

Joint capsule and lateral ligament

Superficial temporal artery

Medial pterygoid

Inferior alveolar nerve and artery

External carotid artery

Body of mandible

Maxillary artery

Lateral pterygoid

Long buccal nerve

Lingual nerve

Fig. 5.34 Lateral aspect of the mandible and skull showing the relationship of structures to the temporomandibular joint: part of the ramus of the mandible has been removed.

Stability

This depends to a large extent on whether the mouth is open or closed, being greater with the mouth closed and teeth occluded.

With the mouth closed, the teeth themselves stabilise the mandible on the maxilla and take any strain if a blow is received on the chin. Furthermore, anterior movement of the condyle is discouraged by the articular eminence and contraction of the posterior fibres of temporalis: posterior movement is prevented by the lateral ligament and contraction of lateral pterygoid.

With the mouth open, the joint is less stable because the condyle has moved anteriorly onto the articular eminence, as well as rotating against the intra-articular disc. Posterior dislocation is opposed again by the lateral ligament and lateral pterygoid, while anterior dislocation is restricted by the articular eminence, tension in the lateral ligament and contraction of masseter, temporalis and medial pterygoid. However, with the mouth open,

there is little to prevent a superior dislocation through the thin roof of the mandibular fossa. In practice, such an injury is extremely rare as a blow to the drooping mandible usually causes the mouth either to close or open more fully.

The most common dislocation is one in which one or both condyles pass anteriorly beyond the articular eminences (anterior dislocation) (Fig. 5.35A): this can occur in yawning or opening the mouth too widely. Reduction of the dislocation is often prevented by spasm of the deep posterior fibres of masseter, which tend to hold the dislocated jaw open because they now pass behind the axis of rotation due to the anterior position of the condyles. To reduce the dislocation, the spasm must be overcome, with or without an anaesthetic. If the dislocation is on one side only, it can be reduced by placing the thumb on the molar teeth of the dislocated side and pushing inferoposteriorly. This releases the condyle, and the mandible springs back into place: care must be taken

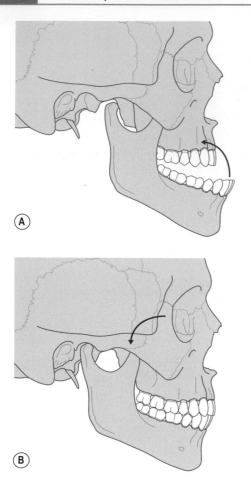

Fig. 5.35 Relationship of the head of the mandible and mandibular fossa at the temporomandibular joint (A) in bilateral dislocation and (B) with the mouth closed.

quickly to remove the thumb. If the dislocation is bilateral, then the angles of the mandible are gripped tightly with one hand and pulled inferoposteriorly, while the other hand pushes the chin superiorly (Fig. 5.35A). On release of the condyles, the mandible should spring back into position (Fig. 5.35B). Occasionally, the dislocation tends to recur, particularly on yawning. With loss of the permanent dentition, the joint is less stable, and anterior dislocation occurs more readily: it is also more easily reduced because of the relative lengthening of the ligaments due to tooth loss.

MOVEMENTS OF THE MANDIBLE

The movements of the mandible are complex, involving the coordinated action of the muscles attached to it.

Because of the nature of the temporomandibular joint, four basic movements of the mandible can be identified:

1. Protraction: pulling the mandible anteriorly so that its head articulates indirectly with the articular eminence of the temporal bone.
2. Retraction: pulling the mandible posteriorly so that its head moves back into the mandibular fossa.
3. Elevation: closing the mouth.
4. Depression: opening the mouth.

Protraction and retraction take place in the superior compartment, while elevation and depression occur in the inferior compartment: side-to-side movements take place in both compartments. Combinations of these basic movements occur in chewing and grinding. Opening the mouth, particularly against resistance (eating sticky foods), also involves the infrahyoid group of muscles to stabilise the hyoid (see Fig. 5.41), by providing a firm base against which mandibular movements can be made.

To understand and appreciate the movements which occur at the temporomandibular joint, some knowledge of the relationship between the upper and lower teeth is necessary. With the teeth in contact (occluded: the upper incisors lie anterior to the lower incisors), there usually is some contact between their opposing surfaces (Fig. 5.36A). When the mouth is opened from this position, the edges of the lower incisors pass inferiorly and anteriorly until the edges of both sets of incisors are directed towards each other. The inferior and anterior movement of the mandible, as in initiating opening the mouth, results from the compound movement of anterior gliding and rotation that occurs at the temporomandibular joint.

The form of the articular surfaces of the joint enables a hinge-like rotation between the condyle and inferior surface of the articular disc in the inferior compartment, while at the same time, the condyle and disc glide anteriorly (and slightly inferiorly) against the mandibular fossa as a single unit in the superior compartment. It is the sinuous form of the mandibular fossa and articular eminence which ensures that the teeth become separated by direct inferior movement of the mandible, as well as by its hinge action.

During the combined gliding and hinge action, the mandible tends to rotate about a transverse axis through the lingulae. The position of this axis is determined by the sphenomandibular and stylomandibular ligaments acting as stays, with various muscles contracting to produce the movements.

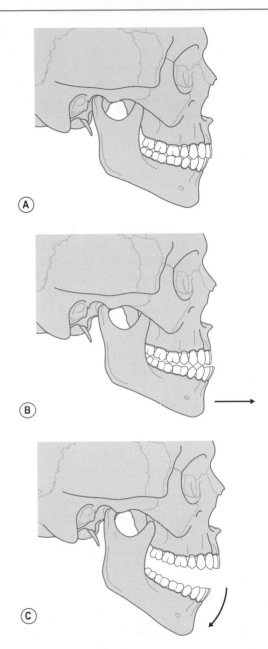

Fig. 5.36 Movements of the mandible: (A) the closed position of the mouth, i.e., retracted and elevated; (B) in protraction; (C) in depression.

Protraction and Retraction

The actions in which the condyle and disc move as a single unit against the mandibular fossa. In protraction, the condyle and disc glide anteriorly so that the condyle rides on the articular eminence (Fig. 5.36B); retraction is the opposite movement in which the condyle is relocated in the mandibular fossa (Fig. 5.36A). The average range of protraction is 6–9 mm (Friedman and Weisberg, 1982) and of retraction 3–4 mm. Protraction is primarily produced by contraction of lateral pterygoid pulling on the disc and neck of the mandible: it is aided by medial pterygoid and the superficial fibres of masseter. Retraction is produced by the posterior, almost horizontal, fibres of temporalis assisted by the suprahyoid muscles. Lateral pterygoid may contract eccentrically during retraction to control the movement.

Elevation and Depression

These movements (Fig. 5.36A and C) of the mandible involve the hinge-like rotation of the condyle against the intra-articular disc in the inferior compartment of the temporomandibular joint. The mouth should be capable of opening sufficiently to enable two or three flexed proximal interphalangeal joints to be inserted into the opening: the distance required for opening ranges from 35 to 50 mm. Closing the mouth (elevation) is a very powerful action produced by the combined action of masseter, medial pterygoid and temporalis: masseter and medial pterygoid hold the mandible in a sling. Temporalis is considered to be the antigravity muscle contracting to keep the mouth closed under normal conditions. Depression of the mandible usually involves eccentric contraction of temporalis to give a controlled opening of the mouth under the influence of gravity. If there is resistance to opening (chewing sticky buns), then geniohyoid, mylohyoid and digastric contract, pulling on the mandible from a fixed hyoid.

Side-to-Side (Grinding) Movements

In chewing and grinding movements, the mandible is alternately protracted and retracted with the two sides usually moving in opposite directions so that one side is protracted and elevated while the opposite side is retracted and depressed. These movements ensure that the mandibular teeth move diagonally across the maxillary teeth, with the intervening food being crushed and ground. Consequently, all of the so-called muscles of mastication are called into action, working rhythmically and alternately. Side-to-side movement has a range of 10–12 mm. Medial pterygoid is of particular importance in this respect as it plays a major role in producing the oblique movement of the mandible. However, to keep the food between the teeth and prevent it from lodging in the vestibule of the mouth or returning to the oral cavity proper, buccinator and the tongue are also working hard: they must be included in any discussion of mastication.

Accessory Movements

A number of accessory movements are possible at the temporomandibular joint; however, only two are described here. With the individual lying supine and the head turned through 90 degrees so that the face looks laterally, an inferiorly directed pressure on the mandibular condyle (using the thumb) causes it to move transversely within the mandibular fossa. Keeping the individual's head in the same position, pressure applied behind the lobe of the ear to the back of the condyle and directed anteriorly produces forward movement of the condyle.

MUSCLES PROTRACTING THE MANDIBLE

Lateral pterygoid
Medial pterygoid (p. 676)
Masseter (p. 674)

Lateral Pterygoid

Lateral pterygoid (Figs 5.34 and 5.37C) has two heads, an upper from the inferior surface of the greater wing of the sphenoid and lower from the lateral surface of the lateral pterygoid plate. From this extensive attachment, the fibres pass posteriorly and slightly laterally to attach to the anterior aspect of the neck of the mandible, capsule and intra-articular disc of the temporomandibular joint.

Innervation

By the mandibular division of the trigeminal (fifth cranial) nerve.

Action

Contraction of lateral pterygoid pulls the head of the mandible, intra-articular disc and joint capsule anteriorly onto the articular eminence, a movement which occurs when opening the mouth. Working with medial pterygoid of the same side, lateral pterygoid produces a slight rotation of the jaw so that the chin swings to the opposite side. When both lateral pterygoids are working, the heads of the mandible are carried anteriorly: there is also slight rotation of the head against the intra-articular disc so that the mouth opens. This is essentially what happens when sleeping with the mouth open. When all four pterygoid muscles contract, the mandible is protruded so that the lower incisors are carried anterior to

the upper incisors (Fig. 5.36B). Lateral pterygoid is the main antagonist to retraction, with its eccentric contraction helping to control the movement.

MUSCLES RETRACTING THE MANDIBLE

Temporalis
Digastric (p. 676)
Geniohyoid (p. 677)

Temporalis

Large, flat, fan-shaped muscle arising from the temporal fossa of the temporal bone and fascia covering it (Fig. 5.37B): the anterior fibres run almost vertically and the most posterior almost horizontally. All fibres converge to a thick tendon which passes deep to the zygomatic arch to attach to the apex and deep surface of the coronoid process and anterior border of the ramus of the mandible. A few fibres may become continuous with buccinator, while other more superficial fibres may fuse with masseter.

Innervation

By the mandibular division of the trigeminal (fifth cranial) nerve, with skin over the muscle supplied mainly by the mandibular branch of the trigeminal nerve and anterior rami of C2 and C3.

Action

The posterior horizontal fibres retract the mandible after it has been protruded. The anterior vertical fibres elevate the mandible and close the mouth: they are constantly active to counteract the effects of gravity.

Palpation

Temporalis can be palpated by applying firm pressure above the zygomatic arch through the temporal fascia over the temporal fossa, particularly when the teeth are firmly clenched together.

MUSCLES ELEVATING THE MANDIBLE

Masseter
Medial pterygoid
Temporalis (p. 674)

Masseter

Flat quadrilateral muscle with deep and superficial parts (Fig. 5.37A). The superficial part arises from the

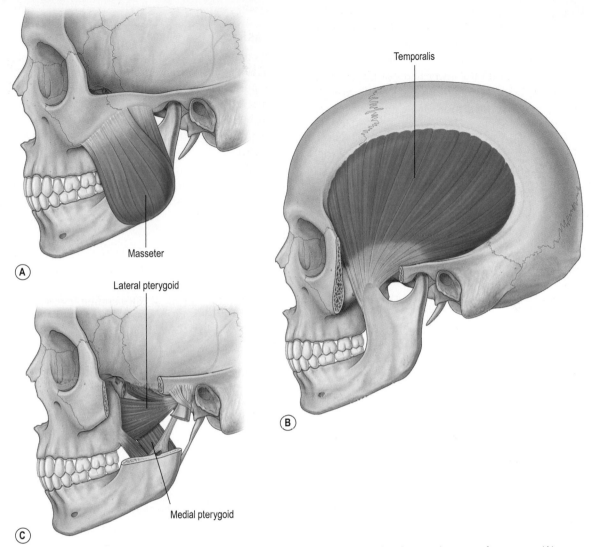

Fig. 5.37 Lateral aspect of the left side of the skull and mandible showing the attachments of masseter (A), temporalis (B) and the pterygoids (C). In (B) the zygomatic arch and in (C) the zygomatic arch and part of the mandible have been removed.

zygomatic process of the maxilla and anterior two-thirds of the zygomatic arch, the fibres running posteroinferiorly to attach to the lateral surface of the angle of the mandible, extending onto the inferior half of the lateral surface of the ramus. The deeper part arises from the deep surface of the zygomatic arch: these fibres run posteroinferiorly to attach to the ramus and coronoid process of the mandible.

Innervation

By the mandibular division of the trigeminal (fifth cranial) nerve, with skin over the muscle supplied mainly by the anterior rami of C2 and C3, and partly by the mandibular branch of the trigeminal nerve.

Action

Masseter elevates the mandible, approximating the upper and lower teeth: the superficial fibres help pull the mandible anteriorly during protraction.

Palpation

Masseter can be palpated by applying pressure through the skin of the cheek below the zygomatic arch when the teeth are clenched together.

Medial Pterygoid

Thick quadrilateral muscle (Figs 5.34 and 5.37C) arising from the medial surface of the lateral pterygoid plate and pyramidal process of the palatine bone: a smaller head arises from the maxillary tubercle. From these two attachments, which surround the lower fibres of lateral pterygoid, the fibres run posteroinferiorly and laterally to attach to a rough triangular impression on the medial surface of the mandible between the angle and mylohyoid line.

Innervation

By the mandibular division of the trigeminal (fifth cranial) nerve.

Action

Medial pterygoid elevates the mandible to close the mouth: because of the direction of the muscle fibres, it also pulls the mandible anteriorly. When the medial and lateral pterygoid of one side contract together, the chin swings to the opposite side. Such movements are important in chewing.

MUSCLES DEPRESSING THE MANDIBLE

Digastric
Mylohyoid

Geniohyoid
Platysma

Digastric

As its name suggests, digastric has two bellies (anterior, posterior) joined by an intermediate tendon (Fig. 5.38). The posterior belly passes anteroinferiorly from the medial surface of the mastoid process in close association with stylohyoid, to an intermediate tendon passing through the attachment of stylohyoid, held by an aponeurotic sling to the superior surface of the hyoid. The anterior belly runs anterosuperiorly to attach to the digastric fossa on the inferior border of the mandible close to the symphysis menti.

Innervation

The posterior belly is supplied by the facial (seventh cranial) nerve and anterior belly by the nerve to mylohyoid from the inferior alveolar branch of the mandibular division of the trigeminal (fifth cranial) nerve.

Action

If the hyoid is fixed, digastric can depress the mandible to assist in opening the mouth, an action required when

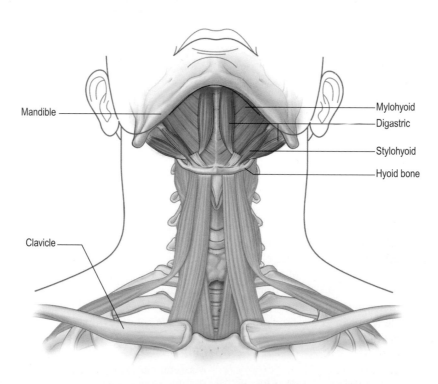

Fig. 5.38 Anterior aspect of the neck showing the suprahyoid muscles.

acting against resistance. With the mandible elevated, digastric also helps in retraction of the mandible. With the mandible fixed, digastric raises the hyoid and, with it, the larynx, an important action in swallowing.

Mylohyoid

Arising from the mylohyoid line on the medial surface of the body of the mandible the fibres of mylohyoid run inferomedially towards the midline to attach to a median fibrous raphe extending from the symphysis menti to the superior surface of the body of the hyoid (Fig. 5.38). The two mylohyoid muscles give rise to a muscular sheet forming the floor of the mouth.

Innervation

By the nerve to mylohyoid from the inferior alveolar branch of the mandibular division of the trigeminal (fifth cranial) nerve.

Action

Mylohyoid can depress the mandible against resistance, elevate the hyoid and also raise the floor of the mouth. In elevating and fixing the hyoid, it helps press the tongue against the roof of the mouth, which is important in swallowing.

Geniohyoid

Small muscle lying deep to mylohyoid, geniohyoid runs from the inferior genial/mental spine on the posterior surface of the symphysis menti to the anterior aspect of the body of the hyoid.

Innervation

By fibres from the anterior primary ramus of C1, which reach the muscle by travelling with the hypoglossal nerve.

Action

Depending upon which end of the muscle is fixed, geniohyoid can elevate the hyoid or depress the mandible. When the hyoid is pulled anterosuperiorly, the floor of the mouth is shortened and the pharynx is widened, ready to receive food.

Platysma

Broad flat sheet of muscle lying in the superficial fascia over the anterior aspect of the neck (Fig. 5.28B), platysma is variably developed in individuals, arising from the skin and superficial part of the chest and shoulder. The fibres cross the clavicle, running superiorly over the anterolateral aspect of the neck to attach to the inferior border of the body of the mandible and fascia of the lower part of the face. In the neck, the platysma of each side is separated by a gap in the midline: just below the chin, the most medial fibres decussate with those of the opposite side.

Innervation

By the facial (seventh cranial) nerve.

Action

Platysma can depress the mandible and help open the mouth; however, as a muscle of facial expression, it can produce expressions of horror by depressing the angle of the mouth and lower lip. When a supreme effort is made, as in weightlifting, platysma can be seen standing out in the neck: similarly, it can be seen standing out in runners after strenuous exertions. In these circumstances, platysma may be acting as an accessory muscle of respiration by pulling on the chest wall. However, it is more probable that the muscle acts to prevent compression of the great veins and the sucking in of the soft tissues of the neck due to the violent respiratory efforts being made. Paralysis of the muscle causes the skin of the neck to fall away in slack folds.

CLINICAL EXAMINATION AND EVALUATION

Different movements occur in each part of the temporomandibular joint: protraction and retraction in the superior compartment, and elevation and depression in the inferior compartment, with side-to-side movements taking place in both compartments.

Protraction, Depression and Lateral Deviation

With the individual seated, stabilise the head and neck to prevent flexion, extension, lateral flexion/bending and rotation. Then either:
- Protract the mandible (Fig. 5.39A).
- Pull the mandible inferiorly to open the mouth (Fig. 5.39B).
- Pull the mandible laterally (Fig. 5.39C).

To assess all the three movements, a plastic rule may be used to measure the distance between the upper and lower incisors. It is important that, in depression, there is no lateral deviation of the mandible.

HYOID

U-shaped bone (Fig. 5.40) deficient posteriorly and suspended in the neck by muscle attachments inferior to the tongue and superior to the larynx (Figs 5.38 and 5.41):

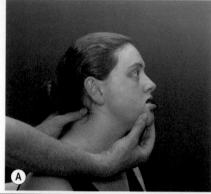

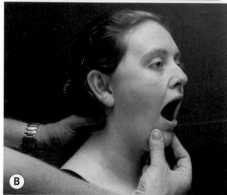

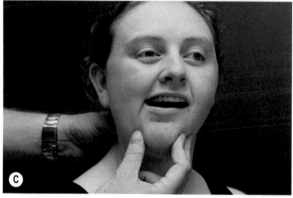

Fig. 5.39 Evaluation of the range of protraction (A), depression (B) and lateral deviation (C) of the mandible.

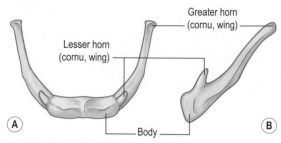

Fig. 5.40 Superior (A) and lateral (B) aspects of the hyoid.

greater horns. The lesser horns and superior part of the body are derived from the second pharyngeal arch, and the greater horns and inferior part of the body from the third pharyngeal arch. The stylohyoid ligament, also from the second arch, attaches to the lesser horn. The hyoid is connected by muscles and ligaments to the tongue, mandible, base of the skull (styloid process), thyroid cartilage and sternum.

Ossification

A pair of ossification centres, which soon unite, appear in the body shortly before birth, as well as a single centre for each greater horn: during the first year centres appear for the lesser horns. The body and greater horns do not fuse until middle age: the lesser horns fusing with the remainder in old age.

Palpation

The two greater horns can be felt through the skin inferior to the mandible if firm pressure is applied between the finger and thumb above the thyroid cartilage of the larynx. In this position, the bone can be moved from side to side. The body can be palpated in the anterior neck about 2 cm above the laryngeal prominence with the chin elevated.

MUSCLES DEPRESSING THE HYOID

Sternohyoid
Sternothyroid
Thyrohyoid
Omohyoid

Sternohyoid

Strap muscle (Fig. 5.41) arising from the medial end of the clavicle, posterior sternoclavicular ligament and posterior surface of the manubrium sterni. The fibres run superiorly and slightly medially to attach to the inferior border of the body of the hyoid.

being attached to the tongue, it moves superiorly and inferiorly during swallowing. Because the hyoid is also firmly attached to the larynx by the thyrohyoid membrane, when the hyoid moves superiorly, it carries the larynx with it. The hyoid consists of a body anteriorly, a pair of greater horns projecting posterosuperiorly from the body and a pair of lesser horns, also projecting posterosuperiorly from the junction of the body with the

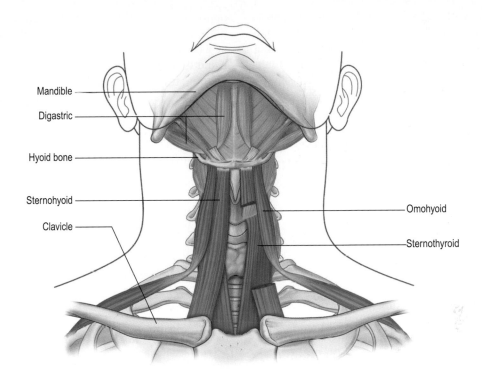

Mandible

Digastric

Hyoid bone

Sternohyoid

Clavicle

Omohyoid

Sternothyroid

Fig. 5.41 Anterior aspect of the neck showing the infrahyoid muscles.

Innervation

By the anterior rami of C1, C2 and C3 via the ansa cervicalis.

Sternothyroid

Smaller than and situated posterior to sternohyoid, sternothyroid (Fig. 5.41) arises from the posterior surface of the manubrium sterni, inferior to the attachment of sternohyoid and first costal cartilage. Broader than sternohyoid, the fibres run superolaterally superficial to the trachea and thyroid gland to attach to the oblique line of the thyroid cartilage.

Innervation

By the anterior rami of C1, C2 and C3 via the ansa cervicalis.

Thyrohyoid

Short muscle running between the oblique line of the thyroid cartilage as a continuation of sternothyroid, and the inferior border of the body and greater horn of the hyoid.

Innervation

By the anterior ramus of C1, which reaches the muscle via the hypoglossal nerve.

Omohyoid

Resembling digastric, omohyoid (Fig. 5.41) has two bellies united by an intermediate tendon. The inferior belly arises from the transverse scapular ligament and adjacent margins of the suprascapular notch on the superior border of the scapula and runs anteriorly and slightly superiorly to an intermediate tendon. From the tendon, the superior belly runs superomedially to attach to the inferior border of the body of the hyoid.

Under cover of sternomastoid, the intermediate tendon is bound down to the clavicle and first rib by a sling of deep cervical fascia, maintaining the angled appearance of the muscle.

Innervation

By the anterior rami of C1, C2 and C3 via the ansa cervicalis.

Action of infrahyoid muscles

The infrahyoid (strap) muscles act to depress the hyoid after it has been elevated during swallowing. Alternatively, by fixing the hyoid, the suprahyoid muscles can act on the mandible to depress it against resistance.

Thyrohyoid acting by itself raises the thyroid cartilage towards the hyoid pulling the larynx superiorly under the root of the tongue. In this way, thyrohyoid is responsible for closing the laryngeal inlet, preventing food from entering the larynx during swallowing. Acting by itself, sternothyroid opens the laryngeal inlet by pulling the thyroid cartilage away from the hyoid. During forced inspiration, sternothyroid probably acts to keep the laryngeal inlet open.

MUSCLES ELEVATING THE HYOID

Stylohyoid
Digastric (p. 676)
Mylohyoid (p. 677)
Geniohyoid (p. 677)

Stylohyoid

Small thin muscle (Fig. 5.41) arising from the posterior part of the styloid process of the temporal bone near its root. It runs inferiorly superficial to the posterior belly of digastric, splitting into two slips, enclosing the intermediate tendon of digastric: the slips unite before attaching to the root of the greater horn of the hyoid.

Innervation

By the facial (seventh cranial) nerve.

Action

Stylohyoid elevates and retracts the hyoid, taking with it the tongue: it lengthens the floor of the mouth.

MASTICATION AND SWALLOWING (DEGLUTITION)

Mastication is the process involved in chewing and grinding food between the molar and premolar teeth to break it down into smaller fragments so that it can be moulded into a softer, more manageable bolus and swallowed. The requisite movements of the mandible occur at the temporomandibular joints (p. 667) and involve opening and closing of the mouth, together with protraction and retraction of the mandible.

Initially, food is bitten off by the incisor teeth by the contraction of masseter, medial pterygoid and temporalis. Chewing movements are essentially produced by the alternate contraction of the pterygoids, first on one side and then the other. The elevators (masseter and medial pterygoid) of the side on which the pterygoids are functioning are also active to keep the teeth opposed. On the opposite side, temporalis retracts that side of the mandible, particularly if the food is sticky: there may also be a contribution from digastric, mylohyoid and geniohyoid to help separate the teeth momentarily when the bolus is sticky. During these swinging movements of the mandible, the food is prevented from escaping between the teeth by the action of other muscles intimately involved in the masticatory process. If food passes into the vestibule of the mouth, it is returned by contraction of buccinator: if it escapes medially into the oral cavity, it is ground against the hard palate and pushed back between the teeth by the action of the tongue. Contraction of mylohyoid helps keep the tongue against the hard palate, while orbicularis oris around the mouth prevents food escaping through the lips.

Once a suitable consistency has been achieved, the bolus of food is collected from the anterior part of the mouth by the tip of the tongue and pressed posteriorly towards the soft palate by mylohyoid, digastric and stylohyoid. At the same time, the elevators of the mandible and mylohyoid contract and the hyoid are elevated, carrying with it the larynx. Geniohyoid then pulls the hyoid anteriorly to widen the pharynx in anticipation of receiving the bolus. The soft palate is raised, closing off the nasopharynx to prevent food entering the nose: elevation of the tongue and hyoid closes the laryngeal inlet so that food does not enter the airway. The food bolus slides over the surface of the epiglottis into the laryngopharynx. Respiration is reflexly inhibited as the constrictor muscles of the pharynx contract successively to push the bolus of food towards the oesophagus. When the bolus has passed the laryngeal inlet, the hyoid and larynx are pulled down to their resting positions by contraction of sternohyoid, sternothyroid and omohyoid. Breathing is once again resumed, and another mouthful can be dealt with.

Swallowing fluids is essentially similar, except that in the initial stages, the tongue forms a gutter. The fluid is then forced posteriorly by the tongue, flowing inferiorly over the sides of the epiglottis, avoiding the laryngeal inlet. See also page 602.

Application

Painful spasm of the muscles of mastication is frequently seen following traumatic overstretching, a situation which can arise during dental extraction. The resulting trismus responds well to gentle heat and soft tissue techniques applied to the muscles.

SECTION SUMMARY

Mandible

- Large U-shaped bone forming lower part of face
- Has a body and two rami, each having a condyle (head) posteriorly and coronoid process anteriorly
- Gives attachment to powerful muscles of mastication

Hyoid

- U-shaped bone with body, greater and lesser horns
- Suspended by muscles connecting it to the tongue, mandible, styloid process, thyroid cartilage and sternum

Temporomandibular Joint

Type	Synovial condyloid
Articular surfaces	Head (condyle) of mandible, mandibular fossa of temporal bone and intra-articular disc
Capsule	Strong, thin loose fibrous capsule completely surrounds joint attaching to articular margins of mandibular fossa and neck of mandible
Ligaments	Lateral, sphenomandibular (accessory) and stylomandibular (accessory)
Stability	By adjacent muscles and ligaments, depends on whether mouth is open or closed
Movements	Protraction and retraction, elevation and depression, lateral deviation (side-to-side)

Movements of the mandible

Movement of the mandible occurs at the temporomandibular joint, with protraction and retraction associated with the superior compartment, and elevation and depression with the inferior compartment. Unless stated, all muscles are supplied by the mandibular division of the trigeminal nerve (V_3).

Movement	Muscles (innervation)
Retraction	Temporalis (V_3)
	Digastric (anterior belly V_3 and posterior belly VII)
	Geniohyoid (C1)
Protraction	Lateral pterygoid (V_3)
	Medial pterygoid (V_3)
	Masseter (V_3)
Elevation	Masseter (V_3)
	Medial pterygoid (V_3)
	Temporalis (V_3)
Depression	Digastric (anterior belly V_3 and posterior belly VII)
	Mylohyoid
	Geniohyoid (C1)
	Platysma (VII)

❓ SELF-ASSESSMENT QUESTIONS

31. What movements are possible at the temporomandibular joint?
32. Which muscles produce the following movements?
    a. Protraction
    b. Retraction
    c. Elevation
    d. Depression
33. Which muscles are included in the infrahyoid group?
34. Which muscles are included in the suprahyoid group?
35. What is the nerve supply of the infrahyoid muscles?
36. What are the attachments of masseter?
37. What attaches to the ramus of the mandible?
38. Name the bony parts of the hyoid bone.
39. What are the articular surfaces involved in the temporomandibular joint?
40. What is the nerve supply to platysma?

▌BRAIN

LEARNING OUTCOMES

By the end of the section, you should be able to:
1. Describe the development of the brain
2. Describe the organisation of the brain into cerebral hemispheres, cerebellum, pons and brainstem
3. Describe the gross organisation of brain tissue into white and grey matter, and what each comprises
4. Describe the lobes of each cerebral hemisphere and their major functions
5. Explain the function of the meninges and the role of the dura mater in protecting the brain
6. Describe the origin, course and distribution of each cranial nerve
7. Describe the arterial supply and venous drainage of the brain
8. Appreciate the influence of pathology and/or trauma on the brain

INTRODUCTION

The central nervous system (CNS) is formed by the aggregation of bundles of axons and clusters of nerve cell bodies. The internal appearance and external form of the CNS reflect the manner in which these components are arranged.

The superficial part of the brain is formed by nerve fibres and cell bodies: such material appears grey in transverse sections. The deep part of the brain consists mainly of myelinated axons: the myelin has a white appearance in transverse sections. Because cell bodies are not myelinated, the ganglia and nuclei form grey matter, and myelinated axons form white matter. Thus areas in the CNS formed mainly by axons are referred to as white matter (Fig. 5.42). In contrast, the cell bodies are not myelinated, so that areas formed mainly by cell bodies appear grey and are referred to as grey matter (Fig. 5.42).

A collection of cell bodies that form a prominent, usually rounded swelling is a ganglion (Fig. 5.43): a cluster of axons that form a recognisable bundle within the CNS is a fasciculus (Fig. 5.43). When bundles of axons form a raised bump or convex contour on the surface of the CNS, typically in the spinal cord, it resembles the external surface of a tube; the elevation is a funiculus.

These terms refer to the topographic appearance of collections of axons or cell bodies without regard to their function: other terms have functional implications. A cluster of axons with a similar function is a tract, while a cluster of cell bodies with a similar function is a nucleus.

Glial Cells

Nerve cells are not the only constituents of the CNS. Interspersed between them are several cell types (glial cells) whose function, in general, is to hold the neurons together. As a whole, glial cells outnumber nerve cells, being almost half the total volume.

Four types of glial cells are found in the CNS: oligodendrocytes, microglia, ependymal cells and astrocytes (Fig. 5.44). Oligodendrocytes are responsible for myelination in the CNS: in addition, because they myelinate several parallel axons, they also serve to hold them together. Microglia are the macrophages of the central system, responsible for removing foreign matter and cellular debris.

Ependymal cells are exclusively found lining the internal surface of the ventricles of the CNS. They are epithelial cells arranged side by side forming a cellular barrier between the nervous system and the cerebrospinal fluid (CSF) in its cavities.

Astrocytes derive their name from their star-shaped appearance consisting of a cell body with long processes

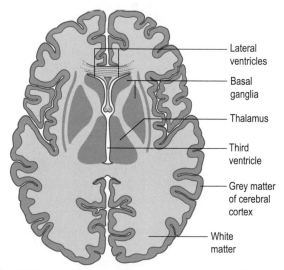

Fig. 5.42 Arrangement of the white and grey matter in the brain viewed in transverse section.

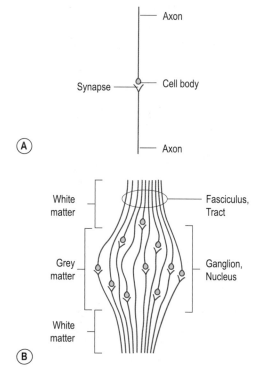

Fig. 5.43 (A) Neurons in the central nervous system are connected in series, with the axon of one neuron synapsing with the cell body of the next neuron; (B) formation of a ganglion/nucleus in the grey matter.

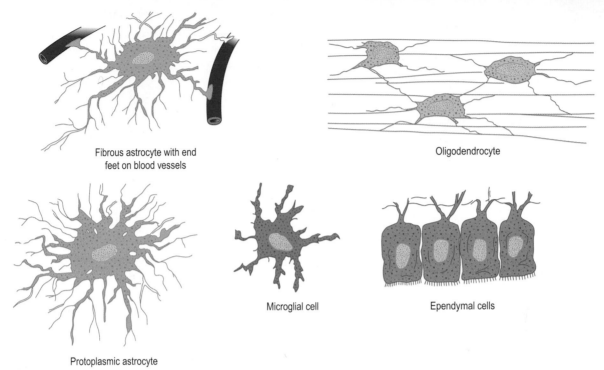

Fibrous astrocyte with end
feet on blood vessels

Oligodendrocyte

Microglial cell

Ependymal cells

Protoplasmic astrocyte

Fig. 5.44 Microscopic appearance of different neuroglial cells.

radiating away from it: two types of astrocyte (fibrous, protoplasmic) can be recognised. Microscopically, protoplasmic astrocytes occur chiefly in the grey matter and have thick processes that branch repeatedly: they weave between cell bodies, collectively holding them together, with some processes attached to small blood vessels (Fig. 5.44). In contrast, fibrous astrocytes are found chiefly in white matter and have fewer, but longer, processes that weave between axons. The principal role of astrocytes is to provide a framework for the CNS by holding the cell bodies and axons in place relative to one another. However, they also play an important role in the nutrition and metabolic activities of neurons by regulating the exchange of chemicals between themselves and blood vessels.

Development

The CNS develops from a single tubular structure (neural tube) which forms along the dorsal surface of the embryo extending from the site of the future head to the tail, with head and tail ends (Fig. 5.45). Because the tube eventually bends in the sagittal plane, during development of the head and brain the terms anterior, posterior, superior and inferior, as used in gross anatomy, cannot be applied to the nervous system without confusion. To

overcome this, different terms of reference are used with respect to the CNS.

The tail end of the neural tube is the caudal end (Fig. 5.45) and the head end is the rostral end irrespective of the direction in which it points with respect to the rest of the body (Fig. 5.45). The surface of the neural tube facing the belly of the embryo is the ventral surface, again irrespective of whether the tube is straight or curved in the sagittal plane: the opposite surface is the dorsal surface. These directional terms are equally applicable to descriptions of the adult CNS.

The neural tube maintains a narrow cavity along its length; however, the thickness of its walls increases as the cells multiply and grow. Most of the caudal part of the neural tube simply grows in length and diameter: its walls get thicker, but its cavity remains narrow. The rostral end undergoes several changes. In various regions, the cavity of the tube expands forming dilations (Fig. 5.45): the walls of the tube surrounding these dilations thicken following nerve cell proliferation. The most rostral end of the neural tube is the prosencephalon, more caudally is the mesencephalon and then the rhombencephalon, which subsequently divides into the metencephalon and myelencephalon. As the walls of the prosencephalon

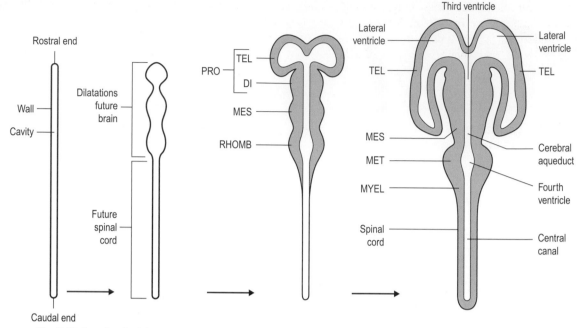

Fig. 5.45 Longitudinal (coronal) sections viewed from a dorsal aspect showing stages in the development of the central nervous system. [PRO, prosencephalon; TEL, telencephalon; DI, diencephalin; RHOMB, rhombencephalon; MES, mesencephalon; MET, metencephalon; MYEL, myelencephalon]

thicken, they expand laterally as the telencephalon, with the contained cavity being the lateral ventricle (Fig. 5.45). The remaining part of the prosencephalon is the diencephalon, which surrounds the third ventricle: the mesencephalon surrounds the cerebral aqueduct and rhombencephalon the fourth ventricle.

Gradually, the telencephalon enlarges and grows in a set pattern: there is some growth rostrally on each side beyond the original rostral limit of the neural tube, but the major growth is laterally and caudally (Fig. 5.45). Cells over the caudolateral aspect of the telencephalon eventually grow forming an extension overlapping the lateral aspect of the main mass of the telencephalon (Fig. 5.46). The lateral ventricles participate in this growth elongating in the directions along which the telencephalon cells proliferate. Overall, the telencephalon and lateral ventricles assume a curved shape, extending laterally and then caudally, eventually curving laterally, ventrally and rostrally. As the telencephalon on each side develops, it covers and buries the diencephalon (Figs 5.45 and 5.46).

Caudal to the diencephalon, the cavity of the neural tube expands to form the diamond-shaped fourth ventricle when viewed posteriorly (Fig. 5.45). The tissue surrounding this ventricle proliferates forming the rhombencephalon (referring to the rhomboid shape of

the fourth ventricle). The rostral part of the rhombencephalon develops into a separate section (metencephalon) (Fig. 5.46). The dorsal portion posterior to the fourth ventricle differentiates into the cerebellum, with the ventral portion of the metencephalon (ventral to the fourth ventricle) forming the pons, a bundle of neurons arching around the ventral surface of the neural tube. The caudal portion of the rhombencephalon (myelencephalon) remains relatively undifferentiated connecting the pons to the spinal cord (Fig. 5.46).

The mesencephalon (Fig. 5.46) between the diencephalon and rhombencephalon does not undergo great proliferation: its walls simply thicken and its cavity (cerebral aqueduct) remains tubular and narrow (Fig. 5.45).

Collectively, the mesencephalon, pons and myelencephalon constitute the brainstem, a single structural unit, connecting the spinal cord to the diencephalon, with the cerebellum attached dorsally.

Nomenclature

The terminology used previously with respect to the subdivisions of the CNS is the most formal nomenclature in use: other systems based on Latin or English are also used. Unfortunately, no single system is used consistently, and certain terms are used only in the most formal circumstances. The different terminologies and their equivalents are shown in Table 5.2: the most commonly used terms are in italics. In general, Latin or English forms are used when nouns are required to refer to various parts, with adjectives usually taking the Greek form.

The term prosencephalon is rarely used. Neither is metencephalon which refers collectively to the pons and

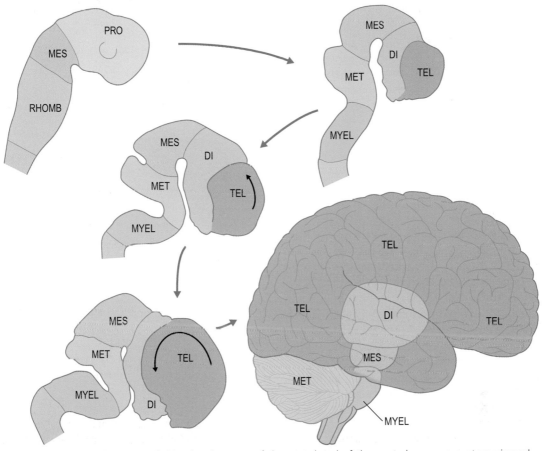

Fig. 5.46 Successive stages in the development of the rostral end of the central nervous system viewed from the right lateral aspect. [PRO, prosencephalon; MES, mesencephalon; RHOMB, rhombencephalon; TEL, telencephalon; DI, diencephalon; MET, metencephalon; MYEL, myelencephalon]

TABLE 5.2 Nomenclature of the Division of the Central Nervous System

Greek system	Latin system	Common English	Related cavity
Prosencephalon		*Forebrain*	
Telencephalon	*Cerebrum*		Lateral ventricle
Diencephalon			Third ventricle
Mesencephalon		*Midbrain*	Cerebral aqueduct
Rhombencephalon		*Hindbrain*	Fourth ventricle
Metencephalon	*Cerebellum*		
	Pons		
Myelencephalon	*Medulla oblongata*		
	Medulla	*Spinal cord*	Central canal

Commonly used terms are in italics

cerebellum. Myelencephalon is almost never used outside an embryological context: it is usually referred to as the medulla oblongata, alluding to the tapering shape of this part of the CNS as it narrows to the diameter of the spinal cord. The terms mesencephalon and midbrain are equivalent and are used interchangeably and with equal frequency.

ADULT MORPHOLOGY

In the fully developed CNS, most subdivisions are clearly recognisable: the spinal cord is long and cylindrical occupying the rostral three-quarters of the vertebral column; the remainder of the CNS lies within the skull (Fig. 5.47). The cerebellum fills the posterior cranial fossa, with the brainstem lying posterior to the clivus: the telencephalon and diencephalon occupy the middle and anterior cranial fossae.

Diencephalon

The diencephalon is not readily apparent in the intact adult brain as it lies deep to the telencephalon. It can be demonstrated in dissections in which the telencephalon and cerebellum have been removed (Fig. 5.48): its largest component is the thalamus, a large collection of nuclei. Each thalamus is continuous caudally with the midbrain and separated from the opposite thalamus by the third ventricle. The functions of the thalamus are diverse including various motor, sensory and emotional processes.

Other components of the diencephalon include the metathalamus, epithalamus and hypothalamus. The metathalamus consists of two prominences projecting from the posterolateral inferior surface of each thalamus (Fig. 5.48A); these are the medial and lateral geniculate bodies involved in certain auditory and visual processes, respectively.

The epithalamus consists of a strip of neural tissue bridging the posterior medial ends of the two thalami (Fig. 5.48B). Projecting from the posterior edge of the epithalamus in the midline is the pineal body (gland), a structure concerned with hormonal regulation, particularly reproductive hormones.

The hypothalamus forms the rostroventral part of the lateral wall of the third ventricle, best seen in sagittal sections (Fig. 5.49). It is a thin layer of tissue hanging from the ventromedial surface of the thalamus, blending with the opposite hypothalamus in the midline, forming a sling of neural tissue across the floor of the third ventricle. Embryologically, the hypothalamus is formed by the ventral and ventrolateral walls of the rostral end

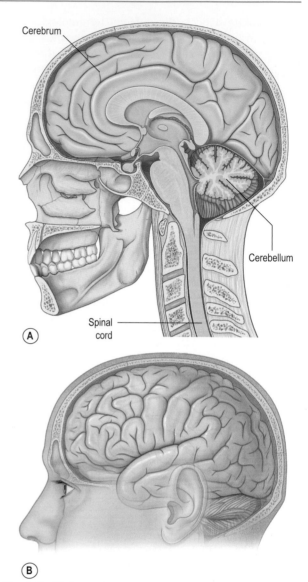

Fig. 5.47 (A) Sagittal section showing the central nervous system within the skull and vertebral canal; (B) left lateral aspect of the brain within the skull.

of the neural tube, while the lateral walls form the thalamus and telencephalon. The rostral end of the hypothalamus is marked by the lamina terminalis, a strip of neural tissue bridging the midline derived from the rostral end of the original neural tube.

Brainstem and Cerebellum

The most obvious feature of the ventral surface of the brainstem is the thick bundle of transversely running

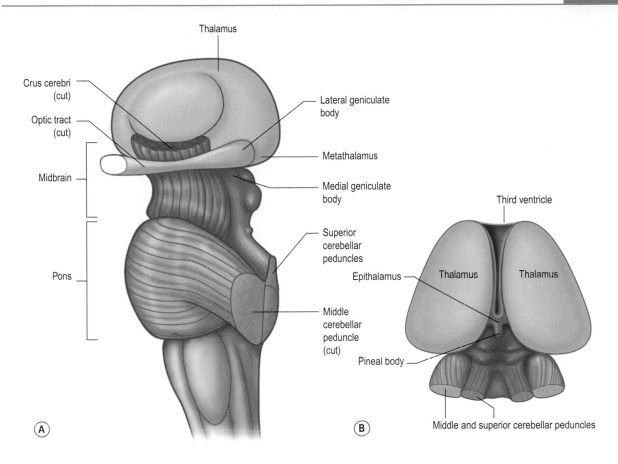

Fig. 5.48 (A) Left lateral aspect of the brainstem and thalamus with the crus cerebri, optic tract and cerebellar peduncles cut; (B) superior aspect showing the thalami either side of the rostral end of the brainstem.

nerve fibres constituting the pons (Fig. 5.50B and C): rostral to the pons is the midbrain and caudal the medulla oblongata.

The ventral surface of the midbrain is marked by two obliquely orientated semicylindrical prominences (crura cerebri/cerebellar peduncle) (Fig. 5.50): the crura cerebri convey motor fibres from the cerebellum to the brainstem.

Fibres of the crura cerebri appear to run deep to the pons, emerging caudal to it on the ventral surface of the medulla oblongata as two longitudinal prominences (pyramids) on either side of the midline (Fig. 5.50): the pyramids convey motor fibres to the spinal cord. A shallow midline cleft (anterior median fissure) separates the pyramids: caudally, this fissure becomes obliterated for a short distance as the fibres in the pyramids cross the midline (pyramidal decussation) before passing into the substance of the spinal cord. The caudal end of the

decussation marks the junction of the medulla oblongata and spinal cord (Fig. 5.50).

Lateral to each pyramid is a rounded prominence (olive) on the surface of the medulla oblongata: cells within the olive are involved in the functions of the cerebellum.

The posterior surface of the midbrain is marked by four rounded projections (colliculi) arranged in pairs with a superior and an inferior colliculus on each side (Fig. 5.50C). The superior colliculi mediate certain reflexes involved in turning the head and eyes in response to visual stimuli, while the inferior colliculi mediate similar responses to auditory stimuli.

The caudal end of the medulla oblongata is marked posteriorly by two rounded elevations on each side of the midline: medially is the nucleus gracilis, and laterally the nucleus cuneatus (Fig. 5.50C). These nuclei are responsible for processing sensory information

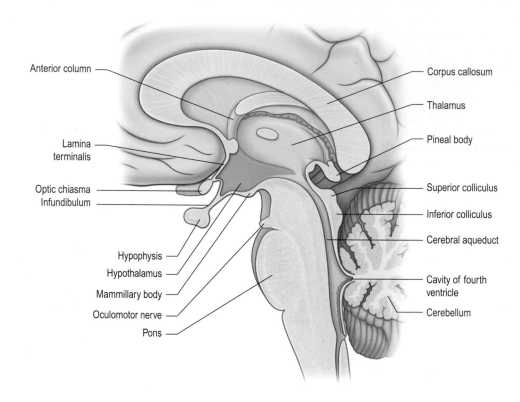

Fig. 5.49 Location of the hypothalamus seen on sagittal section of the brain and brainstem.

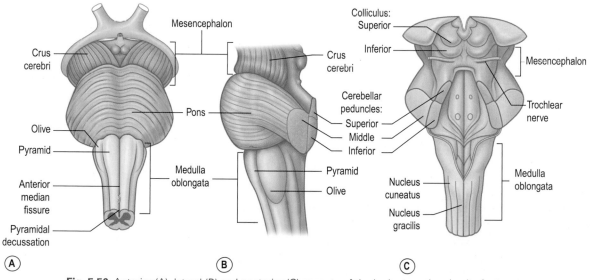

Fig. 5.50 Anterior (A), lateral (B) and posterior (C) aspects of the brainstem showing its features.

concerning pressure, touch and position sense that pass from the spinal cord to the brainstem and thalamus.

The cerebellum is a mass of neural tissue (Fig. 5.49), the principal function of which is the control of posture, repetitive movements and the geometric accuracy of voluntary movements. It is connected to the brainstem by three pairs of structures (cerebellar peduncles) (Fig. 5.50B and C), of which the largest are the middle cerebellar peduncles running around the lateral aspect of the brainstem, being directly continuous with the pons. Passing rostrally from the cerebellum into the dorsal aspect of the midbrain are the superior cerebellar peduncles connecting the cerebellum to the rostral portion of the brainstem and thalamus. Passing caudally from the cerebellum into the dorsolateral aspects of the medulla oblongata are the inferior cerebellar peduncles connecting the cerebellum with the medulla oblongata and spinal cord.

Cerebrum

The cerebrum is divided into left and right halves by a large cleft (longitudinal fissure) (Fig. 5.51A): each half is a cerebral hemisphere. Deep within the longitudinal fissure, the two hemispheres are connected by a large body of transversely running nerve fibres (corpus callosum) (Fig. 5.51B and D). When the two cerebral hemispheres are separated by a midline incision, their medial surfaces are revealed, and the transected surface of the corpus callosum can be seen (Fig. 5.51B and D).

The surface of each cerebral hemisphere is formed by a layer of grey matter (cerebral cortex) varying in thickness between 2 and 5 mm. It contains the cell bodies of neurons responsible for the various functions of the cerebrum. Deep to the cortex, the cerebral hemispheres are formed by a large mass of white matter consisting of the axons of the neurons in the cerebral cortex, together with those that enter the cerebrum from the brainstem and diencephalon.

For descriptive purposes, each cerebral hemisphere is divided into four lobes named according to the bones of the skull to which they are most closely related (Fig. 5.51C). The anterior and posterior end of each cerebral hemisphere tapers to a single prominence (frontal and occipital poles, respectively): similarly, the anterior end of the temporal lobe is the temporal pole.

The surface of the cerebral cortex is thrown into ridges (gyri: singular, gyrus) separated from one another by valley-like depressions (sulci: singular, sulcus). Some sulci and gyri are significant because they subdivide the cerebral hemispheres topographically and functionally (Figs 5.51D and 5.53).

The most obvious sulcus is that separating the temporal lobe from the parietal and frontal lobes (lateral sulcus): from the medial aspect of the temporal pole, it runs posterosuperiorly medial to the temporal lobe, ending at the junction of the temporal lobe with the parietal lobe.

Various transverse sulci cross the frontal and parietal lobes. Located near the middle of the cerebral hemisphere is the central sulcus (Fig. 5.51C and D): it extends from the medial to the lateral surface of each hemisphere, reaching almost as far as the lateral sulcus. Although other sulci may extend onto the medial aspect of the cerebral hemisphere or may reach almost as far as the lateral sulcus, the central sulcus is the only continuous sulcus that does both: it is, therefore, easily recognised.

The central sulcus demarcates the frontal lobe from the parietal lobe: all tissue anterior to the central sulcus constitutes the frontal lobe, with the parietal lobe lying posterior to it. The sulcus running parallel to and anterior to the central sulcus is the precentral sulcus, with the intervening gyrus being the precentral gyrus (Fig. 5.51D). Stimulation of the precentral gyrus results in contraction of voluntary muscles: it is referred to as the motor cortex which contains a detailed topographically organised map (motor homunculus) of the opposite side of the body, with the head represented most laterally and the leg and foot most medially (Fig. 5.52A). The disproportionate representation of body regions (muscles of the face and hands) in relation to their physical size indicates areas capable of finely controlled movements.

Similarly, the sulcus immediately behind the central sulcus is the postcentral sulcus, with the intervening gyrus being the postcentral gyrus (Fig. 5.51D). The postcentral gyrus receives sensory information from the brainstem and thalamus: it is referred to as the sensory cortex which contains within it a topographical map (sensory homunculus) of the opposite side of the body, with the face, tongue and lips represented inferiorly, the trunk and upper limb on the superolateral aspect and the lower limb on the medial side of the hemisphere (Fig. 5.52B).

Posterior to the postcentral sulcus, the medial surface is crossed by a clearly marked transverse sulcus (parietooccipital sulcus) extending onto the superior aspect of the lateral surface of the hemisphere: it demarcates the parietal lobe from the occipital lobe (Fig. 5.51D). Anteriorly, the parietal lobe is separated from the temporal lobe by the posterior end of the lateral sulcus: posteriorly no major topographical feature delineates the junction between the temporal lobe and the parietal and occipital lobes.

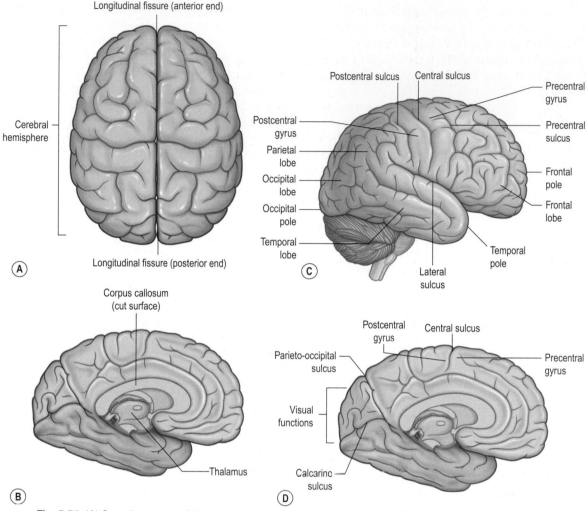

Fig. 5.51 (A) Superior aspect of the brain showing the right and left cerebral hemispheres separated by the longitudinal fissure; (B) medial aspect of the left cerebral hemisphere showing the cut surface of the corpus callosum; (C) right lateral cerebral hemisphere showing its subdivision into lobes and principal sulci; (D) medial aspect of the left cerebral hemisphere showing the principal sulci and gyri.

On the medial aspect of the cerebral hemisphere, the inferior end of the parieto-occipital sulcus merges with the calcarine sulcus (Fig. 5.51D), either side of which the cortex of the cerebrum is responsible for vision.

The occipital lobe is involved in the function of vision. The parietal lobe is, in general, responsible for sensory functions (perception of touch, pressure and position of the body and limbs); however, it is also responsible for more sophisticated functions such as three-dimensional perception, analysis of visual images, language, geometry and calculations (Fig. 5.53). The frontal lobe is involved with motor functions, as well as governing the expression of intellect and personality. The superior part of the temporal lobe opposite the postcentral gyrus is involved in the perception of sound, while the remainder is concerned with memory and various emotional functions.

Base of the Brain

This is formed largely by the ventral surfaces of the frontal, temporal and occipital lobes of the cerebral hemispheres (Fig. 5.54). The medial edge of the most rostral end of the temporal lobe is the uncus, involved in the perception of smell.

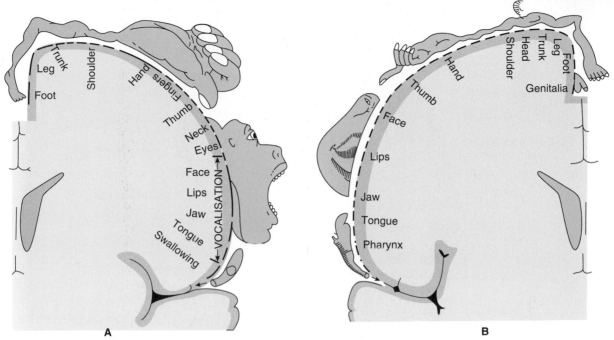

Fig. 5.52 (A) Motor homunculus showing the somatotopical representation in the main motor area; (B) sensory homunculus showing somatotopical representation in the somaesthetic cortex. (From Chapter 10.4: Physiological anatomy and functions of cerebral cortex and white matter of cerebrum. In: Medical Physiology for Undergraduate Students, second ed. (revised and updated edition); pii:B9788131262573000709/f10-04-06-9788131262573; l abel; Figure 10.4-6.)

Anteriorly, neural tissue is absent between the two frontal lobes where they are separated by the longitudinal fissure. Caudal to this space is the floor of the third ventricle, formed by the junction of the hypothalamus from each side. Most posteriorly, the brainstem projects caudally from the inferior (caudal) surface of the diencephalon, which lies deep to the cerebral hemispheres.

Projecting in the midline from the floor of the third ventricle is a funnel-shaped extension of neural tissue (infundibulum), connecting the hypothalamus to the pituitary gland (Figs 5.49 and 5.54): it consists of axons from cells in the hypothalamus which regulate the secretion of oxytocin and antidiuretic hormone by the pituitary gland. Caudal to the infundibulum are two small prominences (mammillary bodies) whose functions are not fully understood (Fig. 5.54).

On the ventral aspect of the diencephalon is an X-shaped structure consisting of two rostral and two caudal limbs: the caudal limbs pass around the crura cerebri to end in the metathalamus (Fig. 5.54). The rostral limbs are the terminal ends of the optic nerves

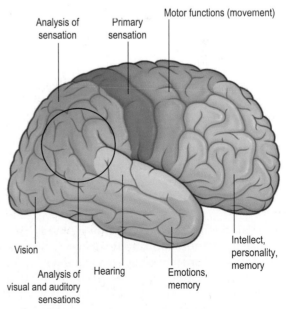

Fig. 5.53 Lateral aspect of the right cerebral hemisphere showing the principal functions of different regions.

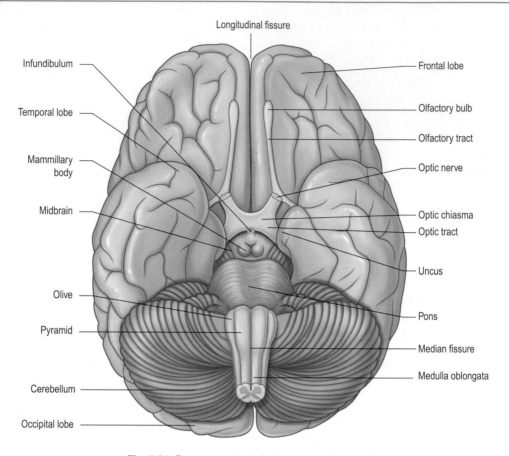

Fig. 5.54 Features on the inferior aspect of the brain.

transmitting visual information from the retina of the eye. The intersecting region (optic chiasma) is where the medial fibres from each optic nerve cross the midline. The caudal limbs (optic tracts) each convey visual information from one-half of the visual field to the ipsilateral lateral geniculate body (Fig. 5.48A).

Internal Structure of the Brain

For introductory purposes, it is sufficient to examine the appearance of simple transections of the CNS.

Brainstem

In general, the brainstem consists of a central core of grey matter (reticular formation) surrounded by white matter formed by motor and sensory tracts and in which are interspersed various nuclei associated with the cranial nerves (Fig. 5.55A). Transverse sections have a diverse appearance because of the variations in external shape and internal contents at different levels. Details

of this internal structure are better addressed when the central system is studied in detail.

Forebrain

The cerebral hemispheres have a characteristic appearance irrespective of whether they are seen in coronal, horizontal or sagittal sections. The cerebral cortex consists of a layer of grey matter extending over the entire external surface of each hemisphere (Fig. 5.55B), the cells of which are responsible for processing information related to the functions of the lobe in which they lie.

Deep to the cortex, white matter forms the main bulk of each hemisphere: it consists of axons of cells in the cerebral cortex that communicate with cells in adjacent, distant and contralateral regions of the cerebrum, as well as with axons that pass out of or into the cerebrum.

Sections through the central parts of the cerebral hemisphere reveal the cavity of the lateral ventricle and large collections of grey matter surrounding the lateral and third ventricles (Fig. 5.55). The large mass adjacent to the third ventricle is the thalamus: the remaining masses are groups of nuclei (basal ganglia) involved in controlling movement.

Meninges

Although the glial cells hold the neurons of the CNS together, providing them with protection against metabolic insults, the CNS is nonetheless a soft cellular mass. As such, it is vulnerable to external mechanical insults which might arise were it freely mobile within the skull or vertebral canal. To protect against such insults, the CNS is surrounded by three membranes (meninges) and bathed in cerebrospinal fluid (CSF).

Intracranial Meninges

The meningeal layers surrounding the spinal cord also surround the brain and brainstem. The pia mater follows every convolution of its surface, extending into the depths of any sulcus or fissure (Fig. 5.56). It is adherent to the underlying neural tissue and endows the CNS with a smooth surface: specimens in which the pia mater has been stripped off have a granulated surface. The arachnoid mater lines the deep surface of the dura mater, forming a network of fine threads bridging the pia and dura mater (Fig. 5.56).

The dura mater forms a mobile sac around the spinal cord, while in the skull it is applied to the internal surface of the cranial cavity where it fuses with the endosteum (Fig. 5.56). At certain sites, it separates from the adjacent bone to form large folds that project towards the centre of the cranial cavity: these folds enclose vascular channels (venous sinuses), which transmit venous blood draining from the CNS, cranium and orbit (p. 696).

The major reflections of the dura mater within the skull are the falx cerebri and tentorium cerebelli (Fig. 5.57A): each fold consists of two layers of dura mater with a free edge and two surfaces. At the attached edge, the two layers are reflected onto the deep surface of the cranium, being continuous with the rest of the dural lining of the cranial bones.

The falx cerebri projects from the roof of the cranium in the median plane from the crista galli anteriorly to the internal occipital protuberance posteriorly (Fig. 5.57A and C), being sickle-shaped in profile: it projects into the longitudinal fissure separating the two cerebral hemispheres. Along its attached margin, it encloses the

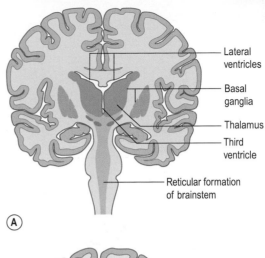

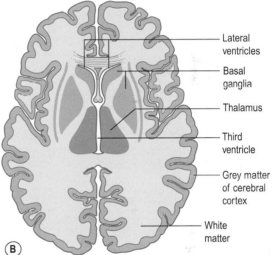

Fig. 5.55 Internal appearance of the brain and brainstem seen in coronal (A) and transverse (B) sections.

superior sagittal sinus, and in its free margin the inferior sagittal sinus (Figs 5.56B and 5.57A and C).

The tentorium cerebelli lies in a transverse plane projecting from the anterior, lateral and posterior walls of the posterior cranial fossa, forming a partial roof to it (Fig. 5.57A): its peripheral attachments are diverse. Anteriorly on each side, it attaches to the posterior clinoid processes and posterosuperior margin of the petrous temporal bone; laterally and posteriorly, it attaches to the margins of the bony sulcus of the transverse sinus. From these attachments, the tentorium cerebelli projects centrally, lying below the basal surface of the occipital and temporal lobes overlying the cerebellum. Centrally, the tentorium forms a U-shaped free

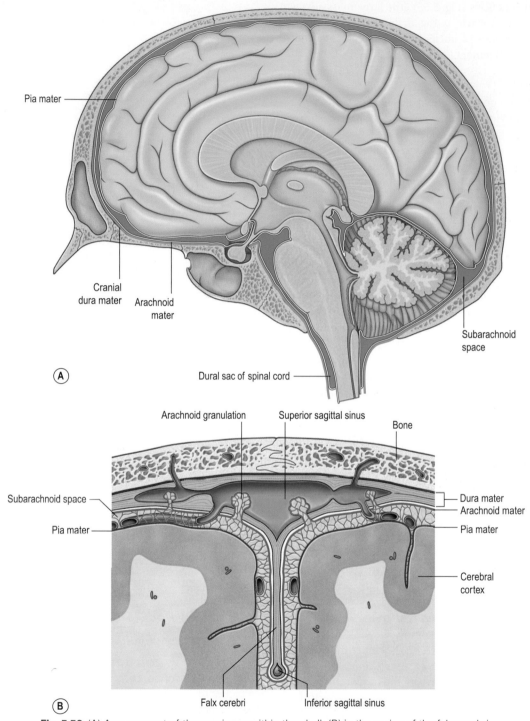

Fig. 5.56 (A) Arrangement of the meninges within the skull; (B) in the region of the falx cerebri.

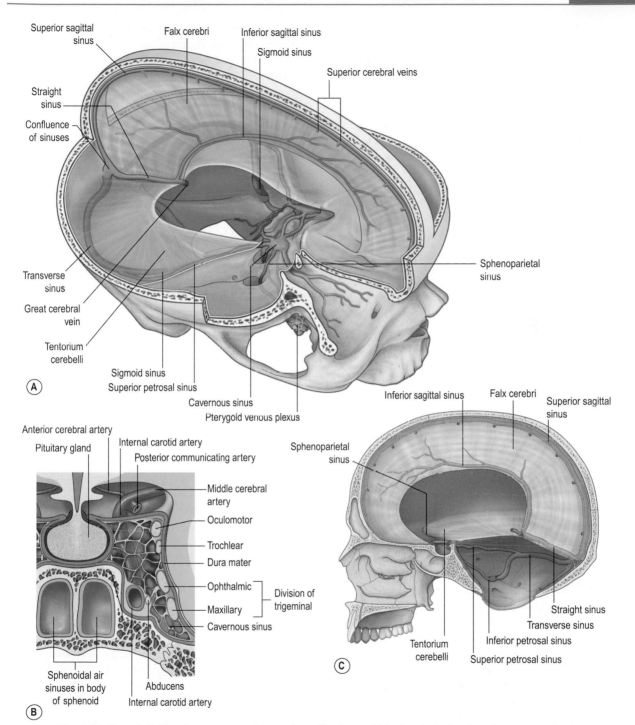

Superior sagittal sinus

Falx cerebri

Inferior sagittal sinus

Sigmoid sinus

Superior cerebral veins

Straight sinus

Confluence of sinuses

Transverse sinus

Great cerebral vein

Tentorium cerebelli

Sigmoid sinus

Superior petrosal sinus

Cavernous sinus

Pterygoid venous plexus

Sphenoparietal sinus

(A)

Anterior cerebral artery

Pituitary gland

Internal carotid artery

Posterior communicating artery

Middle cerebral artery

Oculomotor

Trochlear

Dura mater

Ophthalmic

Maxillary

Cavernous sinus

Division of trigeminal

Sphenoidal air sinuses in body of sphenoid

Abducens

Internal carotid artery

(B)

Inferior sagittal sinus

Falx cerebri

Superior sagittal sinus

Sphenoparietal sinus

Straight sinus

Transverse sinus

Tentorium cerebelli

Inferior petrosal sinus

Superior petrosal sinus

(C)

Fig. 5.57 (A and C) The dura mater and its major reflections within the skull showing the venous dural sinuses; (B) coronal section through the cavernous sinus showing its relationships to the sphenoid, internal carotid artery and III (oculomotor), IV (trochlear), V (trigeminal) and VI (abducens) cranial nerves.

edge which extends from one anterior clinoid process to the other: the notch formed transmits the midbrain from the posterior cranial fossa to the diencephalon. Posteriorly in the midline, the posterior end of the falx cerebri fuses with the superior surface of the tentorium cerebelli and encloses the straight sinus.

Cerebrospinal Fluid

Running between the threads of arachnoid mater and filling the subarachnoid space is cerebrospinal fluid (CSF): it is secreted by strings of capillaries that project into the lateral, third and fourth ventricles. It fills the cavities of the CNS and emerges through the apertures in the roof of the fourth ventricle to fill the subarachnoid space surrounding the brain and spinal cord.

CSF is secreted continuously and reabsorbed into the bloodstream through extensions of the arachnoid mater (arachnoid granulations) that pierce the dura mater of the falx cerebri and project into the superior sagittal sinus (Fig. 5.56B).

Chemically, the CSF protects the CNS by maintaining a constant pH environment, while mechanically it endows it with a cushioning fluid environment. Within the skull, the brain is buoyant in a pool of CSF: within the dural sac the spinal cord is also suspended in a pool of CSF, held centrally within it by denticulate ligaments (p. 568).

Arterial Supply

Derived from the internal carotid and vertebral arteries. The internal carotid artery enters the skull through the carotid canal (Fig. 5.58) and then traverses the foramen lacerum and cavernous sinus (Fig 5.57B). It penetrates the dura and arachnoid mater medial to the anterior clinoid process, entering the subarachnoid space over the ventral surface of the brain where it divides into its terminal branches (anterior and middle cerebral arteries) (Fig. 5.59).

Each anterior cerebral artery curves medially, crossing the optic nerve, to enter the longitudinal fissure (Fig. 5.59). Before doing so, the two anterior cerebral arteries anastomose with one another via the anterior communicating artery. The main trunk of the anterior cerebral artery follows the contour of the corpus callosum, distributing branches to the medial aspect of the cerebral hemisphere (Figs 5.59 and 5.60B).

The middle cerebral artery passes laterally to gain the floor of the lateral sulcus and then runs posteriorly along it. Deep penetrating branches arise from its proximal part, entering the cerebral hemisphere inferiorly to supply the region of the basal ganglia. Superficial branches arise from the middle cerebral artery as it runs in the lateral sulcus: these pass in all directions onto the external surface of the cerebral hemisphere, most notably supplying the motor and sensory regions of the cerebral cortex (Fig. 5.60).

The vertebral arteries pierce the dural sac, entering the subarachnoid space just above the first cervical vertebra. Each passes anterosuperiorly through the foramen magnum joining in the midline anterior to the medulla oblongata forming the basilar artery, which runs superiorly anterior to the pons (Fig. 5.59). Branches of the vertebral and basilar arteries pass laterally to supply the medulla oblongata, pons and cerebellum.

The terminal branches of the basilar artery (posterior cerebral arteries) (Fig. 5.59) pass around the lateral surface of the midbrain to gain the inferior aspect of the temporal lobe of the cerebral hemisphere (Fig. 5.60). Each supplies the posterior parts of the hemisphere, notably the occipital lobe. Branches from the proximal part of the posterior cerebral artery supply the midbrain, thalamus, metathalamus and epithalamus.

On the ventral surface of the brain, each posterior cerebral artery anastomoses with the ipsilateral internal carotid artery through the posterior communicating artery (Fig. 5.59), enabling the vertebrobasilar circulation to communicate with that from the internal carotid arteries. Similarly, the anterior communicating artery permits flow between the two internal carotid arteries. The ring of vessels formed by the anterior communicating, anterior cerebral, internal carotid, posterior communicating, posterior cerebral arteries and the end of the basilar artery is the circle of Willis.

Venous Drainage and Venous Sinuses

Veins draining the internal aspects of the cerebral hemispheres, basal ganglia and thalamus converge to form a large vessel (great cerebral vein) which passes posteriorly to enter the straight sinus. Veins from the external surface of the cerebral hemispheres drain superiorly and inferiorly towards the superior sagittal and transverse sinuses, respectively.

Where the superior cerebral veins pierce the arachnoid and dura mater to enter the superior sagittal sinus (Fig. 5.57A) they can rupture following a blow to the head. If torn at these sites, blood can accumulate between the arachnoid and dura mater, cleaving the two

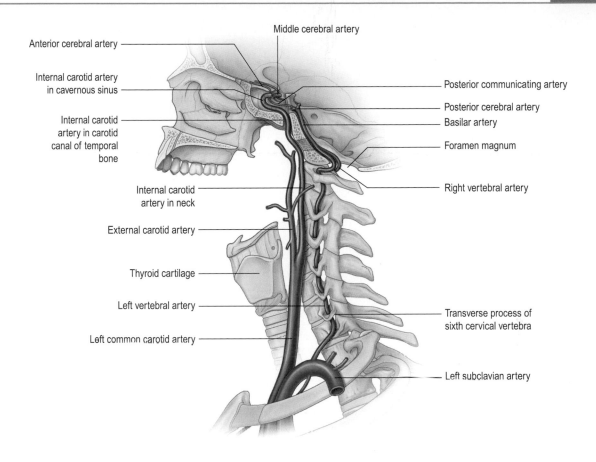

Fig. 5.58 Left internal carotid and vertebral arteries entering the skull to supply the brain.

membranes apart, forming a progressively enlarging collection of blood (subdural haematoma) that slowly compresses the underlying brain.

The dural venous sinuses are vascular channels located at constant sites along the internal surface of the cranium, with most being enclosed by bone on their external aspect and a fold of dura mater internally: others are located wholly within specific folds of dura mater. Some sinuses are small, resembling a small-diameter vein threaded between the dura mater and skull: others are much larger channels. The difference between a sinus and a vein is that a sinus lacks the adventitial and muscular layers normally found in the walls of veins: these are replaced by the bone and dura mater that surrounds the sinus. Consequently, only a layer of endothelial cells separates the blood inside a sinus from its surrounding tissues.

The major venous sinuses of the skull are the paired cavernous, transverse and sigmoid sinuses, the single superior and inferior sagittal sinuses, and the straight sinus (Fig. 5.57A).

The superior sagittal sinus runs posteriorly along the attached edge of the falx cerebri (Figs 5.56B and 5.57A): it drains blood from the external surfaces of the cerebral hemispheres and reabsorbs CSF through the arachnoid granulations. The inferior sagittal sinus is enclosed in the free edge of the falx cerebri.

The straight sinus is enclosed by the dura mater along the line of fusion of the falx cerebri and tentorium cerebelli (Fig. 5.57A): it receives the great cerebral vein and inferior sagittal sinus. The superior sagittal sinus, straight sinus and occipital sinus may meet at the internal occipital protuberance (confluence of sinuses) where the transverse sinuses begin (Fig. 5.57A).

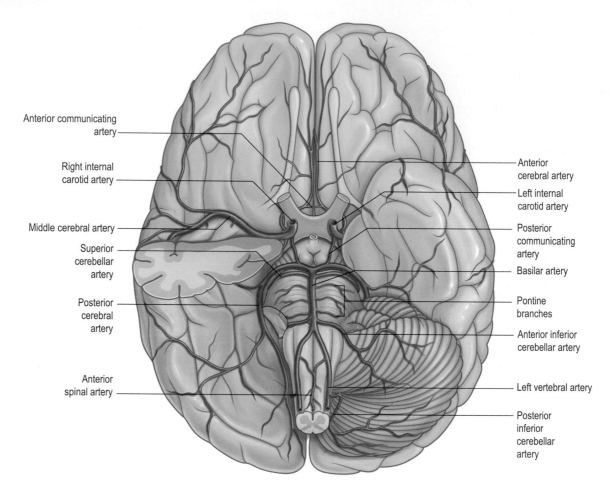

Fig. 5.59 Inferior aspect of the brain and brainstem showing the vertebral and internal carotid arteries and their branches.

From the internal occipital protuberance each transverse sinus runs around the posterior and lateral walls of the posterior cranial fossa in the attached margin of the tentorium cerebelli (Fig. 5.57A). The right transverse sinus is usually a continuation of the superior sagittal sinus, and the left a continuation of the straight sinus. Each receives veins from the surfaces of the cerebral hemisphere and cerebellum as well as the superior petrosal sinus. The transverse sinus is directly continuous with the sigmoid sinus located in a groove on the mastoid portion of the temporal bone. The sigmoid sinus joins with the inferior petrosal sinus, forming the internal jugular vein, to exit the skull via the jugular foramen.

The smaller venous sinuses of the skull are located along the edges of the bones projecting into the middle and posterior cranial fossae (Fig. 5.57A). The superior

and inferior petrosal sinuses run along the respective edges of the petrous temporal bone; the sphenoparietal sinus runs along the lesser wing of the sphenoid; and the occipital sinus along the internal occipital crest.

The cavernous sinus is formed by separation of the dura mater from the lateral surface of the body of the sphenoid on either side of the pituitary fossa (Fig. 5.57B): it is a narrow trabeculated space filled with a dense plexus of venous channels. The third and fourth cranial nerves, and ophthalmic and maxillary divisions of the trigeminal (fifth cranial) nerve pass in the lateral wall of the sinus deep to the dura mater, but external to the endothelium of the sinus. The sixth cranial nerve runs with the internal carotid artery between the endothelium and bony floor of the sinus. The sinus receives venous blood principally from the sphenoparietal sinus and superior ophthalmic vein, which drains the orbit, as well as the middle meningeal vein and veins from the cerebral hemisphere.

Ultimately, the majority of blood in the dural venous sinuses drains to one or other of the internal jugular veins, although some may drain through small emissary veins that penetrate the skull at specific sites to communicate with veins outside the skull.

CRANIAL NERVES

Certain nerves project from the cranial portion of the CNS (within the skull). They connect the brainstem and diencephalon with various structures and tissues in the head and neck, as well as with various thoracic and abdominal viscera. Although inside the skull, these nerves constitute part of the CNS and, as a rule, become peripheral nerves only after they leave the skull. There are 12 pairs of cranial nerves that are known by number or name: the name usually reflects the form, function or distribution of the nerve.

First Cranial Nerve (I: Olfactory)

The olfactory nerve mediates the perception of smell. It is composed of a series of short nerves projecting from the olfactory epithelium in the roof of the nose through the cribriform plate of the ethmoid bone to the olfactory bulb. Because of their small size, they can only be seen in microscopic dissections or histological preparations of the cribriform plate. Each olfactory nerve synapses on cell bodies that form the ipsilateral olfactory bulb, the axons of which constitute the olfactory tract (Fig. 5.54). The olfactory tract ramifies in the anterior end of the hypothalamus where it has diverse connections, the majority of which eventually pass to the uncus.

Second Cranial Nerve (II: Optic)

The optic nerve transmits visual information from the ipsilateral retina to the optic chiasma (Fig. 5.54). Information from both eyes is transmitted by each optic tract to the lateral geniculate body on each side. After processing this information, cells in the lateral geniculate body eventually relay it to the occipital lobes of the ipsilateral cerebral hemisphere through axons that run in the white matter of the cerebral hemisphere.

Third Cranial Nerve (III: Oculomotor)

The oculomotor nerve innervates certain muscles of the eye. It emerges from the ventral surface of the midbrain at the level of the superior colliculus immediately medial

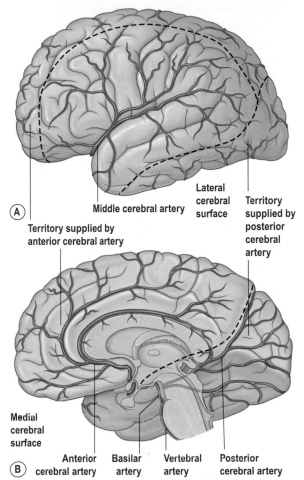

Fig. 5.60 Distribution of the anterior, middle and posterior cerebral arteries on the lateral (A) and medial (B) surfaces of the cerebral cortex.

to the crus cerebri on each side (Fig. 5.61A and B). It reaches the orbit by passing through the cavernous sinus and then the superior orbital fissure.

Fourth Cranial Nerve (IV: Trochlear)

The trochlear nerve innervates superior oblique associated with the eye. It emerges from the dorsal aspect of the midbrain immediately inferior to the inferior colliculus (Fig. 5.61C) and then winds around the crus cerebri to appear on the ventral aspect of the brainstem (Fig. 5.61A and B). It enters the orbit by passing through the cavernous sinus and then the superior orbital fissure.

Fifth Cranial Nerve (V: Trigeminal)

The trigeminal nerve divides into three large divisions (ophthalmic (V_1), maxillary (V_2) and mandibular (V_3)):

it is mainly sensory, with the cell bodies of the sensory fibres located in a swelling on the nerve (trigeminal ganglion) formed at the junction of its three divisions (Fig. 5.61B). The part of the nerve between the ganglion and brainstem is the sensory root: it is attached to the lateral aspect of the pons demarcating the junction of the pons with the middle cerebellar peduncle.

Although the pons and middle cerebellar peduncle are continuous with one another, formed essentially by the same nerves, they are by convention demarcated by an imaginary line passing longitudinally through the point of attachment of the trigeminal root to the brainstem: the middle cerebellar peduncle lies dorsal to this line and pons ventral to it.

The trigeminal nerve projects ventrally onto the superior surface of the petrous temporal bone, with the trigeminal ganglion resting in a shallow depression (cavum trigeminale) on its surface. Beyond the ganglion, the three divisions leave the skull to supply particular regions of the face and skull.

Branches of the ophthalmic division (V_1) enter the orbit through the superior orbital fissure, supplying the ethmoidal air cells, walls of the nasal cavity, cornea and conjunctiva, and skin of the forehead. The maxillary division (V_2) leaves the cranial cavity through the foramen rotundum: its branches are distributed to the nasal cavity, maxillary teeth, hard and soft palates and skin of the face covering the maxilla and zygoma. The mandibular division (V_3) passes through the foramen ovale and supplies the mandibular teeth, temporomandibular joint, tongue and skin overlying the mandible and temporal regions.

Although largely sensory, the trigeminal nerve is accompanied by a small nerve (motor root of the trigeminal nerve), which emerges from the pons just inferior to the sensory root (Fig. 5.61A and B) to join the mandibular division in the foramen ovale: it supplies the muscles of mastication.

Sixth Cranial Nerve (VI: Abducens)

The abducens nerve innervates lateral rectus associated with the eye: it is responsible for abducting it. It emerges from the brainstem at the caudal border of the pons between it and the beginning of the pyramid (Fig. 5.61A and B), entering the orbit through the superior orbital fissure.

Seventh and Eighth Cranial Nerves (VII: Facial and VIII: Vestibulocochlear)

The facial and vestibulocochlear nerves, respectively, emerge as a pair from the lateral aspect of the medulla oblongata immediately inferior to the caudal border of the pons (Fig. 5.61A and B), both entering the internal auditory meatus. The facial nerve is the more medial and, after emerging from the stylomastoid foramen, innervates the muscles of facial expression: it also conveys taste fibres from the anterior two-thirds of the tongue and parasympathetic fibres destined for the lacrimal, submandibular and sublingual glands.

The vestibulocochlear nerve has two components (vestibular and cochlear): the vestibular component innervates the vestibular apparatus of the inner ear and is responsible for the sense of balance; the cochlear

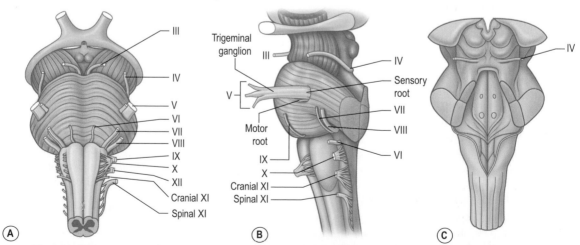

Fig. 5.61 Anterior (A), left lateral (B) and posterior (C) aspects of the brainstem showing the origin of the cranial nerves.

component arises in the cochlea of the inner ear and is responsible for hearing.

9th, 10th and 11th Cranial Nerves (IX: Glossopharyngeal, X: Vagus and XI: Accessory)

These appear as a series of tiny rootlets aligned along the lateral surface of the medulla oblongata (Fig. 5.61A and B). The uppermost rootlets converge to form the ninth cranial nerve (glossopharyngeal); the middle rootlets form the tenth cranial nerve (vagus); the lowest rootlets form the cranial part of the eleventh cranial nerve (accessory). All three nerves leave the skull through the jugular foramen.

The glossopharyngeal nerve supplies stylopharyngeus, but principally is sensory to the pharynx and posterior one-third of the tongue. The vagus nerve has a diverse distribution, including the muscles of the pharynx and larynx, mucosa of the larynx, viscera of the chest and much of the abdomen. The ninth and tenth cranial nerves also innervate the carotid body and carotid sinus and are, therefore, involved in cardiovascular reflexes.

The accessory nerve has two components (cranial, spinal): the cranial accessory nerve is formed by the lowest rootlets from the lateral aspect of the brainstem: the spinal accessory nerve is formed by rootlets that emerge from the lateral aspect of the C1–C5 segments of the spinal cord, which converge forming a single trunk entering the skull through the foramen magnum (Fig. 5.61A and B). The spinal and cranial parts join for a short distance, but the fibres of the cranial part are soon transferred to the vagus nerve through which they are distributed to the muscles of the pharynx, larynx and soft palate. The spinal accessory nerve leaves the skull independently but in company with the glossopharyngeal and vagus nerves passing through the jugular foramen, innervating sternomastoid and trapezius.

12th Cranial Nerve (XII: Hypoglossal)

The hypoglossal nerve supplies the muscles of the tongue (except palatoglossus). It emerges from the brainstem as a series of rootlets attached along the depression between the pyramid and olive on each side (Fig. 5.61A and B) leaving the skull through the hypoglossal canal in the occipital bone.

Nerve Root Sheaths

To reach the peripheral nervous system, the cranial nerves must penetrate the meninges. As they leave the brainstem, their proximal ends and spinal nerve roots are invested by the pia mater (Fig. 5.62): this is one of the morphological reasons for classifying them as part of the CNS. The pia

mater spreads like a tubular extension over the surface of each nerve from its point of attachment to the brainstem as far as where it leaves the skull or vertebral canal.

Generally, the cranial nerves pierce the arachnoid and dura mater at the foramina through which they leave the skull. Here, the dura and arachnoid mater are drawn into the foramen by the exiting nerve: eventually, the meningeal tissues blend with the fibrous sheath of the peripheral part of the cranial nerve (Fig. 5.62). Cranial nerves are, therefore, covered by pia mater and bathed in CSF as far as their respective foramina.

Exceptions to this rule apply to the second to fifth cranial nerves. A dural and arachnoid sheath accompanies the optic nerve as far as the back of the eye, with the nerve covered by pia mater and bathed in CSF up to this point. The third, fourth and fifth cranial nerves pierce the dura mater that forms the cavernous sinus: they run outside the dura along the walls of the cavernous sinus, before passing through the superior orbital fissure. The fifth cranial nerve penetrates the dura mater over the apex of the petrous temporal bone, with its three divisions running extradurally before entering their respective foramina: its sensory and motor roots are covered by pia mater and bathed in CSF as far as the middle of the trigeminal ganglion, which is where the dura and arachnoid mater blend with the nerve.

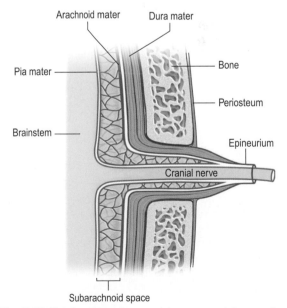

Fig. 5.62 Relationship of a cranial nerve and its meningeal sheath.

SECTION SUMMARY

Brain

- Expanded rostral end of neural tube located within the skull
- Comprises cerebrum, cerebellum and brainstem (pons, midbrain and medulla oblongata); continuous with spinal cord beyond the medulla oblongata
- Contains ventricles (lateral, third and fourth), thalamus and hypothalamus
- The medulla oblongata connects it to the spinal cord: it has an anterior median fissure with pyramids on either side; either side of the midline posteriorly is the nucleus gracilis medially and nucleus cuneatus laterally

Cerebrum

- Separated by longitudinal fissure into right and left cerebral hemispheres, joined by corpus callosum
- Has outer cortex of grey matter (cell bodies) and large inner mass of white matter (axons)
- Cerebral cortex thrown into folds (gyri) and depressions (sulci)
- Central sulcus separates precentral gyrus (motor cortex) and postcentral gyrus (sensory cortex)
- Each hemisphere is divided into four lobes (frontal, parietal, temporal and occipital)
- Temporal and parietal lobes separated by lateral sulcus
- Parietal and occipital lobes separated by parieto-occipital sulcus
- Frontal lobe subserves motor functions and is responsible for expressions of intellect and personality
- Parietal lobe responsible for sensory functions (touch, pressure, position sense), three-dimensional perception, analysis of visual images, language, geometry and calculations
- Occipital lobe is involved in vision
- Temporal lobe is involved in perception of sound, memory and emotion

Meninges

- Three coverings: outer fibrous dura mater, middle arachnoid mater and inner transparent pia mater
- Dura reflected within skull as falx cerebri (in sagittal plane) and tentorium cerebelli (in transverse plane)
- Arachnoid lines deep surface of dura forming network of fine threads bridging gap between dura and pia mater
- Pia mater is adherent to underlying neural tissue
- Subarachnoid space contains cerebrospinal fluid

Cerebrospinal fluid

- Produced by choroid plexus in roof of lateral and third ventricles
- Reabsorbed into venous system through arachnoid granulations

Blood supply

- Arterial supply from right and left internal carotid and vertebral arteries
- Internal carotid divides into anterior and middle cerebral arteries; anterior communicating artery connects anterior cerebral arteries
- Vertebral arteries join forming basilar artery, which terminates as posterior cerebral arteries; posterior communicating artery connects posterior and middle cerebral arteries
- Venous drainage by system of intracranial venous sinuses (superior and inferior sagittal, transverse, cavernous, superior and inferior petrosal and sigmoid) draining into internal jugular vein

Cranial nerves

12 pairs inside skull, form part of CNS: once outside skull are part of peripheral nervous system

- First (I: olfactory) mediates sense of smell
- Second (II: optic) transmits visual information
- Third (III: oculomotor) innervates extraocular muscles (superior, medial and inferior rectus, inferior oblique); conveys parasympathetic fibres to the ciliary ganglion
- Fourth (IV: trochlear) innervates superior oblique
- Fifth (V: trigeminal) divides into three parts: ophthalmic division (V_1) distributed to nasal cavity, cornea, conjunctiva, skin of forehead; maxillary division (V_2) distributed to nasal cavity, upper teeth, hard and soft palates, skin of face; mandibular division (V_3) distributed to lower teeth, tongue, temporomandibular joint, skin over mandible and muscles of mastication
- Sixth (VI: abducens) innervates lateral rectus
- Seventh (VII: facial) innervates the facial muscles; conveys taste from anterior two-thirds of tongue; conveys parasympathetic fibres to the pterygopalatine and submandibular ganglia
- Eighth (VIII: vestibulocochlear) transmits information regarding sense of balance (vestibular part) and auditory information (cochlear part)
- Ninth (IX: glossopharyngeal) innervates stylopharyngeus, sensory to pharynx and posterior one-third of tongue; innervates carotid body and sinus; conveys taste from posterior one-third of tongue; conveys parasympathetic fibres to otic ganglion

❓ SELF-ASSESSMENT QUESTIONS

41. What is the function of cerebrospinal fluid?
42. What are gyri and sulci of the brain?
43. How many cranial nerves are there?
44. Which major blood vessels provide the arterial supply to the brain?
45. Which sense is the lateral geniculate body associated with?
46. What structure connects the two cerebral hemispheres?
47. What are the different types of glial cells?
48. What is the function of the hypoglossal nerve?
49. What separates the cerebral hemispheres from the cerebellum?
50. What are the divisions of the trigeminal nerve?
51. What is the origin of the spinal part of the accessory nerve?
52. Which muscles are supplied by the spinal part of the accessory nerve?
53. What is the function of the frontal lobe of the brain?
54. Stimulation of the precentral gyrus results in what?
55. What does the white matter in the CNS mainly consist of?
56. How many lobes does each cerebral hemisphere have?
57. Which muscle(s) is/are supplied by the glossopharyngeal nerve?
58. What runs in the fixed edge of the falx cerebri?
59. What are arachnoid granulations?
60. Which vessels participate in the circle of Willis?

4. Describe the structural organisation of the inner ear
5. Explain the role of the auditory ossicles in transmitting vibrations of the tympanic membrane to the inner ear
6. Appreciate the influence of pathology and/or trauma on the ear

INTRODUCTION

Not only is the ear responsible for the sensation of hearing by converting sound waves into impulses generated by hair cells in the inner ear, it is also responsible for maintaining balance and equilibrium, again by structures within the inner ear. Although these two functions appear to be separate, both hearing and balance sensations are conveyed to the brain for interpretation by the same cranial nerve (eighth). Loss of hearing can be compensated for with hearing aids; however, the loss of balance can be debilitating, even if it is transitory.

Development

The ear consists of three parts which function together but have different origins. The membranous part of the internal ear originates from the otic vesicle (surface ectoderm origin) during the fourth week *in utero*. The otic vesicle divides into an anterior part which forms the saccule and the cochlear duct, and a dorsal part forming the utricle, semicircular canals and endolymphatic duct. The surrounding bony labyrinth develops from the adjacent mesenchyme. Except for the cochlear duct, from which the organ of Corti (spiral organ) develops, the membranous labyrinth is concerned with maintaining balance.

The epithelial lining of the middle ear (tympanic cavity, mastoid antrum and auditory tube) is derived from the endoderm of the tubotympanic recess of the first branchial pouch. The auditory ossicles develop from the dorsal ends of the cartilages of the first (malleus and incus) and second (stapes) branchial arches.

The external auditory (acoustic) meatus develops from the first branchial cleft and is separated from the

▌EAR

LEARNING OUTCOMES

By the end of the section, you should be able to:
1. Describe the development of the ear
2. Describe the external, middle and inner ear and their function
3. Explain the role of the auditory and vestibular parts of the inner ear

tympanic cavity by the tympanic membrane, which is derived from three sources (ectoderm of the first branchial cleft, intermediate mesodermal layer, endoderm of the first branchial pouch). The external ear (auricle) develops from six mesenchymal swellings around the margin of the first branchial pouch.

COMPONENTS OF THE EAR

The three parts of the ear (external, middle and internal) are all, except for the auricle, found within the temporal bone: the auricle is attached to the tympanic part of the temporal bone. The external ear collects the sounds, conveying them to the tympanic membrane separating the external and middle ear, causing it to vibrate. Vibration of the tympanic membrane is transmitted across the middle ear by the three auditory ossicles (malleus, incus and stapes) to the internal ear. The middle ear communicates with the nasopharynx via the Eustachian (auditory) tube. The internal ear consists of two functionally distinct parts: that concerned with hearing (cochlear part) and that concerned with balance and position sense (vestibular part). The sensory endings of both parts are supplied by the vestibulocochlear nerve (eighth cranial nerve).

External Ear

Consists of the auricle and external auditory (acoustic) meatus (Fig. 5.63A) which collect and convey sound towards the tympanic membrane. The auricle projects posterolaterally from the side of the head, connected to the fascia by three small insignificant muscles. It is a single piece of elastic cartilage, except for the fibrofatty lobule, covered with skin: the named parts are shown in Fig. 5.63A. In adults, its shape is extremely variable, increasing threefold in length from birth to adulthood: it also tends to increase in size and thickness in old age.

The external auditory meatus is 25 mm long, cartilaginous in its lateral third, continuous with that of the auricle, and bony in its medial two-thirds formed by the tympanic part of the temporal bone. The meatus curves superoposteriorly as it passes medially, with the inferior wall being 5 mm longer than the superior because of the obliquity of the tympanic membrane. The skin lining the meatus is firmly attached to the underlying bone, with the lateral third containing numerous ceruminous (wax secreting) cells and hairs. The meatus lies posterior to the temporomandibular joint, with the mastoid air cells being immediately posterior.

Middle Ear

Narrow irregular cavity containing the auditory ossicles immediately medial to the tympanic membrane (Fig. 5.63A). The middle ear can be conveniently viewed as a six-sided space, with that part above the tympanic membrane being the epitympanic recess. The cavity communicates with the nasopharynx via the Eustachian (auditory) tube which opens into the anterior wall, and with the mastoid air cells via the aditus in the posterior wall (Fig. 5.63B). The auditory tube enables the pressure on both sides of the tympanic membrane to be equalised: it is opened during swallowing.

The circular tympanic membrane is concave laterally and consists of three layers (modified skin externally, intermediate fibrous layer and mucous membrane internally). The majority of the membrane is tense; however, there is a small flaccid area (pars flaccida) anterosuperiorly. Between its internal and external layers runs the chorda tympani branch of the facial nerve conveying taste sensations from the anterior two-thirds of the tongue and parasympathetic fibres to the submandibular and sublingual salivary glands.

The auditory ossicles articulate by synovial joints and transmit vibrations of the tympanic membrane to the inner ear. The malleus attaches to the deep surface of the membrane and articulates with the incus, which in turn articulates with the stapes, the oval base of which lies in the oval window. Movements of the malleus and stapes are controlled and reflexly dampened by contraction of tensor tympani and stapedius, respectively, both of which are found within the middle ear. Tensor tympani is innervated by the mandibular division of the trigeminal nerve and stapedius by the facial nerve.

Internal Ear

Situated within the petrous part of the temporal bone, the internal ear consists of a complex series of fluid-filled spaces (membranous labyrinth) occupying a similarly shaped cavity (bony labyrinth). Displacement of fluid in these spaces stimulates the sensory endings of the lining epithelium.

The bony labyrinth consists of three parts: vestibule (containing the utricle and saccule of the membranous labyrinth), semicircular canals (anterior, posterior and horizontal) and cochlea (Fig. 5.64A). The anterior and posterior semicircular canals are at right angles to each other and lie 45 degrees to the sagittal plane, with the anterior being anterior and lateral, and the posterior,

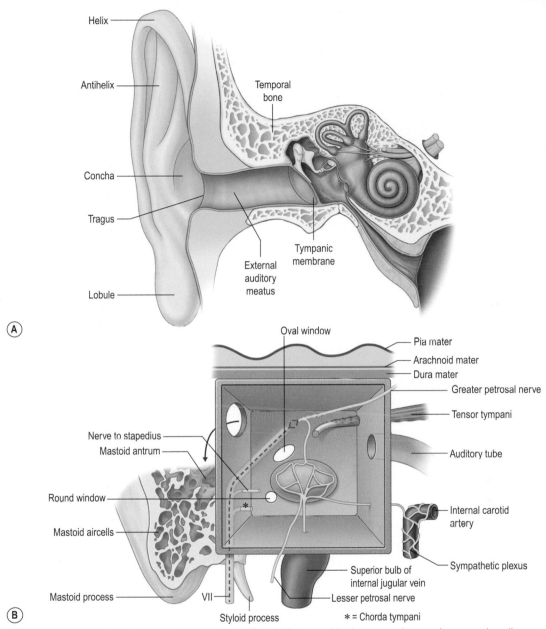

Fig. 5.63 (A) External, middle and internal ear; (B) middle ear with the tympanic membrane and auditory ossicles removed.

posterior and lateral: the lateral semicircular canal lies horizontally. The membranous semicircular ducts are dilated at one end (ampulla) (Fig. 5.64A) in which there is a thickening (ampullary crest), where endings of the vestibulocochlear nerve terminate. The three ducts open into the utricle, which communicates with the saccule, which in turn communicates with the cochlea. Thickenings in both the utricle and saccule (maculae) contain terminations of the vestibulocochlear nerve. The ampullary crests of the semicircular canals convey information about rotatory and angular movements of the head, and the maculae information about linear and

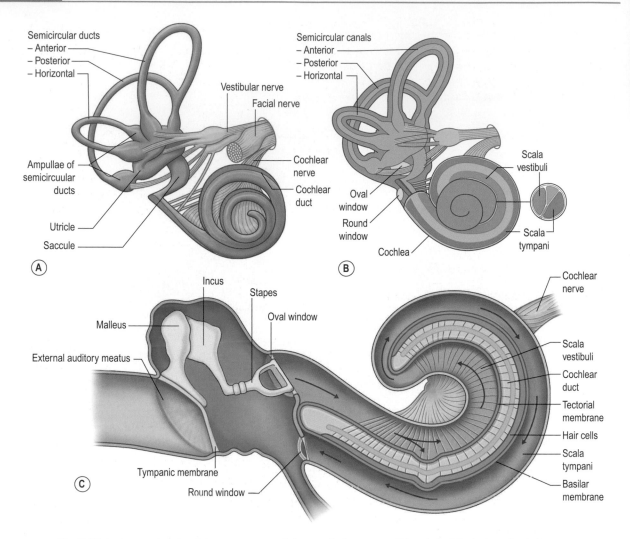

Fig. 5.64 Inner ear showing the arrangement of the vestibular system (A) and the labyrinth and spiral organ (B); (C) conversion of sound waves into mechanical vibrations.

tilting movements. Disease of the semicircular ducts, the utricle and saccule gives rise to giddiness of varying degrees.

The bony cochlea consists of two and three-quarter turns of a spiral, resembling a shell lying on its side. It has a central supporting column of bone (modiolus) to which is attached a thin lamina of bone partially dividing the spiral into two parts: scala vestibuli above, scala tympani below (Fig. 5.64B and C). The membranous cochlear duct lines the bony cochlea and is triangular in cross-section. The outer wall of the triangle is thickened forming the spiral ligament, the inferior part of which is the basilar membrane and superior part the vestibular membrane. The thickened and highly specialised spiral organ (of Corti) lies on the basilar membrane. Pulsations transmitted to the perilymph within the membranous cochlea by movement of the stapes in the oval window pass through the scala tympani and are transmitted to the fluid in the scala vestibuli, adjusted by compensatory movements of the round window, causing movement of the basilar membrane, thereby stimulating the hair cells of the spiral organ (Fig. 5.64C): the result is auditory perception. Low-frequency sounds cause maximum activity in the basilar membrane; high-frequency sounds are limited to the basal portion of the cochlea.

SECTION SUMMARY

The ear consists of three parts (external, middle and inner) each of which has a specific function. As well as being associated with hearing, the inner ear is also important in maintaining balance and equilibrium.

External ear
- Comprises the auricle and external auditory (acoustic) meatus which collect and convey sound towards the tympanic membrane
- Chorda tympani (branch of the seventh cranial nerve) crosses the tympanic membrane between its external and internal layers

Middle ear
- Narrow irregular cavity medial to tympanic membrane containing auditory ossicles (malleus, incus and stapes)
- Ossicles transmit vibrations of tympanic membrane to inner ear
- Communicates with nasopharynx via the auditory tube and mastoid air cells via aditus

Inner ear
- Located within petrous temporal bone comprising bony labyrinth (balance) and bony cochlea (hearing) parts
- Bony labyrinth consists of vestibule (utricle and saccule) and semicircular canals (anterior, posterior and horizontal): movement of perilymph in semicircular ducts detects angular and rotational movements; movement of maculae in utricle and saccule detect linear and tilting movements of head
- Bony cochlea consists of two and three-quarters of a spiral with a central supporting column of bone; movement of stapes in oval window transmits pulsation to perilymph causing movement of basilar membrane, stimulating cells of spiral organ (auditory perception)

❓ SELF-ASSESSMENT QUESTIONS

61. What and where are the auditory ossicles?
62. What structure is located at the medial end of the external auditory meatus?
63. How many pairs of semicircular canals are there?
64. How does the middle ear communicate with the nasopharynx?
65. Which muscle attaches to the malleus to dampen vibrations of the tympanic membrane?
66. Which nerve passes in a canal in the posterior wall of the middle ear?

EYE

LEARNING OUTCOMES

By the end of the section, you should be able to:
1. Describe the development of the eye
2. Describe the structural organisation of eye
3. Explain the functions of the three layers of the eyeball
4. Describe the location and protection of the eyeball within the orbit
5. Describe the role of the extraocular muscles in altering the direction of the gaze
6. Appreciate the influence of pathology and/or trauma on the eye

INTRODUCTION

The eye sits in the orbit supported by the suspensory ligament and surrounded by periorbital fat: each eye faces anteriorly limiting the field of view to approximately 180 degrees; however, by turning the head to the right or left the field of view is enlarged. Images formed on the retina are integrated by the brain to give binocular (stereoscopic) vision. The loss of vision has a major impact on the individual's quality of life.

Development

The eyes begin to develop on either side of the developing forebrain as optic vesicles by the end of the fourth week *in utero*. Continuous with the forebrain, the optic vesicles contact the surface ectoderm and induce development of the lens placode. When the optic vesicle invaginates to form the pigmented and neural layers of the retina, the lens placode also invaginates, forming the lens pit and lens vesicle.

The retina, optic nerve, muscles and epithelium of the iris, and ciliary body are all derived from the neuroectoderm of the forebrain, while the lens and epithelium of the lacrimal glands, eyelids, conjunctiva and cornea all arise from the surface ectoderm. The extraocular muscles and all of the connective and vascular tissue of the cornea, iris, ciliary body, choroid and sclera are of mesodermal origin.

EYEBALL

It consists of three concentric layers: outer fibrous supporting layer (sclera and cornea); middle vascular pigmented layer (choroid, ciliary body and iris); and inner layer of nerve elements (retina). The interior of the eyeball contains fluid under pressure and is divided into anterior and posterior compartments by the lens and its attachments: these contain aqueous humour and the vitreous body, respectively (Fig. 5.65A).

A thin fibrous sheet surrounds the sclera, forming a socket for the eyeball, separating it from the other contents of the orbit. The eyeball is supported inferiorly by the suspensory ligament of the eye and is surrounded

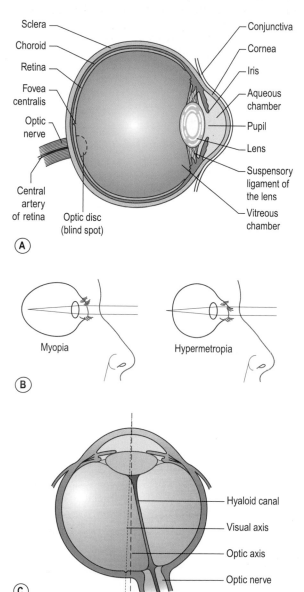

Fig. 5.65 (A) Horizontal section through the eye; (B) representation of myopia (short-sightedness) and hypermetropia (long-sightedness); (C) visual and optic axes of the eye.

and protected by extraocular fat. In adults, the eyeball is almost spherical, having a diameter of approximately 25 mm; however, the anteroposterior diameter may be greater or less than normal giving rise to short-sightedness (myopia) or long-sightedness (hypermetropia), respectively (Fig. 5.65B). Relative to body size, the eyeball is much larger in infants and children as it completes the majority of its growth in the antenatal period: it is also slightly larger in women than men.

The two eyes look forwards: an imaginary line connecting the centre of the corneal curvature (anterior pole) to the centre of the scleral curvature (posterior pole) is the optic axis (Fig. 5.65C). The visual axis is, however, more important and joins the centre of the cornea to the fovea of the retina: it represents the path taken by light from the centre point of vision. When looking at distant objects, the visual axes of the two eyes are parallel: the optic axes are slightly and optic nerves markedly convergent posteriorly.

Outer Fibrous Layer

The sclera is the posterior opaque part of the fibrous layer forming approximately five-sixths of the circumference of the eyeball: the remainder is the cornea. It is approximately 1 mm thick posteriorly and 0.5 mm thick anteriorly and gives attachment to the tendons of the extraocular muscles. The anterior part of the sclera is covered by conjunctiva forming the white of the eye. Posteriorly, the sclera is pierced, 3 mm medial to the fovea, by the optic nerve and accompanying vessels (Fig. 5.65).

The forward-bulging cornea is continuous with the sclera at the corneoscleral junction: it is dense and uniformly thick (1 mm), and covered by conjunctiva. The cornea is avascular but richly innervated by the ophthalmic division of the trigeminal nerve, with abrasion of its surface being extremely painful: its sensitivity to touch forms the basis of the corneal reflex resulting in reflex contraction of orbicularis oculi and closing of the eye.

The majority of refraction of the eye takes place at the surface of the cornea and not at the lens. Irregularities in the curvature of the cornea, which ideally should correspond to a section of a perfect sphere, interfere with the ability to form sharp images on the retina. When the cornea is more curved in one direction than the other, the condition is astigmatism.

The surface conjunctiva and cornea are kept moist and clean by a watery fluid secreted by the lacrimal gland. Constant blinking is an important part of the mechanism of fluid flow across the cornea: drying of the cornea causes serious damage to its surface cells.

Middle Vascular Layer

Often called the uvea, it consists of three parts (choroid, ciliary body and iris) (Fig. 5.65A). The choroid is a thin membrane lining the sclera as far as the corneoscleral junction, loosely connected to the sclera except near where the optic nerve pierces, where it is firmly attached. It consists of two parts: outer pigmented (brown) layer preventing light passing through the sclera and the

scattering of light entering via the pupil, and inner vascular layer which is nutritive to the outer layer of the retina.

The ciliary body is a wedge-shaped ring connecting the choroid to the iris: it contains the ciliary muscle and ciliary processes, lined by the ciliary part of the retina (Fig. 5.66A). The inwardly projecting part of the wedge is directed towards the lens and connected to it by fibres of the suspensory ligament of the lens. The ciliary muscle consists of two sets of smooth muscle fibres (inner oblique and outer radial) both under parasympathetic

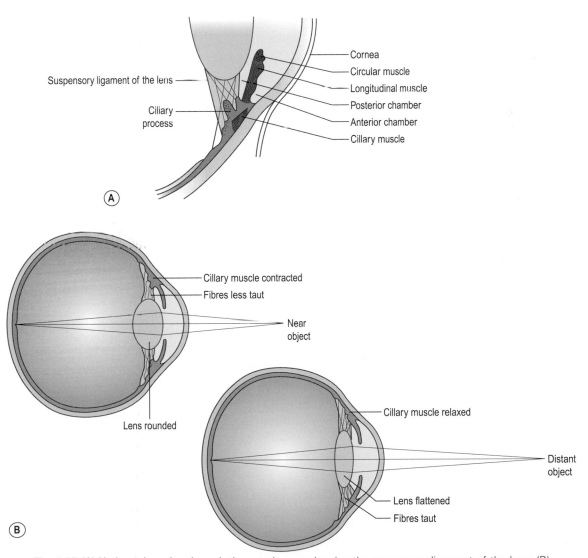

Fig. 5.66 (A) Horizontal section through the anterior eye showing the suspensory ligament of the lens; (B) the process of accommodation.

control. Contraction of the ciliary muscle reduces tension in the suspensory ligament of the lens, allowing its natural elasticity to increase its curvature so that the eye can focus on near objects (process of accommodation). The ciliary processes are 60–80 radiating projections, 2 mm in length, giving attachment to the suspensory ligament of the lens.

The iris is a thin contractile membrane firmly attached at its periphery to the ciliary body, lying anterior to the lens with a central opening (pupil). It contains smooth muscle fibres organised into an inner circular sphincter pupillae and an outer radially arranged dilator pupillae. These two muscles control the size of the pupil and the amount of light entering the eye. Both muscles are under autonomic control, the sphincter pupillae parasympathetic and dilator pupillae sympathetic. The colour of the iris is due to the pigment cells in its posterior layer. In individuals with few pigment cells, and because of the way other elements of the iris absorb and reflect light, the iris appears pale blue: with increasing numbers of pigment cells, the iris darkens and may become dark brown.

Refracting Media

The iris partly divides the region anterior to the lens into anterior (aqueous) and posterior (vitreous) chambers, both of which contain aqueous humour (Fig. 5.65A). This is a clear watery solution formed by the epithelium of the ciliary processes: the fluid is resorbed at the iridocorneal angle into the sinus venosus to re-enter the circulation. Interference with the process of resorption results in increased intraocular pressure (glaucoma) which affects the peripheral part of the visual field due to the pressure on the retina. Posterior to the lens and ciliary body is the posterior chamber containing the vitreous body (transparent, colourless and semi-gelatinous material) (Fig. 5.65A).

The lens is biconvex, approximately 10 mm in diameter and 4 mm thick, becoming thinner in old age. It largely consists of concentric lamellae of lens fibres surrounded by a capsule firmly attached to the ciliary body by the suspensory ligament of the lens. Both the capsule and lens are transparent and elastic. The shape of the lens is modified by the ciliary muscle as the eye focuses on objects at different distances (Fig. 5.66B).

After middle age, the lens becomes less elastic, and the ability to accommodate is gradually lost (presbyopia), so glasses are required for close work. The lens may also become less transparent with increasing age (cataract).

Inner Nervous Layer

Light-sensitive layer (retina) extending onto the ciliary body and iris, but this region contains no nerve elements so is nonfunctioning. The retina is approximately 0.5 mm thick posteriorly, thinning to 0.1 mm anteriorly; however, both the optic disc and fovea centralis are much thinner areas. It comprises two parts: outer pigmented epithelial layer and inner transparent layer containing the light receptors (rods and cones) (Fig. 5.67). The region where the fibres forming the optic nerve converge to pass through the choroid and sclera is the optic disc: it contains no light receptors and is, therefore, insensitive to light (blind spot). Three millimetres lateral to the optic disc is the macula, which has at its centre a depression (fovea centralis) where vision is most acute (Fig. 5.65A).

Within the inner transparent layer, the rods and cones lie closest to the choroid so that light has to pass through most of the retina before reaching them (Fig. 5.67): the cones are used in bright light as well as for colour discrimination. The macula contains only cones so that it functions in detailed vision (when an object is specifically looked at), it is always focused onto the macula. From the macula outwards, the number of cones in the retina rapidly decreases; however,

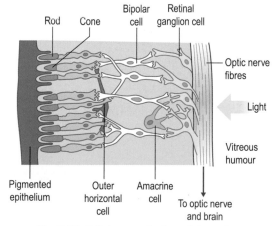

Fig. 5.67 Cellular organisation of the retina.

Medial   Lateral

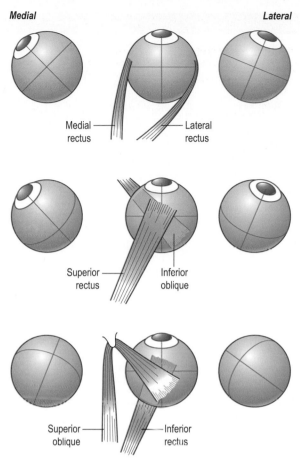

Medial — —— Lateral
rectus   rectus

Superior —— —— Inferior
rectus   oblique

Superior —— —— Inferior
oblique   rectus

Fig. 5.68 Extraocular muscles of the right eye and the action each produces with respect to the direction of gaze.

the number of rods increases: rods are used in dim light. The pigment contained in the rods is bleached out in bright light, but reforms in dim light so that objects previously not visible are seen (dark adaptation). There are six times as many rods as cones in the retina.

The blood supply to the retina is essentially from the central artery of the retina, a branch of the ophthalmic artery, which divides into four branches, each supplying a separate quadrant: because each branch is an end-artery, blockage results in blindness in the associated quadrant. The retina may also become detached from

the choroid, either spontaneously or from a blow to the eye, and vision is impaired. If the retina is torn, fluid passes outside the layer of rods and cones with vision again being lost: in both cases, laser treatment can be used to reattach the retina to prevent further separation.

MOVEMENTS OF THE EYEBALL

The direction of the gaze is controlled by the extraocular muscles: four rectus muscles (superior, medial, inferior and lateral) and the two oblique muscles (superior and inferior). The recti attach posteriorly to a tendinous ring surrounding the optic canal and medial part of the superior orbital fissure, attaching to the sclera 6 mm behind the edge of the cornea. Superior oblique passes anteriorly from the medial wall of the orbit to hook around the trochlea on the frontal bone, then passes posteriorly to attach to the superior surface of the sclera posterior to the equator of the eyeball. Inferior oblique passes laterally from the medial part of the maxilla inferior to inferior rectus to attach to the sclera, again posterior to the equator of the eyeball.

Medial and lateral rectus cause the eye to look horizontally medially and laterally, respectively (Fig. 5.68). However, because of the oblique course of the superior and inferior rectus within the orbit, they tend to pull the eye medially in addition to turning it to look superiorly and inferiorly, respectively (Fig. 5.68). The two oblique muscles tend to pull the eye laterally as well as moving it superiorly and inferiorly (Fig. 5.68): because the oblique muscles attach posterior to the equator, they pull on the posterior aspect of the eyeball. Consequently, superior oblique turns the eye to look inferiorly and laterally, while inferior oblique turns it to look superiorly and laterally. In reality, almost every movement of the eyeball involves at least three muscles. Coordinated movement between the two eyes is controlled by the brain.

Of these muscles, lateral rectus is innervated by the abducens (sixth cranial) nerve, superior oblique by the trochlear (fourth cranial) nerve and the remainder by the oculomotor (third cranial) nerve

SECTION SUMMARY

The eye consists of three layers: the outer fibrous (sclera and cornea), middle vascular (choroid, ciliary body and iris) and inner nervous (retina), surrounding two fluid-filled cavities (anterior and posterior chambers). The visual axis passes between the centre of the cornea and the fovea of the retina.

Outer fibrous layer
- Sclera: anterior part covered by conjunctiva forming white of the eye
- Cornea: continuous with sclera, is avascular but richly innervated

Middle vascular layer
- Choroid is a thin membrane lining the sclera with outer pigmented and inner vascular layers
- Ciliary body connects the choroid to the iris; contains ciliary muscle and processes
- Iris is a thin contractile membrane attached peripherally to the ciliary body; lies anterior to lens

Inner nervous layer
- Retina comprises outer pigmented and inner transparent layers, the latter containing light receptors (rods and cones)
- Optic disc (blind spot) is where optic nerve passes through choroid and sclera; contains no light receptors

Chambers
- Contain clear watery solution within the anterior (aqueous) and posterior (vitreous) chambers
- Lens alters curvature to facilitate changes in focus

Muscles producing movements of eyeball
- To look:
  - directly superiorly: superior rectus and inferior oblique
  - directly inferiorly: inferior rectus and superior oblique
  - laterally: lateral rectus
  - medially: medial rectus

SELF-ASSESSMENT QUESTIONS

67. How many layers does the eyeball have?
68. What is the blind spot?
69. Name the muscles which move the eyeball?
70. Which muscle(s) contract to cause the gaze to be directed towards the left?
71. Which cranial nerve supplies superior oblique?

SELF-ASSESSMENT MULTIPLE CHOICE QUESTIONS

1. How many cervical nerves are there?
   a. 5
   b. 6
   c. 7
   d. 8
   e. 9
2. Which of the following features is NOT associated with the first cervical vertebra (atlas)?
   a. Anterior tubercle
   b. Superior articular facet
   c. Anterior arch
   d. Body
   e. Posterior arch
3. Which of the following muscles is NOT associated with the suboccipital triangle?
   a. Superior oblique
   b. Inferior oblique
   c. Rectus capitis posterior major
   d. Rectus capitis posterior minor
   e. Rectus capitis lateralis
4. Which of the following muscles is NOT involved in rotating the neck?
   a. Trapezius
   b. Semispinalis cervicis
   c. Multifidus
   d. Scalenus anterior
   e. Sternomastoid
5. Which of the following muscles does NOT extend the head on the neck?
   a. Sternomastoid
   b. Rectus capitis posterior major
   c. Rectus capitis posterior minor
   d. Inferior oblique
   e. Superior oblique

6. Which of the following is NOT a paired bone of the skull?
   a. Parietal
   b. Maxilla
   c. Lacrimal
   d. Sphenoid
   e. Temporal

7. Which of the following structures passes through the foramen ovale?
   a. Greater petrosal nerve
   b. Mandibular nerve
   c. Middle meningeal artery
   d. Lesser petrosal sinus
   e. Trochlear nerve

8. The foramen magnum is located in which bone?
   a. Temporal
   b. Parietal
   c. Occipital
   d. Frontal
   e. Sphenoid

9. Through which opening in the base of the skull does the hypoglossal nerve pass?
   a. Anterior condylar canal
   b. Posterior condylar canal
   c. Foramen magnum
   d. Foramen lacerum
   e. Foramen spinosum

10. Concerning the skull, which of the following statements is correct?
    a. The crista galli gives attachment to the tentorium cerebelli
    b. The lambdoid suture is between the parietal and occipital bones.
    c. The frontal bone forms from a single bone.
    d. The maxilla forms the lateral margin of the orbit.
    e. The lacrimal bones form the bridge of the nose.

11. Which of the following muscles does NOT attach to the mandible?
    a. Mylohyoid
    b. Masseter
    c. Lateral pterygoid
    d. Temporalis
    e. Styloglossus

12. Which of the following muscles retracts the mandible?
    a. Masseter
    b. Lateral pterygoid
    c. Medial pterygoid

    d. Temporalis
    e. Buccinator

13. Which of the following muscles is NOT innervated by the mandibular nerve?
    a. Masseter
    b. Temporalis
    c. Posterior belly of digastric
    d. Tensor tympani
    e. Tensor veli palatini

14. Which of the following nerves innervates the skin of the face?
    a. Trigeminal
    b. Facial
    c. Dorsal rami of cervical nerves
    d. Hypoglossal nerve
    e. Ventral rami of cervical nerves

15. Which of the following features is NOT associated with the mandible?
    a. Coracoid process
    b. Body
    c. Lingula
    d. Condyloid process
    e. Neck

16. Concerning the mandible, which of the following statements is NOT correct?
    a. The axis of movement passes through the lingulae.
    b. The head articulates directly with the mandibular fossa of the temporal bone.
    c. Lateral pterygoid is involved in protraction of the mandible.
    d. The inferior alveolar neurovascular bundle runs within the body.
    e. Mylohyoid is attached to the medial surface of each half of the body.

17. Which of the following muscles is NOT attached to the hyoid bone?
    a. Mylohyoid
    b. Stylohyoid
    c. Digastric
    d. Sternohyoid
    e. Thyrohyoid

18. In which part of the brain is the visual cortex?
    a. Temporal lobe
    b. Frontal lobe
    c. Cerebellum
    d. Parietal lobe
    e. Occipital lobe

19. Which of the following nerves innervates lateral rectus?
    a. Oculomotor
    b. Trochlear
    c. Trigeminal
    d. Abducens
    e. Facial

20. Which of the following arteries does NOT supply blood to the brain?
    a. Middle meningeal
    b. Internal carotid
    c. Vertebral
    d. Middle cerebral
    e. Posterior inferior cerebellar

21. Which of the following nerves does NOT pass through the lateral wall of the cavernous sinus?
    a. Oculomotor
    b. Trochlear
    c. Ophthalmic division of the trigeminal
    d. Maxillary division of the trigeminal
    e. Abducens

22. Which of the following structures does NOT pass through the jugular foramen?
    a. Sigmoid sinus
    b. Superior petrosal sinus
    c. Glossopharyngeal nerve
    d. Vagus nerve
    e. Accessory nerve

23. Which of the following runs in the fixed edge of the tentorium cerebelli?
    a. Superior sagittal sinus
    b. Inferior sagittal sinus
    c. Superior petrosal sinus
    d. Inferior petrosal sinus
    e. Transverse sinus

24. Which of the following muscles is attached to the mastoid process?
    a. Temporalis
    b. Posterior belly of digastric
    c. Masseter
    d. Medial pterygoid
    e. Rectus capitis posterior major

25. Concerning teeth, which of the following statements is NOT correct?
    a. The mandibular teeth are innervated by the inferior alveolar nerve.
    b. The teeth are held in place by the periodontal ligament.
    c. In total there are four central incisors.
    d. The tooth above the gum margin is covered by cementum.
    e. The maxillary teeth are innervated by branches of the maxillary nerve.

REFERENCES

American Association of Orthopaedic Surgeons., 1994. Joint Motion: Methods of Measurimg and Recording. In: Greene, W.B., Heckman, J.D. (Eds.), American Associatoin of Orthopaedic Surgeons, Illinois.

Friedman, M.H., Weisberg, J., 1982. Application of orthopaedic principles in evaluation of the temporomandibular joint. Phys. Ther. 62, 597–603.

Youdas, J.W., Carey, J.B., Garret, T.R., 1992. Normal range of motion of the cervical spine: an initial goniometric study. Phys. Ther. 72, 770–780.

Answers to Self-Assessment Questions

PART 1: INTRODUCTION

1. Standing erect with legs together and feet parallel and facing forwards, arms hanging loosely at the sides with the palms facing forwards
2. Proximal
3. Abduction
4. Sagittal/median
5. It lies inferior
6. Sagittal and coronal
7. It lies in front of
8. Turning the palm to face posteriorly
9. Its long axis
10. Bringing the dorsum (top) of the foot towards the anterior aspect of the leg/calf
11. Dermatome, myotome and sclerotome
12. Zygote
13. Somites
14. Two
15. Eight, with each lying above its correspondingly numbered vertebra, except C8 which lies below the seventh cervical vertebra
16. Those of the trunk and neck
17. Lower cervical and first thoracic
18. Anteriorly
19. Between 24 and 26 days after fertilization
20. Three (centrum, two neural arches)
21. Schwann cell
22. Axosomatic, axodendritic and axo-axonic
23. Oligodendrocytes
24. Epineurium
25. Aα and Aγ
26. Efferent fibres are motor fibres: they transmit information away from the central nervous system (CNS)
27. To enable the integration of information in a single neuron from several sources; the result may be excitatory or inhibitory
28. Peripheral and cranial nerves, and sensory receptors
29. A single long process arising from the cell body
30. The gap/space along the length of nerve fibre between successive Schwann cells
31. Epidermis
32. Stratum basale and spinosum
33. Lines reflecting stresses with the skin at rest; incisions along them lead to minimal scarring during healing, while incisions across them may cause scar contraction
34. Eyelids, external acoustic meatus, axillae, areolae and groin
35. Eccrine glands
36. Subcutaneous connective tissue layer
37. Melanin, a subtle red pigment and air
38. Dorsum of the terminal phalanx
39. Stretch
40. Applying moist pads or conducting gel below the site of electrode placement to overcome its electrical resistance due to dryness and natural greasiness
41. Inferior tibiofibular joint: also the interosseous membrane between the radius and ulna, and between the tibia and fibula
42. Secondary cartilaginous joint
43. Epiphysis
44. (a) In the foetus, it forms the temporary skeleton which later ossifies; (b) during growth, it forms the epiphyseal growth plate; (c) in adults, it persists as the cartilage covering articular surfaces
45. White fibrous tissue

46. Trabeculae
47. Intramembranous ossification
48. Flat bones
49. Epimysium
50. Sesamoid bone
51. Monitoring changes in muscle length
52. The junction between a motor neuron and a muscle cell
53. It lengthens
54. They are responsible for producing a specific movement
55. Saddle joint
56. Third class lever
57. The applied load is situated between the fulcrum and resisting force
58. Rotation of one bone with respect to another (the surfaces are usually arranged so that one bone rotates within a fibro-osseous ring)
59. To lubricate and nourish the articular cartilage
60. They are fibrous joints holding the teeth in their sockets in the mandible and maxilla
61. (a) Measuring what you are supposed to be measuring and (b) consistency between successive measurements (under the same conditions)
62. Flexibility generally decreases with age
63. Active movement is produced by the subject, whereas passive movement is produced by the examiner: the range of passive movement is greater than that of active movement
64. Intratester
65. (1) Use well-defined test positions and landmarks; (2) use the same amount of force in passive testing; (3) encourage subjects to exert the same force in active testing; (4) repeat the measurement using the same equipment; (5) have the same examiner take successive measurement

MCQs

1. d. opposes the movement being undertaken.
2. e. provides information about the extensibility of surrounding tissues.
3. c. The epidermis can be considered as a number of distinct layers.
4. c. Contains intercalated discs between individual fibres.
5. a. Osteoblasts remove bone tissue.
6. d. Condyloid
7. c. Direct connection between the articular surfaces

8. e. The joint between the distal ends of the radius and ulna is a syndesmosis.
9. e. Clavicle
10. a. All peripheral nerves arise from the spinal cord.
11. d. Golgi organ
12. b. Muscle
13. e. Helps produce the movement
14. c. Active movement at a joint provides information about the extensibility of the surrounding tissues.
15. d. Isometric contraction involves no change in muscle length.

PART 2: UPPER LIMB

1. Serratus anterior
2. B, pectoralis major
3. Long thoracic nerve (C5, C6 and C7)
4. Coracoclavicular ligament
5. Sternal head of sternomastoid
6. Costoclavicular ligament
7. Interclavicular ligament
8. Joint capsule, posterosuperior aspect of the superior border of the medial end of the clavicle, superior aspect of the first costal cartilage
9. Act as a strut holding the upper limb away from the chest wall; helps transmit the weight of the upper limb to the axial skeleton
10. Rhomboid major, rhomboid minor, pectoralis minor, levator scapulae
11. Plane synovial
12. 60 degrees
13. Just below the root of the spine
14. 15 cm
15. Subclavius
16. Partly from the dorsal scapular nerve (root value C5) and partly directly from the ventral rami of C3 and C4
17. Serratus anterior
18. To provide a connection of the upper limb to the trunk and increase the range of movement of the upper limb
19. Head of humerus and glenoid fossa of the scapula
20. Upper facet, supraspinatus; middle facet, infraspinatus; lower facet, teres minor
21. The angle between the axis of the shaft and that of the head and neck; 135 degrees
22. Synovial ball-and-socket
23. Glenoid labrum

24. Supraspinatus, infraspinatus, teres minor and subscapularis
25. Long head of biceps brachii
26. The three glenohumeral ligaments
27. Axillary nerve, posterior circumflex humeral artery
28. Medial, long head of triceps brachii; lateral, shaft of humerus; inferior, lower border of teres major
29. Supraspinatus initiates movement then deltoid takes over
30. Lower subscapular nerve (C5 and C6)
31. Teres minor, infraspinatus and posterior fibres of deltoid
32. Pectoralis major, anterior fibres of deltoid, long head biceps brachii and coracobrachialis
33. Pectoralis major
34. Dorsal surface of the inferior angle of the scapula and medial lip of the intertubercular (bicipital) groove
35. Extensor, adductor and medial rotator of the arm at the shoulder joint
36. Medial two-thirds of the subscapular fossa and lower facet on greater tubercle of the humerus
37. Serratus anterior
38. Anterior
39. An extension of the prevertebral layer of cervical fascia
40. Anterior
41. Cardinal planes relate to movements from the anatomical position; movements at the shoulder joint can also occur in the plane of the glenoid fossa (anatomical plane)
42. Long head of biceps brachii
43. The angle between a line through the epicondyles of the humerus and the axis of the head and neck when viewed from above
44. Inferior glenohumeral ligament
45. C5, C6 and C7
46. Pectoralis minor
47. As well as their actions on specific movements of the shoulder joint, they act as extensible ligaments aiding stability
48. A vertical line, slightly concave laterally, through a point 1 cm lateral to the apex of the coracoid process
49. Weak flexor of the shoulder joint, powerful flexor and strong supinator of the forearm
50. Capitulum of humerus and radial notch of ulna

51. From anteroinferior aspect of lateral epicondyle to the anterior and posterior margins of the radial notch of the ulna blending with the annular ligament during its course
52. Medially, medial border of pronator teres; laterally, medial border of brachioradialis; superiorly, imaginary line between medial and lateral epicondyles
53. From medial to lateral: median nerve, brachial artery and tendon of biceps brachii
54. A roughened oval area on the middle of the lateral surface of the radius
55. By passing posterior to the medial epicondyle
56. Proximal part of the posterior surface of the olecranon process of the ulna
57. Brachialis
58. Radial nerve, root value C5 and C6
59. Deep fascia of the forearm reinforced medially by the bicipital aponeurosis
60. Long head of triceps brachii
61. Lateral surface of the radius just above the styloid process
62. Biceps brachii
63. Medial (ulnar) collateral ligament
64. Slight abduction and adduction
65. It increases
66. Radial nerve
67. Long head, infraglenoid tubercle; lateral head, superolateral to spiral groove on posterior humerus; medial head, inferomedial to spiral groove on posterior humerus
68. From posterior surface of lateral epicondyle to lateral surface of olecranon and upper quarter of the posterior surface of ulna
69. Supination
70. Pronator quadratus
71. Anterior interosseous nerve (branch of median nerve)
72. Synovial pivot
73. Annular ligament
74. Posterior interosseous nerve (branch of radial nerve)
75. Interosseous membrane
76. Tendon of extensor digiti minimi
77. Inferomedially from radius to ulna
78. 180 degrees
79. 360 degrees
80. Intra-articular disc
81. Supination

82. From the upper two-thirds of the lateral supracondylar ridge of the humerus to the lateral surface of the radius proximal to the styloid process
83. Flexes the elbow putting the forearm into mid pronation/supination
84. Unites radius and ulna; transmits forces from radius to ulna; gives attachment to deep muscles in the anterior and posterior compartments of the forearm
85. Anconeus
86. Inferior
87. Recessus sacciformis
88. Colles' fracture
89. Hamate, capitate, trapezoid and trapezium
90. Humerus, ulna, scaphoid and lunate
91. Capitate
92. Flexor carpi radialis and extensors carpi radialis longus and brevis
93. Flexor retinaculum
94. Proximal and distal rows of carpal bones
95. Plane synovial
96. Flexion 50 degrees, extension 35 degrees
97. 12
98. Extensors carpi radialis longus and brevis
99. Pisiform
100. Flexor carpi radialis
101. Median nerve
102. Ulnar nerve
103. Radial nerve (posterior interosseous branch)
104. Extensor carpi ulnaris
105. Lateral
106. Flexor digitorum profundus (FDP)
107. Gripping
108. From proximal to distal: radial styloid process, scaphoid, trapezium, base of the first metacarpal
109. Thenar muscles (flexor pollicis brevis [FPB], abductor pollicis brevis [APB] and opponens pollicis) and lateral two lumbricals
110. C8 and T1
111. Abduction of the fingers
112. First metacarpal
113. Flexion/extension, abduction/adduction and rotation
114. Synovial hinge
115. Movement of the thumb so that its distal pad is brought against the distal pad of any of the remaining four digits
116. Carpometacarpal joint of the thumb

117. Bases of the medial four metacarpals with the hamate, capitate and trapezoid
118. Three
119. Flexion of the metacarpophalangeal (MCP) joint and extension of the interphalangeal (IP) joints
120. Laterally, the second lumbrical and second palmar interosseous; medially, the third palmar interosseous
121. Flexor digiti minimi, abductor digiti minimi and opponens digiti minimi
122. Radial artery
123. Flexors digitorum superficialis and profundus
124. Increases the phalangeal articular surface area of the MCP and IP joints
125. Posterior, tendons of the dorsal and palmar interossei; anterior, the tendons of the lumbricals
126. From proximal to distal, flexor digitorum superficialis (FDS) lies superficial to FDP, but FDP pierces FDS to reach its attachment to the distal phalanx whilst FDS reaches the middle phalanx
127. Active flexion/extension; passive side-to-side movement
128. Oblique palmar grip
129. Subterminolateral opposition
130. Hook
131. Palmar surface of the base of the distal phalanx of the thumb
132. Over the medial dorsal surface of the radius and dorsal surfaces of the capitate and trapezoid deep to the extensor retinaculum
133. Ulnar nerve
134. Contraction/shortening of the medial part of the palmar aponeurosis and fibrous flexor sheaths of the ring and little fingers
135. The ability to extend the wrist and digits at the MCP and IP joints; gripping
136. Slight flexion/extension
137. Lateral epicondyle via the common extensor origin and lateral collateral ligament of the elbow
138. Either side of the palmar surface of the base of the middle phalanx
139. Musculocutaneous nerve and lateral head of the median nerve
140. C5 and C6
141. Nerve to subclavius and suprascapular nerve
142. Subscapularis and teres major
143. Lateral cord
144. Supinator

145. Deltoid and teres minor
146. Median nerve
147. C6
148. Radial nerve
149. C5, C6 and C7
150. Thoracodorsal nerve
151. Medial pectoral nerve
152. Flexor carpi ulnaris
153. Palmar cutaneous branch of the median nerve
154. Radial and ulnar arteries
155. Lower (inferior) border of teres major
156. Posterior
157. Arch of the aorta
158. Axillary vein
159. Superficial
160. 25–30
161. Pectoral group of axillary nodes
162. Clavipectoral fascia
163. Against the distal border of the radius lateral to flexor carpi radialis

MCQs

1. b. Coracobrachialis
2. e. Protraction
3. c. Triceps brachii attaches to the infraglenoid tubercle.
4. a. The axillary nerve passes through the quadrangular space.
5. d. Flexor pollicis longus
6. b. Ulna
7. d. Pisiform
8. e. Dorsal scapular
9. b. Pronator teres attaches to the medial epicondyle of the humerus.
10. a. Adduction
11. b. Posterior interosseous nerve
12. e. Palmaris longus
13. b. The acromioclavicular joint is a plane synovial joint.
14. e. The medial cord is a direct continuation of the upper trunk.
15. a. Flexor carpi ulnaris and extensor carpi ulnaris
16. a. Median nerve
17. d. The median nerve innervates flexor carpi ulnaris.
18. c. medial and lateral cords
19. b. Condyloid
20. e. Long head of biceps brachii
21. e. Supraspinatus
22. b. Coracoacromial ligament
23. a. Ulnar nerve
24. e. Rhomboid major
25. b. Brachioradialis
26. a. Trochlear notch
27. b. C5, C6 and C7
28. a. Flexor pollicis longus
29. b. Triquetral
30. d. Flexor pollicis brevis
31. e. Adduction of the arm at the shoulder joint
32. c. Median nerve
33. a. Flexion is produced by pectoralis major.
34. b. The radial artery passes deep to the tendon of extensor pollicis longus.
35. c. Brachioradialis can both supinate and pronate the forearm.
36. c. Biceps brachii
37. d. Coracobrachialis
38. a. Abductor pollicis brevis
39. e. Fifth metacarpal
40. b. The profunda brachii artery is a branch of the axillary artery.
41. e. Infraclavicular
42. b. Capitate
43. d. Extensor digiti minimi
44. a. 1st dorsal interosseous
45. c. Median nerve
46. e. Brachioradialis
47. c. Brachioradialis is working concentrically during flexion.
48. c. The ulnar artery passes deep to the flexor retinaculum.
49. b. 2
50. d. Trapezius
51. b. The lateral collateral ligament is not attached to the radius.
52. d. Teres major
53. c. It attaches to the medial lip of the intertubercular groove.
54. a. Serratus posterior superior
55. d. Extensor pollicis longus
56. c. Biceps brachii
57. b. Median nerve
58. c. C5, C6, C7 and C8
59. b. Abductor pollicis longus and extensor pollicis brevis
60. e. The axis for abduction/adduction of the fingers is along the second metacarpal.

PART 3: LOWER LIMB

1. Secondary cartilaginous
2. Sacrotuberous and sacrospinous ligaments
3. Pubis
4. Coronal
5. Tip of transverse process of L5 and posterior part of medial lip of iliac crest
6. The sacral promontory moves superoposteriorly to increase pelvic inlet diameter by 3–13 mm
7. Slipping of one pubic body with respect to the other creating an uneven pubic arch
8. Forward movement of the body of L5 on S1 due to fracture of the pars interarticularis
9. Flexion and extension
10. Interosseous sacroiliac ligament
11. Acetabulum
12. Psoas major and iliacus
13. Fibrocartilaginous
14. Psoas major, iliacus, rectus femoris, sartorius, and pectineus
15. L2, L3 and L4
16. Ischium, ilium and pubis
17. Transverse acetabular ligament
18. Fovea capitis
19. Limits extension, adduction and medial rotation at the hip joint
20. Lateral (outward) twisting of the head and neck with respect to the shaft; it has a value in adults of 10 degrees
21. Centre of the femoral head proximally and midway between the femoral condyles distally
22. Obturator externus
23. Medial
24. Inferior gluteal nerve; L5, S1 and S2
25. Greater trochanter
26. Lower medial facet of the lateral part of the ischial tuberosity to a vertical line on the medial surface of the medial tibial condyle
27. Adduction of the thigh at the hip joint and flexion of the leg/calf at the knee joint
28. Femoral triangle
29. Superior gluteal nerve; L4, L5 and S1
30. Ischial tuberosity to quadrate tubercle halfway down intertrochanteric crest
31. Gemellus superior and inferior
32. Obturator externus and obturator internus
33. Active 20 degrees, passive 30 degrees
34. A fibroelastic fat pad situated within the acetabular fossa
35. Four; longitudinal, oblique and arcuate and the zona orbicularis
36. A line drawn along the upper margin of the obturator foramen and inferior margin of the femoral neck to the medial side of the shaft
37. With the hip flexed 90 degrees, abducted 5 degrees and laterally rotated 10 degrees
38. Gluteus maximus, gluteus medius, gluteus minimus and tensor fascia lata
39. Anterior division of the obturator nerve; root value L2, L3 and L4
40. L1, L2, L3 and (L4)
41. Tendon of biceps femoris
42. Semimembranosus
43. Rectus femoris, vastus lateralis, vastus medialis and vastus intermedius
44. Anterior horn of medial meniscus, anterior cruciate ligament, anterior horn of lateral meniscus, posterior horn of lateral meniscus, posterior horn of medial meniscus and posterior cruciate ligament
45. Lateral
46. (B) intracapsular and extrasynovial
47. Popliteus
48. Quadriceps femoris
49. Sciatic (common fibular/peroneal part) nerve; L5, S1 and S2
50. Ligamentum patellae
51. Lateral epicondyle of the femur superoposterior to the groove for popliteus and lateral surface of the head of the fibula anterior to the apex
52. Semitendinosus, semimembranosus, gracilis, sartorius and popliteus
53. Provides restraint to anterior and medial displacement of the tibia with respect to the femur
54. Increase congruence between the femur and tibia; weight-bearing; aid lubrication; act as shock absorbers
55. Popliteus
56. Popliteal artery
57. Femoral nerve; L2 and L3
58. Medial meniscus moves anterior and lateral meniscus posterior
59. All except the odd facet
60. From the anterior aspect of the body of the pubis and its inferior ramus proximally to a short vertical line on the superior part of the medial surface of the tibial shaft

61. Fibrous (syndesmosis)
62. Oval facet on the head of the fibula and a similar facet on the inferior surface of the lateral tibial condyle
63. Inferolaterally
64. It moves superolaterally and undergoes axial rotation (the direction depending on the shape of the lateral talar surface).
65. Anterior and posterior tibiofibular ligaments; interosseous membrane
66. Common fibular/peroneal nerve
67. Anterior tibial vessels
68. Lateral
69. Tibia
70. Inferolaterally
71. Anteromedially
72. Lateral
73. Anteriorly
74. Medial head from posterior to the medial supracondylar ridge and adductor tubercle on the popliteal surface of the femur, and lateral head to the outer surface of the lateral femoral condyle proximally to middle part of the posterior surface of the calcaneus distally
75. Tibial nerve; S1 and S2
76. Dorsiflexion of foot at ankle joint; inversion of foot
77. Posterior to the medial malleolus
78. Y-shaped, with the stem arising from the superior surface of the calcaneus anteriorly and floor of the sinus tarsi, the upper part attaching to the medial malleolus and lower part blending with the deep fascia on the medial side of the foot
79. Gastrocnemius and soleus
80. Convex anteroposteriorly with a central longitudinal groove bound by medial and lateral lips; the groove and lips make the surface slightly concave transversely
81. Anterior and posterior tibiotalar bands
82. Anterior and posterior talofibular and calcaneofibular ligaments
83. Tibialis anterior
84. Proximal half of the lateral aspect of the posterior surface of the tibia inferior to the soleal line, posterior surface of the fibula between the median crest and interosseous border and covering fascia proximally to navicular tubercle and plantar surface of the medial cuneiform expanding to attach to the plantar surfaces of all tarsal bones except the talus

85. Plantarflexion of the foot at the ankle joint; flexion of the leg/calf at the knee joint
86. Deep fibular/peroneal nerve; L4 and L5
87. Plantarflexion
88. Synovial hinge
89. The mortise is formed by the distal ends of the tibia and fibula (medial and lateral malleoli), and the tenon by the body of the talus
90. A depression on the posteromedial aspect of the lateral malleolus
91. Seven: talus, calcaneus, navicular, cuboid, medial cuneiform, intermediate cuneiform and lateral cuneiform
92. Plane synovial
93. Calcaneus, cuboid and navicular
94. Dorsal surface of the base of the distal phalanx of the hallux
95. Lateral plantar nerve: S2 and S3
96. Adduct the third, fourth and fifth toes towards the second
97. Thick fascia (plantar aponeurosis) in the sole of the foot continuous with the fascia over the heel and on the sides of the foot with the dorsal fascia
98. Superior is the tendon of fibularis/peroneus brevis; inferior is the tendon of fibularis/peroneus longus
99. Tibialis anterior and tibialis posterior
100. Medial plantar nerve; S1 and S2
101. Medial and lateral tubercles of the calcaneus proximally and lateral side of the base of the proximal phalanx of the fifth toe
102. Subtalar joint
103. Proximally calcaneus and talus, distally navicular and cuboid
104. Between the posterior and anterior tubercles of the calcaneus posteriorly and the ridge and tuberosity on the cuboid and bases of the lateral four metatarsals distally
105. Abduction at the subtalar joint and pronation at the transverse (mid) tarsal joint
106. First
107. Tibialis posterior at the level of the navicular and cuboid; fibularis/peroneus longus at the level of the cuneiforms and cuboid; adductor hallucis at the level of the metatarsal heads
108. Deep transverse metatarsal ligament
109. Plantarflexion/dorsiflexion and abduction/adduction

110. Talus, cuboid, medial cuneiform, intermediate cuneiform and lateral cuneiform
111. Flexor hallucis longus
112. Calcaneus
113. Fibularis/peroneus brevis and tertius
114. Tibial nerve; L5, S1 and S2
115. Flexes the metatarsophalangeal joint of the hallux
116. Lateral
117. Proximally the medial, intermediate and lateral cuneiforms and first and third metatarsal bases; distally the proximal phalanx
118. Plantarflexion and dorsiflexion
119. Lateral displacement of the hallux
120. The area immediately below the sinus tarsi
121. L4, L5, S1, S2 and S3
122. Abductor hallucis, flexor digitorum brevis, first lumbrical and flexor hallucis brevis
123. Deep and superficial fibular/peroneal nerves
124. L2 and L3
125. Gluteus medius, gluteus minimus and tensor fascia lata
126. Deep fibular/peroneal nerve
127. Obturator internus and superior gemellus
128. Iliacus
129. Sciatic nerve: long head by the tibial part, short head by the common fibular/peroneal part
130. Fibularis/peroneus longus and brevis
131. L2
132. L5, S1 and S2
133. Lateral plantar nerve
134. Femoral nerve
135. As it passes around the neck of the fibula
136. After passing through the adductor hiatus
137. Lateral and medial plantar arteries
138. Skin below the level of the umbilicus, lower part of anal canal and external genitalia (except testes in males)
139. Posterior to the medial malleolus
140. Profunda femoris
141. Femoral vein
142. By piercing the fascia forming the roof of the popliteal fossa
143. Five: superior medial and lateral genicular arteries; middle genicular artery; inferior medial and lateral genicular arteries
144. Medial
145. Lymphatics

MCQs

1. c. The posterior inferior iliac spine can be palpated.
2. a. It contributes to kyphosis of the thoracic part of the vertebral column.
3. c. has the sacral auricular surface lying entirely on the lateral mass.
4. e. The arcuate pubic ligament strengthens the joint superiorly.
5. b. The lesser trochanter projects posterolaterally.
6. e. The joint capsule is reinforced posteriorly by the iliofemoral ligament.
7. b. Pectineus contributes to flexion at the joint.
8. d. Semimembranosus attaches to the medial epicondyle of the femur.
9. c. Tibialis posterior lies deep to gastrocnemius.
10. b. Flexor accessorius (quadratus plantae) attaches to the tendon of flexor digitorum longus.
11. a. The medial meniscus is of constant width.
12. c. The anterior part of the trochlear surface of the talus is wider than the posterior part.
13. d. L2 and L3
14. c. It leaves the pelvis by passing deep to the inguinal ligament.
15. e. Crosses both the hip and knee joints.
16. a. Tibialis posterior passes behind the lateral malleolus.
17. b. Genitofemoral nerve
18. e. Gluteus medius
19. d. Biceps femoris
20. b. Second
21. c. It is a combined movement at the subtalar and midtarsal joints.
22. a. Popliteus produces medial rotation of the femur on the tibia.
23. d. During extension of the foot at the ankle joint the distal end of the fibula moves laterally.
24. e. The dorsalis pedis pulse can be felt lateral to the tendon of extensor hallucis longus.
25. c. Gluteus medius extends the thigh at the hip joint.
26. e. The great (long) saphenous vein pierces the posterior part of the deep fascia of the thigh.
27. d. S1 and S2
28. b. L2, L3 and L4
29. d. It medially rotates the thigh at the hip joint.
30. c. Quadriceps tubercle
31. b. Lateral malleolus

32. d. Lateral crest
33. b. The calcaneus articulates with the lateral cuneiform.
34. b. Tibialis anterior attaches to both the tibia and fibula.
35. c. Obturator externus lies deep to quadratus femoris.
36. e. Ascending genicular artery
37. c. Middle genicular artery
38. d. Gracilis
39. e. Abductor hallucis
40. b. first lumbrical
41. d. It arises from the anterior divisions of L2, L3 and L4.
42. b. The long axis of the foot is along the third metatarsal.
43. c. Semimembranosus attaches to the ischial tuberosity.
44. a. Soleus
45. c. Rectus femoris
46. d. L5, S1 and S2
47. a. Saphenous nerve
48. e. Sural nerve
49. d. Inferior tibiofibular joint
50. b. 14
51. b. Second
52. d. Bifurcate ligament
53. d. Flexion
54. e. Adduction and lateral rotation
55. c. The obturator nerve divides into anterior and posterior division within the triangle.
56. e. The floor is partly formed by soleus.
57. e. There are no lymph nodes within the popliteal fossa.
58. a. It usually divides into its tibial and common fibular/peroneal components in the proximal third of the thigh.
59. d. Extensor digitorum brevis is innervated by the superficial fibular (peroneal) nerve.
60. b. During flexion of the knee the initial movement of the femur against the tibia is one of gliding.

PART 4: TRUNK

1. Adjacent dorsal rami
2. Facets for the ribs on the body (upper and lower) and on the transverse process
3. Intervertebral disc (IVD)
4. Posterosuperolateral
5. 3
6. Pedicles, laminae, transverse processes and spinous process
7. Rectus abdominis, external oblique, internal oblique, psoas major and psoas minor
8. From lateral two-thirds inguinal ligament, anterior two-thirds iliac crest and thoracolumbar fascia to inferior borders of lower four ribs and rectus sheath
9. T12 and L1–L4
10. From posterior sacrum and fascia covering erector spinae, lumbar mamillary processes, transverse processes of thoracic vertebrae and articular processes of lower four or five cervical vertebrae to spines of all vertebrae from L5 to C1
11. Erector spinae between the posterior and middle layers and quadratus lumborum between the middle and anterior layers
12. An oblique opening in the lower anterior abdominal wall passing through the transversalis fascia and external oblique and inferior to transversus abdominis and internal oblique
13. Extension of the cervical and lumbar spine; stabilizing vertebral column
14. 25%
15. 10 mm
16. Outer annulus fibrosis, inner nucleus pulposus, superior and inferior cartilage end plates
17. IVDs and adjacent margins of vertebral bodies between C2 and S1
18. Synovial
19. From the anterior part of the lower border of the lamina above to the posterior part of the upper border of the lamina below between C1/2 and L4/5
20. Flexion, extension and lateral flexion/bending
21. T7/8
22. Cervical region, vertebral and ascending cervical arteries; thoracic region, costocervical and posterior intercostal arteries; lumbar region, lumbar and iliolumbar arteries
23. Rotation, extension and lateral flexion/bending of the vertebral column at all levels
24. Medial column is spinalis, intermediate column is longissimus, lateral column is iliocostalis
25. Males
26. External oblique
27. Semispinalis capitis, cervicis and thoracis

28. Any three from: carry and support the thoracic cage; give attachment to muscles of the pectoral and pelvic girdles; give attachment to powerful muscles moving the vertebral column; surround and protect the spinal cord; act as a shock absorber; produce accumulated moments of force as well as concentrate and transmit force from other parts of body
29. 24
30. Quadrilateral
31. Heart-shaped
32. Anteriorly, the aponeurosis of external oblique joins with the anterior half of that of internal oblique; posteriorly, the remainder of internal oblique aponeurosis with that of transversus abdominis.
33. S3, S4 and perineal branch of pudendal nerve (S4)
34. Secondary cartilaginous (symphysis)
35. Nucleus pulposus
36. Anterior
37. Its multisegmented arrangement with limited movement possible between adjacent segments
38. Scoliosis
39. Lumbar
40. Lumbar
41. 4 (right and left second and third ribs)
42. Scalenus anterior
43. Primary cartilaginous
44. 14 (first to seventh on each side)
45. Motor, phrenic nerve (C3, C4 and C5); sensory, periphery intercostal nerves, central phrenic nerves
46. Elevates second to fifth ribs during inspiration.
47. T9–T11
48. Inferior vena cava and right phrenic nerve
49. Manubrium, body and xiphoid process
50. Secondary cartilaginous
51. T6 and T7
52. Fifth rib
53. Costotransverse and costovertebral
54. Sternocostal
55. Ribs 11 and 12 as they terminate in the anterior abdominal musculature
56. Intercostal vein, artery and nerve in that order from above down
57. Innermost and internal intercostal muscles
58. Posterior surface of the xiphoid process, lower six ribs and costal cartilages, medial and lateral arcuate ligaments (thickening of fascia over psoas major and quadratus lumborum respectively), right and left crura (anterolateral aspects of bodies of L1–L3 and L1, L2, respectively)
59. 31
60. Ganglion
61. Ventral horn
62. L1/L2
63. Arachnoid and pia mater
64. One anterior and two posterior spinal arteries
65. Sensory
66. S2
67. Acetylcholine
68. III (oculomotor), VII (facial), IX (glossopharyngeal) and X (vagus)
69. T1–L2
70. Ventral horns
71. S2, S3 and S4
72. Preganglionic sympathetic
73. Left pulmonary artery and arch of aorta
74. Interatrial septum
75. Semilunar
76. Ascending aorta
77. Right atrium
78. Left fifth intercostal space 9 cm from midline
79. Right side
80. Aorta
81. Three: superior, middle and inferior
82. With the arm abducted 90 degrees along a line from the T3 spinous process along the medial border of the scapula as far as the mid-axillary line then along the sixth rib and costal cartilage anteriorly
83. Lung root
84. 3 cm above the medial third of the clavicle
85. Upper right
86. Duodenum, jejunum and ileum
87. Store and concentrate bile
88. Two: deciduous and permanent
89. Nephron
90. Anteverted (90 degrees to vagina) and anteflexed (body bent forward with respect to cervix) so that it lies superior to bladder
91. Xiphisternum
92. Communicates with the nervous system to regulate and coordinate body functions

MCQs

1. a. Trapezius

2. d. Foramen transversarium
3. b. Articulates with the bodies of two adjacent vertebrae.
4. b. L1/L2
5. c. S2
6. b. Rectus abdominis is completely enclosed within the rectus sheath.
7. e. External oblique
8. d. L4
9. e. Ninth
10. c. Spinalis is the most well defined column of the erector spinae muscle mass.
11. a. In the thoracic region the range of flexion is greater than that of extension.
12. c. Iliolumbar ligament
13. e. Is unable to transmit forces from one part of the body to another.
14. c. 24
15. a. It consists of two layers.
16. c. Vein, artery and nerve
17. a. Primary cartilaginous
18. e. Manubriosternal
19. d. Above the costal margin it is completely enclosed by the rectus sheath.
20. c. Scalenus posterior
21. b. Symphysis pubis
22. d. The oesophagus passes through the central tendon.
23. b. Levator costarum
24. c. 31
25. e. Each spinal nerve is completely surrounded by the meninges.
26. a. Sympathetic outflow is between the levels of T1 and S2.
27. b. The filum terminale is an extension of the arachnoid mater.
28. a. The brachial plexus is formed by the ventral rami of C5–T2.
29. c. Sympathetic nervous stimulation decreases heart rate.
30. d. It lies in the middle mediastinum.
31. a. The coronary sinus drains into the left atrium.
32. e. The left atrium receives blood from the superior and inferior venae cavae.
33. b. The left lung has three lobes.
34. b. Parietal pleura is firmly adherent to lung tissue.
35. d. The jejunum of the small intestine opens into the ascending colon.
36. c. The pyloric sphincter controls the passage of gastric contents into the ileum.
37. e. The base of the bladder rests on levator ani.
38. c. The round ligament of the ovary passes through the inguinal canal into the labia major.
39. a. Subthalamus
40. e. The phrenic nerve is enclosed within the carotid sheath.

PART 5: NECK AND HEAD

1. Flexion and extension
2. Vertebral artery and vein
3. Seven
4. C1 and C7
5. Three: two lateral atlantoaxial joints and and one median atlantoaxial joint and one median atlantoaxial joint
6. Joints between the lateral margins of adjacent cervical vertebral bodies
7. Three: upper part from anterior tubercles of transverse processes of C3–C5 to anterior tubercle of C1; middle part from anterior bodies C5–T3 to anterior bodies C2–C4; lower part from anterior bodies of T1–T3 to the anterior tubercles of transverse processes of C5 and C6
8. Individually laterally flexes/bends the neck with some rotation to the opposite side, both flex neck; with neck fixed, they steady first rib during inspiration
9. Anterior primary rami of C1 and C2
10. Triangular fibroelastic septum extending between C7 and external occipital protuberance
11. Concave oval facets on the superior surface of the atlas with reciprocally curved occipital condyles on the base of the skull
12. Synovial pivot joint
13. Lesser occipital, greater auricular, transverse cutaneous nerve of the neck and supraclavicular nerves
14. Transverse ligament of atlas
15. Restricted movement between adjacent cervical vertebrae; compression of spinal nerves
16. Investing layer of superficial fascia
17. Tectorial membrane
18. Anterior and posterior atlanto-occipital membranes, ligamentum nuchae
19. Extends head on neck; helps stabilize vertebral column
20. Motor, accessory nerve (XI); sensory, C2 and C3

21. c, maxilla
22. 18 months
23. Occipital, right and left parietal
24. Temporal
25. Foramen magnum
26. Buccinator
27. Frontal lobe
28. Right and left temporal, sphenoid
29. Facial/seventh cranial nerve
30. Orbicularis oculi
31. Protraction, retraction, elevation, depression and side-to-side movements
32. (A) Lateral pterygoid, medial pterygoid and masseter; (B) temporalis, digastric, geniohyoid; (C) masseter, medial pterygoid, temporalis; (D) digastric, mylohyoid, geniohyoid, platysma
33. Omohyoid, sternohyoid, sternohyoid, thyrohyoid
34. Digastric, mylohyoid, stylohyoid
35. C1, C2 and C3 via the ansa cervicalis
36. Lateral surface of the ramus of the mandible and zygomatic arch
37. Lateral aspect, masseter; medial aspect, medial pterygoid; anterior border, temporalis
38. Body, pair of greater horns and pair of lesser horns
39. Head of mandible and mandibular fossa of the temporal bone
40. Facial (seventh cranial) nerve
41. Protects CNS by maintaining a constant pH environment and also cushions the brain against mechanical insult
42. Ridges (gyri) and depressions (sulci) on the surface of the brain
43. 24 (12 pairs)
44. Right and left internal carotid and right and left vertebral arteries
45. Vision
46. Corpus callosum
47. Fibrous astrocyte, protoplasmic astrocyte, oligodendrocyte, microglial cells and ependymal cells
48. Innervates the muscles of the tongue except palatoglossus
49. Tentorium cerebelli
50. Ophthalmic (V_1), maxillary (V_2) and mandibular (V_3) divisions
51. C1–C5 nerve roots
52. Trapezius and sternomastoid
53. Motor functions, expressions of intellect and personality
54. Voluntary muscle contraction
55. Nerve axons
56. Four: frontal, parietal, temporal and occipital
57. Stylopharyngeus
58. Superior sagittal sinus
59. Extensions of arachnoid mater piercing the dura allowing cerebrospinal fluid to drain into the superior sagittal sinus
60. Anterior cerebral arteries, anterior communicating artery, internal carotid arteries, posterior communicating artery, posterior cerebral arteries and basilar artery
61. Small bones (malleus, incus and stapes) found within the middle ear
62. Tympanic membrane
63. Three: anterior, posterior and horizontal
64. Via the Eustachian (auditory) tube
65. Tensor tympani
66. Seventh cranial nerve
67. Three: outer fibrous, middle vascular and inner nervous (the retina)
68. Region where the optic nerve enters the eyeball so that it is devoid of light receptors
69. Superior and inferior oblique; superior, medial, inferior and lateral rectus
70. Left lateral rectus and right medial rectus
71. Fourth (trochlear)

MCQs

1. d. 8
2. d. Body
3. e. Rectus capitis lateralis
4. a. Trapezius
5. d. Inferior oblique
6. d. Sphenoid
7. b. Mandibular nerve
8. c. Occipital
9. a. Anterior condylar canal
10. b. The lambdoid suture is between the parietal and occipital bones.
11. e. Styloglossus
12. d. Temporalis
13. c. Posterior belly of digastric
14. a. Trigeminal
15. a. Coracoid process

16. b. The head articulates directly with the mandibular fossa of the temporal bone.
17. c. Digastric
18. e. Occipital lobe
19. d. Abducens
20. a. Middle meningeal

21. e. Abducens
22. b. Superior petrosal sinus
23. e. Transverse sinus
24. b. Posterior belly of digastric
25. d. The tooth above the gum margin is covered by cementum.

INDEX

Page numbers followed by "*f*" indicate figures, "*t*" indicate tables, and "*b*" indicate boxes.